Psychiatric Mental Health Nursing

Fourth Edition

Psychiatric Mental Health Nursing

Fourth Edition

Noreen Cavan Frisch, RN, PhD, FAAN
University of Victoria
Victoria, BC Canada

Lawrence E. Frisch, MPH
Vancouver Island Health Authority
Victoria, BC Canada

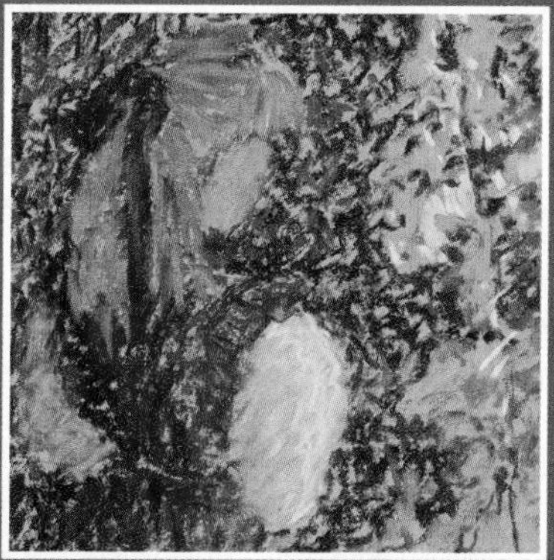

Lea Gaydos, PhD, RN, HN-C
Nurse Artist, Contributor of Chapter Opening Art
University of Colorado
Colorado Springs, Colorado

DELMAR
CENGAGE Learning™

Australia • Brazil • Japan • Korea • Mexico • Singapore • Spain • United Kingdom • United States

DELMAR
CENGAGE Learning™

Psychiatric Mental Health Nursing
Fourth Edition

By Noreen Cavan Frisch and Lawrence E. Frisch

Vice President, Career and Professional Editorial: Dave Garza

Director of Learning Solutions: Matt Kane

Senior Acquisitions Editor: Maureen Rosener

Managing Editor: Marah Bellegarde

Senior Product Manager: Juliet Steiner

Editorial Assistant: Samantha Miller

Vice President, Career and Professional Marketing: Jennifer Ann Baker

Executive Marketing Manager: Wendy Mapstone

Senior Marketing Manager: Michele McTighe

Marketing Coordinator: Scott Chrysler

Production Director: Carolyn Miller

Production Manager: Andrew Crouth

Senior Content Project Manager: Stacey Lamodi

Senior Art Director: Jack Pendleton

Senior Technology Product Manager: Mary Colleen Liburdi

Technology Project Manager: Patricia Allen

Technology Project Manager: Ben Knapp

Production Technology Analyst: Tom Stover

Library of Congress Control Number: 2009925005

ISBN-13: 978-1-4354-0077-1
ISBN-10: 1-4354-0077-1

Delmar
5 Maxwell Drive
Clifton Park, NY 12065-2919
USA

Cengage Learning is a leading provider of customized learning solutions with office locations around the globe, including Singapore, the United Kingdom, Australia, Mexico, Brazil, and Japan. Locate your local office at: **international.cengage.com/region**

Cengage Learning products are represented in Canada by Nelson Education, Ltd.

To learn more about Delmar, visit **www.cengage.com/delmar**

Purchase any of our products at your local college store or at our preferred online store **www.CengageBrain.com**

Printed in the United States of America
Printed by RR Donnelley, Willard, OH, Fourth Ed. 12/2009.
1 2 3 4 5 6 7 12 11 10 09

TABLE OF CONTENTS

CHAPTER 16

THE CLIENT WHO IS SUICIDAL / 369

CHAPTER 17

THE CLIENT WHO ABUSES CHEMICAL SUBSTANCES / 405

CHAPTER 18

THE CLIENT WITH A PERSONALITY DISORDER / 451

UNIT 4

Nursing Interventions and Treatment Modalities / 763

CHAPTER 27

PHARMACOLOGY IN PSYCHIATRIC CARE / 765

CHAPTER 28

INDIVIDUAL PSYCHOTHERAPY / 805

CHAPTER 29

FAMILY THERAPY / 821

CHAPTER 30

GROUP THERAPY / 853

CHAPTER 31

COMMUNITY MENTAL HEALTH NURSING / 871

CHAPTER 32

COMPLEMENTARY AND SOMATIC THERAPIES / 887

UNIT 5
Additional Resources / 905

CHAPTER 33
FRIDAY NIGHT AT THE MOVIES / 907

LIST OF TABLES

LIST OF BOXED FEATURES

CHAPTER OPENING REFLECTIVE BOXES

NURSING ALERT

NURSING TIP

REFLECTIVE THINKING

RESEARCH HIGHLIGHT

CASE EXAMPLE

APPLICATION OF THE NURSING PROCESS

CARE PLANNING GUIDE

NURSING CARE PLAN: NURSING PROCESS FORMAT

NURSING CARE PLAN: CONCEPT MAP FORMAT

FILM CLIPS

CLASSIC ART

CONTRIBUTORS

Genevieve M. Bartol, RN, EdD, HCN
Professor Emeritus
School of Nursing
The University of North Carolina at Greensboro
Greensboro, North Carolina

Arlene Farren, PhD, RN
Assistant Professor
College of Staton Island, City University of New York,
New York

Julia B. George, RN, PhD
Professor Emerita
Department of Nursing
California State University—Fullerton
Fullerton, California

Wanda Horn, RN-C
Psychiatric Unit
Southeast Missouri Hospital
Cape Girardeau, Missouri

Dorothea Hover-Kramer, EdD, CNS, RN
Psychotherapist
Bend, Oregon

Brenda P. Johnson, PhD, RN, MSN
Associate Professor Southeast Missouri State University
Cape Girardeau, Missouri

Vicki Johnson, PhD, MSN, RN
Assistant Clinical Professor
Cleveland State University Cleveland, Ohio

Jane Kelley, RN, PhD
Adjunct Professor
University of Mississippi
Medical Center School of Nursing
Jackson, Mississippi

Chris Paxos, Pharm.D.
Assistant Professor
Northeastern Ohio Universities College of Pharmacy
Rootstown, Ohio

Lynn Rew, EdD, RNC, HNC, FAAN
Professor and Graduate Advisor
School of Nursing
The University of Texas at Austin
Austin, Texas

Karilee Halo Shames, PhD, RN, HNC, CNS
Nurse Educator/Author
Boca Raton, Florida

Marshelle Thobaben, RN, MS, PHN, APNP, PCNP
Professor
Department of Nursing
Humboldt State University
Arcata, California

Wayne Wilson, PD, RPh
Pharmacist Student Health Center Humboldt State
University Arcata, California

Acknowledgment of writers from previous editions of this text whose work on nursing care is contained in current chapters: Dorothea Hover-Kramer and Karilee Halo-Shames (chapter 10), Marshelle Thobaben (chapter 26), and Wayne Wilson (chapter 27).

Acknowledgment of Arlene Farren, PhD, RN of the College of Staton Island, City University of New York, who updated the nursing care plans in this text and to Eileen Greene, MN, RN of Camosun College, Victoria, BC Canada who prepared the learning activities associated with the DVD interviews.

REVIEWERS

Norma Calhoun, RN, BSN
Assistant Professor
Virginia Community College
Big Stone Gap, Virginia

Leona Dempsey, PhD, APNP
Assistant Professor
University of Wisconsin
Oshkosh, Wisconsin

Sue Hendricks, Ed.D., M.S.N., R.N.
Interim Chair of Baccalaureate & Higher Degree Programs
Director for Assessment and Evaluation in Nursing
Associate Professor
Indiana University
Kokomo, Indiana

Theresa Keane, RN, PhD
Assistant Professor
New York City Technical College Brooklyn, New York

YorikoKozuki, PhD, ARNP
Associate Professor
University of Washington School of Nursing
Seattle, Washington

Joanne Lavin, RN, EdD, CS
Professor
Kingsborough Community College
Brooklyn, New York

Glenise McKenzie, RN, PhD
Assistant Professor
OHSU School of Nursing
Portland, Oregon

Marita Terese Peppard, RN, ND, MS
Professor
Austin Community College, Eastview Campus
Austin, Texas

Jeanne F. Saunders, MSN
Associate Professor
Daytona State College
Daytona Beach, Florida

Melodie Stembridge, MSN, ARNP-BC, PhDc
Department of Veterans Affairs Medical Center
Atlanta, Georgia

PREFACE

We continue to be gratified by readers' responses to this work. It has been a pleasure to hear from students how much they enjoy reading the text (because we wrote it to be enjoyed, and we enjoyed writing it). It has been equally rewarding to hear from instructors for whom this text has brought new fun to their teaching. We're delighted this has happened, and we're more delighted you have shared these experiences with us. These authorial pleasures have made lighter the task of revising each of the editions, and they offer further hope that this fourth edition will continue to provide for its readers a welcome mix of knowledge, insight, and pleasure.

In the preface to the previous edition we spoke at length about mental health "carve outs." In an attempt to save costs, managed care insurance companies had "carved out" mental health diagnostic and treatment benefits to organizations that provide only mental health care. The idea behind carving out was that efficiency and perhaps quality might be gained if care for mental illness were taken on by organizations specialized in providing this service. But carve outs were also based on a vision that mental illness and substance misuse treatment are not chronic disorders (like diabetes or heart disease) but are fundamentally different entities largely outside the scope of general medical practice. In the United States had increasingly legislated "parity" for mental health and substance benefits. Parity required that health plans provide the same quantity of benefits for mental or substance disorders compared to physical disorders.

In October, 2008 then-President Bush signed the Mental Health Parity and Addiction Equity Act into law. This federal legislation means that plans must treat mental illness and substance abuse no differently than any other illness: benefits, co-payment, deductibles, must all be comparable across diagnoses. The updated parity legislation (a 1996 federal law had many loopholes) represents a significant change in U.S. thinking about mental illness and substance disorders. Some have suggested that after the terrorist attacks of 9/11, Americans came to recognize that stress, anxiety, depression, and post-traumatic stress could affect anyone, and that there was a real need to have mental health services appropriately accessible when needed. There is also persuasive evidence that providing readier access to mental health care has little overall effect on cost because large expenses associated with crisis and inpatient care are avoided.

Parity legislation is not necessarily inconsistent with carve outs, but it does mean that the decision to carve out or "carve in" mental health benefits ("carving in" means providing mental health and substance care through medical health plans) may be made on the basis of quality and appropriateness rather than solely on cost. Getting high quality mental health care to those who need it remains an important public health priority. The mentally ill need access to health care, and they need *accessible* and *acceptable* high-quality services based on the best available scientifically derived evidence.

An event that we reported in the second edition was the Surgeon General's 1999 report on Mental Illness in the United States. Dr. Satcher produced a report that gave a sharp national focus to mental illness and its treatment. This report greatly influenced the 2008 parity legislation and was based on several important premises:

- The scientific understanding of mental illness and its treatment has made great strides.
- There are still major stigmata associated with mental illness, and these are among a variety of factors that keep many people from receiving helpful diagnosis and treatment.
- There are marked disparities in access to mental health care: the poor and many ethnic minorities seem to have particularly limited access.

- Knowledge of mental illness and its treatment needs to be more widespread, both among health care providers and the public at large.

As readers of this textbook will come to recognize, Dr. Satcher's assessment remains accurate. Our scientific achievements in mental health continue to be impressive; parity legislation reflects the gradual removal of stigmata around mental illness; and great disparities still exist in how effectively we apply what we know to the mental health and substance problems we face. In the third edition, we called attention to *Healthy People 2010,* the national initiative to identify health and public health goals impacting Americans. The two overarching goals for the decade 2000–2010 were 1) to increase quality and years of healthy life, and 2) to eliminate health disparities. There were several focus areas, with one being mental health and mental disorders. The target goals for mental health included: decreasing the suicide rate, decreasing suicidal attempts by adolescents, decreasing the proportion of homeless individuals with serious mental illness, increasing the employment rate for persons with mental illness, reducing relapse rates for persons with eating disorders, increasing the number of persons seen in primary health care who receive screening for mental illness, increasing the proportion of children and adults with mental health problems who receive treatment, increasing the proportion of juvenile justice facilities that screen new admissions for mental health problems, and increasing the proportion of persons with co-occurring substance abuse and mental disorders who receive treatment for both disorders. The fourth edition of this book will come out almost simultaneously with publication of the detailed goals for the next major effort: *Healthy People 2020.* As this preface is being written, there are four proposed over-arching goals for *Healthy People 2020:*

- Achieve health equity, eliminate disparities and improve health for all groups.
- Eliminate preventable disease, disability, injury and premature death.
- Create social and physical environments that promote good health for all.
- Promote healthy development and healthy behaviors across every stage of life.

The last three of these goals are new to *Healthy People,* and they perhaps reflect a change toward a vision of health less focused on disease and more focused on the conditions in which people can lead healthy lives. In some ways these goals echo a vision which this textbook first set out over a decade ago: twin emphases on biological and epidemiological science *and* on the lived experience of mental illness, as illustrated by the many narratives, paintings, and film excerpts included throughout. This emphasis on understanding the client (and his/her "social and physical environment" as well as the illness remains one of our highest priorities. In this spirit, we continue to be inspired by Dr. Samuel H. Barondes' poem entitled "Recapitulation," The final stanzas of which appear below.* With a little page-flipping you will be able to read the entire poem: it begins with "Freud" (in Chapter 3), continues with "Drugs" (Chapter 27), goes on to "Genetics" (Chapter 4), and oddly enough finishes here at the beginning of the book. Lives *are* lived as stories: stories of hope, stories of loss, stories of discovery, stories of despair. They're all part of that ever-expanding world we call psychiatric mental health nursing. Welcome back!

*True to its name, "Recapitulation" is a poetic summary of Dr. Barondes' lucid book *Molecules and Mental Illness* (1999).

IV. STORIES

... For lives are lived as stories
(Though their intrapsychic actors
May play from scripts whose scripting comes
From polygenic factors);
And lives are understandable
In terms of mental rules
(Though they respond, like puppets,
To key protein molecules).
But should a plot develop
That is different than expected,
And should a role have features
That the player wants corrected,
That role may prove refractory
To thespian intention,
While chemicals may constitute
The proper intervention.
So even though our stories are
Intangible, ethereal,
Our mental composition is
Essentially material;
And though we don't experience
This transubstantiation,
To know ourselves requires
Its detailed elucidation.
And not just to design some
More effective medications,
But also to define a view
With wider implications,
Since understanding molecules
That drive us to insanity
Provides a giant window on
The nature of humanity.

Conceptual Approach

Psychiatric Mental Health Nursing was written and designed with the reader in mind. Like no other text currently available, *Psychiatric Mental Health Nursing* Fourth Edition draws readers into the subject matter in a way that is interesting to them. This text conveys the real-life experiences of clients suffering from psychiatric conditions in a manner that will stimulate and keep the reader's attention. Disorders are illustrated through literature, film, and art, then followed by a didactic explanation from the nursing and psychiatric literature, covering etiology, nursing perspectives, theory, nursing process, and sample case studies/care plans. And now, in the fourth edition, video interviews with ten actual clients experiencing disorders are included on the *Study*WARE™ CD-ROM accompanying the text. This exciting new addition to the text is not only engaging and authentic, but it is yet another way this unique approach helps the reader to better understand the experience of psychiatric conditions. As in previous editions, recurring features and an easy-to-follow format offer an approach that is friendly and delivers a wealth of information.

The conceptual approach to this text is based on the following:

- Dual focus combines the best of nursing as the art and science of caring. The use of literature, art, and the human experience, coupled with qualitative and scientific research, emphasizes the need for compassionate nursing care and respect for the lived experience of others. Nursing theory helps readers learn to provide caring and nurturing as part of all interventions while maintaining an emphasis on living with mental illness. The importance of science is evident through the theoretical and epidemiological base underlying conditions.
- Chapter opening reflection boxes help the reader develop critical thinking skills and the ability to deal with moral dilemmas by enticing the reader to enter the world of the mentally ill and by introducing issues of the social and moral implications of treatment. Emphasis is placed on considering first what the client feels and then what the client wants.
- Balanced nursing and medical approaches (NANDA-I, DSM) underscores the importance of nurses working collaboratively with other health care team members with the mutual goal of providing the most appropriate and effective care to clients.
- Focus on self-care encourages nurses to think about and care for themselves as well as their clients. This reflects a fundamental premise that caring for others can be done only if the caregiver is balanced and well-centered.

Readers of *Psychiatric Mental Health Nursing* Fourth Edition will need an understanding of basic nursing skills and the nursing process.

ORGANIZATION

Psychiatric Mental Health Nursing is composed of 33 chapters contained in five units. **Unit 1** outlines the foundations for practice that underlie the psychiatric nursing process. Fundamental principles of nursing, which help the reader understand the importance of the nurse-client partnership in the care of those with psychiatric conditions, are discussed. A unique chapter (Chapter 5) on diagnostic systems outlines scientific bases for care and explains NANDA, DSM-IV-TR, ICD-9, and NIC/NOC, and how they are all used in practice. Chapter 7 on cultural and ethnic considerations highlights the holistic view of the client, and Chapter 8 on epidemiology outlines the scientific and research base for nursing care. Lastly, the chapter on self-care for the nurse remains in Unit 1. This reflects our understanding that self-care is foundational to nursing practice, it is not an "add on," nor is it optional. Nurses must learn to care for themselves in order to sustain their own professional ability. The chapter provides an exploration of self-care modalities discussed in a way that is inviting and uplifting.

Unit 2 highlights specific psychiatric conditions clients may experience. These chapters explore conditions through use of illustrative literature, art, and movie clips, which give riveting examples of clients living with certain psychiatric conditions. These chapters are also key in encouraging the reader to be aware of personal feelings and biases toward mental health and illness, and how these personal opinions may affect interactions with both coworkers and clients.

Unit 3 introduces the reader to special populations needing mental health care. These chapters highlight the needs unique to these populations and discuss how to adapt nursing care to meet these special needs. A unique chapter on treating homeless and incarcerated clients will open doors for many nurses who may not previously have considered these special populations.

Unit 4 covers the diverse interventions and treatment modalities nurses may choose to employ, including psychopharmacology; individual, family, and group psychotherapy; complementary or somatic therapy; and community-based care.

Unit 5 provides special, additional information to the reader. Chapter 33 offers an annotated review of numerous films that can be viewed to help foster understanding of mental health and illness.

SPECIAL FEATURES

There are numerous special features in *Psychiatric Mental Health Nursing* Fourth Edition designed to stimulate critical thinking and self-exploration and to encourage readers to synthesize and apply knowledge presented in the text:

- **Literary excerpts** invite the reader to enter the client's world to better understand the process and impact of a psychiatric condition on an individual's overall health and functioning.
- **Movie boxes and classic art pieces** make the text come alive and help students understand what their clients are experiencing.
- **Chapter opening reflection boxes** set the stage for the chapter by inviting the reader to consider personal experiences with a given topic or to begin thinking about a certain psychiatric condition and the effects it may have on those experiencing it.
- **Reflective Thinking** features encourage readers to examine their own personal views on given topics in order to get and stay in touch with their own feelings, and to understand the varying viewpoints they may encounter in clients and coworkers. These boxes are designed to encourage reflection on an issue from a personal context, to raise awareness, and to stimulate critical thinking and active problem solving.
- **Nursing Tip** boxes encourage the reader to apply basic knowledge to real-life situations and offer helpful hints and shortcuts that will benefit new and experienced nurses alike.
- **Nursing Alert** features indicate life-threatening or serious indications, drug reactions or interactions, or critical precautions that need immediate attention.
- **Case Study/Care Plan** features offer an opportunity for the reader to apply the material presented in the chapter to

a real-life scenario, with an eye to encouraging extrapolation and intuitive thinking. Several case studies are based on the literary excerpts presented in the chapters and invite the reader to apply knowledge presented in text to an actual case example. Case studies are followed by a care plan based on the nursing process, and each concludes with critical thinking foci to challenge readers to revisit the case study to determine what else should be considered in terms of providing thorough, quality care to a client in need.

- **Care Planning Guides** provide additional considerations to planning care for clients. The care planning guides give the reader suggestions of nursing diagnoses, outcomes, and interventions most frequently used for clients with specific diagnoses.
- **Concept Maps** further illustrate priorities in case studies by mapping visually how one issue is related to another. A concept map frequently illustrates a "key" event that becomes the priority of care. We believe that the concept map provides the nurse with one more tool to use in reviewing data and establishing the care plan.
- **Learning Activities** challenge critical thinking by asking open ended questions that require comprehension of the chapter content as well as an ability to demonstrate application and analysis either verbally in class discussions or in thoughtful written responses.

Pedagogical Tools

Psychiatric Mental Health Nursing also includes numerous pedagogical features to promote learning and readability.

- **Competencies** open each chapter and introduce the main areas targeted for mastery in the chapter. They provide a checkpoint for study and tie in to crucial aspects of nursing care.
- **Chapter Outlines** are listed at the start of each chapter and serve as an overview and quick reference for the material to be covered.
- **Key Terms** are listed at the opening of each chapter and are boldfaced and defined at their first use in text.
- **Glossary** at the end of the book offers definitions of key terms used in text and serves as a comprehensive resource for study and review.
- **Appendices** offer important reference information, including DSM-IV-TR and NANDA listings, a critical pathway, and a description of psychological tests in common use.
- **Index** facilitates access to material and also indicates tabular, illustrated, literary, film and art entries.

NEW TO THIS EDITION

In addition to extensive updating throughout the chapters to reflect current research and professional practice, the following have been added to this edition.

- **Chapter 26: Survivors of Violence or Abuse** has been significantly revised to provide a more comprehensive examination of what violence is, what causes violence, and nursing perspectives on violence, abuse, and neglect.
- **Chapter 27: Pharmacology in Psychiatric Care** has been thoroughly updated with common agents and interventions.
- Throughout the text, **updated Care Plans, Case Studies, and Concept Maps** reflect the 2009-2011 NANDA-I Nursing Diagnoses Definitions and Classifications.
- **Research Highlight** features have been updated throughout to provide current research and related discussion of these studies' impact on nursing practice. These boxes can be used in support of developing evidence-based practice skills.
- **NCLEX-Style Review Questions**, a new feature to this edition, provide students with multiple choice questions in this important NCLEX-style format to facilitate assessment and critical thinking skills. With a focus on application and analysis this new feature is an important tool for student and instructor alike.
- ***Study*WARE™ CONNECTION** is a new end of chapter feature that encourages students to use and explore the new, free StudyWARE™ CD-ROM that accompanies this edition. For all chapters, the *Study*WARE™ CONNECTION box encourages use of the glossary games and activities provided. Additionally, for each of the disorders chapters, this box encourages use of the self-assessment quizzes provided on the CD-ROM.
- **Learning Activities using interviews on DVD with real clients.** Selected chapters have incorporated reflective questions for students to answer in response to viewing the *Study*WARE™ DVD providing interviews with real clients having the condition described in the chapter. In these cases, all questions asked of the student are based on chapter content and grounded in the observable material in the actual interview. These interviews provide a structured means for students to observe, think and respond to real client situations.
- **Boxes and most special features have been numbered** to allow for quicker access to desired information.

EXTENSIVE TEACHING/ LEARNING PACKAGE

The complete supplements package was developed to achieve two goals:

1. To assist students in learning the essential skills and information needed to secure a career in the area of nursing.
2. To assist instructors in planning and implementing their programs for the most efficient use of time and other resources.

Instructor Resources

The Instructor's Resource to Accompany Psychiatric Mental Health Nursing, Fourth Edition (ISBN 1-4354-0080-1)

The Instructor's Resource has three components to assist the instructor and enhance classroom activities and discussion.

Instructor's Guide

- **Teaching Methods and Strategies (Helpful Hints):** Ideas and concepts to help educators manage different presentation methods. Suggestions for overall approach to studying and presenting the chapter material are included.
- **Lesson Plans:** Guidelines for incorporating psychiatric nursing into one-semester courses. These are tied into the chapter competencies and include suggestions for different content delivery methods.
- **Learning Experiences:** Categories include theory application, individual activities, group activities, clinical activities, and community application.
- **Answers to Chapter Questions**: Answers and rationales for all end-of-chapter NCLEX style questions are provided.

Computerized Testbank

- Includes 1,000 questions that test students on retention and application of material in the text.
- All questions are now presented in NCLEX style with accompanying answers, rationales, cognitive levels and cross reference to headings in the text to locate supportive content.
- Allows the instructor to mix questions from each of the 32 didactic chapters in order to customize tests.

Instructor Slides Created in PowerPoint

- A robust offering of instructor slides created in PowerPoint outlines the concepts from text in order to assist the instructor with lectures.
- Ideas presented stimulate discussion and critical thinking.

WebTutor Advantage on Blackboard to Accompany Psychiatric Mental Health Nursing (ISBN 1-4354-0082-8) *and* Webtutor Advantage on WebCT to Accompany Psychiatric Mental Health Nursing (ISBN 1-4354-0081-X)

- A complete online environment that supplements the course provided in both Blackboard and WebCT format.
- Includes chapter overviews, chapter outlines, competencies, and reflection exercises.
- Useful classroom management tools include chats and calendars, as well as instructor resources such as the instructor slides created in PowerPoint
- Multimedia offering includes 10 pharmacology 3D animations, and an audio glossary with pronunciations of all terms in the book's glossary.

Online Companion

The Online Companion gives you online access to all the components in the Instructor's Resource as well as additional tools to reinforce the content in each chapter and enhance classroom teaching. Multimedia animations and an audio library are just some of the resources found on this site. To access the site, simply point your browser to http://www.delmar.cengage.com/companions. Select the nursing discipline.

STUDENT RESOURCES

Study Guide to Accompany Psychiatric Mental Health Nursing, Fourth Edition (ISBN 1-4354-0079-8)

A valuable companion to the core book, this student resource provides glossary activities to help drive mastery of information, as well as a excellent selection of challenging critical thinking questions for every chapter. Chapter quizzes have also been updated with additional multiple choice questions allowing the students to test their mastery of concepts in the text. Finally, a comprehensive 100 question final examination is provided, now entirely in NCLEX style, giving students an opportunity to test their comprehension of material in this important testing format.

Online Companion

The Online Companion gives you online access to a range of additional resources to support understanding of the material. An exciting new **Medical Terminology Audio Glossary** is available, providing pronunciations for the book's glossary terms alongside the corresponding definition. Multimedia animations are also available on this site. To access the site, simply point your browser to http://www.delmar.cengage.com/companions. Select the nursing discipline.

ACKNOWLEDGMENTS

The authors are indebted to many individuals and institutions for two lifetimes of learning, stimulation, and challenge. Only a few can be acknowledged in the brief space available to us.

Maureen Rosener, Juliet Steiner, Samantha Miller, Stacey Lamodi, Jack Pendleton, Ben Knapp, Patricia Allen, and Chris Catalina comprise the Delmar Cengage Learning team who helped to make the fourth edition a reality.

We join every reader of this book in thanking Lea Barbato Gaydos, our remarkable psychiatric nurse-artist, for the original paintings that grace the book's front cover and open each chapter. Lea is one of many vibrant members of the American Holistic Nurses Association—an ongoing source of professional inspiration and renewal.

Each of our many contributing authors has brought a unique background and perspective to this book. We greatly appreciate the wisdom with which their efforts have enriched the text. Numerous colleagues offered ideas and support for this project throughout its gestation: The nursing faculty at Cleveland State University School of Nursing, particularly Vicki Johnson, introduced us to the use of concept mapping in setting clinical priorities. Arlene Farren contributed immensely by providing her current knowledge related to care planning and the use of the NANDA-I taxonomy. Ellen Weiss, Nathan Copple, Alan Liu, Vincent Puzick, and fellow Internet webmates from the National Council of Teachers of English led us out of one particularly dark place and into Tennessee (Williams, that is); Alfred Guillaume, Jack Turner, and Beth Amen ably translated correspondence from faraway places. Ton Van Wageningen and his Amsterdam-based sister provided invaluable Dutch-speaking access to museums and art collections in the Netherlands.

Drawings, paintings, and images from movies and drama contribute greatly to this text. We appreciate contributions from the Kobal Collection, the Oregon Shakespeare Festival, and the Folger Shakespeare Library, and from numerous art museums throughout Europe and North America. We owe a special thanks to movie aficionado Ann Kimbrow, who did extensive viewing of many of the films discussed in this text. Also, we owe a special thanks to Dr. Joseph Barley from Akron, Ohio for assistance with movies. The book has benefited greatly from the work of Mary Sherman, Instructor of English at Wichita State University. Her filmography on mental health in the movies has allowed us to offer even more films for your Friday night enjoyment. After having benefited greatly from the monthly psychiatric film evenings in Akron Ohio (with many thanks to Dr. Rob Hermanowski and colleagues), we were delighted to see that Victoria B.C. has its own psychiatric movie Monday. And then there are a whole range of web-based movie sources including Dr. Roland Atkinson's marvelous Psychflix.com, from which we have benefited greatly in our own understanding of film and the experience of mental illness. We found a new contributor to our use of film – we thank Eileen Greene of Camosun College in Victoria for her work to develop learning activities based on the DVD interviews with real clients.

No acknowledgment page would be complete without offering our deepest thanks to the authors, poets, artists, dramatists, and filmmakers whose works bring all of us closer to an understanding of the most profound depths of human experience. The great Russian author and dramatist Anton Chekhov once wrote that "both (the study of) anatomy and (the study of) literature are of equally noble descent; they have identical goals." Following Chekhov, we have tried to include equal measures of literature and anatomy as we pursued our own goal; making both the science and the experience of mental illness come alive for the reader.

For the numerous anatomic images (CT, MRI, and PET) that we have been privileged to include throughout the text, we owe thanks to Drs. John Homan (Mad River Community Hospital), Alex Habibian (St. Joseph's Hospital of

Eureka), Scott Rauch (Massachusetts General Hospital), David Silbersweig (Cornell University Medical Center), Debbye Yurgelun-Todd (McLean's Hospital and Harvard Medical School), and Nancy Andreasen (University of Iowa). Jacqueline Spiegel-Cohen, M.S., of Mount Sinai School of Medicine was uniquely helpful and transferred to us by anonymous FTP more PET scan images than we have been able to use.

Our appreciation still goes to Barbara Georgiana, who spent endless months in the beginning helping us to give the first edition this book its unique character. She did all of the initial tracing of copyrights and obtaining permissions for the literary excerpts, artistic reproductions, and scientific illustrations for this text's first edition, and all before any of us were adept at using the Internet. After more than a decade, this book has her imprint, and we are thankful for her support and perseverance.

And by way of conclusion, the inevitable worry; if we have missed someone important in this lengthy acknowledgment, we offer our humblest apologies. And to our many readers; thank you for letting this text help you grow as a nurse and refine your skills in caring and healing. And of course, our thanks to your teachers who have many excellent textbook choices, but have selected this text because, we hope, it communicates something intangible about the rewards of caring for some of Nursing's most vulnerable clients.

Noreen and Larry Frisch

HOW TO USE THIS TEXT

Subject matter is presented in an innovative, interesting, and engaging manner throughout the text. The following suggests how you can use the features of this text to gain competence and confidence in psychiatric mental health nursing.

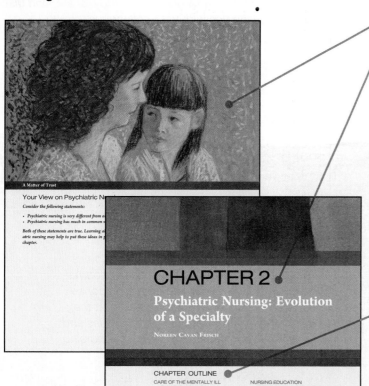

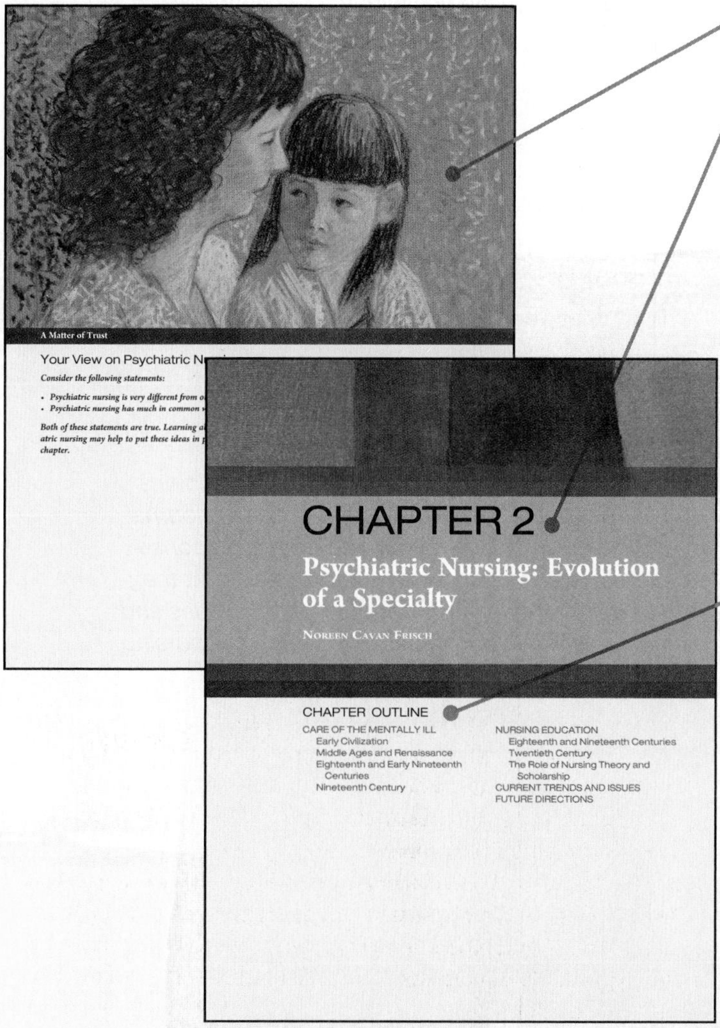

CHAPTER OPENERS

Each chapter opens with questions or statements that challenge you to examine your personal understanding of the psychiatric condition under discussion. These boxes invite you to reflect on your own views of psychiatric nursing and of those individuals who are personally affected by psychiatric conditions.

CHAPTER OUTLINE

These outlines provide a road map for the chapter and are an excellent way to understand how the chapter is organized.

HOW TO USE THIS TEXT (Continued)

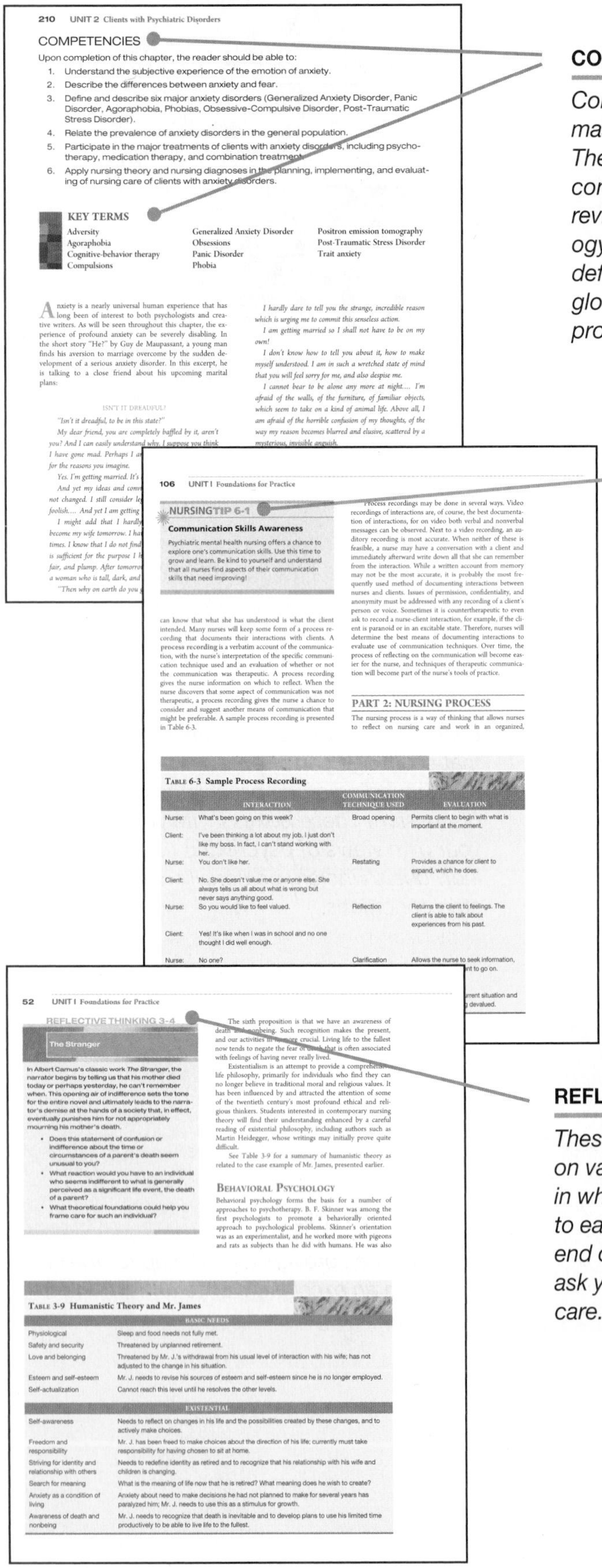

210 UNIT 2 Clients with Psychiatric Disorders

COMPETENCIES

Upon completion of this chapter, the reader should be able to:

1. Understand the subjective experience of the emotion of anxiety.
2. Describe the differences between anxiety and fear.
3. Define and describe six major anxiety disorders (Generalized Anxiety Disorder, Panic Disorder, Agoraphobia, Phobias, Obsessive-Compulsive Disorder, Post-Traumatic Stress Disorder).
4. Relate the prevalence of anxiety disorders in the general population.
5. Participate in the major treatments of clients with anxiety disorders, including psychotherapy, medication therapy, and combination treatment.
6. Apply nursing theory and nursing diagnoses in the planning, implementing, and evaluating of nursing care of clients with anxiety disorders.

KEY TERMS

Adversity	Generalized Anxiety Disorder	Positron emission tomography
Agoraphobia	Obsessions	Post-Traumatic Stress Disorder
Cognitive-behavior therapy	Panic Disorder	Trait anxiety
Compulsions	Phobia	

106 UNIT I Foundations for Practice

NURSING TIP 6-1

Communication Skills Awareness

Psychiatric mental health nursing offers a chance to explore one's communication skills. Use this time to grow and learn. Be kind to yourself and understand that all nurses find aspects of their communication skills that need improving!

PART 2: NURSING PROCESS

Table 6-3 Sample Process Recording

	Interaction	Communication Technique Used	Evaluation
Nurse:	What's been going on this week?	Broad opening	Permits client to begin with what is important at the moment.
Client:	I've been thinking a lot about my job. I just don't like my boss. In fact, I can't stand working with her.		
Nurse:	You don't like her.	Restating	Provides a chance for client to expand, which he does.
Client:	No. She doesn't value me or anyone else. She always tells us all about what is wrong but never says anything good.		
Nurse:	So you would like to feel valued.	Reflection	Returns the client to feelings. The client is able to talk about experiences from his past.
Client:	Yes! It's like when I was in school and no one thought I did well enough.		
Nurse:	No one?	Clarification	Allows the nurse to seek information, ...

52 UNIT I Foundations for Practice

REFLECTIVE THINKING 3-4

The Stranger

BEHAVIORAL PSYCHOLOGY

Table 3-9 Humanistic Theory and Mr. James

Basic Needs	
Physiological	Sleep and food needs not fully met.
Safety and security	Threatened by unplanned retirement.
Love and belonging	Threatened by Mr. J.'s withdrawal from his usual level of interaction with his wife; has not adjusted to the change in his situation.
Esteem and self-esteem	Mr. J. needs to revise his sources of esteem and self-esteem since he is no longer employed.
Self-actualization	Cannot reach this level until he resolves the other levels.
Existential	
Self-awareness	Needs to reflect on changes in his life and the possibilities created by these changes, and to actively make choices.
Freedom and responsibility	Mr. J. has been freed to make choices about the direction of his life; currently must take responsibility for having chosen to sit at home.
Striving for identity and relationship with others	Needs to redefine identity as retired and to recognize that his relationship with his wife and children is changing.
Search for meaning	What is the meaning of life now that he is retired? What meaning does he wish to create?
Anxiety as a condition of living	Anxiety about need to make decisions he had not planned to make for several years has paralyzed him; Mr. J. needs to use this as a stimulus for growth.
Awareness of death and nonbeing	Mr. J. needs to recognize that death is inevitable and to develop plans to use his limited time productively to be able to live life to the fullest.

COMPETENCIES AND KEY TERMS

Competencies list the core concepts you should master after reading and studying each chapter. These are a good way to introduce you to the content in the chapter and are a great study and review tool. Key terms introduce you to terminology covered in the text, and accompanying definitions can be found in both the end of book glossary as well as on the Audio Glossary (link provided on your StudyWARE™ CD-ROM).

NURSING TIPS

In any profession, there are many helpful hints that assist you in performing more efficiently. As a nurse, you will also need to embrace sensitivity in your practice. The wide variety of hints, tips, and strategies presented here will help you to apply your basic knowledge as you work towards professional advancement. Study, share, and discuss these tips with your colleagues.

REFLECTIVE THINKING

These boxes deal with self-reflection and opinions on various topics. It may be useful to keep a journal in which you write down your immediate response to each box on a chapter-by-chapter basis. At the end of each chapter, review your journal entries and ask yourself how your values will affect your nursing care.

HOW TO USE THIS TEXT (Continued)

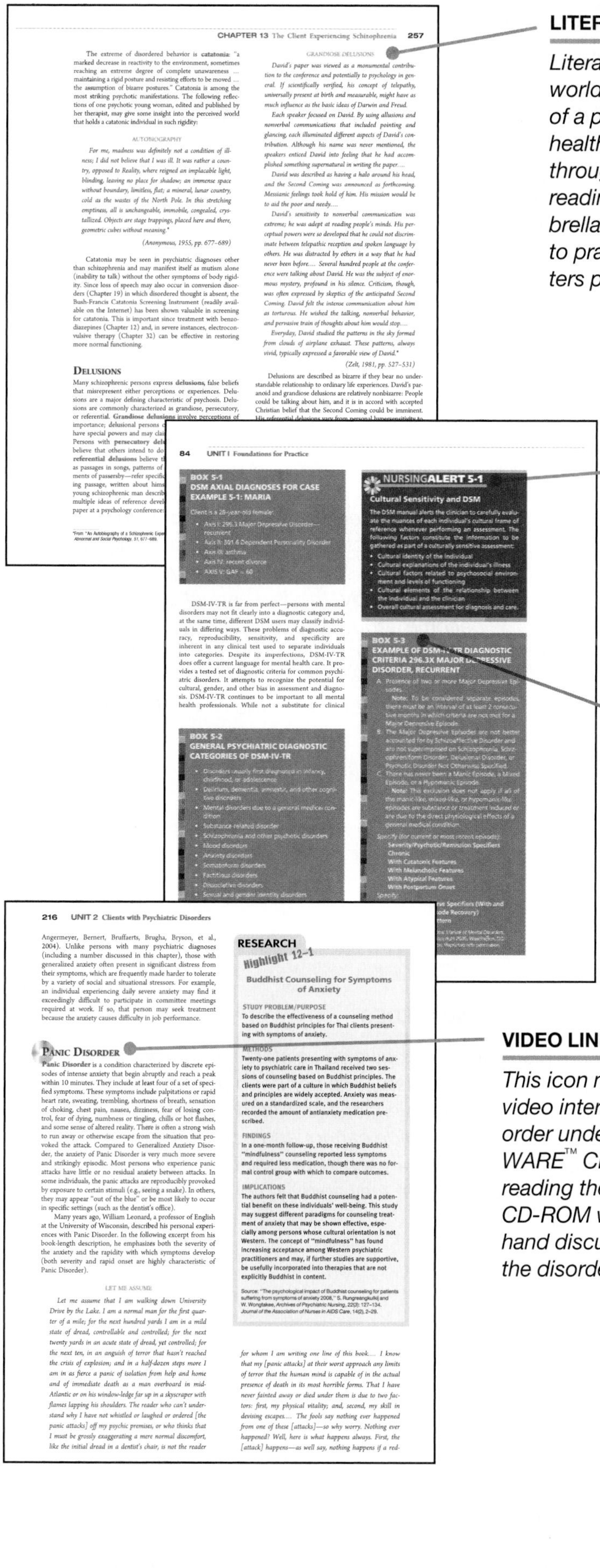

LITERARY EXCERPTS

Literary excerpts invite you to enter the client's world to better understand the process and impact of a psychiatric condition on an individual's overall health and functioning. You may want to browse through a chapter and read the excerpts prior to reading the chapter in its entirety, to get an umbrella view of a given disorder. You may also want to practice writing care plans based on the characters presented through the literature.

NURSING ALERTS

In some situations, you must act immediately in order to ensure the health and safety of your clients. This feature will help you to begin to identify and respond to critical situations on your own, both efficiently and effectively.

BOX

Boxes located throughout each chapter provide valuable additional information that may augment your understanding of core concepts, support successful clinical interactions with clients, or provide additional resources for a wider view of psychiatric mental health nursing.

VIDEO LINK ICONS

This icon next to a heading indicates there is a video interview with a client experiencing the disorder under discussion located on the free StudyWARE™ CD-ROM. Look for this icon as you are reading the text, and go to your StudyWARE™ CD-ROM whenever you see it for real-life first hand discussions of what it is like to experience the disorder.

HOW TO USE THIS TEXT (Continued)

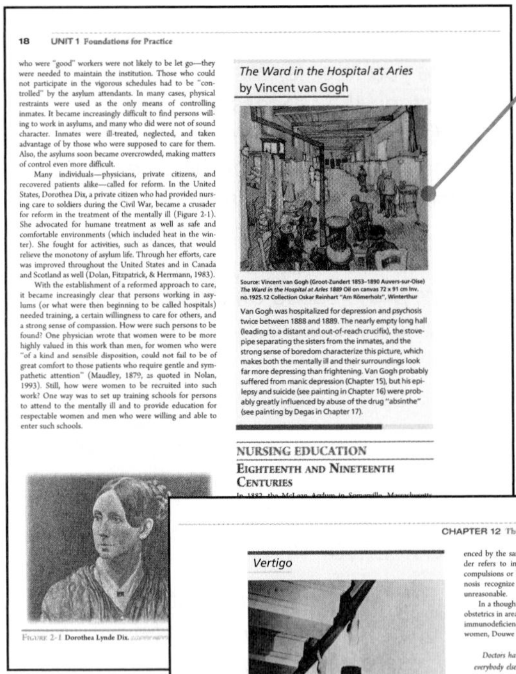

CLASSIC ART

Classic paintings allow you to experience through works of art the fascinating and disturbing worlds of those suffering from psychiatric conditions. The works of many famous artists beautifully illustrate the wide range of emotions and reactions of persons living with psychiatric conditions. As you view these, ask yourself what characteristics of the given disorders seem to be represented in the artwork.

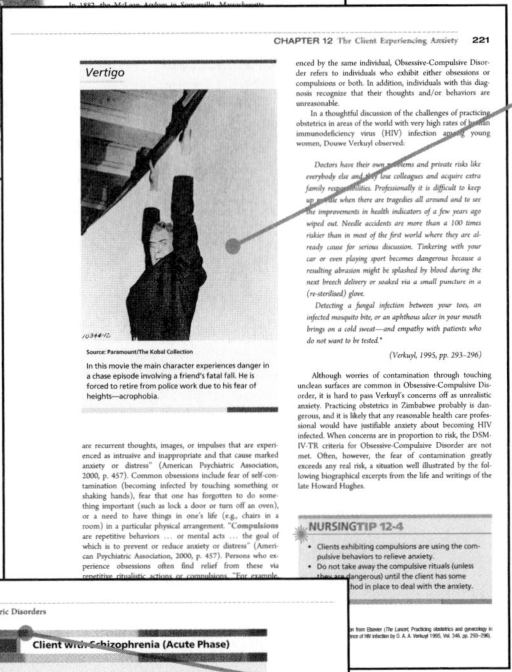

MOVIE CLIPS

We've included photos from popular movies that depict characters who are experiencing the situations you are studying. If you haven't seen these movies already, this is a perfect opportunity to become acquainted with them. Whenever possible, view these films while you are studying the chapter so you can determine what symptoms of a given disorder are embodied in the film's characters.

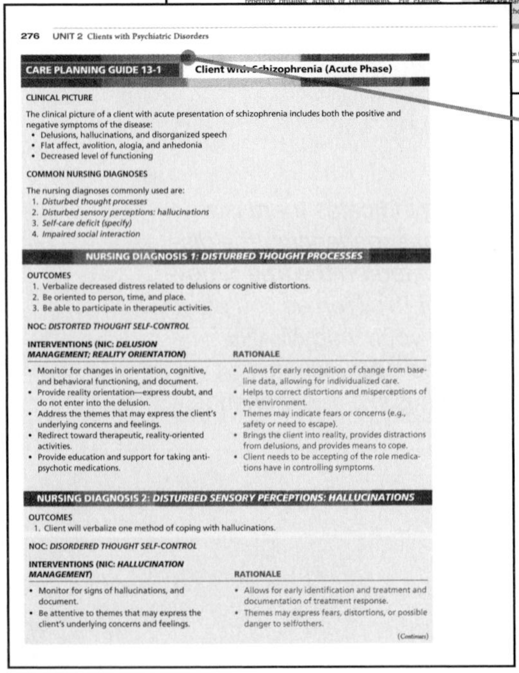

CARE PLANNING GUIDES

Care planning guides give you a start in planning care for a specific client. The common diagnoses, outcomes, and interventions are listed for specified conditions. A guide cannot and does not individualize care for your client, but assists you to think about areas that may apply in your practice plans.

HOW TO USE THIS TEXT (Continued)

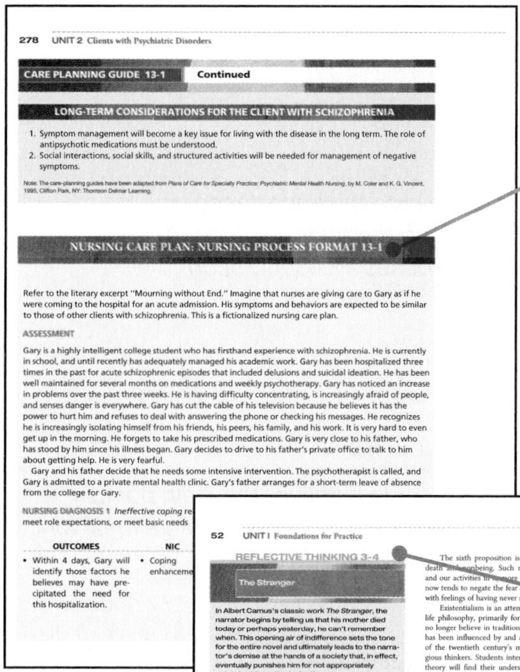

278 UNIT 2 Clients with Psychiatric Disorders

CARE PLANNING GUIDE 13-1 Continued

LONG-TERM CONSIDERATIONS FOR THE CLIENT WITH SCHIZOPHRENIA

1. Symptom management will become a key issue for living with the disease in the long term. The role of antipsychotic medications must be understood.
2. Social interactions, social skills, and structured activities will be needed for management of negative symptoms.

Note: The care-planning guides have been adapted from Plans of Care for Specialty Practice: Psychiatric Mental Health Nursing, by M. Coler and K. G. Vincent, 1995, Clifton Park, NY: Thomson Delmar Learning.

NURSING CARE PLAN: NURSING PROCESS FORMAT 13-1

Refer to the literary excerpt "Mourning without End." Imagine that nurses are giving care to Gary as if he were coming to the hospital for an acute admission. His symptoms and behaviors are expected to be similar to those of other clients with schizophrenia. This is a fictionalized nursing care plan.

ASSESSMENT

Gary is a highly intelligent college student who has firsthand experience with schizophrenia. He is currently in school, and until recently has adequately managed his academic work. Gary has been hospitalized three times in the past for acute schizophrenic episodes that included delusions and suicidal ideation. He has been well maintained for several months on medications and weekly psychotherapy. Gary has noticed an increase in problems over the past three weeks. He is having difficulty concentrating, is increasingly afraid of people, and senses danger is everywhere. Gary has cut the cable of his television because he believes it has the power to hurt him and refuses to deal with answering the phone or checking his messages. He recognizes he is increasingly isolating himself from his friends, his peers, his family, and his work. It is very hard to even get up in the morning. He forgets to take his prescribed medications. Gary is very close to his father, who has stood by him since his illness began. Gary decides to drive to his father's private office to talk to him about getting help. He is very fearful.

Gary and his father decide that he needs some intensive intervention. The psychotherapist is called, and Gary is admitted to a private mental health clinic. Gary's father arranges for a short-term leave of absence from the college for Gary.

NURSING DIAGNOSIS 1 *Ineffective coping* re... meet role expectations, or meet basic needs

OUTCOMES	NIC
• Within 4 days, Gary will identify those factors he believes may have precipitated the need for this hospitalization.	• Coping enhanceme...

NURSING CARE PLAN: NURSING PROCESS FORMAT

The Nursing Care Plan: Nursing Process Format will guide you as you apply the principles of nursing learned in each chapter to a client with the condition under study. Featuring real-world scenarios, the case study feature helps you make the connection between theory and practice more easily. This boxed element will reinforce your knowledge of the nursing process and the steps in the process of assessing, planning care, performing interventions, and evaluating the success of your course of care.

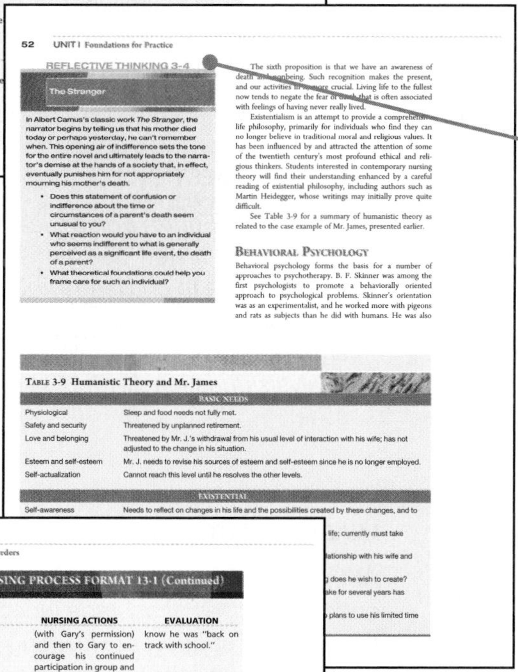

52 UNIT I Foundations for Practice

REFLECTIVE THINKING 3-4

The Stranger

In Albert Camus's classic work *The Stranger*, the narrator begins by telling us that his mother died today or perhaps yesterday, he can't remember when. This opening air of indifference sets the tone for the entire novel and ultimately leads to the narrator's demise at the hands of a society that, in effect, eventually punishes him for not appropriately mourning his mother's death.

- Does this statement of confusion or indifference about the time or circumstances of a parent's death seem unusual to you?
- What reaction would you have to an individual who seems indifferent to what is generally perceived as a significant life event, the death of a parent?
- What theoretical foundations could help you frame care for such an individual?

The sixth proposition is that we have an awareness of death and nonbeing. Such recognition makes the present, and our activities in it, more crucial. Living life to the fullest now tends to negate the fear of death that is often associated with feelings of having never really lived.

Existentialism is an attempt to provide a comprehensive life philosophy, primarily for individuals who find they can no longer believe in traditional moral and religious values. It has been influenced by and attracted the attention of some of the twentieth century's most profound ethical and religious thinkers. Students interested in contemporary nursing theory will find their understanding enhanced by a careful reading of existential philosophy, including authors such as Martin Heidegger, whose writings may initially prove quite difficult.

See Table 3-9 for a summary of humanistic theory as related to the case example of Mr. James, presented earlier.

BEHAVIORAL PSYCHOLOGY

Behavioral psychology forms the basis for a number of approaches to psychotherapy. B. F. Skinner was among the first psychologists to promote a behaviorally oriented approach to psychological problems. Skinner's orientation was as an experimentalist, and he worked more with pigeons and rats as subjects than he did with humans. He was also

TABLE 3-9 Humanistic Theory and Mr. James

BASIC NEEDS	
Physiological	Sleep and food needs not fully met.
Safety and security	Threatened by unplanned retirement.
Love and belonging	Threatened by Mr. J.'s withdrawal from his usual level of interaction with his wife; has not adjusted to the change in his situation.
Esteem and self-esteem	Mr. J. needs to revise his sources of esteem and self-esteem since he is no longer employed.
Self-actualization	Cannot reach this level until he resolves the other levels.
EXISTENTIAL	
Self-awareness	Needs to reflect on changes in his life and the possibilities created by these changes, and to ...
	... life; currently must take ...
	... lationship with his wife and ...
	... does he wish to create? ... ke for several years has ...
	... plans to use his limited time

REFLECTIVE THINKING

Reflective Thinking highlight each of the nursing process steps in the Care Plan. These elements will teach you to look critically at the methods of care suggested in each nursing process section and to look for new ways to provide thorough, quality care to the client under study.

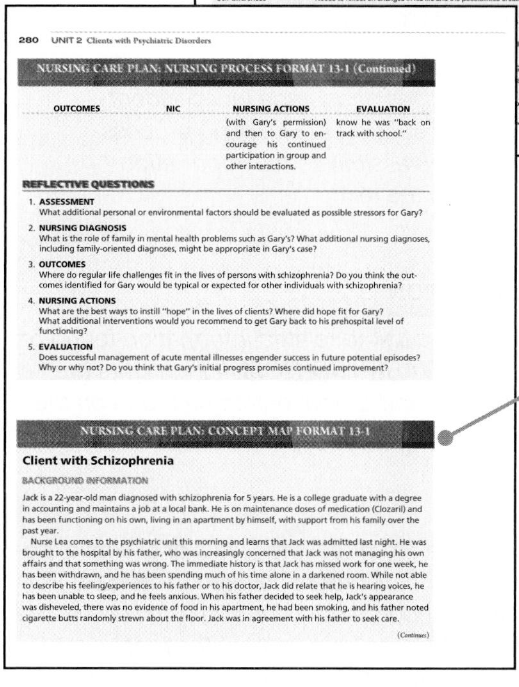

280 UNIT 2 Clients with Psychiatric Disorders

NURSING CARE PLAN: NURSING PROCESS FORMAT 13-1 (Continued)

OUTCOMES	NIC	NURSING ACTIONS	EVALUATION
		(with Gary's permission) and then to Gary to encourage his continued participation in group and other interactions.	know he was "back on track with school."

REFLECTIVE QUESTIONS

1. ASSESSMENT
What additional personal or environmental factors should be evaluated as possible stressors for Gary?
2. NURSING DIAGNOSIS
What is the role of family in mental health problems such as Gary's? What additional nursing diagnoses, including family-oriented diagnoses, might be appropriate in Gary's case?
3. OUTCOMES
Where do regular life challenges fit in the lives of persons with schizophrenia? Do you think the outcomes identified for Gary would be typical or expected for other individuals with schizophrenia?
4. NURSING ACTIONS
What are the best ways to instill "hope" in the lives of clients? Where did hope fit for Gary? What additional interventions would you recommend to get Gary back to his prehospital level of functioning?
5. EVALUATION
Does successful management of acute mental illnesses engender success in future potential episodes? Why or why not? Do you think that Gary's initial progress promises continued improvement?

NURSING CARE PLAN: CONCEPT MAP FORMAT 13-1

Client with Schizophrenia

BACKGROUND INFORMATION

Jack is a 22-year-old man diagnosed with schizophrenia for 5 years. He is a college graduate with a degree in accounting and maintains a job at a local bank. He is on maintenance doses of medication (Clozaril) and has been functioning on his own, living in an apartment by himself, with support from his family over the past year.

Nurse Lea comes to the psychiatric unit this morning and learns that Jack was admitted last night. He was brought to the hospital by his father, who was increasingly concerned that Jack was not managing his own affairs and that something was wrong. The immediate history is that Jack has missed work for one week, he has been withdrawn, and he has been spending much of his time alone in a darkened room. While not able to describe his feeling/experiences to his father or to his doctor, Jack did relate that he is hearing voices, he has been unable to sleep, and he feels anxious. When his father decided to seek help, Jack's appearance was disheveled, there was no evidence of food in his apartment, he had been smoking, and his father noted cigarette butts randomly strewn about the floor. Jack was in agreement with his father to seek care.

(Continues)

NURSING CARE PLAN: CONCEPT MAP FORMAT

Nursing Care Plan: Concept Map Format provides a framework to organize and think about data you have. These concept maps take the information provided and map the relationships between and among concepts. Most often, having completed a concept map, the nurse is faced with a "key" concept, one that impacts on many others or is impacted by many others. This focal concept is often the one to address first in interventions. Examine the concept maps and try one for your own clients and see if you find this a valuable tool in making practice decisions.

HOW TO USE THIS TEXT (Continued)

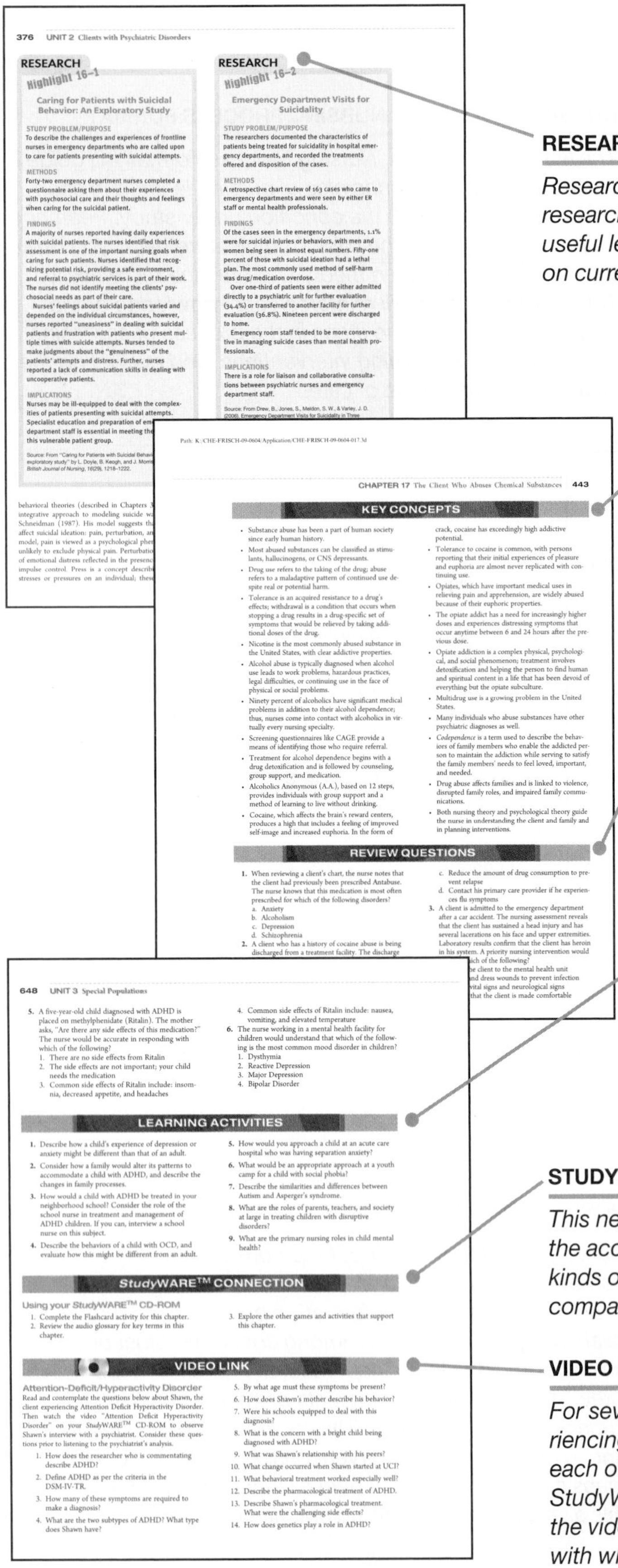

RESEARCH HIGHLIGHTS

Research Highlights emphasize the importance of research in nursing by linking theory to practice. A useful learning tool, these boxes focus attention on current issues and trends in nursing.

KEY CONCEPTS

Key Concepts highlight the main points presented in each chapter and are ideal for study and review.

REVIEW QUESTIONS

New to the Fourth Edition, each chapter provides 10 review questions written in the NCLEX style to challenge your mastery of chapter content while giving you practice answering knowledge, application, and analysis questions written in this important style.

LEARNING ACTIVITIES

At the end of each chapter these open-ended exercises encourage independent thinking and support the learning process by asking you assimilate the information presented in the text.

STUDYWARE™ CONNECTION

This new feature provides a link to related information found on the accompanying StudyWARE™ CD-ROM. It highlights the kinds of activities, quizzes, and animations to be found on the companion CD that relate specifically to the individual chapter.

VIDEO LINK

For several chapters, there are video interviews of clients experiencing different psychiatric disorders covered in the text. For each of these interviews, thought questions are provided in the StudyWARE™ CONNECTION to help you get the most out of the video clip and to connect what you are viewing on the video with what you have read in the chapter.

HOW TO USE THE SOFTWARE

HOW TO USE STUDYWARE™ TO ACCOMPANY PSYCHIATRIC MENTAL HEALTH NURSING, FOURTH EDITION

Minimum System Requirements

- Operating systems: Microsoft Windows XP w/SP 2, Windows Vista w/ SP 1, Windows 7
- Processor: Minimum required by Operating System
- Memory: Minimum required by Operating System
- Hard Drive Space: 500 MB
- Screen resolution: 1024 x 768 pixels
- CD-ROM drive
- Sound card & listening device required for audio features
- Flash Player 10. The Adobe Flash Player is free, and can be downloaded from http://www.adobe.com/products/flashplayer/

Setup Instructions

1. Insert disc into CD-ROM drive. The StudyWARE™ installation program should start automatically. If it does not, go to step 2.
2. From My Computer, double-click the icon for the CD drive.
3. Double-click the *setup.exe* file to start the program.

Technical Support

Telephone: 1-800-648-7450
8:30 A.M.–6:30 P.M. Eastern Time
E-mail: delmar.help@cengage.com

StudyWARE™ is a trademark used herein under license.

Microsoft® and Windows® are registered trademarks of the Microsoft Corporation.

Pentium® is a registered trademark of the Intel Corporation.

Getting Started

Getting started is easy! Install the software by following the installation instructions provided above. When you open the software, enter your first and last name so the software can store your quiz results. Then choose a chapter or section from the menu to take a quiz or explore media and activities.

The StudyWARE™ software helps you learn terms and concepts in Psychiatric Mental Health Nursing, Fourth Edition. *As you study each chapter in the text, be sure to explore the activities in the corresponding chapter in the software. Use StudyWARE™ as your own private tutor to help you learn the material in your* Psychiatric Mental Health Nursing, Fourth Edition *textbook.*

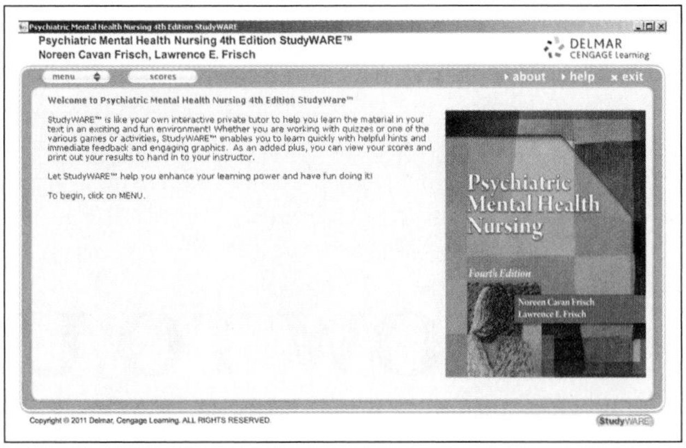

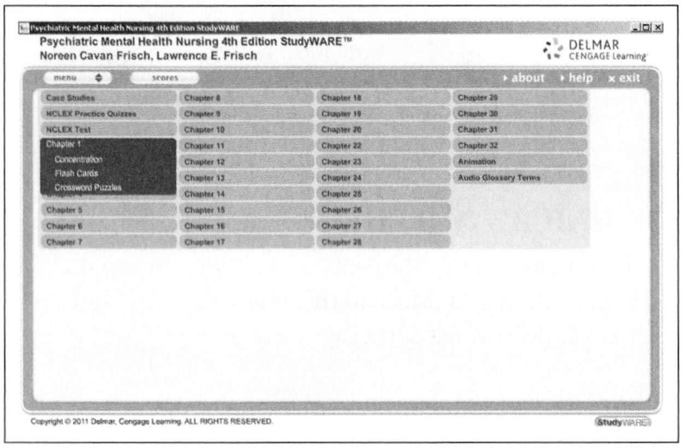

Menu: *You can access the menu from wherever you are in the program. The Menu includes Case Studies, NCLEX Quizzes for major disorders Chapters 12–20, Chapter Activities, Video, Animation, and Audio Glossary Terms. You can also access your scores from the button to the right of the main menu button.*

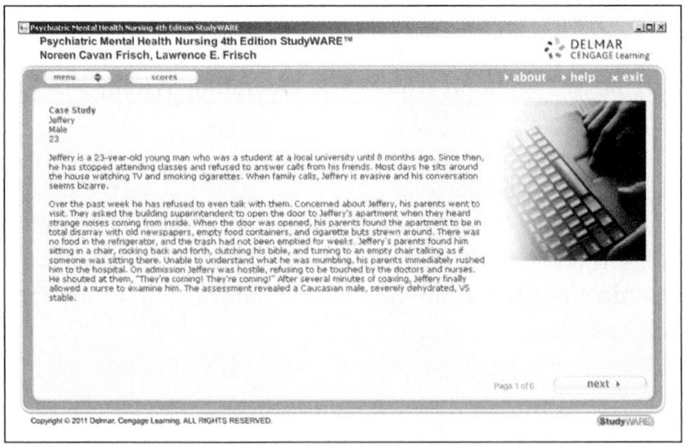

Case Studies: *Twelve case studies are provided to challenge your critical thinking skills and your ability to apply and analyze psychiatric mental health nursing information. Each case study provides background, followed by questions. At any time you can review the initial case study by clicking the Review Case Study button on the lower left hand of the screen. You can check your progress using the score menu to determine how thoroughly you understood the content areas addressed in the case study.*

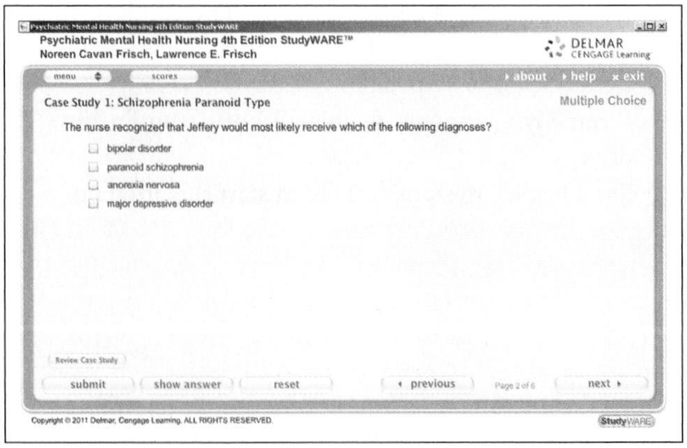

Quizzes: *For the major disorders Chapters 12–20 in* Psychiatric Mental Health Nursing, Fourth Edition, *quizzes are provided to test your understanding of critical concepts. The quiz program keeps track of your answers and a report can be generated at the end of the quiz outlining the questions, your answer, and the correct answer. Once the quiz has been completed, click on the Scores button for these details. Use the questions you missed as topic areas for additional study.*

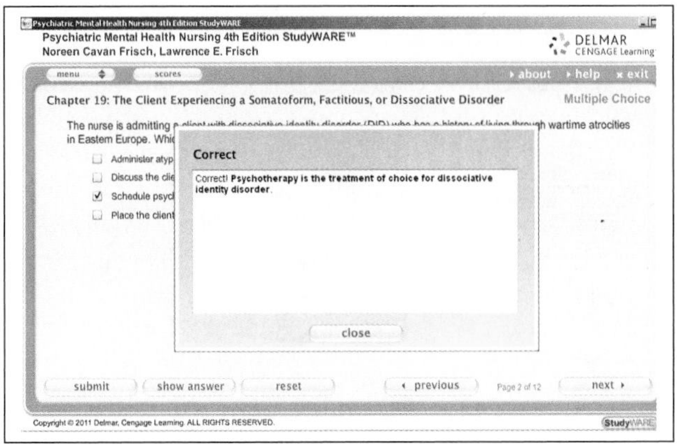

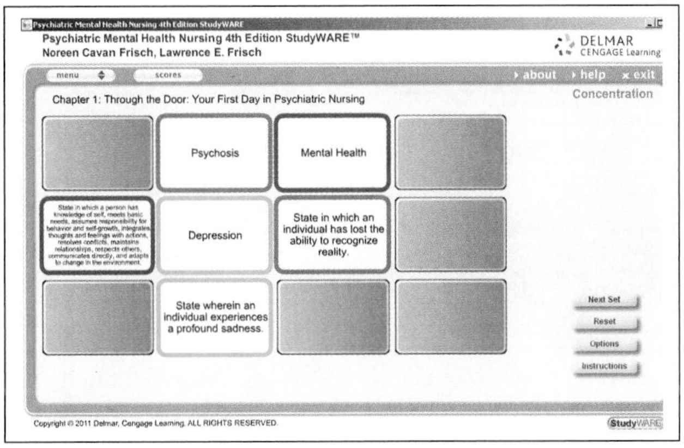

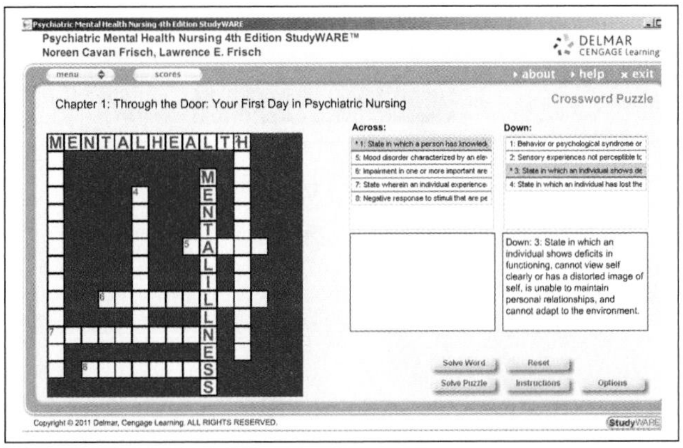

Chapter Activities: *For each chapter from* Pyschiatric Mental Health Nursing, Fourth Edition *with glossary terms, games and activities have been provided to help you master the terminology in a fun and interesting way. Concentration is a memory game that asks you to flip cards to match definitions with their terms. Flash Cards allow you to test your knowledge of a term by reading the term, thinking about the definition, then checking the actual definition. Crossword Puzzles provide definitions of key terms as clues, and you must fill in the appropriate term and clear the board.*

Video: *Throughout* Psychiatric Mental Health Nursing, Fourth Edition, *you will see small DVD icons next to section headings. These icons indicate there is video on the StudyWARE™ disk that further illustrates the disorder under discussion. The Video button is your link to 10 interviews with actual individuals discussing their experience with psychiatric disorders. Click on the disorder you've like to view, then click on the play button on the media viewer in the center of the screen. Questions accompanying each video are located at the end of the related book chapter. Use these questions to better understand the disorder and the client's experience of psychiatric disorders.*

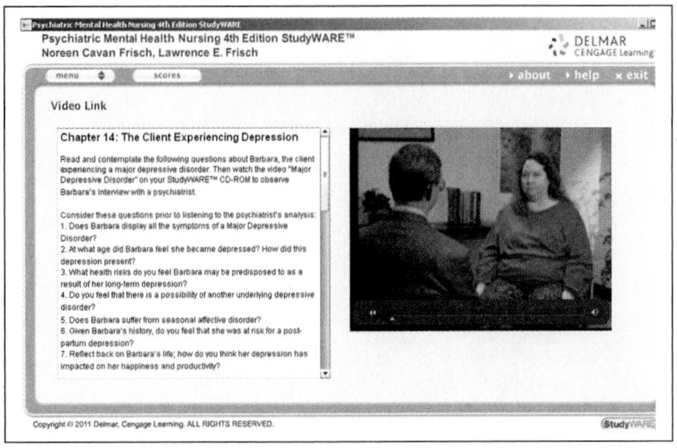

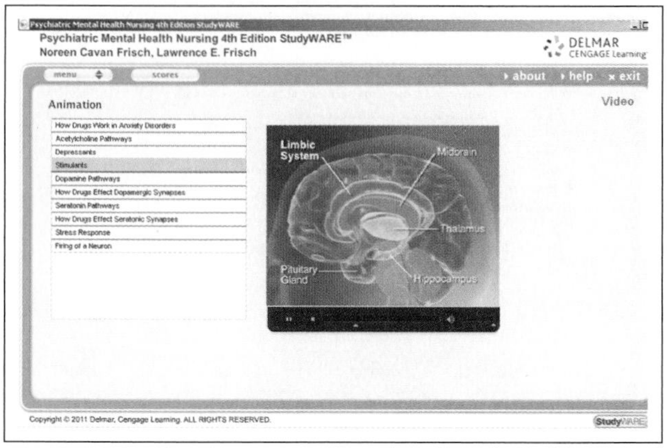

Animation: *This section on your StudyWARE™ CD-ROM provides 10 multimedia animations of biological and pharmacological processes. These animations visually explain some of the more difficult concepts and are an engaging resource to support your understanding.*

Audio Glossary Terms: *This menu selection takes you to a URL that will connect you with a comprehensive audio glossary to accompany* Psychiatric Mental Health Nursing, Fourth Edition. *Once you enter the Cengage Learning podcast site, you'll be able to click on a page for* Psychiatric Mental Health Nursing, Fourth Edition. *From this page you'll have access to correct pronuciations of all terms in the glossary, as well as the related definitions. Use the audio library to practice pronunciation and review definitions. You can browse terms by chapter or search by key word. This resource can be downloaded to any mobile media device for instant access any time, any where.*

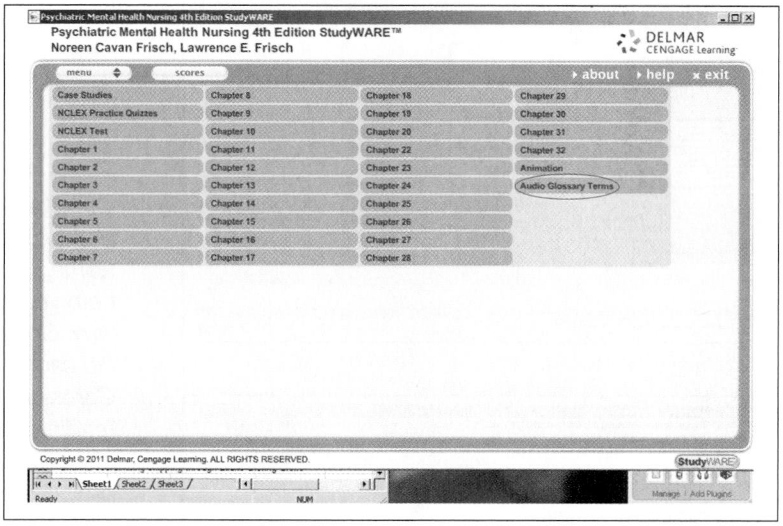

UNIT 1 Foundations for Practice

What is psychiatric mental health nursing? Where does it take place? Does it have a theoretical base? What is the language of psychiatry? How can nurses relate to mentally ill clients? How does culture affect our response to persons with mental illness? What do we know about why a person becomes mentally ill? What are the laws and ethical problems unique to mental health care and psychiatric nursing?

These questions outline some of the Foundations for Practice that are addressed in the next 10 chapters of this text.

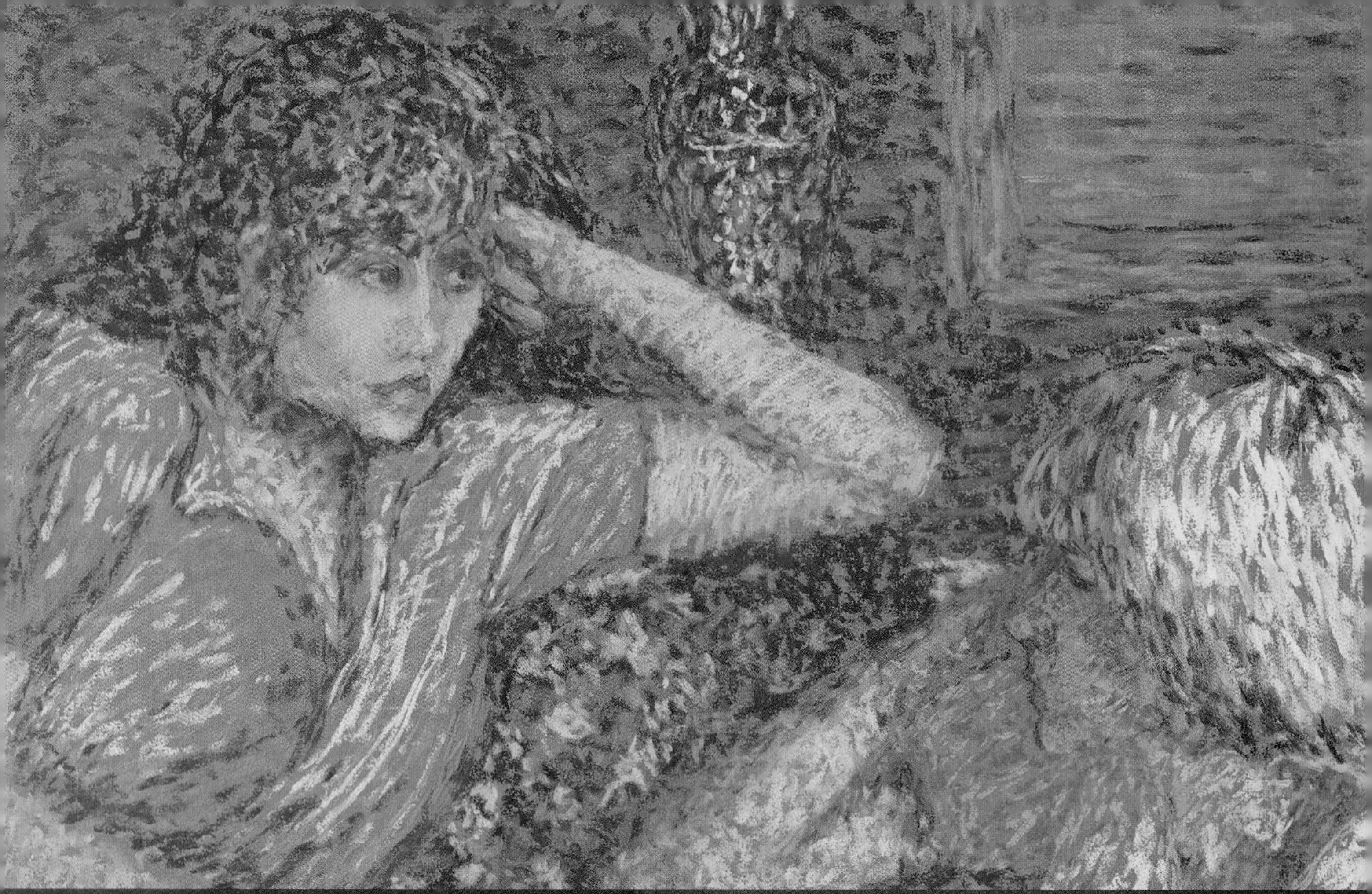

Just Between Friends

Your Own Experience and Feelings

- *What has been your experience with and exposure to psychiatric care? What are your ideas and images of psychiatry and mental health care? Where do they come from?*
- *What are your feelings about taking a course in psychiatric mental health nursing? Are you anxious? Interested? Curious?*

Read this chapter to help prepare for the first day in an exciting and extremely rewarding nursing specialty.

CHAPTER 1

Through the Door: Your First Day in Psychiatric Nursing

NOREEN CAVAN FRISCH
LAWRENCE E. FRISCH

CHAPTER OUTLINE

COMPETENCIES

Upon completion of this chapter, the reader should be able to:

1. Reflect on the experience of a psychiatric nursing course as a rite of passage in the process of becoming a nurse.
2. Describe basic information about the nature and practice of psychiatric mental health care, including:
   - The nature of mental health and mental illness
   - A sense of why a person is hospitalized for psychiatric care
   - Basic job descriptions and education of various mental health workers
   - Concerns and advice from prior students.
3. Interpret the goal of psychiatric care as that of strengthening the healthy portion of the client.
4. Plan your own learning strategies as you enter a course in this specialty.

KEY TERMS

Depression	Hallucinations	Mental Health
Disability	Mania	Mental Illness
Distress	Mental Disorder	Psychosis

You are about to begin your course in psychiatric mental health nursing, an exciting and emotionally rewarding nursing specialty. But, despite the rewards and excitement that we are confident you will find in your psychiatric nursing experience, we would be surprised if you did not feel a bit anxious about what lies immediately ahead. Psychiatric nursing facilities seem very different from the medical-surgical units, from the maternity care units, and from the other clinics students have previously used for their clinical rotations. When you enter the psychiatric unit, often through a locked door, you enter a world significantly different from other health care settings. At first, the differences may seem overwhelming, but there are also many similarities between psychiatric nursing and other areas of nursing. You will learn about similarities and differences between psychiatry and other areas as you experience your course, read the material in the various chapters of this book, and then complete the assignments your instructor has planned for you. A psychiatric course is a good time for reflection and self-examination, so as you begin this new course, take a few moments to reflect with us on what is going to happen and how you feel about it.

RITES OF PASSAGE

Nursing school is a time of growth and learning. Much of the growth is professional; you begin as a very new, novice nurse and leave school with enough background to take a position as a beginning professional. Some of the growth is personal; in nursing, you are exposed to very intimate human experiences, unlike any that are commonly experienced by other college or university students. Many nurses reflect on their time in school as a time of great transitions, of immense learning, and of bonding with other students. Along your path through nursing school and in the transition from new, novice nurse to beginning professional, you will encounter (or perhaps already have encountered) a number of important "rites of passage." Nursing students don special clothing and enter the closed doors of an operating suite to witness the dramatic ritual of modern surgery. They care for persons in pain and offer themselves and their treatments as comfort and support. Each experience marks a significant event, an achievement on the path to becoming a nurse.

For us, the first course in psychiatric mental health care was an experience with many dimensions: anxiety, learning, failure, and growth. We felt, years ago, that something significant happened when we passed through the door separating the psychiatric ward from the rest of the world—not quite sure yet who we really were or what we could do for anyone on the other side. Although locked wards exist today, the majority of clients now are treated through a variety of services in their homes, halfway houses, and clinics. Unfortunately, many chronically mentally ill people are homeless or incarcerated behind prison walls. You will encounter those who are fortunate enough to be treated within a health care service. What you learn from this experience should prepare you to be an advocate for mentally ill people throughout the community and especially for those within your responsibility of care as a nurse.

Caring for the mentally ill and, in the process, growing from student to practicing caregiver, are transitional experiences that anthropologists call rites of passage. A rite of passage occurs when there is a role change; it is often accompanied by a series of accepted rituals, which can reduce the anxiety related to the change in role. Rites represent life transitions; the person going through a rite of passage is transformed and different for having had the experience. As you enter your work in a psychiatric unit, you are going to experience a rite of passage similar to some you have already encountered on your path to becoming a nurse. Remember when you first saw the birth of a baby? This is an experience surrounded by emotion—joy, wonder, and the awe of creation. Remember when you first cared for a person who was dying? Emotions surround this experience as well—sorrow, solemnity, the spiritual sense of grief, and of parting.

The authors believe the experience of caring for and working with persons who are mentally ill to be just as moving, as transformational, as the experiences of birth and death. While caring for the mentally ill, you may confront persons who have great difficulty in communicating and are desperately in need of care. Frequently, the tools you have with which to give care—yourself and your ability to communicate with others—will not work for you as in your past nursing experiences. Approaching and talking with someone who is psychotic or sitting with someone who is profoundly depressed, you will experience a new dimension of nursing that will enrich your abilities to be an effective nurse. You will be challenged to reflect on your own behavior, your own methods of communication, and your own personality. You will have the chance to use this course to study human behavior in general and your own behavior in particular. You may emerge with different views of yourself, of nursing, and of mental health and illness.

But, you may be thinking, "I never wanted to be a psychiatric nurse! I'm taking this course because I have to." That is how many of us started, including most who became psychiatric nurses. However, psychiatric nursing opens up a new world, one that most students have never seen or experienced before, a world of human-to-human interaction, with much room for caring and compassion and excellent nursing. Enter the passage with an open mind and let the experience guide you, and always remember to be yourself.

By way of advice, many former students report that the bonding and support of other students is particularly important in a psychiatric nursing course. Interestingly enough, in many cultures, persons go through rituals or rites of passage as social (rather than solitary) experiences. Like student nurses, people throughout the world often undertake initiation into new roles in the company of valued comrades or friends. In many cultures, people who go through rites of passage together "are considered to be linked by special ties which persist long after the rites have been concluded" (Farb, 1978, p. 406). Value those ties—they are special—and they will be of special help to you when the experiences of the psychiatric unit become intense and challenging.

We have prepared this chapter as a "crash course" to provide you with basic information needed to feel confident and somewhat knowledgeable on your first day(s) in psychiatric mental health work. Of course, information is only a part of what you need. Start by taking an inventory about what you now know about mental illness and where your knowledge came from.

REFLECTIVE THINKING 1-1

Expectations

- What do you expect to see on a psychiatric unit? (List your ideas of what will be there.)
- From where do you think your perceptions came (i.e., what is your source of information about mental illness and psychiatry)?
- Do you have a definition of mental health and mental illness? What influenced your definition?

MENTAL HEALTH AND MENTAL ILLNESS

Members of the general public hold views of mental illness that are negative and stigmatizing. Many fear those who are mentally ill and carry beliefs that all are violent, unpredictable, or in some measure responsible for their own illnesses. Nursing students often enter a psychiatric nursing course with such views, reflecting the attitudes of the public (Emrich, Thompson, & Moore, 2003). Nursing professors know that experience with the mentally ill population can change these attitudes. Such experiences are planned for you in your psychiatric nursing course and will assist you in delivering compassionate care. Begin the course by identifying your views and expectations by answering the questions in the Reflective Thinking box. The information in the next paragraphs provide you with basic knowledge to help you prepare for your clinical work.

A good introduction will begin with some basic definitions and descriptions of concepts of mental health and mental illness. Mental health and mental illness are relative concepts, defined and described in relation to a person's ability to function and, basically, to have a positive self-view.

There is no clear, singular definition of **mental health**. In general, a person is mentally healthy when he possesses knowledge of himself; meets his basic needs; assumes responsibility for his behavior and for self-growth; has learned to integrate thoughts, feelings, and actions; and can resolve conflicts successfully. In relation to others, a mentally healthy person maintains relationships, communicates directly with others, and respects others. Lastly, a mentally healthy person adapts to change in his environment. These characteristics provide a description of mental health but do not fully define mental health. Persons who are mentally ill often possess many of the characteristics of well persons, and mentally healthy persons not infrequently experience symptoms similar to those of mental illness. The difference between sickness and health can be quite arbitrary and is often based on the degree to which characteristics or behaviors affect a person's functioning. Above all, the mentally ill show deficits in functioning; it is usually these deficits that bring them to the facilities where you will encounter them.

Mental illness occurs when an individual is not able to view herself clearly or has a distorted view of self, is unable to maintain satisfying personal relationships, and is unable to adapt to her environment. The American Psychiatric Association defines **mental disorder** as "clinically significant behavior or psychological syndrome or pattern that occurs in an individual and is associated with present **distress** (i.e., negative response to stimuli that are perceived as threatening) or **disability** (i.e., impairment in one or more important areas of functioning) or with a significantly increased risk of suffering, death, pain, disability, or an important loss of freedom" (2000, p. xxxi). Box 1-1 presents possible signs of mental illness, developed by a psychiatric nursing professor. It is important to note that none of these signs, taken in isolation of the individual and his context or life experiences, *necessarily* indicate the presence of mental illness. These signs, however, assist a nurse to begin to understand the nature and experience of mental illness.

BOX 1-1
POSSIBLE SIGNS OF MENTAL ILLNESS

- Marked personality change over time
- Confused thinking; strange or grandiose ideas
- Prolonged severe depression, apathy, or extreme highs and lows
- Excessive anxiety, fear, or suspiciousness; blaming others
- Withdrawal from society; friendlessness; abnormal self-centeredness
- Denial of obvious problems; strong resistance to help
- Thinking or talking about suicide
- Numerous, unexplained physical ailments; marked changes in eating or sleeping patterns
- Anger or hostility out of proportion to the situation
- Delusions (false beliefs that are firmly maintained even though they are not shared by others), hallucinations (perceptual distortions, arising from any of the senses—hearing voices or seeing images that others do not hear or see)
- Abuse of alcohol or drugs
- Growing inability to cope with problems and daily activities such as school, job, or personal needs

From "Possible Signs of Mental Illness," by J. Kozlak, 1996, personal communication. Reprinted with permission.

REFLECTIVE THINKING 1-2

Mental Health

Consider your own behavior and personality. Which traits would you classify as representing mental health? Which seem more representative of mental illness? Are you satisfied with the balance between the two?

Knowing something about symptoms and signs of mental illness is important, but that knowledge represents only the beginning of your passage. To really give nursing care, you will need some sense of what it feels like to be mentally ill, some way to see at least a little way into the suffering within another human being's mind. During your course you will begin to develop the necessary tools of listening, watching, and *being present.* As you interact with clients, some of what you see and hear will seem strange, crazy, and maybe at times a little frightening. If you start from a place of awareness and openness, your skills and confidence will grow each day. Give those skills a try as you read the following excerpt from the writing of a psychiatric client. The writer is responding to the questions, "How did you become mentally ill? What is it like?"

THE PARALLEL UNIVERSE

People ask, How did you get in there? What they really want to know is if they are likely to end up in there as well. I can't answer the real question. All I can tell them is, It's easy.

And it is easy to slip into a parallel universe. There are so many of them: worlds of the insane, the criminal, the crippled, the dying and perhaps of the dead as well. These worlds exist alongside this world and resemble it, but are not in it.

My roommate Georgina came in swiftly and totally. She was in a theater watching a movie when a tidal wave of blackness broke over her head. The entire world was obliterated—for a few minutes. She knew she had gone crazy. She looked around the theater to see if it had happened to everyone, but all the other people were engrossed in the movie. She rushed out, because the darkness in the theater was too much when combined with the darkness in her head.

And after that? I asked her.

A lot of darkness, she said.

But most people pass over incrementally, making a series of perforations in the membrane between here and there until an opening exists. And who can resist an opening?

In the parallel universe the laws of physics are suspended. What goes up does not necessarily come down, a body at rest does not tend to stay at rest, and not every action can be counted on to provoke an equal and opposite reaction. Time, too, is different. It may run in circles, flow backward, skip from now to then. The very arrangement of molecules is fluid: Tables can be clocks, faces, and flowers.

These are facts you find out later, though.

Another odd feature of the parallel universe is that although it is invisible from this side, once you are in it you can easily see the world you came from. Sometimes the world you came from looks huge and menacing, quivering like a vast pile of jelly; at other times it is miniaturized and alluring, a-spin and shining in its orbit. Either way, it can't be discounted.

*Every window on Alcatraz has a view of San Francisco.**

(Kaysen, 1993, pp. 5–6)

The woman writing this excerpt describes mental illness as a parallel universe from which one can see the world of the sane, a place where the predictable laws of our world do not hold—a frightening place. She writes from her current position in "our" world, but the borders between sanity and insanity seem to her only a "membrane" thick. As she reflects on her voyages back and forth across that membrane, it is easy to feel her ambivalence about which world she wants to stay in. There is both fear and a sense of entrapment in the "crazy" world, but it is hard not to sense that a part of her prefers to be there: "most people pass over incrementally, making a series of perforations in the membrane between here and there until an opening exists. And who can resist an opening?" She is describing her experiences, but at the same time she is challenging you, perhaps to see how you will react, whether she can scare you a little. Can you resist an opening? she asks. Come on over, "it's easy." It is not actually easy. Most of us have little chance of becoming psychotic during our lifetimes, but it is easy to get caught up by the expressiveness of her language. This is one way experienced nurses can recognize persons with disordered thought: their own feelings of attraction or intrigue for the world their client reveals to them. While others may not experience mental illness in this highly verbal way, Susanna Kaysen's reflections offer remarkable insight into how a person may feel and may react to the experience of mental illness.

THE PSYCHIATRIC SETTING

Most students want to know who they will encounter in a psychiatric setting (be it a psychiatric unit, clinic, short admission, outpatient/community care, crisis admission, or home care setting), what the setting will look like, and what they can expect from it. Let us begin, then, by describing both clients and staff that the student is likely to encounter.

Clients on an acute psychiatric unit are there because they are ill and in need of supervision. Some, like Susanna, are thought disordered and psychotic. Some are depressed and suicidal; some have been admitted to the unit after an attempt on their lives. Some are manic—they do not sleep, and their energy is boundless. Some have been admitted for drug detoxification or because of a drug-induced depression or psychosis. Each is a unique human being whose mental illness keeps him or her from functioning effectively in society.

Before we go on, we need to introduce some important concepts that will be considered in more depth in subsequent chapters. **Psychosis** means that the individual has lost the ability to recognize reality. A psychotic person may experience **hallucinations**, where he hears voices or sees images of persons or things that others cannot see or hear. A psychotic person is frequently unable to care for his basic needs of safety, security, nutrition, and so on. Such an individual is hospitalized for his own safety and to initiate treatment (usually involving some form of medication) to bring his symptoms under control. A psychotic person may slip into and out of reality much as Kaysen described in her metaphor of parallel universes separated by an easily crossed membrane.

Persons who have a profound **depression** (feeling very sad, despondent, and with no energy and no sense of the future) are in treatment for their own safety, and it is the responsibility of the nursing staff to keep a depressed or suicidal patient from harming himself. Almost every student has some idea of how it feels to be depressed, to be "down," to have no energy and no enthusiasm for activities, but few of us ever reach the profound depths of suicidal depression. Many hospitalized depressed persons are too despondent to talk or communicate except by occasionally echoing the words of others; some are catatonic, holding bizarre and rigid postures despite all attempts to move them. Depression of this degree seems untouchable, unreachable, and its treatment needs all the nurse's resources of presence, patience, and caring.

Other clients may be on the psychiatric unit because they are exhibiting manic behaviors. **Mania** is a condition where the person has excessive energy, exhibits abnormal excitability, and has an exaggerated sense of well-being. The manic client also may exhibit disturbed thinking, most often racing thoughts where she may not be able to concentrate on any one thing for very long. If inadequately supervised, manic clients may injure themselves or others. The manic client is at risk for exhaustion, as is the student assigned to watch, protect, and care for her.

Psychotic, depressed, manic, and drug-dependent clients are generally acutely ill. Their psychiatric illnesses may continue after discharge, but as their symptoms improve, they will likely leave the ward or hospital for the world outside. Other individuals under psychiatric care have long-term chronic mental illnesses. Many of these individuals cannot live outside highly protected environments, and some spend their entire lives in institutions or extended-care facilities for the mentally ill. These persons may be in touch with reality, but often their cognitive skills or coping mechanisms have been severely disrupted. Most have chronic schizophrenia and are unable to work or make choices required for independent living. Some of these persons may have unpredictable behaviors and difficulties controlling aggressive or sexual impulses.

During your psychiatric course you will meet individuals with a variety of acute and chronic psychiatric conditions, and we suspect that some will leave a lasting impression, as they did for us many years ago. You will also meet a variety of staff who work on the psychiatric unit, and hopefully some of these will be among your best teachers and role models. Some of these individuals will have familiar titles and responsibilities, but others may represent unfamiliar disciplines. Table 1-1 presents a brief description of the various persons working in psychiatric facilities. Each person has a different background, and each contributes something different to client care. You are encouraged to learn the specific roles of the various professionals and staff in the facilities where you are assigned to complete your psychiatric rotation in order to better function as a member of an interdisciplinary team.

QUESTIONS STUDENTS USUALLY ASK

Each psychiatric unit and its staff is unique. Your actual experience will be determined by factors unique to the setting in which you work and study. Still, students frequently ask some basic questions as they enter their psychiatric mental health course. We have answered these questions frequently enough that we think many of you may have similar concerns and we thus address them here.

TABLE 1-1 Mental Health Professionals

MENTAL HEALTH STAFF	EDUCATIONAL BACKGROUND	ROLE
Psychiatric nurse	Registered nurse	Manages the inpatient or outpatient nursing care of clients; administers medications; completes assessments on clients, establishes outcomes, writes nursing diagnoses, and implements plan of care, including client/family teaching
Psychiatric nurse, advanced practice, psychiatric nurse practitioner	MSN or DNP with psychiatric nursing specialty	Provides psychotherapy; prescribes psychotropic medications (in most states); manages and coordinates client care
Psychiatrist	MD; has completed a residency program in psychiatry	Manages patient care; admits patients to hospital; prescribes psychotropic medications; may provide in-depth psychotherapy
Psychologist/clinical psychologist	PhD in psychology with an internship in clinical work	Manages care; provides individual or group therapy; skilled in behavioral assessment and interventions
Psychiatric social worker	MSW with background in psychiatric care	Provides care that integrates hospital and community services; skilled in individual and group work
Activity therapist/ recreational therapist	Has completed at least a baccalaureate degree in recreational therapy	Provides recreation, diversional activity aimed at increasing socialization and activity
Occupational therapist	Has completed at least a baccalaureate degree in occupational therapy	Provides vocational counseling and activities designed to prepare clients for job-related skills
Certified addictions counselor	Has completed training and passed a certification exam in addictions-related work	Provides counseling; facilitates group work; gives support to persons with chemical dependency
Psychiatric technician, aide, or assistant	Has completed course work in psychiatric technician work; in some states is certified to work in psychiatric facilities	Provides supervision of clients on inpatient and outpatient units under the supervision of an RN
Student nurse	In school for an RN license	Provides care to selected and assigned clients

Why and How Do Persons Seek Care?

Persons with mental illnesses often seek care for reasons very similar to those who seek care for physical illnesses—they are uncomfortable, in pain, and in need of help. Others seek care because a member of their family or a close friend encourages them to get professional help for problems such as chemical addiction or depression. Still others obtain treatment because they have lost touch with reality and are unable to make judgments. Their deficits in self-care skills bring them to medical or police attention. Some persons become disoriented to person or place and may be brought to a psychiatric hospital or an emergency department for evaluation and treatment.

Will I Be Able to Know the Staff from the Clients?

In most psychiatric facilities nurses and other staff do not wear uniforms, but, rather, wear street clothes. This surprises some students, who are used to the hospital and clinical settings in which uniforms are commonly worn. Students are often concerned about whether they will recognize which persons on a unit are clients and which are caregivers. In almost all settings, the staff wear name tags and can be identified as staff members in this way. You will have an orientation to the unit to which you are being assigned, and after your first day you should feel comfortable that you know who the staff are who will be working with you.

Will Clients' Behaviors Make Me Uncomfortable?

Perhaps yes. In our society, you can walk down the streets of any major city and encounter persons who are mentally ill. You see people actively hallucinating, having conversations with people who are not there, and gesturing wildly. On the streets most of us are made a little anxious by such behaviors and, even if we do not make a point of crossing to the other side, we tend to mind our own business and avoid eye contact. Not so in the psychiatric hospital. No matter how bizarre a client's behavior is, the nursing goal is to establish contact and treat the individual with understanding and compassion. Most nursing students enter psychiatric classes with little or no previous experience working with the mentally ill. Fortunately, staff and instructors are present to offer guidance regarding what to do, what to say, and how to approach a person who is mentally ill. Some ill individuals will prove remarkably approachable; others will resist all efforts. For example, a client experiencing hallucinations may not respond to the nurse's efforts at communication. With time and experience, you will learn how to provide the needed care and grow in your abilities to participate in treatment.

Are Psychiatric Clients Violent?

Yes, some psychiatric clients are violent or have the potential for violence. While there is a risk for violence in psychiatric settings, studies have shown that the incidence of violence among persons with psychiatric disorders is not significantly different from that of the general population. In a psychiatric facility, the staff are experienced in assessing potential for violence and are skilled at recognizing those situations where violence may occur. Also, psychiatric staff know how to remove a client from a setting in which anger is escalating and know how to control a violent client. This experience in management of anger and violence is highly applicable to other settings and is one of the important skills to learn in a psychiatric course. Do be aware that there is a potential for violence in any health care setting, but also be assured that violent outbreaks are not a common occurrence on psychiatric wards and that experienced staff members, not the students, will handle such occurrences.

How Will I Feel without My Regular Nursing Uniform?

It is interesting to observe how closely one can become attached to a nurse's uniform that identifies one as a professional nurse. The uniform provides an identity; to appear on a unit without wearing a uniform makes many feel like something was left behind. Further, nursing in nonpsychiatric settings is easily focused on "doing" things. A nurse takes a blood pressure and uses the need for a blood pressure reading to initiate a conversation with a client. In psychiatric mental health nursing, you must initiate the conversation without the need to take a blood pressure reading. On a psychiatric ward nurses cannot hide behind their uniforms or the physical "tools of the trade." Again, remember that the tools of psychiatric nursing are listening, watching, and being present. As you develop these therapeutic skills, you will come to identify yourself more with your abilities and less with the outward trappings of your nursing identity.

NURSING TIP 1-1

Suggestions for Conversing with a Psychotic Client

The following will help you in interactions with clients who are psychotic or out of touch with reality:

- Introduce yourself to the client.
- Talk to this person as you would other clients.
- Keep conversations concrete (rather than abstract).
- Help the client to stay in touch with reality by focusing on the immediate environment (elements and people in the room).

What Do Psychiatric Clients Think of Student Nurses?

Some clients are too absorbed in their own worlds or troubles to give any special thought to student nurses. However, many clients are very aware of who is coming and going on the psychiatric ward. Susanna Kaysen provides an interesting description of the regular "influx" of student nurses to the hospital unit where she was hospitalized for many months:

STUDENT NURSES

*The student nurses were about nineteen or twenty: our age. They had clean, eager faces and clean, ironed uniforms. Their innocence and incompetence aroused our pity ... it was because when we looked at the student nurses, we saw alternate versions of ourselves. They were living the lives we might be living, if we hadn't been occupied with being mental patients. They shared apartments and had boyfriends and talked about clothes. We wanted to protect them so that they could go on living these lives. They were our proxies ... For some of us, this was the closest we would ever come to a cure.**

(Kaysen, 1993, pp. 90–91)

Kaysen gives us a unique description of nursing students in that she is the same age and sex as many nursing students and was hospitalized for a long enough time period to see students come and go on her unit. Kaysen describes students as different from other hospital staff, as somewhat special. The fact that students are seen as living the lives the clients might live (or want to live) is a powerful idea. Perhaps this description helps you to put your role as a student in perspective.

ADVICE FROM PRIOR STUDENTS

Having taught psychiatric mental health nursing courses for many years, the authors pass along the following recommendations from prior students who wish to provide a bit of advice:

- Get used to a slower pace. You will not be running around a unit trying to get everything done in time for noon medications. Rather, you will be sitting with patients and interacting with them. If you feel you are not being a nurse if you are not busy with activities, you will have an adjustment. Keep in mind the side of nursing that listens, that cares, and that provides presence.
- Be yourself, and interact with clients as real people. The most important tool you have to use as a psychiatric nurse is yourself. If you see yourself as a caring nurse and show respect for other people, both staff and clients will eventually give you their trust.
- Take time to reflect on how you come across to others. You have a unique chance in a psychiatric mental health course to examine your own behaviors. If you sit close to a fellow student, what do they do? If you laugh, how do others respond? Catalog your strengths and weaknesses. What interpersonal situations are you most comfortable in? Which make you most anxious? Do some persons or situations evoke recollections of childhood experiences? How do these recollections affect the way you respond to the persons or situations?
- Emphasize and learn communication skills. Do not be afraid to say the wrong thing. Try out the communication skills you are learning. If you say the wrong thing, you will learn how to do it differently next time. Communication is a skill, and it takes practice to improve and master it. Use this course to practice these skills.
- Use the experience to learn about yourself. When you study psychiatric nursing, you will learn about yourself. For instance, you will read about defense mechanisms in this textbook and subsequently may find yourself using them in a conversation with someone you know! You have probably used such defense mechanisms all your life, but perhaps never recognized them before. Defense mechanisms are normal human responses; it is OK to be normal and to recognize *how* you are normal. You will also read about mental illness and may begin to wonder if you or someone you are close to has some symptoms or characteristics of a certain condition. You probably do: Remember that mental illness is a matter of degree; the vast majority of us are healthy but also have a few characteristics of one psychiatric condition or another. Do not be surprised to find some "abnormal" characteristics in your personality makeup. But *do* seek help if you find any of your discoveries disturbing.

HOW TO GET THE BEST EXPERIENCE AND LEARNING IN YOUR PSYCHIATRIC MENTAL HEALTH NURSING COURSE

Several recent reports of students' experiences in psychiatric nursing courses can help new students understand the unique experiences of such a course. Researchers have found a number of factors that seem to "hold true" for students, and their research findings point to some very specific ways of approaching learning in this specialty. The ideas from this work are summarized in the following discussion.

While few students enter their psychiatric nursing courses with the intention of becoming a psychiatric mental health nurse (Hayman-White & Happell, 2005), experiences in the clinical areas can promote a very positive notion of the specialty. Proactive steps can help the student develop positive learning experiences. For example, students who become actively involved in client care are those that have the most positive experiences of the course (Henderson, Happell, & Martin, 2007). In one study, students found that the structure

*From *Girl, Interrupted* by Susanna Kaysen. Copyright © 1993 by Susanna Kaysen. Used by permission of Turtle Bay Books, a division Random House, Inc.

of inpatient units was more conducive to their learning (Henderson et al., 2007), though this observation did not hold true for other investigations where students were more satisfied with community-based settings (Happell, 2008). That said, there were activities that helped to create positive learning for students: learning to understand mental illness, skill development, dispelling fears, and personal development. In addition, the role of the faculty, preceptor, or mentor cannot be underemphasized. Students found support from other professionals to be essential in creating the learning environment they needed. Thus, students should remain open to developing a relationship with a faculty member or a preceptor who has experience in psychiatric care and who can help to guide the students toward positive learning activities. (The message here is to take the support and help that will be offered.)

There are two other proactive steps that students can take as they begin their courses. First, developing a learning contract with your faculty member may help you as a student gain a sense of autonomy and control over your clinical experiences (Chien, Chan, & Morrissey, 2002). A learning contract is a self-assessment of where you are in ability/confidence in mental health nursing that you use to plan your learning objectives. While it is certainly expected that your faculty member has a set of objectives for you to achieve and competencies that you must meet at the end of the course, a learning contract provides you a beginning plan of where you are now and where you need to go. Also, as you progress, a learning contract can help you set up a step-by-step plan and documentation of your progress, and provides a focus of your communication with your instructor or preceptor. Second, the use of personal reflections on your day-to-day experiences also helps you to put your activities, responses, and thoughts in perspective as you step back and consider what you saw, what you did, and how you and others reacted. Donovan reports that reflection on practice helps students develop self-awareness and helps student themselves see situations where they often "did better" than they thought (2006; 2007). Further, she reports that students needed some time and support to "get the hang of it," but concludes that reflection is an important learning tool.

Finally, advice from the authors is to enjoy your course! Take your time, read the materials we've provided, examine the DVD that accompanies this text, watch a movie or two, and learn.

BEGINNING A NEW COURSE

Beginning with this class, you are in a new phase in your nursing education. Hopefully, you will find this experience challenging and will emerge with different experiences and tools to use in nursing. Enter the course with an open mind, and take information about human behavior and about yourself that is useful to you. Psychiatric care differs from other areas of health care. In order to work as a psychiatric nurse, you must be able and willing to live with a certain amount of ambiguity. Learn and grow from the experience!

Listen to, talk with, and be with the clients on your unit. They will be your best teachers; after a decade or more you may find them as vivid in your memory as they will be the first week. Above all, take time to "smell the flowers." Do not let hard work keep you from connecting with friends, family, nature, music, and the other experiences that make for rich, mentally healthy, and deeply satisfying lives. Now, put your hand on the doorknob, take a deep breath, and walk in.

KEY CONCEPTS

- The study of psychiatric nursing affords an opportunity for the student nurse to perform self-examination of values, feelings, and beliefs.
- Rites of passage in psychiatric nursing refer to expected transitions and learning experiences linking the world of the student and the world of the practicing nurse.
- Mental health is a general concept referring to an individual's positive view of self, others, relationships, and the environment; it must be viewed in terms of degree, as all individuals experience varying degrees of mental health at different times in their lives.
- A mental disorder is presentation of clinically significant behavior or psychological syndrome or pattern as defined by the American Psychiatric Association.
- Familiarity with psychiatric settings and the different types of mental health professionals will ease the transition for the new nurse into the world of psychiatric nursing care.
- Students who are proactive in their learning will probably be more satisfied with the experience of their psychiatric nursing course.

REVIEW QUESTIONS

1. The rite of passage for a nursing student entering psychiatric nursing is which of the following?
   1. The fact that students have more rights.
   2. A role change where the individual is transformed.
   3. The entry of a nursing student into a closed psychiatric unit.
   4. The student's progression to the last semester of the nursing program.
2. The major tool that a student new to psychiatric nursing brings to the experience includes the ability to:
   1. take vital signs
   2. communicate with others
   3. interpret laboratory results
   4. manipulate technical equipment
3. On the first day of the psychiatric nursing clinical experience, a client behaving bizarrely approaches the student nurse. Which of the following would be an appropriate response by the student nurse?
   1. Quickly find the nursing instructor and ask for help.
   2. Grimace and show intolerance for the patient's psychotic behavior.
   3. Establish contact and treat the individual with understanding and compassion.
   4. Tell the charge nurse that the patient needs to be placed in seclusion or restraints.
4. A psychiatric nurse is preparing to interact with a new client. Which of the following tools is necessary to effectively communicate with the client?
   1. Judging
   2. Stereotyping
   3. Being present
   4. Devaluing
5. A major challenge for nursing students entering psychiatric nursing includes which of the following?
   1. Reflecting on own behavior
   2. Reflecting on the client's behavior
   3. Reflecting on the client's personality
   4. Reflecting on the client's method of communication
6. A nurse assessing a client to determine the presence of mental illness would most likely identify which of the following as being present?
   1. Clear and realistic thinking
   2. Moderate use of alcohol or drugs
   3. A strong and confident personality
   4. Inability to effectively cope with problems
7. A client is being discharged from the hospital. Which of the following would indicate that the client has improved?
   1. Low self-esteem
   2. Poor self-concept
   3. Distorted view of self
   4. Ability to set realistic goals

LEARNING ACTIVITIES

1. Differentiate mental health from mental illness and from mental disorder.
2. Reflect back on a time when you experienced a severe threat to your mental health. What were the circumstances? Who was involved? What was your reaction, and what was the resolution?
3. Describe some of the reasons an individual might seek psychiatric care.
4. Discuss some of the professional options for individuals wanting to work in the mental health field and the educational requirements and general scope of practice of each.

*Study*WARE™ CONNECTION

Using your *Study*WARE™ CD-ROM

1. Complete the Concentration activity for this chapter.
2. Review the audio glossary for key terms in this chapter.
3. Explore the other games and activities that support this chapter.

REFERENCES

American Psychiatric Association. (2000). *Diagnostic and statistical manual of mental disorders* (4th ed.-TR) Washington, DC: Author.

Chien, W., Chan, S. W., & Morrissey, J. (2002). The use of learning contracts in mental health nursing. *International Journal of Nursing Studies, 39*(7), 685–694.

Donovan, M. O. (2007). Implementing refection: Insights from pre-registration mental health students. *Nurse Education Today, 27*(6), 610–616.

Donovan, M. O. (2006). Reflecting during clinical placement—discovering factors that influence pre-registration psychiatric nursing students. *Nurse Education in Practice, 9,* 134–140.

Emrich, K., Thompson, T. C., & Moore, G. (2003). Positive attitude: An essential element for effective care of people with mental illness. *Journal of Psychosocial Nursing and Mental Health Services, 41*(5), 44–45.

Farb, P. (1978) *Humankind.* New York: Bantam Books.

Happell, B. (2008). Clinical experience in mental health nursing: Determining satisfaction and the influential factors. *Nurse Education Today, 28*(7), 849–855.

Hayman-White, K., & Happell, B. (2005). Nursing student attitudes toward mental health nursing and consumers: Psychometric properties of a self-report scale. *Archives of Psychiatric Nursing, 19*(4), 184–193.

Henderson, S., Happell, B., & Martin, T. (2007). So what is so good about clinical experience? A mental health nursing perspective. *Nurse Education in Practice, 7,* 164–177.

LITERARY REFERENCE

Kaysen, S. (1993). *Girl, interrupted.* New York: Turtle Bay Books.

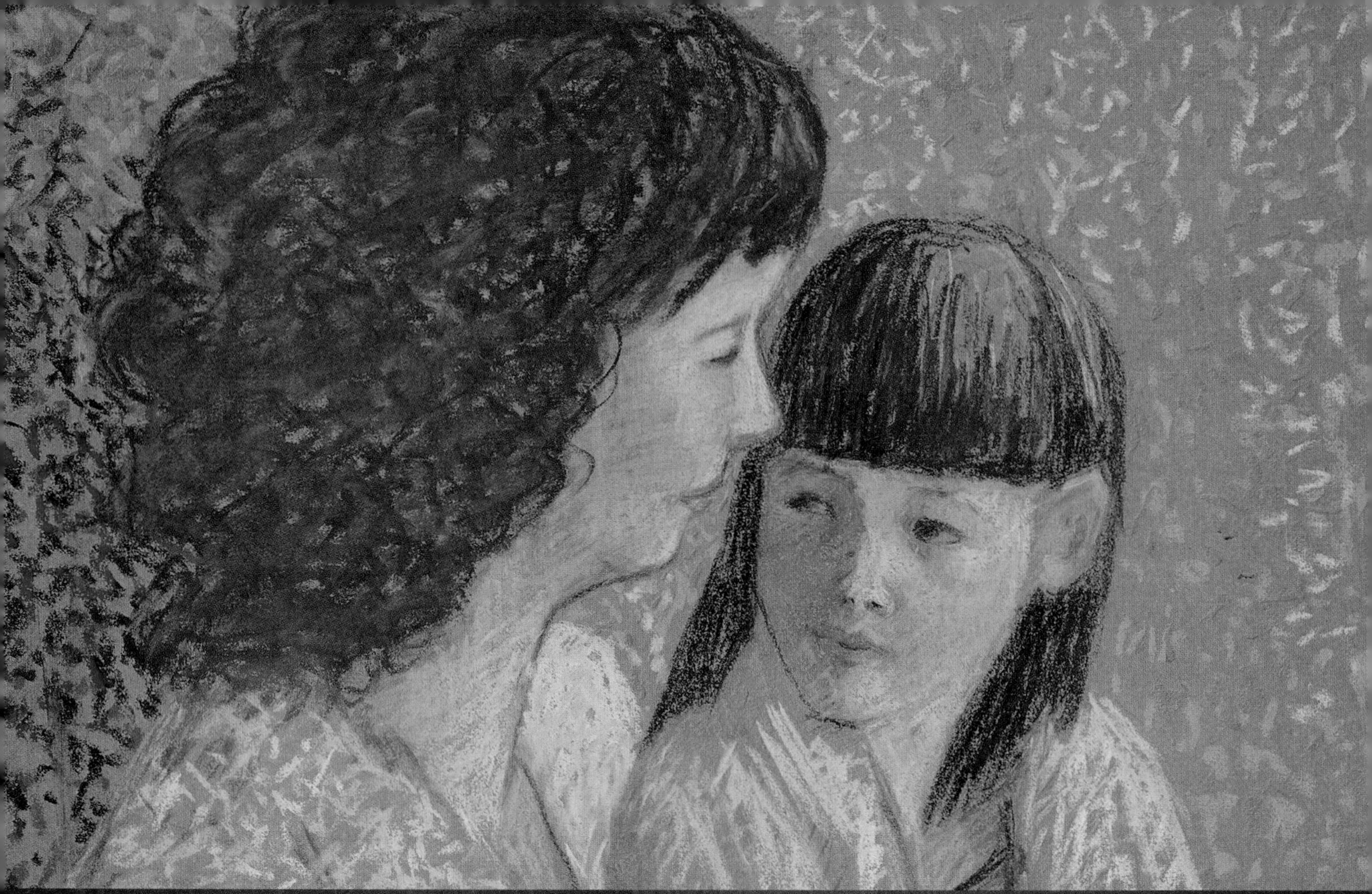

A Matter of Trust

Your View on Psychiatric Nursing

Consider the following statements:

- ***Psychiatric nursing is very different from other nursing specialties.***
- ***Psychiatric nursing has much in common with all areas of nursing practice.***

Both of these statements are true. Learning about the history and development of psychiatric nursing may help to put these ideas in perspective. Reflect on both as you read this chapter.

CHAPTER 2

Psychiatric Nursing: Evolution of a Specialty

NOREEN CAVAN FRISCH

CHAPTER OUTLINE

COMPETENCIES

Upon completion of this chapter, the reader should be able to:

1. Describe societal changes in attitudes toward mental illness, leading to identification of mental illness as a disease.
2. Discuss the medicalization of mental illness in the eighteenth and nineteenth centuries.
3. Explain the reasons why nurses working with the mentally ill in the nineteenth century did not identify with nurses providing physical nursing care.
4. Identify factors that brought nursing of the physically ill and nursing of the mentally ill together.
5. Describe psychiatric nursing's role today as a core subject and content of nursing practice.
6. Identify the evolving role of psychiatric nursing in community settings.
7. Describe the challenges facing psychiatric nursing in today's practice realities.

KEY TERMS

Asylums
Brown Report
National Mental Health Act
Psychiatric Mental Health Advanced Practice Registered Nurse
Psychiatric Mental Health Nurse

Psychiatric nursing in the United States is currently so strongly integrated with the rest of nursing practice it may be hard to believe that 100 years ago general nursing and care of the mentally ill were completely separated. Readers of this textbook have probably assumed that a course in psychiatric mental health nursing would be part of their professional nursing education. Today, we have come to value the basic skills of mental health nursing as important for the nurse in the general hospital or clinic; and we have come to value the basic skills of physical assessment and management of physical health needs as important skills for nurses in both inpatient and outpatient psychiatric settings. However, as nursing schools developed in the nineteenth century, a distinct difference arose between those who studied care for general patients in hospitals and graduated as "nurses" and those who studied care for the mentally ill and graduated to be "mental nurses." Only after several decades of separate education, schools, and employment did the notion that every nurse must have a background in psychiatric mental health care become fully realized in the United States. The purpose of this chapter is to provide a brief history of the evolution of psychiatric nursing and to track the major developments that led to the recognition of psychiatric mental health nursing as an important nursing specialty in the United States. A brief historical overview of the treatment of mentally ill persons is presented, with a discussion of how this treatment evolved to the point where there was recognition that the mentally ill were indeed ill and required both medical and nursing care.

CARE OF THE MENTALLY ILL

Early Civilization

Throughout history, those who were mentally ill have attracted the attention of others. In some societies the mentally ill or the insane were viewed with reverence, and in some they were viewed with repulsion and anger. In primitive cultures where medicine, magic, and religion were not distinct, the insane were treated through magical rituals, prayer, and exorcism. Beliefs in the causes of mental illness ranged from the idea that the ill person was possessed by demons or was ill because of breaking some taboo to the notion that the affected person had had some harmful substance enter his body. Early civilizations, such as the Greek and Roman cultures, developed ideas of body "humors"—blood, black bile, yellow bile, and phlegm—which could influence emotional stability. Hippocrates believed that excesses of black bile caused melancholy and that bloodletting could remove this excess.

Middle Ages and Renaissance

In Europe during the Middle Ages and the Renaissance, mental illness was viewed with fear. Affected persons were thought to be influenced by the moon, thus the term *lunatic* emerged to refer to one controlled by the lunar body. In Europe during this time period, treatment of the mentally ill was influenced by beliefs that the mentally ill were evil, witches, or heretics. The mentally ill were excluded from community life, and, eventually, in order to secure such seclusion, the mentally ill were confined to institutions that housed all those deemed not fit to live in society. Persons were treated as criminals and punished for their behaviors. Care was custodial, and inmates were poorly fed and clothed and were frequently restrained.

Eighteenth and Early Nineteenth Centuries

Throughout the latter part of the eighteenth and early nineteenth centuries, mentally ill persons who were insane were committed to **asylums**; those who committed crimes were put in prison. Care of the mentally ill, by and large, was provided by persons without training or interest in helping others and was often lacking in compassion. In both the United States and England, however, there were a few physicians who began to view the insane as persons suffering from disease and needing some kind of treatment. For example, English physician William Battie had a scientific background and a high social position. His interest in work with the insane ultimately served to elevate mental services to something respectable physicians could do. He believed that there is something powerful about a caring environment and recommended that those who work as attendants and nurses to the insane be carefully selected and trained (Nolan, 1993). Given the very positive influence of his work, it is somewhat ironic that the phrase "going batty" was derived from his name.

During this time period, there were several theories regarding the cause of mental illness, as described in Table 2-1. No one theory was widely accepted, and the views of the physician in charge of an asylum dictated the nature of the care and treatment provided within (Nolan, 1993). Important, however, was the medicalization of the care of the insane. Physicians became those in charge of care; insanity was increasingly viewed as a disease, not a condition of character. In the nineteenth century, physicians began their first attempts to classify mental disorders, and they so described both moral causes of illness (such as jealousy, religious excitement, and disappointment in love) and physical causes (such as epilepsy, injury to the head, overwork, and intemperance or drunkenness; Nolan, 1993).

Table 2-1 Early Nineteenth-Century Theories on Causes of Mental Illness

THEORY	PREMISE
Inheritance theory	Belief that "insanity" is transmitted from one generation to another.
Moral degeneracy theory	Belief that persons are mentally ill by virtue of having bad character.
Miasmic theory	Belief that dirt and putrefaction are the principal causes of ill health. This theory provided justification for removing the ill and insane from the rest of society.
Germ theory	Belief that those who are ill can contaminate others; the insane, therefore, should be segregated.
Septic foci theory	Belief that there is a source of infection that causes insanity; removal of the infection (frequently through surgery) can cure the person.

REFLECTIVE THINKING 2-1

Society's Treatment of Those Who Are Different

All societies have means of dealing with those who are deemed "different" from the norm.

- When reflecting on a society's treatment of the mentally ill, what do you learn about that society?
- Who are the "deviants" in our current society?
- How are our deviants treated? What does that tell you about our modern culture?

In 1846, the term *psychiatry* was first used by asylum doctors in England to identify their work and to further define the medical role in the treatment and cure of the insane. These physicians began to publish *The Journal of Mental Science* to further the legitimacy of psychiatry as a medical specialty (Nolan, 1993).

These physicians in England and their counterparts in the United States were part of a move to build asylums for the treatment and cure of the insane. The asylums were large, public institutions that were to provide humane and rational methods of treatment. The asylums were self-sufficient communities, having their own gardens for food production, their own kitchens, laundry facilities, carpentry shops, and the like. Everything needed for daily living could be found on the asylum grounds. Inmates (as the patients were called) had rigorous daily schedules that included work, time for reading and fresh air, and other activities. These asylums were designed and constructed as short-term hospitals for individuals who were expected to recover and return to society.

Nineteenth Century

Before long, however, the optimistic idea that the mentally ill would recover quickly and return to society broke down. The asylums required productive workers. Therefore, inmates who were "good" workers were not likely to be let go—they were needed to maintain the institution. Those who could not participate in the vigorous schedules had to be "controlled" by the asylum attendants. In many cases, physical restraints were used as the only means of controlling inmates. It became increasingly difficult to find persons willing to work in asylums, and many who did were not of sound character. Inmates were ill-treated, neglected, and taken advantage of by those who were supposed to care for them. Also, the asylums soon became overcrowded, making matters of control even more difficult.

Many individuals—physicians, private citizens, and recovered patients alike—called for reform. In the United States, Dorothea Dix, a private citizen who had provided nursing care to soldiers during the Civil War, became a crusader for reform in the treatment of the mentally ill (Figure 2-1). She advocated for humane treatment as well as safe and comfortable environments (which included heat in the winter). She fought for activities, such as dances, that would relieve the monotony of asylum life. Through her efforts, care was improved throughout the United States and in Canada and Scotland as well (Dolan, Fitzpatrick, & Herrmann, 1983).

With the establishment of a reformed approach to care, it became increasingly clear that persons working in asylums (or what were then beginning to be called hospitals) needed training, a certain willingness to care for others, and a strong sense of compassion. How were such persons to be found? One physician wrote that women were to be more highly valued in this work than men, for women who were "of a kind and sensible disposition, could not fail to be of great comfort to those patients who require gentle and sympathetic attention" (Maudley, 1879, as quoted in Nolan, 1993). Still, how were women to be recruited into such work? One way was to set up training schools for persons to attend to the mentally ill and to provide education for respectable women and men who were willing and able to enter such schools.

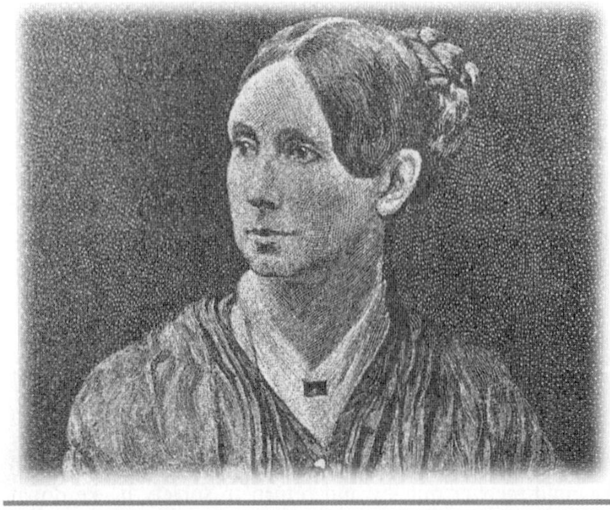

FIGURE 2-1 Dorothea Lynde Dix. (COURTESY AMERICAN NURSES ASSOCIATION.)

The Ward in the Hospital at Aries by Vincent van Gogh

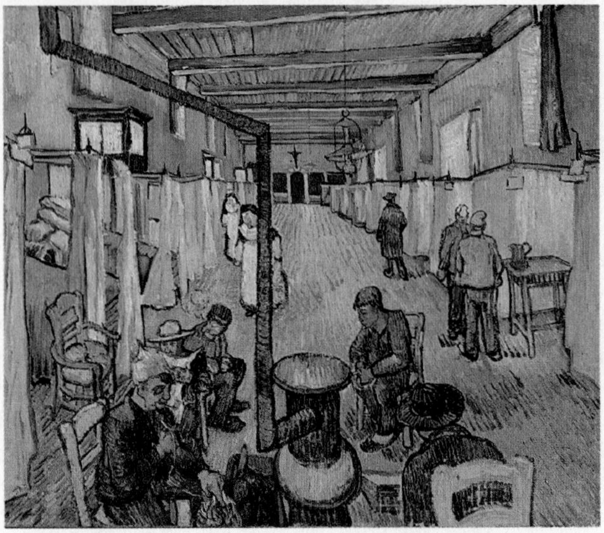

Source: Vincent van Gogh (Groot-Zundert 1853–1890 Auvers-sur-Oise) *The Ward in the Hospital at Arles 1889* Oil on canvas 72 x 91 cm Inv. no.1925.12 Collection Oskar Reinhart "Am Römerholz", Winterthur

Van Gogh was hospitalized for depression and psychosis twice between 1888 and 1889. The nearly empty long hall (leading to a distant and out-of-reach crucifix), the stovepipe separating the sisters from the inmates, and the strong sense of boredom characterize this picture, which makes both the mentally ill and their surroundings look far more depressing than frightening. Van Gogh probably suffered from manic depression (Chapter 15), but his epilepsy and suicide (see painting in Chapter 16) were probably greatly influenced by abuse of the drug "absinthe" (see painting by Degas in Chapter 17).

NURSING EDUCATION

EIGHTEENTH AND NINETEENTH CENTURIES

In 1882, the McLean Asylum in Somerville, Massachusetts, opened the first training school in the world for mental health nurses (Church, 1987). This school graduated its first class of 15 students in 1886 (Figure 2-2). Edward Cowles was the physician superintendent of McLean, and his effort to train nurses was part of his campaign to medicalize care of the insane. He proclaimed that inmates would be called "patients" and that ward attendants would be called "nurses." He believed that the presence of a "nurse" indicated not only that the patient was ill, but also that there was a hope for recovery.

During this same time period, other schools of nursing were opening in the United States. The most notable of these were the Bellevue Training School in New York and the Connecticut Training School in New Haven. These were the first in the country to operate primarily under the

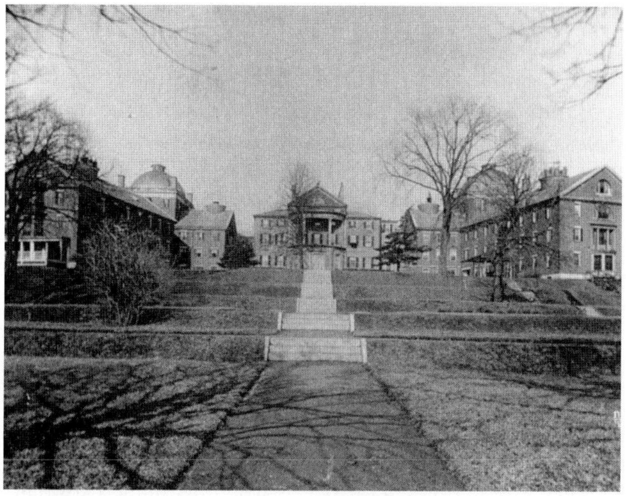

(A)

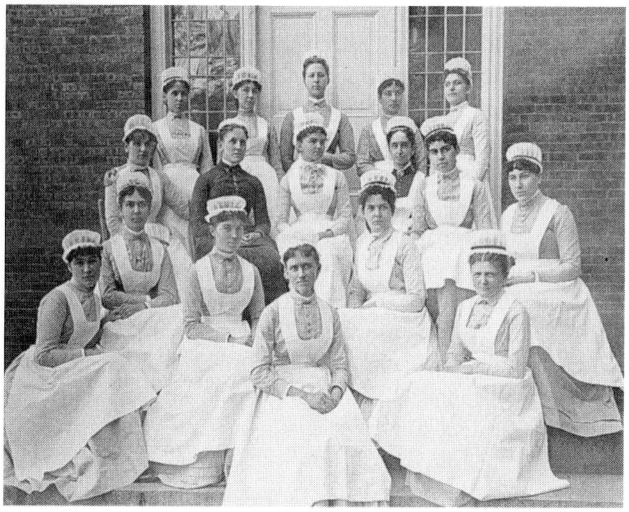

(B)

FIGURE 2-2 **(A) Rear view of McLean Hospital, Belmont, Massachusetts, circa 1890s. (B) America's first psychiatric nurses: The class of 15 women graduated from the McLean Asylum Training School for Nurses in 1886.** (PHOTOS COURTESY OF MCLEAN HOSPITAL, BELMONT, MASSACHUSETTS.)

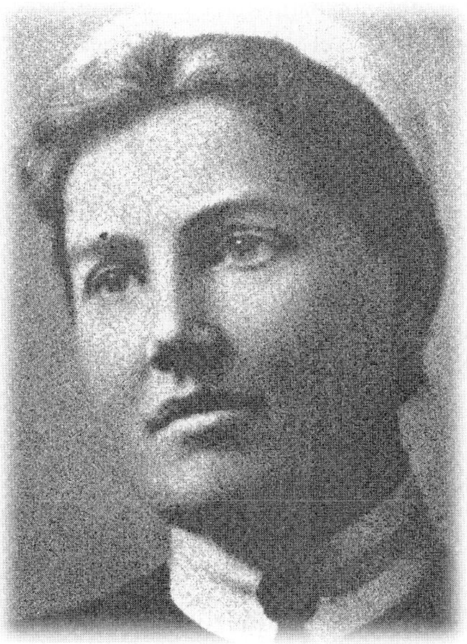

FIGURE 2-3 **Isabel Hampton Robb.** (COURTESY AMERICAN NURSES ASSOCIATION.)

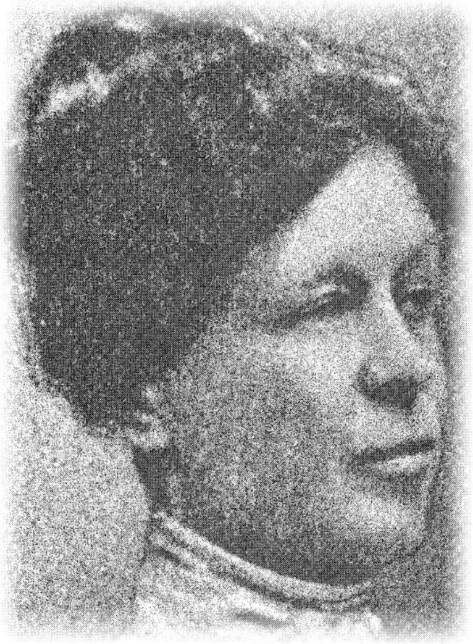

FIGURE 2-4 **Lavinia Lloyd Dock.** (COURTESY AMERICAN NURSES ASSOCIATION.)

Nightingale model, where the training of nurses was accomplished via the tutelage of nurses (rather than physicians). These programs were granted autonomy from the hospital itself, and the education was securely in the hands of the matron or superintendent, who was herself a "trained nurse."

The programs to train the mental nurses were not autonomous in this way. Physicians like Dr. Cowles were in charge of the programs and established the curriculum. Dr. Cowles believed that these nurses needed skills in both physical and mental care and attempted to prepare nurses who could provide both. Ultimately, he designed a program where nurses studied physical nursing for the first year of training and skills in mental care in the second year (Church, 1987).

The year 1893 marked the first meeting of organized nursing in the United States. Nursing leaders met in Chicago at the World's Fair and participated in a formal conference on the state of nursing and nursing training. Various individuals presented papers on these topics, and speakers included national leaders such as Isabel Hampton and Lavinia Dock (Figures 2-3 and 2-4). These women called for clear standards for nursing education and for a clear definition of what it meant to be a "trained nurse" (Hampton, 1949/1893; Dock, 1949/1893). However, care of the mentally ill was not addressed in their proposals. Only one paper at this conference addressed the issues of asylum nursing (May, 1949/1893), and nurses providing care to the physically ill and those providing care to the mentally ill seemed to focus more on their differences than on any similarities that could be identified.

Mental health nurses continued to be trained at asylums, and their training evolved to keep up with new approaches in psychiatric care. These nurses had to care for a wide range of patients. Much of the work still included custodial care and supervision of ward attendants. Staff had to make sure that patients did not harm themselves and did not escape. Treatments such as cold dressings, poultices (hot packs, often made with herbs, applied to a sore or inflamed part of the body), fomentations (lotions or compresses), and enemas were given. Manic behaviors were managed by packing patients in wet sheets (Nolan, 1993). Baths of different kinds were popular treatments: hot baths were used for melancholy, cold baths for mania, and various positive claims were made about Turkish baths. Few drugs were available; however, sedatives such as alcohol and opium might be used sparingly for violent patients (Nolan, 1993).

Twentieth Century

The American Psychiatric Association established a committee on Training Schools for Nurses. This committee submitted a report in 1907 outlining the standards required for nursing, thus marking the physicians' official assumption of control over mental nursing care. In 1913, however, the Johns Hopkins Hospital School, under the leadership of Effie J. Taylor, the nursing director of the Phipps Clinic, included psychiatric nursing in the training of general nurses. This was the first time a hospital program offered training in psychiatric care to all of its students. Taylor's goal was to provide a standard knowledge base for all nursing so that there would be no arbitrary division of the patient's mind and body (Church, 1987). Her reasoning today comes across as the foundation of holistic care.

Over time, other nursing programs adopted a similar model to that of the Johns Hopkins program. Also, other programs developed exchanges where students who were studying to be mental health nurses spent a certain amount of time studying and practicing various aspects of general nursing. The time during and immediately after World War I increased the demand for nurses to provide care to mentally stressed persons. Mental hospitals were overcrowded and understaffed, and the national attitude was to develop increased services to meet the needs of veterans undergoing "shell shock" and other psychiatric disturbances. By 1920, the first psychiatric nursing textbook was published, *Nursing Mental Diseases*. This text was authored by Harriet Bailey, Assistant Superintendent of Nursing at the Johns Hopkins School.

In the 1930s, new approaches to psychiatric care were emerging—mostly somatic therapies that involved treatments such as deep sleep therapy, insulin shock therapy, and ultimately electroshock therapy. The need for nurses trained in the physical care of patients became clearer, and by 1937 the National League for Nursing recommended that all nurses obtain education in psychiatric nursing as part of their basic nursing coursework.

In 1946, the U.S. Congress passed the **National Mental Health Act**, which established the National Institutes of Mental Health (NIMH). This act provided federal funds for research and education in all areas of psychiatric care. This act also provided funds for graduate nursing, assisting universities to establish graduate programs for psychiatric nurses.

During the late 1940s, nursing leaders joined together in a council of 14 nursing organizations and commissioned a study regarding the status of nursing education. Esther Lucille Brown, director of the Department of Studies in the Professions at the Russell Sage Foundation, was selected to carry out this work. She published her findings in 1948 in a document called "The Future of Nursing," better known through the years as the **Brown Report**. Among other recommendations, she advised that psychiatric hospitals be used as agencies for affiliation in nursing programs, rather than having psychiatric hospitals conduct their own schools (Dolan et al., 1983). It was not until 1955, however, that the National League for Nursing required that nursing programs include classroom and clinical experiences in psychiatric nursing in order to receive national accreditation.

The coming of age for psychiatric nursing as a specialty occurred simultaneously with changes in the way those with mental illness were viewed and treated. The mid-twentieth century marked a mental health movement that progressed from the notion of treatment as confinement to treatment based on therapy. The public view became one based more on understanding and sensitivity to the plight of those who were ill. In 1961, President Dwight Eisenhower established a Commission on Mental Illness and Health, and later, legislation was passed that emphasized prevention and rehabilitation.

Congress passed the Community Mental Health Centers Act in 1963, which provided the framework for "deinstitutionalization," or the movement of individuals from psychiatric hospitals to community settings. The idea was to provide treatment for the client in the setting that was the least restrictive alternative. Individuals who could be managed at home, in board-and-care facilities, or who could be supported with day treatment programs, could be released from state mental hospitals and returned to their communities.* This period also marked the era of new perspectives on civil rights and the rights of persons with mental illnesses. Nursing approaches during this time expanded from exclusively hospital-based services to include community mental health services.

The Role of Nursing Theory and Scholarship

Nursing science and scholarship continued to advance in all aspects of nursing. In 1952, nurse theorist Hildegard Peplau published *Interpersonal Relations in Nursing*. This book presented the first nursing theoretical framework for the practice of psychiatric care. The framework is grounded in the interpersonal philosophy of psychiatry and is discussed in some detail in Chapter 3 of this text. Other nursing theorists followed, and some emphasized the interpersonal nature of all nursing care. Ida Jean Orlando published *The Dynamic*

*The relative degree of success of this deinstitutionalization movement became dependent on the degree of funding ultimately provided for the community support services in years following. Chapter 22 of this text deals directly with the issues of those who have "fallen though the cracks" in an imperfect delivery system.

Nurse-Patient Relationship in 1961. This work was the result of a five-year project funded by the NIMH that attempted to identify factors that enhanced or impeded the integration of mental health principles into basic nursing curricula (Leonard & George, 1995). Orlando's theory suggests that all nursing care must be concerned with a patient's need for help (real or perceived) in an immediate situation. She suggested further that nurses help patients through disciplined interaction.

Psychiatric nurses established their own journals to further their work and to share their developing ideas. Two new journals were established in the early 1960s: *Perspectives in Psychiatric Care* and *Journal of Psychiatric Nursing and Mental Health Services*. Both are still published today, with the latter having changed its title to *Journal of Psychosocial Nursing and Mental Health Services*. In the 1970s, specialty certification in psychiatric nursing became available through the American Nurses Association (ANA). With the establishment of certification, the ANA published the first standards of psychiatric and mental health nursing practice. Table 2-2 summarizes the important events in psychiatric nursing history.

TABLE 2-2 Important Events and Trends in Psychiatric Nursing History

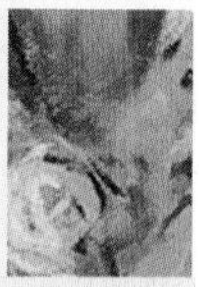

1773	First mental hospital in the United States established in Williamsburg, Virginia
1846	First use of the term *psychiatry* by physicians attempting to upgrade the status of their work with the mentally ill
1882	First school for psychiatric nurses (or mental nurses) established at the McLean Asylum in Somerville, Massachusetts
1913	Johns Hopkins Hospital included psychiatric nursing in the course of study for general nurses
1920	Publication of the first psychiatric nursing textbook, *Nursing Mental Diseases*, by Harriet Bailey
1946	Passage of the National Mental Health Act, which established the National Institutes of Mental Health (NIMH)
1948	Publication of the Brown Report, which recommended that psychiatric nursing be included in general nursing education
1952	Publication of *Interpersonal Relations in Nursing* by nurse theorist Hildegard Peplau
1955	National League for Nursing made psychiatric nursing a requirement for accreditation of basic nursing programs
1963	Passage of the Community Mental Health Act
1960s	Initial publication of psychiatric nursing journals
1970s	Specialty certification of psychiatric nurses
1980s	Differentiation of basic and advanced practice for psychiatric nurses
1990s	Significant advances in biological, genetic, and pharmacological influences on psychiatric disease

CURRENT TRENDS AND ISSUES

Today, scholarship, research, and evaluation of psychiatric nursing have advanced to the point where there is no question that psychiatric nursing is a specialty within nursing. Other, more modern, nursing theories all address the holistic nature of people and emphasize the need to care for a person's mind and body (see Chapter 3). The ANA issued the current *Psychiatric Mental Health Nursing Scope and Standards of Practice* in 2007. These standards document the scope of current practice and two levels of practice (basic and advanced). Box 2-1 summarizes the scope of practice at these two levels. At the basic level of practice, the nurse works with individuals, families, communities, and groups to promote health, assess dysfunction, assist clients to regain or improve coping, and prevent further disability. At the advanced level, the nurse may focus on the full range of activities from mental health promotion to illness care, with additional skills in the diagnosis and treatment of mental disorders.

In the definition of psychiatric nursing, the ANA standards include the idea that psychiatric mental health nursing is a specialized area of nursing practice and that it employs theories of human behavior as its science and purposeful use of self as its art. The preparation for certification at the basic level of practice is a Registered Nurse, who has a baccalaureate degree in nursing and has demonstrated clinical skills within the specialty. The designation **Psychiatric Mental Health Nurse** applies to such a person who has passed a certification exam and is thereby certified within the specialty. At the advanced level is a **Psychiatric Mental Health Advanced Practice Registered Nurse** (APRN), who is a licensed Registered Nurse educationally prepared at the master or doctoral level and nationally certified as a clinical specialist in psychiatric and mental health nursing.

In addition to these levels of practice, there are also clear subspecialties within psychiatric nursing practice. Subspecialization requires education at the graduate level and currently can be categorized by age group addressed (such as child, adolescent, adult, and geriatric) or by a specific disorder (such as addictions, depression, or chronic mental illness). These categories are not mutually exclusive, but they provide a means of identifying a nurse's particular specialization. In some cases, certification is available for the subspecialty; in some cases, it is not. Currently, however, as long as an advanced practice nurse is certified as a specialist in psychiatric nursing, she may practice in a subspecialty.

BOX 2-1
PSYCHIATRIC MENTAL HEALTH NURSING: AREAS OF PRACTICE

BASIC LEVEL FUNCTIONS

- Health promotion
- Intake screening
- Case management
- Milieu therapy
- Self-care activities
- Psychobiological interventions
- Health teaching
- Crisis intervention
- Counseling
- Home visiting
- Community action
- Advocacy

ADVANCED LEVEL FUNCTIONS

- Psychotherapy
- Psychobiological interventions
- Prescriptive authority for drugs (in most states)
- Clinical supervision/consultation
- Liaison nursing

FUTURE DIRECTIONS

In 1990, the ANA acknowledged that the 1990s were a time of increasing interest and knowledge in biological, genetic, and pharmacological treatments of psychiatric disease (ANA, 2000). These advances paralleled an increase in autonomy and professionalization of psychiatric nursing (Boling, 2003). However, these advances present real challenges to the specialty and to its future practice. Advances in the pathophysiological—pharmacological—biological domains hold great promise for treatment; however, they may emphasize these aspects of care to the exclusion of the interpersonal and theory-based components of care. (Cutcliffe, 2008; Clements, 2004). In 2004, Clements commented that even though the increasing technology has provided obvious benefits to clients, there is a concern that our emphasis is shifting away from the recognition that there is a person needing care. The concerns still remain today as we recall our nursing mandate to treat the whole being and take necessary actions to maintain the "art" of nursing in our practice. Nurses in psychiatric care are called on to lead the way for reintegration of physical and psychosocial care for persons with mental illness, though how they will do this is uncertain. The looming shortage of nurses only exacerbates the problem. Many authors have addressed the future of psychiatric nursing and they raise very challenging questions:

- Are psychiatric nurses to become those with complete knowledge of the science of care and the overseers of treatment regimes, medications, side effects, and functioning, or those who provide interpersonal and family-based therapy? (Cutcliffe, 2008)
- Should psychiatric nurses in the community shift their focus from medication administration to psychosocial interventions, case management, family education, and life skills training? (Gillam, 2005)
- In a time of overall nursing shortage, should psychiatric nurses focus on the most severely ill clients and assist in maintaining these individuals to the optimum level of functioning, or should they focus on mental health promotion and the huge issue of alcohol, addiction, and substance abuse? (Brimblecombe & Nolan, 2008)
- Should advanced practice psychiatric nurses take on the role of medication prescription, and is this the best use of nursing skills? (Snowden, 2006)

There are no clear answers to these questions. In an editorial largely devoted to the teaching of psychiatric nursing McCabe (2005) asked, "Would you please tell me which way to go from here?" Like Alice, psychiatric nurses are in a dilemma about the path to follow. McCabe points out that psychiatric disorders account for over 15% of the burden of disease in the United States, and major depressive disorder is the leading cause of disability. Who will care for these patients and how will they be cared for? Are these clients to be served by general duty RNs who have a solid background in mental health? When nurses become specialists in psychiatric mental health care, will they be used as clinical nurse specialists or will they move into "therapist" roles and no longer identify their work as nursing, a concern raised most recently by Hurley and Ramsey (2008). Further, there remains an unquestioned and rather urgent need for nurses with psychiatric nursing skills to provide service to individuals coping with acute and chronic illnesses, terminal diagnoses, effects of stress, societal problems (such as violence), and problems associated with aging, grief, and other serious illnesses or stressful events.

It is clear that psychiatric nursing must be informed by neuroscience as well as behavioral science. The focus of nursing will certainly adapt due to the explosion of scientific knowledge (discussed in Chapter 4) leading to highly sophisticated technology, diagnostics, and pharmacologic treatments. However, the future provides challenging work for those interested in combining knowledge of neuroscience with an understanding of human behavior and their relationship to social and environmental conditions affecting people.

Mental health services are delivered today within a philosophy of managed care and cost containment. Today, many persons may be underdiagnosed and untreated. For example, data have suggested that barely half of the persons with depression receive treatment, and that less than half of that treatment is judged to be adequate based on number and timing of follow-up visits (Kessler et al., 2003). Those who are severely ill may be hospitalized for a very limited time, stabilized on medication, and discharged with unrealistic plans for follow-up care. There is an increasing need for psychiatric specialists in home care. At the same time, the notion of prevention is not being fully realized in most aspects of health. Mental health is no exception, and programs such as those that promote healthy parenting, stress reduction, or avoidance of addictive substances are underfunded and/or nonexistent in many communities. Contemporary issues such as domestic violence, addiction, homelessness, and poverty create environments where psychiatric care cannot remedy individuals' problems without addressing larger social issues. It appears that much of the delivery of mental health care and almost all of preventive mental health care must be done in community-based settings such as schools, homes, religious institutions, or halfway houses. As a majority of nursing care moves from the hospital to the community, there will be an increasing need for psychiatric nurses to use all of their creativity and skill to provide needed services in the most effective way possible. Psychiatric nurses are taking on many additional roles in the community, including psychiatric home health care, prevention of mental illness and stress, and direct services to specific populations. Box 2-2 presents many of the psychiatric nurse's community-based roles and lists the chapters in this text that present detailed information on each.

There are several nursing organizations that support psychiatric nursing, and these will continue to play a role in public education and forming professional alliances to advocate for individuals' access to care. The resource list at the chapter's end provides information on each.

BOX 2-2
COMMUNITY-BASED ROLES IN PSYCHIATRIC NURSING HOME HEALTH PSYCHIATRIC CARE

- Case management for persons who live alone and are in need of supervision; care of the elderly and demented (see Chapter 25)
- Care for individuals with medical illnesses for which there is a strong emotional response (see Chapter 21)
- Ongoing care for the chronic mentally ill who live at home or in alternative care settings such as group homes/halfway houses (see Chapters 12 and 13)
- Participation in crisis response teams (see Chapter 11)

COMMUNITY-BASED CARE

- Family preservation, care of families at risk for violence, abuse, and dysfunction (see Chapters 23, 24 and 26,)
- Care of the homeless (see Chapter 22)
- Care of the incarcerated (see Chapter 22)
- Psychiatric nursing in the community (see Chapter 31)

KEY CONCEPTS

- Mental illness was not always viewed as illness, which led to inhumane treatment of the ill until the mid-1900s.
- In the eighteenth and nineteenth centuries, a number of physicians became interested in the care of the mentally ill. Their work served to medicalize mental illness such that mental illness could be seen as a disease requiring medical treatment and nursing care.
- In the nineteenth century, nurses who were trained to work with the mentally ill were educated by physicians; nurses who were trained to work with the physically ill were educated by nurses.
- Several factors in the twentieth century led to the integration of psychiatric mental health nursing with general nursing.
- Psychiatric mental health nursing today is a core subject on which the professional practice of nursing is based.
- The current shift to community-based care has created new roles for the psychiatric nurse in managed care, primary and secondary prevention, and care of vulnerable populations.

REVIEW QUESTIONS

1. During the eighteenth and early nineteenth centuries, there was the belief that dirt and putrefaction were the principal causes of ill health. This belief is based on which of the following theories?
   1. Germ theory
   2. Miasmic theory
   3. Septic foci theory
   4. Inheritance theory

2. Many believe the major challenge for psychiatric nursing in the twenty-first century is which of the following?
   1. Caring for individuals with mental illness who are currently incarcerated in legal detention centers.
   2. Having an excess of both undergraduate and graduate students enrolled in psychiatric nursing programs.

3. Keeping a nursing focus in a field that is rapidly changing on the basis of new discoveries of science, genetics, and technology.
4. Expanding psychiatric nursing to include the care of children and adolescents who are severely impaired by mental health illness.

3. In what year did nursing leaders meet at the World's Fair in Chicago to discuss the state of nursing and nursing training?
1. 1825
2. 1893
3. 1924
4. 1957

4. When was the first psychiatric nursing text published?
1. 1793
2. 1865
3. 1920
4. 1949

5. A major difference between the beginning nurse and the Advance Practice Registered Nurse (APRN) is that the APRN can do which of the following?
1. Health teaching
2. Intake screening
3. Conduct psychotherapy
4. Perform crisis intervention

6. A somatic therapy for the treatment of mental health problems, introduced in the 1930s, included which of the following?
1. Chemotherapy
2. Light therapy
3. Radiation therapy
4. Electroshock therapy

7. The National Mental Health Act of 1946 provided for which of the following?
1. Funds for preventive health care services
2. Guidelines for certification of the mentally ill
3. Funds for research in all areas of psychiatric care
4. Assistance to individuals experiencing mental health problems of an acute nature

LEARNING ACTIVITIES

1. Explain the reasons early societies did not view the mentally ill as ill.
2. Describe the process by which care of the mentally ill was medicalized.
3. What was the original purpose of constructing large asylums to care for the mentally ill?
4. How did Dorothea Dix reform services and care?
5. What was nursing training like for those who became mental nurses in the nineteenth century?
6. What factors led to the integration of general nursing and mental nursing?
7. Examine the current standards and scope of practice for psychiatric mental health nursing, and suggest how this work supports the development of nursing as a profession.
8. Describe the community-based role of psychiatric nursing in your home community.

*Study*WARE™ CONNECTION

Using your *Study*WARE™ CD-ROM

1. Complete the Crossword activity for this chapter.
2. Review the audio glossary for key terms in this chapter.
3. Review the audio glossary for key terms in this chapter.

REFERENCES

American Nurses Association (ANA). (2000). *A statement of psychiatric-mental health clinical nursing practice and standards of psychiatric-mental health nursing practice*. Washington, DC: Author.

American Nurses Association (ANA). (2007). *Psychiatric mental health nursing scope and standards of practice*. Co-published by the American Psychiatric Nursing Association. Washington, DC: Author.

Boling, A. (2003). The professionalization of psychiatric nursing: From doctors' handmaiden to empowered professionals. *Journal of Psychosocial Nursing and Mental Health Services, 41*(10), 26–40, 52–53.

Brimblecombe, N., & Nolan, P. (2008). Mental health nursing in Europe: What is the future? *Mental Health Practice, 11*(6), 18–22.

Church, O. M. (1987). The emergence of training programmes for asylum nursing at the turn of the century. In C. Maggs (Ed.), *Nursing history: The state of the art* (pp. 107–123). London: Croom Helm.

Clements, P. T. (2004). Guest editorial: Three-dimensional psychiatric nursing. *Journal of Psychosocial Nursing and Mental Health Services, 42*(3), 4–5.

Cutcliffe, J. (2008). The die has been cast: Rediscovering the essence of psychiatric nursing. *British Journal of Nursing, 14*(2), 88–91.

Dock, L. L. (1949/1893). Relation of training schools to hospitals. In I. A. Hampton, et al. (Eds.), *Nursing of the sick* (pp. 13–23). New York: McGraw-Hill.

Dolan, J. A., Fitzpatrick, M. L., & Herrmann, E. K. (1983). *Nursing in society: A historical perspective* (15th ed.). Philadelphia: WB Saunders.

Gillam, T. (2005). The changing role of the community psychiatric nurse. *Mental Health Practice, 9*(1), 14, 16.

Hampton, I. A. (1949/1893). Educational standards for nurses. In I. A. Hampton, et al. (Eds.), *Nursing of the sick* (pp. 1–12). New York: McGraw-Hill.

Hurley, J., & Ramsay, M. (2008). Mental health nursing: Sleepwalking towards oblivion? *Mental Health Practice, 11*(10), 14–17.

Kessler, R. C., Berglund, P. I., Demier, O., Jin, R., Koretz, D., Merkargas, K. R., et al. (2003). The epidemiology of major depressive disorder: Results of the National Comorbidity Survey Replication Study (NCS–R). *Journal of the American Medical Association, 289*, 3095–3105.

Leonard, M. K., & George, J. (1995). Ida Jean Orlando. In J. George (Ed.), *Nursing theories, the base for professional nursing practice* (pp. 159–178). Norwalk, CT: Appleton & Lange.

May, M. E. (1949/1893). Nursing of the insane. In I. A. Hampton, et al. (Eds.), *Nursing of the sick*. New York: McGraw-Hill.

McCabe, S. (2005). "Would you please tell me which way to go from here?" *Perspectives in Psychiatric Care, 41*(3), 130–132.

McCabe, S. (2000). Bringing psychiatric nursing into the twenty-first century. *Archives of Psychiatric Nursing, 14*(3), 109–116.

Nolan, P. (1993). *A history of mental health nursing*. London: Chapman & Hall.

Orlando, I. J. (1961). *The dynamic nurse-patient relationship: Function, process and principles*. New York: GP Putnam's Sons.

Peplau, H. (1952). *Interpersonal relations in nursing*. New York: Putnam Press.

Snowden, A. W. A. (2006). Nurse prescribing in mental health. *Nursing Standard, 20*(29), 41–46.

RESOURCES

ORGANIZATIONS

American Psychiatric Nurses Association
Association of Child and Adolescent Psychiatric Nurses
National Consortium of Chemical Dependency Nurses
National Nurses Society on Addictions
Society for Education and Research in Psychiatric-Mental Health Nursing

JOURNALS

Archives of Psychiatric Nursing
Hospital and Community Psychiatry
Issues in Mental Health Nursing
Journal of Psychosocial Nursing and Mental Health Services
Journal of the American Psychiatric Nurses Association
Journal of Psychiatric and Mental Health Nursing
Perspectives in Psychiatric Care

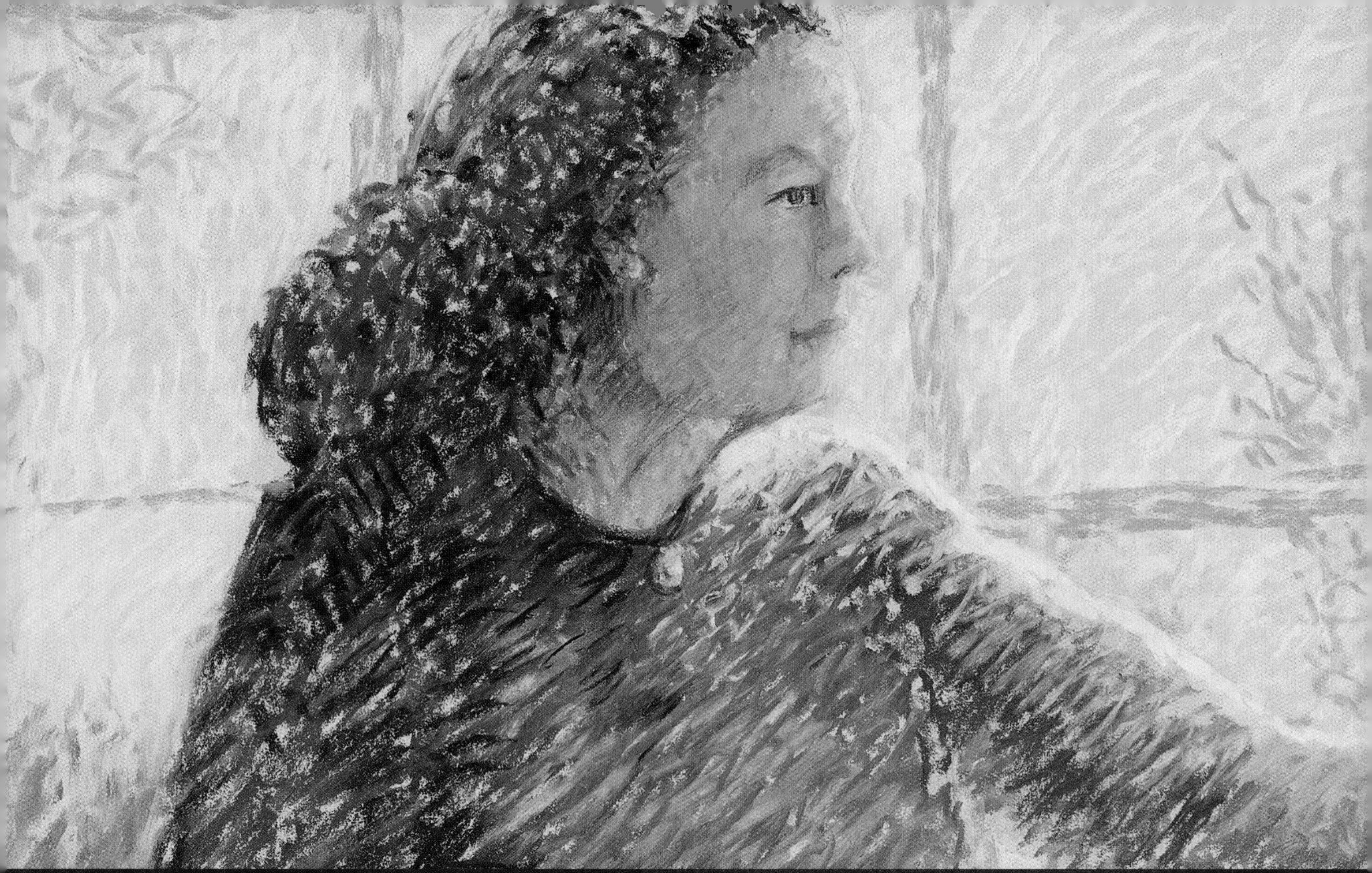

Nobody's Fool

What Is a Theory?

The term, or word, "theory" is often used in everyday conversation. For example, a person might say, "I have a theory about why Susanna didn't come to class today."

- ***What does a person mean when making such a statement?***
- ***What do you think the word "theory" means in a discipline?***

Having your own answers to these questions may be helpful before thinking about how theory might influence nursing practice.

CHAPTER 3

Theory as a Basis for Practice

JULIA B. GEORGE

CHAPTER OUTLINE

COMPETENCIES

Upon completion of this chapter, the reader should be able to:

1. Discuss the relationship between psychiatric mental health nursing practice and theory.
2. Define terminology related to theory.
3. Identify the major components of selected nursing theories.
4. Discuss psychosocial theories from other disciplines useful in psychiatric nursing practice.
5. Consider various theories as a guide to nursing practice.

KEY TERMS

Adaptive Potential
Choice Point
Cognator Subsystem
Cognition
Concepts
Conceptual Framework
Created Environment
Culture
Culture Care
Culture Care Accommodation/Negotiation
Culture Care Preservation/Maintenance
Culture Care Repatterning/Restructuring
Ego
External Environment
Extrapersonal
Fixation
Generic or Folk Care Activities
Helicy
Id
Integrality
Internal Environment
Interpersonal
Intrapersonal
Modeling
Nursing Agency
Nursing System
Orientation
Professional Care-Cure Practices
Regression
Regulator Subsystem
Resonancy
Role-Modeling
Self-Care
Self-Care Agency
Self-Care Deficit
Superego
Termination
Theory
Therapeutic Self-Care Demand
Working Phase

Nursing differs from other health care professions such as medicine, physical therapy, and pharmacy in many important ways; among these is the prominent place given to theory in both the teaching and the practice of nursing. If you have friends who are students or practitioners of pharmacy, medicine, or occupational therapy, you may find them surprised to hear you talking about theory, because it is uncommon for theoretical concepts to be explicitly discussed in these fields. In contrast, many nursing curricula and practicing nurses consistently use theory on a daily basis to help them understand and explain the basis for nursing care. Nurses are by no means alone in their adoption of theory-based practice. Theory is very important to the work of anthropologists, sociologists, and psychologists. Most scientists, in both the natural sciences and the social sciences, use theory to help guide their daily work. Physicists are, of course, among the best-known theory users. Even as non-physicists, most of us have heard of the big bang theory, the grand unified theory, and the theory of relativity, to name only a few. We may not know much about the details of any of these physical theories, but we do know enough about the enterprise of physics to believe that theories are important for guiding thought and experimentation. Theory is also important to nursing and perhaps especially so to psychiatric nursing. The authors of this book believe strongly in the usefulness of theory for nursing practice, but they also recognize that acquiring a theory base is hard for beginning nurses. This is true for several reasons:

- The meaning and use of theory are not fully intuitive, and it can be difficult for a nurse to reach an understanding of what theory is and precisely how it can be useful. Courses in theory may come near the end of nursing studies, so the nursing student may have completed almost all of the required clinical courses, such as this one, before acquiring a formal grounding in theory.
- Individual theories are often difficult to understand, at least initially. The language is technical, the ideas are abstract, and the theory frequently contains a variety of new words.
- Theory may seem highly abstract in contrast to work with clients in one's clinical rotation, in which there are real individuals with pressing physical and emotional needs. It is sometimes hard to see how the abstractions of theory can be of practical help in providing care to individual clients, especially in the real world, where there never seems to be enough time to complete the day's pressing tasks.

Theory really is understandable and practical. However, learning and applying theory are not things that can happen quickly. Rather, they are like learning a new language: First comes the vocabulary, then the grammar, then simple applications, and only after all of these are assimilated does the whole structure become easy to use. The purpose of this chapter is not to make the reader an expert in either theory or any of the individual theories that are briefly discussed. This will take time and further study. Instead, the chapter provides an overview of theory and theories. The author has tried to show throughout the chapter how a nurse might use the individual theories to better understand a specific client, who has been called Mr. James. In each of its clinical chapters, this text incorporates examples from a variety of these nursing theories. The reader may wish to return to this chapter or to some of the chapter's references when encountering the application of theory later in the course.

WHAT IS THEORY?

First, what is **theory**, and how is it used? Theory is a way to abstract or generalize knowledge so that it can be applied to a variety of individual circumstances. In this way, theories can be tested by observation and experimentation. Theory may be defined as a set of interrelated concepts that provide testable relationships and direction or prediction. As abstractions, theories generate further hypotheses or research questions that can take the form of a series of logical propositions: "If this theory is true, then we predict that A follows. We have shown that A is true, so then theory predicts that B should also follow. Is B true? Let's try to find out." Theories are highly tentative structures and are constantly open to modification or replacement. A theory that correctly predicts a variety of phenomena is certainly strengthened by such predictions, but it can never be proven "true." To understand this better, consider a theory predicting that "all clovers have three leaves." While every three-leaf clover we find may seem to strengthen this theory, it should not be long before we find a two-leaf clover. On close examination we conclude that this clover began its life with three leaves but subsequently lost one. We may need to modify our theory as a result of finding a two-leaf clover, but the theory need not be abandoned. In contrast, finding a four-leaf clover, while lucky in folk belief, represents a potentially disastrous problem for the three-leaf theory. Theories are somewhat strengthened by observations that seem to confirm their validity, but they are seriously threatened or disproven by any observation that contradicts them. The finding of a four-leaf clover may lead to a change in the theory statement to "clovers typically have three leaves."

Theories are not discovered but instead are created by experienced practitioners and scientists who can make abstractions from a large store of facts, concepts, and conceptual frameworks. Concepts are the basic building blocks of theory. **Concepts** are words and abstractions that represent reality. For example, the word "nurse" is a concept that represents the reality of the person who is being identified as a nurse. Concepts may be grouped together to form conceptual frameworks. A **conceptual framework** is a group of concepts that are linked together to provide a way of organizing or viewing something. The conceptual framework for this chapter includes the concepts of theory, nursing theory, psychiatric/psychological theory, and sociocultural theory. The major difference between a conceptual framework and a theory is that a theory is more precise and developed such that the relationships contained within the theory can be tested. The relationships in a conceptual framework are organized, but they are not developed to the extent that they can be tested. A theory is used in nursing practice to describe what happens, to explain relationships or responses, to predict results of nursing actions, or to control outcomes through the selection of appropriate nursing actions. The nurse whose practice is based in theory can identify why certain behaviors are more appropriate in a given situation than other behaviors would be, can transfer knowledge and experience from one circumstance to another, and can communicate about nursing practice to others.

THEORY AND PRACTICE

Theory-based nursing practice may use both theories of and theories for nursing (Barrett, 1991; Phillips, 1990). Theories of nursing are theories basic to nursing, about nursing, and derived for nursing by nurses. They are original to nursing and deal with the phenomena of interest to nursing. Theories for nursing are theories that are developed in other disciplines but that inform and are applicable to nursing practice. Examples of theories of and for nursing are included in this chapter.

A word about the relationship among theory, practice, and research. Nursing is a practice discipline in which the practice is derived from theory that has been developed through or tested by research. The relationships among theory, practice, and research are continuously intertwined. We have already defined theory as a set of testable interrelated concepts. Theory provides a systematic way of looking at the world in order to describe, explain, predict, or control it. Practice, in terms of this text, is the delivery of nursing care to those who have psychiatric or mental health needs. Research is the planned and organized search for knowledge, either new knowledge (basic research) or knowledge whose implementation is being tested in practice (applied research). Research is conducted to answer research questions or test hypotheses. Both questions and hypotheses can be derived from practice situations or from relationships suggested by theory. The results of research may provide direction to practice and may lead to the development of new theory or modification of existing theory. Practice may be based on theory and may be modified by the application of research results. Theory may be derived from practice or from research. Thus, practice may be shaped by theory or research, theory may be developed from practice or research, and research may grow from practice or theory. Or all of these may occur simultaneously! Theory, practice, and research are forever linked together.

REFLECTIVE THINKING 3-1

About Theory

- Why is theory important to nursing practice?
- What is the difference between theory of and theory for nursing?
- How does the approach to practice vary when using different theories as a base for practice?

NURSING THEORY

Nursing theory may guide and inform specific steps of the nursing process in psychiatric care or may supply a general approach to providing care. The nursing theories to be summarized include those of Hildegard Peplau, Dorothea Orem, Martha Rogers, Callista Roy, Betty Neuman, Jean Watson, Rosemarie Rizzo Parse, Madeleine Leininger, Helen Erickson, Margaret Newman, and Anne Boykin and Savina Schoenhofer. Nursing theories have been classified in a variety of ways. For the purposes of this text, the nursing theories discussed will be classified as focusing on relationships (Peplau and Erickson), caring (Watson, Leininger, and Boykin and Schoenhofer), energy fields (Rogers, Parse, and Newman), or when nursing is needed (Orem, Roy, and Neuman). In discussing these theories, the term *patient*, rather than *client*, will be used when that is the term used by the theorist. These theories are presented in summary form. For greater detail and understanding, the reader is referred to the original works cited at the end of this chapter.

NURSING THEORIES BASED ON RELATIONSHIPS

Some nursing theorists have identified that relationship is central to the practice of nursing. For some clients the relationship with a nurse may extend over years, whereas for others it may occupy only a few moments. Theories based on relationship recognize that no matter how lengthy or brief the human interaction and no matter what the content is of that interaction, a relationship is inevitably established between the nurse and client. The form and content of that relationship may have a significant and long-lasting effect on both individuals.

Hildegard Peplau

Hildegard Peplau was a psychiatric nurse leader who was also an important pioneer in the development of nursing theory. Peplau describes nursing as a therapeutic interpersonal relationship that provides a growth opportunity for both the nurse and the patient. The primary components of this relationship are two persons (a nurse and a patient, or client), professional expertise, and client need (Peplau, 1992). The interpersonal relationship identified by Peplau (1988) initially had four distinct phases: orientation, identification, exploitation, and resolution. In 1997, Peplau combined identification and exploitation into the working phase and renamed resolution "termination." During **orientation**, the nurse and patient meet, get to know each other, identify and clarify the patient's need(s) (previously felt but not necessarily identified by the patient), and progress toward patient comfort in a helping environment. In the **working phase**, the patient begins to respond selectively to those who can help meet the felt need. In this phase, the patient begins to experience an increased sense of belonging as well as a developing capability for problem solving alone and

CASE EXAMPLE 3-1

Mr. James

The following case study will be used in examples of application of theory to practice. As several nursing theories are discussed, each will be applied to the situation of Mr. James, a 60-year-old man whose company downsized 4 months ago. In the process of downsizing, Mr. James's position of consulting engineer was eliminated; he was given a golden handshake and early retirement. He had no plans for retirement, having thought he would not retire until between ages 65 and 70 and "there was plenty of time to plan what he would do." His golden handshake provides him with the income he would have had should he have retired at the planned time. Mrs. James continues with her full-time employment. They own their own home and at the present time have no serious financial concerns. Both of their children are married and live with their spouses and children in other cities in the same state. The entire family gets together three or four times a year and keeps in touch via telephone and e-mail.

Mr. James reports that since his retirement he is not sleeping well, he feels tired all the time, and he does not really have much interest in food. In fact, he has lost 10 pounds in the last 4 months. He says he feels useless and, at times, hopeless.

with others. The patient takes advantage of available services to meet the felt needs and begins to gain a greater sense of control. Patients in this phase have not yet been fully restored to health and may manifest varying degrees of both independence from and dependence on their nursing caregivers. The latter part of the working phase is a transition period and may at times be difficult for both patient and nurse. It is important that the nurse maintain the therapeutic relationship in a nonjudgmental atmosphere while this transition is occurring. In the third and final phase, **termination**, the therapeutic relationship is terminated after the patient's needs have been met. Conflicts and uncertainties found in the working phase have been resolved, and the patient is ready to gain full independence, at least for the time being. Both nurse and patient will have gained from the experience.

Peplau (1992) indicates that her theory of interpersonal relations is particularly appropriate for psychiatric nursing practice because psychiatric patients often have problems with communication and with relating to others. Psychiatric nurses in particular may find that tracking their position in Peplau's scheme may help them understand both how to help their clients and how to respond to frictions that develop between them and their clients, especially in the working phase. Peplau's theory is relatively simple and accords easily with commonsense notions of human relationships. This simplicity and lack of complex concepts and terms make empirical testing of the theory difficult, but a number of psychiatric nurses have found Peplau's theory useful in generating testable hypotheses.

Helen Erickson, Evelyn Tomlin, and Mary Ann Swain

Helen Erickson, Evelyn Tomlin, and Mary Ann Swain (1983) developed the theory of modeling and role-modeling. This theory owes some of its key concepts to the work of psychiatrist Milton Erickson and as a consequence is also easily adapted to working with psychiatric clients. Like Peplau's theory, modeling and role-modeling theory emphasizes the nurse's interpersonal and interactive skills. The theory provides a formalized process through which those interpersonal skills can be applied in daily practice. The process begins with the concepts of modeling and role-modeling.

Modeling involves nursing assessment (Erickson et al., 1983). The goal is for the nurse to develop an understanding of the client's world from the client's perception of that world—to understand the client's subjective experience. Modeling requires empathy to understand the client's view of the current situation, and in this way it differs substantially from the nursing assessment as traditionally incorporated in the nursing process. Traditional nursing assessment is factually oriented. The nurse's role is to obtain details of the client's life, illness, and perceived needs so that these can be synthesized into a care plan. Modeling requires a more holistic approach in which the nurse attempts to explicitly understand how the client sees his world. This worldview may be very different from the nurse's own and may be importantly influenced by cultural perceptions, prior experiences, and, for psychiatric clients, even thought disorders such as delusions or hallucinations. In the modeling process, it is the nurse's role to avoid objectification and judgment and instead to develop a clear concept of how the client views his or her life and personal needs. **Role-modeling** consists of developing an individualized plan of care based on the client's worldview. Role-modeling proposes that nursing interventions be guided not by the nurse's abstract perceptions of what the client needs but by the model that he or she has formed of the client's worldview. Role-modeling is not based solely on the nurse's model of the client's world but also incorporates a variety of theoretical constructs that are further aspects of the theory. Among these are aims of intervention, self-care knowledge, affiliated individuation, and adaptive potential.

Erickson et al. (1983) identified five principles and associated aims of intervention that relate to similarities among human beings. The first principle is that of building trust: "The nursing process requires that a trusting and functional relationship exist between nurse and client" (p. 170) with the associated aim of building trust through the use of therapeutic communication skills. The second principle is that of promoting a positive orientation to increase the client's self-worth and hope: modeling and role-modeling theory assumes that a healthy state "is dependent on the individual's perceiving that he or she is an acceptable, respectable, and worthwhile human being" (p. 170). The third principle is that of promoting perceived control. Modeling and role-modeling theory postulates that individuals do not readily achieve physical or emotional health unless they have a sense of control over their lives: "Human development is dependent on the individual's perceiving that he or she has some control over his or her life, while concurrently sensing a state of affiliation" (p. 170). The fourth principle is that of focusing on client strengths. Every individual, no matter how ill or troubled, has a repertoire of strengths that can be called on to lead to a healthier state. Modeling and role-modeling theory postulates that "there is an innate drive toward holistic health that is facilitated by consistent and systematic nurturance" (p. 170). Such holistic health is achieved by emphasizing the client's strengths so that ill health can be overcome or compensated for. The fifth principle is based on the concept that, working together, nurse and client can set mutual goals directed toward health enhancement. Modeling and role-modeling theory assumes that each individual has an innate drive toward health. The nurse's role is to work with the client to develop goals so that the innate drive can move the individual as rapidly as possible toward an enhanced state of health: "Human growth is dependent on satisfaction of basic needs and facilitated by growth-need satisfaction" (p. 170).

Having established a model of the client's world, the nurse working in this theory will attempt to focus care in a way such that each of the five aims of intervention is given an emphasis. That emphasis is further influenced by the three related concepts of self-care knowledge, affiliated individuation, and adaptive potential. Self-care knowledge is perhaps the most intuitive of these three concepts since modeling and role-modeling theory postulates that most clients know what they need to do to improve their health. The nurse's job is to help the client express that knowledge and to act on it through the development of personalized self-care resources. Over the centuries, poets and songwriters have expressed continuously the modeling and role-modeling principle of affiliation when they write about the importance of wanting and needing "somebody to love." Modeling and role-modeling theory uses the concept of affiliated individuation to emphasize that humans have the need to both feel attached to other individuals (affiliation) and separate from those individuals (individuation). Wanting and needing to love and be loved are important aspects of affiliated individuation, but health also requires an element of independence from entangling relationships.

Adaptive potential is the capacity of a person to respond to stressors—to utilize resources to cope. Erickson et al. (1983) propose the adaptive potential assessment model, which includes equilibrium (adaptive or maladaptive), arousal, and impoverishment. Equilibrium is a non-stress state, which will be adaptive or maladaptive. In adaptive equilibrium, all of the client's subsystems are in harmony. In maladaptive equilibrium, one or more of the client's subsystems are placed in jeopardy to maintain equilibrium. In either state of equilibrium, the client perceives no need to change. However, the client in maladaptive equilibrium requires interventions that help create a desire to change. Arousal is a stress state in which the individual has difficulty mobilizing resources. The client in the arousal state requires more support for individuation than for affiliation. Assistance for this client is directed at helping mobilize resources through guidance, direction, and teaching in relation to self-care. Impoverishment is a stress state in which the individual's resources are diminished or depleted. The client who is impoverished requires help in meeting affiliation needs, promoting internal strengths, and identifying or accessing external resources.

The theory of modeling and role-modeling can be very useful in the practice of psychiatric nursing as well as in a variety of nonpsychiatric nursing settings. Nurses may practice modeling a client's world as an empathic therapeutic technique without employing the entire theory. The concepts of adaptive potential may be found useful in conceptualizing a client's adaptive state even if the nurse is not explicitly using other aspects of the theory. Modeling and role-modeling theory is sometimes criticized for being overly simple and lacking explicit definitions and theoretical constructs. Some view this simplicity as one of the theory's strengths, whereas others view it as a weakness. In this chapter, the student will find the theory applied to the case of Mr. James. Modeling and role-modeling theory is also used to analyze several other cases later in the book. From these analyses, the student can begin to decide whether relative simplicity, the theory's major strength, is also a significant liability.

See Table 3-1 for a summary of relationship nursing theories as related to the case example of Mr. James, presented earlier.

Nursing Theories Based on Caring

Theories based on caring recognize the importance of the relationship between nurse and client, with emphasis on the nurse's role in providing support through the means of human caring. This chapter considers three caring-based theories: those of Jean Watson, Madeleine Leininger, and Anne Boykin and Savina Schoenhofer. These three theories have substantial differences, and Leininger's theory is uniquely focused on caring across cultural boundaries. Each theory has elements that the nurse may find useful in approaching clients both in the practice of psychiatric mental health nursing and in the broader domain of nursing practice.

Jean Watson

Initially, Jean Watson (1979, 1988) differentiated between nursing and medicine by stating that curing is the domain of medicine, and caring is the domain of nursing. From her original discussions of holistic human caring, her thoughts have evolved to a model of the Transpersonal Caring Relationship (Watson, 1999, 2002, 2005). Basic premises of transpersonal caring include the following:

1. Being human is more than a physical body; it includes a spirit in that body (embodied spirit); a consciousness that supports sharing between persons and beyond persons; a unity of mind, body, and spirit, which Watson expresses as mindbodyspirit; and a connected oneness of the person, nature, and the universe.
2. There is a human-environment energy field that includes caring-healing consciousness.
3. Consciousness is energy, and forgiveness and surrender are the highest level of consciousness.
4. Caring increases the possibility of healing and wholeness.
5. Modalities that arise from caring-healing involve the mind, the hands, the heart, and the soul.
6. The processes and relationships linked with caring-healing are sacred, and the nurse can provide a sacred healing environment.
7. Viewing the connectedness of all (subject, object, environment, person, and all living things) is unitary consciousness; unbroken wholeness is the ultimate form of healing, and transcendence is love.

Watson (1996) indicates the transpersonal caring relationship depends upon a moral commitment to human dignity, wholeness, caring, and healing. It also depends on (1) the nurse's orientation to affirming the significance of the person; (2) the nurse's ability to realize, detect, and connect with the spirit of another; (3) the nurse's ability to realize the other's state of being-in-the world—and to feel a union with that other; (4) caring, healing modalities to potentiate comfort, wholeness, and harmony, including promoting inner healing; and (5) the nurse's own life history and ability to care for self. In 2005 Watson expanded self-care to include the ability to forgive self and others, to be grateful for life and its blessings,

TABLE 3-1 Relationship Nursing Theorists and Mr. James

PEPLAU	
Orientation	Nurse explores with Mr. J. what his felt need is. After discussion, they conclude that he needs to feel needed and useful and has not felt this way since his forced retirement. Since his wife has continued working and has essentially not changed her lifestyle, he is uncertain how to continue feeling useful to others and an important part of his wife's life.
Working	The nurse and Mr. J. explore how he can communicate these needs to his wife; they also explore where in the community he could use his skills to provide assistance to others and increase his sense of usefulness. Mr. J. initiates a conversation with his wife in which she assures him that she values his ability to do repairs around the house and loves him for himself, not for the job he held. He also contacts community agencies about volunteer work and selects two to visit. In the process, he learns about a community organization of retired businesspeople who provide support and advice to persons beginning new business ventures; he contacts them and discovers they have been seeking someone with his background and skills.
Termination	Mr. J. reports that he is sleeping better, his appetite is back, he is exercising regularly, and he has been called to consult with two new businesses. It is time to conclude the nurse-patient relationship.
ERICKSON, TOMLIN, AND SWAIN	
Building trust	Nurse seeks to learn about Mr. J. to model his world. He shares that he had not planned to retire and had no plans for what to do after he retired. He feels at loose ends and is depressed.
Affiliated individuation; positive orientation	Mr. J. states he feels that he is a burden to his family now; he used to feel that he was a productive member of society. He felt good about what he did and saw himself as the provider for his family.
Sense of control	The nurse explores with Mr. J. what activities might help him feel useful again (self-care knowledge).
Nurturance	The nurse explores what would reassure Mr. J. that his family still cares for him. He identifies that feedback from others that he has been helpful makes him feel good (self-care knowledge and self-care resources).
Client strengths and mutual goals for growth	With encouragement from the nurse, Mr. J. identifies and explores opportunities to use his professional skills in helping others through volunteering and consulting (self-care action).

and to surrender and let go of ego, and accept experiences without seeking control.

On her website (Watson, 2007) she lists her clinical caritas processes as follows:

- Practice of loving-kindness and equanimity within context of caring consciousness
- Being authentically present and enabling and sustaining the deep belief system and subjective life world of self and one-being-cared-for
- Cultivation of one's own spiritual practices and transpersonal self, going beyond ego self
- Developing and sustaining a helping-trusting, authentic caring relationship
- Being present to, and supportive of, the expression of positive and negative feelings as a connection with deeper spirit of self and the one-being-cared-for
- Creative use of self and all ways of knowing as part of the caring process; to engage in the artistry of caring-healing practices
- Engaging in genuine teaching-learning experience that attends to unity of being and meaning, attempting to stay within the other's frame of reference
- Creating healing environment at all levels (physical as well as nonphysical, and the subtle environment of energy and consciousness), whereby wholeness, beauty, comfort, dignity, and peace are potentiated
- Assisting with basic needs, with an intentional caring consciousness; administering "human care essentials," which potentiate alignment of mindbodyspirit, wholeness, and unity of being in all aspects of care; and tending to both embodied spirit and evolving spiritual emergence
- Opening and attending to the spiritual-mysterious, and the existential dimensions of one's own life-death; soul care for self and the one-being-cared-for

The caring occasion or caring moment is an experience that is difficult to describe due to limitations in language. It is a transpersonal experience of the nurse and other in a human-to-human interaction, at a particular moment in their life histories with the connection existing in a dimension not bounded by space or time. The manifestations of the caring moment include healing, harmony, diversity, and wholeness.

Watson (2002) provides some suggestions for how to cultivate and activate your intentional caring-healing practice. First is to begin each day with a spiritual practice of your choosing, including establishing intentions about what you can control and letting go of what you cannot control. Second is to be mindful of nursing as a spiritual, spirit-filled practice. Third is to develop sensitivity in your daily activities seeking to be grounded in the spirit. Fourth is to seek to identify the spirit-filled person behind each client or colleague. Fifth is to use all experiences, both joyful and dark, as lessons to help you "grow more deeply into your own humanity" (p. 18). This includes seeking help and guidance when you need it. Sixth is to commit yourself to practicing your heartfelt intentions daily to the best of your ability. Seventh is to offer gratitude at the end of the day. Eighth, and last, is to "create your own intentions and your own authentic practice to cultivate caring consciousness and meaningful intentionalities" (p. 19).

While Watson's emphasis on caring is not unique, the strength of her emphasis on the embodied spirit is. She sets a very high standard for nurses to follow and brings into her work a number of important concepts. Watson's curative approach is deeply involved with spiritual concepts and with the philosophical concepts of existentialism and phenomenology, subjects more abstract than some nurses wish to pursue. However, Watson's theory continues to evolve and to attract the attention of many, as nurses are drawn to the holistic and spiritual nature of the theory. Watson's theory is studied by nurse researchers and is often involved in qualitative studies.

Madeleine Leininger

Madeleine Leininger's (1991; Leininger & McFarland, 2002, 2006) theory is titled culture care diversity and universality. She bases this theory on the belief that across cultures there are health care practices and beliefs that vary (diversity) and that are similar (universality). A nurse must have an understanding of the client's culture in order to give culturally appropriate care. **Culture** includes values, beliefs, norms, and lifeways that are learned and shared within a particular group. These guide the thinking, decisions, and actions of members of that group in a way that creates patterns specific to the group. **Culture care** involves those facets of culture that deal with individual and group health and well-being, including efforts to improve on the human condition or to deal with illness, handicaps, or death. The practices for culturally related care are shaped by a number of aspects of the culture, including kinship, cultural values, political and legal factors, and language.

Leininger presents her theory pictorially in what she has labeled the "Sunrise Enabler." This enabler further explicates the elements of culture that will contribute to the nurse's knowledge of the client. These elements are factors associated with technology, religion, philosophy, kinship and social relationships, politics, law, economics, and education, as well as the cultural values, beliefs, and lifeways. All of these elements influence the care practices and expressions of care in a culture through language, environment, and history and help shape and define health or well-being within a culture.

Leininger and McFarland (2006) identify three concepts involved in providing care. These are generic or folk care, professional care-cure practices, and nursing care practice. **Generic or folk care activities** are those culturally based acts for responding to apparent or anticipated needs related to living, health, well-being, handicaps, or death. **Professional care-cure practices** are those acts based on a formal preparation for dealing with health, illness, and wellness, generally within a multidisciplinary setting that is designed to serve consumers. Nursing is "a learned, humanistic, and scientific profession and discipline focused on human care phenomena and caring activities in order to assist, support, and facilitate or enable individuals or groups to maintain or regain their health or well-being in culturally meaningful and beneficial ways, or to help individuals face handicaps or death" (Leininger & McFarland, 2002, p. 46).

Nursing care decisions and actions are defined as **culture care preservation/maintenance** (actions that help people keep and preserve their culture, for example, supporting one's need for prayer), **culture care accommodation/negotiation** (reshaping the way in which values are enacted to support well-being, for example, supporting the use of a culturally based healing ritual as complementary to biomedical recommendations for treatment), and **culture care repatterning/restructuring** (encouraging change in culturally based practices, for example, the way in which food is prepared) (Leininger & McFarland, 2006). Any nursing decisions or actions should be sensitive to the beliefs, values, norms, and lifeways of the culture with which the individual, family, group, community, or institution identifies. Leininger warns against cultural imposition, in which the nurse functions as though the client's culture is the same as the nurse's. She also alerts us to the possibility of culture shock, in which the nurse is so surprised by cultural differences that she cannot function appropriately.

Madeleine Leininger urges us to begin by having an understanding of the client's culture. Nurses need to recognize that illness, and especially mental illness, occurs within a cultural framework. Culturally related issues are further considered in Chapter 7 of this text.

Anne Boykin and Savina Schoenhofer

Anne Boykin and Savina Schoenhofer developed an abstract theory of nursing as caring, which may be used in combination with other theories, for example, one of the relationship theories of nursing. The details of this theory are complex and derive in part from the study of philosophical existentialism (Boykin & Schoenhofer, 1993).

Boykin and Schoenhofer describe caring as a process of living rather than as an end product. Caring involves knowing, rhythm (moving closer and farther away), patience, honesty, trust, humility, hope, and courage. Humans are innately caring, but not all acts are caring acts. Humans, at any moment, are complete and growing in completeness and are enhanced through participation in nurturing relationships with caring others. The capacity for caring grows throughout life. As a caring practice, nursing is both a discipline and a profession. The discipline of nursing is a response to a unique social call that unifies the science, art, and ethic of practice and involves being, knowing, living, and valuing concurrently. The profession of nursing arises from an understanding of the need on which that social call is based and the development and use of the body of knowledge needed to create the discipline response. Boykin and Schoenhofer (1993) describe the relationship between nursing and nursed as caring between, which occurs in the nursing situation and enhances the personhood of both. The focus of nursing is living caring and growing in caring specific to the individual practice situation.

In psychiatric nursing, Boykin and Schoenhofer's theory calls on the nurse to empathize with clients and to provide unconditional acceptance to clients who may not express caring or consideration of others in return. The nurse is challenged to provide nurturing and express caring so that the client may accept human care and initiate growth of self.

See Table 3-2 for a summary of caring nursing theories as related to the case example of Mr. James, presented earlier.

Nursing Theories Based on Energy Fields

A variety of nursing theories are based on the concept of a human energy field. The reader will recall a prior definition of the term *concept* as "words and abstractions that represent reality." The reality represented by the concept of a human energy field is that human interactions are complex beyond our ability to understand them fully. While there is little doubt that we respond directly to others through our senses of sight, hearing, smell, and touch, many highly intuitive persons feel that human interaction involves more subtle and intangible factors. The concept of human energy fields tries to capture this intangible essence in a way that allows it to fit into a theory of nursing practice. Theories based on energy fields share a common view of the person as an irreducible whole comprising a physical body surrounded by an aura. Some persons claim to be able to see auras, but the concept of energy fields does not require an aura to be visible (or perhaps even that it really exists in the way that the reality of a magnetic field can be shown by bringing a compass into its path). The concept represents theorists' assumption that humans are more than their physical bodies and that their interpersonal influence extends beyond the scope of sight or sound. Accepting the concept of energy fields demands that the nurse take on a broader and highly holistic view of human existence than is implicit in the more traditional biopsychosocial view. Three nursing theories based on the concept of energy fields are described below. These theories are highly abstract and are presented in brief. Again, the reader wishing more detail is referred to the original works and to other readings cited at the chapter's end.

While energy-based theories have not generally been applied in psychiatric care, the complementary intervention of therapeutic touch (Krieger, 1979) is grounded in the concept and has been used to produce a relaxation response that can be helpful in psychiatric mental health nursing (see also Chapter 32).

Martha Rogers

According to Martha Rogers (1990, 1992), the science of nursing is the Science of Unitary Human Beings. In this theory, humans are irreducible, indivisible, pandimensional energy fields bearing recognizable patterns and are greater than the apparent sum of their physical parts. In Rogers's view, humans are in constant interaction with the environment. Thus, human life is a continual interplay between a person and that person's environment. In reflecting on this idea, one must remember that Rogers's view of both an individual and the environment is energy based. Rogers believed that the human and environmental fields are continual and without boundaries. (Her term for this is **integrality**, meaning that the energy fields of the human being and of the environment are each part of the other's.) Rogers views the human energy field as having a kind of physical resonance (her term is **resonancy**, and she describes this in terms of wave patterns) that interacts constantly with the environmental field. Rogers further views these changing interactions as a homeodynamic process characterized by an inevitable movement toward increasing complexity (Rogers's term for this is **helicy**). From these concepts, Rogers (1970) presents five assumptions about human beings:

1. Humans are unified wholes who are indivisible and cannot be identified as a sum of their parts.
2. Humans and their environments are in a constant exchange of energy and matter.
3. The life process of humans evolves irreversibly but unpredictably in one direction only.
4. The wholeness of humans is reflected in their energy patterns.
5. Humans are capable of imagery, thought, abstraction, language, sensation, and emotion.

Unlike some other theorists, Rogers neither makes nor implies a specific definition of health or of the process of nursing. She states that health is defined by each person as a personal value. Nursing participates in the process of human individual evolution and tries to understand how a person and his or her environment have previously interacted. Since life evolves in one direction only (that of increasing complexity and diversity), nursing interventions cannot return clients to their previous state of health but can only work to move them forward toward more complex human states. Because of the mutual interaction between the individual and the environment, the nurse works *with* the client to achieve maximum potential, as opposed to working *to* or *for* the client, as in many other theories.

Rogers's theory can seem divorced from reality. However, for many nurses it serves as a stimulus to rethink simplistic assumptions about human nature and, in

Table 3-2 Caring Nursing Theorists and Mr. James

WATSON	
The nurse will seek to develop a transpersonal caring-healing relationship with Mr. J. Examples involving the clinical caritas processes include the following:	
Loving kindness	Recognizing the value he places on feeling needed.
Belief system	Identifying how he can help others and meet his value to be needed, and how he needs to experience and express his faith belief system.
Spiritual practices	By exhibiting sensitivity to Mr. J., the nurse can help him regain his sensitivity to others.
Helping-trusting relationship; authentic caring	Developing a trusting relationship with Mr. J. will help him regain his confidence in his ability to trust in and help others.
Expression of feelings	Mr. J. has made a first step in expressing his feelings to the nurse; he needs to consider how to express his feelings to his family.
Creative use of self	Mr. J. has scientific problem-solving skills but needs problem-solving assistance in applying them to himself and his situation, e.g., where can his skills be used to help others so he will once again feel needed and useful?
Teaching-learning	Mr. J. has knowledge to share: Where and how can he share it most effectively?
Healing environment	Nurse supports Mr. J. in seeking answers to the questions raised above.
Embodied spirit	Finding ways to feel useful: volunteering, consulting.
Soul care	Nurse recognizes the choices are Mr. J.'s; he must be the one to make decisions about what he will seek to do.
LEININGER	
Gather information about the following:	
Technology	Mr. J. is an engineer; he is comfortable with a variety of technologies, including business use of computers.
Philosophy	The man of the household should be the provider.
Society	Mr. J. lives in a society that values self-care and self-direction.
Political/legislative	Policies allowed for forced early retirement.
Education	Mr. J. has a master's degree in business administration.
Environment	Mr. J. was in a busy office; now he is primarily home alone during the day.
Religion	Protestant; Mr. J. does not attend church regularly.
Kinship	Most important family members are his wife, children, and grandchildren. He has no living siblings.
Cultural values	He considers himself true-blue American.
Economic	Mr. J. has no major financial concerns but still would like to see himself as the primary provider for his family.
Language	English is Mr. J.'s primary language.
Generic or folk care	Mr. J. takes 2 tsp. of Grannie (golden raisins soaked in gin) daily for arthritis; he believes pain and constriction of motion have decreased significantly since he began this practice.
Professional care-cure practices	Mr. J. had an annual physical while working and has no major health problems; now he relies on health practices insurance from his wife's employment.
Nurse identifies with his need to feel useful again and chooses to provide culturally congruent care through repatterning/restructuring. The goal is to assist Mr. J. in changing from seeing his work as the primary source of his feeling useful to gaining a sense of usefulness from other sources. They explore ways in which he can use his engineering and business skills as a volunteer in a culturally congruent manner.	

(Continues)

Table 3-2 (Continued)

BOYKIN AND SCHOENHOFER	
Nursing situation	Being: The nurse meets and talks with Mr. J., encouraging him to direct the conversation as he wishes. Knowing: The nurse seeks to understand and to help Mr. J. understand what his concerns are. Living: The nurse and Mr. J. together explore the avenues of opportunity that are available to him (such as volunteering). Valuing: Mr. J. decides what he wants and chooses ways in which he can feel useful (care).
Nurture him in living caring	Identify Mr. J.'s ways of living caring (helping others and feeling useful) and growing in caring
Enhance personhood of both	Both the nurse and Mr. J. grow and change as they explore the choices available to him and as he chooses volunteer activities in the community.
Response to social call for nurturance	The nurse, in aspiring to grow in caring, has a commitment to recognize and nurture caring. Mr. J.'s caring is demonstrated in his concern for his family and his desire to help others.

consequence, to understand the client and self in clinically useful ways.

Rosemarie Rizzo Parse

Rosemarie Rizzo Parse (1981, 1992, 1998) developed her human becoming school of thought from existential phenomenology and the initial work of Martha Rogers (1970). Initially she labeled her work a theory, but in 1998 changed that to a "school of thought." Parse (1995) extends Rogers's theory and gives it a much denser philosophical underpinning.

Parse (2007) writes of humanbecoming and humanuniverse to emphasize the concept of indivisible cocreation. Using this language, Parse's assumptions include that humanuniverse is coconstituting rhythmical patterns, including patterns of relating; open and freely choosing meaning and being responsible for decisions; transcending limitlessly with the possibles; and that becoming is humanuniverse health, rhythmically coconstituting the humanuniverse process, the patterns of relating value priorities, an intersubjective process of transcending with the possibles, and the humanuniverse's emerging.

Parse believes that people create reality for themselves through the choices they make at many levels. People reflect their reality through spoken words, silence, movements and being still (languaging), living based on personal beliefs (valuing), and knowing both specifically and implicitly (imaging).

Parse sees paradoxes within human interactions: revealing-concealing, enabling-limiting, and connecting-separating. For example, as one chooses to reveal something, one must also conceal something else; one cannot reveal both one's face and one's back simultaneously—one is concealed when the other is revealed. As one enables an action, one also limits choices at the same time. One who chooses to go to the movies with friends cannot be in the library studying at the same time. As two people connect, they also will separate. In practice, the nurse does not seek to control or shape the actions of the client or family but, rather, helps them recognize their own experience through a process of equal partnership—individuals coming together to examine and understand the meaning of life's experiences. Parse describes three processes for using her theory. These are explicating or putting into words what is occurring; dwelling with or being open to connecting and separating in the relationship with another; and moving beyond or seeking opportunities for change. Parse's theory can help link theories of energy fields with theories of caring, especially for the nurse who relishes a very high degree of philosophical and linguistic complexity.

Margaret Newman

Margaret Newman developed her theory through her efforts to describe health beyond Martha Rogers's definition. The result is Newman's theory of Health as Expanding Consciousness (Newman, 1994). As noted previously, Rogers indicated that each individual has a personal definition of health, and Parse, in her focus on human becoming, supports Rogers's statement. Newman's definition of health may be seen as a perplexing paradoxical formulation by some. Health, Newman states, includes both the condition of being well (an ordinary definition of health) *and* the condition of being ill. Because health is seen, in ideas deriving from Rogers and others, as the evolving process of expanding consciousness, becoming ill may paradoxically be a manifestation of health. Newman proposes that those states that we identify as sickness may be needed to achieve something an individual has desired but been unable to achieve otherwise—an idea that may be seen as in agreement with classical psychoanalysis. She further adopts from Rogers the concept of unitary human beings and concludes that if beings are truly unitary, they cannot be either ill or well but instead must at all times manifest some synthesis of the two conditions.

Newman's view of health has strong implications for how nursing is practiced. The client is not seen as having an illness to cure or care for but as manifesting patterns that themselves provide information about the whole person. Often the nurse will come in contact with a person when that person's patterns have been disrupted and activities that had been successful in the past are not effective in handling the disruption. Newman describes this as the person having reached a **choice point**. Recognizing these patterns, the nurse then seeks to relate to the unfolding of the individual's life pattern. Newman (1994) indicates that one's flexibility in responding to one's own illness or stress determines whether or not the result will be disabling. She strongly encourages that we accept our experiences as ours no matter how they differ from what we had planned or wished for. "The important factor is to be fully present in the moment and know that whatever the experience, it is a manifestation of the process of evolving to higher consciousness" (p. 68).

Newman's theory is, of course, more complex than outlined here and includes extensive consideration of the role of time and rhythms in human experience. For some, Newman's theory is a challenge to understand and apply, while others who are attracted to paradox and complexity may find themselves especially interested in Newman's work.

See Table 3-3 for a summary of nursing theories based on the concept of energy fields.

Nursing Theories Based on the Concept of "When Nursing is Needed"

Several nursing theories have evolved to answer questions something like the following: How do we know that, or when, any specific individual needs nursing care? These theories offer the attraction of addressing fairly concrete and practical questions and seek to identify the specific needs people have that they cannot meet for themselves and thus seek to meet through nursing care.

Dorothea Orem

Dorothea Orem (2001) proposed a general Self-Care Deficit Theory of Nursing, composed of three constituent theories—self-care, self-care deficit, and nursing systems—that are themselves based on six central and one peripheral concept. The central concepts are self-care, self-care agency, therapeutic self-care demand, self-care deficit, nursing agency, and nursing system. The peripheral concept is that of basic conditioning factors (Orem, 1995). **Self-care** includes those activities that human beings perform for themselves (or for dependent others) to maintain life, health, and well-being. **Self-care agency** is the ability to perform self-care and is influenced by the basic conditioning factors of gender, age, socioeconomic status, developmental level, and health; health care system factors such as available diagnostic and treatment facilities; family; environment; living patterns; and the availability of adequate resources, as well as by the self-care requisites. Self-care requisites may be universal, developmental, or health deviation requisites. Universal self-care requisites relate to life processes and maintaining the integrity of structure and function, including such things as air, water, and elimination. Developmental self-care requisites relate to needs that arise from developmental processes and may include adjusting to life changes or learning to get along with peers. Health deviation self-care requisites are those that arise from illness, injury, or disease or from medical measures taken to diagnose or treat such diseases. **Therapeutic self-care demand** consists of all the activities needed to meet self-care requisites to fulfill self-care agency. **Self-care deficit** occurs or exists when the therapeutic self-care demand is greater than the person's capacity to meet the demand (Orem, 1995). Thus, nursing is needed when the person can no longer provide self-care. Nursing activities to help the person may include doing for the person, teaching, guiding, supporting, or managing an environment to be developmentally supportive. **Nursing agency** is that complex characteristic gained through formal preparation and experiences that allows nurses to act for others in meeting therapeutic self-care demands through exercising or developing self-care agency.

After a self-care deficit is identified, the nurse designs the appropriate **nursing system** (Orem, 2001). The type of nursing system needed is defined by the type of self-care deficit that exists. A wholly compensatory system is needed when the patient is incapable of or should not be engaging in deliberate actions focused on meeting self-care needs. Incapability may be physical, mental, emotional, or some combination of these. In contrast, those who can perform some but not all aspects of self-care activities require a partially compensatory nursing system. In this system, both nurse and patient are active participants. Finally, those who can perform all self-care actions but need assistance with gaining new knowledge or skills, making decisions, or achieving behavior control require a supportive-educative or supportive-developmental system.

Orem's theory has proven popular with both practicing nurses and academicians. Many studies have tested hypotheses derived from Orem's work. In contrast to Newman's theory discussed previously, Orem's concept of health is related to human structure and function, while well-being is related to perceptions of existence. Her view of the nursing systems may seem somewhat one-sided when viewed from the perspective of a theory such as modeling and role-modeling. Further, Orem's theory has little explicitly to say about psychiatric care or the issues of caring addressed in Watson's theory. Nonetheless, because it is concrete and widely known, Orem's theory has potential utility in approaching the unique challenges of psychiatric nursing care.

TABLE 3-3 Energy Field Nursing Theorists and Mr. James

ROGERS	
Integrality	Mr. J. is in continuous process with his environment; change in his employment status has changed the physical environment from a mix of office and home to primarily home.
Resonancy	The length and frequency of Mr. J.'s wave patterns have changed; his level of activity was much higher and changed more often when he was working. His own description of himself indicates much slower change.
Helicy	The direction of change for Mr. J. continues to be toward increasing diversity and complexity. He has not lost the business knowledge he had, but he has not been using it for the last 4 months.
Mr. J. needs to balance his exchange with his environment (integrality) to regain a wave pattern (resonancy) that is acceptable to him and supports his increasing diversity and complexity (helicy). One outcome that could emerge from the nurse-client process is for Mr. J to volunteer in the community, thus increasing the diversity of the environments in which he functions, causing more frequent change in his patterns, and providing additional learning for him, which will support increasing his diversity and complexity.	
PARSE	
Explicating	The nurse and Mr. J. explore the meaning of the situation to him and attempt to make a connection between his current feelings of despair and his forced retirement.
Dwelling with	The nurse and Mr. J. become involved in the struggle of connecting-separating. Mr. J. was forced to separate from his employment and has not experienced equivalent connecting. What connecting would be of interest to him?
Moving beyond	The nurse supports Mr. J. in planning for changing patterns, identifying choices for connecting (volunteering), and making choices.
NEWMAN	
Choice point	Mr. J. was forced to retire and does not have past experience in how to handle the situation. He has identified that staying at home does not meet his needs, and he wants to find new ways of behaving.
Movement	Mr. J.'s movement is less than it was 4 months ago; he seeks new ways to increase his movement.
Time	Time is moving slower in association with decreased movement.
Space	The space Mr. J. has been occupying has been smaller than before.
Consciousness	Mr. J. has experienced a decreased exchange of new information.
Patterns	His patterns have changed without his control; he seeks a transformation in which he regains control of his choices and activities.
Health	As a reflection of the whole and examples of underlying patterns, Mr. J. indicates his current patterns are not satisfactory to him.
Search for patterns	Mr. J. has had a change in pattern from Monday–Friday work to retirement; he is searching for new acceptable patterns.
Information	Mr. J. provides information about his feelings of uselessness.
Body-dynamic energy field	Sleeplessness and weight loss indicate reaching a choice point.
Data indicate that Mr. J. has reached a choice point. Selecting volunteer activities that get him out of the house and allow him to feel useful again will change his patterns and indicate expanding consciousness.	

Callista Roy

The four essential elements of the Roy adaptation model, developed by Callista Roy, are humans as adaptive systems (individual or group), environment, health, and the goal of nursing (Roy & Andrews, 1999). Humans are seen as holistic adaptive systems that respond to stimuli from the environment. When adaptation occurs, health may be present. Health is defined as both a state and a process in which the person is being and becoming integrated and whole and is apparent when the person is able to meet goals of survival, growth, reproduction, mastery, and gaining higher levels of adaptation.

The person processes the environmental stimuli through coping mechanisms identified as the cognator and regulator subsystems. The **cognator subsystem** processes are related to higher brain functions such as information processing, judgment, emotion, and perception. The **regulator subsystem** processes are related to chemical, neural, and endocrine responses such as those of the autonomic nervous system. The processes within these subsystems are not seen directly but, rather, are identified through psychomotor behaviors within four adaptive modes (Roy & Andrews, 1999).

These modes are named physiological, self-concept, role function, and interdependence (Roy & Andrews, 1999). The physiological mode includes oxygenation, nutrition, elimination, activity and rest, protection, senses, fluids and electrolytes with acid-base balance, neurological function, and endocrine function. The self-concept mode relates to the spiritual and psychological aspects of the person and includes the physical self (body sensation and body image) and the personal self (self-consistency, self-ideal, and moral-ethical-spiritual self). The role function mode includes the behaviors that are expected of a person in interaction with another. The interdependence mode includes interpersonal relationships with both individuals and groups. Affectional needs are met in this mode.

Responses to environmental stimuli may be either adaptive or ineffective (Roy & Andrews, 1999). Adaptive responses are those that support the integrity of the system and help fulfill goals of survival, growth, reproduction, mastery, and higher adaptation levels. Ineffective responses are those that do not support integrity or help fulfill goals.

Roy's nursing process has six steps: assessment of behaviors, assessment of stimuli, nursing diagnosis, goal setting, intervention, and evaluation (Roy & Andrews, 1999). The first level of assessment focuses on behaviors that are responses to environmental stimuli and results in identifying those behaviors that are adaptive and those that are ineffective. The second level of assessment focuses on ineffective behaviors and those adaptive behaviors that need nursing support. This assessment includes identifying the stimuli that have led to the behaviors. The stimuli may be identified as focal (making the major contribution to the identified behavior), contextual (also contributing to the identified behavior), or residual (possibly contributing to the identified behavior but not yet verified). Roy also indicates the nurse is to assess the pooling of the internal stimuli or adaptation level in order to identify the life processes as integrated (functioning appropriately), compromised (not functioning in a way to lead to adaptive behaviors), or compensated (seeking to return the system to adaptive behaviors).

After assessment comes diagnosis. Roy recommends stating the diagnosis by listing the observed behavior along with the most influential stimuli (focal and possibly contextual). The nursing diagnosis may also be stated as the adaptive responses or behaviors that are sought.

The goal of nursing is to promote adaptive responses (Roy & Andrews, 1999). Thus, goal setting will include identifying those behaviors that, when observed, will indicate the person has achieved adaptive responses as well as the time frame for these changes. Nursing interventions will seek to alter or manage the stimuli so adaptive responses can occur. Evaluation requires that patient behaviors be compared to goal behaviors to identify whether adaptive responses are present.

Roy's model is discussed here as a theory of when nursing is needed, but in reality it is both more and less than this. Roy presents her work as a model rather than a theory, and technically this makes her work somewhat less than a theory. The distinction is somewhat arbitrary, but models are often taken to be descriptions of practice out of which theories are abstracted. Like theories, models may be used to generate testable hypotheses, so Roy's model has many of the features of other theories considered in this chapter. In addition to considering when nursing is needed, Roy's model presents a comprehensive view of the overall nursing process. Roy challenges the nurse to follow assessment with a nursing diagnosis using specific qualifiers and offers opportunities for assessing diagnostic accuracy between observers. She further challenges the nurse to assess clinical outcomes by setting and monitoring desired behavioral outcomes. With Roy's emphasis on diagnosis, qualifiers, and observed outcomes, her model may have considerable applicability to psychiatric care.

Betty Neuman

Betty Neuman's systems model is based on concepts related to stress and reaction to stress (Neuman, 2002). The system in the model may be an individual, a family, a group, a community—any of which can be identified as an open system. Open systems function with repeating cycles of input, throughput, output, and feedback exchanges with the environment. Forces, or stressors, from both within and outside of the system seek to disrupt system balance or stability. Stability is present when the energy available to deal with these forces exceeds that which is being used by the system. Neuman indicates that reactions to stressors may be positive or negative and either possible (not yet occurring) or actual (identifiable).

The Neuman systems model includes the physiological, psychological, sociocultural, developmental, and spiritual variables at all levels of the system (Neuman, 2002). The physiological variable deals with the body and its structures and functions. The psychological variable deals with mental relationships and processes. The sociocultural variable deals with those functions of the system that involve social and cultural interactions and expectations. The developmental variable deals with developmental processes and needs that vary as the system matures. The spiritual variable deals with the system's spiritual beliefs and their influence and is, according to Neuman, the least understood despite its importance.

The core of the system is the basic structure or central core that represents basic survival factors. The system core is surrounded by the lines of resistance (Neuman, 2002). The function of the lines of resistance is to protect the system core and basic functions. These lines are activated when stressors invade the normal line of defense. Effective responses by the lines of resistance protect the system and allow for reconstitution, or return to system stability. Reconstitution is apparent through an increase of energy in reaction to the stressor. Ineffective responses lead to depletion of energy resources and even to death. The next layer of protection is the normal line of defense. The normal line of defense represents the system's usual level of wellness, or system stability. This stability is not fixed but dynamic; it changes over time as the system copes with various stressors. When stressors invade the normal line of defense, the system reacts in the form of illness. The outer boundary of protection is the flexible line of defense. This is the initial protection, the portion of the system that is first encountered by the stressor. Neuman describes the flexible line of defense as an accordion-like cushion or buffer that protects the normal line of defense. The greater the distance between the flexible line of defense and the normal line of defense, the greater the protection available to the system.

The system has an environment. Neuman (2002) defines three types of environment—internal, external, and created. The **internal environment** consists of those forces, factors, and influences that occur completely within the boundaries of the system. The **external environment** consists of those forces, factors, and influences that occur outside the system boundary. The **created environment** symbolizes system wholeness, exemplifies the exchange between the internal and external environments, and represents the unconscious mobilization of all system variables, particularly the sociocultural and psychological variables.

Stressors are those factors or stimuli that place a demand on the system, create system tension, and have the potential for leading to system instability (Neuman, 2002). Stressors may be **intrapersonal**, or from within the system boundary; **interpersonal**, or from outside the system boundary but proximal to the system; or **extrapersonal**, or from a greater distance outside the system boundary. At any moment, the system may be dealing with one or more stressors.

Neuman (2002) labels the interventions that may be taken to assist the system in retaining, attaining, or maintaining system stability as primary, secondary, or tertiary prevention. Primary prevention occurs before stressors invade the normal line of defense and seeks to strengthen the flexible line of defense through prevention or reduction of risk factors. Examples of primary preventions include health promotion activities and immunizations. Secondary prevention occurs after the system has reacted to the invasion of a stressor; secondary prevention deals with existing symptoms. The focus of secondary prevention is to strengthen the internal lines of resistance to protect the system core and energy resources. Tertiary prevention occurs after secondary prevention has begun to be successful and seeks to support system reconstitution through protecting client strengths and conserving client energy.

Neuman's theory was not explicitly derived from a mental health perspective, but its emphasis on stressors and on psychological, sociocultural, developmental, and spiritual variables would certainly seem to suggest psychiatric applicability. Neuman claims that her theory is useful over the entire range of nursing practice and even outside the field of nursing. This would further suggest applicability to psychiatric mental health nursing.

See Table 3-4 for a summary of nursing theories based on the concept of when nursing is needed as related to the case example of Mr. James.

PSYCHIATRIC/PSYCHOLOGICAL THEORY

Just as nurses need to identify the theoretical bases of their practice, it is helpful to understand the theoretical bases of practice of others in health care. In psychiatric nursing, the interdisciplinary team is of particular importance and may include psychiatrists, psychologists, social workers, and counselors as well as nurses. Each of these individuals, including nurses, may use psychological theories as the basis for their practice. Knowledge of representative psychological theories will enhance the nurse's ability to communicate with other members of the team.

Psychoanalytic Theory

The psychoanalytic theories to be reviewed here are those of Sigmund Freud, Erik Erikson, and Harry Stack Sullivan. Freud's focus was on psychosexual development, Erikson's on psychosocial development, and Sullivan's on the development of interpersonal relationships. All are stage theorists, that is, the developmental process they each describe is envisioned as occurring in discrete stages or steps rather than continuously.

Freud and Psychosexual Development

Sigmund Freud is best known for two sets of concepts: those related to personality (id, ego, and superego) and those related to stages of psychosexual development (oral, anal, and phallic or oedipal). Freud initially described the **id** as the unconscious and identified it as the most primitive part of the personality. The goal of the id is to minimize pain and maximize pleasure—otherwise known as the pleasure principle. Freud (1965a/1920) viewed pleasure as the release of tension and suggested that frustration and psychological symptoms might occur when the release of tension was repressed, or blocked. The id also contains impressions and impulses that have been repressed into it and thus are not accessible to the conscious mind. Because the goal of the id is to release tension, it also includes forces of aggression and destruction. The id is not logical; thus, when it seeks to reduce tension, it does not consider the consequences of pleasure-seeking actions, even when those might result in serious harm to someone or something the person needs or loves.

The **superego**, or conscience, serves to delay the immediate impulse generated by the id and to bring rationality into consideration before the **ego**, or self, acts.

TABLE 3-4 When Nursing Is Needed: Nursing Theorists and Mr. James

	OREM
Basic conditioning factors	Gender: male Age: 60 Socioeconomic status: middle class Development: retired (not by choice) Health: generally good by history; currently not sleeping well, losing weight Health care system factors: has insurance and a primary physician Family: wife; two married children, four grandchildren Environment: lives in own home Living patterns: change in these in last 4 months
Universal self-care requisites	Air: occasional rapid breathing Food: available, decreased appetite Water: met Elimination: occasional constipation Activity/rest balance: significant decrease in activity in last 4 months, sleep disturbed Solitude and social interaction: decreased social interaction, increased solitude over last 4 months Promotion of human functioning: decreased functioning over last 4 months Hazard prevention: no identified environmental hazards; potential hazards related to feelings of uselessness
Developmental self-care requisites	Retired, not by own choice; had made no plans for activities postretirement
Health deviation self-care requisites	None identified at this time
Therapeutic self-care demand	Need to feel useful greater than current ability to meet the need; thus self-care deficit exists
Nursing system design	Supportive-educative nursing system needed; key components are to help Mr. J. identify skills he has to offer others and ways in which he can use these skills: work at home, community volunteering, connecting with programs at church
	ROY
First-level assessment	Physiologic mode: oxygenation, protection, senses, fluids and electrolytes, neurologic, endocrine, all show adaptive responses. Ineffective responses seen in nutrition (lack of appetite and 10 lb. weight loss over 4 months), elimination (occasional constipation), and activity and rest (sleeplessness). Self-concept mode: body image shows adaptive responses; ineffective responses in personal self (feels useless and worthless). Role function mode: secondary roles show adaptive responses; primary roles show ineffective responses in relation to development stage of retirement; tertiary roles show ineffective responses in lack of development of hobbies and other non-work-related activities Interdependence mode: may have ineffective responses in interdependence with wife; more data needed
Second-level assessment	Focal stimulus: forced retirement Contextual stimuli: no plans for retirement, major changes in his life with little apparent change in lives of family members

(Continues)

TABLE 3-4 (Continued)

	Residual stimuli: concerns that he will die if he is not employed
Nursing diagnosis	Stress and depression related to early retirement
Goal setting	Establish activities that are effective in enhancing sense of self within 2 months
Intervention	Nurse and Mr. J. identify activities in which he would be interested and locate places where he can carry out these activities; for example, serving as a consultant to new small businesses
Evaluation	Successful if Mr. J. is once again sleeping well, his appetite has returned, his weight has stabilized, and he is feeling useful and needed
	NEUMAN
Person	Physiological: loss of system stability seen in change in eating and sleeping patterns
	Psychosocial: loss of system stability demonstrated in feelings of uselessness
	Sociocultural: loss of system stability seen in lack of contact with previous business associates
	Developmental: loss of system stability seen in view of retirement as unplanned and forced
	Spiritual: loss of system stability seen in feelings of uselessness
Flexible line of defense and normal line of defense	Both flexible and normal lines of defense invaded
Lines of resistance	Activated as seen by symptoms of sleeplessness, loss of appetite, weight loss, and feelings of uselessness, and in his seeking help with these
Stressor	The major stressor identified is Mr. J.'s change in employment status (an interpersonal stressor)
Primary prevention	Planning for retirement did not occur
Secondary prevention	Symptoms are present, so this level of prevention is needed; plan and seek ways to be occupied and useful—volunteering, home repairs, church activities
Tertiary prevention	Once sleeping and eating well again and feeling useful (system stability restored), develop plans for continued involvement, potentially including development of hobbies that he and his wife can enjoy together when she retires

In Freud's view, the ego both represses and derives its own energy from the id; consequently, it seeks to achieve a balance among the demands of three masters—the id, reality, and the superego. The ego is subject to anxiety associated with concerns about meeting the demands of each of these masters. Anxiety occurs when there is concern about controlling the impulses of the id. Moral anxiety is associated with meeting the expectations of the superego, and realistic anxiety occurs in response to dangers in the external world.

Freud's theories of personality remain of interest to psychoanalysts, literary critics, and writers, as well as some nurses. They seem to accord fairly well with the way we perceive our behavior to be influenced by conscience and impulse. It is not clear to what extent these theoretical concepts explain common psychopathology, and many psychologists believe that Freud's theories of personality have very little empirical support. They have remained influential because, until recently, Freudian psychoanalysis was the dominant model of treatment for mental illness. As a more biomedical model has evolved in recent years, the Freudian viewpoint has lost influence.

This decreased influence also extends to Freud's concepts of psychosexual development. The stages of development, according to Freud (1905), are based on sexual feelings (defined as anything that produces pleasure) and occur in a sequence of stages. Freud's general term for sexual energy is libido, and when this energy becomes focused on a part of the body through the process of cathexis, that area of the body is known as an erogenous zone. The stage sequence occurs as the zone that is the focus of the child moves from the mouth (oral) to the anus (anal) and finally to the genital region (phallic or oedipal). The oral stage is divided into two parts. The first part occurs during the first 6 months of life, in which sucking provides not only nutrition but also pleasure in its own right. Freud called finding gratification through one's own body autoerotic and described the young infant as objectless, or having no conception of differentiation between self and others. The infant's focus is primarily inward and was identified by Freud as a state of narcissism. At about 6 months of age, the infant enters the second part of the oral stage and begins to be aware of the mother as a separate being. Because the infant identifies the mother as necessary, anxiety is often exhibited when she leaves the room or house. The infant is at this time developing teeth and the urge to bite. Few mothers will tolerate being bitten during nursing, so the infant is faced at this early stage with two conflicting urges: biting and feeding.

The anal stage occurs between approximately ages 6 months and 3 years, when, according to Freud, children become increasingly aware of pleasurable sensations associated with bowel movements. As they gain maturational control, Freud felt, children might deliberately delay having a bowel movement in order to heighten the pleasure through increasing pressure on the rectal mucosa (Freud, 1905). There is little evidence that such delay actually occurs, but this has not kept the concept of anality from enjoying popular recognition. Toilet training does require that the child delay defecation, but the reward for this outcome is probably praise or a sense of mastery rather than anal pleasure. In the conflicts that arise around the period of toilet training, Freud (1959/1908) saw the origins of certain personality characteristics, one of which he termed anal retentiveness Freud saw the anal retentive personality as manifesting excessive interest in cleanliness, order, and reliability along with resentment of authority that is often expressed passive aggressively. While some psychoanalysts still adhere to such Freudian descriptions of personality types and disorders, many other psychiatrists separate out the obsessive-compulsive and the passive-aggressive personalities as distinct (but indeed related) entities. It is by no means universally agreed on that personality aberrations derive from early toileting experiences. This book discusses common disorders of personality in Chapter 18.

The phallic, or oedipal, stage occurs between about 3 and 6 years of age and applies primarily to boys. According to Freud, an oedipal crisis begins with a boy's interest in his penis. This interest leads to a desire to compare his organ to those of other males, of animals, and of girls and women. His fantasies often involve being the heroic lover of his primary love object—his mother. He quickly learns that the behaviors required to carry out his fantasies are not viewed by others as acceptable. He discovers that he cannot marry his mother and may even be offered less physical contact with the mother than before, either because (likely more in Freud's time than now) such contact was felt to be developmentally inappropriate or because other children have subsequently been born and require more of the mother's time. In Freud's view, the boy observes that his father has seemingly unlimited access to physical contact with the mother, and this observation leads to the Oedipus complex, in which the little boy views his father as a rival for his mother's affection. (The reader will remember that in ancient Greek tradition, Oedipus unwittingly killed his father and married his mother.) The young boy may become frightened by his wishes to see his father out of the way since, after all, he loves and needs his father too. More importantly, the boy may also begin to fear castration, especially if threatened when caught masturbating. Freud associated the fear of castration with the boy's realization that females do not have penises and the boy's belief that they once had penises that were cut off. If this happened to females, it could happen to him! These predicaments are typically resolved through a series of defensive actions (Freud, 1989/1923). Repression, or burial of any sexual feelings toward the mother, is used to fend off incestuous desires and to identify his love for his mother as a higher, purer love. Resolving the Oedipus complex, the boy seeks to identify with his father, to join him rather than fight him. He also internalizes a superego or takes on his parents' moral prohibitions as his own. In this way, Freud was able to explain a striking range of psychological phenomena, especially the emergence of conscience, or the superego.

Freud was less specific about the Oedipus complex for girls. He stated that at about the age of 5, girls become disappointed in their mothers (Freud, 1965b/1933). He associated this disappointment with feelings of deprivation since she no longer receives the level of love and attention she received as a baby (especially if another baby has entered the family); irritation about her mother's prohibitions, especially in relation to masturbation; and anger that she does not have a penis (penis envy). Feminine pride is regained as the little girl begins to appreciate the attentions of her father. As with the little boy, she will discover that she cannot lay sole claim to her father and may see her mother as a rival (Freud termed this the Electra complex). While the boy's primary motivation to resolve the Oedipus complex is the fear of castration, Freud was unable to find a comparable motivator for girls but did not deny that women also develop superegos. Freud believed, however, that a girl's superego is weaker than the boy's because the girl's motivation to resolve the conflict is weaker. This belief accorded with popular nineteenth-century views that women were morally inferior to men and were less capable of repressing sexual impulses. Freud seems to have based his view of woman's superego on theory alone rather than on any empirical data. This is a good example of the ability of a theory to gain acceptance even when evidence might be obtained that would call it seriously into question.

With the development of the superego and its associated defenses against oedipal impulses, the child enters the latency stage. This stage lasts from ages 6 to 11. Freud (1905) described this stage as one in which the sexual feelings and memories from the previous three stages are repressed. Thus, the latency period is relatively calm, and energies are directed into socially acceptable activities.

Latency has been described as the lull before the storm. Puberty begins around age 11 in girls and 12 in boys. In puberty, sexual energy rises to adult levels and threatens the previously established defenses. Freud (1965a/1920) described the individual's task from now onward as that of "freeing himself from the parents" (p. 345). This task involves releasing the tie to the parent of the opposite sex and finding a mate of one's own. Freud (1905) noted that human struggles for independence from parents are never easy and rarely result in complete independence.

While Freud carefully described each of the stages of normal psychosexual development, he also recognized (1905) that not all persons pass uneventfully through each. He concluded that an individual might become fixated at a stage or regress from one stage to a previous one. **Fixation** occurs when we maintain a preoccupation with the pleasures associated with a stage, even though we have advanced beyond that stage. For example, in the Freudian model, those who are fixated at the oral stage are often preoccupied with food or suck or bite on objects such as pencils. **Regression** occurs when one reverts to the pleasures of an earlier stage during times of frustration. For example, a child may seek comfort in thumb sucking when very upset, or an adult may seek comfort in food when depressed. Freud (1965a/1920) believed that more serious fixations and/or regressions resulted in serious emotional disorders. For example, the psychotic individual with delusions of grandeur who believes him or herself to be God may be considered as having regressed to a primary narcissism in which the boundaries between self and the external world are once again blurred. While an excellent example of Freud's imaginative inventiveness, once again no empirical evidence supports this contention. Even many supporters of Freudian psychoanalysis feel that Freud's theories apply better to minor psychological abnormalities than they do to major psychotic illness. A summary of Freud's stages of development can be found in Table 3-5.

This text discusses psychoanalysis in Chapter 28, where more of Freud's ideas are considered along with his therapeutic techniques. His ideas have exerted a huge influence on twentieth- and twenty-first-century culture and society. While Freud continues to have many adherents over 50 years after his death, nurses should regard his theories as fascinating but still largely unproven.

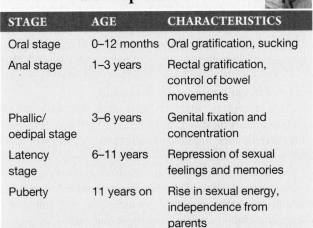

TABLE 3-5 Freud's Stages of Development

STAGE	AGE	CHARACTERISTICS
Oral stage	0–12 months	Oral gratification, sucking
Anal stage	1–3 years	Rectal gratification, control of bowel movements
Phallic/oedipal stage	3–6 years	Genital fixation and concentration
Latency stage	6–11 years	Repression of sexual feelings and memories
Puberty	11 years on	Rise in sexual energy, independence from parents

Psychosocial Development

Erik Erikson developed a theory of child development that emphasizes social growth over Freud's sexually related conflicts. Also a stage theory, Erikson's description took from Freud the concept of a series of personal crises that led the child from stage to stage. In Erikson's view, the successful resolution of one stage will have a positive effect on the person's ability to be successful in the next stages. Biological maturation and social forces compel the individual to move through all of the stages whether or not a given stage has been resolved successfully (Crain, 1985). As in Freud's theory, the failure to resolve a stage may lead to psychological symptoms either in childhood or in adulthood.

The first stage deals with trust versus mistrust and occurs between birth and age 1½ years. The focus here is to develop a healthy ratio between trust and mistrust. Infants seek to meet their needs through interactions with caregivers. When the caregiver's responses are consistent, predictable, and reliable, the baby begins to develop a basic trust in the caregiver. The alternative is a sense of mistrust that develops based on unpredictable and inconsistent responses from the caregiver (Erikson, 1950). Infants also must learn to trust in themselves. Erikson (1950) states that when the teething child learns to regulate chewing and biting urges to suck without nipping, that child begins to view him or herself as "trustworthy enough so that providers will not need to be on guard lest they be nipped" (p. 248). The developing sense of trust is demonstrated in the infant's behavior. Erikson states the first sign of trust in the mother is seen when the infant is willing "to let her out of sight without undue anxiety or rage" (p. 47). Trust must be balanced with an appropriate amount of mistrust: "The human infant must experience a goodly measure of mistrust in order to trust discerningly" (Erikson, 1976, p. 23). Erikson (1950) emphasized that the development of trust in the infant is dependent on the confidence of the caregivers and indicates that it is culturally important that we believe that what we do for our children is good. Trust is seen as an ego strength that enables the delay of gratification, which is an important psychological tool for success in adolescence and adulthood.

The second stage, autonomy versus shame and doubt, occurs between 1½ and 3 years of age. Erikson identified the basic modes of this stage as holding on and letting go, thus exercising choice. This exercise of choice is associated with a sense of autonomy. The developing sense of autonomy is further supported by developing abilities to walk, feed oneself, and talk. It is a common experience that a 2 year old says "no" much more frequently than "yes," thus seeking to exercise self-determination. Autonomy comes from within as the child grows and develops. Shame and doubt occur as a result of social pressures—the efforts of parents and family to teach the child culturally defined proper behavior. Shame occurs with concern about being looked on favorably by others; doubt is associated with questioning one's ability to perform. This conflict between autonomy and shame and doubt is successfully resolved when the child's experiences with shame and doubt do not overwhelm the initial sense of autonomy. Those who do not resolve this conflict successfully are likely to have lifelong feelings of shame and doubt when they seek to respond to their urges toward self-determination.

The third stage, initiative versus guilt, occurs between the ages of 3 and 6 years. Erikson's (1950) term for the primary mode of this stage is intrusion, which he uses to describe the sense of exploration and daring exhibited by children of this age. Developing physical and mental abilities allow the child to intrude physically and verbally through activity, locomotion, talking, and other methods of exercising curiosity. Initiative is also intended to indicate forward movement. In developing initiative, the child demonstrates the ability to plan, set goals, and seek to carry out the plans to meet the goals. The crisis occurs when children realize they cannot achieve their biggest goals, those described by Freud in the oedipal phase as the desire to possess one parent and thus rival the other. The discovery of the social taboos associated with these goals leads to the development of the superego and the production of guilt. Erikson (1950) recognizes the necessity of the superego for socially acceptable behavior but views the development of a superego also as a loss since it often stifles imagination and initiative.

The fourth stage, industry versus inferiority, occurs from about 6 to 11 years of age. This is a period of mastery of social and cognitive skills. Socially, the child now focuses skill development outside of the family to the wider culture. This is a time of development of peer relationships. It is also a time fraught with the danger of failure, which may result in feelings of inadequacy and inferiority. Erikson felt that such a sense of inferiority is likely to be greatest in those who developed more doubt than autonomy and in those who believe themselves to be viewed as inferior by those outside of the family.

The fifth stage, identity versus role confusion, is associated with adolescence (11–12 years to 18–20 years). Erikson's theory was one of the first to recognize the developmental stage of adolescence and to emphasize its association with the growth of personal autonomy. Erikson claimed that the conflicts in this stage are related to the adolescent's great increase in energy, dramatic physiological changes, and the evolution of new social conflicts and demands. The primary task is to develop identity—a sense of who one is and how one fits into the larger social order. The physical changes that occur in adolescence are dramatic and visible. These changes can lead the adolescent to identity confusion—a sense of hardly recognizing oneself. This, in turn, leads to concerns about looking attractive to others, meeting others' expectations, and establishing a vocational role. Erikson observed that adolescents often delay making commitments in an effort to avoid "identity foreclosure" or, instead, make decisions before all of the options are known. The uncertainty about who they are leads adolescents to associate with groups, which helps provide them with identity and clear-cut good/bad views of the world. In Erikson's view, identity is developed through identification with those whom we admire as well as through our accomplishments. The search for identity, and thus the time spent in role confusion, may be a long and painful one but can lead to higher levels of personal integration and to social innovations (Crain, 1985).

The Eriksonian period for young adulthood (ages 18 to 25) is labeled intimacy versus isolation. The adolescent is too self-absorbed to develop real intimacy with another. This becomes the task of the young adult, who has developed enough of a sense of identity to be able to lose him or herself in mutuality with another (Crain, 1985). Those who are unable to attain such mutuality experience isolation and, often, self-absorption. Adulthood (ages 21 to 45) is described as involving generativity versus stagnation. Once two people have achieved intimacy, they are ready to look beyond themselves. Generativity involves the production of both children and success at work. Erikson focused more heavily on the creation of and care for children than on the contributions made at work. Note that in Erikson's theory, the mere creation of children does not satisfy the definition of generativity. Generativity involves productivity through caring for and guiding children, whether one's own or those of others. Those who do not achieve generativity will experience stagnation and impoverishment of the personality. Erikson suggested that the person who cannot achieve generativity may have had such an empty childhood that he or she cannot envision parenting in a more enriched fashion.

In contrast with the general social view of old age as a period of decline, Erikson (1950) sees this period (ages 45 years to death) as one with potential for growth and wisdom. He labeled the crisis of this period ego integrity versus despair. Rather than focus on the external adjustments related to the series of physical and social losses experienced by the elderly, Erikson focused on an internal struggle. As death approaches, people begin a life review that involves deciding whether or not their lives have been worthwhile. This opens them to the ultimate despair—the view that their lives have not been what they could or should have been and now it is too late to do anything about it. The resulting disgust is actually contempt for themselves (Erikson, 1959). Facing such despair invokes the search for ego integrity. Ego integrity involves "the acceptance of one's one and only life cycle as something that had to be and that, by necessity permitted no substitutions" (Erikson, 1950, p. 268). It includes accepting that mistakes were made (perhaps unavoidably) while recognizing the good things that were accomplished, developing a sense of the inevitable order of the past. It also involves a feeling of companionship "with the ordering ways of distant times and different pursuits" (p. 268) or a detached, philosophical wisdom about life in general rather than only one's own in particular. See Table 3-6 for a summary of Erikson's stages of development.

Half a century after its publication, Erikson's theory seems at times a bit dated, and, like Freud's, it was developed with relatively little formal empirical basis. Erikson was, however, among the first popular psychologists to recognize that human development did not stop in childhood but proceeded over an entire lifetime. Whether or not Erikson's stages are real milestones that apply to every individual, they still offer a relatively useful view of the challenges that each of us pass as we move from childhood to productive adult roles.

TABLE 3-6 Erikson's Stages of Development

STAGE	AGE	CHARACTERISTICS
Trust versus mistrust	0–18 months	Development of trust
Autonomy versus shame and doubt	18 months–3 years	Exercise of choice and self-determination
Initiative versus guilt	3–6 years	Exploration and daring
Industry versus inferiority	6–11 years	Mastery of social and cognitive skills
Identity versus role confusion	11–20 years	Development of identity
Intimacy versus isolation	18–25 years	Mutuality and intimacy with another person
Generativity versus stagnation	21–45 years	Productivity through caring for and guiding children
Ego integrity versus despair	45 years to death	Internal struggle and life review

Sullivan's Interpersonal Theory

Harry Stack Sullivan was a leader in emphasizing the importance of interpersonal relationships. He sought to decrease what he perceived to be an emphasis on heredity in assigning cause to psychiatric conditions and to increase recognition of the importance of environment, especially the sociocultural environment. His approach has been described as holistic and interactional (Mullahy, 1970). In Sullivan's view, no one can become fully human without "the support and nurture of the social environment" (Mullahy, 1970, p. 128). All human processes occur in interrelationships; none occur in isolation. Sullivan identified three life processes: genetic organization, communal existence, and functional activity. Genetic organization determines the type of organism, innate individual differences, instincts, and the general course of development. Genetic organization provides the possibilities and boundaries for development and in general prescribes the sequence for maturation but does not determine the development itself. Communal existence includes those processes that connect the human with his or her environment. The interaction between human and environment is ever present, although the boundaries between human and environment are often not clear-cut. Functional activity in general is associated with the accumulation of "free energy" and activity to maintain life. Mentally, functional activity represents mental processes such as imagining, learning, desiring, thinking, perceiving, and sensing.

Sullivan viewed humans as essentially social beings and believed childhood development should be understood in terms of interpersonal relations as influenced by culture. In earliest infancy, the prevailing activity is sleeping followed by the taking of nourishment and those activities associated with relieving distress not connected to hunger. Like Freud, Sullivan viewed sucking as a form of oral behavior, which he thought both met the need for nourishment and helped to use excess energy.

Infancy ends and childhood begins with the development of articulate speech. The variety of total activities increases as cultural forces begin to make themselves felt. The juvenile period begins as the child develops the need to interact and play with other children. This is "the period of growth of egocentric sociality and of the elaboration of social personality. If real playmates are not available, the youngster creates imaginary playmates" (Mullahy, 1970, p. 125).

The next interpersonal relation that develops is the beginning of a new kind of attachment to another; this attachment, when it prospers, is love. A new need, the need for interindividual affection, arises and replaces the egocentricity of the juvenile. The ability to love, according to Sullivan, moves the development of the personality into its "ultraimportant phase" of growth. During this phase of early adolescence (initially termed preadolescence by Sullivan), boys and girls tend to participate in gender-specific organized groups or gangs. Those whose personal or social circumstances do not support the development of these interpersonal relationships will not experience this phase of development and may never experience love.

In Sullivan's view, true adolescence begins with the development and psychosocial management of overt sexual impulses. This stage is followed by adulthood, a life situation that includes one or two other persons in "a total activity, prevailingly sexual in character, the resolution of which is complete, in the sense that it does not proceed into disturbing situations, which in turn would require resolution" (Mullahy, 1970, p. 126). Entering adulthood requires successfully passing through all the previous stages.

Each stage or phase of development prepares the personality for the principal development of the next stage. In Sullivan's view, failure to successfully achieve the activities of a stage can severely limit one's personality development and chances for a normal, successful life. Sullivan shared this determinative view of stage theory with Erikson and Freud. Clearly, Sullivan had much in common with Erikson but tended to emphasize social and interpersonal determinants more than strictly psychological ones. Both were concerned with the factors that lead to healthy psychological development from infancy into adulthood.

Cognitive Development Theory

Cognition, the process of thinking, knowing, and perceiving, is of particular interest to psychiatric nursing, as alterations in this ability are often the first indications of psychiatric concerns. Jean Piaget was among the first psychologists to describe and define stages of child cognitive development. Piaget's pioneering work was expanded by Perry (1970) and, with regard to females, by Belenky, Clinchy, Goldberger, and Tarule (1986). Together, these writers have offered a still largely valid view of the way in which cognitive skills come to maturation. These cognitive skills are thought to develop in much the same staged way as do the more explicitly interpersonal or psychodevelopmental skills described by Freud, Erikson, and Sullivan.

Jean Piaget

Piaget developed a stage theory of cognitive development largely by empirically observing the sequence in which infants and young children acquire skills. While Erikson, Freud, and Sullivan were careful observers of childhood development, Piaget designed psychological experiments to try to assess when and how children become able to make specific cognitive distinctions. Piaget established what he felt to be an accurate sequence of cognitive stages that all children progress through on their way to maturity. He believed that children move through each of these stages at various paces but will always do so in the same order. Piaget's stages are based on the belief that children themselves develop their cognitive structures. They must interact with the external environment to do so, but neither the environment nor anything in it constructs the changes in cognition (Crain, 1985). This interaction with environment comprises what Piaget termed assimilation, accommodation, and organization. Assimilation involves taking in the experiences from the environment. Accommodation occurs when what is taken in from the environment does not match a person's existing structure and the person changes the structure to match the new information. Organization is the process of placing one's ideas into a coherent state or order.

Piaget proposed several multistaged periods of development. The first period of development is entitled the sensorimotor intelligence period and occurs approximately from birth to 2 years of age. During this period, babies organize their physical actions and reactions to deal with the environment that immediately surrounds them. The first stage, from birth to 1 month of age, deals with the use of reflexes; the inborn reflexes are the first pattern of action. The most conspicuous reflex is sucking, which occurs whenever the infant's lips are touched or brushed. These reflexes begin as passive activity but soon develop into self-initiated activity. The second stage, from ages 1 to 4 months, is called primary circular reactions. A circular reaction is when an infant seeks to repeat a new experience. Piaget's (1974) example is that of thumb sucking. The infant encounters the experience of thumb in mouth and seeks to repeat this experience. Coordination is such that initial efforts to again insert thumb in mouth are not successful—body movements are not yet coordinated by individual parts. Instead, the entire body moves as a whole. In Piaget's terms, the infant is not yet able to make the accommodations needed to assimilate the hand into the sucking scheme. Eventually, after many efforts, the infant is successful and thumb sucking becomes part of the scheme. The third stage, from ages 4 to 10 months, is identified as secondary circular reactions. These reactions involve repeating an event that occurs outside the infant's body, such as making a mobile move. This typically involves a single action and a single result, such as the baby kicking and causing the mobile to move. Awareness of objects as separate from self is beginning in this stage. Children will look where an object has fallen and can find partly hidden objects. They can also find objects they have put aside but cannot find something that has been completely hidden by another person.

The fourth stage, from ages 10 to 12 months, involves the coordination of secondary schemes. In this stage, the infant learns to coordinate two schemes to achieve a desired result. For example, the child may push aside a cereal bowl to reach a piece of fruit that is behind the bowl. This involves the schema of pushing and grasping. It also demonstrates some understanding of space and time, as the infant has demonstrated a sense that some objects are in front or back of others and that some events or actions must precede or follow others (Ginsberg & Opper, 1979). In this stage, object permanence begins. The child can find a completely hidden object, for example, a toy covered by a blanket or cushion. The fifth stage, from ages 12 to 18 months, is designated tertiary circular reactions, which involve using different actions for different results. In this stage, the child explores the world without adult teaching, encouraged by an intrinsic curiosity. Examples include pounding upon a hollow object with varying levels of intensity to obtain different sounds or splashing water from different angles to direct the water toward different objects. In Stage 5, a child can follow a series of displacements so long as he or she has observed those displacements. The sixth stage, from ages 18 months to 2 years, marks the beginning of thought. In Stage 5, the child explores the world through physical action; in Stage 6, there is more apparent thinking before acting. Piaget's (1974) example involved his daughter and her efforts to remove a chain from a matchbox. Her initial, and unsuccessful, efforts were to turn the box over and to try to stick her finger in a slit in the box. She then paused, concentrated on the slit, and opened and closed her mouth several times. After this "thought process," she proceeded to open the box and remove the chain. In Stage 6, the child can follow invisible displacements such as detouring around a chair to find a ball that has rolled under the chair.

The second and third periods are those of preoperational thought, from ages 2 to 7, and concrete operations, from 7 to 11 years of age. Preoperational thought marks the beginning use of symbols and requires reorganization of thinking. This reorganization takes some time and effort, as is evidenced by the child's thinking being unsystematic and illogical during this stage. The use of symbols allows make-believe play and rapid development of language. While some believe that language mastery enhances the development of logic, Piaget disagrees. His belief is that a child organizes his or her world from the beginning in a logical manner. To demonstrate the organization, Piaget used a series of scientific tasks with children as young as 4. The most famous of these relates to the conservation of continuous quantities of liquid. The child is shown two tall, slender glasses that are filled to the same level. When asked if they contain the same amount, the child usually agrees that they do. Then, the liquid from one glass is poured into a shorter, wider glass and the child is again asked if the two contain the same amount of liquid. The child in the preoperational stage answers in two substages. In the first substage, the child fails to conserve and states that the amounts are not equal; one or the other has more because it is higher or because it is wider. The use of a single dimension of measurement overcomes the logic that they must still be the same. In the second substage, the child is moving toward but has not yet reached conservation. The child's response may first be that one has more because it is taller, and then the response is changed to that the other has more because it is wider. Finally, the child becomes confused. This demonstrates intuitive regulations—a beginning consideration of two dimensions that does not yet include reasoning about both dimensions at the same time. About the age of 7, the child enters the period of concrete operations and recognizes that equal amounts of liquid are in both glasses.

A second task relates to the conservation of number. In this task, Piaget gave children a row of egg cups and several eggs. The children were asked to take just enough eggs to fill the cups. Preoperational children in the first substage made rows that were equal in length with no consideration for the number of cups or the number of eggs. They were consistently surprised they had more eggs than cups when asked to place the eggs in the cups. At the second substage, children lined one egg up with each cup. However, if either row was bunched up or spread out, the children claimed that now one row had more in it, as they equated length with quantity. Some did begin to waver in their reasoning between thinking there was more because a row was longer and there was more in the other row because it was denser. In concrete operations, children again recognized the number did not change with changes in length.

Just as preoperational children seem unable to take into consideration two dimensions of an object simultaneously, they seem unable to consider a perspective other than their own. Piaget called this inability egocentrism. An interesting example can be found when listening to preoperational children talking. Two preoperational children may appear to be having a conversation, but if you listen closely, you will discover that each is talking about what is of personal interest. These "conversations" are known as collective monologues. As children enter concrete operations, they become more concerned about and interested in the viewpoints of others, and conversations with an exchange of ideas begin.

Piaget's fourth period is entitled formal operations; it begins at about age 11 and continues through adulthood.

TABLE 3-7 Piaget's Stage Theory of Cognitive Development

STAGE	AGE
Sensorimotor intelligence	0–2 years
Preoperational thought	2–7 years
Concrete operations	7–11 years
Formal operations	11 years to adulthood

The child operating at the level of concrete operations can think systematically and logically as long as the thought is related to tangible objects. Formal operations involves the ability to organize and work with ambiguity and multiple meanings.

Piaget's theories are complex, challenging, and of abiding interest to the study of childhood cognitive development. New theories about language acquisition have called into question some of Piaget's work, but his efforts remain among the important contributions of twentieth-century developmental psychology.

See Table 3-7 for a list of the stages of Piaget's theory of cognitive development.

Adult Cognition

While differing with each other and with Freud in significant details, Erikson and Sullivan carried Freud's view of stage theory beyond adolescence and into adulthood. Perry accomplished much the same task by expanding on Piaget's conceptions. Unsatisfied with the idea that formal operations represents the final stage of human cognitive development, Perry (1970) studied young men during their years as undergraduate students at Harvard University. His focus was on how their perception of nature and the nature of knowledge evolved during their college experience. As a result of his study, Perry identified positions, or stages, of knowing that he described as linear, or occurring in a specific order, with each succeeding position dependent upon the previous one. The first position is dualism, in which the knower sees him or herself as passive and authorities as all-knowing. The view

REFLECTIVE THINKING 3-2

Responses of Children

How would the responses of children in concrete operations and in formal operations differ for the following question: How many meanings can you identify for the statement "The duck is ready to eat"?

of the world is one of dichotomies—right or wrong, black or white, and good or bad. The student perceives that there is one right answer to every question or human dilemma. The next position is multiplicity, in which the knower recognizes that authorities may not always have the right answer and that the knower can have a personal opinion. There is a tendency to believe that any one opinion is as good as any other opinion. The third position is relativism, in which the individual comes to understand that any apparent truth is valid primarily in a particular context. As the context changes, so may the likelihood of a given position being true. In this position, the knower recognizes that knowledge is constructed rather than given, contextual rather than absolute, and mutable rather than fixed. This recognition extends into all aspects of life. While Perry's theory was first developed in a longitudinal study of men, the theory has been tested and used by others in numerous college populations of both men and women (Knefelkamp, Widick, & Parker, 1978). These studies confirm that Perry's studies, while derived from a unique Harvard male sample, are probably applicable to a wide range of young adults. Clearly, not all adults complete the transition from dualism to relativism, and perhaps even a majority of adults remain concrete dualistic thinkers. This has important implications for nursing and teaching in all disciplines as well as for the psychiatric nurse trying to convey difficult or novel information to a client.

Belenky, Clinchy, Goldberger, and Tarule (1986), concerned that Perry's positions may not reflect the ways in which women learn, conducted a similar study with a group of women drawn from academic institutions and the "invisible colleges"—human service agencies that serve women who are parents. Building on Perry's scheme, they identified five perspectives from which women know or view the world. These perspectives are not linear, and the knower may shift from one perspective to another. The first perspective is silence, in which the knower sees self as mindless, voiceless, and subject to authority in all its whims. The second perspective is received knowledge, in which the knower sees self as capable of receiving knowledge as well as of reproducing it. This knowledge comes from authorities, and the knower is not capable of creating knowledge. The received knower listens to the voices of others. The third perspective is subjective knowledge, in which the knower sees knowledge as personal, private, and intuitive. The subjective knower listens to an inner, intuitive, subjective voice and seeks to know self. The fourth perspective is procedural knowledge, in which the knower is invested in learning and applying information empirically; information is both obtained and communicated. The procedural knower seeks a voice of reason and experiences knowledge as that which is both autonomous (separate) and in relationship with others (connected). The fifth perspective is constructed knowledge, in which knowledge is seen as contextual; the knower views self as capable of creating knowledge, and both objective and subjective strategies for knowing are valued. The constructed knower seeks to integrate the voices and blend both that knowledge that is intuitively considered personally important and that which is learned from others.

Belenky et al. (1986) have made a potentially important contribution to the study of adult development by suggesting that women's cognitive maturation develops differently from that of men. Their conceptualization is clearly different from that of Perry, and it remains to be seen how useful the Belenky model will prove for understanding how women come to see the adult world or even if this conceptualization should be limited to women.

See Table 3-8 for a summary of developmental theories as related to the case example of Mr. James, presented earlier.

Humanistic Theory

Other schools of thought that are applicable to psychiatric nursing include basic needs theories, existential philosophy, and behavioral theories. Basic needs theories are represented by Abraham Maslow, general propositions of existential philosophy are presented, and the work of psychologist B. F. Skinner is summarized to represent the behavioral theories he pioneered.

Basic Needs Theories

Maslow (1970) proposed a hierarchy of needs to explain motives for human behavior. His hierarchy has five levels. The bottom two levels represent basic needs, and the upper three represent growth needs. The first level is physiological needs for food, air, water, sleep, sex, and so on. The second is safety and security. The third level (the first growth need level) is love and belonging. The fourth level is esteem and self-esteem. The fifth level is self-actualization. Maslow indicated that persons seek levels 3 to 5 only after more basic needs have been satisfied. The primary focus of his work was on the highest level, self-actualization. He identified the characteristics of the self-actualized person as being tolerant, even welcoming, of uncertainty; being self-accepting, with an inner directedness; being spontaneous, creative, and autonomous; demonstrating caring for others; being capable of intense interpersonal relationships; having a sense of humor and an open attitude to life; as well as needing solitude and privacy. Maslow's work is frequently cited by other theorists, and his hierarchy of needs has been a consistently useful conceptual framework for thinking about human sociocultural development. However, this hierarchy was developed primarily through studying males, and questions have been raised about its generalizability across genders and cultures.

Existential Philosophy

Many authors have contributed to the development of existential philosophy, a philosophical movement of the latter half of the twentieth century that has strongly influenced the language and content of several important nursing theories. The basis of existential philosophy, sometimes referred to as existentialism, is a view of human beings as continually changing or becoming. Corey (2000) presents a summary of six major existential propositions. The first is that the capacity for self-awareness allows us to reflect and make

TABLE 3-8 Developmental Theories and Mr. James

Freud	No stage beyond puberty.
Erikson	Ego integrity versus despair: involves external adjustments associated with physical and social loss. Mr. J.'s current loss is primarily social in the loss of his status as an employed person and of the social interactions associated with that employment. Mr. J. is involved in life review: what has been worthwhile in his life (primary identification with his work), and how his life can continue to be worthwhile. He experiences despair and self-contempt if he views himself as no longer capable of doing worthwhile things. If he faces any despair associated with his change in status, accepts his mistakes (e.g., not planning for retirement and not seeking other activities during the last 4 months), and recognizes his capacity for good (ability to contribute to others), he will regain ego integrity.
Sullivan	Adulthood: a total situation that involves one or two others. Mr. J. has isolated himself from his wife in seeing his retirement as primarily creating change for him. He needs to resolve the changes with his wife, not by himself.
Piaget	As a consulting engineer, Mr. J should have demonstrated cognition at the formal operations level. He has not been demonstrating the ability to organize and work with ambiguity since his retirement and needs to reactivate formal operations cognition in relation to his own life.
Adult cognition	If thinking is relativistic, he will see situations as contextual. Retirement could be seen as good or bad. If seen as the end of a productive life, then it is bad. If seen as an opportunity to be productive in new and different ways, then retirement is good.

choices. As our awareness increases, so do the possibilities for freedom. Increasing awareness includes being cognizant of a series of apparent human realities. Among these are the following realizations:

- Life is finite (there is a limit to the time we have to accomplish what we want to do).
- We have the potential to act or not to act (taking no action is a decision).
- We choose our actions and thus influence our destiny.
- Existential anxiety is essential to living.
- As awareness of choice increases, so does our sense of responsibility for the effects of these choices.
- We are subject to multiple feelings (e.g., loneliness, meaninglessness, emptiness, isolation, and guilt).
- We are basically alone while having the opportunity to relate to others.

Second, we have freedom and responsibility. While we did not choose to be born, the choices we make shape the way in which we live. This freedom for making choices is connected to the need to accept responsibility for the outcomes of those choices. Existential guilt occurs when we evade a commitment, choose not to make a choice or take an action, or allow others to make choices for us.

The third proposition is that we are striving for identity and relationship to others. This involves the courage to be, the experience of aloneness, and the experience of relatedness. As humans, we are simultaneously seeking to maintain our uniqueness and establish relationships with others and with nature. As humans, we depend on relationships with others as part of our fulfillment. Once we are comfortable with our aloneness, we can seek the fulfillment associated with interaction with others.

The fourth proposition relates to the search for meaning, which includes discarding old values, experiencing meaninglessness, and creating new meaning. This creative act continues throughout our lives; it is never finished. Meaning is not found by searching for it directly; rather, it is found through an activity known as engagement. Engagement is the person's commitment to creating, loving, working, and building—to living a fully involved life.

The fifth proposition is that anxiety is a condition of living. The efforts to survive, to have personal identity and relationships with others, and to identify meaning lead to normal anxiety. This anxiety can be a stimulus for growth. In fact, Corey (2000) indicates that existential anxiety is a form of normal anxiety that can stimulate growth because it arises from an increased awareness of our freedom to make choices and the associated necessity of accepting the consequences of either accepting or rejecting that freedom.

REFLECTIVE THINKING 3-3

Developmental/Psychoanalytic Theories

How do developmental/psychoanalytic theories help you understand the behavior of people of various ages?

REFLECTIVE THINKING 3-4

The Stranger

In Albert Camus's classic work *The Stranger*, the narrator begins by telling us that his mother died today or perhaps yesterday, he can't remember when. This opening air of indifference sets the tone for the entire novel and ultimately leads to the narrator's demise at the hands of a society that, in effect, eventually punishes him for not appropriately mourning his mother's death.

- Does this statement of confusion or indifference about the time or circumstances of a parent's death seem unusual to you?
- What reaction would you have to an individual who seems indifferent to what is generally perceived as a significant life event, the death of a parent?
- What theoretical foundations could help you frame care for such an individual?

The sixth proposition is that we have an awareness of death and nonbeing. Such recognition makes the present, and our activities in it, more crucial. Living life to the fullest now tends to negate the fear of death that is often associated with feelings of having never really lived.

Existentialism is an attempt to provide a comprehensive life philosophy, primarily for individuals who find they can no longer believe in traditional moral and religious values. It has been influenced by and attracted the attention of some of the twentieth century's most profound ethical and religious thinkers. Students interested in contemporary nursing theory will find their understanding enhanced by a careful reading of existential philosophy, including authors such as Martin Heidegger, whose writings may initially prove quite difficult.

See Table 3-9 for a summary of humanistic theory as related to the case example of Mr. James, presented earlier.

Behavioral Psychology

Behavioral psychology forms the basis for a number of approaches to psychotherapy. B. F. Skinner was among the first psychologists to promote a behaviorally oriented approach to psychological problems. Skinner's orientation was as an experimentalist, and he worked more with pigeons and rats as subjects than he did with humans. He was also

Table 3-9 Humanistic Theory and Mr. James

	BASIC NEEDS
Physiological	Sleep and food needs not fully met.
Safety and security	Threatened by unplanned retirement.
Love and belonging	Threatened by Mr. J.'s withdrawal from his usual level of interaction with his wife; has not adjusted to the change in his situation.
Esteem and self-esteem	Mr. J. needs to revise his sources of esteem and self-esteem since he is no longer employed.
Self-actualization	Cannot reach this level until he resolves the other levels.
	EXISTENTIAL
Self-awareness	Needs to reflect on changes in his life and the possibilities created by these changes, and to actively make choices.
Freedom and responsibility	Mr. J. has been freed to make choices about the direction of his life; currently must take responsibility for having chosen to sit at home.
Striving for identity and relationship with others	Needs to redefine identity as retired and to recognize that his relationship with his wife and children is changing.
Search for meaning	What is the meaning of life now that he is retired? What meaning does he wish to create?
Anxiety as a condition of living	Anxiety about need to make decisions he had not planned to make for several years has paralyzed him; Mr. J. needs to use this as a stimulus for growth.
Awareness of death and nonbeing	Mr. J. needs to recognize that death is inevitable and to develop plans to use his limited time productively to be able to live life to the fullest.

more concerned with getting these animals to perform specific tasks through a system of rewards than with understanding specific human behavioral motivations. Nonetheless, Skinner's work provided a framework for subsequent efforts that have changed the way in which psychotherapy is done. One of the most successful current therapeutic approaches is titled cognitive-behavioral therapy, in acknowledgment of the debt its conception owes to the work of Skinner and his followers.

Skinner believed that the focus of psychological study should be behavior and the ways in which behavior is affected by environment. He rejected psychological studies and theories about developmental stages, perception, cognition, personality, and a number of other areas that had tended to interest psychologists. Instead, he focused exclusively on operant behavior, or behaviors that are repeated by experimental subjects who have been rewarded for that repetition. For example, a rat that successfully runs through a maze and is then fed will be likely to work hard to repeat its maze-running success. Behaviorists call this process of modifying behavior by providing rewards "operant conditioning." Skinner defined a variety of terms and concepts describing elements of conditioning as he observed them in a variety of experimental studies. These elements included reinforcement, extinction, discriminative stimuli, shaping, behavior chains, schedules of reinforcement, and negative reinforcement, or punishment.

Reinforcement occurs, Skinner taught, when the consequence of the behavior is satisfying to the person. Primary reinforcers are those that have "natural" reinforcing properties, for example, food or comfort. Conditioned reinforcers develop in association with primary reinforcers and are usually connected to responses from others such as smiles or approval. The closer in time the reinforcement occurs to the behavior (immediacy), the greater the reinforcement effect. Extinction of undesirable behaviors is a result of withdrawal of attention from those behaviors. Behaviors that have been extinguished may show spontaneous recovery and need to be extinguished again. While the emphasis is on behavior and consequences rather than on stimulus and response, Skinner does recognize that there are discriminative stimuli that will encourage or discourage a behavior. For example, we are more willing to approach someone who is smiling than someone who is frowning. Shaping of behavior is the process of reinforcing closer and closer approximations of the desired behavior. This process happens bit by bit as each new aspect is developed. The child learning to play the piano may first gain approval for proper posture, then for appropriate hand placement, then for identifying the correct key for the desired note, and so on. Behavior chains develop as each step in such a bit-by-bit sequence begins to serve as a reinforcer for the previous step as well as a stimulus for the next one (Crain, 1985).

Behavior is rarely reinforced continuously but, rather, receives intermittent reinforcement. Skinner discovered by experiments with animals that certain patterns of intermittent reinforcement were associated with very good long-term adherence to the desired behavior. Behavior that has been intermittently reinforced appears to be harder to extinguish than that which has been continuously reinforced. These observations suggest that the best way to achieve a desired behavior quickly is to begin by reinforcing the behavior continuously; after the behavior has been well established, switching to an intermittent schedule of reinforcement will increase the likelihood of persistence.

Positive reinforcement strengthens responses by providing positive consequences. Negative reinforcement, or punishment, is an effort to extinguish behavior rather than reinforce it and does not always work. Punishment, according to Skinner (1953), typically provides only a temporary suppression of the undesired behavior and often produces unwanted side effects. While Skinner's experiments were largely involved with animals, he also spoke and wrote about child rearing. His and his followers' ideas about punishments and rewards have greatly influenced contemporary views of managing human behavior.

See Table 3-10 for a summary of behavioral theory as related to the case example of Mr. James, presented earlier.

TABLE 3-10 Behavioral Theory and Mr. James

Observation of behavior	Mr. J. has been sitting at home since his retirement.
Operant conditioning	His wife does not like his behavior change and chooses to use operant conditioning to improve the situation. She uses extinction by no longer commenting on his staying at home and discriminating stimuli by smiling when he makes an effort to do something new. She provides pamphlets on community agencies that could use his skills and reinforces his positive behavior of seeking more information about an agency by telling him how pleased she is.
Example	A behavior chain she might reinforce by positive comments, smiles, and such would be Mr. J. reading a pamphlet about a community agency, calling the agency for information, visiting the agency, agreeing to go back one day to help out, and gradually increasing his volunteer time at the agency. Mr. J. will also gain reinforcement from the satisfaction he receives from once again being helpful to others.

REFLECTIVE THINKING 3-5

Sociocultural Perspectives

- What theories in this chapter reflect, include, or are congruent with a sociocultural perspective?
- What theories focus so completely on the individual that they ignore the potential influence of society and culture?

REFLECTIVE THINKING 3-6

Is Mental Illness Real?

Not all agree with the concept of psychiatric diagnoses. One author in particular, Thomas Szasz (1974), argues that mental illness is a myth. His arguments are summarized as follows:

- Strictly speaking, disease or illness can affect only the body; hence, there can be no mental illness.
- Mental illness is a metaphor. Minds can be "sick" only in the sense that jokes are sick or economies are sick.
- Psychiatric diagnoses are stigmatizing labels phrased to resemble medical diagnoses and applied to persons whose behavior annoys or offends others.
- Those who suffer from and complain of their own behaviors are usually classified as "neurotic"; those whose behaviors make others suffer and about whom others complain are usually classified as "psychotic."
- Mental illness is not something a person has but something he or she does or is.
- If there is no mental illness, there can be no hospitalization, treatment, or cure for it. Of course, people may change their behaviors or personalities with or without psychiatric intervention. Such intervention is nowadays called "treatment," and the change, if it proceeds in a direction approved by society, is called a "recovery" or "cure."
- The introduction of psychiatric considerations into the administration of criminal law—for example, the insanity plea and verdict, diagnoses of mental incompetence to stand trial, and so forth—corrupts the law and victimizes the subject on whose behalf they are ostensibly employed.
- Personal conduct is always rule following, strategic, and meaningful. Patterns of interpersonal and social relations may be regarded and analyzed as if they were games, the behaviors of the players being governed by explicit or tacit game rules.
- In most types of voluntary psychotherapy, the therapist tries to elucidate the inexplicit game rules by which the client conducts him or herself and to help the client scrutinize the goals and values of the life games he or she plays.
- There is no medical, moral, or legal justification for involuntary psychiatric interventions. They are crimes against humanity.

What do you believe and why?

SOCIOCULTURAL THEORY

While the influence of social factors on personal behavior has been recognized for many years, the movement of social psychiatry has only fairly recently provided a conceptual framework for understanding the relation of society and culture to human behavior. Schwab and Schwab (1978) suggest that the following eight questions or concepts are important for understanding the basis of social psychiatry:

1. Social causation: How much do sociocultural processes (e.g., poverty and child abuse) alone and intertwined with genetic and other influences contribute to mental health or illness?
2. Community and family causation: How much do group and familial processes, including an individual's social role and economic status, contribute to mental illness?
3. Treatment and rehabilitation: Should the individual be treated alone, or must the family and other social groups be involved?
4. Prevention: How do interdisciplinary efforts to deal with "political, economic, environmental, and ethical issues" (p. 18) influence the protection or attainment of mental health?
5. Governmental and community programs: How do these provide treatment and rehabilitation for mental illness?
6. Cultural influences: How does culture (of the therapist as well as the person being treated) influence both the definition of mental illness and the treatment outcome?
7. Social control mechanisms: What are the means used by society to maintain social order?
8. The possible existence of a sick society: Is it possible that it is society rather than the person that is ill?

KEY CONCEPTS

- A theory is a group of concepts linked together that give a nurse a way of understanding phenomena.
- Nurses use theories of nursing and theories for nursing.
- Nursing theories can be grouped as those focusing on relationships, caring, energy fields, or the notion of when nursing is needed.
- Relationship theories include Peplau's Theory of Interpersonal Relationships and Erickson, Tomlin, and Swain's Modeling and Role-Modeling Theory.
- Caring theories include Watson's Theory of Transpersonal Relationship, Leininger's Culture Care Diversity and Universality Theory, and Boykin and Schoenhofer's Theory of Nursing as Caring.
- Energy field theories include Rogers's Science of Unitary Human Beings, Parse's Humanbecoming School of Thought, and Newman's Theory of Health as Expanding Consciousness.
- Theories based on the notion of when nursing is needed include Orem's Self-Care Deficit Theory, Roy's Adaptation Model, and Neuman's Systems Model.
- Each nursing theory gives the nurse a different way of perceiving, interpreting, and understanding his or her client's condition.
- Psychiatric and psychological theories also inform psychiatric nursing practice; these theories were developed to assist in understanding human behavior.
- Theories grounded in psychoanalysis include Freud's theory of psychosexual development, Erikson's theory of psychosocial development, and Sullivan's Interpersonal Theory.
- Theories of human cognitive development include Piaget's stage theory of the cognitive development of children, Perry's theory of young adult cognitive development, and Belenky et al.'s theory of the way women know.
- Humanistic theories are exemplified by the basic needs theory and existential philosophy.
- Behavioral theory focuses on overt behavior and ways in which the environment and changes in it affect behavior.
- Sociocultural theory suggests that all human behavior must be understood from within the society and culture in which the person lives.

REVIEW QUESTIONS

1. A nurse assesses a family and identifies a disruption in the communication patterns of the family system. Because of the ineffective communication pattern, the system cannot function effectively. This nurse's approach to client care is most likely influenced by which of the following nurse theorists?
   1. Jean Watson
   2. Dorothea Orem
   3. Martha Rogers
   4. Betty Neuman

2. A client diagnosed with catatonic schizophrenia is admitted to the psychiatric unit. The client is unable to feed himself or address his hygienic needs. According to the theory of Dorothea Orem, the client is experiencing which of the following?
   1. Self-care deficit
   2. Altered body image
   3. Ineffective coping
   4. Distorted sense of self

3. A psychiatric client is extremely agitated and confused. The nurse interviews the client in a quiet room to avoid excessive stimulation. The nurse is addressing which component of Betty Neuman's systems model?
   1. Internal environment
   2. External environment
   3. Created environment
   4. Social environment

4. The psychiatric nurse has based her practice on the work of Martha Rogers. The nurse's primary concern would focus on which of the following?
   1. Disruption of energy fields
   2. The client's ability to perform self-care activities
   3. The relationship between nurse and client
   4. Impact of the client's culture on behavior

5. An advanced practice nurse is assessing a 3-year-old child who was admitted to the hospital due to possible physical abuse. The nurse allows the child to play with a set of dolls. The child begins to use the father doll to hit the little girl doll. The principles of which theorist has the nurse implemented in her assessment?
   1. Jean Piaget
   2. Sigmund Freud
   3. Abraham Maslow
   4. Harry Stack Sullivan

6. According to psychoanalytic theory, a client experiencing depression would exhibit which of the following?
   1. Strong id, strong ego, weak superego
   2. Weak id, week ego, punitive superego
   3. Weak id, strong ego, weak superego
   4. Strong id, strong ego, punitive superego

7. A nurse provides close observation of a patient who is depressed and expressing feelings of worthlessness and hopelessness. The nurse is concerned that the client is having suicidal ideations. Close observation of the client is addressing which of the client's basic needs based on Maslow's Hierarchy of Needs theory?
   1. Physiologic
   2. Safety and security
   3. Love and belonging
   4. Self-actualization
8. A nurse provides positive reinforcement to clients who achieve successes during their psychiatric treatment. The nurse's behavior is based on which approach to psychiatric treatment?
   1. Psychoanalytic
   2. Humanistic
   3. Existential
   4. Behavioral
9. A nurse graduated from her nursing program six months ago. She has refused to take the NCLEX-RN examination out of fear she will fail. Without completing and passing the exam, she will not obtain an RN license or be able to secure a job as a professional nurse, which has been her lifelong dream. According to existential theory, the nurse's problem falls in which of the following domains?
   1. Self-awareness
   2. Freedom and responsibility
   3. Search for meaning
   4. Anxiety as a condition of living
10. The nurse caring for a client, who has recently immigrated to the United States, recognizes the importance of including the family in the planning process. The nurse is sensitive to the client's culture and the role of the family when addressing health issues. The nurse is most likely influenced by which of the following theorists?
   1. Betty Neuman
   2. Madeleine Leininger
   3. Sigmund Freud
   4. Harry Stack Sullivan

LEARNING ACTIVITIES

1. What is theory?
2. How are theory, practice, and research related in a practice discipline such as nursing?
3. What are the phases of interpersonal relationships described by Peplau?
4. How and why does the nurse model and role-model, according to Erickson, Tomlin, and Swain?
5. What is the difference between caring and curing? How is a transpersonal relationship achieved?
6. What is culturally congruent care? Can you provide an example?
7. What do Boykin and Schoenhofer indicate is involved in caring?
8. According to Rogers, what is the relationship between the person and the environment?
9. How does Newman define health?
10. According to Orem, when is nursing needed?
11. In the Roy adaptation model, what is the goal of nursing?
12. Describe primary, secondary, and tertiary prevention.
13. Select an age between birth and 12 years, and compare the developmental expectations of that age as outlined by Freud, Erikson, Sullivan, and Piaget.
14. In what ways are the two theories of adult cognition alike, and in what ways are they different?
15. What is the basis of existentialism? What are the major propositions of existentialism?
16. What is the difference between positive and negative reinforcement?
17. Why is culture important in understanding mental illness?

*Study*WARE™ CONNECTION

Using your *Study*WARE™ CD-ROM

1. Complete the Concentration activity for this chapter.
2. Review the audio glossary for key terms in this chapter.
3. Explore the other games and activities that support this chapter.

REFERENCES

Barrett, E. A. M. (1991). Theory: Of or for nursing? *Nursing Science Quarterly, 4,* 48–49.

Belenky, M. F., Clinchy, B. M., Goldberger, N. R., & Tarule, J. M. (1986). *Women's ways of knowing: The development of self, voice, and mind.* New York: Basic Books.

Boykin, A., & Schoenhofer, S. (1993). *Nursing as caring: A model for transforming practice.* New York: National League for Nursing.

Corey, G. (2000). *Theory and practice of counseling and psychotherapy* (6th ed.). Pacific Grove, CA: Brooks/Cole.

Crain, W. C. (1985). *Theories of development: Concepts and applications* (2nd ed.). Englewood Cliffs, NJ: Prentice-Hall.

Erickson, H. C., Tomlin, E. M., & Swain, M. A. P. (1983). *Modeling and role modeling: A theory and paradigm for nursing.* Lexington, SC: Pine Press.

Erikson, E. H. (1950). *Childhood and society* (2nd ed.). New York: Norton.

Erikson, E. H. (1959). *Identity and the life cycle: Psychological issues* (Vol. 1). New York: International Universities Press.

Erikson, E. H. (1976). Reflections on Dr. Borg's life cycle. *Daedalus, 105,* 1–28.

Freud, S. (1905). *Three contributions to the theory of sex: The basic writings of Sigmund Freud* (A. A. Brill, Trans.). New York: Modern Library.

Freud, S. (1959/1908). Character and anal eroticism. In *Collected papers* (Vol. II, J. Riviere, Trans.). New York: Basic Books.

Freud, S. (1965a/1920). *A general introduction to psychoanalysis* (J. Riviere, Trans.). New York: Washington Square Press.

Freud, S. (1965b/1933). *New introductory lectures on psychoanalysis* (J. Strachey, Trans.). New York: Norton.

Freud, S. (1989/1923). *The ego and the id* (J. Riviere, Trans., J. Strachey, Ed.). New York: Norton.

Ginsberg, H., & Opper, S. (1979). *Piaget's theory of intellectual development* (2nd ed.). Englewood Cliffs, NJ: Prentice-Hall.

Knefelkamp, L., Widick, C., & Parker, C. (1978). Applying new developmental findings. In L. Knefelkamp, C. Widick, & C. Parker (Eds.), *New directions in student services* (No. 4). San Francisco: Jossey-Bass.

Krieger, D. (1979). *Living the therapeutic touch: Healing as a lifestyle.* New York: Dodd, Mead.

Leininger, M. (1991). *Culture care diversity and universality: A theory of nursing.* New York: National League for Nursing Press.

Leininger, M., & McFarland, M. R. (2002). *Transcultural nursing* (3rd ed.). New York: McGraw-Hill.

Leininger, M. M., & McFarland, M. R. (2006). *Culture care diversity and universality: A worldwide nursing theory.* Boston: Jones & Bartlett.

Maslow, A. (1970). *Motivation and personality* (Rev. ed.). New York: Van Nostrand Reinhold.

Mullahy, P. (1970). *Psychoanalysis and interpersonal psychiatry: The contributions of Harry Stack Sullivan.* New York: Science House.

Neuman, B. (2002). The Neuman systems model. In B. Neuman & J. Fawcett (Eds.), *The Neuman systems model* (4th ed). Upper Saddle River, NJ: Prentice Hall.

Newman, M. A. (1994). *Health as expanding consciousness* (2nd ed.). New York: National League for Nursing.

Orem, D. E. (1995). *Nursing: Concepts of practice* (5th ed.). St. Louis, MO: Mosby.

Orem, D. E. (2001). *Nursing: Concepts of practice* (6th ed.). St. Louis, MO: Mosby.

Parse, R. R. (1981). *Man-living-health: A theory of nursing.* New York: Wiley.

Parse, R. R. (1992). Human becoming: Parse's theory of nursing. *Nursing Science Quarterly, 5,* 35–42.

Parse, R. R. (Ed.). (1995). *Illuminations: The human becoming theory in practice and research.* New York: National League for Nursing.

Parse, R. R. (1998). *The human becoming school of thought.* Thousand Oaks, CA: Sage.

Parse, R. R. (2007). A humanbecoming perspective on quality of life. *Nursing Science Quarterly, 20,* 308–311.

Peplau, H. E. (1988/1952). *Interpersonal relations in nursing.* New York: Springer.

Peplau, H. E. (1992). Interpersonal relations: A theoretical framework for application in nursing practice. *Nursing Science Quarterly, 5,* 13–18.

Peplau, H. E. (1997). Peplau's theory of interpersonal relations. *Nursing Science Quarterly, 10,* 162–167.

Perry, W. G. (1970). *Forms of intellectual and ethical development in the college years.* New York: Holt, Rinehart, & Winston.

Phillips, J. R. (1990). Nursing: A basic or an applied science? *Nursing Science Quarterly, 3,* 144.

Piaget, J. (1974/1936). *The origins of intelligence in children* (M. Cook, Trans.). New York: International Universities Press.

Rogers, M. E. (1970). *The theoretical basis of nursing.* Philadelphia: Davis.

Rogers, M. E. (1990). Space-age paradigm for new frontiers in nursing. In M. E. Parker (Ed.), *Nursing theories in practice.* New York: National League for Nursing.

Rogers, M. E. (1992). Nursing science and the space age. *Nursing Science Quarterly, 5,* 27–34.

Roy, C., & Andrews, H. A. (1999). *The Roy adaptation model.* Norwalk, CT: Appleton & Lange.

Schwab, J. K., & Schwab, M. E. (1978). *Sociocultural roots of mental illness: An epidemiologic survey.* New York: Plenum.

Skinner, B. F. (1953). *Science and human behavior.* New York: Macmillan.

Szasz, T. S. (1974). *The myth of mental illness* (Rev. ed.). New York: Harper & Row.

Watson, J. (1979). *Nursing: The philosophy and science of caring.* Boston: Little, Brown.

Watson, J. (1988/1985). *Human science and human care: A theory of nursing.* New York: National League for Nursing.

Watson, J. (1996). Nursing, caring-healing paradigm. In D. Pesut, *Capsules of comments in psychiatric nursing.* Chicago, IL: Mosby Year Book.

Watson, J. (1999). *Postmodern nursing and beyond.* New York: Churchill-Livingston.

Watson, J. (2002). Intentionality and caring-healing consciousness: A practice of transpersonal nursing. *Holistic Nursing Practice, 16*(4), 12–19.

Watson, J. (2005). *Caring science as sacred science.* Philadelphia: Davis.

Watson, J. (2007). Theory evolution. Retrieved June 5, 2009, from http://www.nursing.ucdenver.edu/faculty/jw_evolution.htm as accessed 6/5/2009

SUGGESTED READINGS

Chinn, P. L., & Kramer, M. K. (2008). *Integrated theory and knowledge development in nursing* (7th ed.). St. Louis, MO: Mosby.

Fawcett, J. (2005). *Contemporary nursing knowledge: Analysis and evaluation of nursing models and theories* (2nd ed). Philadelphia: Davis.

Fitzpatrick, J., & Whall, A. (2005). *Conceptual models of nursing: Analysis and application* (4th ed.). Upper Saddle River, NJ: Prentice Hall.

George, J. B. (Ed.). (2002). *Nursing theories: The base for professional nursing practice* (5th ed.). Norwalk, CT: Appleton & Lange. (Note: 6th ed. is in press.)

Meleis, A. I. (2006). *Theoretical nursing: Development and progress* (4th ed.). Philadelphia: Lippincott, Williams and Wilkins.

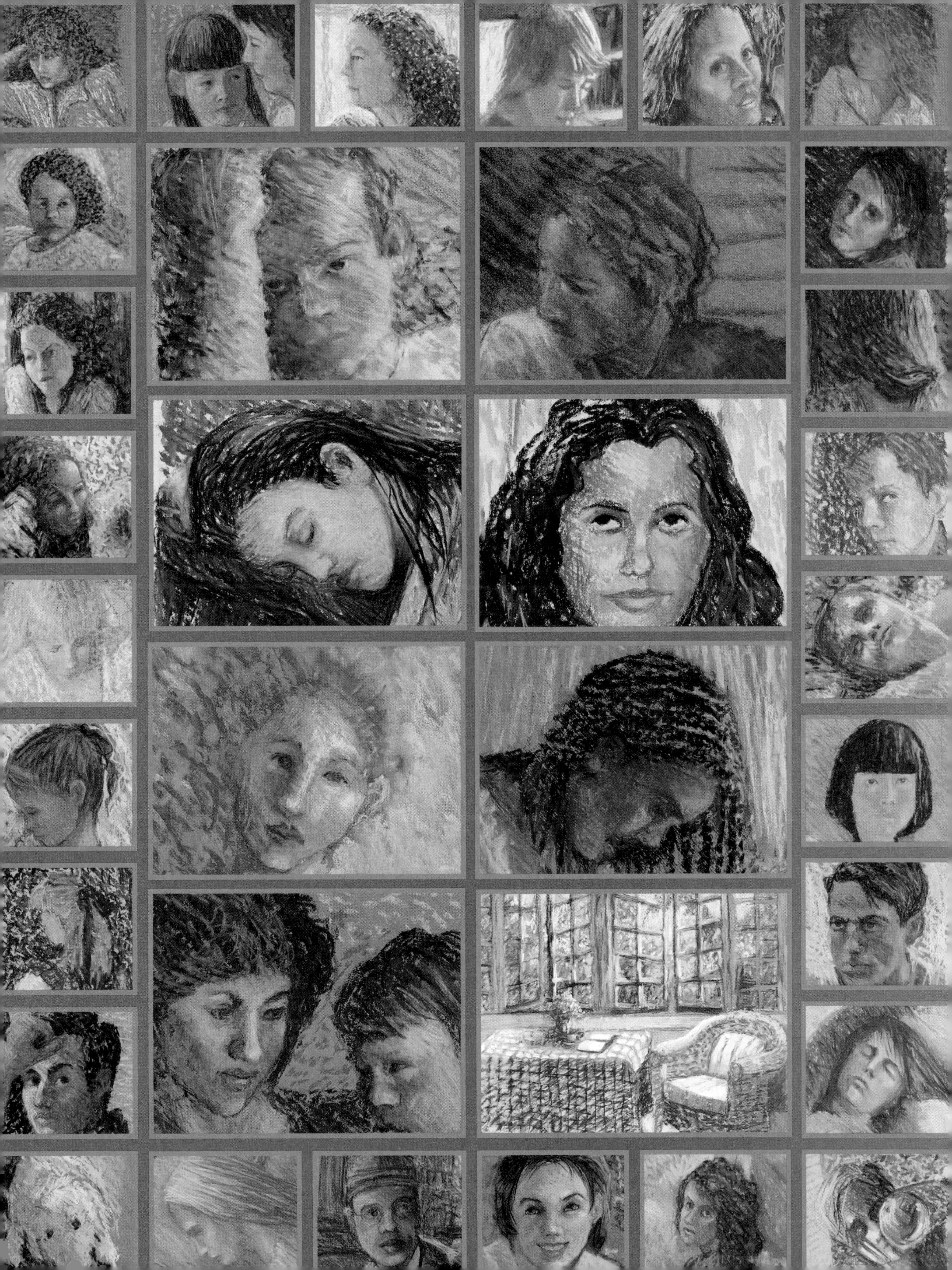

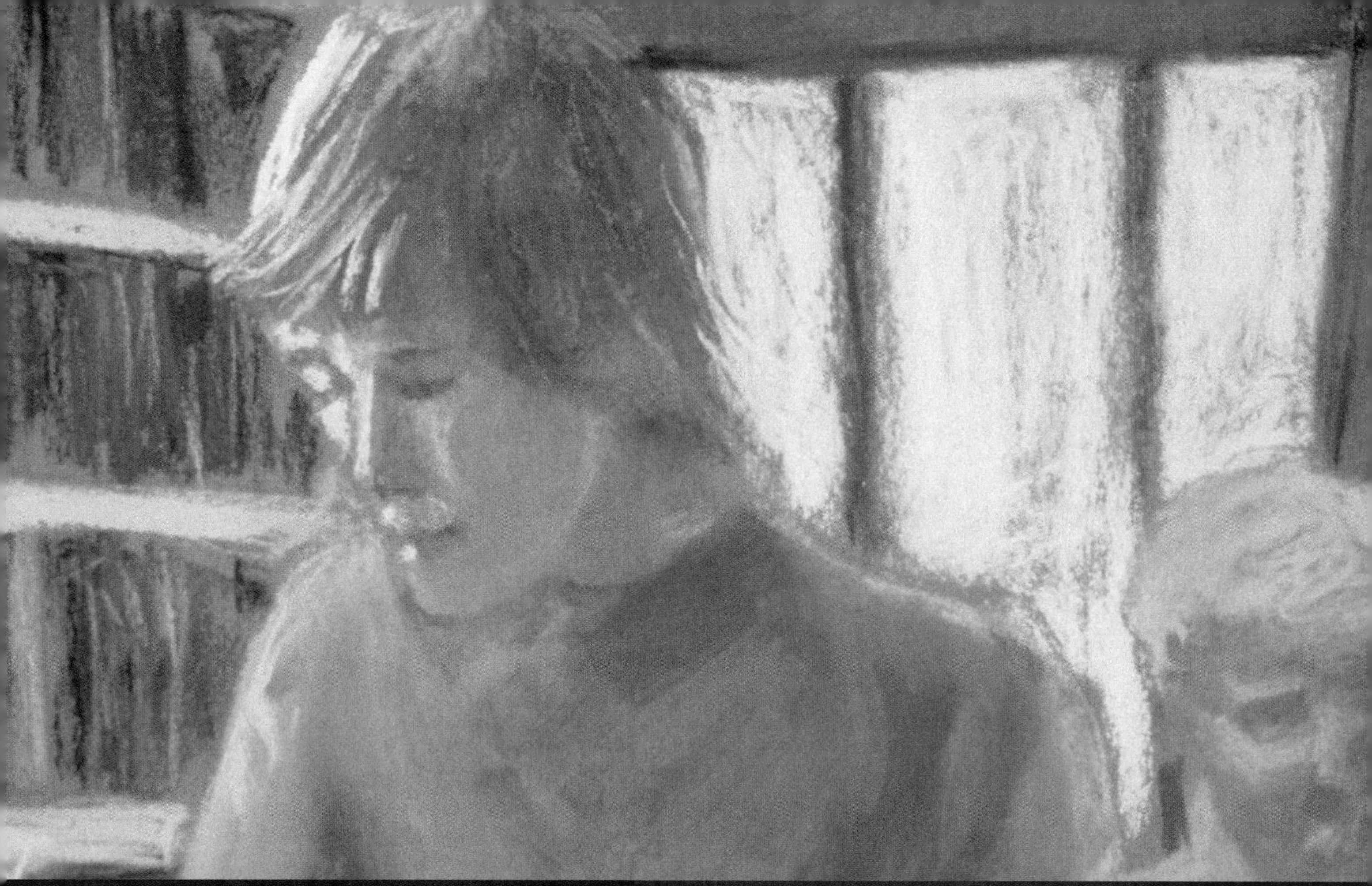

I Think, Therefore I Am?

Neuroscience and Thoughts

Consciousness, thoughts, emotions, memory, and intuition are all concepts we know and understand in some way. They are part of the subjective human experience. When we study neurobiology, we must consider how these and other mental phenomena are related to, and perhaps caused by, an array of biochemical and neurophysiological processes. When exploring the neurobiology of mental illness, we work on the assumption that our minds and consciousness are phenomena that arise out of the complex neurochemical workings in the brain that take place from moment to moment. The processes that give rise to mental life are open to investigation. In this chapter, we review the means we have for such investigations and the emerging body of knowledge of biopsychophysiological theory.

CHAPTER 4

Neuroscience as a Basis for Practice

LAWRENCE E. FRISCH

CHAPTER OUTLINE

COMPETENCIES

Upon completion of this chapter, the reader should be able to:

1. Discuss the emerging model of biopsychophysiological theory as an explanation of emotions and behaviors.
2. Explain the major functions of the cerebral lobes and the diencephalon.
3. Describe modern brain-imaging techniques.
4. Explain the role of neurotransmitters, membrane receptors, and messenger-signaling systems.
5. Discuss the role of genetics in understanding and possible treatment of psychiatric disorders.

KEY TERMS

Computerized Tomography (CT)
Cortex
Deoxyribonucleic Acid (DNA)
Diencephalon
Genetic Markers
Genome
Hypothalamus
Magnetic Resonance Imaging (MRI)
Neurotransmitter
Positron Emission Tomography (PET)
Synapses
Thalamus

BIOPSYCHOPHYSIOLOGICAL THEORY

The biopsychophysiological theory of mental illness is quite different from the other theories described in Chapter 3, for it assumes that mental illness occurs because something has gone wrong with fundamental physiological processes in the brain. What actually "goes wrong" can vary widely depending on diagnosis. In some instances, the problem may stem from a fixed anatomical abnormality such as a loss of brain cells; in others, it may stem from a maldistribution of critical neurotransmitters; while in yet others, it may derive from abnormal functioning of some critical enzyme or biochemical pathway. The biopsychophysiological theory does not place any limits on how such specific brain abnormalities came to be: They may be due to genetics, acquired brain injury, interpersonal or psychological experiences, or some combination of the above. The theory does not exclude an interpersonal, psychodevelopmental, or environmental causation of mental symptoms. It does say, however, that in whatever way mental illness is originally caused, the resultant symptoms can be associated with some abnormality in neuroanatomy or neurophysiology (or both).

The word "biopsychophysiology" seems relatively intuitive: Psychological phenomena are explained by neurobiological events within the brain. While it is unlikely that anyone actually claims the entire title of biopsychophysiologist, in recent years the study of mental disorders has been greatly enriched by the convergence of research interests that this word implies. Psychiatrists, physiologists, and neuroscientists have grown more sophisticated in their biochemical understanding as biologists have brought exceptionally powerful new tools to bear on the various neurotransmitters, receptors, and genetic encodings relevant to healthy and diseased brain functioning. In conditions such as schizophrenia, bipolar disorder, and obsessive-compulsive disorder (all addressed in this book), there is an evolving certainty that the illnesses result from specific biochemical, neuroanatomical, or genetic processes.

At the root of the current strong interest in exploring the neurobiology of mental illness is a basic assumption that we sometimes forget to see as a theoretical assumption: the concept that our minds and our consciousness are phenomena that arise out of the complex neurochemical workings of the brain. For hundreds of years, philosophers and theologians have believed that the mind (or what Aristotle and others have termed the soul) had some sort of unique existence. It certainly feels to us as if our minds are real entities, quite independent of our brains: That is more or less what the philosopher René Descartes meant more than 350 years ago when he wrote, "I find myself thinking, therefore I must exist." (In reality, he wrote more simply, *cogito ergo sum*: "I think, therefore I am.") Francis Crick, best known for his discovery with James Watson of the DNA double helix, summarizes the biopsychophysiological position as follows: "'You,' your joys and your sorrows, your memories and your ambitions, your sense of personal identity and free will, are in fact no more than the behavior of a vast assembly of nerve cells and their associated molecules" (Searle, 1995, p. 62).

In some ways, Crick has reversed Descartes' epigram: *sum ergo cogito*, "I am, therefore I think." But however one interprets Crick's statement (and in one form or another, his ideas are shared by many leading neuroscientists), he is making a dramatic claim: Mental phenomena—how we feel and act—are somehow caused by an array of biochemical and neurophysiological processes that take place from moment to moment in the brain. In this view, the mind is most decidedly not a soul and not fundamentally distinct from the body itself. In Crick's view, consciousness owes its existence to processes or forces that someday will be described in a physiology laboratory. While the biopsychophysiological view does not mean that we will necessarily ever have a "brain in a box" or in a test tube, it does say that the processes giving rise to consciousness, mental life, and mental illness are open to investigation using the tools of modern biology.

The great twentieth-century Anglo-Irish poet William Butler Yeats once asked rhetorically, "Who can distinguish darkness from the soul?" Yeats believed that the goals of art and poetry are to elevate human thought toward the rarified spiritual realm in which the soul was conceived, was nurtured, and finally—with death—returns. Yeats believed that poetry and art were the "star-lit ... flames begotten of flame" that distinguished the soul from darkness. Neuroscientists might assign a comparable role to electrical action potentials in neurons of the brain, but most neuroscientists are neither poets nor philosophers, and few think of themselves as developing or even working with a biological macrotheory. Most practicing scientists resist speculation, restricting their investigative efforts to observable phenomena: for example, the interaction between membrane proteins and cyclic AMP, the distribution of haloperidol among the various brain pathways, and the measurement of hippocampal size in brain scans from individuals with different psychiatric disorders. Observations based on such studies may generate their own theories (strictly speaking, hypotheses) such as the theory that the hippocampus of schizophrenic individuals is smaller than that of unaffected persons. Such "microtheories" require some belief in the larger assumptions underlying the biopsychophysiological theory, whether or not this dependency is explicitly acknowledged by scientists.

There are several concepts and ideas underlying the biopsychophysiological theory. These are summarized below where the following topics are addressed: brain anatomy and function, brain imaging, electrophysiology and neurochemistry, and genetics. Readers wishing more detailed treatment of these topics should consult a major textbook (e.g., Kandel et al., 2000) or a shorter "essentials" version (e.g., Kandel et al., 1995). Dr. Kandel, the Nobel Prize–winning first author of these texts, has also written *In Search of Memory*, a wonderful autobiography that describes how his own major contributions to biopsychophysiological theory developed out of a love affair with psychoanalysis (or, perhaps more accurately, with the daughter of a famous psychoanalyst) and became over many decades a love affair with science about which he communicates with great warmth and passion (see Kandel, 2006).

Brain Anatomy and Function

Of the four major divisions of the central nervous system (spinal cord, brain stem, diencephalon, and cerebral hemispheres; see Figure 4-1—where the hemispheres are the large structures in orange, blue, pink, and green), this review focuses only on the last two because virtually all major functions having to do with consciousness can be localized to the diencephalon and cortex (cerebral hemispheres).

Psychiatric disorders generally involve emotional experience, and through many years of experimentation on animals and humans, emotions have been closely mapped to specific brain regions. Most of us have a commonsense view of how

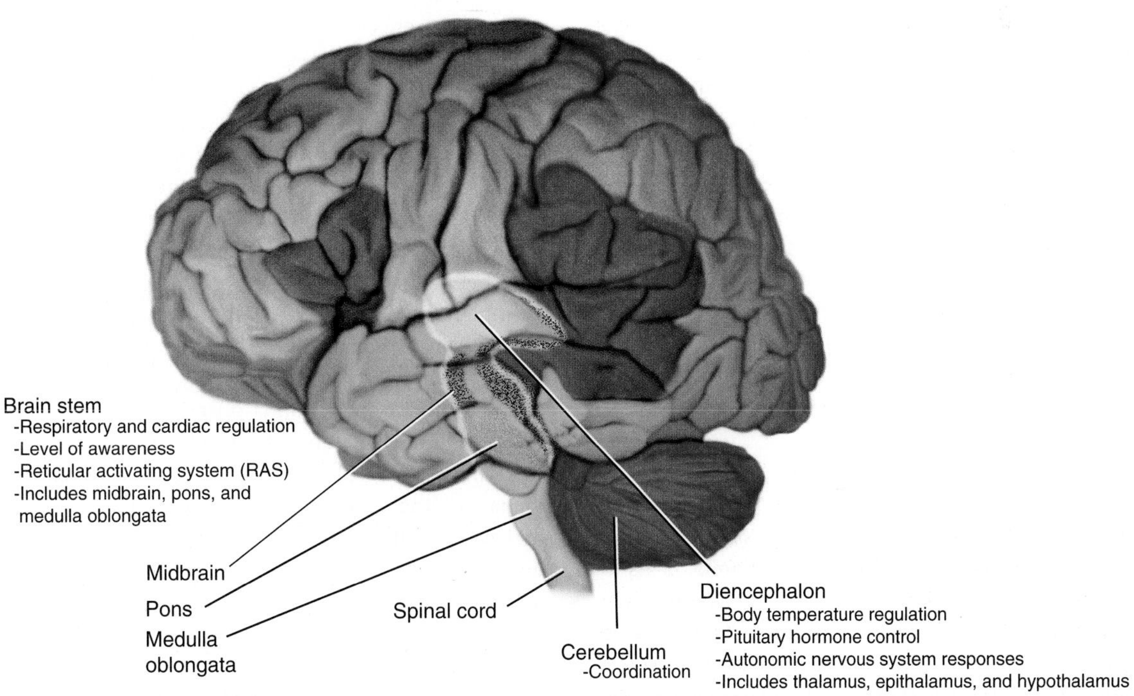

Figure 4-1 Locations and functions of the cerebral lobes, brain stem, and cerebellum. (DELMAR/CENGAGE LEARNING.)

emotions develop: For example, we generally assume that people cry because they experience something sad, we expect that people get angry because someone offends them, and we believe that people become sexually aroused because they see (or think about, or remember, or otherwise focus their attention on) someone who attracts them. As with many such "commonsense" views, careful scientific study shows that this intuitive understanding of emotional responses is not quite correct. Stated most simply, we do not experience our emotions solely because of events in the "real world"; instead, we experience the internal signals of emotional responses and then *associate* them with those outside events.

The difference is subtle but important. Let us look at an example: Someone who rear-ends us when we have stopped our car at an intersection of course makes us angry. But this experience of anger is generated deep in the brain and is then cognitively associated with the car accident only in the highest areas of the association cortex. The brain assembles the two experiences (the visceral sense of anger and the sights and sounds of the collision) in such a way that it seems to us that the accident has caused our emotion.

In the example just discussed, a car accident has set off the biologically programmed anger response, but sometimes the response occurs without a real-world cause and for no clearly understood reason. This phenomenon is commonly seen in a number of mental disorders, perhaps more clearly with emotions other than anger or rage. For example, depressed persons (see Chapter 14) frequently assume they feel sad because something bad has happened to them or feel guilty because they have done something wrong. But in reality nothing bad has happened and they have done nothing wrong. The biopsychophysiological theory suggests that in these persons, the association cortex takes the "raw" emotional perception of sadness or guilt and associates it with previously learned behavior ("at other times when I felt guilty I had done something bad, so this time ..."). The resulting inaccurate perception of guilt or misfortune is, for many, a fundamental experience of depression. Other psychiatric conditions may involve similar cognitive misperceptions, such as in panic disorder (see Chapter 12), where, for no discernible reason, diencephalic and limbic "fear centers" produce such strong autonomic stimuli that the conscious cortex falsely assumes some terrible physical catastrophe has taken place. Having addressed some of the general features of the biopsychophysiological theory (including its relationship to some aspects of depression and panic), it is time to look more explicitly at relevant brain anatomy.

The Diencephalon

The **diencephalon** consists of two major structures: the thalamus and the hypothalamus. The hypothalamus is a single midline organ. The thalami (there are two, one on each side) are exceptionally important brain regions that serve to relay a wide range of sensory inputs to the cerebral cortex. The **thalamus** is a critical structure for maintaining consciousness and processing visual information (Reinagel, 2007), but its function is still incompletely understood. In contrast, it has long been known that the hypothalamus participates in a wide range of regulatory functions, especially those that relate to emotion. These are discussed in the following paragraphs.

The brain has been shown to possess a set of stereotyped emotional responses that may be triggered by a variety of factors: drugs, environmental or interpersonal stimuli, or even electrical stimulation. These responses are produced in and adjacent to the hypothalamus and are communicated by neural pathways to higher brain centers, where cortical association systems attempt to link the emotional responses to perceived or remembered stimuli.

The **hypothalamus**, perhaps amazingly for such a small part of the brain, also exerts control over both the autonomic nervous system and the endocrine system—two systems that affect the way we perceive emotion. For example, most of the symptoms of anxiety are mediated through the autonomic nervous system: rapid heart rate, racing thoughts, and increased respiration. Direct stimulation of the hypothalamus can act on the autonomic nervous system to change vital signs of pulse, respiration, and blood pressure. The endocrine system is also involved in emotion. The hypothalamus controls pituitary function by releasing hormones that flow through the pituitary portal venous system. Although psychiatrists still disagree on precisely how this endocrine control affects emotions, depressed individuals sometimes have measurable abnormalities of the hypothalamic-pituitary axis, often manifested as elevations of serum cortisol (directly from hypothalamic stimulation of the pituitary). These endocrine abnormalities have no proven clinical significance, but persons with profound endocrine derangements (such as Cushing's disease or hyperthyroidism) may have significant psychiatric symptoms as part of their illnesses. Without question the hypothalamus affects the way we feel and behave through its effect on the autonomic nervous system; its control of the endocrine system is vitally important for regulating our metabolism and may subtly influence our psychological state as well. But this is only part of the hypothalamic role in emotion. Over 60 years ago, in a Nobel Prize–winning series of experiments, Walter Hess showed that highly localized hypothalamic stimulation of animals' brains reproducibly evoked a range of stereotypical physical and behavioral responses: for example, rage or sexual excitement (Hess, 1949). When appropriately chosen hypothalamic sites were electrically stimulated, Hess' cats displayed the behavior that we know precedes a "catfight": The spine arches, and the hair stands on end. His work demonstrates that the diencephalon is by itself capable of generating stereotypical states of behavior—and, by inference from that behavior, the emotions and feelings that accompany such behavior—without any intervention from higher brain centers. Without a doubt, the diencephalon has a powerful direct and indirect effect on the way we feel and behave.

The Cortex

Most of the brain is composed of the **cortex**, which is, in turn, divided into four lobes: frontal, temporal, parietal, and occipital. The best-understood cortical functions are the processing of sensory data and the organization of motor behavior; much of the parietal, temporal, and occipital lobes is devoted to sensory and motor functioning. A great deal of the remainder of the cortex is made up of association areas, of which the temporal association cortex and the closely related limbic cortex are by far the most important for the present review.

Temporal association areas are strongly involved with emotion and with memory. Memory clearly is of great importance to normal mental health: Persistent unpleasant memories, as in post-traumatic stress disorder, can play a central role in psychopathology. Such recollections represent long-term memories, whereas short-term memory (lost in many dementias) is essential for conducting activities of daily life. Memory is not highly localized in the brain, but the temporal association areas play a major role in organizing the process of long-term memory storage.

Deep in the temporal lobe is a complex set of structures known as the limbic system. The limbic system is intimately connected with the hypothalamus and consists of several highly important structures: the amygdala, the hippocampus, and the cingulate gyra. These are all very near the center of the brain, and together they form a loop encircling the thalamus. The limbic system seems to be important in the first weeks of memory storage; after this period, memories either are lost or are transferred back into the cortex for very long-term storage. While memory processing is clearly a highly important limbic and temporal lobe function, the limbic system has an equally significant role in the experiencing of emotion.

Recent research on the generation of emotions assigns an increasingly major role to a previously little-known member of the limbic system: the amygdala. The word "amygdala" means "almond," referring to the appearance of this small but critical brain region. Experiments confirm that the amygdala is involved in a wide variety of emotions and emotionally mediated behaviors: for example, fear, apprehension, sexual response, and feeding and sucking behaviors. The amygdala has direct connections to and from the hypothalamus, and many of the hypothalamic responses discovered by Hess (Hess, 1949) may actually have their origins in the amygdala.

Brain Imaging

"Imaging" is a generic word to describe a range of remarkable techniques to visualize internal organs. Although imaging can be applied to nearly any structure from the knee to the eye, this section focuses on imaging of the brain (Malhi & Lagopoulos, 2008; Konarski et al., 2007; Broderick, 2005).

Computerized Tomography

Computerized tomography (CT) scanning was among the first of the current techniques to be developed (Figure 4-2). The CT scan uses conventional X-rays to form an image, but

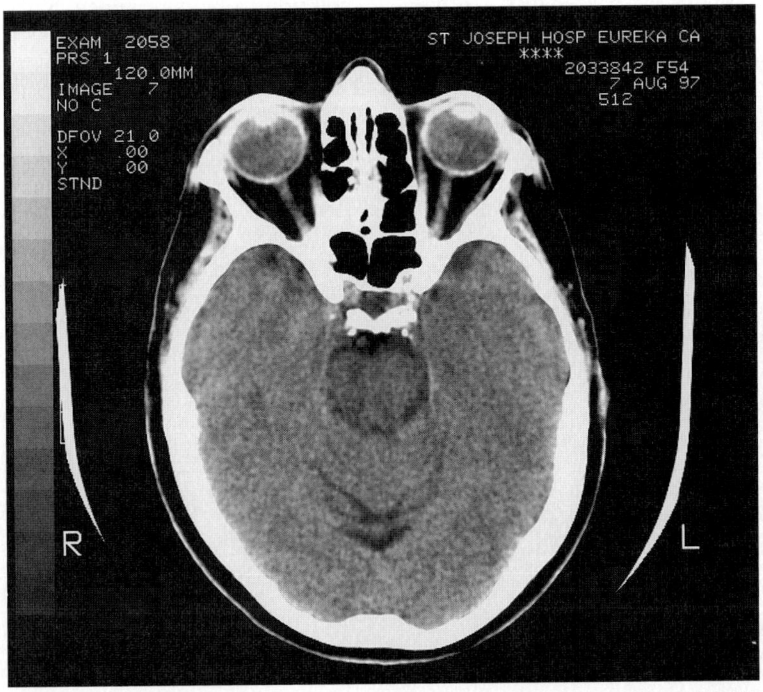

Figure 4-2 CT scan of the normal human brain. This CT scan reproduces a "slice" of the human brain at the level of the orbits. The eyes (with the tip of the nose visible in between) can be clearly seen at the top of the illustration. The lens of the eye appears white, and the optic nerves are clearly visible, passing superiorly and medially from the rear of each eye. The small black areas between the orbits are portions of the sinuses. The white and gray matter of the brain forms a large mass within the (white) margins of the skull. Some brain detail is visible on the particular slice, and greater contrast of structures can be obtained by injecting "contrast material" into the client's vein. The CT scan can easily delineate a tumor or bleeding within the homogeneous brain substance. A full CT study includes many separate "slices" taken at intervals of several millimeters and in different orientations. (REPRINTED COURTESY OF ALEX HABIBIAN, MD, HUMBOLDT COUNTY, CALIFORNIA ST. JOSEPH HEALTH SYSTEM,.)

the image is reconstructed from hundreds of X-rays taken at varying angles. Since X-ray beams are absorbed differently by different body structures, averaging this absorption over many angles can allow very powerful computers to generate an image of the underlying tissue. Prior to CT scanning, X-rays could generally give useful information only about bones or about soft tissues that were highlighted by radio-opaque "contrast material." The CT scan allowed remarkable views of soft-tissue structures, especially the brain. Although CT images are reconstructions from multiple X-ray images, modern scanners record images at very low radiation levels so that the total dose is not much different (or may even sometimes be lower) than that of conventional X-rays.

Magnetic Resonance Imaging

Magnetic resonance imaging (MRI) (Figure 4-3) is an imaging technique that uses no ionizing radiation (X-rays) at all. Instead, a portion of the body, such as the head or the knee, is placed into a very powerful magnetic field. Hydrogen atoms respond strongly to magnetic fields, and the body has many magnetically active hydrogen atoms, primarily in water molecules. If a brief pulse of radio-frequency energy is passed through water-containing tissue exposed to a strong magnet, the hydrogen atoms will release energy that can be measured by detectors. Through a complicated series of computer reconstructions, this energy can be converted into visual images that bear a remarkable resemblance to true tissue anatomy. The MRI images often can separate out features, especially in the brain, that cannot be visualized by CT scans. The technique of functional MRI (fMRI) further allows the anatomy visualized by standard structural MRI to be superimposed on an MRI-based measure of blood flow. fMRI identifies brain areas with increased blood flow in response to various psychological stimuli. The technique for identifying increased blood flow is called "blood oxygen level–dependent contrast," or BOLD.

Positron Emission Tomography

Positron emission tomography (PET) has been a major advance in research studies on a variety of psychiatric disorders. The PET-scanning techniques are not fundamentally different from those used in CT scanning, with one important addition: The PET scan requires the injection of a small amount of radioactive isotope that is localized in brain tissue. The PET scan allows the location of that isotope to be traced while a subject performs certain tasks. This emphasis on task is critical because, unlike CT and MRI, which largely focus on brain structure, PET scanning assesses brain function.

As implied in its name, PET scanning uses positrons as radioactive tracers, or, more precisely, uses positron-generating tracers that are bound to molecules (including glucose and certain neurotransmitter analogues). Positrons are a form of antimatter: electrons with a positive charge. When antimatter and matter (in this case, an electron) meet, they are both annihilated and produce two gamma particles traveling in nearly opposite directions. This production of two diverging particles allows the precise location of the original collision to be determined. Since human tissues (like nearly

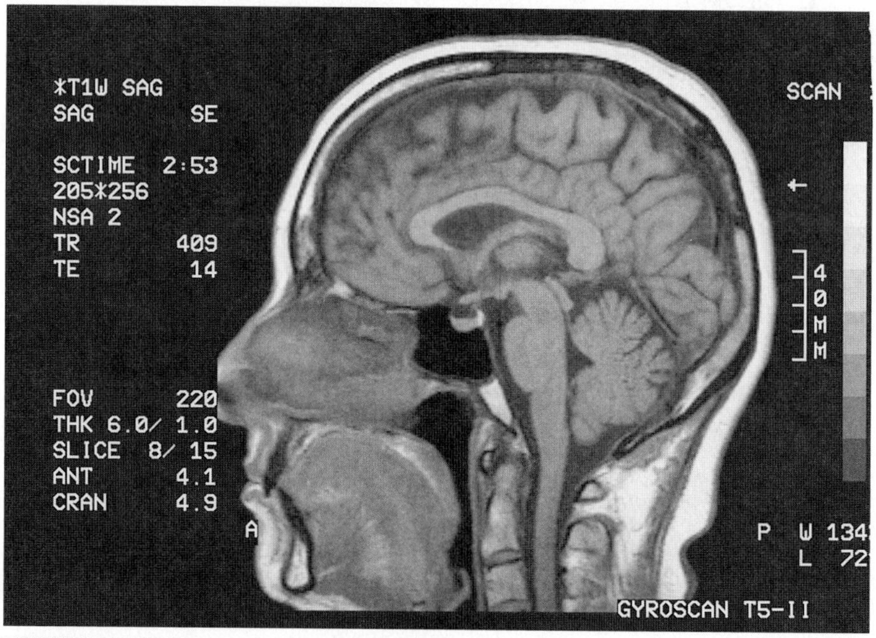

FIGURE 4-3 MRI scan of the normal human brain. This MRI image is a "sagittal" view taken as if the client's brain had been sliced from top to bottom by a sharp knife. The "slice" has occurred at about the midline. The mouth is visible at the lower front end just above the lowest letter "A." To the right of this "A" is the large gray mass of the tongue. The brain structures are seen in remarkable detail. Students familiar with neuroanatomy will easily recognize the midbrain, pons, cerebellum, diencephalon, corpus callosum, and cerebral hemisphere. Even the pituitary gland is visible, extending slightly into the black nasoparyngeal cavity, which is seen just behind the tissues of the nose. The eyes cannot be seen on this midline slice, but would be imaged in a full MRI study, which includes a dozen or more similar images taken in different planes or orientations. (REPRINTED WITH PERMISSION COURTESY OF ALEX HABIBIAN, MD, HUMBOLDT COUNTY, CALIFORNIA ST. JOSEPH HEALTH SYSTEM,.)

all matter) are full of electrons, the collision occurs very close to the site at which the positron-generating substance was concentrated. The PET scan allows scientists to map functions such as the flow of blood within the brain, the uptake of glucose, and the binding of neurotransmitters to synaptic membranes, all in response to *specific real-time behaviors*. For example, studies with PET (Figure 4-4) show that in normal individuals, there are major differences in where brain functions localize depending on whether an individual does the following activities:

- Looks at a word: The metabolic activity is limited to the visual cortex.
- Listens to a word: The metabolic activity is limited to parts of the temporal cortex.
- Speaks a word: The metabolic activity is limited to the medial frontal cortex.
- Thinks about word meaning: The metabolic activity is widely spread over areas of the association cortex.

The PET scan provides a remarkable confirmation of aspects of the biopsychophysiological theory: Brain functions do link to mental processes and are highly localized within the cortex. Throughout this text, the nurse will see how PET scanning can provide images of brain functioning, not just in health but also in various psychiatric disorders.

Newer Scanning Techniques

Two new MRI-derived scanning techniques, magnetic resonance spectroscopy (MRS) and diffusion tensor imaging (DTI), have recently been developed. MRS does not produce visual brain images, but it allows scientists to determine which neurotransmitters and other chemicals are present at specific brain sites. DTI is an extension of MRI that allows brain white matter fibers—previously invisible to imaging—to be recognized. It remains very much a limited research tool at the time of this writing. Figure 4-5 provides a summary of the major forms of imaging in current use.

Electrophysiology and Neurochemistry

A defining characteristic of higher organisms is that they consist of numerous cells that have highly complex interconnections with each other. This is especially true for neural tissue, whose primary purpose is to pass signals from cell to cell. The brain consists of billions of cells (neurons) arranged in complex anatomical structures and connected by axons, dendrites, fibers, and tracts. Most nerve cells have axons, relatively long fibers that serve to conduct electrical impulses from the body of the cell to some other cell lying as close as 0.1 mm and as far away as a person's full height. Dendrites receive signals from the axons of other nerve cells and may be short, long, single, or very richly branched, depending on their locations within the nervous system. Fibers and tracts are collections of axons all traveling together as in an electrical cable. Tracts usually connect areas of the nervous system that are physically separated. Tracts travel within nerve substance but are clearly devoted to one function. Tracts differ from nerves in that the latter typically pass out of the nervous system into adjacent connective tissue, whereas tracts stay within the brain. The nervous system contains many nonnerve cells known as glial cells, which protect, nourish, and sheathe neural tissue so that it can effectively carry on its communication and signaling functions. (Figure 4-6 illustrates parts of a nerve cell.)

Physiologists have learned that electrical impulses called action potentials travel down the substance of neural axons.

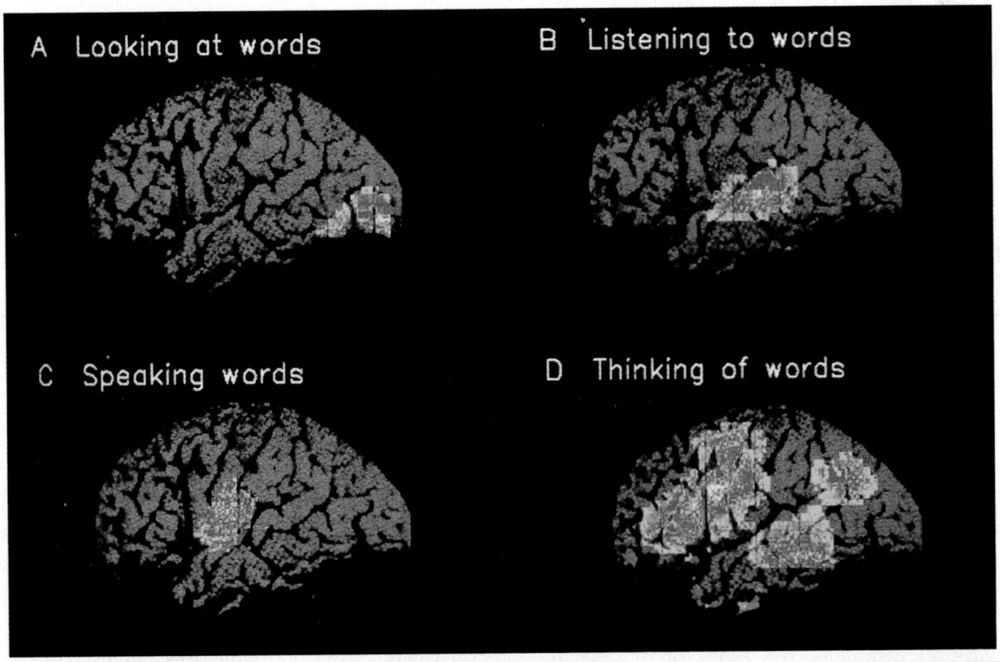

FIGURE 4-4 **PET scans illustrating changes in blood flow within the brain based on subject's activities: looking at a word, listening to words, speaking words, and thinking of words.** (FROM KANDEL, E. R., SCHWARTZ, J. H., & JESSELL, T. (1995). *ESSENTIALS OF NEURAL SCIENCE AND BEHAVIOR.* STAMFORD, CT: APPLETON & LANGE. REPRINTED WITH PERMISSION OF APPLETON & LANGE, MCGRAW, HILL, AND DR. ERIC R. KANDEL, MD, NEW YORK CENTER FOR NEUROBIOLOGY & BEHAVIOR.)

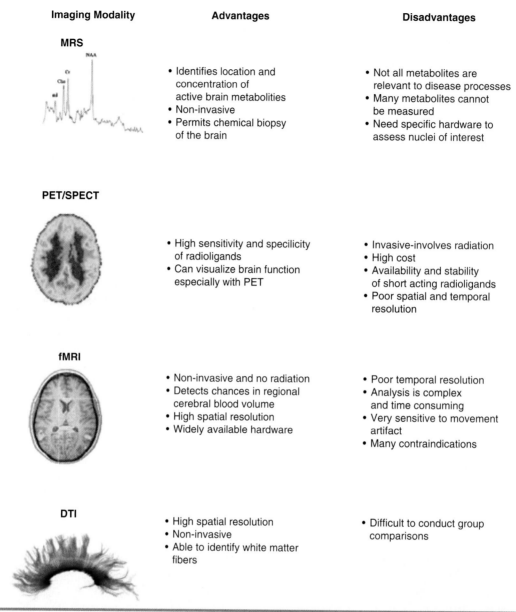

Imaging Modality	Advantages	Disadvantages
MRS 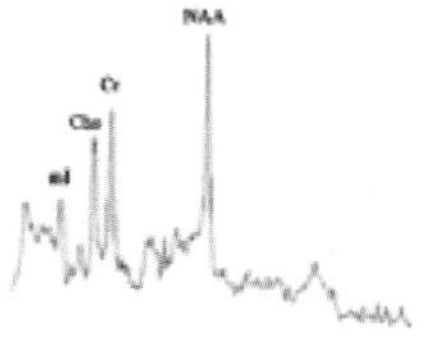	• Identifies location and concentration of active brain metabolities • Non-invasive • Permits chemical biopsy of the brain	• Not all metabolites are relevant to disease processes • Many metabolites cannot be measured • Need specific hardware to assess nuclei of interest
PET/SPECT 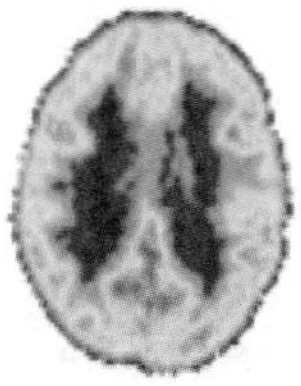	• High sensitivity and specilicity of radioligands • Can visualize brain function especially with PET	• Invasive-involves radiation • High cost • Availability and stability of short acting radioligands • Poor spatial and temporal resolution
fMRI 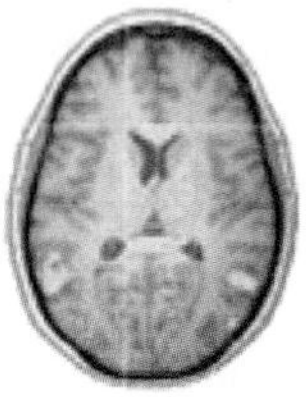	• Non-invasive and no radiation • Detects chances in regional cerebral blood volume • High spatial resolution • Widely available hardware	• Poor temporal resolution • Analysis is complex and time consuming • Very sensitive to movement artifact • Many contraindications
DTI 	• High spatial resolution • Non-invasive • Able to identify white matter fibers	• Difficult to conduct group comparisons

FIGURE 4-5 **Summary of the major forms of imaging in current use. This figure provides a visual display of the actual data output obtained from magnetic resonance spectroscopy (MRS), positron emission tomography (PET), functional MRI (fMRI), and diffusion tensor imaging (DTI) neuroimaging modalities. The output for MRS takes the form of a spectral graph that depicts the relative concentration of metabolites present in the region of the brain sampled. PET output consists of a slice of whole brain at a specified level that depicts the uptake of radioligands via a gradation of color. Warm colors such as red/orange depict increased uptake, whereas cooler colors such as blue/green indicate little or no uptake. The fMRI output is depicted by an MRI slice with the coregistered BOLD activations present and indicated in red/yellow. Finally, DTI tractography shows the actual arrangement of white matter fibers.** (REPRINTED WITH PERMISSION FROM MALHI, G. S., & LAGOPOULOS, J. (2008). MAKING SENSE OF NEUROIMAGING IN PSYCHIATRY. *ACTA PSYCHIATRICA SCANDINAVICA*, 117(2), 100–117.)

When the action potential reaches the end of the axon, communication is made with the body of another cell, usually through that cell's dendrites (if it is a nerve cell) or through a motor end plate (if it is a muscle cell). Within the central nervous system, virtually all axons end on the dendrites of other nerve cells. Communication between those cells occurs in one of two ways. Occasionally, the axons of one cell lie very close to the dendrites or the cell body of another. The connection between these cells is termed a gap junction and is formed so that the membranes of each cell come close together and form a point of contact. When an action potential builds up electrical charge on one side of a gap junction, multiple hexagonal pores in the membranes open up and allow the free flow of a wide range of chemical compounds between the cells. Simple ions such as sodium, potassium, and chloride flow freely, but pores are also large enough that relatively large organic molecules can occasionally get through as well. After the action potential passes, the pores close and the cells are once again physically isolated. This kind of direct depolarization through a gap junction is usually

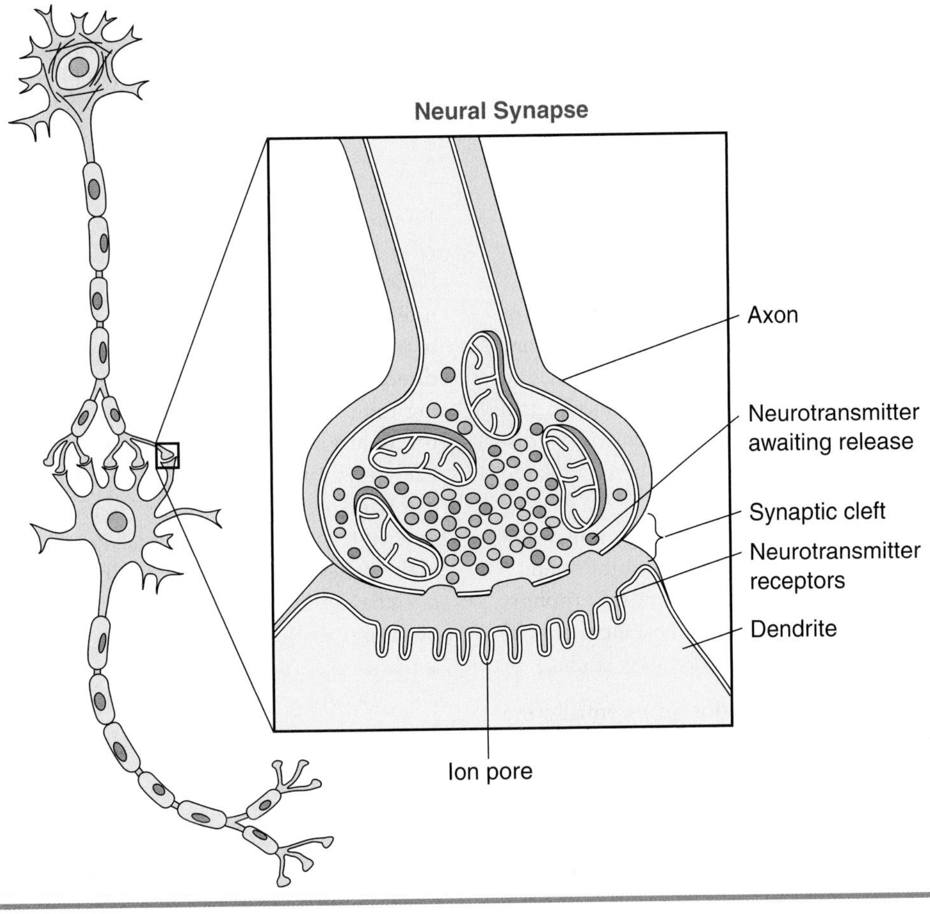

FIGURE 4-6 **Microanatomy of a neuron.** DELMAR/CENGAGE LEARNING

bidirectional and is most frequently seen in motor nerves, where very rapid muscle responses are required. In the human brain, most nerve cells communicate with each other through **synapses** rather than gap junctions. Synapses are special structures formed where axons and dendrites come together. The separation between cells across synapses is much wider than at gap junctions, and, as a result, no direct flow of ions or other nonspecific cellular chemicals occurs across synapses. Instead, the synapse is specialized to allow a unique chemical messenger, called a **neurotransmitter**, to pass from the axon of one cell to the dendrite of the other across the synaptic cleft separating the cells. Once on the other side of the cleft, the neurotransmitter interacts with the dendrite's cell wall to cause the opening of channels, which, in turn, allows ions (typically sodium) to pass into the dendrite. Finally, the neurotransmitter returns to the axon from which it was originally released; cellular processes lead to reuptake of the neurotransmitter back into the cytoplasm of the axon. When the neurotransmitter is taken back up out of the synaptic cleft, the channel pores close and ion flow stops. Signaling across synapses is in one direction only and can be very precisely controlled by a range of factors including the mix of neurotransmitters released: Some *stimulate* the dendrite, whereas others *inhibit* it. In summary, direct conduction across a gap junction is a physiologically simple process, but synaptic transmission is far more complex, involving neurotransmitter release, channel opening, ion flow, and, finally, neurotransmitter reuptake. Since most psychiatric medications exert their pharmacological effects directly at the nerve synapse, it is particularly important for nurses to develop an understanding of synaptic transmission and of neurotransmitters. Neurotransmitters and their receptors are discussed in the following sections.

Neurotransmitters

Neurotransmitters are substances that:

1. Are released by presynaptic axon membranes,
2. Cross the synaptic cleft,
3. Interact with receptors on an adjacent postsynaptic neuron, and
4. Are quickly removed from the synaptic cleft by a biochemical process specific to the individual neurotransmitter.

Neurotransmitters have yet another important property: Their actions at postsynaptic neurons are directly mimicked when they are given as drugs, most commonly by parenteral injection. The doses required for such systemic action are generally quite large, but the effects are indistinguishable from those that occur during natural synaptic release.

Most known neurotransmitters belong to one of a limited number of chemical families: biogenic amines, amino acids, acetylcholine, and purines. Each of these chemical substances or families contains an active nitrogen group that facilitates binding to the appropriate neurotransmitter receptor in the postsynaptic membrane (see the section on receptors, following).

- Biogenic amines are a group of substances (dopamine, epinephrine, histamine, norepinephrine, and serotonin) synthesized either from a common amino acid (tyrosine or histadine) or from one of the other biogenic amines.
- Amino acids: While tyrosine and histadine are neurotransmitter precursors but not themselves neurotransmitters, two other amino acids (glycine and glutamic acid) do function as neurotransmitters. Gamma amino butyric acid (GABA), a very important neurotransmitter widely distributed throughout the nervous system, is closely related to glutamic acid.
- Acetylcholine is the major neurotransmitter in all muscles; it also is widely distributed at synapses throughout the brain.
- Purines include adenine, guanine, and adenosine triphosphate (ATP). Most of these chemical substances should be familiar to the nurse from past biochemistry studies.

Almost all neurotransmitters function in essentially the same manner: An action potential propagated along an axon causes release of the neurotransmitter across the synaptic cleft. After receiving a neurotransmitter "message" across the synaptic cleft, the postsynaptic neuron has two choices: It can either fire its own action potential to communicate with other cells to which it is connected, or it can fail to respond to the message. Which of these two "choices" the postsynaptic cell makes depends on whether it receives an excitatory or an inhibitory stimulus across its membrane. Excitatory stimulation will continue the action potential on its way to the next cell(s), whereas inhibitory stimulation will decrease the likelihood that the postsynaptic cell will fire its own action potential. Most cell-to-cell communication is very complex, and cells may receive synaptic signals from up to 10,000 other neurons, some excitatory, others inhibitory. The receiving cell sums up all its inhibitory and excitatory inputs, and then "decides" to fire its own action potential depending on the overall balance of excitation and inhibition. Inhibitory synapses are often located near the receiving cell's body, where their effects are more pronounced. In contrast, excitatory synapses are more likely to be relatively far out along dendrites. As a result, whether or not a given cell "fires" is not just a "counting" of the number of inhibitory and excitatory signals it receives; some signals are given more "weight" than others. Inhibitory and excitatory synapses function very similarly, but they are actually distinguishable when viewed through an electron microscope. Not only are there structural differences between these synapses, but also their neurotransmitters are typically different: GABA and glycine are the commonest brain inhibitory transmitters, whereas glutamic acid (very closely related to GABA) is an excitatory transmitter. Most, if not all, neurotransmitters consistently act either in an inhibitory or in an excitatory role, but not both. Nothing is more important to understanding how the brain works than recognizing that each neuron continuously receives hundreds upon thousands of competing inputs; it then fires (or fails to fire) its own action potential to multiple other cells (depending on whether excitatory or inhibitory stimuli were more strongly expressed on its membrane).

Membrane Receptors

For nearly 100 years, scientists have recognized that the specific functions of neurotransmitters, hormones, and other biologically active molecules occur because these molecules interact with receptors that "recognize" one specific hormone or neurotransmitter. Recognition occurs through a direct chemical bond between the receptor and its stimulating molecule. The relationship of neurotransmitter to receptor is just like that of key and lock; usually only one fits. (There is another important similarity: Just as a locksmith can often make a "master key" that opens a lock without being exactly the same as the usual key, so pharmacologists can make drugs that act on receptors even though the drugs are not chemically identical with the natural neurotransmitter or hormone. Without such an ability to produce useful receptor-active drugs, modern nursing practice would be very different.) Receptors recognize only one specific molecule, and binding of that molecule to the receptor site sets up a chain of other chemical reactions analogous to the opening of a door when a key is turned in a lock. When a neurotransmitter binds to a specific receptor, either of two outcomes may result, depending on the nature of the receptor site:

- An influx of ions or other small molecules into the cell: Ion influx occurs because nearly all membrane receptors are protein molecules that bridge the cell membrane, partly outside the cell and partly inside. Some such receptors have central "ion channels" that open when a neurotransmitter is bound and close when the neurotransmitter leaves to return to its presynaptic site. This direct gating results in very rapid interneuron signaling, as ion flows are very quick.
- The activation of another signaling system—the "second messenger." Other receptors are more complex: These receptors activate another signaling system that brings about intracellular changes. Neurotransmitters interact with receptors that, in turn, bind to a G protein on the inside of the membrane. The G protein turns on an enzyme called adenyl cyclase, which quickly produces a large quantity of the substance cyclic AMP. Cyclic AMP itself activates other intracellular enzyme systems that bring about metabolic change within the cell. The "first messenger" in this system is the neurotransmitter; cyclic AMP is the second messenger and is activated indirectly by the interaction of neurotransmitter and cell-surface receptor. Second-messenger effects are somewhat slower than those produced by direct gating, and they may continue briefly after the neurotransmitter dissociates from the membrane receptor. Cyclic AMP is the best-understood second messenger, but other substances may act as second messengers within cells.

Many of the neurotransmitters important in psychiatric disorders act through second messengers, including the biogenic amines, GABA, glutamate, and many neuropeptides (see the section on neuropeptides following). However, GABA is one of a number of neurotransmitters that has both directly gated receptors ($GABA_A$) and G-protein-type receptors ($GABA_B$).

Receptor Subtypes

Many neurotransmitters can exert their effects at more than one receptor. For example, the first major discovery of twentieth-century pharmacology was that peripheral acetylcholine receptors are of two kinds: muscarinic and nicotinic. Acetylcholine acts on both types of receptors, but specific drugs (muscarine and nicotine) exist that will activate only one receptor and not the other. Recent studies have revealed unexpected variety in receptor numbers and types. The development of "atypical" neuroleptic drugs such as clozapine (used to treat symptoms of psychosis) has helped document the existence of at least five such receptor subtypes for the neurotransmitter dopamine (D_1–D_5). Drugs that block the D_2 receptor are very effective at relieving symptoms of psychosis such as delusions and hallucinations. They are also quite likely to produce symptoms of Parkinson's disease or other movement disorders. (Persons with movement disorders have difficulty in coordinating their movements and may have repetitive unexpected activity of muscle groups—either tremors or choreoathetosis.) That symptoms of Parkinson's disease might appear when the D_2 receptor is blocked should not be surprising given that this disorder is due to insufficient dopamine in certain brain centers, and treatment with dopamine-enhancing drugs often causes psychosis as a side effect. So, too much stimulation of the D_2 receptor causes psychosis, and too much inhibition causes movement disorders such as Parkinson's disease! Clozapine has the remarkable property that it greatly improves symptoms of psychosis, but it has no tendency to produce movement disorders. It now appears that clozapine has little effect on the D_2 receptor, but its major actions occur at the D_4 receptor, a previously unknown biochemical structure. Apparently, drugs that act uniquely on this receptor can effectively control symptoms of psychosis without producing debilitating motor side effects.

Neuropeptides and Intracellular Modification of Synaptic Signals

Most neurons receive simultaneous signal inputs from a number (sometimes thousands) of other neurons. Some inputs are excitatory, others inhibitory. The receiving cell sums up its many input signals, and when the sum is excitatory, it responds with an action potential; when the sum is inhibitory, there is no action potential sent on to the next cell. Nerve cells share with computers this basic "binary" function: they are either *on* or *off*; the action potential either fires or does not fire. While the sum of inhibitory and excitatory synapse inputs is a major factor in determining whether any particular cell fires, there are other important influences on the firing behavior of neurons. Among the most important of these influences is a group of chemicals called neuropeptides.

Peptides are relatively small chains of amino acids that are generally smaller than proteins and so typically lack the folded configuration that gives most proteins their functions. Nurses are very familiar with many common biological peptides, including insulin, vasopressin, adrenocorticotropic hormone (ACTH), thyrotropin (TSH), and calcitonin. While better known as hormones, each of these peptides has been shown to act on the nervous system as well. There are several dozen neuropeptides that, like the examples given, either are hormones or are active within the gastrointestinal tract (or both).

Neuropeptides seem to have an important effect on the way in which emotions and sensations are perceived. Stress responses and perceptions of pain are strongly influenced by neuropeptides. The neuropeptide endorphins act to moderate the perception of pain and emotion in the central nervous system; synthetic opiates such as morphine, heroin, and methadone act at endorphin receptor sites. Prolactin seems to have an effect on maternal behavior, and cholecystokinin may mediate the sensation of "being full" after a large meal.

One of the most interesting findings in recent years has been that in addition to peptides, there is yet another set of brain chemicals that modify the way in which synapses respond to electrical stimulation. These substances are called "cannabinoids" and are associated with two special cannabinoid receptors located respectively in the brain and nervous system. Cannabinoid release blocks the inhibiting effects of GABA on synapses. By releasing cannabinoids, nerve cells can allow their own action potentials to "fire" by reducing the amount of GABA secreted at synapses to which they are connected. In this manner, cannabinoids are unique in that their action is "retrograde"—passing from cell to cell in a direction opposite to that of the action potential; this is a form of signaling that is not otherwise known to occur in the adult nervous system. The active chemical substances in marijuana bind to cannabinoid receptors, and in turn receptor activation is responsible for the psychological effects produced by marijuana. Once again, as with the opium poppy (the source of most of the psychoactive drugs that bind to opioid receptors), nature has produced in the plant world a "key" tailored to the cannabinoid receptor "locks" in our brains (Nicoll & Alger, 2004).

Genetics

DNA

Deoxyribonucleic acid (DNA) is a highly variable molecule that consists of two strands that wrap around each other so that they resemble a pair of entwined ladders (Figure 4-7). The ladder sides are made up of sugars, whereas the rungs connecting the two sides consist of matched pairs of "bases." Bases, in turn, are either purines or pyrimidines, relatively simple organic molecules that contain nitrogen rings. The DNA carries a "genetic code" in its sequence of bases: The base adenine pairs only with thymine, and cytosine pairs only with guanine. From this very simple set of rules, the entire genome is generated.

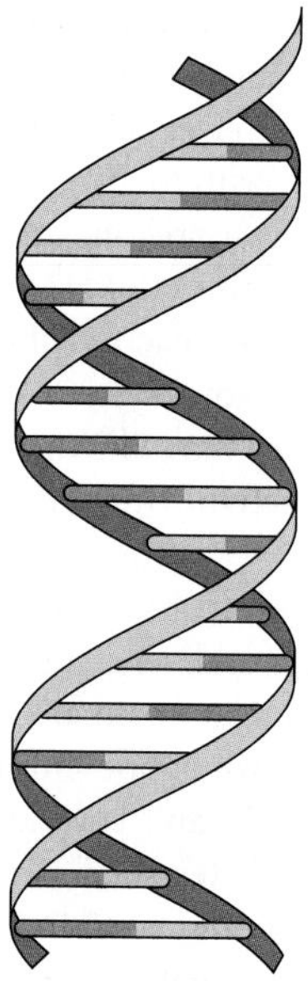

FIGURE 4-7 **Deoxyribonucleic acid (DNA).** DELMAR/CENGAGE LEARNING

Chromosomes and Genes

The human **genome** (the entire complement of heritable information) contains 20,000 to 30,000 genes, each of which is formed from a defined length of DNA localized to one of 24 chromosomes. Chromosomes typically contain 100 million or more base pairs, and the entire human genome consists of about 3 billion base pairs. Amazingly, only about 10% of the genome is actually genetic information. Ninety percent of all human DNA is contained in intron sequences that separate genes. Some introns clearly serve to provide signaling functions so that DNA can be accurately transcribed into RNA for the production of proteins. Remarkably little is known about the function (if any) of the majority of human intron DNA.

A great deal is known, however, about the 10% of DNA that codes for genetic material. Nurses will be familiar with the transcription and translation processes that lead to unfolding of DNA, transcription into RNA, and, finally, translation into protein on the surface of cytoplasmic ribosomes. The primary purpose of DNA is to code for the amino acid structure of proteins. Three base pairs are required to code unambiguously for each amino acid, and as a result, the average protein of about 1,000 amino acids requires 3,000 base pairs to code.

Chromosomes are far from mere collections of DNA; rather, they contain nearly identical quantities of DNA and protein. When chromosomes are stained with certain dyes, a complex banding pattern is revealed (Figure 4-8). This banding reflects large-scale variations in the number of base pairs. Sometimes banding studies can be used to identify mutations in DNA, particularly where chromosomes have been broken and rejoined (translocations) or where pieces of chromosomes are missing (deletions). Most mutations result from subtle DNA changes, often at the level of a single base pair, and cannot be detected by visual examination of chromosomes.

Genetic Linkage

While some mutations have been identified by directly sequencing proteins, the major recent breakthroughs in

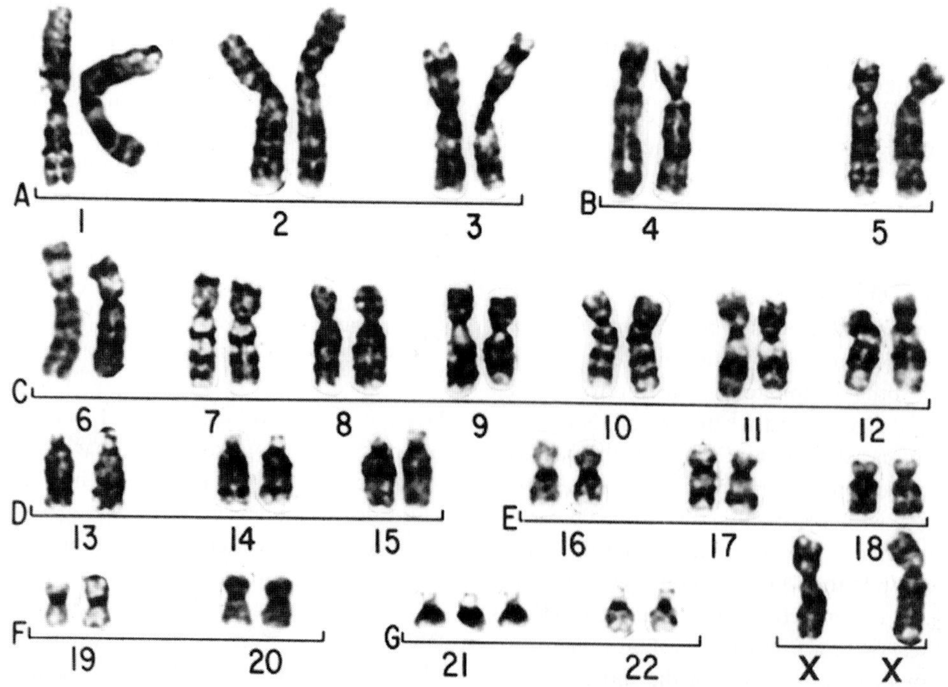

FIGURE 4-8 **Chromosomes.** DELMAR/CENGAGE LEARNING

genetic understanding have come from studies of genetic linkage. Linkage studies require the identification of one or more **genetic markers**. Markers are identifiable patterns of DNA structure that can be readily confirmed by laboratory analysis. In most cases, markers are unambiguous sequences of DNA base pairs, but certain highly repetitive areas of DNA allow other characteristics (such as DNA length) to occasionally be used as markers. Linkage studies are done by observing how frequently two markers are inherited together. Since recombination (breakage and reassembly of DNA occurring between two DNA chains, one from each of two parents) is a common genetic process, the farther apart two markers are on a chromosome, the more likely it is that a recombination process will separate them. (This separation leads, for example, to a maternal marker sequence being replaced by a paternal sequence through the process of recombination.) When two markers are located very close to one another on a chromosome, they are very likely to be passed together from a parent to the offspring. When markers are so close that they are nearly always passed together, this is termed *tight linkage*. Two markers are defined as being 1 cM (cM = centimorgan, named after Thomas Morgan, a famous geneticist) apart if they are separated by recombination 1% of the time. Further studies show that a separation of 1 cM is roughly equal to 1 million base pairs. (The reader should note that a centimorgan bears absolutely no direct relationship to the similarly abbreviated centimeter. While the centimorgan is functionally a measurement of DNA length, it is not a physical measurement and is in no way related to the metric system.)

By the end of the twentieth century, the human genome had been mapped to a resolution of about 5 million to 7 million base pairs. While this is much finer resolution than is possible with banding studies on chromosomes, it is still quite crude compared to the basic mutation level of one base pair. While linkage has proved a very powerful tool for genetic understanding, recent completion of the full human genome map will eventually open new vistas on our understanding of psychiatric disorders.

Chromosome Mapping

More precise understanding of chromosome structure has come from techniques of physical mapping. Chromosome banding, discussed earlier, is a crude form of physical mapping that can provide gross detail of the microscopic appearance of chromosomes but is limited in its resolution to the identification of regions visible in the light microscope, about 10 million base pairs (10 cM). Increasingly precise mapping can be done using the techniques involving DNA restriction enzymes. Restriction enzymes can be thought of as miniaturized "DNA choppers" able to cut the large molecules of DNA found in chromosomes into much smaller fragments. Many different restriction enzymes have been isolated (mostly from bacteria, where they serve to protect against invading viruses by destroying foreign DNA), and each is able to reduce DNA to fragments of differing sizes. Depending on the choice of restriction enzymes, large strands of DNA can be converted to a few long fragments containing millions of base pairs or, more usefully, a myriad of small fragments each containing only hundreds or thousands of base pairs.

For restriction analysis to be useful, it is first necessary to separate individual chromosomes from each other. This is accomplished via a remarkable technique known as flow sorting, in which laser-guided equipment successfully identifies and separates individual chromosomes from each other. Once the chromosomes are separated, restriction enzymes can reduce them to a "library" of different-sized fragments (each size produced by interaction with a separate restriction enzyme). The process of building DNA fragment libraries is laborious, but once fragments have been produced, they can be amplified by processes such as polymerase chain reaction (PCR) to produce quite large quantities of each fragment. The fragments can then be ordered by matching regions on different overlapping fragments. Once again, the process is tedious, but the results are quite powerful, at least for understanding small areas of chromosomes.

DNA Sequencing

Even more powerful mapping strategies come from techniques of DNA sequencing, which have led to mapping of the entire human genome. Sequencing requires that very large quantities of DNA fragments be produced, often by splicing these fragments into the genome of microorganisms, growing the microorganisms in large quantities, and then extracting the microbial DNA containing the fragments of human (or other higher-animal) DNA. This procedure can provide nearly limitless quantities of specific DNA, as can the process of PCR, mentioned in the previous paragraph. Polymerase chain reaction is a remarkable technique that can produce very large quantities of any DNA fragment in a "test tube" after only a few hours of incubation. Current PCR techniques can amplify a single DNA target by 1 million times in only an hour.

RECAPITULATION

III. Genes

The problem solved by Mendel was
Why yellow peas, or green,
Could be either smooth or wrinkled,
Which he understood to mean:
That the color and the texture
Each reflects a different gene.
But far beyond the reach of even
Mendel's intuition,
There lurked the well-kept secrets of
Genetic composition:
The nature of the stuff used in
Genetic fabrication;
And the nature of the rules that rule
Genetic replication.
But behold nucleic acids, and

The secret is exposed,
And the rules of replication can be
Finally proposed,
And the meaning of base pairing
Can be rapidly revealed,
Since the bases tell the story
(That was cunningly concealed).
For the code of replication is
Determined by the places
That are copied in transcription
(By touching all four bases),
In that A and T, or G and C
Perform a clever trick,
By being complementary
(As Watson is to Crick).
And three of them, in order,
Lead to literal translation
In amino acid language
That transmits this declamation
To a hundred thousand proteins
That complete the transmutation
From the sequence of the bases
Into protein conformation.
But beware a single error
In the linear array
Of As and Ts, or Gs and Cs,
Whose orderly display
Is absolutely needed
Lest there be a misquotation
That causes odd behavior
From molecular mutation.
For instance, in a fruit fly
If the error is in per
It dysregulates some rhythms
So the wings won't rightly whir;
And a mutant human enzyme
Can bring total devastation
To the elegant progression
Of our cerebral formation.
So, given these examples,
The task becomes to seek
(By proper application
Of molecular technique)
The genes that cause such problems
As obsessional neurosis,
Severe agoraphobia,
Delusional psychosis.
For once a gene's discovered
And is captured in a clone,
The protein that it codes for is
Immediately known,
Unleashing all the power of
Molecular biology
To exorcise the demons of
Behavioral pathology.
IV. Stories
The problem that remains is that,
Despite these revelations,
A science based on molecules
Has latent limitations
That limit its capacity
To serve as a notation
*For thoughts that we experience in our imagination.**

(Barondes, 1999, p. 207)

Once large quantities of the desired DNA have been produced, automatic analyzers are capable of analyzing the base-pair sequences of the DNA. While often fully automated, this sequencing process remains slow and costly.

The result of all this effort will soon be a detailed physical map of the human genome. Such a map would tell scientists where the genes for specific inherited disorders are located and would potentially allow further understanding of—and perhaps therapy for—genetically related disorders. Since many psychiatric and mental health disorders have important inherited components, understanding the human genome better may have highly important implications for the diagnosis and treatment of psychiatric conditions.

Summary

Biopsychophysiological theory is based on the premise that consciousness (and the whole range of mental and emotional activity that accompanies it) not only is a psychological phenomenon but also derives in some as-yet-unknown way directly from processes of brain functioning. The processes that "produce" consciousness rely on the complexities of brain anatomy and on the principles of neurophysiology. Among the most important neurophysiological principles is the concept that neurons receive input from a variety of cells and that the neuron's "decision" to discharge an action potential results from summation of a range of excitatory and inhibitory stimuli and modulatory factors such as the effect of one or more neuropeptides released into synaptic clefts along with neurotransmitters. Brain structure can be imaged with remarkable detail by CT and MRI scanning, but PET scanning allows function to be localized within the brain. The PET scan offers the potential for important insights into brain functioning in psychiatric disorders. Finally, many psychiatric mental health disorders have important genetic components. Some are inherited in precisely known genetic patterns; others just "tend to run in families." There have been great advances in genetics in the past decades, and

*From *Molecules and Mental Illness*, by S. H. Barondes, Copyright © 1999, New York: Scientific American Library.

these have allowed the localization of some psychiatric disorders to specific points on a chromosome. Regardless of whether such discoveries will truly lead the way to revolutionary forms of "gene therapy," they certainly allow increasingly more profound understanding of the brain and its function in health and disease.

KEY CONCEPTS

- Mental phenomena, how we think and act, are somehow caused by an array of biochemical and neurophysiological processes that take place from moment to moment.
- All major functions having to do with consciousness can be localized to the diencephalon and cortex of the brain.
- Emotional responses are triggered by a variety of factors (e.g., drugs, environmental or interpersonal stimuli, and electrical stimuli) and are produced in and adjacent to the hypothalamus.
- The best understood of brain cortical functions include processing sensory data and the organization of motor behavior.
- Temporal association areas of the brain are strongly involved with emotion and memory.
- Brain-imaging techniques such as CT scans, MRIs, and PET scans permit visualization of the brain. CT scans and MRIs focus on brain structure, whereas PET scans can assess brain functions.
- Neurotransmitters are substances that serve as chemical messengers; neurotransmitters are released by a presynaptic cell and cross the synapse to stimulate or inhibit the postsynaptic cell.
- Membrane receptors are cells to which a neurotransmitter binds, resulting in either an influx of ions (or other small molecules) into the cell, or the activation of a "second messenger" producing an additional biochemical reaction.
- Study of human genetics and detailed mapping of the human genome could tell scientists where genes for inherited disorders are located and permit better understanding of genetically related disorders.

REVIEW QUESTIONS

1. The nursing assessment of a client with Schizophrenia reveals that the client is actively hallucinating and delusional. The client is withdrawn and the client's affect is flat. The nurse would hypothesize that these alterations in the client's consciousness is involves which structure of the brain?
   1. Hypothalamus
   2. Thalamus
   3. Medulla oblongata
   4. Cerebellum

2. A nurse caring for a Schizophrenic client reviews the client's laboratory results. Which result is common for clients with Schizophrenia?
   1. Increased dopamine levels
   2. Increased serotonin levels
   3. Decreased dopamine levels
   4. Decreased serotonin levels

3. A nursing student asks her instructor, "Which body systems are controlled by the hypothalamus. The instructor would be correct if which body systems were identified?
   1. Muscular system and Circulatory system
   2. Circulatory system and Nervous system
   3. Nervous system and Endocrine System
   4. Endocrine System and Muscular system

4. A nurse is caring for a client who has overdosed on a drug and requires frequent monitoring of vital signs. The nurse's care is based on the understanding that changes in vital signs are controlled by which portion of the brain?
   1. Hypothalamus
   2. Thalamus
   3. Medulla oblongata
   4. Cerebellum

5. The nurse caring for clients with substance abuse problems would assess which of the following when reviewing laboratory results?
   1. Dopamine
   2. Serotonin
   3. Epinephrine
   4. Norepinephrine

6. The nurse caring for a client with depression would hypothesize that the client has which of the following?
   1. Increased serotonin, norepinephrine, and dopamine
   2. Decreased serotonin, norepinephrine, and dopamine
   3. Increased GABA, increased serotonin, and increased epinephrine
   4. Decreased GABA, decreased serotonin, and increased dopamine

7. A client with Schizophrenia who is exhibiting disturbances in thought process is scheduled for a PET scan. The nurse would hypothesize that the PET scan would most likely show changes in which lobe of the brain?
   1. Frontal lobe
   2. Parietal lobe
   3. Temporal lobe
   4. Occipital lobe

LEARNING ACTIVITIES

1. Describe how emotions and behavior can be understood in terms of physiological processes in the brain.
2. Describe basic brain anatomy and the functions of each component of the brain.
3. Discuss the differences among CT scans, MRIs, and PET scans. What kind of information is provided by each?
4. What is the difference between a gap junction and a synapse?
5. What is meant by "second messengers"?
6. What is the potential impact of genetic discoveries on psychiatric disease?

*Study*WARE™ CONNECTION

Using your *Study*WARE™ CD-ROM

1. Complete the Concentration activity for this chapter.
2. Review the audio glossary for key terms in this chapter.
3. Explore the other games and activities that support this chapter.
4. Review the Animation: Firing of Neurotransmitters

REFERENCES

Barondes, S. H. (1999). *Molecules and mental illness.* New York: Scientific American Library.

Broderick, D. F. (2005). Neuroimaging in neuropsychiatry. *Psychiatric Clinics of North America, 28*(3), 549–566, 564.

Estes, M. E. (2010). *Health assessment and physical examination* (4th ed.). Clifton Park, NY: Delmar Cengage Learning.

Hess, W. (1949). The central control of the activity of internal organs. *Nobel Prize Lecture.* December, 12. Retrieved June 6, 2009, from http://nobelprize.org/nobel_prizes/medicine/laureates/1949/hess-lecture.html.

Kandel, E. (2006). *In search of memory: The emergence of a new science of mind.* New York: Norton.

Kandel, E. R., Schwartz, J. H., & Jessell, T. (1995). *Essentials of neural science and behavior.* Stamford, CT: Appleton & Lange.

Kandel, E. R., Schwartz, H., & Jessell, T. M. (Eds.). (2000). *Principles of neural science* (4th ed.). New York: McGraw-Hill/Appleton & Lange.

Konarski, J. Z., McIntyre, R. S., Soczynska, J. K., & Kennedy, S. H. (2007). Neuroimaging approaches in mood disorders: Technique and clinical implications. *Annals of Clinical Psychiatry, 19*(4), 265–277.

Malhi, G. S., & Lagopoulos, J. (2008). Making sense of neuroimaging in psychiatry. *Acta Psychiatrica Scandinavica, 117*(2), 100–117.

Nicoll, R. A., & Alger, B. E. (2004). The brain's own marijuana. *Scientific American, 291*(6), 68–75.

Reinagel, P. (2007). The inner life of bursts. *Neuron, 55*(3), 339–341.

Searle, J. R. (1995). The mystery of consciousness. *New York Review of Books, 42*(17), 60–67.

SUGGESTED READINGS

Damasio, A. R. (2000). *The feeling of what happens.* New York: Harvest Books.

Faracone, S. U., Tsuang, M. T., & Tsuang, D. W. (1999). *Genetics of mental disease.* London: Guilford.

Functional brain imaging: Twenty-first century phrenology in psychobiological advance for the millennium? (Editorial). (1999). *American Journal of Psychiatry, 156,* 671–673.

Hyman, S. E. (2000). The genetics of mental illness: Implications for practice. *Bulletin World Health Organization, 78*(4), 455–463.

Kandel, E. (2006). *In search of memory: The emergence of a new science of mind.* New York: Norton.

Leader, D. (2008). *The new black: Mourning, melancholia, and depression.* London: Hamish Hamilton.

LeDoux, J. E. (2000). Emotion circuits in the brain. *Annual Review of Neuroscience, 23,* 155–184.

Pinker, S. (1997). *How the mind works.* New York: Norton.

Siegel, D. J. (1999). *The developing mind: Toward a neurobiology of interpersonal experience.* New York: Guilford.

Siegel, D. J. (2001). *The developing mind: How relationships and the brain interact to shape we are.* New York: Guilford.

Synder, S. J., & Ferris, C. D. (2000). Novel neurotransmitters and their neuropsychiatric relevance. *American Journal of Psychiatry, 157*(11), 1738–1751.

Zeman, A. (2008). *A portrait of the brain.* New Haven, CT: Yale University Press.

LITERARY REFERENCE

Barondes, S. H. (1999). *Molecules and mental illness.* New York: Scientific American Library.

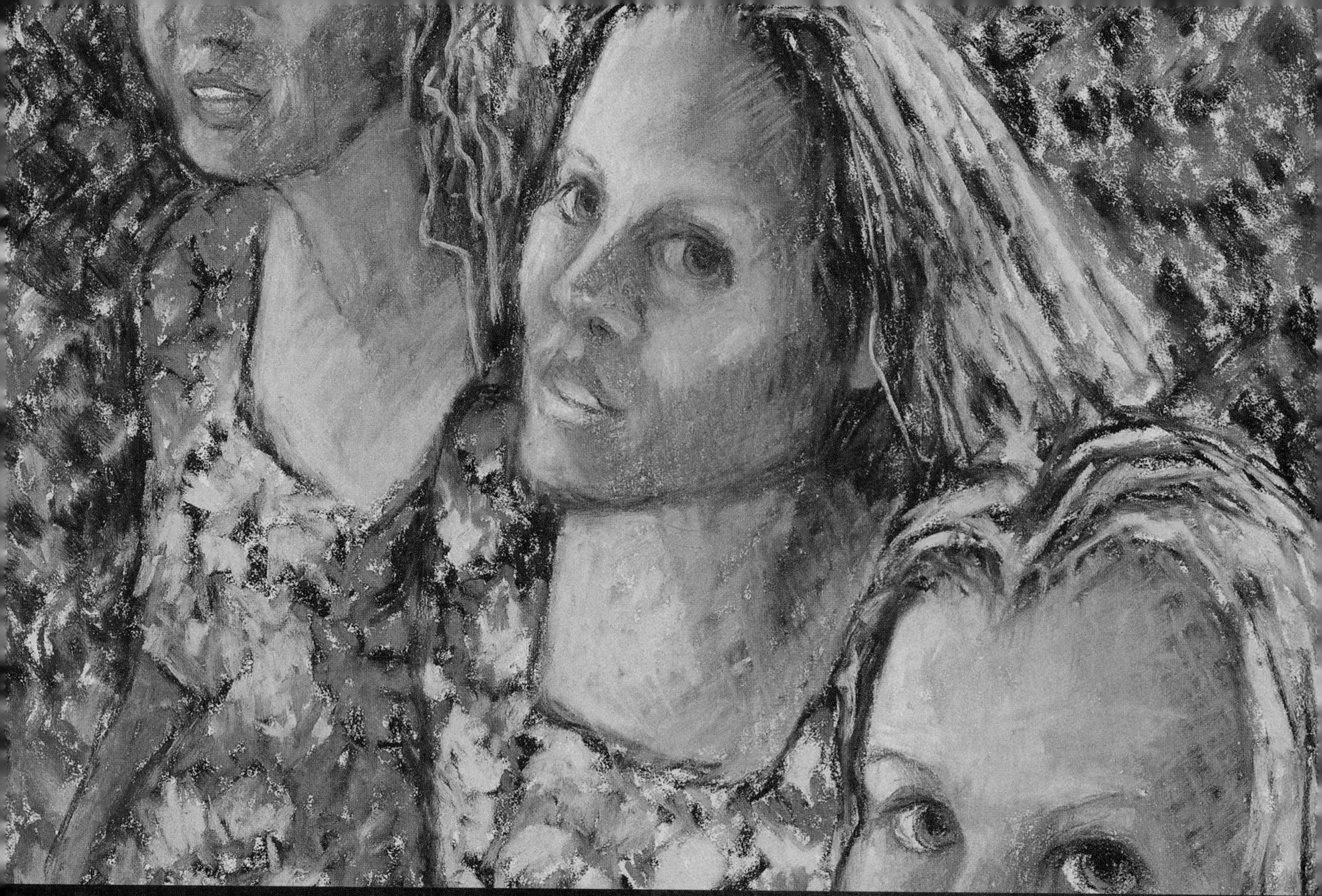

Variations on a Theme

What's in a Name?

Consider the following phrases:

- *Type 1 diabetes*
- *Carcinoma in situ*
- *Risk for infection*
- *Insomnia*
- *Upper respiratory infection*
- *Decreased cardiac output*
- *Major depressive disorder*

These words are labels that clearly identify certain signs, symptoms, or client conditions. For nurses, these labels bring to mind specific physiological, emotional, or environmental conditions.

- *Imagine if or how we could practice nursing without such language.*
- *Try to identify how you learned the language of health care professionals and how knowing that language affects your thinking and behavior.*

This chapter focuses on the languages used in psychiatric practice. Think about how our language affects communication and care.

CHAPTER 5

Diagnostic Systems for Psychiatric Nursing

Noreen Cavan Frisch
Lawrence E. Frisch

CHAPTER OUTLINE

COMPETENCIES

Upon completion of this chapter, the reader should be able to:

1. Define a diagnostic system and the meaning of a diagnostic taxonomy.
2. Explain the ICD system of medical diagnoses.
3. Explain the DSM diagnostic system, including the meaning of each axis.
4. Explain the use of the NANDA-I taxonomy in psychiatric mental health nursing.
5. Explain the use of the current *Nursing Interventions Classification*.
6. Describe how information systems affect psychiatric nursing care.

KEY TERMS

Classification
DSM-IV-TR
Health Insurance Portability and Accountability Act (HIPAA)
International Classification of Diseases (ICD)
International Classification of Nursing Practice (ICNP)
NANDA
Nursing Interventions Classification (NIC)
Nursing Minimum Data Set (NMDS)
Systematized Nomenclature of Medicine (SNOMED)
Unified Medical Language System (UMLS)

Fascination with naming and classifying has been part of human experience from earliest times. Noah was careful to include representatives of all animal species on his ark, and by Aristotle's time, the passion for categorization had reached seemingly modern proportions. Jorge Luis Borges seems gently amused by such human efforts to impose order on a stubbornly chaotic world. Borges invents a "comprehensive" classification of animals that he fancifully attributes to an ancient encyclopedia, the *Celestial Emporium of Benevolent Knowledge*. He offers his readers a selection from the *Emporium*:

CELESTIAL EMPORIUM

*On those remote pages it is written that animals are divided into (a) those that belong to the Emperor, (b) embalmed ones, (c) those that are trained, (d) suckling pigs, (e) mermaids, (f) fabulous ones, (g) stray dogs, (h) those that are included in this classification, (i) those that tremble as if they were mad, (j) innumerable ones, (k) those drawn with a very fine camel's hair brush, (l) other, (m) those that have just broken a flower vase, (n) those that resemble flies from a distance.**

(Borges, 1964, p. 103)

It doesn't take much effort to see that Borges's intriguingly imaginative categories are completely arbitrary: Category (h) adds no new animals to the list, whereas category (l) seems to add an exceedingly large number. And then there is the seeming irrelevance of flower vases and flies. At their core, are all classification schemes as absurd as the Celestial Emporium? Borges might wish us to think so, but few modern experts would agree. Good classification is not easy, and many categories are arbitrary, perhaps sometimes almost as arbitrary as the Celestial Emporium's. However, despite such shortcomings, classification has important uses in clinical practice, especially in psychiatric and mental health nursing.

Classification is a system of categorization that allows useful distinctions to be established, distinctions that may lead to deeper understanding of natural phenomena. Colors and shapes are part of the ways in which we perceive differences among persons and objects around us. These differences can be investigated further through observation and experiment. Assessing similarities and differences can help us understand the nature of objects and phenomena. For example, acute viral hepatitis, liver failure from isoniazid, and cirrhotic end-stage liver disease all share jaundice as a major manifestation. This jaundice identifies them each as diseases of the liver, but not all conditions resulting in jaundice are liver disease; in fact, hemolytic disease of the newborn is typically associated with profound jaundice in the presence of completely normal liver function. Increasingly sophisticated understanding of pathophysiology has allowed medical phenomena to be categorized in ways that bring out *differences* between superficially similar categories and *similarities* between conditions that superficially seem unrelated.

In recent years, the science of epidemiology has contributed greatly to such knowledge of health and illness. Epidemiology is the study of factors that lead to the occurrence of disease in a population of people. Epidemiological

*From *The Analytical Language of John Wilkins*, 1964, by Jorge Luis Borges, translated by Ruth L. C. Simmons. Austin: University of Texas Press.

investigation begins with a careful definition of clinical phenomena so that their incidence and prevalence can be compared between groups of individuals who differ in defined ways. While epidemiological investigations have given rise to many important insights into human health and illness, enthusiasm for classification and for the epidemiological approach to understanding human experience is not universal. Many modern scientists share Borges's mistrust of epidemiological methods based on categorization and description; they prefer to seek causes of phenomena in molecular and neurochemical processes that can be measured in the laboratory. Fortunately, the study of mental illness today benefits from both laboratory insights and insights that derive from classifications. Take, for example, Borges's category (i), "those that tremble as if they are mad": Some of these trembling animals in Borges's *Celestial Emporium* (the human ones, at least) may have hyperthyroidism, whereas others will have anxiety disorders (generalized, post-traumatic, panic, and phobias). There is much to be gained from establishing and steadily refining such categories.

This chapter discusses important formal categorizations relevant to psychiatric nursing practice, particularly the *International Classification of Diseases* (ICD), each associated with a unique numerical code; the *Diagnostic and Statistical Manual*, Fourth Edition-Text Revision (DSM-IV-TR), the NANDA International (NANDA) taxonomy, the *Nursing Interventions Classification* (NIC), and the *Nursing Outcomes Classification* (NOC). To illustrate each of these classification systems, Case Example 5-1 will be used. The reader will see that each of the diagnostic classification systems will provide a different view of Maria's case. Each system gives one a perspective from which to think and from which to plan Maria's care.

INTERNATIONAL CLASSIFICATION OF DISEASES (ICD)

The **ICD** is published by the World Health Organization and consists of a comprehensive listing of clinical diagnoses, each associated with a unique numerical code. Each revision of the ICD carries a new number, the ICD-9 (ninth revision) being currently used in the United States. The numerical codes of ICD resemble library book call numbers and serve to uniquely identify each of many possible physical and psychiatric diagnoses. ICD codes are most commonly three-digit numbers followed by a decimal point and a single digit. A typical ICD-9 code might be 296.2 (Major Depressive Disorder single episode). Similar disorders are grouped together so that similar-appearing codes usually refer to closely related conditions. For example, 296.2 and 296.3 are, respectively, Major Depressive Disorder—single episode and Major Depressive Disorder—recurrent. ICD utilizes codes so that diagnoses can be evaluated by computer and closely related diagnostic categories can be "lumped" for data analysis. Because ICD codes are so valuable for epidemiological analysis, it is very important that they be both specific and descriptive. There was strong feeling in the United States that the original ICD-9 codes were not fully applicable to American medicine and its specialist-oriented diagnostic categories. In consequence, soon after the release of ICD-9, the U.S. National Center for Health Statistics published a "clinical modification" of ICD-9 (ICD-9-CM). This modification added a fifth digit to many codes in order to accommodate more complex diagnostic codings. The four basic ICD digits

CASE EXAMPLE 5-1

Maria

Maria is a 28-year-old woman who has recently been divorced from her husband of 5 years. She has the history of one admission to a psychiatric hospital at age 22 years for depression and suicidal ideation. After that hospitalization, she was followed for 6 months of individual and group therapy. She works as a teller in a bank, where she has been employed for 7 years.

She is now seeking care in a mental health clinic because of feelings of severe depression, sadness, and inability to concentrate at work. She is having increasing trouble thinking of herself as independent; she states, "I can't handle life alone." She reports that her coping style had been such that her former husband would "take care of things" and "tell me what to do." She did not want the divorce and identifies the divorce as the event that precipitated her current state.

Past medical history indicates adult-onset asthma, which she controls with inhaled medication. Other medical history is unremarkable.

She lives alone, reports feeling isolated from others, and states she wishes she had more social contact with others. She has very few friends and has begun to experience conflicts with others at work because she isn't "doing her share." She has lost her appetite and doesn't prepare meals for herself at home. She has lost about 10 pounds over the past few weeks. Her parents are a source of support to her, but they live in the family home, about 2 hours' drive from the city in which Maria lives.

were unchanged so that ICD-9-CM is more detailed than its international predecessor but otherwise compatible. Despite the subsequent release of ICD-10 in 1992 and its widespread use in other countries including Canada, ICD-9-CM will remain the diagnostic standard in the United States until the release of ICD-11.

The ICD classification lists the name of the clinical condition, for example, Major Depressive Disorder, without further definitions of the diagnostic label. Therefore, as a coding system, ICD can be used to label a diagnosis but has limited ability to describe clinical symptoms such as sleep disturbances, laboratory abnormalities, or other nondiagnostic information (such as client lifestyle or social conditions such as homelessness). Current versions of ICD have been expanded to include health status, disability, and some clinical procedures. Despite these additions, ICD is strongest in the coding of diagnoses. Its primary scientific uses have been for epidemiological studies and tracking of illnesses. Insurance coverage and reimbursement for services are linked to ICD and all billed clinical services must be associated with an ICD diagnosis in order for a clinic or hospital to receive payment.

For Maria's case, the appropriate ICD-9 diagnosis would be Major Depressive Disorder—recurrent (296.3). Her asthma could be identified according to ICD-9 as well, with indication that her asthma is controlled at the present time.

DIAGNOSTIC AND STATISTICAL MANUAL FOR MENTAL DISORDERS (DSM)

The first version of a diagnostic classification for mental disorders, DSM, was published in 1952 as *Diagnostic and Statistical Manual: Mental Disorders.* DSM-IV, the fourth revision, appeared 42 years after its parent. The DSM is published by the American Psychiatric Association. The first version, now known as DSM-I, was adapted from the post-World War II edition of *International Classification of Diseases* (ICD-6), one of the first such classifications to include psychiatric diagnoses (American Psychiatric Association, 2000). The first version of DSM offered little guidance on making accurate and reproducible psychiatric diagnoses, as it was patterned after the model of ICD. The authors of DSM-I assumed that psychiatrists knew how to diagnose mental disorders and that no further guidance was necessary for diagnostic success. There was little real change between DSM-I and DSM-II, but by the time DSM-III was published in 1980, much had changed. DSM-III included explicit criteria for making psychiatric diagnoses, and these criteria have been increasingly validated by careful epidemiological study. Thus, DSM-III was the first classification system to clearly define the criteria needed to confirm a diagnosis. New to DSM-III was a multiaxial system that allowed developmental and other disorders to be considered along with psychiatric diagnoses of more recent onset. This axial system involves assessment of different domains that help the mental health clinician understand an individual client's situation and plan appropriate care. There are five axes:

- Axis I identifies clinical disorders.
- Axis II identifies personality disorders and conditions of mental retardation.
- Axis III identifies general medical conditions.
- Axis IV identifies psychosocial and environmental problems.
- Axis V identifies a global assessment of functioning.

In practice, the axial system facilitates comprehensive evaluation and provides a format for organizing clinical information and for describing the unique character of a client's condition. The axial system requires that the clinician evaluate all five domains and record information regarding each. The DSM manual clearly presents diagnostic criteria that must be met for a client to receive a diagnosis on Axis I or II. Axis III conditions, that is, general medical conditions, are diagnosed according to ICD-9. Axis IV is used for reporting psychosocial and environmental problems that may affect the diagnosis, treatment, and outcome of the mental disorders diagnosed on Axes I and II. For example, homelessness is a social and environmental problem that would undoubtedly affect the treatment of Major Depressive Disorder. Therefore, should the condition of homelessness exist, it would be documented in Axis IV. Axis V, the global assessment of functioning, is based on the clinician's judgment. DSM-IV provided the Global Assessment of Functioning (GAF) Scale, which suggests criteria for assigning points on a scale of 0 to 100. Table 5-1 presents the GAF Scale, so the reader may see how the numbers on Axis V are assigned.

For the case example of Maria, the DSM-IV diagnoses are listed in Box 5-1. The reader is encouraged to examine these diagnoses and to consider how the multiple axes provide comprehensive information. Compared to the ICD-9 diagnosis, it is clear that DSM-IV provides an expanded view of the client's situation.

In July 2000, the American Psychiatric Association updated DSM to **DSM-IV-TR**. The "TR" stands for "text revision" and emphasizes the incremental changes in the newest version. The TR version has not changed any of the diagnoses in DSM-IV or any criteria for making them, but it has changed some of the accompanying descriptions of diagnoses. Areas of most extensive revision in DSM-IV-TR include schizophrenia (with special emphasis on new knowledge derived from imaging studies and neuropsychological testing), autism, and alcohol-related disorders.

A very important advantage of DSM is the avoidance of controversies about what causes psychiatric conditions. Much of American and British psychiatry in the middle twentieth century had been dominated by psychoanalysis, and psychoanalytic theories of etiology were complex and rooted in subjective interpretations of reported memories, experiences, and dreams. The great achievement of DSM-III was to describe the *phenomena* of mental disorder without taking sides in the controversies of causation. This neutrality opened the way both for the widespread acceptance of DSM

TABLE 5-1 Global Assessment of Functioning Scale

Consider psychological, social, and occupational functioning on a hypothetical continuum of mental health–illness. Do not include impairment in functioning due to physical (or environmental) limitations.

Code	(**Note:** Use intermediate codes when appropriate, e.g., 45, 68, 72.)
91–100	**Superior functioning in a wide range of activities, life's problems never seem to get out of hand, is sought out by others because of his or her many positive qualities. No symptoms.**
81–90	**Absent or minimal symptoms** (e.g., mild anxiety before an exam), **good functioning in all areas, interested and involved in a wide range of activities, socially effective, generally satisfied with life, no more than everyday problems or concerns** (e.g., an occasional argument with family members).
71–80	**If symptoms are present, they are transient and expectable reactions to psychosocial stressors** (e.g., difficulty concentrating after family argument); **no more than slight impairment in social, occupational, or school functioning** (e.g., temporarily falling behind in schoolwork).
61–70	**Some mild symptoms** (e.g., depressed mood and mild insomnia) **OR some difficulty in social, occupational, or school functioning** (e.g., occasional truancy or theft within the household), **but generally functioning pretty well, has some meaningful interpersonal relationships.**
51–60	**Moderate symptoms** (e.g., flat affect and circumstantial speech, occasional panic attacks) **OR moderate difficulty in social, occupational, or school functioning** (e.g., few friends, conflicts with peers or co-workers).
41–50	**Severe symptoms** (e.g., suicidal ideation, severe obsessional rituals, frequent shoplifting) **OR any serious impairment in social, occupational, or school functioning** (e.g., no friends, unable to keep a job).
31–40	**Some impairment in reality testing or communication** (e.g., speech is at times illogical, obscure, or irrelevant) **OR major impairment in several areas, such as work or school, family relations, judgment, thinking, or mood** (e.g., depressed man avoids friends, neglects family, and is unable to work; child frequently beats up younger children, is defiant at home, and is failing at school).
21–30	**Behavior is considerably influenced by delusions or hallucinations OR serious impairment in communication or judgment** (e.g., sometimes incoherent, acts grossly inappropriately, suicidal preoccupation) **OR inability to function in almost all areas** (e.g., stays in bed all day; no job, home, or friends).
11–20	**Some danger of hurting self or others** (e.g., suicidal attempts without clear expectation of death; frequently violent; manic excitement) **OR occasionally fails to maintain minimal personal hygiene** (e.g., smears feces) **OR gross impairment in communication** (e.g., largely incoherent or mute).
1–10	**Persistent danger of severely hurting self or others** (e.g., recurrent violence) **OR persistent inability to maintain minimal personal hygiene OR serious suicidal act with clear expectation of death.**
0	**Inadequate information.**

Note: The rating of overall psychological functioning on a scale of 0–100 was operationalized by Luborsky in the Health-Sickness Rating Scale in "Clinicians' Judgments of Mental Health," by L. Luborsky, 1962, *Archives of General Psychiatry*, 7, pp. 407–417. Spitzer and colleagues developed a revision of the Health-Sickness Rating Scale called the Global Assessment Scale (GAS) in "The Global Assessment Scale: A Procedure for Measuring Overall Severity of Psychiatric Disturbance," by J. Endicott, R. L. Spitzer, J. L. Fleiss, and J. Cohen, 1976, *Archives of General Psychiatry*, 33, pp. 766–771. A modified version of the GAS was included in DSM-III-R as the Global Assessment of Functioning (GAF) Scale.

Source: Reprinted with permission from the *Diagnostic and Statistical Manual of Mental Disorders*, Fourth Edition-Text Revision, Copyright 2000, Washington, DC: American Psychiatric Association.

and for new, increasingly "biological" approaches to the understanding of mental illness.

DSM-IV-TR defines a set of general psychiatric diagnostic categories presented in the accompanying box. Within each of these categories is a group of psychiatric diagnoses, each typically characterized by explicit diagnostic criteria. The box on major depressive disorder is presented as an example of diagnostic criteria; it lists the criteria for major depressive disorder. For many DSM-IV diagnoses, there are more diagnostic criteria given than are necessary to make the diagnosis. This means that individuals with any given diagnosis may differ significantly in their clinical presentations. Some diagnoses have a set of *required* criteria followed by optional ones. In most cases, a number (usually the majority) of the optional criteria must be present for a diagnosis to be made. Some criteria are strongly influenced by culture and are said to apply only to some cultural groups and not necessarily to others.

BOX 5-1
DSM AXIAL DIAGNOSES FOR CASE EXAMPLE 5-1: MARIA

Client is a 28-year-old female:

- Axis I: 296.3 Major Depressive Disorder—recurrent
- Axis II: 301.6 Dependent Personality Disorder
- Axis III: asthma
- Axis IV: recent divorce
- AXIS V: GAF = 60

DSM-IV-TR is far from perfect—persons with mental disorders may not fit clearly into a diagnostic category and, at the same time, different DSM users may classify individuals in differing ways. These problems of diagnostic accuracy, reproducibility, sensitivity, and specificity are inherent in any clinical test used to separate individuals into categories. Despite its imperfections, DSM-IV-TR does offer a current language for mental health care. It provides a tested set of diagnostic criteria for common psychiatric disorders. It attempts to recognize the potential for cultural, gender, and other bias in assessment and diagnosis. DSM-IV-TR continues to be important to all mental health professionals. While not a substitute for clinical

BOX 5-2
GENERAL PSYCHIATRIC DIAGNOSTIC CATEGORIES OF DSM-IV-TR

- Disorders usually first diagnosed in infancy, childhood, or adolescence
- Delirium, dementia, amnestic, and other cognitive disorders
- Mental disorders due to a general medical condition
- Substance-related disorder
- Schizophrenia and other psychotic disorders
- Mood disorders
- Anxiety disorders
- Somatoform disorders
- Factitious disorders
- Dissociative disorders
- Sexual and gender identity disorders
- Eating disorders
- Sleep disorders
- Impulse-control disorders
- Adjustment disorders
- Personality disorders

NURSINGALERT 5-1

Cultural Sensitivity and DSM

The DSM manual alerts the clinician to carefully evaluate the nuances of each individual's cultural frame of reference whenever performing an assessment. The following factors constitute the information to be gathered as part of a culturally sensitive assessment:

- **Cultural identity of the individual**
- **Cultural explanations of the individual's illness**
- **Cultural factors related to psychosocial environment and levels of functioning**
- **Cultural elements of the relationship between the individual and the clinician**
- **Overall cultural assessment for diagnosis and care**

BOX 5-3
EXAMPLE OF DSM-IV-TR DIAGNOSTIC CRITERIA 296.3X MAJOR DEPRESSIVE DISORDER, RECURRENT

A. Presence of two or more Major Depressive Episodes.
Note: To be considered separate episodes, there must be an interval of at least 2 consecutive months in which criteria are not met for a Major Depressive Episode.
B. The Major Depressive Episodes are not better accounted for by Schizoaffective Disorder and are not superimposed on Schizophrenia, Schizophreniform Disorder, Delusional Disorder, or Psychotic Disorder Not Otherwise Specified.
C. There has never been a Manic Episode, a Mixed Episode, or a Hypomanic Episode.
Note: This exclusion does not apply if all of the manic-like, mixed-like, or hypomanic-like episodes are substance or treatment induced or are due to the direct physiological effects of a general medical condition.

Specify (for current or most recent episode):
Severity/Psychotic/Remission Specifiers Chronic
With Catatonic Features
With Melancholic Features
With Atypical Features
With Postpartum Onset

Specify:
Longitudinal Course Specifiers (With and Without Interepisode Recovery)
With Seasonal Pattern

REFLECTIVE THINKING 5-1

Pros and Cons of a Psychiatric Diagnostic System

Pros

- Observable behaviors are identified as necessary to make a diagnosis.
- Diagnoses are standardized and bias is removed.
- Practitioners are held accountable for language used.
- Records can be computerized.

Cons

- Human experience is reduced to a diagnostic label.
- Some clients will not easily fit into a predefined category.
- Some persons with differing presentations and differing needs will carry the same diagnosis.

Given the above:

- What do you think the nurse's role should be in using psychiatric diagnoses?
- Evaluate the use of DSM diagnoses in a clinical facility. What are the benefits you can observe?
- Can you identify an alternative to our current system?

judgment and diagnostic skill, DSM-IV-TR serves as the current "gold standard" for making mental health diagnoses. Few health care fields have such a gold standard, and for the foreseeable future, DSM makes a landmark contribution to progress in mental health care.

After three years of preliminary discussions, groups of psychiatrists began to meet formally in 2007 to plan the new DSM-V that is currently scheduled for release in May 2012. Some experts feel that the new version needs to move away from symptoms to a focus on brain structure (imaging) and function. Others argue for a shorter, less complex manual (Bell, Sowers, & Thompson, 2008). To date, there have been 13 international conferences held to work on the revisions and updates. In addition, there are workgroups of experts evaluating the strengths, problems, and currency of the DSM-IV (http://www.psych.org/dsmv.asp).

NANDA CLASSIFICATION OF NURSING DIAGNOSES

Most nurses are familiar with the **NANDA** nursing diagnoses. The term NANDA originally stood for the "North American Nursing Diagnosis Association." Over the years since its inception in the 1970s, NANDA became an increasingly international organization, extending far beyond North American boundaries. Eventually, NANDA became NANDA–I which stands for NANDA-International, a worldwide organization that is committed to development and support of nursing diagnoses that represent the totality of nursing's phenomena of concern. The NANDA classification has been developed and published by NANDA or NANDA-I and has been in general use in nursing for more than three decades. The NANDA classification can be used with DSM criteria to document nurse-specific concerns, or can be used as the sole method of documenting nurse-specific concerns related to the psychiatric mental health client. As published, the NANDA-I diagnoses list is a tool in naming and describing phenomena of concern to all nurses and in all of nursing's specialties. Nurses must recognize, however, that the list is a "work in progress." The current list, having more than 200 diagnoses, is always being reviewed, revised, and expanded (Herdman, 2009). Some authors question if the number of diagnoses is too limiting and suggest that these terms cannot fully represent all of the phenomena upon which nurses act (Muller-Straub, Lavin, Needham, & van Achterberg, 2006).

While the NANDA-I taxonomy is the most commonly used system of nursing diagnoses in the United States, nurses should know that there are other diagnostic systems developed for nursing practice. Through collaborative efforts of nurses internationally and under the auspices of the International Council of Nursing (ICN), there is an **International Classification of Nursing Practice (ICNP)** combining North American and other systems to develop a universal reference terminology for practice (Muller-Straub, Lavin, Needham & van Achterberg, 2007; Coenen, Marin, Park, & Bakken, 2001). Other nursing diagnostic systems exist as well, for example: the Saba system, the Omaha system, and the Perioperative Nursing Data Set. For purposes of this text, however, the NANDA-I taxonomy will be used to identify and name nursing concerns for the psychiatric mental health specialty.

History of NANDA

In 1973, a group of nurses met in St. Louis, Missouri, and organized the First National Conference for the Classification of Nursing Diagnoses. This meeting began a formal effort to develop a list of diagnoses that addressed the independent role of the professional nurse in client care. Nurses were acutely aware of the fact that without diagnoses to name the phenomena of concern specifically to nursing, the nurse's role in client care was largely identified as one of carrying out physician orders and working in collaboration with other health care professionals. Nurses observed that much of what we might call the "essence" of nursing remained undocumented and unnoticed. For example, a nurse understood that certain nursing care was considered critical in preparing a client for surgery (preoperative medications had to be given and vital signs needed to be taken and recorded), but the *caring* aspect of nursing was unnoticed and undocumented. In a hypothetical situation, a preoperative nurse might well assess that the client who is to receive the preoperative medications is anxious and/or fearful of the surgical procedure. Upon making a further assessment of the client's fear, the nurse might learn that the client is waiting for his aunt to arrive and that this aunt is the primary support person for the client. Before surgery, then, the nurse assesses that the client expresses anxiety and fear, is in a state of isolation from support persons, and wants to ask the nurse questions about the surgical procedure and outcome itself. These aspects of nursing care—*care* of the client experiencing anxiety, fear, sense of isolation, and need for information—would have been met by a professional nurse in the 1960s or 1970s (or earlier), but without a nursing language to communicate and document these aspects of care, they would very likely have gone unnoticed in the work setting.

In the 1970s, nurses began to recognize that without language to state the "essence" of nursing, such aspects of nursing care would be known and understood only by nurses. Further, nurses realized that without such language it would be difficult to communicate nursing knowledge about a client to another nurse. Thus, the group meeting in St. Louis began the process of naming that which "is" nursing for the purpose of giving nursing a language of its own.

REFLECTIVE THINKING 5-2

What Is Unnamed Is Unnoticed

Psychiatric nurse Wendy admits a client, Harold, to her unit at 2:00 A.M. Harold is depressed, with suicidal ideation. He has been homeless for about 6 weeks. He is fatigued, with no affect. He is in touch with reality. He was brought to the hospital for evaluation because the police found him wandering the city streets. He is crying and states he is at the "end of his rope." The psychiatrist's evaluation includes the DMS-IV-TR diagnosis of Major Depressive Episode with suicidal ideation.

Nurse Wendy assesses Harold during the night and determines that Harold is demonstrating the defining characteristics of the nursing diagnoses of *chronic low self-esteem*, *powerlessness*, and *disturbed sleep pattern*.

- **What if Wendy provides care for all three diagnoses but does not label and document the nursing diagnoses? Does that affect the care Wendy gives?**
- **Will her nursing care be valued more or less through such documentation?**
- **In the facility in which you work, is Wendy's care for above-noted nursing problems expected? Reinforced? How do you know?**

In 1974, Gebbie and Lavin identified four steps that they believed were necessary for the development of a classification system for nursing:

1. Identify all those things that nurses locate or diagnose in patients.
2. Reach some agreement about consistent language that can be used to describe the domain of nursing as identified in Step 1.
3. Group the identified diagnoses into classes and subclasses so that patterns and relationships among them can emerge.
4. Substitute numbers or abbreviations for the terminology that evolves so that data related to the various diagnoses can be assessed and manipulated easily.

In one way or another, each of these steps has been followed to devise the current NANDA-I list (NANDA-I, 2007).

There have been 16 biannual conferences on the development and classification of nursing diagnoses. The process for accepting new diagnoses has been refined over the years. Currently, there are written guidelines for the submission and review of diagnoses, and a new diagnosis is now accepted based on information presented formally to the Diagnosis Review Committee. Diagnoses are staged on the basis of how well developed they are, so that diagnoses reaching the third stage have research bases that document the relevance and applicability of the diagnoses to nursing practice.

Organization of the diagnoses was first proposed after a series of conferences with nurse theorists. After some time, the concept of human response patterns was adopted as a means of organizing the diagnoses. The human response patterns were used as a means of organizing or grouping a series of diagnoses, though not included in taxonomy II. Clearly, the notion of human response patterns was derived from the American Nurses Association's (1960) early definition of nursing as "the human response to actual or potential health problems," first introduced in the 1960s. This concept of the "human response" assisted nurses in their thinking about what nursing is and how nurses could identify that which was truly important in their work. In 2004, the nursing diagnoses were reclassified into a structure that is consistent with the National Library of Medicine's coding structure for health care terminologies. Later, the diagnoses were registered with Health Level Seven (HL-7) a health care informatics standard. Currently, the diagnoses are organized according to domains (spheres of activity), classes (subdivisions of the domains), and nursing diagnoses (NANDA-I, 2007). Box 5-4 lists the domains and classes.

There is currently a list of over 200 diagnoses that have been placed within the taxonomy under a domain. A NANDA-I diagnosis consists of a name (or diagnostic label), a definition, defining characteristics, and related factors. The definition is simply a statement of what the label means. The defining characteristics provide the observable criteria that must be present to make the diagnosis. For example, for the nursing diagnosis *hopelessness*, the definition is "a subjective state in which an individual sees limited or no alternatives or personal choices available and is unable to mobilize energy

BOX 5-4
DOMAINS AND CLASSES OF NURSING DIAGNOSES

FUNCTIONAL DOMAIN

- Activity/exercise
- Comfort
- Growth and Development
- Sexuality
- Sleep/rest
- Values/beliefs

PHYSIOLOGICAL DOMAIN

- Cardiac Function
- Elimination
- Fluid/electrolyte
- Neurocognition
- Pharmacological Function
- Physical Regulation
- Reproduction
- Respiratory Function
- Sensation/perception
- Tissue Integrity

PSYCHOSOCIAL DOMAIN

- Behavior
- Communication
- Coping
- Emotional
- Knowledge
- Roles/relationships
- Self-perception

ENVIRONMENTAL DOMAIN

- Health Care Systems
- Populations
- Risk Management

From *Nursing Diagnoses: Definitions and Classifications 2009–2011*, by H. Herdman (Ed.), Copyright 2009, Oxford: Wiley-Blackwell. Reprinted with permission.

on own behalf" (Herdman, 2009, p. 184). The defining characteristics include "passivity, decreased affect, and verbal cues (such as "I can't" and sighing), lack of involvement in care, lack of initiative, and decreased appetite (Herdman, 2009); for the nursing diagnosis of *chronic low self-esteem,* the definition is "long-standing negative self-evaluation/feelings about self or self-capabilities" (Herdman, 2009, p. 194) and defining characteristics include "evaluations of self as unable to deal with events; expressions of uselessness, expressions of helplessness, indecisive behavior, self-negating verbalizations, and nonassertive behaviors (Herdman, 2009). Diagnoses are staged on the basis of supporting evidence. Those with names, definitions, and risk or related factors are staged as level 1; those meeting level 1 criteria with the addition of references from the literature, consensus studies, and completed concept analyses are staged as level 2, and those with level 2 criteria with the addition of clinical validation studies are staged as level 3.

In examining the NANDA-I list, it is important to note that over half of the approved/accepted nursing diagnoses address nursing concerns in the psychosocial-spiritual realm of client care. This fact underscores that the essence of nursing has been defined over a 30-year period to include meeting the mental health, emotional, and spiritual needs of clients. Whether or not a nurse works in a psychiatric mental health setting, attention to these needs and concerns stands out as nursing's unique contribution and nursing's unique role.

The current NANDA-I list has several important features that advance the progress and support the use of nursing diagnoses. These include the use of seven axes that improve the flexibility and use of the diagnostic concepts. The seven axes of the NANDA-I list follow, with an example from psychiatric care (see Box 5-5). A nursing diagnosis is constructed by combining values from Axis 1 (concept) with Axis 2 (subject) and Axis 3 (the nursing judgment about the condition). In addition, the five other axes may be used for clarity and specificity. Axis 3 is the area where the nurse must use professional knowledge and skill to determine if the concept is limited or best described by a number of adjectives (for example, disturbed, dysfunctional, impaired, or ineffective). Nurses are cautioned that while the multiaxial system provides flexibility, diagnostic statements should be constructed on the basis of nursing knowledge, common sense, and ability to test and validate nursing's work (Herdman, 2009). To illustrate the use of axes in writing a diagnostic statement, Figure 5-1 provides the general relationship among the axes and Figure 5-2 provides an example for the diagnosis of *coping* at an individual level.

BOX 5-5
AXES OF NURSING DIAGNOSIS

1. The Diagnostic Concept (*sensory perception*)
2. Subject of the Diagnosis (individual)
3. Judgment (*disturbed* or *impaired*)
4. Location (*visual*)
5. Age (adult)
6. Time (intermittent)
7. Status of the Diagnosis (actual)

(Note: The diagnostic statement *intermittent impaired sensory perceptions (visual hallucinations)* could be written to provide clarity about the nurse's concerns; alternatively, the diagnostic statement could be written as *impaired sensory perceptions related to visual hallucinations, intermittent.)*

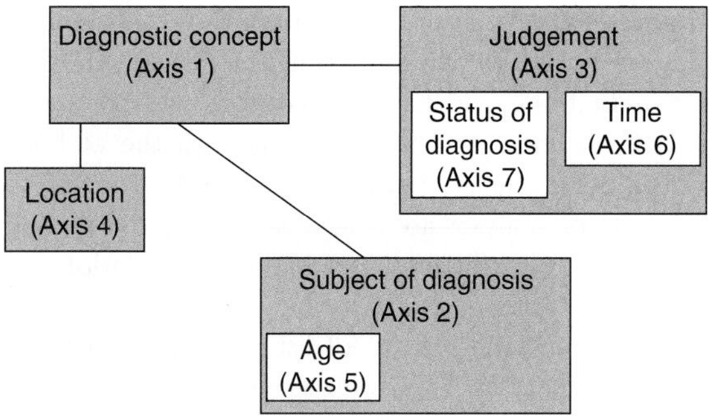

FIGURE 5-1 The NANDA-I Model of a Nursing Diagnosis. REPRINTED WITH PERMISSION FROM H. HERDMAN (ED.) (2009). NURSING DIAGNOSES: DEFINITIONS AND CLASSIFICATIONS 2009–2011. OXFORD: WILEY-BLACKWELL.)

In publishing the current NANDA-I taxonomy, a comprehensive effort was undertaken to identify and list diagnoses that had been developed to evidence criterion at level 2.0 and beyond so that listed nursing diagnoses had clearly developed definitions, defining characteristics, risk factors, related factors and references, as well as initial concept analyses and consensus studies. In addition, other diagnoses were included, but identified as those needing further development. One can easily applaud the rigor sought in the development and staging/listing of diagnoses. The result, however, poses some important challenges for nurses in the psychiatric mental health specialty. For example, the nursing diagnosis of *self-care deficit* that in previous editions of the NANDA list referred to situations where the client was unable to meet health-related goals is now on the NANDA-I list as a cluster of diagnoses quite specifically related to health care needs such as bathing/hygiene, toileting, grooming, and feeding. Nurses dealing with clients who experience thought disorders and/or suicidal ideations recognize immediately that these clients face deficits in their own self-care agency, and, thus, psychiatric nurses still need to make a diagnosis of *self-care deficit* to identify the nursing role in protection and supervision of these clients. Similar cases can be made for use of diagnostic concepts of *sleep patterns* and *thought processes.* Thus, psychiatric nurses, students, and their faculty can take the approach that any diagnostic concept as defined in Axis 1 can and should still be used coupled with the descriptor in Axis 3 to identify the real client need and nursing phenomena of concern in the context of psychiatric nursing as long as nursing knowledge and good judgment guide the nursing care plan. In turn, the use of these diagnoses in the psychiatric specialty need to be directed to the NANDA-I taxonomy committee for further consideration, revision, and updating of the current list. For purposes of this textbook, any nursing diagnostic concept appearing on the NANDA-I Axis 1 list is recommended for use, coupled with an Axis 3 descriptor that promotes clarity for use of the diagnosis in the context of the psychiatric mental heath specialty.

Box 5-6 lists the nursing diagnoses most likely to be used by the nurse in psychiatric mental health practice. Following that, Box 5-7 lists the Axis 3 descriptors to be used in nursing diagnostic statements (see also Chapter 6).

Returning to the case of Maria, use of nursing diagnoses provides a clear and concise statement of nurses' focus on her care. The accompanying box lists the NANDA diagnoses

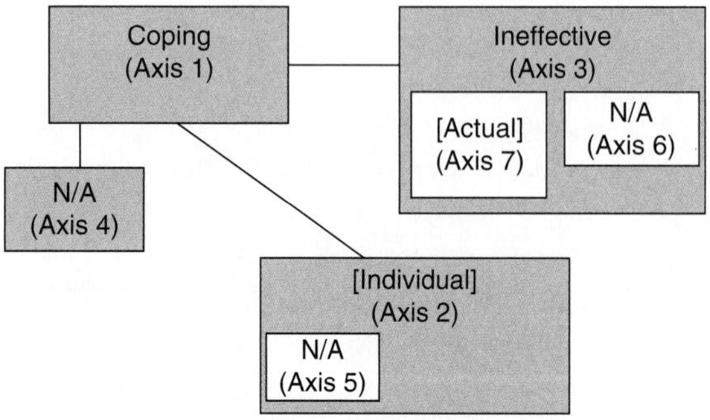

FIGURE 5-2 The NANDA-I Nursing Diagnosis Model: (Individual) Ineffective Coping. (REPRINTED WITH PERMISSION FROM H. HERDMAN (ED.) (2009). NURSING DIAGNOSES: DEFINITIONS AND CLASSIFICATIONS 2009–2011. OXFORD: WILEY-BLACKWELL.)

BOX 5-6
SELECTED NURSING DIAGNOSES FREQUENTLY USED IN PSYCHIATRIC MENTAL HEALTH CARE

- *Anxiety*
- *Body image*
- *Caregiver role strain*
- *Confusion*
- *Environmental interpretation syndrome*
- *Family processes*
- *Fear*
- *Hopelessness*
- *Loneliness*
- *Moral distress*
- *Personal identity*
- *Post-trauma syndrome*
- *Powerlessness*
- *Relocation stress syndrome*
- *Risk for injury*
- *Risk for violence*
- *Risk for self-mutilation*
- *Risk for suicide*
- *Self-care*
- *Self-esteem (chronic or situational)*
- *Sensory perception (hallucinations)*
- *Thought processes*
- *Verbal communication*

From *Nursing Diagnoses: Definitions and Classifications 2009–2011*, by H. Herdman (Ed.), Copyright 2009, Oxford: Wiley-Blackwell, Reprinted with permission.

BOX 5-7
AXIS 3 DESCRIPTORS REPRESENTING NURSING JUDGMENT ABOUT THE DIAGNOSTIC CONCEPT

anticipatory	enhanced
compromised	excessive
decreased	imbalanced
defensive	impaired
delayed	ineffective
disabled	interrupted
disorganized	low
disproportionate	organized
disturbed	perceived
dysfunctional	readiness for
effective	situational

From *Nursing Diagnoses: Definitions and Classifications 2009–2011*, by H. Herdman (Ed.), Copyright 2009, Oxford: Wiley-Blackwell, Reprinted with permission

BOX 5-8
NURSING DIAGNOSES FOR CASE EXAMPLE 5-1: MARIA

- *Social isolation*, related to absence of satisfying personal relationships, as evidenced by expressed feelings of loneliness and statements that she feels removed from others and wishes more social contacts
- *Chronic low self-esteem*, related to feelings that she cannot function on her own, as evidenced by self-negating verbalizations
- *Imbalanced nutrition: less than body requirements*, related to psychological factors, as evidenced by loss of appetite and recent weight loss

that could be made for Maria. Note that use of the NANDA list places emphasis on particular aspects of care (e.g., social isolation) that might not be addressed by using only the ICD or DSM labels.

CHOOSING A DIAGNOSTIC SYSTEM

A clear question that emerges from the information presented thus far is which diagnostic system a nurse should use. Table 5-2 presents the diagnoses made for the case example of Maria. One can see that each system provides a different perspective on Maria's care. Examine the table and reflect on how each system allows the nurse to document and think about the client's condition.

REFLECTIVE THINKING 5-3

Are Nursing Diagnoses Useful?

Consider the following comments, made by experienced nurses:

- "I work in a home health agency following mental health clients. We only get paid for what we can document by ICD-9 codes. I don't use nursing diagnoses because it only takes up my time and doesn't help us with reimbursement."
- "I work in psychiatric home health care, too. I do much more than provide care based on medical problems described in ICD. When I document that my client has hopelessness, I remind myself and others to care for the whole person and to provide true nursing care."
- "I'm a holistic nurse, and I think diagnosis is putting labels on real people; it reduces human experience to a title. I don't make any diagnoses."
- "I'm a member of NANDA, and I joined the organization to promote the development of diagnoses. I think nurses need to identify what they do that is nursing's unique contribution to care."
- "I'm a psychiatric nurse, and I need to communicate with other mental health professionals—DSM-IV is our common language. I have no use for nursing diagnoses."
- "At the mental health clinic where I work, the focus is on outcome of care. We are developing critical pathways and care maps that identify what must be done within a certain amount of time. Nursing diagnoses aren't needed, because we only care about outcome of care."
- "My hospital administrator said we don't need the number of registered nurses we have because the tasks of care can be provided by psychiatric technicians."

Each of these comments represents a different perspective on the use and benefit of nursing diagnoses. In many discussions with nurses across the country, the authors have heard nurses making such comments.

- What do you think affects the use of nursing diagnoses? The decisions to use or not use them?
- Describe how the use of nursing diagnoses can both help and hinder professional nursing.

In many settings, the psychiatric nurse uses the DSM-IV-TR diagnoses because the clinical setting requires that

Table 5-2 Diagnoses from Three Systems for Case Example 5-1: Maria

ICD-9	DSM-IV	NANDA
Major Depressive Disorder, Recurrent Asthma, controlled	Axis I: Major Depressive Disorder, Recurrent Axis II: Dependent Personality Disorder Axis III: asthma Axis IV: recent divorce Axis V: GAF = 60	*Social Isolation* *Chronic Low Self-esteem* *Imbalanced Nutrition: Less Than Body Requirements*

care be documented by all care providers in the same manner. Because DSM was developed for use by all mental health workers, nurses certainly find that it is a useful means of identifying client problems and planning appropriate care. However, the DSM-IV-TR diagnoses do not take into account all of the activities that may be specific to nursing, for example, assistance with self-care deficit or interventions directed at enhancing client communication. The nursing classifications are clearly more specific to the realm of what a nurse actually assesses and does.

In making a decision about which classification system to use, the nurse must remember that each of these systems was developed with one major purpose in mind: Any classification system should facilitate understanding and enhance communication about its content area. If we are to enhance communication between nurses, the NANDA-I system is helpful, simply because diagnoses are discipline specific and advance communication within the discipline. If we are to enhance communication among nurses, psychologists, psychiatrists, and psychiatric social workers, the DSM system is the common language. If we are to enhance communication between the psychiatric nurse and a medical internist who is called in to evaluate a physically ill client, the ICD-9 diagnoses are clearly appropriate. Advice from the authors is to use each of these diagnostic systems as tools to enhance communication and understanding. Practicality of current health care reimbursement systems has dictated that, in many instances, ICD-9 must be used in order to establish diagnoses and document care consistent with the diagnosis to gain reimbursement for care. A nurse must gain an appreciation for each of the diagnostic systems and use the tool or tools that are most effective to accomplish nursing's work. Further, institutional requirements may dictate that a nurse use, for example, the ICD-9 system simply because that system is clearly linked to reimbursement.

Throughout this text, the authors have presented information from both the DSM-IV-TR and the NANDA-I classifications. DSM-IV-TR is of major importance in understanding psychiatric diagnoses for clients who are admitted into care. The NANDA-I diagnoses have been used to identify the part of care that is unique to nursing. It is hoped that the case studies presented using NANDA-I diagnoses will assist the nurse who is already familiar with nursing diagnoses to move her practice into the specialty of psychiatric mental health nursing.

NURSING INTERVENTIONS NURSING OUTCOMES CLASSIFICATIONS

A discussion of classification systems in a nursing text is not complete without reference to the ***Nursing Interventions Classification*** (NIC). First published in 1992, the NIC is a list of nursing interventions. The purpose of such a classification is to identify and document those activities that nurses carry out to assist client status or behavior. The widespread use of the nursing diagnostic language has increased nurses' awareness of the need for standardized classifications of nursing activities (Dochterman & Bulechek, 2004), for if nurses can identify those situations for which nursing care is needed, the next step is to clearly define what nurses actually do in providing that care.

The current NIC is the fifth edition, and there are 542 interventions on this list (Bulechek, Butcher, & Dochterman, 2008). This list serves as a public statement that the activities described are widely accepted within the nursing profession as being within the domain of nursing practice. Further, the NIC provides the standardized language for nurses to use when researching which interventions are most likely to produce positive outcomes in particular client situations.

Of interest to psychiatric nurses is the wide range of nursing interventions dealing with psychosocial interventions with clients. A selection of these are in Box 5-9. Of note as well is that the Society for Education and Research in Psychiatric-Mental Health Nursing is one of the many nurse specialty groups that participated in the development and validation of the NIC. The NIC itself provides the reader with the name of the nursing intervention, its definition, and

BOX 5-9
SELECTED NURSING INTERVENTIONS ADDRESSING PSYCHOSOCIAL NEEDS

- Active listening
- Anger control assistance
- Anxiety reduction
- Assertiveness training
- Behavior management
- Body image enhancement
- Caregiver support
- Communication enhancement
- Delusion management
- Eating disorders management
- Grief work facilitation
- Hallucination management
- Impulse control training
- Milieu therapy
- Mood management
- Patients' rights protection
- Role enhancement
- Sleep enhancement
- Smoking cessation assistance
- Spiritual support
- Substance abuse: prevention and treatment
- Suicide prevention
- Teaching

the nursing activities involved in carrying out the nursing care (Bulechek et al., 2008).

In addition to this work on nursing interventions, a research team at the University of Iowa has developed a classification of patient outcomes sensitive to nursing treatment. The Nursing Outcomes Classification (NOC) provides another tool to assist nurses to relate three aspects of nurses' work: diagnosis, interventions, and outcomes. The current classification, now in its fourth edition, is a list of 385 outcomes with definitions, indicators, and measurement scales. Outcomes are for use at individual, family, and community/population levels. There are seven domains used to categorize the outcomes on the list. Domain III—Psychosocial Health describes outcomes related to psychological and social functioning. For example, nursing outcomes describing emotional health (body image, depression, mood), psychosocial adaptation (coping, adjustment), self-control (abusive behavior, aggression, impulse control), and social interaction (role performance, social involvement, social support) are listed under this domain and are of specific relevance to psychiatric mental health nurses (Moorhead, Johnson, Maas, & Swanson, 2008).

DIAGNOSTIC SYSTEMS AND COMPUTERIZED HEALTH RECORDS

Several important developments promise to significantly affect diagnostic practice during the next century and will likely have an impact on the practice of mental health nursing. First, there is an increased interest in computerized health records. Computerized records permit documentation of diagnoses and outcomes of care, permit epidemiological evaluation of populations, and facilitate the management of care based on data. All computerized records require use of a diagnostic or classification system coded in a manner that allows one to trace diagnoses knowing that the diagnoses have been made using clear criteria. Computerized records will make use of one or all of the diagnostic and classification systems described earlier. Further, currently work is being completed that attempts to link all of these systems together, both for use in computerized records and for use in a universal medical/health care database that will allow a comprehensive literature search to obtain current information on any condition. Some highlights of this work are summarized in the following discussion.

In 1991, the U.S. Institute of Medicine released its landmark report strongly endorsing the universal adoption of computerized patient records in health care (Dick & Steen, 1991). The institute's report highlighted numerous deficiencies in U.S. health care that directly or indirectly derived from the inefficiencies of paper-based records systems. These included the frequent unavailability of records either within a single institution or between health care institutions. This unavailability results in unnecessary delays, costly and unneeded repetition of tests when data are inaccessible, complete loss of important information, and inability to provide appropriate coordination and continuity of care.

Preventive health care (such as immunizations or Pap smears) is difficult to trace and document in cumbersome paper records and, following the course of chronic physical or mental illness, is frequently impossible. The American population at the century's beginning is characterized both by high mobility and by an increasingly large numbers of elderly. Paper-based records cannot easily be transferred as individuals move, and health care documentation becomes complex for an aging population due to the greater number of health problems identified in this population. Both of these factors add to the urgency of finding automated record-keeping solutions. As the institute report observed, technology to implement automated records has been available at least since the 1980s. Missing have been leadership, motivation, and an adequate set of diagnostic and coding standards to incorporate into new records systems. Since *managing* care requires hard data, the dramatic growth of managed-care organizations has increased motivation for automated records.

Widespread adoption of computerized clinical records will likely come within the first decade of the twenty-first century, and most readers of this text will find their professional lives much influenced by automated records systems. For this reason, important definitions and issues are described next.

Information systems are typically computer-based systems used by managers to assess the efficiency or effectiveness of their activities and to increase their strategic advantage in a competitive market. Hospital information systems may be used to optimize patient flow, length of stay, reimbursement, staffing, and resource utilization. These types of information systems are typically regarded as management investment, and their goal is to reduce costs or increase revenue.

Computer-based records are systems for recording and storing on computers important aspects of the clinical encounter. These systems may be as "simple" as scanning existing records and storing them as images on large computer discs. Such storage increases availability, ensures that multiple users can access records when needed, and usually prevents loss or tampering. Imaging of records does not allow easy searching for data, does not improve problems of readability, and does not allow data to be readily graphed or otherwise presented in useful summary form. But because such imaging solves some of the problems of paper records, it is being adopted as an interim system by many hospitals and medical centers.

True computer-based patient records utilize direct data entry, often by the primary caretaker at the point of service. For example, nurses will often use computers on a ward, or even in a client's home, to enter data about the individual's course and care. In some systems, data may be dictated or entered as "free-text" narrative, but in most applications, the care provider enters discrete information (most often specific observations, diagnoses, or interventions). These are then coded and stored for later display or analysis. In most cases, preexisting coding schemes such as ICD or NIC are used to classify diagnoses or interventions. When the automated record is used both in the hospital and in primary care practice, it is sometimes referred to as the computer-based *health* record to reflect its more general basis. The principles remain the same: structured data entry based on diagnostic and procedural coding, longitudinal record-keeping throughout an individual's lifetime, and widespread access for authorized users in multiple settings.

Issues of Privacy and Confidentiality

Clearly, such widespread access to health records raises important issues of confidentiality and privacy. Clients are currently concerned about the privacy of their records, particularly when these reflect some of the highly sensitive personal disclosures that may occur in mental health and psychiatric practice. Inappropriate disclosure of medical or psychiatric data may threaten individuals' employment, community status, or general future prospects. Inappropriate disclosure may occur when data are shared for reasons other than a client's personal interest or the protection of others, and, of course, any disclosure without the client's consent is inappropriate. Issues of privacy and confidentiality are being addressed by experts who are designing systems with password-protected access to records and strictly enforced policies regarding access and use of information.

In 1996, Congress passed the **Health Insurance Portability and Accountability Act (HIPAA)**, which explicitly required that medical record privacy legislation be passed within 3 years. Subsequently, Congress failed to enact the legislation within the 3-year time frame, so the 1996 law required the federal Department of Health and Human Services (HHS) to issue regulations for medical record privacy. Such regulations were first announced in October 1999, opening a national debate on how matters of privacy could and would be addressed. Initially, the HHS regulations were controversial and misunderstood by many. The "final" rules for medical record privacy were announced by President Bill Clinton on the last days of his administration, and President George W. Bush postponed their implementation for 60 days (Lehman, 2001). These rules addressed privacy of all records, both paper and electronic. The regulations required health care institutions to develop systems for training staff and for implementing privacy protections. After considerable discussion and review, the HIPAA regulations were amended and fully implemented in April 2003. The American Psychiatric Association was generally supportive of the provisions of HIPAA, noting that psychiatric records contain exceedingly private information, but it expressed concerns over provisions for consent that might preclude meaningful consents for all uses of information (Lehman, 2001). The regulations do include a provision for client consent to release medical information and a separate client authorization to release psychotherapy notes. Originally, the rules required separate forms for consent to release information for treatment, payment, or peer review and for authorization to release information for all other disclosures, including requests for client records to be disclosed to the client's attorney (American Psychiatric Association, 2002). However, an amendment to the original rule permits consent for disclosure for treatment, payment, and health care operations, which is implied by the client's willingness to begin treatment.

Nurses should recognize that the area of confidentiality and privacy in practice is an important one in which there will be changes over the next few years. It is hoped the end result will truly be better protection of privacy, and at the same time, the continuing ability to appropriately use clinical data for research that enhances our understanding of illness and its optimal management.

Diagnostic Coding

The primary focus of diagnostic coding is to ensure that all descriptions make maximum use of a "controlled vocabulary." A controlled vocabulary means the use of words that have well-established descriptive and diagnostic meaning. Readers of this text will recognize that *depression,* while a useful informal clinical term, is not a DSM-IV-TR concept. DSM-IV-TR refers to mood disorders, depressive symptoms, and depressive disorders, but it does not formally use the term *depression*. The goal of diagnostic coding is to ensure that clinical encounters can be described using controlled (and hence codeable) terms.

ADVANCES IN DIAGNOSTIC NOMENCLATURE

Over the years there have been major developments in coding and computer tools for organizing clinical terms and codes. These developments are complex and beyond the scope of this text; however, three ideas merit mention. The **UMLS** is the **Unified Medical Language System** that has been developed by the national Medical Library (Humphreys, 1994). The core of UMLS is a "Metathesaurus," a listing on CD-ROM of all terms included in existing taxonomies. Terms from the ICD, DSM, NANDA list, and NIC are included. The purpose of UMLS is to organize codes into a semantic network so terms can be linked and relationships identified. Since its inception, the UMLS has grown steadily and now it is the largest existing collection of medical terms containing over 1.3 million concepts derived from more than 100 databases (Chen, Perl, Geller, & Cimino, 2007). A use of the UMLS, for example, would be to link terms such as *Major Depressive Disorder* to terms such as *hopelessness* and *powerlessness*, so that one could ultimately evaluate in what situations (or in how many cases) individuals diagnosed with Major Depressive Disorder are also treated by nurses for the condition of *hopelessness*. In another example, a medical diagnosis such as "cancer" could be linked to the nursing diagnosis of *powerlessness* to further study and evaluate the nursing contribution to a particular aspect of client care.

A related effort is called **SNOMED**, the **Systematized Nomenclature of Medicine** (Henry, Holzemer, Reilly, & Campbell, 1994), now retitled to Systematized Nomenclature of Medicine Clinical Terms (SNOMED-CT; Giannangelo, 2006). SNOMED is a coding system that is far more inclusive than ICD-9, as it includes nursing diagnoses and nursing interventions as well as multiple axes that identify causative factors of illness and related functional deficits and social factors. To one way of thinking, SNOMED is a system that patterns ICD after the axial system in DSM and includes nursing taxonomies as well. In 2006, SNOMED was identified as a preferred terminology in electronic health care records (Giannangelo, 2006). SNOMED is designed to capture clinical information "behind the scenes" for use in computerized health care records. Incorporation of SNOMED into the UMLS system, along with NANDA, NIC, and NOC, which it contains, has become the de facto diagnostic language for U.S. health care.

Lastly, nurses should be aware that there is a recognized **Nursing Minimum Data Set (NMDS)** that identifies the minimum information necessary to meet information demands of nursing practice (Werley & Lang, 1988). Box 5-10 lists the items originally included in the NMDS. This list is nursing's attempt to clarify the factors that must be recorded to show nursing's contributions to client care. For all practical purposes, the NMDS has not changed since its inception. In 2006, Delany reported that the key elements and the definitions had not changed, however there is a committee in the United States that is discussing possible revisions (Helper, 2006). Currently, the NMDS is driving data collection and is being used in the United States, Canada, and a number of other countries including Thailand, Belgium, and Switzerland

REFLECTIVE THINKING 5-4

Where Will Nursing Be in an Era of Computerized Records?

If computerized records do not include nursing classification systems:

- Will professional nursing be needed?
- Who will notice if nursing care is provided or not?

If computerized records do include nursing classification systems:

- Are nurses ready to measure outcomes of care based on defined categories of diagnoses?
- Are nurses ready to be accountable for measuring the outcomes of their care?

BOX 5-10
ELEMENTS IN THE NMDS

1. NMDS: identifies the minimum set of data items necessary to meet information demands of nursing practice
2. Nursing care items
   - Nursing diagnosis
   - Nursing interventions
   - Nursing outcomes
   - Intensity of care
3. Client demographics
   - Personal identification
   - Date of birth
   - Sex
   - Race or ethnicity
   - Residence
4. Service time
   - Unique facility or service agency number
   - Health record number
   - Registered nurse provider number
   - Episode admission or encounter date
   - Discharge or termination date
   - Disposition of client
   - Expected payer of bill

From *Identification of the Nursing Minimum Data Set*, edited by H. Werley and H. Lang, Copyright 1988, New York: Springer. Reprinted with Permission.

(Helper, 2006). For psychiatric nurses, use of the NMDS on computerized records permits evaluation of the unique aspects of care provided under a strictly nursing model.

If psychiatric nurses choose to document their care under a DSM model, nursing's contributions become incorporated into a larger set of contributions made by all mental health professionals. While there may be benefits to this interdisciplinary approach, some are concerned that nursing could be undervalued by systems that do not identify nursing. Over the next decade, the challenges facing psychiatric nursing will be threefold: providing the best care possible; documenting and evaluating that care; and maintaining a presence amidst computerized systems so that nursing contributions can be noticed, valued, and remunerated.

KEY CONCEPTS

- Classification systems provide language by which to define, describe, and record phenomena and allow health professionals to document the differences and similarities between conditions.
- ICD is a classification system of medical diagnoses. The coding of ICD-9 permits computerized data entry and tracking.
- DSM defines mental disorders and is multiaxial, allowing the classification system to take several domains into account.
- The NANDA taxonomy is a listing of phenomena of concern to nursing and permits one to identify client concerns as nursing diagnoses.
- The NIC is a classification of nursing interventions.
- DSM, NANDA, and NIC all have use in psychiatric mental health nursing practice.
- Evolving information systems that will ultimately track nursing diagnoses, interventions, and outcomes are based on the classification and coding systems that can be computerized and will influence how care is delivered, documented, evaluated, and reimbursed.

REVIEW QUESTIONS

1. A client is admitted to the psychiatric unit with a diagnosis of major depression. An assessment revealed that the client has lost more than 30 pounds in the last month and has not had any interaction with friends since the death of her mother. Laboratory results reveal that the client is severely anemic. The nursing student assigned to the client is developing a care plan that would identify which domain of the nursing diagnosis as priority?
   1. Comfort
   2. Nutrition
   3. Health promotion
   4. Growth and Development

2. A nursing student is assigned to a client who is interested in learning about strategies to prevent developing cancer. Together they develop a teaching plan and strategies that will address the client's lack of knowledge regarding cancer prevention. A priority nursing diagnosis for this client would involve which domain?
   1. Comfort
   2. Nutrition
   3. Health promotion
   4. Growth and Development

3. A nurse working in a pediatric outpatient clinic assesses that a toddler has not achieved certain milestones as identified by Erick Erikson. A priority nursing diagnosis would most likely be in which of the following domains?
   1. Comfort
   2. Nutrition
   3. Health promotion
   4. Growth and Development

4. A nurse newly hired for a position on a psychiatric nursing unit wants to understand the major characteristics of the different types of schizophrenia. When she asks the nurse manager for possible resource, which response by the manager would be most appropriate?
   1. "Just read the charts of the clients admitted with schizophrenia."
   2. "You should be familiar with the types of schizophrenia from your psychiatric nursing course."
   3. "The best resource would be to review the *Diagnostic and Statistical Manual*, 4th edition (DSM-IV-TR) published by the American Psychiatric Association."
   4. "A good reference source for you to review is the Nursing Outcomes Classification (NOC) System."

5. A nurse begins to discuss a client's diagnosis and prognosis in front of family members of another client. The nurse is in violation of which of the following?
   1. Nurse Training Act
   2. Mental Health Fair Treatment Act
   3. Community Mental Health Centers Act
   4. Health Insurance Portability and Accountability Act

6. A nursing instructor requests that each student develop nursing interventions that will appropriately meet the needs of their assigned clients. It would be most helpful for the students to review which of the following documents once they have identified their nursing diagnoses?
   1. NIC
   2. NOC
   3. NANDA
   4. DSM-IV-TR

7. A nurse who recently transferred to the mental health unit of her hospital has been assigned to develop the care for a client recently admitted. When deciding on appropriate outcomes the nurse should focus on the nursing diagnosis that she identified and review which of the following?
   1. NIC
   2. NOC
   3. NANDA
   4. DSM-IV-TR

LEARNING ACTIVITIES

1. Examine three client records in a psychiatric mental health facility. Look for DSM diagnoses and explain the axial system and what information is provided.
2. Choose appropriate NANDA diagnoses for the same three clients. Write these nursing diagnoses, including the diagnostic statement with a "related to" clause.
3. Compare the information and nursing care planned on the basis of the DSM and NANDA diagnoses assigned for the same three clients.
4. Examine the use of coding systems in the psychiatric mental health facility. Inquire whether computerized records are being used or planned for use. Explain reasons behind the answer you receive.

*Study*WARE™ CONNECTION

Using your *Study*WARE™ CD-ROM

1. Complete the Concentration activity for this chapter.
2. Review the audio glossary for key terms in this chapter.
3. Explore the other games and activities that support this chapter.

REFERENCES

American Nurses Association (ANA). (1960). *A social policy statement.* Kansas City, MO: Author.

American Psychiatric Association. (2000). *Diagnostic and statistical manual* (4th ed.-TR). Washington, DC: Author.

American Psychiatric Association (Ed.) (2002). More on the privacy rule. *Psychiatric News, 37*(3), 24.

American Psychiatric Association. Retrieved July 2008, from http://www.psych.org/dsmv.asp.

Bakken, S., Warren, J. J., Lundberg, C., Casey, C., Konicek, D., & Zingo, C. (2002). An evaluation of the usefulness of two terminology models for integrating nursing diagnostic concepts into SNOMED clinical terms. *International Journal of Medical Informatics, 68,* 71–78.

Bell, C. C., Sowers, W., & Thompson, K. S. (2008). American Association of Community Psychiatrists' views on general features of DSM-IV. *Psychiatric Services, 59*(6), 687–689.

Bulechek, G. M., Butcher, H., & Dochterman, J. M. (2008). *Nursing interventions classification* (5th ed.). St. Louis: Mosby.

Chen, Y., Perl, Y., Geller, J., & Cimino, J. (2007). Analysis of a study of users, uses and future agenda of the UMLS. *Journal of the American Informatics Association, 14*(2), 221–231.

Coenen, A., Marin, H. F., Park, H., & Bakken, S. (2001). Collaborative efforts for representing nursing concepts in computer-based systems: International perspectives. *Journal of the American Medical Informatics Association, 8*(3), 202–211.

Dick, R. S., & Steen, E. B. (Eds.). (1991). *The computer-based patient record: An essential technology for health care.* Washington, DC: National Academy Press.

Dochterman, J. M., & Bulechek, G. M. (2004). *Nursing interventions classification (NIC)* (4th ed.). St. Louis: Mosby.

Gebbie, K., & Lavin, M. A. (1974). Classifying nursing diagnoses. *American Journal of Nursing, 74,* 250–253.

Giannangelo, K. (2006). Making the connection between standard terminologies, use cases and mapping. *Health Information Management Journal, 25*(3), 8–12.

Helper, A. (2006). Interview: Data element – Nursing Minimum Data Set (NMDS). *Online Journal of Nursing Informatics, 10*(3). 3p. Item number: 2009508886.

Henry, S. B., Holzemer, W. L., Reilly, C. A., & Campbell, K. E. (1994). Terms used by nurses to describe patient problems: Can SNOMED III represent nursing concepts in the patient record? *Journal of the American Medical Informatics Association, 1,* 61–74.

Herdman, H. (Ed). (2009). *Nursing diagnosis: Definitions and classifications: 2009–2011.* Oxford: Wiley-Blackwell.

Humphreys, B. L. (Ed.). (1994). *UMLS knowledge sources: Fifth experimental edition documentation.* Bethesda, MD: National Library of Medicine.

Lehman, C. (2001). APA leaders deliver mixed verdict on federal patient-privacy regulations. *Psychiatric News, 36*(3), 1.

McCloskey, J., & Bulechek, G. M. (2000). *Nursing interventions classification (NIC)*, 3rd ed. St. Louis: Mosby.

Moorhead, S., Johnson, M., Maas, M., & Swanson, E. (2008). *Nursing Outcomes Classification (NOC)* (4th ed.). St Louis: Mosby.

Muller-Straub, M., Lavin, M. A., Needham, I., & van Achterberg, T. (2007). Meeting the criteria of a nursing diagnosis classification: Evaluation of ICNP, ICF, NANDA, & ZEFP. *International Journal of Nursing Studies. 44*(5), 702–713.

Muller-Straub, M., Lavin, M. A., Needham, I., & van Achterberg, T. (2006). Nursing diagnosis, interventions and outcome—application and impact on nursing practice: Systematic review. *Journal of Advanced Nursing, 56*(5), 514–531.

North American Nursing Diagnosis Association. (2009). *NANDA-I nursing diagnoses: definitions and classifications 2009–2011.* Indianapolis, IN: Wiley-Blackwell.

U.S. Department of Health and Human Services. (1994). *International classification of diseases (ICD-9-CM)*. (DHHS Publication No. PHS94-1260). Rockville, MD: Author.

Werley, H., & Lang, H. (Eds.). (1988). *Identification of the nursing minimum data set.* New York: Springer.

LITERARY REFERENCES

Borges, J. L. (1964). The Analytical Language of John Wilkins, pp. 101–105 in *Other Inquisitions, 1937–1952.* trans. Ruth L.C. Simms, Austin: University of Texas Press.

SUGGESTED READINGS

Bowker, G. C., and Star, S. L. (1999). *Sorting things out: Classification and its consequences.* Cambridge: MIT Press.

Giannangelo K. (Ed.). (2006). *Healthcare code sets, clinical terminologies, and classification systems.* Chicago: AHIMA.

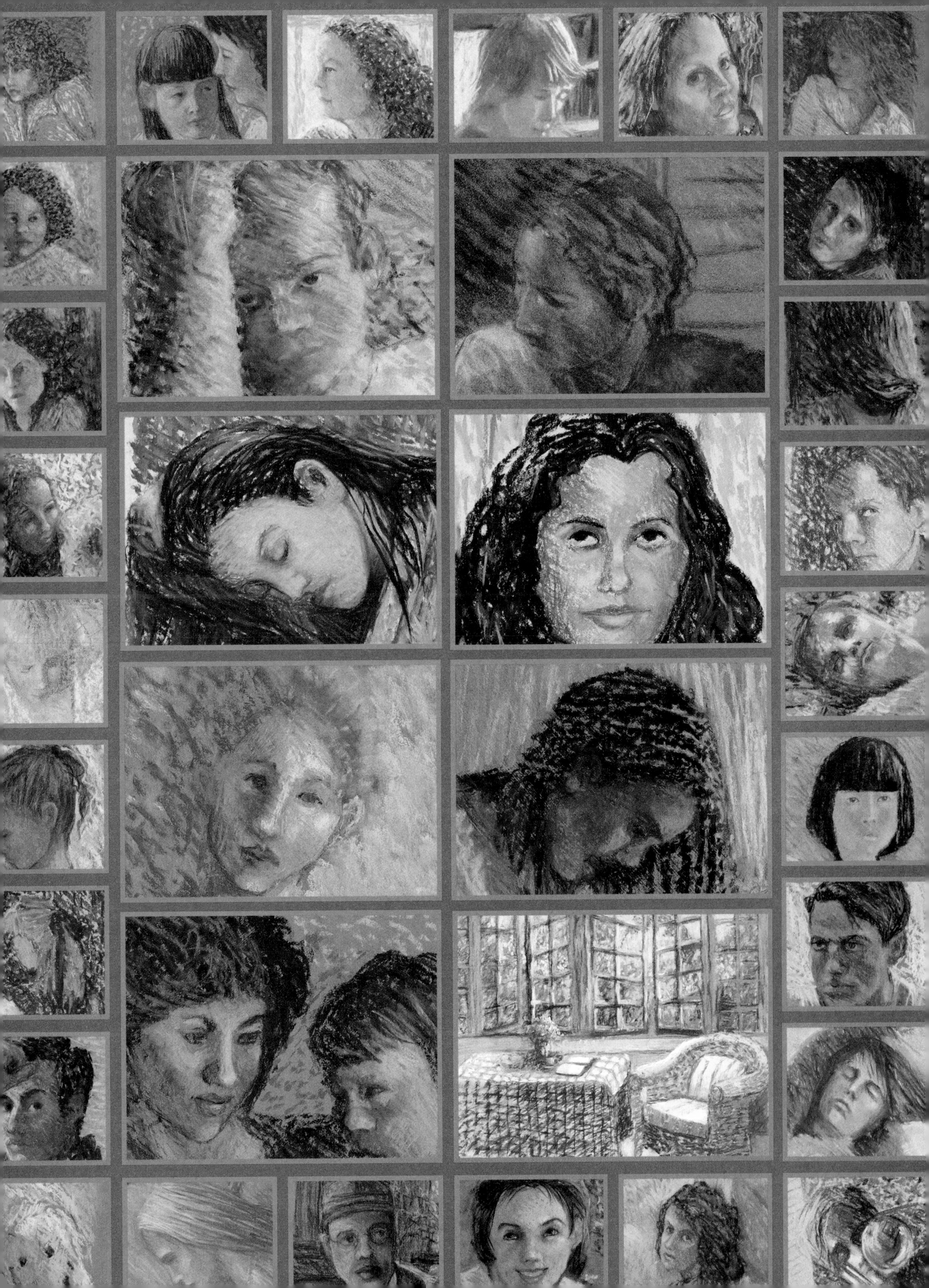

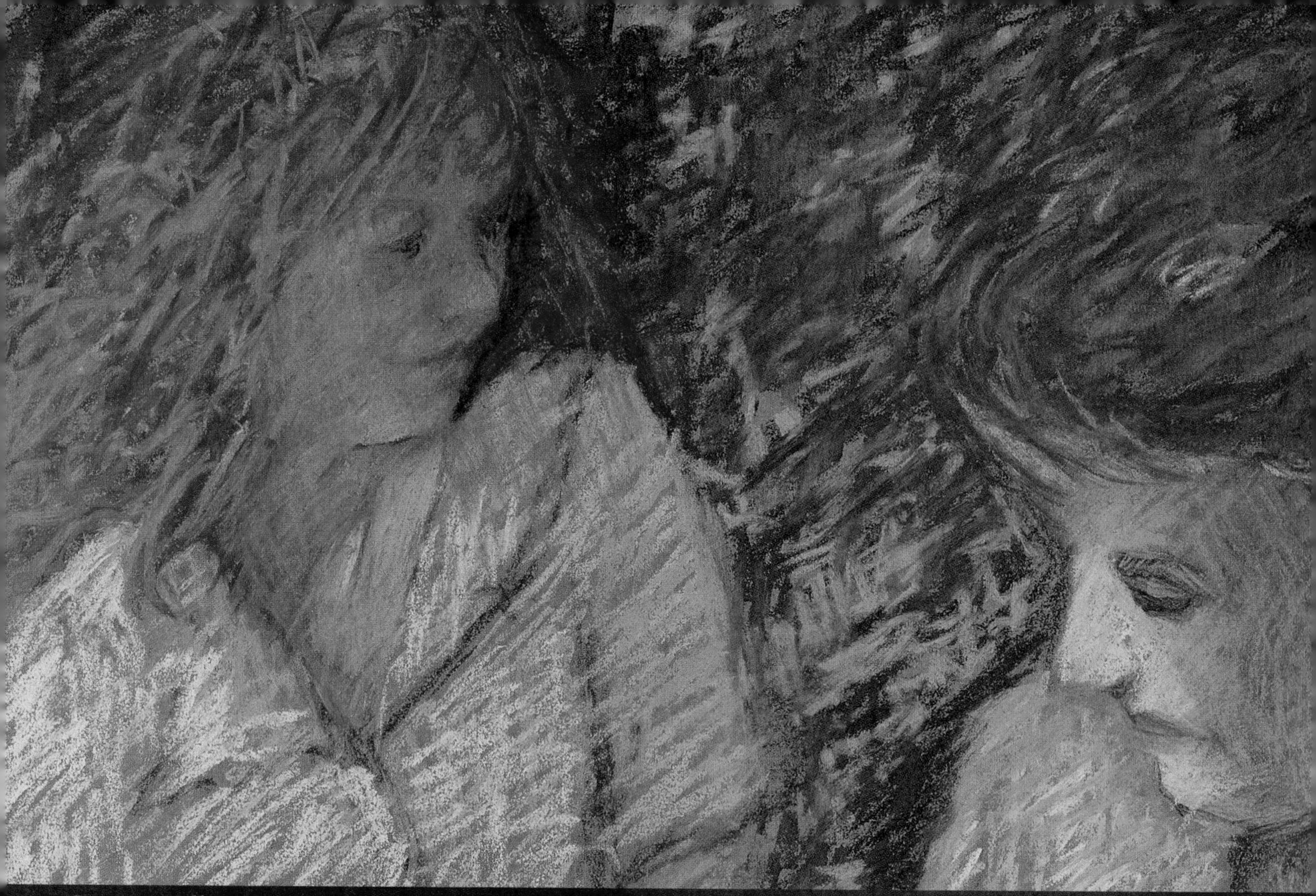

Can We Talk?

Using ''Self'' in a Therapeutic Manner

- *Can you identify a time in your past when you wanted and/or needed the presence of another person to help you with something?*
- *How have you benefited from experiencing silence with another?*
- *Can you identify an individual you would seek out for support at a time of crisis? If yes, what qualities does that individual have?*
- *How do you see yourself in a helping role with others?*
- *Reflect on your activities when reaching out to others for the purpose of giving emotional support and/or comfort; which activities seem most effective?*
- *How do you express caring to others, especially those with different lifestyles, abilities, cultural backgrounds, and languages than your own?*

Reflecting on answers to each of these questions will help you to understand how to give and receive support and how to develop a positive and supportive nurse-client relationship.

CHAPTER 6

Tools of Psychiatric Mental Health Nursing
Communication, Nursing Process, and the Nurse-Client Relationship

VICKI D. JOHNSON
NOREEN CAVAN FRISCH

CHAPTER OUTLINE

COMPETENCIES

Upon completion of this chapter, the reader should be able to:

1. Describe what is meant by therapeutic use of self.
2. Define verbal and nonverbal communication, giving examples of each.
3. Utilize skill of therapeutic communication in interactions with clients.
4. Identify various techniques of therapeutic communication and state when each could be helpful in interactions.
5. Evaluate own communication with clients.
6. Apply the nursing process in psychiatric settings, emphasizing nursing diagnoses frequently seen in psychiatric care.
7. Describe how to document the nursing process using a nursing care plan.
8. Describe how to document the nursing process using concept mapping.
9. Utilize a method of selecting priorities of care for psychiatric clients.
10. Identify phases of the nurse-client relationship.
11. Use the nursing process and a therapeutic nurse-client relationship to establish care.

KEY TERMS

Concept Map
Defense Mechanisms
Feedback
Nonverbal Communication
Nursing Care Plans
Orientation
Process Recording
Termination
Therapeutic Communication
Working

Nurses working in acute-care facilities have several "tools of the trade" (stethoscopes, thermometers and other measuring instruments, IV pumps, computers) that assist them in providing care. Further, nurses in acute-care facilities exert a great deal of control over the care environment—the clients are usually in bed, furniture in client rooms is arranged by the nursing staff, and nurses arrange objects/tools needed for necessary nursing care (bandages, IV tubing, etc.). In acute-care nursing, there is usually an immediate focus on the client's physical needs related to illness or injury. Many nurses find that when they go into a psychiatric or mental health facility or on a psychiatric home visit for the first time, they feel something is "missing." There are no physical objects to become the focus of care—dressings, IVs, or blood pressure cuffs. The psychiatric hospital environment is quite different from the general hospital setting: the staff and care providers do not wear uniforms; the clients are not confined to bed; and the environment may look more like a residence hall than a health care facility. New psychiatric nurses frequently report feeling somewhat "lost," sometimes with the sense of "I don't know what to do!" and "I don't know how to be here!" The purpose of this chapter is to review the tools of psychiatric nursing to help the novice psychiatric mental health nurse begin a new area of practice.

The psychiatric nurse uses tools of self and of knowledge as the basis for care. The psychiatric nurse needs well-developed communication skills, knowledge of nursing and psychological/psychiatric theory, and knowledge of resources for community referrals. The nurse, using this set of skills and knowledge, has the ability to offer interactions to the client that are compassionate and empathetic, that offer hope and a sense of future, and that provide clients with the ability to see their current situations in a new light and to focus on their strengths and abilities. These abilities help to meet the goals of psychiatric care: control of symptoms, provision of a therapeutic relationship, identification of nursing problems, and provision of nursing interventions that assist in returning the client to the best state of health that is possible. This chapter is divided into three sections: communication, the nursing process, and the nurse-client relationship.

PART 1: COMMUNICATION

Nurses learn early in their careers that there are certain ways to communicate with clients, regardless of setting, and that they must present a professional and helpful stance in interactions. For example, the professional nurse will approach a new client, introduce herself, and then let the client know that she will be the nurse in charge of the client's care that day. Part of this professional communication includes the requirement that the nurse present congruous verbal and nonverbal cues that the nurse is kind, accepting of the nursing role to provide care, and competent to do so.

Nurses must also understand the role that culture plays in professional communication. Experienced nurses are aware that transcultural differences may create barriers to verbal and nonverbal communication that, in turn, can negatively affect client outcomes (Munoz & Luckmann, 2005). By recognizing that these barriers may exist and continually striving for cultural competence, nurses can increase the likelihood of effective communication with individuals who identify with another culture or ethnic group. Chapter 7 explores cultural and ethnic factors that affect nurse-client interactions.

In psychiatric nursing, the nurse must build on already solid skills of professional communication and develop expertise in the techniques of **therapeutic communication**. Therapeutic communication is the purposeful use of dialog to bring about the client's insight, control of symptoms, and/or healing. To accomplish therapeutic communication, the nurse needs a thorough understanding of communication theory and of how to build a positive nurse-client relationship; both of these are discussed next.

Communication Theory

Communication theory suggests that there are two roles in any interaction: the communicator (the person sending a message) and the receiver (the person receiving the message). For communication to be effective, the meaning of the message received should be the same as the meaning of the message sent. To evaluate communication skills and use communication as a therapeutic tool, the nurse must have knowledge of verbal and nonverbal communication and must know how to interpret feedback from clients regarding what is being communicated.

Feedback is the response of the receiver of a message to the communicator. Feedback serves to let the communicator know that his message was understood, or in the opposite circumstances, feedback is a clue that the message was not interpreted correctly. In interactions between two persons, there is always some type of feedback occurring. The nurse must become skilled in looking for and interpreting the client's feedback to her messages, so that she can deal directly and immediately with any misperceptions that may have occurred. Further, in psychiatric mental health nursing practice, many of the clients with whom nurses interact have a history of poor and ineffective communication with others. For example, some clients may not know that they are sending feedback to others that discourages interactions or that makes others feel intimidated. The nurse who is alert to understanding communication can use her observations of the communications sent, received, and interpreted to assist clients in developing better skills.

Nonverbal Communication

While most of us think of communication as a verbal interchange, there is much about communication that is nonverbal. **Nonverbal communication** refers to all of the messages sent by other-than-verbal or written means. It has been estimated that well over half of all messages communicated are nonverbal, for they include behaviors, cues, and presence (such as proximity) that send a message. Consider the following two scenarios:

Student Alice goes to her instructor's office because she is having trouble completing an assignment. The instructor has given her the office building and room number and has told the class she has office hours today from 3 to 5 P.M. Alice walks down the hall and finds the room number. The door to the room is barely open, but Alice can see into the room. Instructor Smith is sitting behind a rather large, dark, wooden desk that is situated in the middle of the room, almost directly in front of the door. Ms. Smith has a computer on the top of the desk and is busy reading something on the computer screen. Alice knocks on the door, but there is no answer. Almost immediately, the telephone rings, and Ms. Smith picks up the phone and begins to have a rather loud and animated discussion with someone. Alice waits about 5 more minutes, unnoticed, and then retreats to her dorm with a resolve to try and complete the assignment without help.

Across town, student Barry is having trouble with an assignment given him by his instructor. Instructor Jones has provided his class with his office building, room number, and office hours (which occur today). Barry finds the room and sees that the door is wide open. Mr. Jones has a desk pushed up against a wall, to one side of the door. Mr. Jones is sitting in a chair at the desk, allowing him to have a clear view of the door. Mr. Jones is talking on the phone and gestures immediately for Barry to wait a minute so the two can talk. Barry waits, and soon initiates discussion with his instructor.

In these student-instructor scenes, each instructor provided the student with nearly identical verbal cues regarding office hours and availability. However, the nonverbal cues influenced interaction greatly. Which instructor met the needs of the student seeking help? Did each instructor purposefully set up the nonverbal cues? One finds that many persons (instructors included!) have little understanding of the nonverbal messages they send. The following components of nonverbal communication may greatly influence interactions.

Physical Space

The physical space between two individuals, as well as the design of the room and the furniture that contributes to the environment, have great meaning in communication. Space between two persons gives a sense of their relationship and, like all aspects of communication, is linked to cultural norms and values. In general, studies of interactions between and among people in North America indicate that a person has four zones of interaction defined by the space or distance between two persons (Hall, 1959). Public space, or approximately 12 feet, is comfortable for most persons in public

REFLECTIVE THINKING 6-1

Nonverbal Communication in Your Life

Take time today to observe and reflect on the nonverbal communication of those around you:

- If at school, what nonverbal messages are sent to you by your classmates when you walk into your class?
- What nonverbal messages do students in your class send your instructor when it is 5 minutes before the end of the scheduled lecture time?
- When you have an informal conversation with a friend, what messages let you know that it is time to end the conversation and do something else?
- At home, what nonverbal messages are sent to you and your family members/housemates at the dinner table? At the end of the work day? Before people in the household leave for an activity?

Noticing nonverbal communication will help you develop skills in therapeutic communication.

REFLECTIVE THINKING 6-2

Physical Space and Interaction

1. Observe your own level of comfort on a psychiatric unit. For instance, when you sit next to a client, what seating arrangement is most comfortable for you?
   - At a table (e.g., playing cards)
   - On a couch
   - Other
2. In what settings are most clients likely to approach you?
   - When you are at the nurses' station
   - When you are at a meal table during dinner
   - When you are sitting in a day room
3. How do you interpret the social space on the unit?
   - How is the physical space in the unit arranged? Sketch the furniture/space arrangement.
   - How do you think the physical space contributes to communication and interaction between and among people?
   - What changes would you suggest to enhance communication?

activities, such as giving a talk in a classroom. Social space is about 9 to 12 feet and is a comfortable distance in social settings, for example, walking down a street or being seated at a restaurant. Personal space ranges from 18 inches to about 4 feet and refers to the space between persons with some sense of connection: fellow students seated in a classroom, for example. Intimate space is space closer than 18 inches and is reserved for those with whom a person has a close relationship, such as family and personal friends.

A nurse can use her knowledge of the meaning of space and distance between two persons to understand and interpret nonverbal behaviors. Some clients are comfortable sitting next to the nurse in "social" space; others may get up and walk away. The nurse can use these cues to understand that, for some, social interactions may feel too invasive and be uncomfortable, while for others, the contact within social space may provide a source of comfort and be interpreted as support. In some situations, the nurse may find that a client moves in "too close" for the nurse to feel the interaction can be professional and appropriate. A nurse may find that a passive, dependent client always sits next to her on a couch such that the client chooses to be within 12 to 18 inches of the nurse. Further, the same client may follow the nurse this closely down the hall. In such cases, the nurse will understand that the client may need to develop boundaries and a stronger sense of self in order to establish the social skills necessary to initiate communication with others. When appropriate in the nurse-client relationship, the nurse will use observations to let the client know how the client's nonverbal messages come across to others.

Room and space design (e.g., the design of an instructor's office) can also send messages about how inviting interaction may be. Chairs can be spaced to invite personal and social interactions. Desks can be placed to provide barriers to interactions. Observations of where persons choose to sit and where they put furniture provide many cues as to the desire and need for interactions.

Actions or Kinetics

Actions refer to movements, expressions, gestures, and posture that accompany interactions and influence communications. They convey messages of intent and mood and can support or contradict a verbal message. For instance, an instructor who is frequently glancing at a clock during a student conversation conveys a different message than one who is looking directly at the student. While actions during speech have significant meaning, these actions are almost always culture-bound, and interpreted meaning must be understood within the sociocultural context of the speaker.

Paralinguistic Cues

Vocal cues are parts of spoken language other than words. These include tone, pitch, emotions expressed verbally (such as anxiety or anger or fear), sounds of hesitation, nervous laughter, and nervous coughing. These cues provide the context in which the words are delivered, and they influence meaning directly. As the actions during speech convey messages based on social and cultural norms, so do paralinguistic cues. The nurse is cautioned to interpret vocal cues within the context of the client's cultural and social/familial norms.

Touch

Touch is a form of communication used almost daily by nurses providing direct physical care and support to clients. Touch can convey warmth, positive regard, support during silence, and reassurance that the nurse is fully present and caring. Touch has many meanings, however. Psychiatric mental health nurses often use touch—for example, reaching out and holding a client's hand—as a means to extend support. However, like other forms of nonverbal communication, touch may be interpreted in many ways. The nurse must take her cues from the patient as the therapeutic value of touch is dependent upon the client perceiving the intended message. Nurses must always be aware of the meaning touch has for any particular client and use touch only in a way that is therapeutic (Figure 6-1).

Verbal Communication

Verbal communication is the use of words, written and spoken, to send messages to another. For communication to be most therapeutic, it must convey a respectful attitude, one that supports the individuality and self-esteem of both the client and the nurse. There are identified techniques of communication that allow one to learn *how* to convey such an attitude and also allow one to step back and reflect on the nurse-client interaction. These techniques are summarized in Table 6-1 and are discussed next.

Listening

Listening is perhaps the most important communication technique, for it involves being fully present for another while obtaining information needed to truly understand the client. While it is sometimes difficult to listen, it is essential that the nurse learns to give the client every chance to be heard.

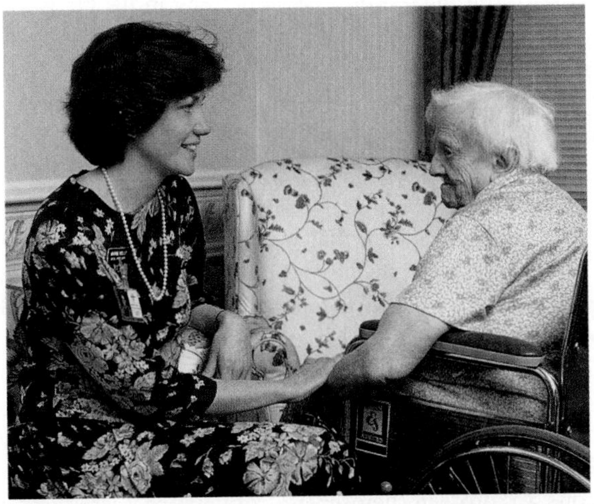

Figure 6-1 Touch can be a valuable means of extending therapeutic support and comfort to a client. (DELMAR/CENGAGE LEARNING.)

Silence

Silence is the ability to wait, to pause, to refrain from using language, giving the client and nurse time to reflect, respond, and feel emotions. Silence is effective in letting the client lead the way, for silence is waiting for the client to direct the communication. The nurse's silence encourages the client to feel and explore emotions and may foster self-awareness. Silence can be active or passive. To be therapeutic, silence must be active; that is, the nurse must be fully present.

Broad Openings

Broad openings are words that permit the client to decide the manner of the response. Comments such as "Tell me about that" or "What do you think about that?" or "What's on your mind today?" are all broad openings. Such statements let the client know the nurse wants to listen and permit the client a wide range of responses. The client will choose the topic, as well as the degree to which he will open up to disclose inner feelings. The broad opening allows the nurse to get the conversation started without making demands that the client talk about one particular subject.

Restating

Restating is a technique whereby the nurse repeats the main message the client has expressed. Restating, also called paraphrasing, permits the nurse to verify understanding of the client's message and also permits the client to reflect on the statement and emotion expressed. Restating lets the client know that the nurse is truly listening and making every attempt to understand.

Clarification

Clarification is a technique whereby the nurse tries to put the client's ideas into a simple statement and asks the client if the nurse's understanding is correct. The nurse might say, "Are you saying that ..." and fill in the messages she has heard to check her understanding and to make the client's thoughts or feelings explicit.

Reflection

Reflection is, as its name implies, reflecting or interpreting back to the client what has been heard and understood. Reflection may be a statement such as "It sounds like you got mad when your roommate left the kitchen dirty," reflecting on the situation and the client's feelings. Reflection is a powerful tool to bring out important aspects of the client's feelings and to put them in the context of when and where they occur. Different from restating, reflection allows the nurse to describe a theme that the client has not identified verbally. Therefore, reflection must be used when the nurse has a good understanding of what is important to the client, so that the nurse does not come across as implying that she knows the client's feelings better than the client does. Reflection must be used sparingly and works best in those situations where the nurse intends to underscore a theme that seems important to the client.

TABLE 6-1 Summary of Therapeutic Communication Techniques

TECHNIQUE	EXAMPLE	PURPOSE
Listening	Silence, eye contact, attitude of being fully present	Permits the client to be heard; conveys interest in what the client is saying
Silence	Not breaking the quiet	Provides time for nurse and client to gather thoughts, to reflect
Broad openings	"What's been going on?" "Tell me what's been on your mind."	Initiates conversation; puts the client in control of the content
Restating	"Are you saying you were angry when your wife had to work late?"	Provides feedback, letting the client know that the nurse understood the message; lets the client know that the nurse is attentive
Clarification	"Are you saying you want to move out of your apartment?"	Puts client's ideas into a simple statement; makes the client's ideas explicit
Reflection	"So you start feeling depressed when no one calls you over the weekend."	Presents themes that have emerged through a series of interactions
Focusing	"Let's go back to the situation at school, where you felt uncomfortable in class."	Directs conversation back to an area of importance; explores a topic in depth
Informing	"The medication must be taken every day."	Provides facts or recommendations
Suggesting	"Have you considered the alternative of a self-help group for weekly support?"	Presents new ideas; assists client to consider alternative options
Confronting	"You say you're upset, but you are laughing."	Presents contradictions and inconsistencies

Focusing

Focusing is a technique in which the nurse directs the conversation to focus on a topic of particular importance or relevance to the client. Here, the nurse asks questions about one theme that has emerged or is emerging in the client interactions. The purpose is to draw the client's attention to the theme—its meaning and significance in the client's life and adjustments. An example of focusing would be "Let's talk some more about…"

Informing

Informing is the nursing skill of providing information, when needed. Informing, used by nurses in the nurse-client education role, refers to simply giving facts and information. In psychiatric mental health nursing, the client often needs information about his illness, the etiology and genetic basis of his disease, the legal aspects of care, and alternatives for medication and treatment. "The medication will not have an effect for two weeks…" is an example of informing.

Suggesting

Suggesting is used to encourage a client to consider alternatives, for example, suggesting or questioning whether the client has considered a specific option, or asking the client to consider an alternate means of coping with a particular situation. For suggesting to be therapeutic, the nurse must not tell the client what to do or implicitly take responsibility for the decision and the outcome away from the client.

Confronting

Confronting is communication that points out inconsistencies or incongruencies between feelings, thoughts, and actions. For example, the nurse might state, "You say you are upset about the degree of drinking in your family, but you smile as you say so and ask others to party with you on Saturday night." Used correctly, confrontation encourages clients to explore maladaptive behaviors. To use confrontation as a therapeutic tool, the nurse must use a friendly but firm approach and recognize that a client may deny or become angry with the suggestion that something in his life is inconsistent. Nonetheless, in using confrontation, the nurse must remain patient and know that confrontation may be the only way to encourage the client to examine his own dysfunctional behaviors.

In addition to these techniques of communication, the nurse should also evaluate her choice of words and whether or not the messages she has sent are being understood by the client. Clear, precise language is always preferable. Simple words that convey the meaning intended are better than complicated phrases and difficult vocabulary.

DEFENSE MECHANISMS

Defense mechanisms are unconscious responses used by persons to protect themselves from internal conflicts and external stressors. A nurse skilled in therapeutic communication will notice when a client is using one or more of these mechanisms. When a nurse concludes that her client is using a defense mechanism to avoid dealing with certain subjects, the nurse can use this knowledge to guide interactions, knowing that the defense mechanism indicates the presence of psychologically significant material. In interviews, the nurse may choose to pursue additional information on the topic, but the nurse will also realize that the client may not be able to answer direct questions about related issues. Table 6-2 presents examples of common defense mechanisms.

EVALUATING COMMUNICATION

The nurse must always evaluate whether communication was therapeutic or nontherapeutic. A course in psychiatric nursing is a time for self-examination, a time to look carefully at how one as a nurse comes across to others, and a time to look at how one's own communication skills and behaviors impact others.

Use of therapeutic communication techniques does not, in and of itself, mean that communication will be therapeutic. There is judgment involved in deciding when to be silent, when to probe or question, when to restate, when to ask for clarification. After the communication has taken place, one can determine if it was therapeutic. A therapeutic communication is one that builds a trusting relationship and helps to give the client insight and tools to become independent and regain or attain health.

There are several ways of evaluating communication. First and foremost, the nurse should take the time to get feedback from the client that he understands what the nurse has said. Second, the nurse should provide feedback so she

TABLE 6-2 Common Defense Mechanisms

MECHANISM	DESCRIPTION	EXAMPLE
Denial	Negation of reality of threatening situations, despite factual evidence	The client refuses to admit to anger, even though the situation warrants it and the client's voice indicates anger.
Projection	Attribution of one's own thoughts, feelings, or impulses to others	"I'm not attracted to him. My best friend is."
Repression	Unconscious blocking from awareness material that is threatening or painful	"I never got angry at my father; our family lived in harmony and love" (when such descriptions of the family life would not fit with anyone else's interpretation of the events).
Rationalization	Intellectual explaining away of threatening circumstances	"The test had too many trick questions; I really know all the material; our instructor was out to get me."
Introjection	Incorporating, without examination or thought, the qualities or attitudes of others	The adolescent who takes on all the values and styles of an admired teacher.
Displacement	Transfer of feelings or reactions evoked by one topic or event to another that is less threatening	The husband who is angry at his wife and yells at the family dog rather than deal directly with his anger.
Reaction formation	Expression of a feeling that is the opposite of one's authentic feeling or of feelings that would be appropriate in the situation	A client who brings gifts to the nurse at whom he is really mad.
Regression	Retreat to a previous developmental level	A child starts to suck his thumb (after 2 years of not thumb sucking) when admitted to the hospital.
Suppression	Conscious or unconscious attempt to keep threatening material out of consciousness	Failure to remember a significant childhood event, such as the death of a grandmother.
Sublimation	Channeling of socially unacceptable impulses into socially acceptable activities	A young man who is dealing with aggression by playing socially acceptable activities
Symbolization	Use of an object, idea, or act to express emotion that is not expressed directly	The client who leaves the nurse a flower rather than directly saying she cares about the nurse.

NURSINGTIP 6-1

Communication Skills Awareness

Psychiatric mental health nursing offers a chance to explore one's communication skills. Use this time to grow and learn. Be kind to yourself and understand that all nurses find aspects of their communication skills that need improving!

can know that what she has understood is what the client intended. Many nurses will keep some form of a process recording that documents their interactions with clients. A **process recording** is a verbatim account of the communication, with the nurse's interpretation of the specific communication technique used and an evaluation of whether or not the communication was therapeutic. A process recording gives the nurse information on which to reflect. When the nurse discovers that some aspect of communication was not therapeutic, a process recording gives the nurse a chance to consider and suggest another means of communication that might be preferable. A sample process recording is presented in Table 6-3.

Process recordings may be done in several ways. Video recordings of interactions are, of course, the best documentation of interactions, for on video both verbal and nonverbal messages can be observed. Next to a video recording, an auditory recording is most accurate. When neither of these is feasible, a nurse may have a conversation with a client and immediately afterward write down all that she can remember from the interaction. While a written account from memory may not be the most accurate, it is probably the most frequently used method of documenting interactions between nurses and clients. Issues of permission, confidentiality, and anonymity must be addressed with any recording of a client's person or voice. Sometimes it is countertherapeutic to even ask to record a nurse-client interaction, for example, if the client is paranoid or in an excitable state. Therefore, nurses will determine the best means of documenting interactions to evaluate use of communication techniques. Over time, the process of reflecting on the communication will become easier for the nurse, and techniques of therapeutic communication will become part of the nurse's tools of practice.

PART 2: NURSING PROCESS

The nursing process is a way of thinking that allows nurses to reflect on nursing care and work in an organized,

TABLE 6-3 Sample Process Recording

	INTERACTION	COMMUNICATION TECHNIQUE USED	EVALUATION
Nurse:	What's been going on this week?	Broad opening	Permits client to begin with what is important at the moment.
Client:	I've been thinking a lot about my job. I just don't like my boss. In fact, I can't stand working with her.		
Nurse:	You don't like her.	Restating	Provides a chance for client to expand, which he does.
Client:	No. She doesn't value me or anyone else. She always tells us all about what is wrong but never says anything good.		
Nurse:	So you would like to feel valued.	Reflection	Returns the client to feelings. The client is able to talk about experiences from his past.
Client:	Yes! It's like when I was in school and no one thought I did well enough.		
Nurse:	No one?	Clarification	Allows the nurse to seek information, yet encourages client to go on.
Client:	Yeah, my parents, friends, they made me feel like I was no good.		
Nurse:	This current situation at work, it is similar to feelings you've had before.	Reflection	Returns focus to current situation and the theme of feeling devalued.

systematic manner. Many nurses have criticized the nursing process as unhelpful in providing holistic care (Jones & Brown, 1993). It is important, however, to remember that there are, and have always been, two definitions of the nursing process (Erickson, Tomlin, & Swain, 1983). The first is that the nursing process is a step-by-step, linear process of assessment, diagnosis, outcome identification, planning/interventions, and evaluation. As such, it is a problem-solving technique. The second, more basic definition is that the nursing process is a means of reflecting on the entire process of the nurse-client interaction. In this second definition, one is reminded that *process* means a series of actions leading to an end. If one views nursing as an interactive encounter, the nursing process is the means by which the nurse-client interaction takes place (Frisch, 1994). Experienced nurses know that one never really applies the nursing process in a step-by-step fashion. One does not assess, then diagnose, then devise outcomes, then plan, provide, and evaluate care in that order. One is diagnosing while one is assessing. As soon as a nurse begins an interaction with a client, the nurse is intervening, because the nurse's words, actions, and presence serve as an intervention and are part of nursing care. A nurse is constantly evaluating; one knows that evaluation does not come only at the end of a detailed care plan. As a nurse provides care in the psychiatric mental health setting, it is important to recognize that the nursing process is a complex process—it is more circular than linear—and that the idea of the step-by-step analysis of the nursing process can help one to understand and reflect on the nursing care more than it actually reflects activities as they are experienced in real life. Figure 6-2 presents two views of the nursing process, the linear view and the circular view. The nurse is encouraged to consider the meaning of the nursing process in a setting in which interaction and use of self are the most important nursing tools.

For purposes of learning, it is useful to consider the steps of the nursing process in order and then apply the steps to the psychiatric mental health setting. A discussion on each step follows.

Steps of the Nursing Process

Assessment

A nurse will always begin by gathering data from the client (and his family/significant others) to develop an understanding of the client's reason(s) for seeking help and to determine the client's specific needs. Assessment in psychiatric nursing begins with knowledge obtained from a basic psychiatric history and a mental status assessment. The purpose of such an initial assessment is to:

1. Document the client's presenting problem and/or the precipitating event (mental health history).
2. Evaluate whether the client is in touch with reality (mental status examination).
3. Determine whether the client is in danger such that he needs protection or whether the client is likely to injure others (critical decisions related to safety).

In many cases the initial evaluation will be done by a psychiatrist, and results of the evaluation will be available to the nurse. The nurse can complete her own assessment, based on a nursing model; that is, the nurse may gather data relevant to a nursing theory or functional health patterns (Gordon, 1994) or on the basis of the human response patterns). Table 6-4 lists the elements contained in a psychiatric history (Mabbett, 1996). Although all mental health professionals use data obtained to write DSM diagnoses, the nurse will also use information to identify specific nursing problems that can be written as nursing diagnoses.

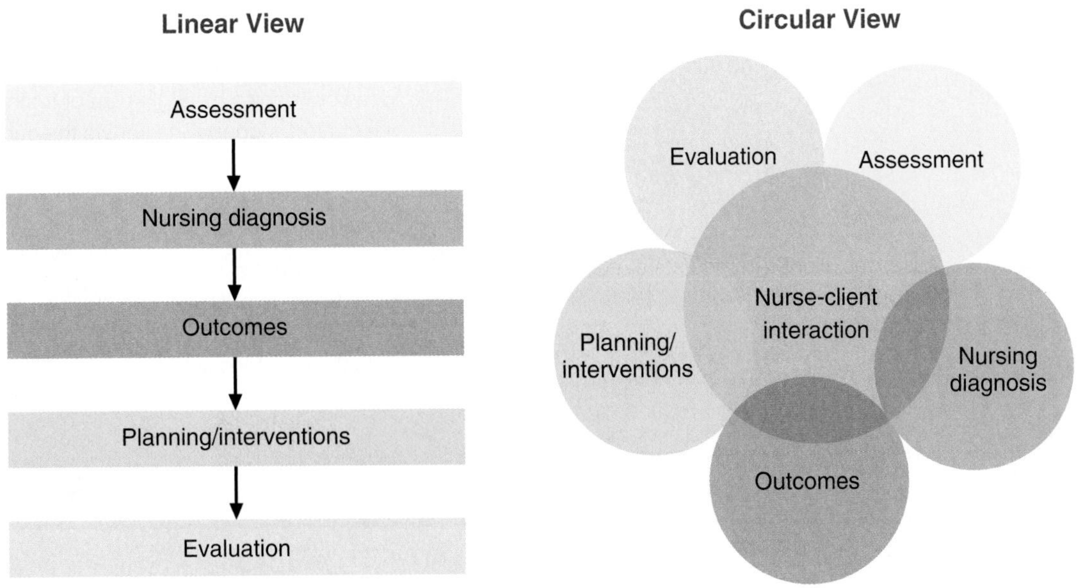

FIGURE 6-2 **Two views of the nursing process.** DELMAR/CENGAGE LEARNING.

Table 6-4 Elements of a Psychiatric History

ELEMENT	DESCRIPTION	EXAMPLE
Identifying data	Summarizes the case, including information about previous hospitalizations or treatment and some indication of the current problem.	This is one of numerous psychiatric admissions for this 45-year-old woman, who is readmitted at this time for recurrence of paranoia, auditory hallucinations, and suicidal ideation.
Chief complaint	Describes the client's perception of the current problem.	"The voices are telling me to kill myself and I can't get away from them."
Present illness history	Describes events leading to admission or seeking of psychiatric help.	The client was discharged from hospital 1 month ago. She attended day treatment, but took her medication inconsistently. Over the past 3 days, she has become preoccupied with suicide. She states she has recently discovered that her husband is having an affair, and she thinks he wants to leave her. She blames herself for difficulties in her marriage.
Past medical history	Outlines medical conditions, including laboratory or diagnostic data.	There are no known medical conditions.
Developmental and psychosocial history	Outlines circumstances that are significant for understanding the current problems. Includes such information as marital status, children, significant relationships, work or school history, relationships with family members, and developmental stage.	Client was the middle child in a family of three children. Her parents had an intact marriage, although there was a great deal of hostility between them. She has flashbacks of her mother and father yelling at each other in the night. She is currently married, with no children. She has completed college, with a liberal arts degree. She is employed part time in a local decorating business.
Mental status examination	Evaluates the client's mental and emotional functioning, including appearance, behavior, and attitude; characteristics of speech; affect and mood; thought content (delusions, illusions, ability to concentrate); orientation (oriented to person, time, place, and self); memory; intellectual level; and suicidal ideations.	The client is cooperative with the interviewer. Her mood and affect are depressed and anxious. She became tearful throughout the interview. Her flow of thought is coherent, and her thought content reveals feelings of low self-esteem as well as auditory hallucinations that are self-demeaning. She admits to suicidal ideas but denies having a plan or intent. Her orientation is good. She knows the current date, place, person. Recent and remote memory are good. She shows some insight and judgment regarding her illness and need for help.
Critical Decisions	Assesses client's immediate status and risk factors.	• Is the client suicidal? • Is there a potential for suicide in the near future? • Is the client violent?

Note: The content of examination for suicide and violence is covered in detail in Chapter 16.

From *Instant Nursing Assessment: Mental Health,* by P. D. Mabbett, Copyright 1996, Clifton Park, NY: Thomson Delmar Learning. Adapted with permission.

Nursing Diagnosis

More often than not, the nurse will obtain data over a period of time. Most clients will not be willing to disclose very personal information to a nurse they do not know. Further, many clients will present in a state of emotional excitement or depression such that they are unable to sit and answer many questions. The nurse must focus on the client's immediate needs, take steps to develop trust, and build a positive nurse-client relationship. Over time and the course of interactions, it will become clear that a client has particular needs that the nurse will be able to address.

Many of the nursing diagnoses in the human response patterns emphasized in psychiatric care cannot be made on the basis of direct observation or objective evidence alone. For example, the nursing diagnosis of *social isolation* cannot be made unless the client provides subjective evidence that he experiences feelings of aloneness imposed by others (Herdman, 2009). Similarly, the nursing diagnosis of *situational low self-esteem* is made only by assessing that the client has negative feelings about self or self-capabilities in response to a current situation (Herdman, 2009). Thus, the nurse must have a rapport with the client to the degree where the client will disclose information about his perceptions and feelings. Further, the nurse can make diagnoses and address these as nursing concerns only after discussion with the client that these are areas the client wishes to pursue with the nurse. When the nurse and client agree that a particular area is a nursing concern, the nurse can make a nursing diagnosis and begin to plan care directed toward the concern. Table 6-5 lists the NANDA-I diagnoses most frequently seen in psychiatric care.

Outcome Identification

For every nursing diagnosis, the nurse must identify specific outcomes that can reasonably be expected as a result of nursing and psychiatric care. Outcomes will be both short term and long term. Outcomes should be clearly stated and be discussed with the client so that the nurse and client have a stated, mutual goal of their work together.

For example, if the initial assessment indicates that the client is feeling depressed, alone, and isolated, and that he wishes more interactions with others, the nurse may list the following as a short-term outcome: The client will form a one-on-one relationship with the nurse such that the client will talk with the nurse for 30 minutes daily. A more long-term outcome might be: The client will build relationships with others in his environment and will interact socially with others at least two times throughout the day by 3 months' time. Further, another longer-term goal for this client might be: Within 1 month, the client will interact in a social setting with another person, at least twice per week. With these specific outcomes in mind, the nurse will plan interventions with this client aimed at establishing a nurse-client relationship first and extending that relationship to others by increasing the amount of social interaction the client will have with others in his environment.

TABLE 6-5 NANDA-I Diagnoses Frequently Seen in Psychiatric Care According to a Human Response Pattern Framework

HUMAN RESPONSE PATTERNS	DIAGNOSES
Exchanging	Risk for injury
Communicating	Impaired verbal communication
Relating	Impaired social interaction
	Social isolation
	Risk for loneliness
	Ineffective role performance
	Impaired parenting
	Sexual dysfunction
	Interrupted family processes
	Dysfunctional family processes: alcoholism
	Caregiver role strain
	Ineffective sexuality pattern
Valuing	Spiritual distress
	Moral distress
Choosing	Ineffective coping
	Risk-prone health behavior
	Defensive coping
	Ineffective denial
	Compromised family coping
	Ineffective therapeutic regimen management
	Decisional conflict
	Disabled family coping
	Parental role conflict
	Relocation stress syndrome
	Stress overload
Moving	Self-care deficit (specify)
Perceiving	Disturbed body image
	Situational low self-esteem
	Disturbed personal identity
	Hopelessness
	Powerlessness
	Disturbed sensory perception (specify)
	Chronic low self-esteem
Knowing	Deficient knowledge (specify)
	Acute confusion
	Chronic confusion
	Disturbed thought processes
	Impaired memory

(Continues)

TABLE 6-5 (Continued)

Feeling	Grieving Complicated grieving Risk for violence: self-directed or other-directed Self-mutilation Post-trauma syndrome Rape trauma syndrome Chronic sorrow Death anxiety Anxiety Fear

Consulting the NOC (particularly Domain 5, which covers psychological health) as described in Chapter 5 will assist the nurse in selecting nurse-sensitive outcomes related to the care of psychiatric mental health clients.

Planning/Interventions

After the nurse has made nursing diagnoses and identified outcomes of care, the nurse will plan interventions directed at each nursing diagnosis. These interventions may be autonomous or collaborative. Autonomous nursing interventions are those that the nurse is licensed to perform independently. Collaborative interventions are those that the nurse must work with another professional (e.g., psychiatrist, medical doctor) to carry out. Collaborative problems are further defined as situations that nurses monitor to detect symptom onset or changes in status (Carpenito-Moyet, 2007). In planning care for any client, the nurse must consider both types of interventions to determine the priority nursing role. For example, if the client is admitted to an inpatient unit and the nurse has made the diagnosis of *social isolation*, the nurse will plan autonomous nursing interventions to help alleviate the client's feelings of aloneness, planning a certain amount of time to be with the client one on one and then assisting the client to engage in interaction with another client over a game of cards. The nurse may then support the client in social activity by inviting him to participate in a ward activity with a different client. In these interactions, the nurse is attempting to teach the client a means of becoming socially involved and is meeting the client's affiliation needs so that his feelings of aloneness and isolation can be diminished.

The NIC (described in Chapter 5) is an excellent source on nursing interventions, as it presents a list of commonly accepted nursing activities with a wide range of nursing interventions in the psychosocial domain.

Collaborative Nursing Interventions

In addition to the independent nursing role, psychiatric nurses will participate in a multidisciplinary treatment plan. This is a collaborative nursing role whereby the nurse will

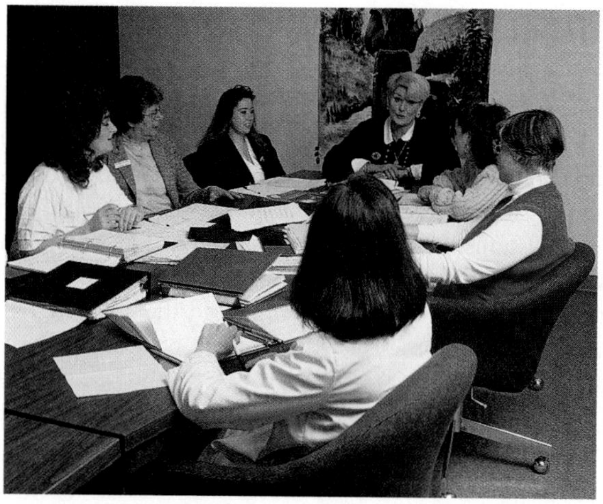

FIGURE 6-3 **Nurses often work in collaborative teams to plan client care.** (DELMAR/CENGAGE LEARNING.)

collaborate with other health professionals to meet clients' needs (Carpenito-Moyet, 2007). Two major areas of collaborative care arise in the care of most clients: (1) medication/direct services provided by other professionals such as occupational therapists, and (2) services in the community provided by identified volunteer or self-help groups. The nurse has an important collaborative role in each (Figure 6-3).

To administer medications, the nurse must be fully aware of the drugs used, the reasons for their prescription, the dose, and the client's individual response. As in all situations of administering medications, the nurse is fully responsible for the safe administration and the evaluation of the client's response. Chapter 27 provides a detailed description of the major medications used in psychiatric care; the nurse will also need to consult with appropriate drug references for medications, as needed. Managing and evaluating the safe administration of psychotropic drugs and teaching the client and family about the medications ordered are critically important nursing interventions. Given that a majority of chronic psychiatric clients are readmitted to inpatient units as a result of poor compliance and/or inappropriate knowledge of medications, nurses must consider their role in medication administration of very high priority.

When the individual client is receiving care from another professional, for example, an occupational therapist (OT), the nurse has a role to know and understand the goals the OT has for the client's care and to support those goals in her own interaction with the client. Chapter 1 details the roles of various health professionals. It will suffice here to reaffirm that the nurse will support the work of other professionals during their interactions with the client. Lastly, because a nursing goal is to return the client to the community and to help the client achieve a maximum state of health, the nurse will almost always have a role in referring the client to community resources.

Nursing Theory to Guide Interventions

Some nurses still find it difficult to initiate interventions with psychiatric clients. Following guidelines of established

BOX 6-1
FIVE AIMS OF INTERVENTION

- Build trust
- Promote positive orientation
- Promote perceived control
- Promote strengths
- Set mutual goals that are health directed

From *Modeling and Role-Modeling: A Theory and Paradigm for Nursing*, by H. Erickson, E. Tomlin, and M. A. Swain, 2009, Tenth Printing. Printed with permission, EST Company: Cedar Park, TX 78613.

nursing theory will help the new nurse feel confident in initiating care. The authors recommend basing interactions on the five aims of intervention described by Erickson, Tomlin, and Swain (1983), listed in Box 6-1. The five aims help one to focus interventions on goals that are universal and appropriate for psychiatric clients. (The Modeling and Role-Modeling Nursing theory is described in detail in Chapter 3.) The nurse may find that she needs additional assessment data to meet the five aims; for example, she may need to know more about the client's strengths. Thus, following the five aims gives the nurse insight as to when additional information is needed and provides goals that nursing interventions can address.

Evaluation

The final step of the nursing process is to evaluate the outcomes of the nursing actions. In most cases, nurses evaluate care by comparing projected or anticipated outcomes against observed outcomes. As all health care moves to outcome-based evaluations, psychiatric nurses need to demonstrate that their interventions with clients result in positive outcomes. Returning to the example cited previously, consider that the client expresses social isolation, feels aloneness that he perceives to be imposed by others, and tells the nurse this is uncomfortable for him. The nurse plans specific interventions and implements them. The nurse must seek the client's evaluation of his own feelings of social isolation to monitor the degree of success achieved, as every diagnosis and intervention must be clearly evaluated. Further, when all health care must account for outcomes achieved, nurses will need to demonstrate that there is some significance in the outcomes of nursing care. For example, nurses may be asked to explain why it is important for clients to feel engaged with others rather than isolated. While it may appear self-evident that social interactions are positive, nurses will be challenged to explain why and how that is so. Evaluating care, then, means documenting that care had or did not have intended outcomes and demonstrating that the outcomes of care had significant positive effects.

Documentation of the Nursing Process

Nursing Care Plans

Nurses have used **nursing care plans** as tools to document activities described in the nursing process. Traditional care plans have provided nurses and students with a means to record assessment data, provide a list of nursing diagnoses drawn from the data, record anticipated outcomes of nursing interventions, and present a plan of care that is a statement of nursing interventions to be used. Finally, the nursing care plan provides documentation of the observed outcome, which can then be compared to the anticipated outcome. While there are a variety of formats used for nursing care plans, almost all utilize a template, where columns are presented for at least the final phases of the nursing process and data are filled in as the care is provided. For students, additional data regarding etiology of conditions leading to diagnoses, references for abnormal findings on assessments, and references or justifications for interventions are not unusual, as the student is often required to use such a format to demonstrate the thinking that goes on behind the care that is being given. As students know well, many clients have more than one nursing diagnosis, and one characteristic of a nursing care plan is that each diagnosis is addressed separately.

Concept Maps

In recent years, many nurses have found that a different technique, called a **concept map**, is a useful, perhaps superior, method of documenting the nursing process. Simply stated, a concept map is a diagrammatic representation of organized knowledge. This representation is contextually based, meaning that it is drawn out of real-life experiences or situations. More accurately, perhaps, one would state that a concept map is one individual's interpretations of certain real-life experiences or situations. Thus, a concept map of the nursing process will be a diagrammatic representation of the nursing assessment data put in the context of the client, the nurse, and the condition in which they find themselves. The concept map permits a nurse to review assessment data and their associated nursing diagnoses in an "all-at-once" manner, rather than viewing each data bit and each diagnostic characteristic one at a time. Further, the concept map permits the nurse to think through all data and the relationships between and among areas of nursing concerns. This "thinking through" assists nurses to develop priorities of care in situations where the nurse concludes that one diagnosis or issue is a focal point of all of the diagnoses or issues observed.

The interest in concept maps for documentation of the nursing process stemmed from use of concept maps in education, particularly in teaching science. Research has indicated that students using concepts maps learn scientific knowledge at a higher level than do students who do not use them (Cliburn, 1990; Jegede, Alaiyemola, & Okebukola, 1990; McCagg & Dansereau, 1991). In nursing education, several authors have suggested that students learn to think critically when called upon to use concept maps in planning care (Baugh & Mellott, 1998; King & Shell, 2002; Pesut & Herman, 1999; Schuster, 2008). The textbook authors have also observed that the use of concept maps greatly assists many in establishing priorities of care.

For purposes of this text, documentation of the nursing process is presented in both formats at the end of each chapter's content in Unit 2. The care plans presented utilize the nursing care plan model providing the student with the client case and the pertinent assessment data, followed by the priority nursing diagnoses, outcomes, planning/interventions, and evaluation. The critical thinking questions are a learning tool to ask the student about items of further concern related to the case. Answering the critical thinking questions gives the student a chance to consider "what next" or "what else" could be included in the client's plan of care. The exemplars from practice/concept maps provide examples of the alternative method of documenting care. The exemplars from practice/concept maps present the cases and the initial reflections and statements of nursing diagnoses. Then a concept map is drawn to illustrate the connections and relationships, and the focal issues are selected as the priorities of care. The authors believe that the most useful function of a concept map is in establishing the priority of care and identifying the steps to be taken first. Box 6-2 illustrates the format for the documentation of the nursing process in this text: the care plan and the concept map.

PART 3: THE NURSE-CLIENT RELATIONSHIP

A nurse-client relationship evolves over time, as do relationships between any two individuals. There is an **orientation** phase—a time for getting to know each other, for establishing trust; a **working** phase—implementing nursing interventions to achieve outcomes; and a **termination** phase—an end to the relationship because the client has achieved independence from the nurse and can maintain health or stability without the nurse's care.

In the orientation phase, the nurse assumes responsibility for initiating and sustaining the relationship. To establish trust, the nurse must demonstrate respect, caring, and consistency. The nurse must keep all appointments or promises and will always follow through on any activity she said or implied she would do. Further, the nurse will provide a supportive environment in which the client can feel free to express his feelings and thoughts. The nurse will convey an attitude that is accepting and nonjudgmental.

In the working phase, the nurse identifies and implements interventions that facilitate positive changes for the client. The client accepts the nurse's caring and may discuss concerns with the nurse that he has been unable to discuss with others. He listens to the nurse's reactions and, with the nurse's guidance, explores his methods of interaction and coping. He may tentatively try out new ways of responding to situations, and evaluate the effects. The working phase of the relationship can become extremely rewarding, and it is not uncommon for the client to become emotionally attached to the nurse during this time.

Table 6-6 Relationship of the Nursing Process with the Phases of the Nurse-Client Relationship

STEPS OF THE NURSING PROCESS	PHASES OF THE NURSE-CLIENT RELATIONSHIP
Assessment	Orientation phase
Diagnosis	
Outcome identification	Working phase
Planning/interventions	
Evaluation	Termination phase

The termination phase occurs when the nurse and client evaluate progress and determine that the client is ready to move on, to establish new patterns of interacting without the nurse. Termination is part of a professional relationship, because there is no expectation that the nurse and client will become friends or continue a relationship beyond that period of time when the client needs the nurse's assistance. Successful termination may mark the beginning of other relationships for the client. Peplau referred to this termination phase as a "freeing process," in which the client can let go and move on with other aspects of his life and with other relationships (Peplau, 1991).

The phases of the nurse-client relationship follow the steps of the nursing process. The orientation phase is also the assessment phase—the time of getting to know each other and gathering information. The working phase begins with mutually establishing goals and setting plans for nursing care. The termination phase comes about during evaluation, when it becomes clear that initial goals are met and there are no further goals that need to be established to continue the work. Table 6-6 illustrates the relationship.

Case Example 6-1 illustrates the phases of the nurse-client relationship.

The nurse must use all of the skills described in this chapter to initiate client care in the psychiatric setting. First, skills of therapeutic communication are needed to establish interactions with the client, and good communication skills are necessary to begin the nursing process. The nurse must be able to communicate in a manner that puts the client at ease and gives the client enough comfort to disclose information about self. The nurse-client relationship is based on

BOX 6-2
ALTERNATE FORMATS FOR DOCUMENTATION OF THE NURSING PROCESS: CARE PLAN AND CONCEPT MAP

CARE PLAN
Case summary, followed by an assessment of issues that stand out as important for care

Statement of nursing diagnosis with "related to" clause

Outcomes (anticipated outcomes of nursing care)	Nursing Actions (nursing activities to achieve outcomes)	Evaluation (data permitting the nurse to compare anticipated outcomes with observed outcomes)

Critical Thinking Questions (questions for further consideration)

CONCEPT MAP
Background data on the client
Initial Assessment and Reflection, based on the data
Initial Review of Nursing Diagnoses
Concept map diagram depicting relationships between and among issues

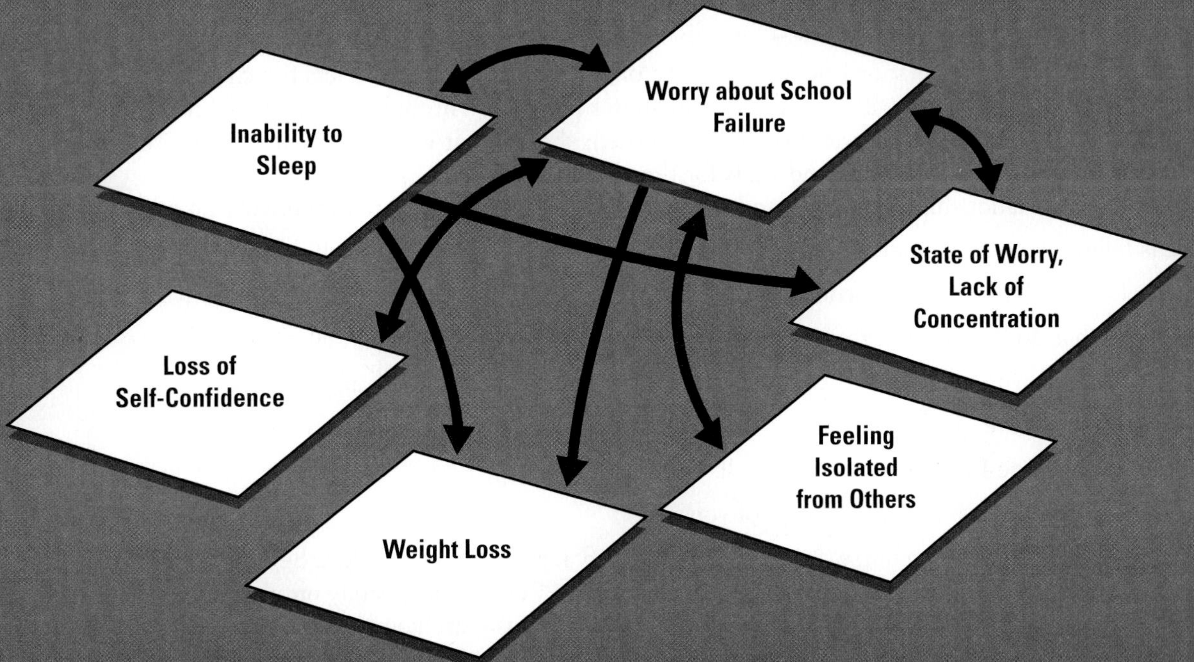

Nursing diagnosis, with rationale for priority setting
Nursing Interventions
Evaluation

trust and caring. All communications (verbal and nonverbal) must demonstrate this caring and show that the nurse is trustworthy. New psychiatric nurses find that the best way to begin their work is to approach a client sincerely and begin interactions. With experience, nurses find that positive nurse-client relationships require time and energy; some clients are easier for some nurses to engage than for others. Continual self-exploration helps the nurse assess her own limitations and abilities. The nurse-client relationship helps both nurse and client to grow, to engage, and to learn about self.

CASE EXAMPLE 6-1

Mrs. Rose M

Rose M. is a 50-year-old woman who was married for 27 years. She has one grown son in college. She and her former husband have just obtained a divorce. Her husband has moved out of their home, and Rose now lives alone. Rose has become depressed, finds herself crying often, and lacks energy. She came to a mental health clinic for help and was assigned to nurse Maria.

Maria initiates interactions so to build trust and establish a working relationship with Mrs. M. On their first encounter, the interactions included the following:

Nurse: I understand that you came here to the clinic because you have been troubled recently. Tell me about your situation.

Rose: I am at the end of my rope. I cry a lot and don't feel that I can function on my own. I feel ugly; I've never been strong, and now I don't know what I will do. This is worse than I've felt before.

Nurse: Tell me about what's happened before and how this is different.

Rose: You don't really want to know all about me. It doesn't matter.

Nurse: I have time to talk with you. I'm interested in exploring how I might assist you. You are upset now. That's why you came in. I am here to listen to you.

During this initial (orientation) phase, the nurse offers herself to the client, lets the client know she has time and interest to speak with her, and demonstrates patience. Through her nonverbal messages, Nurse Maria demonstrates she is attentive and concerned; she looks at Rose, offers herself by sitting at Rose's level and leaning toward her, and waits for the client to respond.

Later, as the relationship between Rose and Nurse Maria evolves, they are in the working phase. Rose is telling the nurse about experiences within her life that contributed to self-doubt:

Rose: I always had to be independent as a young girl. I never could rely on anyone, but I wanted to.

Nurse: What does that mean to you in terms of your current life?

Rose: If I am divorced, I have to be independent. I have to rely on myself, and I'm not so sure.

Nurse: Not so sure of what?

Rose: Not so sure I can take care of myself.

Nurse: What does it mean to take care of yourself?

In the working phase, the nurse assists Rose to identify feelings and to explore her life. Nurse Maria presents the reality of the situation to Rose. Maria learns that Rose is successfully employed as a secretary, is able to live on her own, but feels emotionally vulnerable. Rose is searching for stability and support. With Maria's referral, Rose joins a women's support group in the community. Rose continues to see Maria for several weeks, as her social supports in the community increase. At this point, Maria and Rose enter into the termination phase:

Nurse: Rose, you seem to have built many supports in the community. How are you feeling about this?

Rose: I am better. I have a friend to call if I am lonely. I have people who will listen to me and care about me.

Nurse: Perhaps now you need only come and see me once a month—to check in. You are quite independent now, compared to when we first met.

Rose: Yes, I think that is good. We can meet the first week of next month; then we'll see what I need.

Nurse: I have enjoyed getting to know you, and I am pleased that you seem happier than you were a few weeks ago.

Maria suggests that Rose may not need the nurse-client relationship on an ongoing basis. By suggesting that Rose come to see her next month, Maria is terminating the relationship over time to prevent any sense of abandonment. Rose's response indicates that she, too, feels that termination is appropriate.

KEY CONCEPTS

- Psychiatric mental health nurses use tools of self and tools of knowledge in their work.
- Well-developed skills in communication are essential to effective psychiatric nursing care. These include awareness of verbal and nonverbal communication techniques.
- The nurse should evaluate her own communication skills, identifying therapeutic and nontherapeutic techniques.
- The nursing process can be viewed in both a linear and a circular fashion as a tool to help nurses assess clients, identify appropriate outcomes, plan and implement effective care, and evaluate outcomes of nursing interventions.
- Several NANDA-I nursing diagnoses are seen frequently in the psychiatric mental health setting and help to identify the nursing role in care.
- Effective nursing interventions are grounded in a positive nurse-client relationship and address specific nursing diagnoses.
- The nurse-client relationship can be viewed as having three phases: orientation, working, and termination.

REVIEW QUESTIONS

1. A nurse has been treating an inpatient client for depression after the loss of her spouse. As the patient is being discharged, she attempts to schedule weekly outings with the nurse. The client also expresses a desire to call the nurse several times a week. Which of the following is the most appropriate action by the nurse?
   1. Continue to see the client socially, to insure that no relapses occur.
   2. Continue to see the client socially, because the nurse is the client's only friend.
   3. Terminate the nurse client relationship as scheduled in order to facilitate client growth and independence.
   4. Refuse any communication after the client has been discharged, and tell the client never to speak to her again.

2. In her first meeting with an agitated client, the nurse decides to use a tape recorder so she will not forget the client's responses. In the three subsequent meetings with the client, the nurse is unable to gain rapport and trust with the client. The most likely reason that rapport and trust has not developed is which of the following?
   1. The client has established a bond with the nurse, but is unable to express it.
   2. The client is unable to establish rapport with anyone, and the nurse should simply continue on without it.
   3. The client has an unfounded dislike for the nurse and prefers to be assigned to another nurse.
   4. The client may be defensive and closed because the nurse has never requested the client's consent to record their conversations.

3. The nurse has assessed each of her assigned clients. Which action should the nurse take next?
   1. Collaborate with each client to develop a set of outcomes.
   2. Ask the client for a list of outcomes the client wishes to achieve from treatment and rely exclusively on those. The client knows what is best for self.
   3. Have the client's family and friends develop a list of outcomes for treatment, since they have known the client longer than the nurse.
   4. Create a list of outcomes for the treatment and instruct the client that this is what he will be working on, because only the nurse knows what is in the best interest for the client.

4. The nurse admits a new client to the psychiatric unit where she works. Which of the following communication approaches would be most therapeutic in initiating a relationship with the client?
   1. "My name is Susan and I will be your nurse."
   2. "Why were you admitted to the hospital?"
   3. "Would you like a short tour of our unit?"
   4. "You are lucky to get admitted. The hospital has been very busy."

5. A client is admitted with a diagnosis of depression. The client is very withdrawn and sits in a chair in the dayroom saying very little to the staff or other clients. An appropriate nursing intervention would include which of the following?
   1. Allow the client her privacy.
   2. Ask some of the other clients to participate in an activity with the individual.
   3. Sit with the client to initiate a nurse-client relationship.
   4. Demand that the client interact with others on the unit.

6. A client who was admitted to the hospital for chemical dependence tells the nurse that he could control his use of drugs if he wanted to. The nurse assesses that the client is using which defense mechanism?
   1. Denial
   2. Projection
   3. Displacement
   4. Reaction formation
7. A client was sexually abused by a family member but is unable to recall the abuse. The nurse understands that which of the following defense mechanisms is active?
   1. Denial
   2. Repression
   3. Regression
   4. Suppression
8. A nurse is assigned to administer medications to all clients. Upon receiving his medications, one of the clients states, "You really look good! I'm being discharged tomorrow and would like to take you to dinner at a nice restaurant." The most therapeutic response by the nurse would be which of the following?
   1. Ignore the client's remark because the nurse is married.
   2. Clarify the relationship and set limits on inappropriate behavior.
   3. Ask the nursing supervisor if it is okay to date a former client.
   4. Request that another nurse be assigned to passing medications in the future.
9. A toddler is admitted to the hospital diagnosed with cancer. When the nurse enters the child's room, she finds the mother sobbing uncontrollably. The mother states, "It's my fault my baby has this disease. I must have done something wrong during my pregnancy." Which response by the nurse would be most therapeutic?
   1. "Do you want to talk about it?"
   2. "Does your husband blame you for the child's illness?"
   3. "This must be a difficult time for you. I will sit with you for a while."
   4. "Don't worry, your child will be fine. We have very good doctors here."
10. One of the nurse's clients has been diagnosed with AIDS. During a conversation with the nurse the client states, "Am I going to die?" Which statement by the nurse is most therapeutic?
    1. "What do you think?"
    2. "We all must die at some time."
    3. "You need to ask your doctor that question."
    4. "You should have thought of that before you had unprotected sex."
11. Driving to work, a nurse is assaulted and her purse is stolen. After completing the police report, she continues on to work and arrives more than an hour late. The supervisor meets the nurse at the elevator and reprimands her for being tardy. The nurse tries to explain why she is tardy, but the charge nurse just yells, "There are no excuses!" When the nurse enters a client's room, the client begins to complain about his breakfast. The nurse replies in an angry voice, "I'm not the cook, don't complain to me!" The nurse's response to the client indicates the use of which defense mechanism?
    1. Projection
    2. Displacement
    3. Reaction formation
    4. Rationalization

LEARNING ACTIVITIES

1. Identify ways that you can approach a client with the intention of establishing a positive nurse-client relationship.
2. Describe nonverbal interactions between yourself and another over a 5-minute period (or between two other persons you can observe).
3. Complete a process recording.
4. Explain the value of the nursing process in understanding client needs.
5. Use the NANDA-I diagnostic categories for a psychiatric mental health client; identify the independent nursing role and the collaborative nursing role.
6. Identify the phases of the nurse-client relationship as you initiate interaction with clients, as you enter the working phases, and as you plan for termination.

*Study*WARE™ CONNECTION

Using your *Study*WARE™ CD-ROM

1. Complete the Concentration activity for this chapter.
2. Review the audio glossary for key terms in this chapter.
3. Explore the other games and activities that support this chapter.

REFERENCES

Baugh, J., & Mellott, K. (1998). Clinical concept mapping as preparation for student nurses' clinical experiences. *Journal of Nursing Education, 37*(6), 253–256.

Carpenito-Moyet, L. J. (2007). *Handbook of nursing diagnosis* (12th ed.). Philadelphia: Lippincott, Williams & Wilkins.

Cliburn, J. W. (1990). Concept maps to promote meaningful learning. *Journal of College Science Teaching, 19*, 212–217.

Erickson, H., Tomlin, E., & Swain, M. (1983). *Modeling and role-modeling: A theory and paradigm for nursing*. Englewood Cliffs, NJ: Prentice Hall.

Frisch, N. (1994). The nursing process revisited. *Nursing Diagnosis, 5*, 51.

Gordon, M. (1994). *Nursing diagnosis: Process and application* (3rd ed.). St. Louis: Mosby.

Gordon, M. (2002). *Manual of nursing diagnosis* (10th ed.). St. Louis: Elsevier Mosby.

Hall, E. (1959). *The silent language*. New York: Doubleday.

Herdman, H. (Ed). (2009). *Nursing diagnosis: Definitions and classifications: 2009-2011*. Oxford: Wiley-Blackwell.

Jegede, O., Alaiyemola, F., & Okebukola, P. (1990). The effect of concept mapping on students' anxiety and achievement in biology. *Journal of Research in Science Teaching, 27*(10), 951–960.

Jones, S., & Brown, L. N (1993). Alternative view on defining critical thinking through the nursing process. *Holistic Nursing Practice, 7*(3), 71–75.

King, M., & Shell, R. (2002). Teaching and evaluating critical thinking with concept maps. *Nurse Educator, 27*(5), 214–216.

Mabbett, P. D. (1996). *Instant nursing assessment: Mental health*. Clifton Park, NY: Thomson Delmar Learning.

McCagg, E., & Dansereau, D. (1991). A convergent paradigm for examining knowledge mapping as a learning strategy. *Journal of Educational Research, 84*(6), 317–324.

Munoz, C., & Luckmann, J. (2005). *Transcultural communication in nursing* (2nd ed.). Clifton Park, NY: Delmar Cengage.

Peplau, H. (1991). *Interpersonal relations in nursing*. New York: Springer.

Pesut, D., & Herman, J. (1999). *Clinical reasoning: The art and science of critical and creative thinking*. Clifton Park, NY: Thomson Delmar Learning.

Schuster, P. M (2008). *Concept mapping: A critical-thinking approach to care planning* (2nd ed.). Philadelphia: F. A. Davis.

SUGGESTED READINGS

Munoz, C., & Luckmann, J. (2005). *Transcultural communication in nursing* (2nd ed.). Clifton Park, NY: Delmar Cengage.

Schuster, P. M. (2008). *Concept mapping: A critical thinking approach to care planning* (2nd ed.) Philadelphia: F.A. Davis.

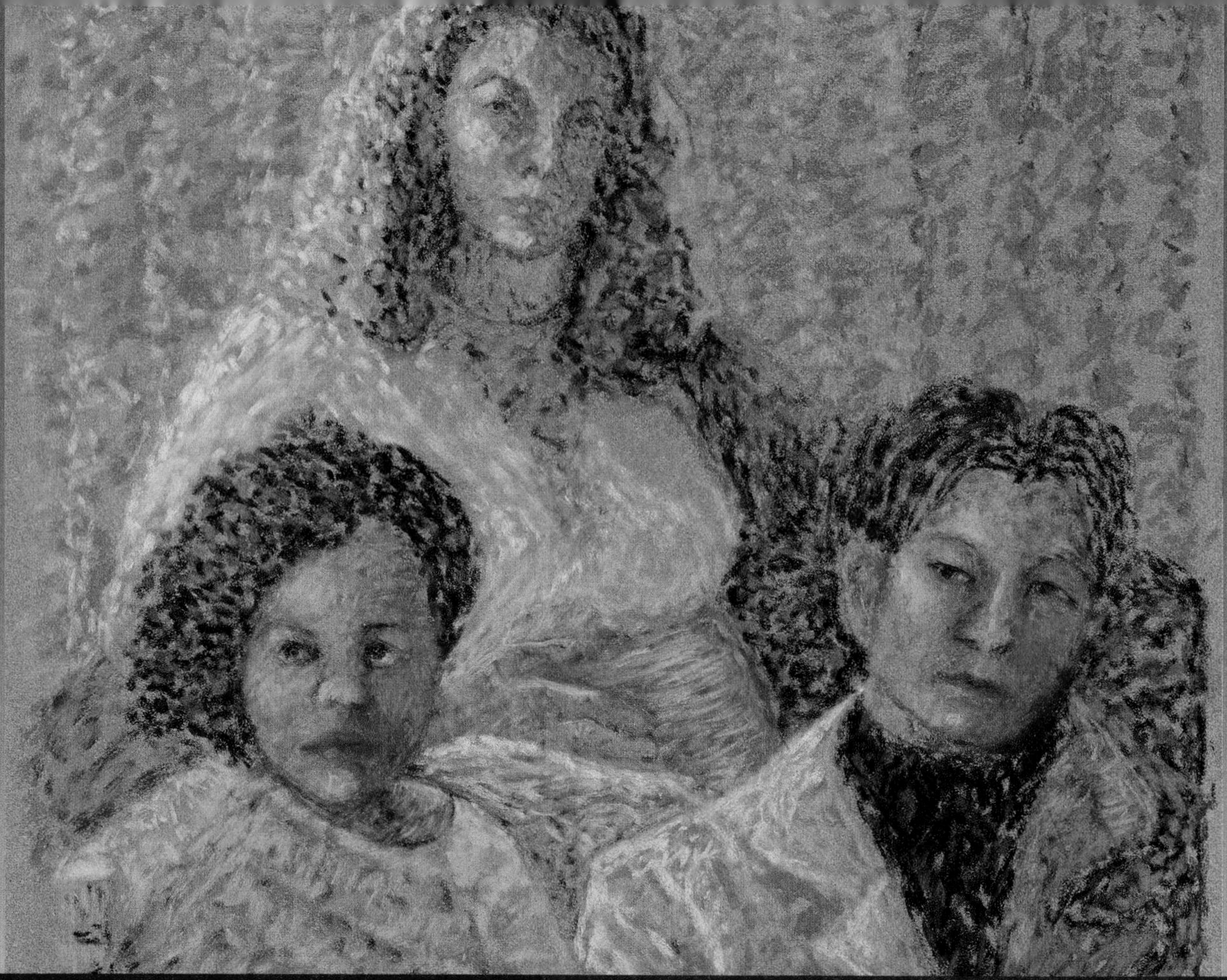

Categorically Speaking

Know Your Own Culture

To understand the culture of others, what do I have to know about myself? We can see the culture of others because of the different behaviors, customs, and beliefs. But we do not see our own culture unless we learn about it. Why? Because we experience our own culture as the way things really *are. Our reality is an exotic* other culture *to others! So, what must you know about yourself to provide skillful care to persons of different cultures? You must examine those aspects of your own behaviors, customs, and beliefs that are drawn from your culture. Andrews suggests that a critical element of cultural self-knowledge is recognizing the cultural groups that a person views negatively or positively, and recognizing the tendency to stereotype persons from cultures viewed negatively (Andrews & Boyle, 2008). Think about your own culture as you study this chapter.*

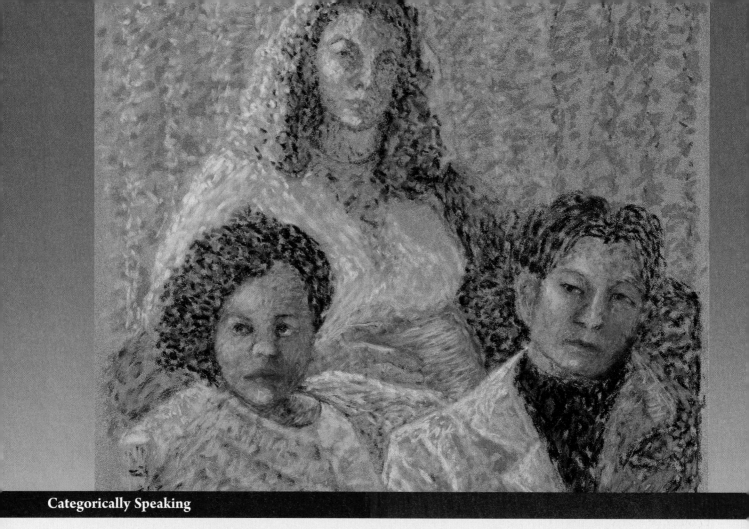

CHAPTER 7

Cultural and Ethnic Considerations

JANE KELLEY

CHAPTER OUTLINE

COMPETENCIES

Upon completion of this chapter, the reader should be able to:

1. Define *culture* as it applies to psychiatric mental health nursing.
2. Discuss the importance of understanding cultural variation when planning and implementing care.
3. Recognize, when caring for clients, ways in which clients may vary in their beliefs about the health care system and their attitudes about seeking appropriate care, especially mental health care.
4. Analyze verbal and nonverbal communication factors that affect transcultural interactions between nurse and client.
5. Describe the effect of cultural and ethnic variation on therapeutic management of psychiatric mental health care, including pharmacologic and behavioral elements.

KEY TERMS

Cultural Blindness
Cultural Facilitator/Broker
Culture
Culture Shock
Ethnicity
Ethnocentrism
Norms
Stereotype
Values

In recent years there has been an enormous increase in the number of cultures represented in the U.S. population. The challenge to mental health care has grown along with the changing population. This challenge includes the responsibility of mental health professionals to become culturally competent in delivering mental health care through understanding the cultural factors that affect mental health and mental health care. As noted by Saldana (2001, p. 3), "Developing culturally sensitive practices can help reduce barriers to effective treatment utilization."

The role of culture in mental health is difficult to isolate because every human lives within a cultural context. However, our beliefs and behaviors and the way we communicate these interpersonally are culturally based. The variation among cultures can create misunderstandings and misinterpretation of behaviors and communications when interacting individuals are unfamiliar with each other's culture. The purpose of this chapter is to identify the components of culture that can affect the therapeutic relationship and to determine how psychiatric mental health nurses can incorporate this knowledge to provide culturally competent care.

Interpersonal relationships, verbal and nonverbal communication, value orientations, religion, social systems, diet, and health- and illness-related beliefs are all culturally based and directly or indirectly affect psychiatric mental health care. Given that culture affects our thoughts and behaviors to such a pervasive extent, it can be concluded that nurses who deal with peoples' thoughts and/or behaviors must understand the role of culture.

The primary tool of the psychiatric mental health nurse is interpersonal communication. Because culture is intrinsic to communication, and because interpersonal communication is an interaction of two cultures (client's and nurse's), it is essential that the nurse understand how culture affects verbal and nonverbal communication and how to modify communication skills to appropriately interact with a variety of clients. Culture and its expression through group and individual norms, values, and behaviors must be understood and used to assess client status and to plan and implement appropriate care.

CULTURE DEFINED

Culture has been defined in many different ways, but is still not well understood. One classic and comprehensive definition is that of Tylor (1871), which describes culture as the complex whole, including knowledge, belief, art, morals, law, custom, and any other capabilities and habits acquired by man as a member of society. Culture comprises every verbal or behavioral system that transmits meaning. Culture is learned, shared, and ever-changing. It is learned through socialization, shared by all group members, and associated with adaptation to the environment.

The traditional definition of culture describes it to be static or near static. Agar (1994) has proposed a different definition that incorporates the ever-changing, dynamic nature of culture. He proposes that culture is malleable like clay, and any interaction by persons from different cultures modifies the cultures of both participants.

For Agar, culture serves as an ever-changing frame for interpreting information and understanding how the world works. Agreeing with Hermans, Kempen, and Van Loon (1992), Agar sees the self as "dialogical," a product of all past stories and multicultural experiences, producing multiple identities interacting within the same individual. In this view, psychological processes are influenced by and develop from this dynamic interaction of culture and history. Therefore, in Agar's view, one cannot talk about a person's culture as though it can be shared by all members of a group and transmitted as a whole from one generation to the next, as is implied in more traditional definitions of culture.

Culture, itself, is universal in that humans cannot exist apart from culture. In this traditional view of culture, the culture defines **values** (learned beliefs about what is held to be good or bad in a culture) and **norms** (learned behaviors that are perceived to be appropriate or inappropriate in a culture). Therefore, in a given society, culture defines the roles, relationships, rights, and obligations of its members. It is through the lens of culture that profound questions of existence and being are addressed, such as the essence of human nature, the purpose of human existence, and the relationship of humans to one another, to nature, and to the divine or eternal. The worldview is drawn from and reflects the total integration of the group's beliefs and practices, flowing from the culture.

The worldview that each of us forms based on our own culture becomes for us reality. Unless we have come to recognize that many cultures have different worldviews, we are often not aware that other people might have a different perception about what is right and true. This perception that our worldview is the only acceptable truth and that our beliefs, values, and sanctioned behaviors are superior to all others is called **ethnocentrism**.

Many individuals are aware that other cultures exist and that they have different beliefs, values, and accepted behaviors. However, many persons do not understand that great variation exists within any cultural group. When this variation is not recognized, individuals tend to **stereotype** all members of the particular culture, expecting the group members to hold the same beliefs and behave the same way.

NURSINGTIP 7-1

What is Culture?

Remember the many points related to culture:

- Transmits meaning
- Is learned
- Is shared
- Is ever-changing
- Is "dialogical"
- Defines values
- Defines norms for:
    - Roles, relationships
    - Rights and obligations
    - Beliefs and practices or behaviors
    - Defines worldview

CULTURAL SENSITIVITY

Much has been written on the need for nurses to become skilled at incorporating transcultural concepts into nursing care. Campinha-Bacote's (1998, 2003, 2008) model described in *The Process of Cultural Competence in the Delivery of Healthcare Services* has five elements: cultural desire, cultural awareness, cultural knowledge, cultural skill, and cultural encounter. The elements interact to depict an ongoing process "in which the healthcare professional continuously strives to achieve the ability and availability to work effectively within the cultural context of the client (individual, family, community)" (2003, p. 14). The author defined each element in 1998 and again in 2003. *Cultural desire* represents the motivation to "want to" engage in becoming culturally competent (p. 15); *cultural awareness* represents self-examination and in-depth exploring of one's own cultural background (p. 18); *cultural knowledge* involves seeking and obtaining a sound educational base about culturally different groups (p. 27); *cultural skill* reflects the ability to collect cultural data about the client's presenting problem and also accurately perform a culturally based physical assessment (p. 35); and *cultural encounters* encompasses the process that encourages the professional to directly engage in face-to-face interactions with culturally varied clients (p. 49).

Campinha-Bacote (2003, p. 14) lists assumptions on which the model is based:

1. Cultural competence is a process; not an event.
2. The process of cultural competence consists of five inter-related constructs [as noted].
3. The key and pivotal construct of cultural competence is cultural desire.
4. There is more variation within cultural groups than across cultural groups (intracultural variation).
5. There is a direct relationship between a healthcare professional's level of cultural competence and "the" ability to provide culturally responsive healthcare services.
6. Cultural competence is an essential component in rendering effective culturally responsive care to all clients (Campinha-Bacote, 2003).

Cultural assessment assumes that the nurse adopts a cultural perspective for providing nursing care. Such a cultural perspective includes three interacting viewpoints: objective, subjective, and contextual (Lipson, 1996a). The context referred to is the context of the cross-cultural encounter, which includes the broader cultural, socioeconomic, and political influences operating within the health care system and affecting the client and nurse. Objective components include the client's, family's, nurse's, and community's cultural and social characteristics, communication patterns, and worldviews. The subjective components are the nurse's personal and cultural characteristics and cultural self-awareness.

Cultural assessment can only be accomplished skillfully when the nurse has acquired sufficient knowledge of his or her own culture and a variety of other cultures to avoid stereotyping and ethnocentrism. Leininger (1978, 1991) and

Leininger and McFarland (2002, 2006) urge nurses to avoid seeing all individuals as being alike and to adopt a broad, open, objective attitude toward cultural variation and toward individuals from the various cultural groups. Another behavior to avoid is **cultural blindness**, which is the attempt to treat all persons fairly by ignoring differences and acting as though the differences do not exist. Such cultural blindness can be perceived as insensitivity just as readily as are stereotyping and ethnocentrism.

Cultural assessment in any health care setting must address the many sources of within-group variation that result from influences other than culture. First, cultural assessment usually includes elements often identified as racial, based on biological differences such as disease susceptibility and genetic variation. (Incidentally, studies of biological variation show no clustering of characteristics that would support a biological basis for race.) Cultural assessment includes variation resulting from **ethnicity**, which is identification with a "socially, culturally, and politically constructed group of individuals that holds a common set of characteristics not shared by others with whom its members come in contact" (Lipson, 1996b, p. 8). Such characteristics as common ancestry, sense of historical continuity, common language, religion, and intergroup interaction are elements of ethnicity. These characteristics may not be shared by any but one subgroup of a larger cultural group.

Other cultural assessment components not directly related to culture are socioeconomic status and social class. Circumstances of minority status or recent immigration may be thought to be inseparable from low socioeconomic status and social class, but much variation can be found within any cultural or ethnic group. However, a challenge for the nurse undertaking a cultural assessment is separating the effects of these four influences on health and health care. Often, the effect of low socioeconomic status on health and seeking care is greater than that of other cultural or ethnic influences (Saraceno, Levav, & Kohn, 2005; Williams & Collins, 1995). Careful assessment will seek to distinguish between cultural and socioeconomic influences or the interactions of the two. It is important to note that most cultural or ethnic groups within the United States have some members who are in high socioeconomic categories and high social class. The nurse must recognize that variation within cultural groups may be great.

Several approaches to cultural assessment have been developed by and for nurses. A framework for cultural assessment by Giger and Davidhizar (2003; 2008) addresses six cultural variables having an effect on health and illness behaviors: (1) communication, (2) space, (3) social organization, (4) time, (5) environmental control, and (6) biological variations.

Andrews and Boyle (2003) provide a comprehensive guide for transcultural nurses to assess cultural manifestations relevant to nursing. Categories to be assessed include (1) biocultural variations and cultural aspects of the incidence of disease; (2) communication (language; fluency in English; verbal and nonverbal communication styles; comfort with health care provider of different culture, social class, gender, age); (3) cultural affiliations; (4) cultural sanctions and restrictions; (5) developmental considerations; (6) educational background; (7) health-related beliefs and practices; (8) kinship and social networks; (9) nutrition; (10) religious affiliation; and (11) values orientation, and economics (2008, pp. 453–457). The importance of these two sets of cultural variants to psychiatric mental health nursing will be examined. For purposes of this chapter, categories to be assessed and around which culturally sensitive mental health care can be planned include (1) beliefs about mental illness and related care, (2) interpersonal interaction, (3) verbal and nonverbal communication, (4) diet and food habits, and (5) biological variation.

Beliefs about Mental Illness and Care

Health and illness states are not universally perceived. Culture defines what is considered to be normal or abnormal with regard to physical and psychological health: "It is culture not nature that defines disease, although it is usually culture and nature which foster disease" (Hughes, 1978, p. 153).

Many variations in culturally based beliefs and behaviors affect care, specifically care for clients with mental aberrations. Beliefs about causation of illness or disease vary greatly across cultures. There is a close integration of these beliefs with other institutions of the society, such as religious and social structures (Hughes, 1978). In less industrialized societies, and to some extent in fully industrialized societies, these beliefs about causation fall into five basic categories: (1) sorcery; (2) breach of taboo; (3) intrusion of a disease object; (4) intrusion of a disease-causing spirit; or (5) loss of soul (Clements, 1932, as discussed in Hughes, 1978). Usually the major belief pattern in a society will emphasize one or more of the categories. For instance, Eskimos emphasize soul loss or breach of taboo as causes of illness, while many African groups attribute disease to sorcerers or witches. The ancient Greeks emphasized the role of interaction with others and the environment. They attributed illness more to a disharmony in the relationship with the universe. The Native American belief system is more aligned with the Greek belief in that illness is believed to result more from

REFLECTIVE THINKING 7-1

Cultural Identity

Consider the dominant culture in which you live. What are the values and beliefs (i.e., time, money, family, honesty, productivity, wisdom, and the like) that seem most important in this culture? Which of these values do you most closely espouse? If your values come into conflict with those of the dominant culture or with the value system enforced by the institution where you work, how do you decide which set of values to follow?

moral transgression (thought or action) against the norms of society, creating an imbalance in mind, body, spirit, and environment (Hughes, 1978).

If the client's belief system differs from that of the usual Western psychomedical beliefs, then the effect of the type of treatment and its method of delivery must be considered before interventions can be determined. Otherwise there may be no therapeutic effect or the intervention could actually produce harm for the client or for the client's family.

To provide culturally safe and effective care, the nurse needs to understand the potential variations in the who, what, and when of care seeking. In a given cultural group, and specifically for a particular client, the nurse needs to determine:

1. What behaviors, feelings, or states would be considered abnormal, depending on subgroup (age, gender, or other designation)
2. At what point or in what circumstances the individual would seek care and from whom care would be sought
3. What care or treatment would be acceptable.

Normal vs. Abnormal Behavior

One behavior often cited as an example of cultural variation in the perception of normal versus abnormal behavior is *pibloktog*, seen in Eskimo women, also called "Arctic hysteria." Under certain circumstances, the women exhibit unrestrained, bizarre behavior such as running naked through the snow. The condition is not considered to represent abnormal behavior in the Eskimo culture (Parker, 1977).

Even in cultures as closely related as the American Anglo culture and the British culture of England, what is considered normal and abnormal behavior differs. The behaviors that lead to the diagnoses of depression and anxiety differ enough for an American who is vivacious, talkative, and energetic to be diagnosed as anxious or manic in England and for an English man or woman who is only slightly more reserved in demeanor than is average to be diagnosed as depressed in the United States (Dasen, Berry, & Sartorius, 1988).

Care Seeking and Acceptable Care

As noted in the following chapter on epidemiology of mental illness, even within the dominant cultures of the United States, there is variation in care seeking for mental illness. Often, immigrant and minority individuals seek mental health care only or initially from a traditional practitioner such as a medicine man, herbalist, curandero or santero, voodoo priest, or other traditional healer. Sue and Sue (1990) reported studies that found that Native Americans, Asian Americans, African Americans, and Hispanics use mental health services substantially less or terminate therapy after only one contact at a rate much higher than European Americans. Reasons for the differences are thought to be: few minority professionals; a one-to-one counseling style in the counselor's office; an emphasis on social-emotional needs rather than on vocational and educational needs; and the verbal focus, which is difficult for those with nonstandard English or an accent. Other suggested barriers include:

Big Raven by Emily Carr

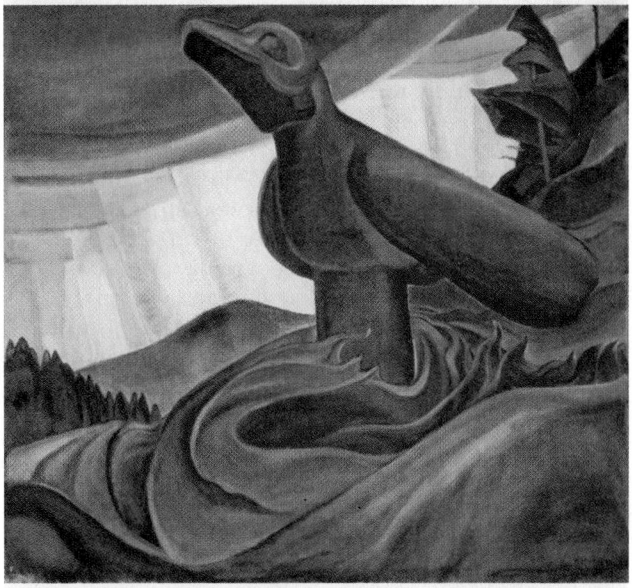

Source: Emily Carr, *Big Raven*, 1931, Oil on Canvas, 87.0 × 114.0 cm, Vancouver Art Gallery, Emily Carr Trust, VAG42.3 11 (Photo: Trevor Mills)

This well-loved Canadian painter returned throughout her long life to paintings and carvings of the Northwest Indian villages. Of this painting she wrote: "Here I wanted to paint not so much . . . what they looked like as what they felt like." It is unlikely that Carr ever saw totems of this monumental size, but the Raven's spiritual power—and that of the culture that created him—stirred the painter's imagination. The painting is a powerful depiction of a culture's physical and psychospiritual environment as seen through the sympathetic eyes of an outsider.

1. Monocultural assumptions of mental health
2. Negative stereotypes of pathology for minority lifestyles
3. Ineffective, inappropriate, and antagonistic counseling approaches to the values held by minorities.

Another example of cultural beliefs producing a barrier to professional care seeking for mental illness is described by Ho, Rasheed, & Rasheed (2003). Ho noted that a central Asian belief is that "the best healing source lies within the family" and seeking help from outside (such as counseling and therapy) is nonproductive and against dictates of Asian philosophy. Since balance is the Asian ideal, and mental as well as physical illness is thought to be associated with imbalance, traditional healers and Chinese medicine would be the care options of choice to many Asians. "The Chinese have characteristic ways of dealing with mental illness in the family, starting with a protracted period of intrafamilial coping with even serious psychiatric illness, followed by recourse to friends, elders, and neighbors in the community, consultation with traditional specialists, religious healers, or general

REFLECTIVE THINKING 7-2

Culturally Inappropriate Therapy

You are caring for Michael Wong, an Asian American student who reveals that he is from a "very traditional" Chinese family from San Francisco. He is a student at your university and comes to the student health center when he becomes very stressed by his studies. The psychologist, based on her assessment that Michael is under great family pressure to make high grades in his science major, uses an approach encouraging Michael to express his true feelings of anger and frustration toward his parents.

1. Why are you not surprised that Michael has returned to the health center even more depressed and withdrawn than before the therapy?
2. How could the therapy techniques be clashing with traditional Chinese cultural values?
3. What could the nurse do to improve the situation?

physicians, and finally, treatment from Western specialists" (Andrews & Boyle, 2008, p. 242).

Other ethnic groups within the United States seek folk or popular health care systems before entering the Western, institutionalized system. Many do so out of contrasting beliefs about cause of illness. Others do so because they are intimidated by the impersonal and technological environment, lengthy history taking, and invasive diagnostic procedures. Traditional, alternative, or complementary health care techniques are also rapidly increasing in popularity among members of the educated mainstream U.S. culture.

The role of spirituality and religion cannot be omitted from a discussion of mental illness and care. Modern psychology and psychiatry have developed mostly in Western cultural settings, and, therefore, many of the concepts and ideas for achieving psychological health are based on Western culture and theology. However, beliefs about the role of psychic forces in mental status have a cultural and theological basis. Because spiritual concerns are deeply entwined with self-perception and perception of the world around us, the nurse providing care must understand the client's beliefs with regard to self, others, and God or a transcendent being and how these beliefs may affect care. As noted by Andrews and Boyle (2003, p. 291), "use of psychiatric resources is discouraged by professionals' intolerance for magical and religious orientations and practices, which is common when science and systems of symbolic beliefs and faith compete."

INTERPERSONAL INTERACTION

Culture is an important variable to be incorporated into therapeutic interpersonal interactions. In addition to verbal and nonverbal communication, to be discussed in the next section, other components of interpersonal interaction vary across cultures and affect personal relationships, therapeutic relationships, and care for psychiatric mental health clients. Examples of cultural values that may be reflected in interpersonal interaction include: (1) acceptance of inequality of status and power among its members; (2) acceptance of collectivism versus individualism; (3) favoring of masculine versus feminine cultural traits; and (4) the level of need to avoid uncertainty (Pedersen & Ivey, 1993).

Differences in these cultural values relative to interpersonal interaction can affect care. For instance, persons from cultures that accept inequality of status and power among its members may expect different levels of care for more or less powerful persons, and they may specify decision-makers among family or group members who will need to be consulted. Persons from collectivist cultures will determine the individual to be less important than the group, and dependent or self-sacrificing behaviors must be interpreted within the cultural belief system. In group-oriented societies, the concept of self is not well defined; self-actualization as a goal or psychoanalysis as a therapy would not be acceptable in such a cultural setting. Persons from cultures valuing masculine traits will focus on achievements, assertiveness, competitiveness, and toughness, and social gender roles will be distinctly separated. Such persons will be less likely to seek health care, especially mental health care, because of its association with weakness.

Pedersen and Ivey (1993) noted that within a given culture, certain behaviors are interpreted to communicate attributes, such as being friendly, unfriendly, trusting, mistrustful, interested, or bored. However, the associated behaviors that clearly communicate given attributes will differ across cultures. When people of two quite different cultures interact, the behaviors exhibited may not be the behaviors expected in each other's culture to convey the attribute. For instance, in one culture, interest is conveyed by direct eye contact, while in another culture, no eye contact is interpreted to indicate interest and direct eye contact may indicate boredom (Pedersen & Ivey, 1993).

NURSINGTIP 7-2

Storytelling

Could storytelling be used as a way of bridging the cultural gap for persons from cultures in which self-disclosure is not acceptable or is not valued? Narayan (1991), in a chapter entitled "According to Their Feelings: Teaching and Healing with Stories," tells of the use of folklore stories to heal, to decrease pain, or to increase endurance. These stories are well-known folklore transformed to meet the needs of the occasion. He describes the use of symbols and symbolic meaning in Hindu, Oriental, Islamic, and Amerindian stories. Perhaps sharing the story with input from the client may elicit feelings and provide understanding without the client having to directly reveal personal details or emotions. (Read Narayan in Witherell and Noddings, 1991, *Stories Lives Tell: Narrative and Dialogue in Education*, pp. 113–135.)

Because we tend to assume that others are similar to us, differences such as these can result in enormous communication barriers. People from outside a cultural group may not know the cultural rules of that group. It is easy to see where a client and nurse or counselor from different cultures may misunderstand each other. One may be restrained and formal, the other animated. One may be soft-spoken, the other loud. One may internalize stress, the other externalize it. In each case, the person is likely behaving in a manner appropriate to his or her culture, but may be conveying a very different meaning because the behaviors do not meet the expectations of the other's culture.

It is important for a nurse to communicate effectively with a client; to do so, the nurse must be able to interpret the meaning of more than the words used. The nurse must be conscious of the patterns, expectations, meanings of behaviors, and the likely barriers to communication: "When two culturally different parties misattribute each other's behavior, this misattribution is likely to result in a negative chain reaction of escalating hostility" (Pedersen & Ivey, 1993).

VERBAL AND NONVERBAL COMMUNICATION

When the client and nurse do not speak the same language, a potentially challenging communication barrier must be overcome. As can be surmised from the preceding discussion and from the discussion to follow about nonverbal communication, more than mere words must be interpreted if effective communication is to occur. It is for this reason that persons designated as "translators" or "interpreters" must know more of the culture than just the oral or written language to adequately meet the need in a health care setting. A **cultural facilitator** or **broker**, who can interpret the language, the client's culture, and the health care culture, is the ideal person to serve as interpreter (Jezewski, 1993). If such a person is unavailable and a language interpreter must be used, then certain criteria should be considered. Avoid selecting an interpreter from a rival faction or group; from a sex, age, or socioeconomic group that would prevent open communication; or from among family members when status would affect disclosure. When using an interpreter, the nurse should speak in his or her own language directly to the client, not to the interpreter. This direct approach conveys much more than just the content of the words.

If no interpreter is available even for word translation, then approach the client in a calm, friendly manner using pantomime as necessary, and construct a picture board to which the client can point to communicate basic needs until an interpreter can be found. One source of interpreters is a telephone company. Some telephone companies, such as AT&T, offer immediate interpreting services.

Communication is the primary tool of psychiatric mental health nursing. In order to understand the client's situation as the client does, the nurse needs to be able to understand the meaning of the words used and the implication of the behaviors demonstrated or described by the client. Mutually understandable communication between nurse and client will facilitate a working, collaborative relationship.

There are many components of communication that may serve as barriers to conveying the message intended by the sender. Nurses must recognize the areas of verbal and nonverbal communication that can serve as barriers and use this knowledge to facilitate understanding. Andrews and Boyle (1999) divide nonverbal components of communication into five categories: vocal cues (pitch, tone, and quality of voice); action cues (posture, facial expression, and gestures); object cues (clothing, jewelry, and hair style); care of belongings and use of personal and territorial space; and touch (use of personal space and action; p. 35). In addition to oral and written language, the relevance of tone of voice, eye contact, facial expressions, use of gestures, use of silence, proxemics (touch and comfortable distance), courteous social behavior, dress, and associated gender differences will be discussed as areas of potential miscommunication.

An example of variation in the cultural norm for tone of voice is described by Thiederman (1991, video). A Middle Eastern mother and baby were passengers on an airplane. The mother approached Dr. Thiederman and said, "Give me your newspaper." The woman's voice was relatively harsh, forceful, and to the point, not asking "please" or "may I." As an American raised in the predominant culture of the American middle class, Dr. Thiederman's first reaction was negative and resentful. But as a consultant for cultural variation, Dr. Thiederman recognized that the Middle Eastern woman was using the polite and normal requesting style of her culture. Had the woman asked in the American style of "Could you let me have your newspaper, please?" it would have sounded to her as if she were saying, "Would it be possible for you to graciously let me have your newspaper, please?" This would sound overly solicitous to our ears, just as our courteous request would sound overly solicitous to a Middle Easterner.

Eye Contact

Eye contact has many implications in different cultures and is probably the most variable of the nonverbal communicators. Whether or not to maintain direct eye contact, with whom, and for how long are all variables to consider. Gender differences are also to be considered, because eye contact is tied to expression of modesty and intimacy. Persons from certain Middle Eastern, Asian, Native American, and Appalachian backgrounds consider direct eye contact to be impolite or aggressive, and Hispanic Americans may use downcast eyes to indicate appropriate deference and respect toward others based on age, sex, social position, economic status, or position of authority (Andrews & Boyle, 2003, p. 27). As clients, these individuals may avert their eyes when talking, but in their cultures, such behavior indicates paying close, respectful attention to what is being said. Often African Americans will avert their eyes when being spoken to but use direct eye contact when speaking, and some use eye rolling when asked a question that is perceived to be ridiculous (Andrews & Boyle, 2003, pp. 27–28). This pattern is perceived by European Americans to represent inattention or disrespect. The effect of differences in rank or gender may result in reluctance to maintain direct eye contact or to interpret the nurse's eye contact pattern to be insulting or disrespectful. If the nurse maintains the level of direct eye contact considered professionally therapeutic in American nursing, the client may interpret the behavior to be sexual in nature. In many cultures, the only women who smile at men in a public place are prostitutes (Andrews & Boyle, 2008, p. 25).

Proxemics (Space and Distance)

Proxemics, or how close we stand to another individual for social or professional conversation and what is considered to be culturally appropriate regarding touch, varies greatly across cultures. Social events that include guests from a variety of cultures are often used to illustrate social distance. When European Americans and persons of Arabic, European, or Hispanic origin begin a conversation, the American tends to take a step back, the person from the other culture moves closer, the American moves back, the other moves closer, and on and on, until the American is against the wall! In international circles, this has been referred to as the "cocktail party two step."

Touch

Touch is such an important part of the therapeutic role of the nurse, in providing hands-on care, in healing through therapeutic or healing touch, and in conveying comfort. Extreme care must be exercised when using touch with persons from different cultures. For instance, whether or not to touch a baby has major implications. Touching or examining a baby's head requires parental permission or should not be done at all in some Southeast Asian cultures. A perceived affliction that is feared in various parts of the world, particularly among the Hispanic population, is called *mal ojo*, whereby a child is thought to become ill if given excessive admiration by another person (Andrews & Boyle, 2003, p.157). However, there is even variation within cultures. In some parts of Mexico, looking at and admiring a child without touching is considered to be the source of illness; in other parts of Mexico, touching itself if done by a stranger is considered to be the source of illness. And then there is touch between adults. Physical touch by health care professionals is acceptable only between clients and professionals of the same sex in some Islamic and Hispanic societies. Even within middle-class American society, some individuals (caregivers or clients) are uncomfortable with touching or being touched by another. It may be necessary to discuss expectations of touch with a client to prevent misunderstanding and miscommunication.

Silence

Silence is both a nonverbal behavior and a component of the qualities of verbal expression patterns. In both senses, the use of silence varies across cultures. Trompenaars (1993, 1994) contrasted speech patterns of European Americans, Hispanic Americans, and Asian Americans and described the discomfort of each group with the alternate patterns of the other two. In a conversation between two European Americans, when one stops speaking, the other starts. Among Hispanic Americans, there is overlap so that before one is finished, the other person begins. Among Asian Americans, when one stops speaking, the other waits in silence for a few moments before beginning to speak. These patterns are characteristic of polite, interested conversation in the respective cultures. If a European American interrupts or remains silent when the other person stops speaking, it usually indicates rudeness or disinterest or some other undesirable intent. If a Hispanic American either does not enthusiastically jump in with comments before the other person finishes or remains silent, disinterest or distrust is being conveyed. The Asian American remains silent in order to allow processing of the comments and to formulate a thoughtful, respectful reply.

Other uses of silence also convey meaning. For instance, silence may convey respect for privacy among English and Arabs; a sign of agreement among French, Spanish, and Russians; or a sense of absurdity if asked what is perceived to be a ridiculous or senseless question (Andrews & Boyle, 2008, p. 25). But silence used in a manner not considered positive in the respective culture produces discomfort or other negative feelings.

REFLECTIVE THINKING 7-3

Use of Silence

Have you ever been caring for a client from a cultural background different from your own and experienced awkwardness with the use of silence? In the dominant American culture, silence is often viewed as uncomfortable, and you may feel an urge to jump in and fill the silence. As a nurse, you must remember that silence can be a very valuable therapeutic tool when used to allow a client to gather thoughts, reflect on statements or situations, or check emotions.

NURSINGTIP 7-3

Cultural Awareness

Analyze a conversation with another person, preferably one from a culture different from your own, and list the similarities and differences in your approaches to silence, time, proxemics, body language, and eye contact.

Social Behavior

Behavior is culturally based. The level of formality in human relationships varies markedly, from the informality of American social interaction, wherein people of different age groups and economic or social positions often call each other by first name, to the formality of Asian cultures, wherein a rigid system exists for interactions between people of different ages or ranks. Accepted methods for greeting each other are defined by the culture as well. In Latino cultures and some European cultures, kissing on both cheeks is expected for females who know each other and, often, for males who know each other, and hugs between same-sex friends or colleagues are expected. Handshaking is the norm and may accompany cheek kisses in some cultures. Who offers a hand first and to whom also varies among cultures.

Time Orientation

Orientation to time is another cultural factor that influences interpersonal behavior. There are two aspects of time orientation that can affect psychiatric mental health care: (1) emphasis on past, present, or future time orientation, and (2) organization of activities either sequentially or synchronically.

In cultures emphasizing the present, for instance, keeping appointments may be a low priority. Whatever is going on in the present is perceived to be of greater importance than a future good, so if one is involved in something pleasing or important, then the appointment will be dealt with later. Delaying gratification is not perceived to be of great benefit because future outcome is not the focus. In some cultures, such as American and Northern European ones, time is perceived to move in a straight line. In other cultures, time is often perceived to be moving in a circle, with the past and present mixed together with future possibilities (Trompenaars, 1993, 1994).

The expected way of organizing activities varies across cultures and can produce miscommunication. Sequentially organized persons complete a task before moving to the next one. Synchronically organized persons can skillfully carry out two or more tasks at the same time. Trompenaars (1993, 1994) describes this difference and the misunderstanding that can result. An example describes major misunderstanding resulting from a Korean man entering an office when his American colleague is talking on the telephone. Having just arrived in America, the Korean expects the American to be able to continue the conversation while eagerly welcoming him. Instead, the American barely acknowledges his entrance until ending the telephone conversation, at which time he enthusiastically greets the Korean. But the greeting is perceived to be too late and, therefore, insincere.

Sequential people tend to be punctual and keep to an agenda, characteristics less common among synchronous people. Again, several other cultural values compete with punctuality. Obviously, sequentiality and synchronicity are associated with the different time orientations of past, present, or future.

> **NURSINGTIP 7-4**
>
> **Time Orientation**
>
> In the mainstream American culture, time is a very valued commodity (after all, "time equals money!"). When caring for clients of different cultural backgrounds, be sensitive to the fact that they may well place a different value on time than what you are accustomed to. If a client is late for an appointment or seems to want to spend more time discussing a certain topic than you feel is warranted, be careful not to jump to the conclusion that the client is lazy or disrespectful of your time. Instead, take a moment to step back from the situation and ask yourself what value this client might place on time and consider how you might meet the client's needs as well as your own.

Diet and Food Habits

There is much variation in diet and food habits across cultures. These differences are readily noted in the many ethnic cookbooks at bookstores. Many variations exist even in the United States. New England food differs from Southern food, and both differ from California cuisine. But of greatest importance to psychiatric care is the interaction of certain foods with medications or mood. More detail is provided on these variations in the chapters where conditions and medications are discussed.

Biological Variation

Biological variation is important to consider for psychiatric mental health care because certain physical and genetic characteristics affect the epidemiology of diseases and the effects of medications. The epidemiology of psychiatric conditions is discussed in another chapter. A brief overview of ethnopharmacology is included here.

The effects of genetic, environmental, and behavioral differences across cultural groups must be considered when administering medications. Differences in pharmacokinetic and pharmacodynamic properties of medications have been compared for individuals of Asian, African, Hispanic, Native American, and European descents (Campinha-Bacote, 2000). Important findings suggest that Asian Americans are slow metabolizers as compared to African Americans and European Americans (reviewed in Andrews & Boyle, 1999). The basis for this finding may be the association between smoking, drinking alcohol, and increased drug metabolism (evident in African Americans and European Americans) and between a low-protein, high-carbohydrate diet and slow metabolism (characteristic of Asian Americans). Andrews and Boyle (2008) provide a table of cultural difference related to drugs (pp. 47–48).

Examples of the cultural variation seen in psychotropic and tranquilizing medication according to Andrews and Boyle (2008) include the following:

- Arab Americans may need lower doses.
- Asian/Pacific Islanders need lower doses and may need only half the usual dose for tricyclic antidepressants (TCAs).

REFLECTIVE THINKING 7-4

Institutional Culture Shock

There is a culture in every work environment. Persons not a part of the work group culture can experience the same reactions as they would to negotiating a foreign culture, with its own language, meanings, and assumptions about acceptable behavior. Employees and clients who have to learn the routines and language of an institution often experience this culture shock. Since all clients who have not previously been admitted to a mental health facility are subject to institutional culture shock, how would you modify the assessment for a client from a culture different from your own? What approaches would convey caring and sensitivity, despite cultural differences?

- Blacks have increased extrapyramidal side effects to TCAs. Up to 20% may also metabolize Valium (diazepam) poorly.
- Jewish North Americans and other Ashkenazi may develop agranulocytosis when clozapine is used for schizophrenia (Andrews & Boyle, 2008, 47–48).

"The misdiagnosis" and overmedication of African Americans for psychosis is thought to be associated with cultural behaviors that are diagnosed as abnormally violent by non-African American caregivers (Andrews & Boyle, 1999). Further, as noted by Lin, Poland, and Lesser (1986), "Asians, especially Chinese, require significantly smaller doses of neuroleptics, tricyclic antidepressants (TCAs), and lithium than do whites, sometimes one-half the dose." Not all researchers have found consistent racial differences in neuroleptic dosage requirements (Sramek, Sayles, & Simpson, 1986). Similar differences have been reported between Indian or Pakistani clients and white clients (Andrews & Boyle, 1999). Lin, Smith, and Ortiz (2001) provide a review of ethnic variations in psychotropic metabolism and effects. Because of these metabolic and behavioral differences, care should be taken to base medication dosages on serum levels and culturally relevant clinical observations rather than on culturally biased norms.

THE CULTURALLY COMPETENT MENTAL HEALTH NURSE

When a client enters a mental health facility, the culturally competent nurse will have some knowledge of the central beliefs and behaviors of the client's culture of origin. The

CASE EXAMPLE 7-1

Clash of Cultures

Anita, a 26-year-old female from Honduras, was traveling by bus to visit relatives in the United States. While traveling through the Midwest, Anita began to demonstrate mannerisms that concerned other passengers. They reported to the bus driver that Anita was reaching into the air and talking unintelligibly. At the next stop, the bus driver called the police, who took Anita to the emergency room of the local hospital for an evaluation.

A psychiatrist and a psychiatric nurse attempted to interview Anita, but recognized that Anita spoke limited English; an adequate psychiatric examination was not possible without an interpreter. Because of her unexplained mannerisms, the psychiatrist and the nurse determined that Anita might not be in touch with reality and might not be able to safely care for herself. The psychiatrist decided to admit Anita to the psychiatric unit on an emergency admission and to request that an interpreter be called to assist with further evaluation.

The hospital staff learned that Anita was responding to and interacting with "spirits." She denied seeing the spirits, but reported that she knew they were present. The staff also learned that Anita's aunt lived in the vicinity, and the aunt was notified of Anita's admission and asked to come to the hospital to assist.

Anita's aunt attended a staff conference. After assisting with interpretation among the psychiatrist, nurse, and Anita, Anita's aunt explained that Anita had become exhausted from traveling and was communicating with spirits, asking their assistance to relieve the stress and anxiety of travel in a strange land where she could hardly make herself understood to meet even basic needs. The idea of spirits was part of her cultural background, and the behaviors she demonstrated were appropriate and expected in her culture. The staff quite readily decided to discharge Anita.

This case example illustrates the idea that there is no universal definition for mental illness. Each society defines what it will accept as "normal." In the assessment of any client, cultural background has to be considered. The behaviors being evaluated must be examined from the client's cultural perspective. Obviously, cultural differences and poor English language skills are not appropriate reasons for admission to a psychiatric setting. They are not symptoms of mental illness.

nurse will verify the client's level of integration and identification with that culture and with the dominant culture of the society where care is being given. The nurse will be aware of similarities and differences among the dominant culture, the client's culture, and the nurse's culture; will assess areas that may produce miscommunication or conflict; will discuss these areas with the client; and will work with the client to plan culturally sensitive care.

If the client has only recently arrived in the country or entered a cultural setting different from her culture of origin, the nurse will assess for signs of **culture shock**. Culture shock occurs when a person is overwhelmed or even immobilized by cultural differences in expectations, communication, and general habits between the culture of origin and a new culture to which the individual is trying to assimilate. Feelings of helplessness, anger, or acute discomfort are usual. Entry into an institution of the health care culture can produce this reaction in persons who share the culture of origin of the caregivers but who do not share the institutional or professional culture. The professional routines and language differ substantially and can result in culture shock. For persons whose cultures differ from the caregivers' cultures of origin, the culture shock will be that much greater, and the culturally competent nurse will take this into consideration as diagnoses, status, and care are assessed and planned.

Understanding broad cultural patterns is a good first step to providing sensitive care, but broad generalizations about any client based on his or her culture of origin can lead to cultural misunderstanding. It is not the culture of origin but the person's level of integration into or identification with the culture that influences beliefs and behaviors (Helman, 2000). Within any culture there are groups that differ from the broader culture in one or many ways. There are differences even among group members who have a high level of identification with the culture. And constant fluctuations and small variations of culture in the individual based on personal experiences must be considered. For culturally competent care to be provided, the client's level of integration and identification with both the culture of origin and the dominant culture of the society in which he or she is residing must be determined.

KEY CONCEPTS

- Culture (classic definition) comprises all that is learned through socialization, shared by all group members, and associated with adaptation to the environment. Culture includes knowledge, beliefs, art, morals, law, and customs.
- Culture, as used by those facilitating intercultural communication, is defined to be malleable and changes slightly during interpersonal interactions between persons from different cultures.
- Stereotyping clients from different cultures can lead to unsafe care.
- Culture pervades thoughts and behaviors associated with value orientations, interpersonal relations, communication, religion, social systems, diet and food habits, and health and illness beliefs.
- When assessing and providing care, the nurse must consider cultural and ethnic influences on beliefs about mental illness and care, interpersonal interaction, verbal and nonverbal communication, diet and food habits, and biological variation.
- All aspects of verbal and nonverbal communication are culturally based and often serve as barriers to communication.
- A cultural facilitator or culture broker is the best person to assist with interpreting for a non-English-speaking client. A translator or interpreter who translates only words is unable to interpret the many cultural components of the communication.
- What are considered to be normal versus abnormal behaviors, feelings, or states reflecting mental states vary across cultures.
- Genetic, environmental, and behavioral differences affect pharmacological and behavioral aspects of medicating clients of different cultures.
- There is much variation in the level of integration into or identification with a specific culture among members of that cultural group. Careful assessment of the level of integration and identity is necessary.

REVIEW QUESTIONS

1. A nurse has been employed on a psychiatric unit where the client population is very diverse. In order to provide individualized nursing care for each client, the nurse must do which of the following?
   1. Communicate her values to each client
   2. Provide care that demonstrates cultural competence
   3. Accept the ethnocentricities of each of her clients
   4. Identify cultural factors which differentiate each of her clients

2. A new graduate nurse has decided to seek a position on a psychiatric unit at a local hospital. The hospital staff and clients are very culturally diverse. To be

effective in this new position, a priority for the nurse would be which of the following?
   1. Examine own cultural beliefs and values regarding mental health and mental illness
   2. Learn everything possible about the culture and beliefs of the staff and clients
   3. Provide care to the clients based on her cultural values and beliefs
   4. Treat everyone the same because there are no differences between people

3. The nurse is admitting a client who recently emigrated from Mexico and speaks very little English. Unfortunately the nurse only speaks English and German. Which of the following would be a priority action for the nurse to take?
   1. Ask one of the client's relatives to translate
   2. Request a hospital translator to assist with the interview
   3. Refer the client to a hospital where the nurses speak the client's language
   4. Ask another client on the unit to translate

4. A client who has recently immigrated to the United States is brought to the clinic for evaluation. The most important data for the nurse to obtain is which of the following?
   1. Subjective data from the client
   2. Subjective data from the family
   3. Subjective data about the culture
   4. Objective data about the culture

5. The nurse is working in a crisis center located in a diverse community. The nurse understands that a critical component of crisis intervention is determining whether the individual has a support system to assist with resolving the crisis in a healthy manner. The nurse would hypothesize that which of the following clients is least likely to have a strong family support system available:
   1. An African American woman living with her parents
   2. A Mexican American male living with his sister and her family
   3. An international student who is attending the local university on scholarship
   4. A Filipino American student who lives in the dormitory and whose parents live in the next county.

LEARNING ACTIVITIES

1. Define culture.
2. Describe the importance of integrating concepts of cultural variation into planning and implementing psychiatric mental health nursing care.
3. Discuss ways in which clients may differ in beliefs about what are normal or abnormal behaviors, feelings, or states associated with mental status.
4. What are the dangers of stereotyping, ethnocentrism, and cultural blindness? What steps should nurses take to ensure that they provide sensitive nursing care?
5. Plan methods for adapting communication skills to effectively communicate with a client from a culture other than your own. Begin by verifying the client's level of identification with the culture; then work to find out the values held by the client and how they may complement or differ from your own.

*Study*WARE™ CONNECTION

Using your *Study*WARE™ CD-ROM

1. Complete the Concentration activity for this chapter.
2. Review the audio glossary for key terms in this chapter.
3. Explore the other games and activities that support this chapter.

REFERENCES

Agar, M. (1994). The intercultural frame. *International Journal of Intercultural Relations, 18*(2), 221–237.

Andrews, M., & Boyle, J. (1999). *Transcultural concepts in nursing care* (3rd ed.). Philadelphia: J. B. Lippincott.

Andrews, M., & Boyle, J. (2003). *Transcultural concepts in nursing care* (4th ed.). Philadelphia: Lippincott, Williams & Wilkins.

Andrews, M., & Boyle, J. (2008). *Transcultural concepts in nursing care* (5th ed.). Philadelphia: Lippincott, Williams & Wilkins.

Campinha-Bacote, J. (1998). *The process of cultural competence in the delivery of healthcare services: A culturally competent model of care* (4th ed.). Cincinnati, OH: Transcultural C. A. R. E. Associates.

Campinha-Bacote, J. (2000). Ethnic psychopharmacology: A neglected area of cultural competence in mental health. In *Readings and resources in transcultural health care and mental health* (12th ed.). Cincinnati, OH: Transcultural C. A. R. E. Associates.

Campinha-Bacote, J. (2003). Ethnic psychopharmacology: A neglected area of cultural competence in mental health. In *Readings and resources in transcultural health care and mental health* (12th ed.). Cincinnati, OH: Transcultural C. A. R. E. Associates.

Campinha-Bacote, J. (2008). Transcultural C.A.R.E. Web site. Available at: http://www.transculturalcare.net.

Dasen, P., Berry, J., & Sartorius, N. (Eds.). (1988). *Health and cross-cultural psychology*. Newbury Park, CA: Sage.

Giger, J., & Davidhizar, R. (2003). *Transcultural nursing: Assessment & intervention* (4th ed.). St. Louis: Mosby.

Giger, J., & Davidhizar, R. (2008). *Transcultural nursing: Assessment & intervention* (5th ed.). St. Louis: Mosby.

Helman, C. G. (2000). *Culture, health and illness: An introduction for health professionals* (4th ed.). London: Wright.

Hermans, H., Kempen, H., & Van Loon, R. (1992). The dialogical self: Beyond individualism and rationalism. *American Psychologist, 47*(1), 23–33.

Ho, M. K., Rasheed, J., & Rasheed, M. (2003). *Family therapy with ethnic minorities* (2nd ed.). Newbury Park, CA: Sage.

Hughes, C. (1978). Medical care: Ethnomedicine. In M. Logan and E. Hunt (Eds.), *Health and the human condition*. Belmont, CA: Wadsworth.

Jezewski, M. (1993). Culture brokering as a model for advocacy. *Nursing and Health Care, 12*(2), 78–85.

Leininger, M. (1978). *Transcultural nursing: Concepts, theories and practices*. New York: John Wiley & Sons.

Leininger, M. (1991). *Culture care diversity and universality: A theory of nursing*. New York: National League for Nursing.

Leininger, M., & McFarland, M. (2002). *Transcultural nursing: Concepts, theories, research and practice* (3rd ed.). New York: McGraw-Hill.

Leininger, M., & McFarland, M. (2006). *Culture care diversity and universality: A worldwide nursing theory* (2nd ed.). Sudbury, MA: Jones & Bartlett.

Lin, K. M., Poland, R. E., & Lesser, I. M (1986). Ethnicity and psychopharmacology. *Cultural Medicine and Psychiatry, 10*(7), 151–165.

Lin, K. M., Smith, M. W., & Ortiz, V. (2001). Culture and psychopharmacology. *Psychiatric Clinics of North America, 24*(3), 523–538.

Lipson, J. (1996a). Culturally competent nursing care. In J. Lipson, S. Dibble, & P. Minarik (Eds.), *Culture & nursing care: A pocket guide* (pp. 1–6). San Francisco: UCSF Nursing Press.

Lipson, J. (1996b). Diversity issues. In J. Lipson, S. Dibble, & P. Minarik (Eds.), *Culture & nursing care: A pocket guide* (pp. 7–10). San Francisco: UCSF Nursing Press.

Narayan, K. (1991). "According to their feelings": Teaching and healing with stories. In C. Witherell & N. Noddings (Eds.), *Stories lives tell: Narrative and dialogue in education* (pp. 113–135). New York: Teachers College, Columbia University.

Parker, S. (1977). Eskimo psychopathology in the context of Eskimo personality and culture. In D. Landy (Ed.), *Culture, disease and healing: Studies in medical anthropology* (pp. 349–358). New York: Macmillan.

Pedersen, P., & Ivey, A. (1993). *Culture-centered counseling and interviewing skills: A practical guide*. Westport, CT: Praeger.

Saldana, Delia. (2001). *Cultural competence: A practical guide for mental health service providers*. Hogg Foundation for Mental Health. Available http://www.hogg.utexas.edu/PDF/saldana.pdf

Saraceno, B., Levav, I., & Kohn, R. (2005). The public mental health significance of research on socio-economic factors in schizophrenia and major depression. *World Psychiatry, 4*(3), 181–185.

Sramek, J. J., Sayles, M. A., & Simpson, G. M. (1986). Neuroleptic dosage for Asians: A failure to replicate. *American Journal of Psychiatry, 143*(4), 535–536.

Sue, D., & Sue, D. (1990). *Counseling the culturally different* (2nd ed.). New York: John Wiley & Sons.

Thiederman, S. (1991). *Bridging cultural barriers: Managing ethnic diversity in the workplace* (videotape). Irwindale, CA: Barr Films.

Trompenaars, F. (1993, 1994). *Riding the waves of culture: Understanding diversity in global business*. Burr Ridge, IL: Irwin.

Tylor, E. B (1871). *Primitive cultures* (Vols. *1 and 2*).London: Murray.

Williams, D., & Collins, C. (1995). U.S. socioeconomic and racial differences in health: Patterns and explanations. *Annual Review of Sociology, 21*, 349–387.

Witherell, C., & Noddings, N. (Eds.). (1991). *Stories lives tell: Narrative and dialogue in education*. New York: Teachers College Press.

SUGGESTED READINGS

American Academy of Nursing. (1992). Culturally competent health care. *Nursing Outlook, 40*(6), 277–283.

Burk, M., Wieser, P., & Keegan, L. (1995). Cultural beliefs and health behaviors of pregnant Mexican-American women: Implications for primary care. *Advances in Nursing Science, 17*(4), 37–52.

Campinha-Bacote, J. (2002). *Readings and resources in transcultural health care and mental health* (13th ed.). Cincinnati, OH: Transcultural C. A. R. E. Associates.

Campinha-Bacote, J. (2003). *The process of cultural competence in the delivery of health care services* (4th ed.), p.13, Cincinnati, OH: Transcultural C.A.R.E. Associates.

Foster, S. (1990). The pragmatics of culture: The rhetoric of difference in psychiatric nursing. *Archives of Psychiatric Nursing, 4*, 292.

Frackiewicz, E. J., Sramek, J. J., Herrera, J., Kurtz, N., & Cutler, N. (1997). Ethnicity and antipsychotic response. *Annals of Pharmacotherapy, 31*(11), 1360–1369.

Galanti, G. (1997). *Caring for patients from different cultures* (3rd ed). Philadelphia: University of Pennsylvania Press.

Gaw, A. (1993). *Culture, ethnicity, and mental illness*. Washington, DC: American Psychiatric Press.

Hofstede, G. (1991). *Cultures and organizations: Software of the mind*. London: McGraw-Hill.

Lipson, J., Dibble, S., & Minarik, P. (Eds.). (1996). *Culture & nursing care: A pocket guide*. San Francisco: UCSF Nursing Press.

Meleis, A., Isenbery, M., Koerner, J., & Stern, P. (1995). *Diversity, marginalization, and culturally competent health care: Issues in knowledge development*. Washington, DC: American Academy of Nursing.

Purnell, L., & Paulanka, B. (2003). *Transcultural health care: A culturally competent approach* (2nd ed.). Philadelphia: F. A. Davis.

Qureshi, B. (1994). *Transcultural medicine: Dealing with patients from different cultures*. (2nd ed). Newbury, UK: Kluwer Academic.

Rooda, L. (1992). Attitudes of nurses toward culturally diverse patients: An examination of the social contact theory. *Journal of National Black Nurses Association, 6*(1), 48–56.

Spector, R. (2008). *Cultural diversity in health & illness* (7th ed.). Upper Saddle River, NJ: Prentice Hall.

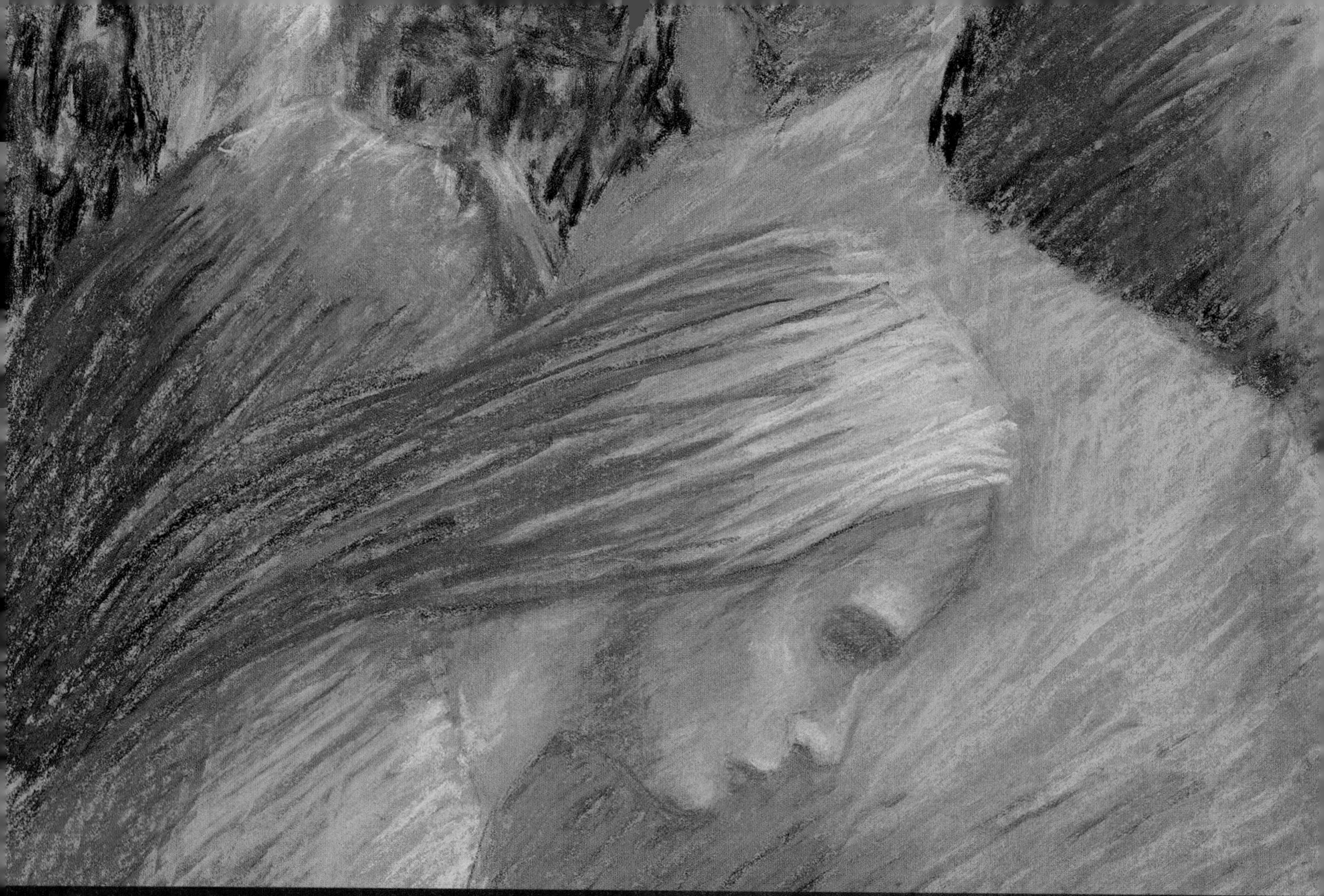

Against the Grain

Planning Services and Guiding Public Policy

- *If you had to tell your city planners what services were needed in your community to care for those with mental disorders, what would you say?*
- *As a nurse, you will have opportunities to be involved in helping plan policy (writing letters, serving on committees, being involved in civic organizations); think about what areas of nursing care and public policy interest you the most.*
- *There is specific information required to intelligently guide decisions regarding care facilities and servicing clients. Have you ever considered how health professionals gather this information?*

Epidemiology is important for all public health policy. In this chapter you will explore its role in mental health.

CHAPTER 8

Epidemiology of Mental Health Illness

LAWRENCE E. FRISCH

CHAPTER OUTLINE

COMPETENCIES

Upon completion of this chapter, the reader should be able to:

1. Define epidemiology and describe the major types of epidemiological studies related to mental health.
2. Explain the basic tools of epidemiology, including research tools of descriptive studies, case-controlled studies, and meta-analysis.
3. Discuss the challenges of standardized definitions in mental health.
4. Describe the development of the *Diagnostic and Statistical Manual* as a means to standardize definitions of psychiatric diagnosis.
5. Present data from early epidemiological studies and the Epidemiologic Catchment Area Study to provide insight regarding the incidence and prevalence of mental disease in the United States.

KEY TERMS

Blinded Clinical Trial
Case-Control Studies
Cohort Study
Control Group
Controlled Clinical Trials
Descriptive Study
Double-Blinded Trial
Endemic
Epidemic
Epidemiology
Experimental Group
Incidence
Interrater Agreement
Interrater Reliability
Intrarater Reliability
Longitudinal Study
Meta-Analysis
Placebo
Prevalence
Quasi-Experimental Study
Reliability
Risk Factors
Validity

Epidemiology is the study of the causes and distribution of injuries and diseases in a population. Many people think that epidemiology is the study of epidemics, but this is only partly true. The word ***epidemic*** is well known in nursing practice and describes a disease or condition that spreads or circulates within a population. In 1861, Florence Nightingale, referring to the spread of diseases such as diphtheria and scarlet fever, wrote of "children's epidemics," and similar use of the word can be traced back to Shakespeare's time. While the tools of epidemiology are very important in understanding epidemics, most diseases that we face in modern life are not epidemic. More typically, they are **endemic**, meaning that they are constantly or regularly found in the population. Epidemiology also includes the study of such endemic diseases: their causes, their treatment, and their prevention and control.

Most mental disorders are endemic or sporadic—while they may be common in most communities, they seem to occur largely without pattern. This lack of pattern has ensured that the causes and treatment of mental illness have been of continuing concern in history and imaginative literature. In the Old Testament, only the music of David's harp could rouse Saul from his deep depression. Robert Burton's *Anatomy of Melancholy* is an important seventeenth-century work filled with classical quotations on mental illness and written to keep its lonely author's mind off his own severe depression. It is now more clearly understood that Alexander the Great suffered from alcoholism. As one of the greatest soldiers and conquerors of the ancient world, surely Alexander's struggles with alcohol have profoundly influenced history. While epidemiology rarely concerns itself directly with the illness or struggle of an individual, epidemiology is very much the study of how diseases of all kinds manifest themselves in populations (Kessler, 2000). Depression, alcoholism, and other mental disorders are important epidemiological concerns that affect both individuals and populations. The epidemiologist's goal is to better understand how frequently diseases occur in a population, in whom they are most likely to occur, and what is their natural history.

WHY STUDY EPIDEMIOLOGY?

Epidemiology is of value because it allows one to understand how illnesses affect a population. Only through epidemiology can we know accurately how many cases of a given illness occur, who is likely to become ill, and what the impact of that illness is likely to be. Through epidemiological study, researchers may be better able to determine possible causes for disease and can often detect **risk factors**, such as age, race, or gender, that predispose persons to a disease. Epidemiology may guide public policy that leads to the prevention of illness. For example, national and international programs for immunization grew out of classic epidemiological investigations and are among the greatest public health successes of the modern era.

In addition to exploring disease causation and prevention, epidemiology can also examine health care outcomes. Effective health care is now available for many illnesses, but often at great cost. It is essential to know what the natural, or untreated, course of an illness is likely to be if no treatment is given. The outcome of differing treatments can then be compared to see which treatment is better and whether any offer improved outcome over the untreated course of the disease. Many studies of outcomes are done as **controlled clinical trials**, evaluations in which neither clients nor their caregivers are allowed to know exactly what treatment is being given. Box 8-1 provides an example of a controlled clinical trial. Epidemiology allows us to study the outcomes both of disease and of treatment. In this way, the study of illness in a population may translate to improved health care for an individual who is ill with a disease.

BOX 8-1
WHAT IS A CONTROLLED CLINICAL TRIAL?

Controlled clinical trials are epidemiological studies conducted like true experiments. Each trial has at least one **experimental group** (persons receiving treatment or having a given condition or disease under study) and at least one comparison or **control group** (persons receiving no treatment or being free of a given condition or disease under study). Controlled trials are usually conducted to test a type of treatment, and treated individuals are assigned to the experimental group while untreated individuals make up the controls. A true clinical trial is **blinded**, which means that the subjects in the trial do not know whether they are receiving the active treatment or a **placebo** treatment that is thought to have no specific effect on the expected outcome. In a **double-blinded trial**, neither the subjects nor the persons evaluating the outcome know whether any subject is receiving active treatment or placebo.

EXAMPLE

To determine the effect of treatments for depression, cognitive-behavioral therapy, interpersonal psychotherapy, antidepressant medication (imipramine), and placebo treatments were compared in a study of 155 clients. Clients were assigned to one of four groups: Group 1 received cognitive behavioral therapy, Group 2 received interpersonal psychotherapy, Group 3 received medication with clinical management, and Group 4 received a placebo with clinical management. Study findings indicated that 40% of the clients recovered with placebo and 60% recovered with one of the specific treatments. Also, the study results suggested that the specific treatments were more powerful in the more severely affected clients. It was noted that cognitive and interpersonal therapies are of benefit and particularly helpful for persons who cannot or do not wish to take drugs.

Example taken from "National Institute of Mental Health Treatment of Depression Collaborative Research Program: General Effectiveness of Treatments," by I. Elkin, T. Shea, and J. Watkins, 1989, *Archives of General Psychiatry*, *46*, 971–983.

HOW IS EPIDEMIOLOGY DONE?

Epidemiologists may be equally at home studying insects in a tropical rain forest as poring over century-old records of births and deaths. They may use pencils and pocket calculators or the latest techniques in molecular biology and computerized biostatistics. Some epidemiologists interview and examine clients; others look only at medical records or at public archives. Important epidemiological work may be done through written or telephone-based questionnaires. Epidemiologists may measure concentrations of toxins and pollutants, they may examine the latest data on genetic linkages, or they may read and analyze already published data using complex statistical tools such as **meta-analysis**, a form of statistical analysis in which the results of several separate clinical studies are combined. The epidemiologist is concerned both with the phenomena of disease, illness, and treatment, and with public policy. Epidemiologists study natural occurrences of illness, but they also study the effectiveness of treatments and the effects of political and social decisions on the health and living circumstances of groups and individuals.

Epidemiologists use a specific vocabulary to define aspects of their work. They typically begin their work by defining the condition or disease of interest, the population at risk for illness, and the potential risk factors to be examined. They then decide what data to collect and how to examine it. In some cases the data are preexisting, either in public archives or in medical records. Often new data collection is required, either by interviews with clients or in some other manner. When new data are needed from clients, the epidemiologist must decide whether to use a previously established data instrument (often a questionnaire) or to develop a new instrument specifically for the purpose. Established instruments generally have known **validity** and **reliability** (they determine accurately and reproducibly what the epidemiologist believes them to measure), but they may not be designed to answer the question needing investigation. For this reason and despite the extra work required to pretest and validate questionnaires, new instruments are often developed for major epidemiological research undertakings.

Many epidemiological studies are **descriptive**. This means that the study documents describe the condition under study. Often the goal of descriptive work is to determine the incidence or prevalence of a disease or condition.

Incidence refers to the number of *new* cases of an illness, condition, or injury that begin within a certain time period. **Prevalence** refers to the number of persons in a population who are living with a disease or disorder at any time. Prevalence measures both new cases *and* old cases, whereas incidence measures only new cases. Incidence is the most important measurement for serious acute problems such as heart attacks; prevalence may be a more important measure for disorders such as depression, which may begin almost unnoticed but may cause severe symptoms for many years.

While descriptive studies are important, other epidemiological studies are analytical or **quasi-experimental**, meaning that a population is studied before and after some event such as the introduction of a new service or a new law. In these studies the epidemiologist usually studies both a set of cases and a set of controls. **Case-control studies** compare two groups: In one group (the cases) all members have the given disease or condition; in the other group (the controls) all members are free of the disease or condition. By comparing these groups, the epidemiologist tries to determine what factors are likely causes of the condition. Sometimes cases and controls come from the same population, and this population is observed over time to see who develops a disease or other outcome. These population-based studies are known as **longitudinal** or **cohort** studies. Some cohort studies have followed specific groups of clients for 25 years or longer. This long follow-up is difficult to achieve when clients (or epidemiologists) move periodically from place to place, change interests, or drop out of the study.

Once data are collected, epidemiologists may use complex biostatistical analysis to interpret their data. However, much epidemiological data are presented using simple rates and percentages. Many important epidemiological questions can be answered with basic descriptive statistics; other questions require complicated mathematical modeling or techniques. Thus, many epidemiologists maintain a high level of mathematical proficiency.

EPIDEMIOLOGY AND MENTAL DISORDERS: DEFINING DISEASE

One of the important contributions that epidemiology makes to the understanding of diseases and disease processes is its insistence on standardized definitions. The question of case definition is so important that a complete book entitled *What Is a Case?* has been written on this question alone (Wing, Bebbington, & Robins, 1981). Defining a case when studying mental disorders initially proved difficult for epidemiologists for two reasons. First, psychiatrists tended to diagnose mental disorders without using any standardized criteria. Consequently, two psychiatrists seeing the same client may disagree completely on diagnosis, echoing the confusion faced by Alice in the Looking-Glass world: "'When I use a word,' Humpty Dumpty said, 'it means just what I choose it to mean—neither more nor less.'" (http://www.sabian.org, retrieved August 2009). While obviously troubling for the client, any difficulty in getting **interrater agreement** between psychiatrists evaluating the same client meant that epidemiologists could never accurately determine the incidence or prevalence of the conditions the psychiatrists were diagnosing. This problem of nonstandardized definitions was found to be serious wherever epidemiologists studied mental disorders.

Second, at one time many psychiatrists and therapists felt that for a variety of mental disorders there was no clear dividing line between normal and disease. This too was troubling for epidemiologists who usually do not have much trouble defining diseases. It is generally not difficult to know whether or not a person has measles, for example. It would seem nonsensical to say that "she's just a little more 'measly' than normal" when we mean she has a mild case of measles. The diagnosis of a mental disorder is much more complicated, however. Most persons feel blue or depressed some days, or after a personal disappointment, and nearly all normal persons have a period of profound mourning after the death of close friends or family. How does the disease "depression" differ from these normal feelings? Or, as an epidemiologist might put it, "What is a *case* of depression?" Many psychiatrists felt that they could best answer this question by carefully interviewing an individual, but often two psychiatrists would interview the same client and still disagree on whether or not the person was depressed.

THE DIAGNOSTIC AND STATISTICAL MANUAL OF MENTAL DISORDERS

Fortunately for epidemiology, psychiatrists and other therapists were also troubled by these difficulties with definition, and in the 1950s, leaders in the American Psychiatric Association began to develop a standardized set of criteria on which to base psychiatric diagnosis (American Psychiatric Association, 2000). After lengthy discussion and debate, the first version of these criteria, DSM-I, was published in 1952. By 1980, the third edition (DSM-III) had been published, and the validity of using DSM to make standardized diagnostic assessments had been widely accepted. In 1987, DSM-III was further revised, in 1994 DSM-IV was released, and in 2000, DSM-IV-TR was released. The *Diagnostic and Statistical Manual* offers a series of diagnoses, and for each diagnosis it provides a list of symptoms and diagnostic criteria. To be diagnosed, a client must meet a specified minimum number of the listed criteria or symptoms. The number of criteria (and their type) varies for each diagnosis, but the process is similar and similarly standardized. Multiple studies have established that when made by trained professionals, DSM diagnoses have substantial agreement between different evaluators (**interrater reliability**) and on different examinations by the same evaluator (**intrarater reliability**) (American Psychiatric Association, 2000). While the multiple revisions since DSM-I suggest that there has been much to improve in DSM, the widespread adoption of DSM criteria among mental health providers has allowed standardized case definition.

Assessing the Epidemiology of Mental Disorders

One of the reasons for DSM's success is that despite being authored by the American Psychiatric Association, DSM does not require diagnoses to be made only by a psychiatrist. The level of acceptance that DSM has achieved has been remarkable in large part because DSM can be effectively used by all well-educated mental health professionals. More important from the epidemiological perspective, many of the psychiatric disorders listed in DSM have diagnostic criteria that can be readily assessed by asking persons a series of questions on a standardized questionnaire. These questions need not be asked by a highly trained mental health professional. This means that specially trained nonprofessionals can survey large numbers of persons using standardized written questions, and while the results may not have full psychiatric validity, they are likely to correspond fairly closely to diagnoses that would have been made by a skilled psychiatrist or psychiatric nurse directly interviewing the same patient.

Disorders in DSM-IV-TR

In DSM-IV-TR there is an extensive number and range of diagnoses, many of which are treated in more detail throughout this textbook. To understand the epidemiology of mental disorders, it is necessary to have some understanding of psychiatric terms. The following discussion is very brief and touches on only a few general DSM diagnoses. For more detail, the reader can consult either the appropriate chapter in this text or a copy of DSM-IV-TR (American Psychiatric Association, 2000).

MOOD DISORDERS. **Mood disorders** are most often characterized by feelings of depression. The most common mood disorder in DSM is Major Depressive Disorder, which is diagnosed when a set of symptoms associated with depression (feeling "blue, sad, or depressed," losing interest in previously pleasurable activities, and/or having thoughts about death or suicide) have been present for 2 weeks or more. Other important diagnostic criteria may include weight change and sleep disturbance. In addition to Major Depressive Disorder, important mood disorders include Dysthymia (characterized by significant sadness most days for at least 2 years) and Bipolar Disorder (commonly called manic-depressive disorder and characterized by episodes of excitement and racing thoughts, often, but not always, alternating with episodes of depression).

REFLECTIVE THINKING 8-1

Labeling Diseases

Some professionals are concerned over the consequences of giving clients labels, such as "depressed" or "schizophrenic." Labels seem to stigmatize clients and turn them from real human individuals into objects of scientific description. The ANA standards of performance require a nurse to be nonjudgmental and nondiscriminatory. How do you respond to this concern, knowing there is a need for standardization in language?

SCHIZOPHRENIA. Schizophrenia is a major psychiatric disorder characterized by symptoms of psychosis or loss of touch with reality. These symptoms include delusions (such as beliefs that other persons can read one's mind or are controlling one's thoughts or movements) and hallucinations (most commonly hearing "voices"). The diagnosis of schizophrenia also requires that a person have deteriorated from a previously more normal level of functioning and that symptoms have been present for at least 6 months.

SUBSTANCE ABUSE DISORDERS. This category includes abuse of both alcohol and a variety of other substances. The DSM-IV-TR criteria require that a person show evidence of dependence on drugs or alcohol to be classified as having a drug- or alcohol-related disorder. Substances considered potentially abusive in DSM-IV-TR include sedative drugs (among them Valium and other benzodiazepines), opioid drugs (including heroin), amphetamines, cocaine, hallucinogens, marijuana, and alcohol.

ANXIETY DISORDERS. The common DSM-IV-TR diagnoses in this category include Obsessive-Compulsive Disorder, phobias, Generalized Anxiety, and Panic Disorder. In DSM-IV-TR, obsessions are defined as "persistent ideas, thoughts, impulses, or images that cause marked anxiety or distress." A common obsession might be that one's hands are dirty even though they have been recently washed. Compulsions are "repetitive behaviors the goal of which is to prevent or reduce anxiety or distress ... that accompanies an obsession or to prevent some dreaded event or situation." Common compulsions include washing hands repeatedly or counting objects ritually. Phobias are "unreasonable" fears of specific situations such as heights, closed spaces, or going out of the house alone. Since most people are afraid of dangerous situations, to qualify as phobic such fears need to be severe and to occur in situations where the average person would probably not have any significant anxiety. Generalized Anxiety is defined as "unrealistic or excessive anxiety or worry ... about two or more life circumstances" in the absence of other DSM-IV-TR diagnoses that can cause anxiety. Symptoms must also be present for a specified period of time. Panic Disorder is a condition in which one experiences brief, intense feelings of anxiety associated with physical symptoms (such as rapid heart rate, sweating, or dizziness) in the absence of a definable physical diagnosis. The diagnosis is made only when a certain number of episodes occur within a specified period of time.

There are numerous other DSM-IV-TR diagnoses, and the diagnostic criteria listed previously are also far from complete. Nonetheless, this very brief introduction to psychiatric terminology should allow the reader to understand some of the actual accomplishments of recent studies of the epidemiology of mental disorders.

EPIDEMIOLOGICAL STUDIES OF MENTAL DISORDERS

EARLY STUDIES

As early as the 1950s, three important studies were carried out (Robins & Regier, 1991): the Stirling County Study in Nova Scotia, Canada (Murphy, Laird, Monson, Sobol, & Leighton, 2001); the Midtown Manhattan Study in New York; and the Baltimore Morbidity Study. Each of these studies interviewed about 1,000 residents of a community for evidence of mental disorder and made important contributions to the understanding of mental illness in the community. These studies are all considered groundbreaking efforts because they marked the first actual studies of entire communities. They were all carefully designed by sophisticated epidemiological thinkers, they used highly trained interviewers and carefully researched interview protocols, and each tried to assess the prevalence of psychiatric symptoms and disorders. Previous investigations had looked only at persons under psychiatric or psychological care, but the Nova Scotia, Manhattan, and Baltimore studies chose people at random living in the community and interviewed them for the presence (or absence) of psychiatric symptoms.

In some ways the most important outcome of these three studies was the highly different conclusions that they reached (Robins & Regier, 1991). The Stirling County Study found that 57% of the people interviewed had at some time in their lives met DSM diagnostic criteria for a mental disorder and 24% of people at one time had severe impairment of the ability to function at work and home as a result of mental disorder. Strikingly, 90% of all these people were experiencing symptoms of mental disorder and severe functional impairment at the time of the Stirling County interviews. In contrast, the Baltimore study found only 11% of the population to qualify for a current DSM diagnosis and only 2% to have moderate to severe functional impairment. The Midtown Manhattan Study reported findings much closer to those of rural Nova Scotia, with significantly impaired functioning in 23% of the population. These three studies suggested that some form of mental illness was widespread in the general population. Because of the differences in findings among the studies and the difficulties in directly comparing any of them, epidemiologists and psychiatrists recognized the need for solid epidemiological data to determine the true national prevalence of mental illness and functional impairment due to mental disorder.

THE CARTER COMMISSION AND THE EPIDEMIOLOGIC CATCHMENT AREA STUDY

Concerns about the results of these important studies led President Carter's Commission on Mental Health to push for a multisite comprehensive epidemiological survey in 1978. One of President Carter's first official actions was to appoint a President's Commission on Mental Health under the supervision of his wife, Rosalyn. Among the achievements of this commission was the recognition that many important basic epidemiological facts about mental illness were unknown. The President's Commission listed the following questions it thought important:

1. What is the prevalence of mental illness in the overall U.S. population?
2. Does the prevalence and type of illness vary in differing parts of the country?
3. Is there variation in type and severity of illness depending on race or socioeconomic status?
4. Among people who have ever had mental illness, how many are currently affected by this illness?
5. How much difficulty does mental illness cause?
6. What is the outcome of mental illness?
7. What percentage of persons with past and current mental illness are receiving treatment, and from what sources?
8. Does treatment for mental illness change outcome?
9. What are the causes of mental illness?
10. Can mental illness be prevented?

In reviewing these and similar questions, the President's Commission and the National Institutes of Mental Health (NIMH) recognized that there was a more important question underlying epidemiological study of mental health: How is mental illness to be defined? Studies in the 1960s had shown marked differences between the United States and England in frequency of hospitalization for several psychiatric diseases. Further evaluation of these studies showed, however, that these differences in hospitalization rates had little to do with real differences between clients or services, but were explained almost completely by consistent differences between how clients were diagnosed in the two countries. The certainty sought by the President's Commission required that the definition of mental disorders be sufficiently standardized so that information collected was equivalent and comparable regardless of in which city or state it was collected. This led to a landmark project known as the *Epidemiologic Catchment Area (ECA) Study*.

Planning and Execution

The ECA Study had several purposes (Robins & Regier, 1991). One purpose was to establish prevalence data for major psychiatric diagnoses. By 1980, DSM-III had been published, but as DSM had come to maturity, there were no data on how frequently the increasingly sophisticated DSM-III diagnoses were found in the population at large. A second purpose was to seek out subgroups in the U.S. population who had unusually high or low rates of mental disorder. It was hoped that finding any such differences might provide useful clues to the causes of these disorders.

The first ECA task was to design a screening questionnaire based on DSM-III. This questionnaire had been completed by 1981 and was called the *NIMH Diagnostic Interview*

Schedule (DIS). The DIS was 25 pages long and consisted of several sections. The first section included general information about education, work, household income, and marital status/family structure. The next section included questions about use of health and mental health treatment services. The remainder of the DIS asked questions designed to suggest probable diagnoses of a range of mental disorders perceived likely to be most common and selected from among the 122 included in DSM-III. Questions were designed to elicit diagnoses of mood disorders (called affective disorders in DSM-III), schizophrenia, substance use disorders (including alcohol abuse or dependence), and anxiety disorders. Eight other diagnoses including Pathological Gambling, Tobacco Use Disorder, and several disorders of sexual functioning were also covered in the questionnaires. While DSM does not specifically include the diagnosis of "cognitive impairment," questions designed to determine an individual's level of intellectual functioning were also included in the DIS.

The next step in carrying out the ECA Study was to decide how many subjects needed to respond to the DIS questionnaire. Determining needed sample size is one of the most important tasks in epidemiology because if too few people participate in a study, it may not be valid to apply results to a larger population, and its results may not be convincing enough to justify its cost; however, large sample sizes greatly increase cost. The ECA Study planners decided that the DIS should be given to 20,000 persons in communities throughout the United States. Because some of the conditions about which the DIS asked were rare enough that even a sample of 20,000 would likely turn up few affected persons, the ECA Study planners decided that a small number of the persons studied would be residents in institutions (including nursing homes, psychiatric hospitals, and prisons). The rarer disorders were thought likely to occur more commonly among institutionalized individuals.

While no professional credentials were required of DIS interviewers, all interviewers were trained uniformly. Five sites were selected: St. Louis; Durham, North Carolina; Los Angeles; Baltimore, Maryland; and New Haven, Connecticut. The DIS was tested for interrater reliability using studies in which the test was given by an interviewer and by a psychiatrist; the same client was then freely interviewed by a second psychiatrist. Reliability was said to be "much better than chance." By the time the "first wave" of the ECA Study was completed, a total of 19,182 persons had been interviewed; 17,803 were living at home or had lived at home during the preceding year, and the remainder were living in institutions (primarily nursing homes or prisons).

General Results

The ECA Study results (Robins & Regier, 1991) showed that 32% of all persons surveyed had, at some time in their lives, symptoms that would have assigned them a DSM psychiatric diagnosis. More strikingly, 20% of persons had symptoms that would have qualified them for some kind of psychiatric diagnosis within the preceding year:

- Alcohol abuse/dependence and phobias were by far the most common diagnoses discovered by the ECA Study, with anxiety, depression, and drug abuse also fairly prevalent.
- In the year preceding the ECA Study, 3% to 4% of people reported symptoms that would qualify for a DSM diagnosis of anxiety, depression, or drug abuse.

One of the most important ECA findings was that gender correlated strongly with the types of symptoms found:

- Women were overall twice as likely as men to suffer from phobias, depression, or panic disorder.
- In contrast, men were five times more likely to receive a diagnosis of alcoholism.

Another major ECA Study finding was that mental disorders are significant problems for young and middle-aged Americans:

- Cognitive impairment (not a DSM diagnosis) was, not surprisingly, much more common in persons over 50 years of age. However, nearly all other symptoms of psychiatric disorder were evident in young persons.
- For those whose symptoms indicated a psychiatric diagnosis sometime in their lives, the median age of onset of symptoms was 16 years.
- Over 75% of those with psychiatric diagnoses had developed their symptoms by age 24, and over 90% by age 38.

Social factors were also shown to be related to symptoms of mental disorder:

- Almost all diagnoses studied were more common among persons who were less well educated or who had been multiply divorced or separated.
- Persons unemployed or on welfare had significantly higher rates of diagnosed disorder, although it was not possible to say how financial and mental states were related. For example, researchers could not determine whether poor financial status was a stress that led to mental illness or whether the impairments of mental symptoms made an individual less able to get and hold employment.

The contributions of race were more complex. The study had relatively few Hispanic participants (nearly all were in the Los Angeles catchment area) and virtually no participants who were Native American or of Asian origin. In contrast, African Americans were well represented among study participants, and though their rate of mental disorder did exceed that of whites, the difference was largely attributable to excess cognitive impairment in older males. What role earlier educational deficits and social deprivation may have played in skewing these men's responses was not determined by the study.

In some ways, the most striking ECA Study findings involved the relationship between symptoms and treatment (Robins & Regier, 1991):

- Only 20% of persons who reported symptoms diagnostic of a psychiatric disorder within the preceding year reported receiving any kind of treatment.
- Only 2.4% of the population had ever been hospitalized for psychiatric reasons.

The Tip-of-the-Iceberg Phenomenon

The Stirling County Study was explicitly based on a "tip-of-the-iceberg" concept (Leighton, 1985). The study's authors recognized that many more persons in a community have symptoms of mental disorder than actually seek health care. This concept that *many persons have symptoms but few seek help* became known as the tip-of-the-iceberg phenomenon, because an iceberg may show only a small tip above water, while most of it is invisible below the waterline. The Stirling County Study estimated that 20% of the population had significant symptoms of mental illness and hence were "part of the iceberg." The ECA Study findings seemed to corroborate these earlier conclusions:

- In the ECA Study sample, 20% had symptoms of a DSM psychiatric disorder within the preceding year, yet only one in five of these reported having sought professional help.

A concern related to the tip-of-the-iceberg phenomenon is that many people who *do* seek mental health care may be less troubled or ill than their neighbors who "tough out" their symptoms without looking for, or at least without finding, help.

- Of the people who completed the ECA Study and *had no evidence of a psychiatric diagnosis*, 4% were currently receiving some form of mental health treatment.
- Ten percent of persons with a past history of mental disorder *but with no present symptoms* were currently in treatment. (It is, of course, possible that without treatment they would have significant symptoms.)

Arctic Landscape by Frederick H. Varley

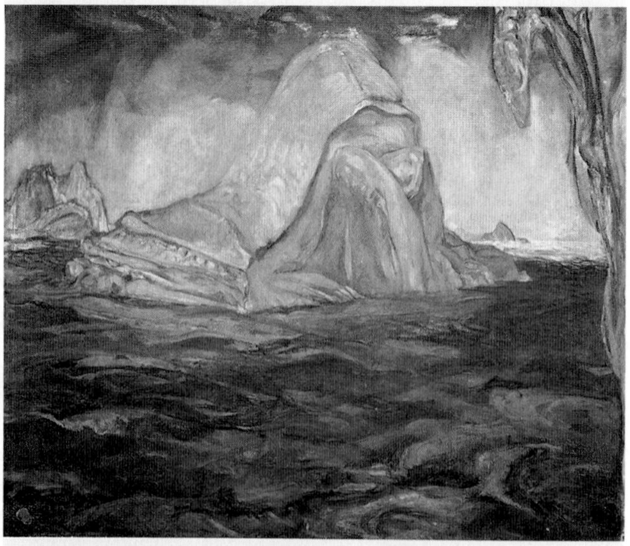

Courtesy: National Gallery of Canada, Ottawa.

Epidemiologists like to talk about the tip-of-the-iceberg phenomenon. Canadian F. H. Varley illustrates an iceberg in his painting *Arctic Landscape*.

This tip-of-the-iceberg concept is of the utmost importance to nursing and to the general delivery of health care.

- While much education for mental health professionals takes place in inpatient and outpatient facilities for mental health care, the majority of persons with symptoms of significant mental disorders do not seek care for these symptoms. They are more likely to be encountered at home while giving care to ill friends or family members or in general medical facilities. Some clients who seek mental health care have symptoms of mental illness but may not meet criteria for a psychiatric diagnosis. Some of these may be less "sick" than clients not receiving care or services.
- Clients hospitalized for mental illness represent only the tip of the iceberg of those with symptoms. The ECA Study found that even for schizophrenia, among the most serious of all psychiatric diagnoses, only 40% of sufferers had ever been admitted to a hospital. Only about 1% of schizophrenic persons were hospitalized at the time of the study. Twice as many were in nursing homes. In the ECA Study sample, as many schizophrenic persons were found in prisons as in mental hospitals.
- Because of the high prevalence of mental symptoms, most persons will have one or more friends, acquaintances, or family members with significant mental illness.
- Alcohol and substance abuse are pervasive problems in our society and are generally underrecognized by health care providers.
- While not a specific DSM diagnosis, cognitive impairment is common and often unrecognized in older individuals.
- Anxiety (including phobias) and depression are among the most common of mental disorders. Many clients suffer from anxiety, fear, and despair without revealing their suffering to caregivers. Unless nurses explicitly ask about these symptoms, clients are unlikely to reveal them or to seek help.

Importance of the ECA and Other Related Studies

The ECA Study was a costly undertaking, and it is unlikely that a comparable effort to define the prevalence or causes of mental illness will be made again for many years, and there has been no attempt to replicate this study at this time. This chapter has discussed only the most general conclusions of the ECA Study. The ECA Study findings have been reported for many specific DSM diagnoses, and summaries of this epidemiologic data along with more detailed consideration of these diagnoses can be found later in this text. Knowing how common a disorder is and who is most likely to be afflicted can certainly help nurses in performing assessments and providing care. This is undoubtedly one of the contributions of the ECA Study and of psychiatric epidemiology in general. There are differences between DSM-III (the diagnostic criteria used by the ECA Study) and DSM-IV-TR. These differences make it somewhat more difficult to apply the ECA Study to the diagnostic categories that are currently accepted. Nonetheless, the ECA Study remains important both for what it has taught us and for what it failed to determine.

The ECA found that alcohol and substance use are among the most prevalent mental health disorders. To

REFLECTIVE THINKING 8-2

The Tip of the Iceberg

One finding of the ECA Study is that many people who have severe symptoms of mental disorders do not seek help:

- **What are the barriers to obtaining psychiatric help in your community?**
- **How can a nursing organization influence availability of services, or the acceptance of services?**
- **How are nurses and other mental health professionals reaching the needy population?**
- **What do you think should be done to ensure that psychiatric care is available to those who need it?**

further explore this important area, the National Institute on Alcohol Abuse and Alcoholism (NIAAA) has conducted the National Epidemiologic Survey on Alcohol and Related Conditions (NESARC). "Wave 1" of this study occurred in 2001–2002 and "Wave 2" in 2004–2005. NESARC has generated more than 100 publications so far, and its results are complex. NESARC confirms the widespread prevalence of alcohol and substance use, along with many regional differences in that use. It is likely that many NESARC findings will be used to change how mental health providers classify alcohol and substance use within DSM-V when the new version emerges in 2012 (Li et al., 2007; Lynskey & Agrawal, 2007).

Another important epidemiological study was the National Comorbidity Study (NCS). Whereas comorbidity (the simultaneous occurrence of two or more conditions or diagnoses) was considered by the ECA, the NCS set out to investigate the frequency and significance of comorbidity in a population of 8,000 persons. The results showed that comorbidity was strikingly common. Nearly 90% of persons who reported recent severe symptoms met DSM criteria for three or more disorders. For example, depression and panic disorder commonly occurred together as did social phobia and a variety of mood disorders (Kessler et al., 1994).

As various psychiatric conditions are considered in this text, it will be seen that effective treatments are currently available for mood disorders, Obsessive-Compulsive Disorder, and some other manifestations of anxiety disorders. The ECA Study showed that each of these conditions is widespread in the population and probably both underrecognized and largely untreated. This underrecognition and undertreatment are major health care challenges that, at least for depression, have begun to be addressed. The NCS emphasized that psychiatric disorders rarely occur in isolation, but that many diagnoses tend to cluster together. The most recent revision of the NCS, the National Comorbidity Study Replication (NCS-R), confirms the high prevalence and relatively low frequency of effective treatment and frequent association with other DSM-IV diagnoses that were seen in the original NCS (Kessler et al., 2003).

For many other high-prevalence conditions, such as substance abuse, treatment is costly and of unproven benefit. The ECA Study clearly shows the prevalence of these conditions, but it does not point the way to effective treatment. In addition, the ECA Study has not offered new insights into the prevention of mental disorders. Like many other major accomplishments, the ECA Study has taught much but leaves many questions unanswered. Both these questions and the partial answers gained from the ECA Study will surface many times in the remaining chapters of this book.

KEY CONCEPTS

- Epidemiology is the study of causes and distribution of diseases in a population.
- The goal of epidemiology is to better understand how frequently diseases occur in a population and in whom they are most likely to occur, and to document the natural history of the diseases.
- Many epidemiological studies in mental health are descriptive, that is, they seek to evaluate the incidence and prevalence of a disorder.
- Standardization of definitions of mental disorders posed challenges to any significant epidemiological study, as there were no standard or agreed-upon definitions of mental disorders until the *Diagnostic and Statistical Manual,* 1st ed. (DSM-I), was published in 1952.
- The *Diagnostic and Statistical Manual,* 4th ed. (DSM-IV), is now widely recognized and used and has served to standardize definitions.
- Three early epidemiological studies in mental health were the Stirling County Study in Nova Scotia, Canada, the Midtown Manhattan Study, and the Baltimore Morbidity Study. These early studies suggested that some form of mental illness might be widespread in the general population.
- In 1978, President Carter commissioned the Epidemiologic Catchment Area (ECA) Study, a multisite comprehensive study in the United States, which showed that mental illness was more common than most people were aware of; for example, 32% of persons surveyed had symptoms that would have assigned them a psychiatric diagnosis according to DSM.
- The most common diagnoses discovered by the ECA were alcohol abuse/dependence and phobias, with anxiety and depression also being fairly common.
- The ECA also indicated that only 20% of persons who reported symptoms diagnostic of a psychiatric disorder reported receiving any kind of treatment.

REVIEW QUESTIONS

1. A graduate nursing student is interested in obtaining information regarding people's perception of mental illness. Her research proposal is approved and she identifies two groups of individuals. The first group consists of students who have a friend or family member diagnosed with a mental health problem, and a second group consists of students who do not have a friend or family member with a mental health disorder. The graduate student's study could be classified as which type of study?
1. Experimental
2. Case control
3. Longitudinal
4. Quasi-experimental

2. A graduate psychiatric nursing student develops a questionnaire to be used in her research project. She sends the questionnaires to four expert nurses to determine if she has identified the best questions that will address the information she is attempting to obtain. By sending the questionnaire out to these individuals, the student is attempting to determine which of the following?
1. Validity
2. Reliability
3. Interrater reliability
4. Intrarater reliability

3. A psychiatric nurse epidemiologist performs a statistical analysis in which the results of several separate clinical studies are combined. The nurse researcher is conducting which type of study?
1. Cohort
2. Case-control
3. Meta-analysis
4. Quasi-experimental study

4. A nurse epidemiologist wants to conduct a study to identify characteristics of individuals who seek mental health treatment. The study would most likely have which of the following research designs?
1. Descriptive
2. Ethnographic
3. Experimental
4. Historical

5. A nurse epidemiologist wants to determine the number of new cases of schizophrenia identified in a small community. The nurse epidemiologist is attempting to determine which of the following?
1. Incidence rate
2. Morbidity rate
3. Mortality rate
4. Prevalence rate

6. A nurse epidemiologist wants to determine the number of cases of schizophrenia identified in a small community. The nurse epidemiologist is attempting to determine which of the following?
1. Incidence rate
2. Morbidity rate
3. Mortality rate
4. Prevalence rate

LEARNING ACTIVITIES

1. Define *epidemiology.*

2. Differentiate between epidemic and endemic.

3. Provide an example of how one could conduct a controlled clinical trial for some aspect of mental health care.

4. Differentiate between incidence and prevalence.

5. Discuss the challenges of standardization of definitions in psychiatric care.

6. Describe the most prevalent mental conditions in the United States.

7. All epidemiological studies indicate that a large number of Americans are suffering from mental illness. How does this information impact nursing in the general hospital? In mental health care clinics? In home health care?

*Study*WARE™ CONNECTION

Using your *Study*WARE™ CD-ROM

1. Complete the Concentration activity for this chapter.
2. Review the audio glossary for key terms in this chapter.
3. Explore the other games and activities that support this chapter.

REFERENCES

American Psychiatric Association. (2000). *Diagnostic and statistical manual of mental disorders.* (4th ed.) (DSM-IV). Washington, DC: Author.

Elkin, I., Shea, T., & Watking, J. (1989). National Institute of Mental Health Treatment of Depression Collaborative Research Program: General Effectiveness of Treatments. *Archives of General Psychiatry, 46,* 971–983.

Kessler, R. C. (2000). Psychiatric epidemiology: Selected recent advances and future directions. *Bulletin of the World Health Organization 2000, 78*(4), 464–474.

Kessler, R. C., Berglund, R., Demler, M. S., Jin, R., Koretz, D., Merikangas, K., et al. (2003). The epidemiology of major depressive disorder. *Journal of the American Medical Association, 289,* 3095–3105.

Kessler, R. C., McGonagle, K. A., Zhao, S., Nelson, C. B., Hughes, M., Eshelman, S., et al. (1994). Lifetime and 12 month prevalence of DSM-III-R psychiatric disorders in the United States, results of the National Comorbidity Study. *Archives of General Psychiatry, 5*(1), 8–19.

Leighton, A. (1985). The initial frame of reference of the Stirling County study: Main questions asked and reasons for them. In J. E. Barrett & R. M. Rose (Eds.), *Mental disorders in the community: Progress and challenge.* New York: Guilford.

Li, T. K., Hewitt, B. G., & Grant, B. F. (2007). The Alcohol Dependence Syndrome, 30 years later: A commentary. The 2006 H. David Archibald lecture. *Addiction, 102*(10), 1522–1530.

Lynskey, M. T., & Agrawal, A. (2007). Psychometric properties of DSM assessments of illicit drug abuse and dependence: Results from the National Epidemiologic Survey on Alcohol and Related Conditions (NESARC). *Psychological Medicine, 37*(9), 1345–1355.

Murphy, J. M., Laird, N. M., Monson, R. R., Sobol, A. M., & Leighton, A. (2001). Incidence of depression in the Stirling County study: Historical and comparative perspectives. *Psychological Medicine, 30*(3), 505–514.

Robins, L. N., & Regier, D. A. (Eds.). (1991). *Psychiatric disorders in America: The epidemiologic area study.* New York: Free Press.

Wing, J. K., Bebbington, P., & Robins, L. N. (1981). *What is a case? The problem of definition in psychiatric community surveys.* London: Grant McIntyre.

SUGGESTED READINGS

Kessler, R., & Ustun, T. B. (2008). *The WHO mental health surveys: Global perspectives on the epidemiology of mental disorders.* Cambridge, UK: Cambridge University Press.

Last, J. M. (Ed.). (1988). *A dictionary of epidemiology.* New York: Springer-Verlag.

Robins, L. N., & Regier, D. A. (Eds.). (1991). *Psychiatric disorders in America: The epidemiologic area study.* New York: Free Press.

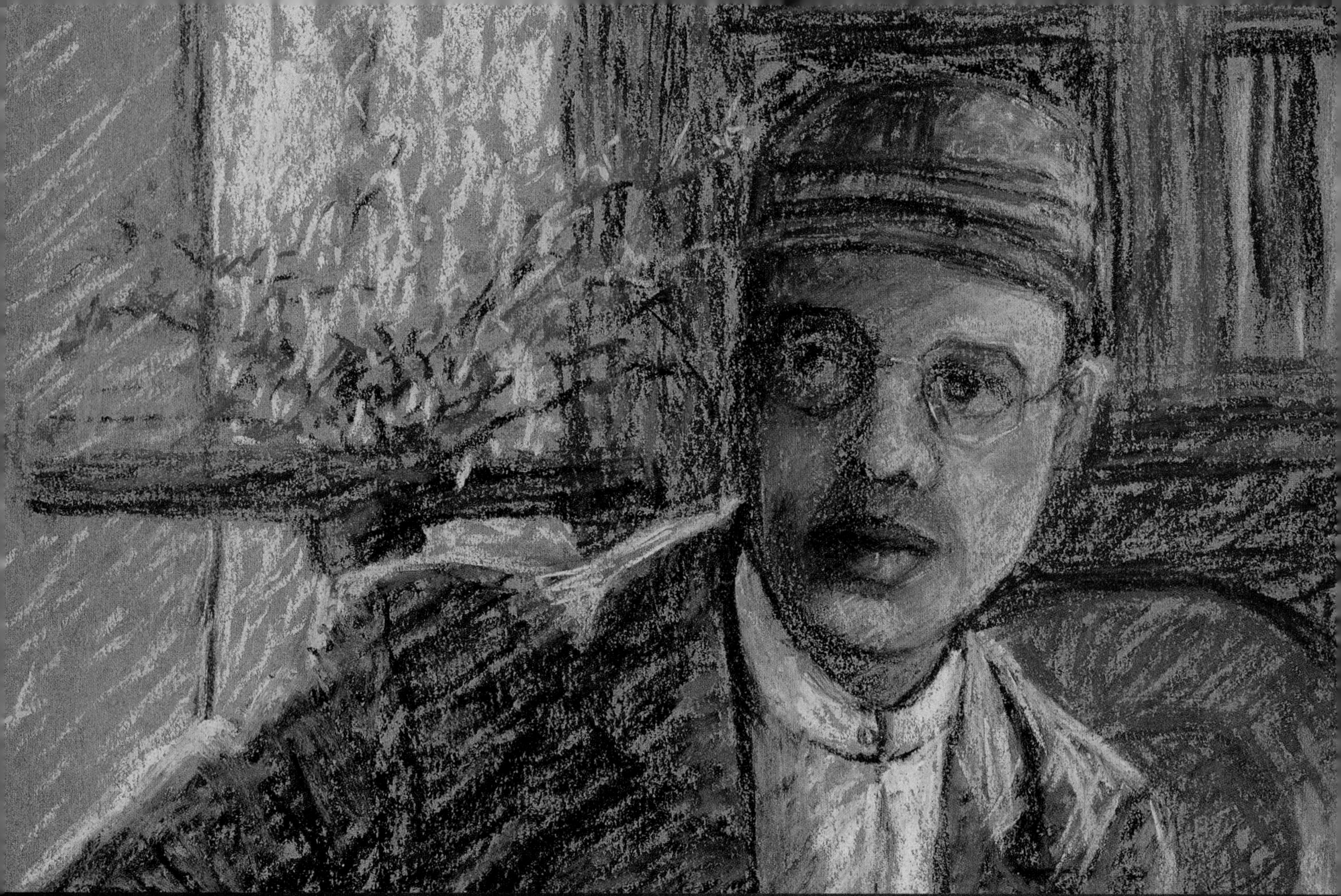

Pride and Prejudice

Power and Control

Individuals usually seek nursing care when they are ill, at risk for illness, or dependent in some way. Thus, nurses continually encounter clients who are vulnerable and in need of protection. Consider the following:

- ***When you provide care to compensate for a client's self-care deficit, what kind of power do you have over that client?***
- ***When you participate in decisions regarding a psychiatric client's treatment plan, what kind of control do you have over the client?***

Professional nurses are in a position of power and control over other human beings—those clients under their care. The nurse is generally regarded by the public as compassionate—the health care professional who is present to care for and support others.

Nurses must forever maintain the public trust and, to do so, must continually examine the roles of power and control in nursing practice. As you read this chapter, take time to reflect on these issues in your day-to-day work. Keeping a journal that identifies situations of either power or control may be particularly helpful in encouraging you to reflect on moral, ethical, and legal behaviors.

CHAPTER 9

Ethical and Legal Bases for Care

LAWRENCE E. FRISCH

CHAPTER OUTLINE

COMPETENCIES

Upon completion of this chapter, the reader should be able to:

1. Describe the legal parameters and nursing responsibilities related to:
   - Clients' rights
   - Confidentiality
   - Psychological competence
   - Informed consent
   - Right to refuse treatment
   - Involuntary hospitalization
   - Professional negligence
   - Violent or self-destructive clients
2. Define the ethical theories of utilitarianism and deontology.
3. Identify the principles that guide practice decisions in psychiatric mental health nursing, including autonomy, beneficence, fidelity, justice, and non-maleficence.
4. Use the Value Analysis Model for evaluation of ethical dilemmas.

KEY TERMS

Abandonment
Autonomy
Beneficence
Civil Commitment
Code of Ethics
Competency to Stand Trial
Conservator
Deontology
Emergency Hospitalization
Ethics
Fidelity
Incompetence
Justice
Least Restrictive Alternative
Malpractice
M'Naghten Test
Negligence
Nonmaleficence
Normative Ethics
Physical Restraints
Probate Proceedings
Seclusion
Tarasoff Duty to Warn
Utilitarianism

Every working day, nurses confront a variety of ethical and legal issues that arise in the course of providing care that respects each client as an individual. Nursing actions in psychiatric care must be consistent with the Nurse Practice Act of the state in which the nurse is practicing and also with laws governing clients' rights and society's interests should the two come into conflict. The purpose of this chapter is to review ethical principles and legal issues applied to psychiatric care so that the nurse will have additional tools to analyze situations and make considered and defensible judgments. The chapter is divided into two parts, covering first the ethical and then the legal perspectives on practice.

ETHICAL ISSUES IN PSYCHIATRIC MENTAL HEALTH NURSING

Many real-life situations are highly emotional and people cannot always assess their options and choices dispassionately. Even when truly dispassionate reflection is possible, reasonable individuals do not always come to the same decision. Philosophers have long recognized the difficulties posed by complex decisions involving alternative courses of action and competing personal and group interests. Such decisions, difficult as they are, must be made every day in health care as well as in other fields. In recent years, ethicists have tried to define rules and procedures useful in providing guidance for human decisions and actions. This philosophical effort is often called the study of **normative ethics**. Normative ethics is a core discipline for nursing education, and nowhere is it more important than in the field of psychiatric mental health nursing.

NORMATIVE ETHICS

Ethics is the branch of philosophy that considers how behavioral principles guiding human interactions can be analyzed and set. Normative ethics tries to establish parameters and guidelines for making human moral decisions. The study of ethics can help uncover guiding principles that allow one to describe and value differing human interactions, but individuals must still rely on moral and religious guidance as they decide how to react when confronted with various ethical dilemmas. Although many persons may live most of their lives without confronting a major ethical dilemma or decision, this is not true for nurses, who typically confront such issues on virtually any working day. Nurses are sometimes frustrated to discover that ethical study cannot tell them precisely how to behave in any given situation, but understanding the basic principles of ethics can help with responsible ethical decision-making.

Many of the dilemmas that nurses face are encountered as legal problems; for example, the nurse wanting to mandate treatment for a homeless person finds that there are laws prohibiting her from forcing the individual into treatment. Legislators have already confronted these dilemmas and in an effort to ensure "right" behavior have constructed laws. While laws often originate as an attempt to promote ethical behavior, law and ethics are quite separate concepts. Law most commonly involves what are called negative duties—duties that dictate what persons must *not* do. Ethical principles dictate positive duties—those activities one *should* do. The familiar "golden rule" is a generalized statement of the importance of positive duties: "Do unto others as you would have them do unto you." These kinds of positive statements of what persons should do are more commonly found in codes of ethics.

The American Nurses Association (ANA) published a **code of ethics** for nurses in the 1960s, covering all aspects of nursing practice, and in 2001, the ANA Congress of Nursing Practice and Economics approved a revision, which can be viewed online at http://www.nursingworld.org.

Also, in 1995, the American Holistic Nurses' Association (AHNA) published the *Code of Ethics for Holistic Nurses* and has recently revised that code to become its current *Position Statement on Holistic Nursing Ethics* (see Box 9-1). The AHNA statement includes many of the principles of other nursing ethical codes (responsibilities toward clients and coworkers and protection of the client from harmful acts). In addition, this code adds provisions for nurses' responsibilities toward self and the environment and their behavior toward other nurses.

The ANA Council on Psychiatric and Mental Health Nursing, in collaboration with the American Psychiatric Nursing Association, have set standards of professional performance, which guide psychiatric nursing practice (ANA, 2007). The core of these standards is that the relationship between a nurse and client is therapeutic and professional. The standards further specify that the nurse performs in an ethical manner, maintains confidentiality, functions as a client advocate, and is nonjudgmental and nondiscriminatory. The purpose of the following discussion is to highlight how nurses in psychiatric mental health practice can maintain behaviors that are both professional and ethical.

REFLECTIVE THINKING 9-1

Considerations of Homelessness and Well-Being

Harold is a man about 30 years old who lives in a small community in California. He is homeless and lives on the streets, in camps in a forest outside of town, or on the beach. He is frequently seen pacing in town during the day; many in the community know him by name. He often responds to voices that others do not hear and talks and gestures as if someone is present although there is no one with him. He gets food from a food bank some of the time, but he is often observed picking through discarded food in public garbage cans.

Harold has never committed an act of violence (to anyone's knowledge). He appears to have no family or friends, as he is always alone. A community social worker has been able to arrange for Harold to receive support from various community agencies from time to time. She has offered to take Harold to see a mental health worker for evaluation and possible treatment, but Harold refuses to go. The district public health nurse has also approached Harold and offered basic health care services, including a physical assessment. Again, Harold has refused treatment.

The social worker and nurse are both concerned for Harold's well-being. They would like to have him evaluated and treated. The nurse has stated that she believes any moral society would ensure that Harold had treatment, care, shelter, and food.

- **What ethical principles come into conflict when considering Harold's case?**
- **What do you think is the best action for society to take in a case such as this?**

ETHICAL THEORIES

There are two broad ethical theories that can guide the development of professional ethics: the theories of utilitarianism and deontology. **Utilitarianism** is based on the principle that an ethical decision serves to produce the greatest good for the greatest number of persons involved. While many ethical theorists endorse utilitarian thinking, many nursing ethicists find deontological analysis more helpful in approaching common clinical dilemmas. **Deontology** looks at human duties to others and tries to analyze the principles on which these duties are based. The basic deontological principles are autonomy, beneficence, fidelity, justice, and nonmaleficence. **Autonomy** refers to the client's right to self-determination and independence. **Beneficence** is the view that all treatments must be for the client's good. **Fidelity** is an individual's obligation to be faithful to commitments and contracts. **Justice** is the principle ensuring fairness, equity, and honesty in decisions. **Nonmaleficence** is the view that, above all, care providers must do no harm. Biegler provides a deontological analysis of decision-making in the treatment of depression that offers an instructive view of how the principles of autonomy and beneficence apply to mental health treatment (Biegler, 2008) He argues convincingly that

BOX 9-1
AMERICAN HOLISTIC NURSES' ASSOCIATION POSITION STATEMENT ON HOLISTIC NURSING ETHICS

Holistic nurses hold to a professional ethic of caring and healing that seeks to preserve wholeness and the dignity of self and others. (Standards of Holistic Nursing, Core Value 1.3)

CODE OF ETHICS FOR HOLISTIC NURSES

The fundamental responsibilities of a nurse are to promote health, facilitate healing, and alleviate suffering. Inherent in nursing is the respect for life, dignity, and the rights of all persons. Nursing care should be given within a context mindful of the holistic nature of humans, understanding the body-mind-spirit connection. Nursing care is unrestricted by considerations of nationality, race, creed, color, age, sex, sexual preference, politics, or social status. Given that nurses practice in culturally diverse settings, professional nurses must have an understanding of the cultural background of clients in order to provide culturally appropriate interventions.

Nurses provide services to a diverse array of clients that may include individuals, families, groups or communities. Each client should be treated as an active participant in his or her health care and should be included in all nursing care planning decisions.

When providing services to others, each nurse has a responsibility towards the client, co-workers, nursing practice, the profession of nursing, society, and the environment.

NURSES AND SELF

The nurse has a responsibility to model health care behaviors. Holistic nurses strive to achieve harmony in their own lives and assist others striving to do the same.

NURSES AND THE CLIENT

The nurse's primary responsibility is to the client needing nursing care. The nurse strives to see the client as whole and provides care that is professionally appropriate and culturally consonant. The nurse holds in confidence all information obtained in professional practice and uses professional judgment in disclosing such information. The nurse enters into a relationship with the client that is guided by mutual respect and a desire for growth and development.

NURSES AND CO-WORKERS

The nurse maintains cooperative relationships with co-workers in nursing and other fields. Nurses have a responsibility to nurture each other and to assist nurses to work as a team in the interest of client care. If a client's care is endangered by a co-worker, the nurse must take appropriate action on behalf of the client.

NURSING AND NURSING PRACTICE

The nurse carries personal responsibility for practice and for maintaining continued competence. Nurses have the right to utilize all appropriate nursing interventions, and have the obligation to determine the efficacy and safety of all nursing actions. Wherever applicable, nurses utilize research findings in directing practice.

NURSES AND THE PROFESSION

The nurse plays a role in determining and implementing desirable standards of nursing practice and education. Holistic nurses may assume a leadership position to guide the profession towards holism. Nurses support nursing research and the development of holistically oriented nursing theories. The nurse participates in establishing and maintaining equitable social and economic working conditions in nursing.

NURSES AND SOCIETY

The nurse, along with other citizens, has the responsibility for initiating and supporting actions to meet the health and social needs of the public.

NURSES AND THE ENVIRONMENT

The nurse strives to create a client environment that is one of peace, harmony, and nurturance so that healing may take place. The nurse considers the health of the ecosystem in relation to the need for health, safety, and peace of all persons.

treatment decisions (for example, choice of psychotherapy vs. medication) can and should be made after considerations of the benefits each treatment might afford to patient autonomy. Biegler provides an interesting perspective in that he suggests that psychotherapy provides people with depression a positive level of autonomy in decisions and action, and concludes that patient autonomy should be given weight and have greater influence in treatment choices than it currently does.

Ethical principles assert that mental health professionals adopt an attitude of respect for persons, ensure that clients make their treatment decisions without coercion (the principle of autonomy), and work for their clients' well-being (the principle of beneficence). Ethical standards typically endorse the importance of professional behavior and responsibility (the principle of fidelity). Certain activities—for example, sexual relationships with clients—are prohibited as being explicitly unethical because these activities could bring harm to the client (the principle of nonmaleficence). The principle of justice is less prominent in professional codes of ethics than are the other principles. Perhaps this is because in American society, neither health nor mental health care has been defined to be a universal right.

Ethics and the Law

Nurses should recognize that conflict between the law and ethics may be unavoidable. Involuntary psychiatric commitment, a seemingly essential means to prevent harm to a mentally ill individual or others around him, is provided for by the laws of every state but flagrantly violates the principle of autonomy. Autonomy establishes that a person can make free choices even if those choices result in personal harm. Commitment law is based on the premise that if there is reason to doubt an individual's ability to make fully rational decisions, the principle of beneficence takes priority over that of autonomy.

Ethical conflicts and dilemmas are often accompanied by highly emotional circumstances that may not be fully conducive to patient and rational consideration. The very presence of conflict or emotion suggests the likelihood of an ethical dimension. When faced with such a crisis, the nurse should reflect on the ethical principles: Autonomy, beneficence, and nonmaleficence are usually the critical principles to consider. When doubt arises, nurses often use techniques in helping them consider all aspects of the ethical dilemma. One such technique, the Value Analysis Model, is discussed next.

REFLECTIVE THINKING 9-2

Autonomy

Your neighbor has been judged to be unable to make rational decisions. He is 80 years old, lives alone, and has appeared "forgetful" to you. He is about to be placed in a nursing home against his expressed wishes.

- **How do you feel about this situation?**
- **At what point is commitment acceptable to you? What behaviors make it so?**

Making Ethical Decisions

Many approaches have been used to assist nurses and nursing students to gain analytical skills and confidence in making ethical decisions (Numminen & Leino-Kilpi, 2007). Current evidence suggests that reflective models that assist one to engage with simulated experiences and find meaning in one's own time are beneficial (Kyle, 2008). The Value Analysis Model is a classic model for use in evaluating a dilemma and is presented here as one approach (Coombs & Meux, 1971). This model is a formal method of analysis to assist individuals in making value judgments when facing ethical dilemmas. The model emphasizes the need for careful evaluation and weighing of facts prior to drawing conclusions regarding ethical problems. The model requires the nurse to complete six steps of analysis before drawing conclusions regarding the issue. The steps are presented in Box 9-2. The initial steps of the analysis force the nurse to articulate the value questions and assemble facts regarding the question. Thus, the nurse must search for data supporting claims regarding action. Next, the nurse must judge assembled facts according to their truth or validity as well as determine whether the arguments presented by others have relevance for the situation at hand. The nurse must give plausible and rational arguments for each decision. Completing the analysis of facts, the nurse must arrive at a tentative value decision and go on to test the value principle implied in that decision by hypothetically putting self in the position of all persons involved with the decision. It is recommended that the nurse complete the entire process before attempting conclusions about the issue. The reader is encouraged to think about moral and ethical judgments that arise in psychiatric mental health practice and use this model in analyzing the dilemmas that arise, as the model has proved helpful to many.

Alternatively, other authors (Gray & Gibbons, 2007) present four questions that assist one in considering morally correct choice when confronted with ethical dilemmas:

- Is the situation we see an ethical dilemma?
- If so, what is the dilemma?
- How do existing ethical frameworks help us deal with this situation?
- What, if anything, do our codes of ethics say about this situation?

In general, those who consider ethical situations and conflicts in advance of encountering them in practice feel more able to respond in the actual situation. Students are encouraged to use the previous principles and models throughout their studies.

BOX 9-2
STEPS OF VALUE ANALYSIS MODEL

1. Identify and clarify the value question.
2. Assemble purported facts.
3. Assess the truth of purported facts.
4. Clarify the relevance of the facts.
5. Arrive at a tentative value decision.
6. Test the value principle implied by the decision.
    - Does the value principle fit in the current situation?
    - Does the value principle fit in other, similar situations?
    - Would the value principle fit if the client were your mother? Your father? Your spouse? Your child?
    - Would the value principle fit if you were the client?

Ethical Actions for the Social Good

Nurses may occasionally disagree with specific laws or with the ethical analysis underlying them. For example, the nurse may believe that health professionals should have the right to medicate clients who are delusional and unable to function fully in society because the nurse believes that medication will lead to a more positive adjustment and quality of life for the client. In such a case, the nurse may choose to work actively to identify those specific situations where the nurse believes the law should change and may take action to bring about a change in the law. There are certainly instances in which nurse activists and nurse legislators have brought about legal changes that greatly benefit their clients. Occasionally, such changes may require actions of civil disobedience. Nurses and other mental health professionals risk being judged guilty of unethical behavior if they violate laws, even laws they judge to be against the interests of their clients.

LEGAL ISSUES IN PSYCHIATRIC MENTAL HEALTH NURSING

Law has relevance in nearly all aspects of nursing practice, but in no other area of nursing is the law more intimately involved than in psychiatric mental health nursing. Psychiatric clients may:

- Be placed in treatment against their will
- Pose a risk to themselves
- Have been judged to have committed a crime while legally insane
- Be unable or unwilling to consent to treatment
- Be incapable of fully understanding medication risks
- Require restraint for their safety or that of others
- Make threats that obligate their caretakers to warn potential victims
- Undergo forensic evaluation that requires the nurse to testify in court

In each of these circumstances, the client's rights and society's interests may, and often do, come into conflict. In such cases, laws ideally act to clarify the conflicting interests involved. Unfortunately, at times the laws themselves seem contradictory on the subject of mental health treatment. Some statutes ensure that clients cannot be forced into treatment; others require that treatment be offered to certain subgroups of the mentally ill but not to others. To a nurse practicing psychiatric mental health nursing, such contradictions are visible every day. For example, in most communities, the practicing mental health nurse will find no shortage of untreated mentally ill clients who have access to care but choose to exercise their legal right of refusal. At the same time, most nurses encounter individuals actively seeking mental health assistance who are denied care because they lack satisfactory insurance coverage (Sturm & Wells, 2000). Laws attempt to provide for the public good and public safety, but rarely do the laws offer comprehensive solutions to social problems such as how a community is to support a homeless individual who is mentally ill and refusing treatment. Instead, laws set out series of rules and procedures and often penalize those who fail to follow those procedures. The following sections, while not intended to make the reader an expert in mental health law, will provide a general introduction. Experience in local clinical placements will help nurses become acquainted with the specific regulations and procedures that apply in their communities.

Clients' Rights

While the law is based on the complementary social concepts of responsibilities (duties) and rights (privileges), many Americans have come to view laws almost exclusively in terms of rights rather than responsibilities. The last half of the twentieth century saw a remarkable extension of legal rights to groups and individuals who had previously been inadequately protected. Among the groups who benefited most from this extension of rights were the mentally ill. Not only has national and local legislation been drafted to protect the mentally ill from unwanted treatment and other loss of personal liberty, but a number of voluntary agencies have attempted to define appropriate treatment standards. For example, the American Hospital Association has issued a statement of Patients' Bill of Rights, which many health care agencies have adopted. The American Psychological Association has published a Mental Health Patient's Bill of Rights (www.apa.org) that focuses almost exclusively on managed care and insurance issues. This managed care focus is mirrored in the National Patient's Bill of Rights that emerged from divisive election-year legislative squabbles in a form that seemed to serve politics better than patient rights. Although the insured certainly need protection against managed care cost-savings efforts that threaten their well-being, traditional categories of patient rights protections remain important, especially in mental health practice. These are considered in more depth in the following section.

Right to Privacy

Privacy is the right of any client to keep personal information secret. Thus, any client has the right to keep the fact that he is in treatment to himself. He may not wish for his spouse, employers, friends, or others to know that he is receiving care. In honoring that right, professional codes of behavior frequently state that confidentiality must not be breached. Laws, however, rarely state that the nurse *must* maintain confidentiality, as laws more commonly define negative rather than positive duties. Thus, it is generally recognized that the nurse has an obligation to maintain confidentiality, and in any situation where a client can show that a breach of confidentiality has caused the client damage (e.g., damage to his reputation), the client may sue the nurse in civil court for inappropriate disclosure of professional, confidential information.

While laws in every state differ, most states have laws that do allow the nurse to discuss a client case with a supervisor or with other members of the treating team. However, nurses and other mental health providers cannot release information to a client's family members without explicit permission, and this information includes disclosing that their family member is in the hospital or is being seen at the mental health clinic. Further, nurses may not disclose client information to other nurses or other health professionals who are not involved with direct care or service to that client. If such disclosure occurs, the nurse is legally liable for any resulting harm experienced by the client. For example, a psychiatrist was successfully sued for revealing information to a client's spouse when that information appeared to contribute to a subsequent divorce (*MacDonald v. Clinger*, 1982).

Partly to address the disparities in privacy protection afforded by different states, Congress enacted the Health Insurance Portability and Accountability Act and then required the secretary of the Department of Health and Human Services (DHHS) to create regulations protecting the public's privacy under the act. Known as HIPAA regulations, these rules came into effect in 2003 and provide civil and criminal penalties when patient information is released inappropriately. The rules are complex, but they can be summarized as follows:

- Any nurse who works for a "covered entity" must comply with HIPAA regulations. Almost all health care is currently provided by covered entities. Any mental health facility that exchanges billing or insurance eligibility data by electronic means is considered to be a covered entity.
- All employees, volunteers, and trainees working in covered entities must receive training in privacy procedures adopted by the organization.
- Privacy procedures must include: (1) client notification of privacy policies—usually with a posted notice and a signed privacy description given to each client; (2) a log of all information releases documenting to whom the information was given and by which employee; (3) a procedure for review of privacy complaints; and (4) clear restrictions—governed by clients' specification in writing—on which parts of a clinical record can be released and to whom.
- HIPAA does not prevent sharing clinical information with persons who are providing care to an individual and have a clear "need to know" about the client—even without a client's explicit permission. However, HIPAA limits information to be shared to that which might be reasonably thought to be important for clinical care.
- HIPAA does not limit the nurse's right or obligation to release information necessary to save life or to comply with the law. For example, if a nurse suspects child or elder abuse, she is still required by law to report this to appropriate authorities. Similarly, if a client tells the nurse that she or he plans to murder another individual, in most states the nurse has a duty to warn (see following section on Tarasoff Duty to Warn) that is not affected by HIPAA (even though warning might be thought to violate the potential murderer's privacy rights).

An important disclaimer from the authors: This summary is only an informal interpretation of a complex law. Most organizations will have hired consultants and health care attorneys to advise them on the details of HIPAA compliance. If the agency where you work implements HIPAA regulations differently from those implied in the preceding paragraphs, it is best to assume that that agency's policies are a more accurate interpretation of the law than is given here. (See additional discussion of HIPAA in Chapter 5.)

The release of mental health information that does not follow HIPAA regulations may have detrimental effects if it is released to employers, insurance carriers, or others whose interest is not primarily therapeutic. Nurses must ensure and document that their clients have considered and are able to understand any risks that might occur as a result of the client's authorization for records release. In most cases the client should be allowed (or even encouraged) to see the contents of any records being released. If for some reason

REFLECTIVE THINKING 9-3

Releasing Information

You are a nurse working on a chemical dependence unit, and you answer the telephone at the nurses' station. A woman who tells you she is Mrs. Anderson is calling. Mrs. Anderson states that her son, Joe, was admitted to your unit last night, and she is very concerned about his condition. She is asking you for an update on his status. Joe Anderson is a 20-year-old young man who was admitted during the night.

- **What do you tell Mrs. Anderson?**
- **What do you say if the caller says, "I'm from the Police Department and need to know if Joe Anderson, who is wanted for arrest, is at the hospital"?**

this cannot be done, it is important that the nurse be certain of the client's intent that specific records be released and to document the reason for that certainty.

As noted before, there are several situations in which laws related to privacy and confidentiality allow different actions than discussed in the previous paragraph. These are described following:

1. Mental health evaluations done for reasons other than direct client care: Examples of such evaluations include court-ordered exams, disability determinations, and employment physicals. These examinations are done for the benefit of a third party, and the reports are sent to this third individual or agency. By agreeing to participate in the evaluation, the client waives some confidentiality rights. The client should be told at the onset of the evaluation who will see the completed report and that confidentiality may not be fully ensurable.
2. The case of minors: Parents can usually be given details of their child's mental health treatment. However, older adolescents living on their own are usually considered "emancipated," and parents may not have a right to information concerning their mental health. These issues are usually treated in mental health statutes, which vary from state to state. Nurses should be sure they understand laws that apply to the care of minors in their respective states and can usually obtain information from the administrators and/or legal counsel of the psychiatric facility in which they work.
3. Issues of violence and safety: Confidentiality can (and must) be breached in certain situations where the nurse has reason to suspect child abuse, elder abuse (see Chapter 26), or that an individual may be at risk to harm specific other persons. The latter situation, involving "duty to warn," is discussed in more detail later in this chapter.

Right to Keep Personal Items

When a client enters treatment in a facility—hospital, board-and-care home, halfway house, or nursing home—the client still maintains rights to his personal property. When storage of items becomes difficult, the client can be asked to leave some of his items at home. However, if a client has items of value, the nurse is obligated to document the items and store them in the safe or other secure place. Removing items from a client may be considered theft if the nurse takes them away and either loses them or refuses to return them. In situations where the nursing staff have professional justification to remove potentially harmful objects such as knives, guns, or scissors, the nurse must recognize that the objects are still owned by the client and can be removed only during the time of hospitalization or treatment.

Right to Enter into Legal Contracts

A client maintains his legal rights as a citizen. Thus, if an adult, the client has a right to vote, get married, sign for a mortgage, write a personal last will and testament, and manage personal financial affairs or control personal funds.

There are some situations, however, when a client is deemed not responsible (hence not accountable) for his own actions. In these cases, mental health professionals are often called on to assess individuals' competence both in and outside of mental health care settings. Judgments of competence may have important consequences in determining whether an individual can continue to manage his own finances, whether he should be placed in a nursing home or other supervised living environment against his will, or whether he can appropriately make decisions about his own medical and psychological treatment. At times, competence judgments are required to assess whether an accused person can stand trial or was sane at the time a crime was committed. While the issues in each of these situations are similar, the details of competency assessments vary between them and from individual to individual.

Probate proceedings are often carried out to establish a judicial ruling that an individual is or is not competent to manage activities. These are court proceedings wherein a judge hears evidence on the individual's ability to function and makes a judgment of "competence" or "incompetence." **Incompetence** is a legal term reflecting that the individual has a mental disorder, the disorder causes inability to make judgments, and the disorder renders the person unable to handle his or her own affairs. Such probate proceedings can result in the appointment of a conservator of the person or a **conservator** of the estates for persons whose mental status makes them unable to care for their daily needs or to handle their financial affairs. Many mentally ill, retarded, or demented individuals will need conservators, and some states allow an individual to select his or her own conservator (subject to court approval). Limited conservatorships may be defined to act in certain specific areas, leaving the person some residual personal or financial responsibilities without explicit oversight. Nurses may be asked to testify in such proceedings.

A ruling of incompetence means that the individual cannot enter into contracts and further deprives the person of rights such as voting and, in some cases, driving. Such rights may be restored to the individual only through another court hearing.

A related concept of relevance to the psychiatric nurse is **competency to stand trial**. Competence to stand trial requires that an individual be able to understand the nature of legal proceedings and be able to cogently tell his own story to his attorney and the court. At times, mental health professionals must assist the court in judging whether an individual was sane at the time a crime was committed. While successful insanity defenses are often highly publicized, less than 1% of criminal defendants are judged legally insane (Swenson, 1993, p. 214). Such judgments usually involve the **M'Naghten test**, sometimes also called the M'Naghten rule. This legal definition was put forth after a famous nineteenth-century murder trial in which Daniel M'Naghten was found not guilty by virtue of insanity. As any reader of Charles Dickens knows, public opinion in Victorian England was strongly in favor of vigorous punishment for wrongdoing. M'Naghten's commitment to a mental hospital, in lieu of execution, caused a huge public outcry, and the queen ordered a judicial reexamination of the basis for the insanity defense (Swenson, 1993, p. 215). This judicial review established two criteria for legal responsibility that are still used over 150 years later. The M'Naghten test requires that if a defendant either does not know the significance of her action or does not know it was wrong, then she cannot be held legally accountable. While the M'Naghten test remains important and useful, it fails to apply to the mentally ill individual who, for any of a variety of reasons, lacks the ability to control his behavior even if he knows that behavior is wrong and harmful. In recent years, courts have expanded the "insanity defense" to apply also to acts seemingly not within an individual's control. Across the country, there have been controversies over the use of the "insanity defense," and since 2000 a number of states have introduced a "guilty but mentally ill" (GBMI) verdict that declares the individual guilty of the crime committed, but mentally ill and entitled to receive psychiatric treatment while serving time for the crime. Should the individual recover from the psychiatric illness while being treated, the person is still required to serve out his prison sentence before being released (see PBS, http://www.pbs.org/wgbh/pages/frontline/shows/crime/trial/history.html, retrieved 2008).

Right of Habeas Corpus

Habeas corpus is a right protected by the U.S. Constitution that permits a speedy legal hearing and evaluation for any individual who claims he is being detained illegally. In such a hearing, a judge (and at times a jury as well) hears evidence and makes a determination of whether or not the individual may be released or detained for psychiatric treatment.

Right to Informed Consent

Informed consent is fundamental to all medical treatment and must be obtained whenever there is a potential for harm from any therapeutic intervention. Clients have the right to be given clear information about treatment options, risks, benefits, and alternatives. They may have the right to refuse treatments that are offered to them. Informed consent presumes that clients are mentally competent, as defined previously. It is important to recognize that individuals may be judged legally competent to consent to (or refuse) treatment despite elements of irrational thought or behavior (Merz & Fischoff, 1990). To give consent, an individual must be alert and oriented, must understand the procedure or treatment being offered, and must freely (without coercion) accept the treatment. Courts frequently regard consent as informed when clients can actively communicate their choice of therapies and can show that they understand information provided to them (Simon, 1992, p. 126).

To obtain informed consent, the standards of communication of risk to psychiatric clients do not differ from those applying to any other clients; that is, major risks need to be described, but there is no need to be exhaustive in listing all possible harms from a therapy (DHHS, 1982). The importance of communicating risks is greatest when alternative treatments are available that may be safer.

Informed consent is a legal requirement in all states, but the nature of the required consent may differ among states. Under some circumstances the law requires written consent, and in most cases it is highly prudent for clinicians to obtain written consent for treatments that have any risk of adverse outcome. There are several situations in which the requirement for consent may be waived or significantly modified. For example, in a genuine emergency, physicians and other licensed caregivers are obligated to do whatever is required to treat or protect a client. For example, if any individual is brought to an emergency room comatose and in need of life-saving treatment, the emergency department staff are expected to provide immediate care. It is important to define emergencies with accuracy. Some states have statutory definitions of emergencies that clarify when informed consent can be dispensed with. Even in the absence of such definitions, it is risky to forgo informed consent unless the client's safety and/or well-being would be threatened by any necessary delay in treatment.

Documented consent is of utmost importance for somatic treatments, especially hospitalization, the prescription of drugs, and the administration of electroshock.

Right to Refuse Treatment

Of clients' legal rights, the right to refuse treatment is among the most important. No different than other clients, psychiatric clients have the right to consent to treatment, to refuse specific treatments, and, where consent has been given, to withdraw consent. To threaten to give treatment or to actually force treatment without consent leaves the nurse criminally liable for charges of assault and battery.

An issue of particular importance to psychiatric nursing is consent to take medications. There are legally identified situations where clients may not have the right to refuse psychiatric hospitalization. However, once hospitalized, the law generally gives individuals the right to decide whether or not to be treated with medication. Psychiatrists have, not surprisingly, expressed their concern about a "legal system that orders people into mental hospitals and then orders psychiatrists not to treat them" (Stone, 1981, p. 358). This concern is made even more acute because not only do mental health providers risk liability if they treat a client against his wishes, but they may also (rarely) be sued for *not* treating a client who refuses such treatment (*Whitree v. State*, 1968).

Most treatment refusals focus on antipsychotic medications and are based on real concerns that use of these medications may lead to permanent neurological disability (most commonly tardive dyskinesia, discussed in Chapters 14 and 27). In a well-known case, the New York Supreme Court ruled that under certain conditions, medication could be given to clients against their will when four considerations were explicitly taken into account:

1. The client's liberty interests (freedom to travel, right to autonomy)
2. The client's best interests
3. The benefits of treatment
4. The available less intrusive alternative treatments (*Rivers v. Katz*, 1986)

RESEARCH

Highlight 9–1

Patients' Views and Readmissions 1 Year After Involuntary Hospitalization

STUDY PROBLEM/PURPOSE

To assess patients' retrospective views of involuntary admissions to psychiatric care and to identify factors associated with those views.

METHODS

A national observational prospective study with 1-year follow-up was conducted in the United Kingdom. Seven hundred and seventy-eight patients were interviewed on admission to hospital as baseline and 51% of these (N = 396) were followed up at 1 year. Demographic data, along with ICD diagnosis, measures of perceived coercion, perceived risk to self and others, and satisfaction with treatment were collected. At 1-year follow-up, patients were interviewed and asked if they believed their involuntary admission had been justified. Readmissions during that 1 year were also recorded, as were basic indicators of functioning.

FINDINGS

Only 40% of patients who had been involuntarily admitted felt in retrospect that their original admission was justified. The researchers noted that patients who expressed lower satisfaction with hospital care during the first week of involuntary treatment are more likely to be readmitted within one year and are also less likely to believe that their involuntary admission was justified. Poor global functioning at time of involuntary admission was associated with a more positive assessment of that admission later. Living alone is linked with lower involuntary readmission rates and more positive retrospective views of the admission. Other factors, such as being on social assistance and being African and/or Caribbean were associated with higher readmission rates at 1-year follow-up.

IMPLICATIONS

Many earlier studies have indicated that up to 80% of patients involuntarily admitted for psychiatric treatment felt retrospectively that their admission had been justified. The current report finds a significantly lower number, possibly attributed to the fact that the follow-up was done after 1 full year. Information on factors associated with a positive view of the involuntary admission can give direction to those providing care. Since the data show that satisfaction with treatment in the first week of care has an impact on later perceptions and readmissions, nurses and others need to focus on communications and actions that work to engage the client in positive relationships with care and care providers immediately after admission.

Source: "Patients' views and readmissions 1 year after involuntary hospitalization," by S. Priebe, C. Katsakou, T. Amos, M. Leese, R. Morriss, D. Rose, T. Wykes, and K. Yeeles. 2009. *British Journal of Psychiatry*, *194*, 49–51.

These considerations may not apply in other states, but do provide fairly clear guidelines for medication decision-making.

Issues of treatment refusal are, in some cases, being addressed by psychiatric advance directives. Here, while well, a client may indicate the conditions under which he would consent to treatment should he become ill and unable to make decisions (Atkinson, 2007). For example, a client with bipolar disorder may indicate that, should he become manic, he would consent to hospitalization, medication, or other specified treatments. Should such advanced directives be in place, both clients and providers may be able to avoid some of the most difficult legal and ethical issues of care; however, the actual implementation of such a process remains unclear.

Another very difficult situation in psychiatric care occurs when a client refuses treatment for a physical condition based on thought processes that are part of the psychiatric illness, for example, a client who refuses to go to the dentist because the client believes that dental tools carry evil radio waves harmful to them. In such cases, the client's family can petition a court for power of attorney to give consent for treatment. In all cases, however, the much-preferred approach is to work with the client over time so that he may give consent for care himself.

Individuals committed for psychiatric care because of criminal behavior raise a particularly difficult societal problem. Such persons would seem to lose some liberties because the purpose of their commitment should be rehabilitative. Some court decisions have allowed involuntary medication of committed persons following crimes (*Stensvad v. Reivitz*, 1985). A more recent U.S. Supreme Court case, *Washington v. Harper* (Applebaum, 1990), allowed medication against an incarcerated person's will when the individual was a danger to himself or others and when the proposed medications were clearly in the person's best interests. In this decision, the court seemed to endorse the use of professional review

REFLECTIVE THINKING 9-4

Right to Refuse Treatment

Mrs. Wenzel is a middle-aged woman diagnosed as having schizophrenia, paranoid type. She lives with her daughter Wendy and son-in-law and is generally happy with her living arrangement. She is independent in her daily activities. She does take medication for her schizophrenia and has monthly visits with her psychiatrist. She helps with the housework and cooking and volunteers some of her time to do filing and office work at a local community recreational center.

Over the past month, Wendy has noticed that Mrs. Wenzel has a skin lesion on her left forearm that is raised and dark in color and has not been noticed before. At Wendy's urging, Mrs. Wenzel agrees to see the family doctor about this lesion. Dr. Percens immediately raises strong concerns that the lesion could be a melanoma and recommends that the lesion be biopsied and removed. Dr. Percens explains that the lesion could be a form of skin cancer and that without treatment this cancer could lead to metastases and death.

Mrs. Wenzel refuses treatment, stating, "I don't like needles!" She and Wendy go home, and Wendy again urges her mother to reconsider having the lesion treated. At this point, Mrs. Wenzel becomes agitated and anxious and says, "This spot is nothing. Doctors just want money and tell us to do things we don't need to do!" She goes on to say, "If you take off this spot, I will lose my soul—I don't want to lose my soul." The more Wendy raises the issue, the more upset and agitated Mrs. Wenzel becomes.

Wendy, concerned for her mother's health, makes an appointment to talk with Dr. Percens regarding her mother's refusal of the treatment. Dr. Percens explains that the lesion very likely is a melanoma, but also explains that Mrs. Wenzel has the right to either consent to or refuse the biopsy.

Wendy then contacts Mrs. Wenzel's psychiatrist regarding her mother's refusal of treatment, her agitation, and her delusion that removing the lesion is connected with her soul. Psychiatric evaluation indicates that Mrs. Wenzel is alert and oriented, able to talk coherently about her reasons for refusing treatment, and able to state that she understands that Dr. Percens believes this "spot" could be a cancer.

- Does Mrs. Wenzel have a life-threatening condition?
- What do you think Wendy and the physicians should do?
- Do you think there are grounds for court-ordered treatment?

panels within the hospital to decide whether or not to medicate against a client's wishes. The court observed that such panels generally provide adequate constitutional protection and are more likely to decide in the client's interest than are medically naive judges. This argument may eventually have some impact on procedures for decision-making in medication refusal situations, but at present these decisions almost always end up being made in a courtroom.

LEGAL ISSUES IN HOSPITALIZATION AND INPATIENT TREATMENT

A client may be admitted to a hospital voluntarily or through a court-ordered commitment. About half of the admissions to psychiatric hospitals are voluntary and occur when a client seeks treatment of his own free choice. For admission to be voluntary, the client must have knowledge of the facility, its appearance, and the conditions of his hospitalization there, and must be informed of alternatives to hospital care.

For the other half of admissions to psychiatric hospitals, clients are admitted involuntarily through proceedings of emergency hospitalization or civil commitment. **Emergency hospitalization** is the power of states to detain a person in an emergency situation for a limited time until further evaluation and court proceedings can occur. Emergency hospitalization is usually for a short period only, typically 48 to 72 hours, and allows the need for longer inpatient treatment to be assessed. In most jurisdictions, emergency hospitalization is legally based in police powers and can generally be invoked only when an individual is judged potentially harmful to himself or others.

After the 48- to 72-hour period has lapsed, legally empowered mental health providers (usually psychiatrists) can petition the court for a lengthier period of hospitalization. This lengthier involuntary hospitalization is known as **civil commitment**. Procedures for approving or denying civil commitment vary from state to state, but almost always involve a court hearing. In such hearings the court may use a standard of "clear and convincing evidence," which is lower than the "beyond a reasonable doubt" standard used in criminal cases. Once an individual is committed to involuntary mental hospitalization, periodic judicial case reviews are required on a regular basis, but no less than yearly. Long-term commitment almost always requires evidence that the individual remains dangerous either to self or to others (Simon, 1992, p. 157).

A recent development in mental health care is that a number of states have passed laws requiring certain mental health clients to obtain mandatory outpatient therapy (MOT). These laws have been a reaction to high profile cases that resulted in harm to innocent parties. The American Psychiatric Nurses Association (APNA) states in their code of ethics that MOT does have a place in the mental health treatment continuum and is appropriate for some cases. APNA recommends that MOT be considered a last resort for treatment and protection of the public (APNA, 2004). Certainly, nurses should investigate the laws and regulations in their own state.

Depending on where they work, psychiatric nurses may also encounter clients who have been involuntarily hospitalized through the criminal justice system. These individuals have been judged either guilty of crimes or not guilty by reason of insanity, and they have been criminally committed for treatment. This form of involuntary hospitalization is very different from involuntary commitment initiated by a psychiatrist, as the client is in the criminal justice system, not the health care system. (Refer to Chapter 22 for specific information on care of the incarcerated.)

Involuntarily hospitalized clients do not lose their civil rights and are not presumed legally incompetent solely because they have been committed. As noted earlier, most clients retain their right to refuse treatment, especially with potentially dangerous psychiatric medications. However, the law also provides that judicially committed individuals have a right to receive psychiatric treatment. Applicable state laws stipulate very little about the content or quality of mandated treatment in the community, and often the right to treatment applies only to inpatient settings. Hospitalized clients have a variety of other rights, such as those to visitation, control of funds, and privacy that can only rarely be abridged and then only in the client's interests. Quite different ethical issues arise, however, when nurses and other professionals provide care to incarcerated clients. As discussed in Chapter 22, persons with mental illness are commonly found within the prison system. Some have committed serious crimes, whereas others may be incarcerated for public disturbances related to alcohol or to mental illness itself. Mental health providers in prison settings necessarily serve both the client and the institution, and in consequence sometimes face ethical role conflicts in providing care for these individuals. Echoing earlier work by Appelbaum (Appelbaum, 1997), Sen and colleagues propose that the principle of promoting justice should take primacy over other considerations in providing that care (Sen, Gordon, Adshead, & Irons, 2007).

Legal Issues Related to Care in the Community

There are specific legal obligations for psychiatric nurses practicing in the community. These involve both informed consent and the concept of professional abandonment.

Many experts feel informed consent is required for individuals beginning psychotherapy (Simon, 1992, p. 135), for psychotherapy is a treatment, and a client must understand what psychotherapy is before granting consent. Informed consent to begin psychotherapy requires that the client be provided information about what is to be expected in the therapy sessions, how long the therapy may take, the fact that there will be records kept of the therapy visits, and how the bill for service is expected to be handled. Some clinicians assume that consent requires a client's signature on specially prepared

REFLECTIVE THINKING 9-5

Informed Consent

Mrs. Roebuck is a 50-year-old, married woman with a history of depression. Today, she was brought to the emergency room by her husband, who found her at home this afternoon. She has self-inflicted, superficial cuts on each wrist and states she has been drinking both beer and wine today. She is crying, stating, "I don't care what happens to me." She requires treatment (stitches) for the wounds on her wrist, although the bleeding has stopped. The emergency room physician has requested a psychiatric consult for possible admission to the mental health unit.

Mrs. Roebuck is oriented to reality and states that she understands the hospital staff and her husband want to help her, but she says, "I'm too much trouble—I don't want your help." Further, she states, "I don't want anything! Just let me be, I don't want to live."

Mr. Roebuck says, "Please help us, she is not herself today."

- **Under the circumstances, do you think Mrs. Roebuck gave informed consent for her treatment?**
- **Can the emergency room staff provide treatment for the wounds on her wrists, given her comment that she does not want help?**
- **Can the hospital staff and Mr. Roebuck hospitalize Mrs. Roebuck on the mental health unit without her consent?**

REFLECTIVE THINKING 9-6

Informed Consent and the Community Health Nurse

At a team meeting, a group of community health nurses were discussing client families they had been visiting in their maternal-child program. Several of the families they were seeing had stress in the home following the birth of a baby, and the nurses offered education, support, and counseling during the home visit.

Community health nurses in this setting visit any mother with a new baby, and they frequently continue visiting during the postpartum period. When a nurse's assessment indicates stress in the home, increased numbers of visits are offered. Nurses keep records in the health department office to document the visits.

Janette, a new nurse to the health department, inquired if the families were all informed that records were kept at the health department office. Further, she asked if the clients knew the content of the records.

- **Do nurses need to inform clients that written records are kept in this situation?**
- **How can conditions of informed consent be met in this situation?**

consent forms, and indeed such a signature may document informed consent. However, a chart note describing what the clinician told the client and the clinician's perception of the degree of understanding and free choice involved is probably more important than a client's signature. In ideal practice, both a signature and a chart note would be completed.

All mental health professionals have an obligation to provide continuing care to their clients and to arrange appropriate follow-up care in the provider's absence. These clinicians make an implicit contract with their clients at the time of initiating care that they will provide continuing service. Failure to do so constitutes a breach of contract and could lead to accusations of **abandonment**, a form of negligence that stems from leaving a client in need without alternatives for treatment. At times, clinicians may choose to terminate care for one or more clients, either because the clinician is changing jobs or affiliations, or because she finds the course of the client encounter unsatisfactory. Codes of conduct require that in such circumstances the clinician provide clear interpretation of her intent to the client and continue to see the client for a reasonable time until other care arrangements have been worked out. Failure to ensure such follow-up can leave the clinician open to a legal charge of abandonment. Nurses providing group or individual psychotherapy in any setting potentially risk an accusation of abandonment by the nature of their contract to provide continuing care to their clients.

Professional Negligence

Professional negligence in mental health care is a problem that all nurses need to understand and prevent. **Negligence** means either behaving in a way that a prudent individual would not have behaved or failing to use the diligence and care expected of a reasonable individual in similar circumstances. In situations where negligence has occurred, the nurse may be faced with a **malpractice** lawsuit, that is, a lawsuit where the client seeks recovery for damages caused by the nurse's negligent actions. It is probable that all health care providers are negligent on occasion, but most negligent events do not lead to serious client harm either through good fortune or because a colleague recognizes and corrects the negligent error. Negligence that results in harm to a client or that allows a client to harm someone else may involve the nurse in a lawsuit. Although lawsuits against psychiatrists and psychotherapists may be more common than those against nurses, certain situations likely pose a particular risk for all mental health professionals.

Failure to Prevent Dangerous Client Behavior

Mental health professionals have increasingly been held to high standards of accountability in predicting and preventing client danger. Thus, in situations in which a client discloses that he is likely to inflict harm on himself or on others, the mental health professional is obligated to take action to prevent that harmful action.

All nurses should be aware of the **Tarasoff Duty to Warn** potential victims of violence that might be directed against them. In most states, if a mental health professional has any reason to believe that a client harbors thoughts of harm toward a specific individual or individuals, then she has a legal obligation to ensure that the potential victim is warned so that protection may be sought. In the Tarasoff case, a client informed his psychologist that he intended to kill a young woman acquaintance. The psychologist informed the police, who interviewed the man, but neither psychologist nor police warned the woman of the potential risk to her life. She was subsequently murdered by the client, and her parents brought successful suit for failure to warn. The Tarasoff Duty to Warn potential victims takes precedence over the duty to protect client confidentiality. Even if the client does not name a specific victim, warning is required if the therapist can reasonably deduce who is at risk. Lawsuits continue to occur over failure to warn, and while few, if any, have involved nurses, there is no reason to believe the Tarasoff Duty does not extend to the psychiatric nurse.

One of the corollaries of the Tarasoff Duty is that therapists are held accountable for their ability to correctly predict when a client is likely to be lethally violent. Prediction of any behavior is difficult, and clinical predictions of violence are generally not particularly accurate (Bednar, Bednar, Lambert, & Waite, 1991). The clinician is legally required to take threats very seriously and to be alert for historical data, such as poor impulse control, use of stimulant drugs, and prior violence that might substantially increase the likelihood of recurrent violence. While courts do not require unreasonably accurate prediction, they may judge a nurse or other clinician negligent if due caution is not taken to assess, record, and act on potential warnings and risk factors for subsequent violent behavior.

Clinicians may also be held negligent if they fail to recognize suicidal risk. As with violence, this is a particularly difficult task because suicidal behavior is notoriously difficult to predict. Relatively few successful malpractice lawsuits are brought because of a client's suicide. Nonetheless, the nurse will always use her best skills to assess suicidal risk (see Chapter 16) and to contract with a potentially suicidal client. Providing and documenting information about 24-hour telephone support (usually through community hotlines) are

REFLECTIVE THINKING 9-7

Abandonment

Psychiatric nurse Linda has been providing individual and group therapy to clients in her community for 5 years. Linda is moving to another city and will be closing her practice.

- **How do you think Linda should make this move, leaving about 20 active clients in her practice and many others whom she has not seen in several months?**
- **How does Linda leave her clients in a manner that is ethically and legally responsible?**

helpful to clients and serve as evidence of careful clinical practice. Periodically assessing and documenting a client's mental competence will help detect delusions or other bizarre thought processes that might lead to suicide and will help provide evidence regarding the client's competency and state of mind in the event of a subsequent accusation of negligence.

Lawsuits are not an inevitable consequence of negligent care. Many clinical errors are not followed by lawsuits, even when considerable damage results. Suits seem to occur more frequently when clients fail to develop close, therapeutic relationships with their caregivers and feel residual anger—anger that is increased by unfavorable clinical occurrences. The nurse who cultivates professionally appropriate, but close and nurturing, relationships with clients very likely reduces the risk of being sued, while at the same time increases satisfaction with the practice of psychiatric mental health nursing.

Sexual Involvement with Clients

The ANA *Standards of Psychiatric-Mental Health Clinical Nursing Practice* explicitly prohibits intimate or sexual relationships with present or former clients. Such prohibitions are part of virtually all codes of behavior for other mental health professionals, and sexual liaisons between therapist and client are prohibited by statute in a number of states. Violation of such statutes may result in loss or suspension of one's professional license. Despite this widespread prohibition, sexual relationships between client and therapist do occur. One author summarizes known data reporting that sexual attraction is quite a common phenomenon among mental health professionals (probably between 70% to 90% of practitioners report having been sexually attracted to at least one client), however, the incidence of sexual involvement with clients in very low (1% or 2%) and may be declining (Fisher, 2004).

Breaching Confidentiality

Issues related to confidentiality have been discussed in a previous section. Whether purposefully or by accident, if a nurse reveals information given to her in clinical confidence, the client may bring suit. Clearly, the nurse must avoid any release of confidential information without explicit authorization from the client.

Failure to Honor Individual Rights

Clients may bring suit against mental health professionals for wrongful commitment to a psychiatric hospital, failure to obtain appropriate consent, wrongful restraint, or a variety of other perceived assaults on personal autonomy. Following appropriate guidelines for commitment, restraint, and medication treatment can significantly protect against successful lawsuit.

Control of Violent or Self-Destructive Behaviors

Violent or self-destructive clients are frequently committed involuntarily to psychiatric hospitals. When violent or self-destructive behavior is overt or thought highly probable, the nurse's primary focus is on protecting the client and those around him. Suicidal or potentially violent individuals may refuse medication or other potentially useful treatments. Under conditions of true emergency, treatment without permission is occasionally justified. When urgency is less but treatment is clearly in a refusing individual's best interest, an attempt should be made to obtain court-ordered treatment, usually through a declaration of judgmental incompetence.

Either because appropriate treatment is refused or because insufficient time has elapsed for treatment to be effective, hospital staff must sometimes make special efforts to ensure a client's safety. These efforts may include one-to-one staffing, use of on-site police or other guards, **seclusion** (putting someone in a usually empty or padded room or cell by themselves), or **physical restraints** (apparatus that significantly inhibit mobility). Seclusion and restraints are treatments that could violate the important treatment principle of the **least restrictive alternative**. This principle is a legal doctrine that requires that clients be treated with the least amount of constraint of liberty consistent with their safety. Clearly, seclusion and restraints should be used only when required to prevent imminent harm to self or others (Lion & Soloff, 1984). While some institutions may use restraints to prevent agitated individuals from inflicting physical damage on hospital facilities, this use of restrictive treatments is hard to justify unless all other options for behavioral control have been exhausted.

Some states have explicit laws regulating or prohibiting the use of restraints and seclusion. Nurses should be aware of the laws that apply in their respective states and be careful to ensure that care complies with these regulations. It is of course important that seclusion and restraint not be used as substitutes for close nursing attention and supervision. Since seclusion and restraint are often used for agitated clients, the

NURSINGTIP 9-1

Prudent/Appropriate Nursing Behaviors

1. Present self as trustworthy to clients:
   - Tell the truth
   - Establish rapport.
2. Know your state laws.
3. Use techniques to de-escalate client anger (speak in a calm voice, acknowledge that anger is an appropriate emotion but that it must be controlled, remove the client who is getting angry from excess stimulation).
4. Do not rush in your interactions with clients or your explanations to clients.
5. Carefully document all assessment data.
6. Carefully record all treatments, interventions, and procedures followed when giving care.

nurse should be absolutely confident that the agitation is not due to some undiagnosed medical condition for which treatment is necessary, perhaps urgently. Perhaps influenced by pressure from accrediting agencies, many hospitals and units have worked actively to severely limit the use of restraints whenever possible (Swauger & Tomlin, 2000).

Many institutions still use neuroleptic medications as "chemical restraints" to sedate agitated individuals. This use of medication has historically been particularly common in the elderly. Chemical restraint is currently regarded as unethical unless antipsychotic medication is used to treat a diagnosed psychotic disorder that is causing agitation. While there are undoubtedly justified exceptions that allow the cautious use of neuroleptics in the nonpsychotic, these are rare. The short-term and well-monitored use of physical restraints is generally preferable to medicating clients with either neuroleptics or respiratory-depressing sedatives.

Other risks for negligence that psychiatric nurses face are similar to those confronted in nonpsychiatric nursing practice: errors in medication administration, failure to prevent nonintentional physical injury, violation of privacy, and failure to provide needed treatment. Nurses who practice psychotherapy or prescribe medications may be found negligent in these activities in much the same way as a physician.

KEY CONCEPTS

- Nurses are responsible for knowing and following all laws relevant to their work.
- There are specific legal issues central to psychiatric mental health nursing: confidentiality, clients' rights, psychological competence, informed consent, involuntary hospitalization and treatment, violent or self-destructive behaviors, and professional negligence in mental health care.
- Ethical theories of utilitarianism and deontology give the nurse a moral guide to practice.
- Ethical principles of autonomy, beneficence, fidelity, justice, and nonmaleficence may be used to guide decisions.
- The Value Analysis Model gives the nurse a method of evaluating an ethical dilemma before drawing conclusions about an issue.

REVIEW QUESTIONS

1. Administering a medication to a client without first reviewing the benefits, side-effects, and risks of such medications and subsequently getting the clients permission is a violation of which ethical principle?
   1. Caring
   2. Informed consent
   3. Nurse patient confidentiality
   4. The Nurse Practice Act

2. One of the key criteria for determining whether an involuntary commitment is warranted in the case of a mentally ill person is to ask which of the following questions?
   1. Does the person's behavior go against the traditional norms of society?
   2. Does the person express beliefs that are completely out of touch with reality?
   3. Can the person no longer work in the field/profession in which he/she was trained?
   4. Is the person is a threat to self or others, or unable to care for self?

3. A client on the psychiatric unit refuses his 6 P.M. dose of Haldol. Which action should the nurse take next?
   1. Contact the physician immediately.
   2. Contact the nursing supervisor on call.
   3. Hold the medication and chart the client's refusal.
   4. Have the client restrained so that an intramuscular (IM) dose of the medication can be given.

4. A client refuses his 6 P.M. dose of Haldol. The nurse requests that other staff members assist her in restraining the client, so that the medication can be given IM. Because of this action, the nurse can legally be charged with which of the following?
   1. Assault
   2. Battery
   3. Libel
   4. Slander

5. A client is admitted to the unit from the emergency room after a physical altercation with the police. When the client arrived on the unit, the nurse was passing medications and only had a chance to do a cursory search for contraband. Later that evening, the client used a razor that had been hidden in his shoe, to cut another patient. The client's nurse can be charged with which of the following?
   1. Negligence
   2. Malpractice
   3. Assault
   4. Battery

6. A client is admitted to the psychiatric unit of the local hospital after treatment for an acute psychotic episode. Several days later, after being treated with medication the client states to the nurse, "I'm only

here because of a neighbor. She is the nosiest person I have ever seen. When I get out of here, I'm going to take care of her permanently. No one will ever miss her." The client's statement requires the nurse to address which of the following legal issues:
   1. Habeas corpus
   2. Duty to warn
   3. Breach of confidentiality
   4. Right of privacy

7. A client is brought to the emergency department by the police. The client is admitted involuntarily to the psychiatric hospital because he is believed to be homicidal. On the third day of admission, the client demands to be discharged. What should the nurse do next?
   1. Allow the client to leave on his own will.
   2. Contact the nursing supervisor on call.
   3. Request that the client sign a Voluntary Admission form.
   4. Explain to the client that he was admitted on an involuntary admission and she is unable to discharge him at this time.

8. Which of the following legal rights is available to a client who believes he is being detained in a psychiatric unit against his will?
   1. Right to privacy
   2. Right of Habeas Corpus
   3. Right to informed consent
   4. Right to enter into a legal contract

9. A nurse and a client have created a contract to meet every morning to discuss issues of interest to the client. Yesterday the nurse was absent due to illness. Today the nurse is extremely busy and cannot meet with the client. The nurse's behavior has the potential of violating which ethical principle?
   1. Beneficence
   2. Fidelity
   3. Justice
   4. Nonmaleficence

10. A nurse is a member of her community's Mental Health Council. During a business meeting, the council decides to close four of their 10 mental health outpatient clinics to save costs. Upon reviewing the list of clinics, the nurse realizes that the clinics to be closed are the only four located in areas where the populations are predominantly poor and minority. The nurse decides to file a complaint against the council based on their violation of which ethical principle?
   1. Beneficence
   2. Fidelity
   3. Justice
   4. Nonmaleficence

LEARNING ACTIVITIES

1. You are working in a geriatric psychiatric unit where a client who is in touch with reality is yelling at others for hours at a time. His behavior is disruptive to the overall unit environment. At what point do you think the client's right to autonomy is overridden by the utilitarian notion of greater good for the greater number? How do you decide? What is your state law? Could you or would you administer chemical restraints?
2. Give an example of a situation where you would violate a client's right to confidentiality and disclose psychiatric information to another person. Explain why.
3. Does your psychiatric institution have a client bill of rights? If yes, how does this bill of rights ensure that clients' legal rights are being met?
4. What procedures are taken at your psychiatric facility to obtain informed consent for hospitalization, medications, treatments, and outpatient care?
5. Identify a client who has been hospitalized under 48/72-hour emergency hospitalization proceedings. What were the factors that led to commitment?
6. Define the concept of least restrictive alternative.
7. What is the Tarasoff Duty to Warn?
8. Apply the Value Analysis Model either to a situation you have observed in practice or to a hypothetical situation in which you think it would be difficult to decide what to do.

*Study*WARE™ CONNECTION

Using your *Study*WARE™ CD-ROM

1. Complete the Concentration activity for this chapter.
2. Review the audio glossary for key terms in this chapter.
3. Explore the other games and activities that support this chapter.

REFERENCES

American Holistic Nurses' Association. (2008). *Position statement on holistic nursing ethics and code of ethics for holistic nurses.* Flagstaff, AZ: Author.

American Nurses Association (ANA). (2001). *Code of ethics.* Washington, D.C.: Author.

American Nurses Association (ANA)/American Psychiatric Nurses Association (APNA). (2007). *Psychiatric mental health nursing—Scope and standards of practice.* Washington, DC: Author.

American Psychiatric Nurses Association (APNA). (2004). American Psychiatric Nurses Association Position Statement on Mandatory Outpatient Therapy. *Journal of the American Psychiatric Nurses Association, 19*(5), p. 251.

Applebaum, P. S. (1990). *Washington v. Harper:* Prisoners' right to refuse antipsychotic medication. *Hospital and Community Psychiatry, 41,* 731–732.

Appelbaum, P. S. (1997). A theory of ethics for forensic psychiatry. *Journal of the American Academy of Psychiatry and the Law, 25*(3), 233–247.

Atkinson, J. (2007). *Advance directives in mental health: Theory, practice and ethics.* London: Jessica Kingsley Publishers.

Bednar, R. L., Bednar, S. C., Lambert, M. J., & Waite, D. R. (1991). *Psychotherapy with high-risk clients: Legal and professional standards.* Pacific Grove CA: Brooks/Cole.

Biegler, P. (2008). Autonomy, stress, and treatment of depression. *BMJ, 336*(7652), 1046–1048.

Coombs, J. R., & Meux, M. (1971). Teaching strategies for values analysis. In L. Metcalf (Ed.), *Values education* (pp. 29–74, 41st Yearbook). Washington, DC: National Council for the Social Studies.

Department of Health and Human Services (DHHS). (1982, October). *President's Commission for the Study of Ethical Problems in Medicine and Biomedical and Behavioral Research: Making health care decisions: A report on the ethical and legal implications of informed consent in the patient-practitioner relationship.* (Vol 1: Report). Washington, DC: Superintendent of Documents.

Fisher, C. D. (2004). Therapist self-disclosure of sexual feelings. *Ethical Issues in Therapy, 14*(2), 105–121.

Gray, M., & Gibbons, J. (2007). There are no answers, only choices. *Australian Social Work, 60*(2), 222–238.

Kyle, G. (2008). Using anonymized reflection to teach ethics. *Nursing Ethics, 15*(1), 6–16.

Lion, J. R., & Soloff, P. H. (1984). Implementation of seclusion and restraint. In K. Tardiff (Ed.), *The psychiatric uses of seclusion and restraint* (pp. 19–34). Washington, DC: American Psychiatric Press.

Merz, J. F., & Fischoff, B. (1990). Informed consent does not mean rational consent: Cognitive limitations on decision-making. *Journal of Legal Medicine, 11,* 321–350.

Numminen, O., & Leino-Kipli, H. (2007). Nursing students' ethical decision-making: A review of the literature. *Nurse Education Today, 27*(7), 796–807.

Public Broadcasting Service (PBS). *From Daniel M'Naugten to John Hinckley: A brief history of the insanity defense.* Retrieved August 2008, from http://www.pbs.org/wgbh/pages/frontline/shows/crime/trial/history.html

Schwartz, H. I., Vingiano, W., & Perez, C. B. (1988). Autonomy and the right to refuse treatment: Patients' attitudes after involuntary medication. *Hospital and Community Psychiatry, 39,* 1049–1055.

Sen, P., Gordon, H., Adshead, G., & Irons, A. (2007). Ethical dilemmas in forensic psychiatry: Two illustrative cases. *Journal of Medical Ethics, 33*(6), 337–341.

Simon, R. I. (1992). *Clinical psychiatry and the law.* Washington, DC: American Psychiatric Press.

Stone, A. A. (1981). The right to refuse treatment. *Archives of General Psychiatry, 38,* 358–362.

Sturm, R., & Wells, K. (2000). Health insurance may be improving—but not for individuals with mental illness. *Health Services Research, 35*(1, Pt. 2), 253–329.

Swauger, K. C., & Tomlin, C. (2000). Moving toward a restraint-free patient care. *Journal of Nursing Administration, 30*(6), 325–329.

Swenson, L. C. (1993). *Psychology and law for the helping professions.* Pacific Grove, CA: Brooks/Cole.

SUGGESTED READINGS

Fisher, C. B. (2003). *Decoding the ethics code.* Thousand Oaks: Sage.

Koocher, G., & Keith-Spiegal, P. (2008). *Ethics in psychology and the mental health professions.* Oxford: Oxford University Press.

Radden, J. (2004). *The philosophy of psychiatry: A companion.* New York, NY: Oxford University Press.

COURT CASES

MacDonald v. Clinger, 84, A.D.ed 482, 446, N.Y.S.2d 801 (N.Y. App. Div. 1982).

Rivers v. Katz, 67 N.Y.2d 485, 504 N.Y.S.2d 74, 495 (N.E.2d 337, 1986).

Stensvad v. Reivitz, 601 F Suppl. 128 (W.D. Wis. 1985).

Whitree v. State, 56 Misc. 2d 693, 290 N.Y.S.2d 485 (N.Y. Sup. Ct. 1968).

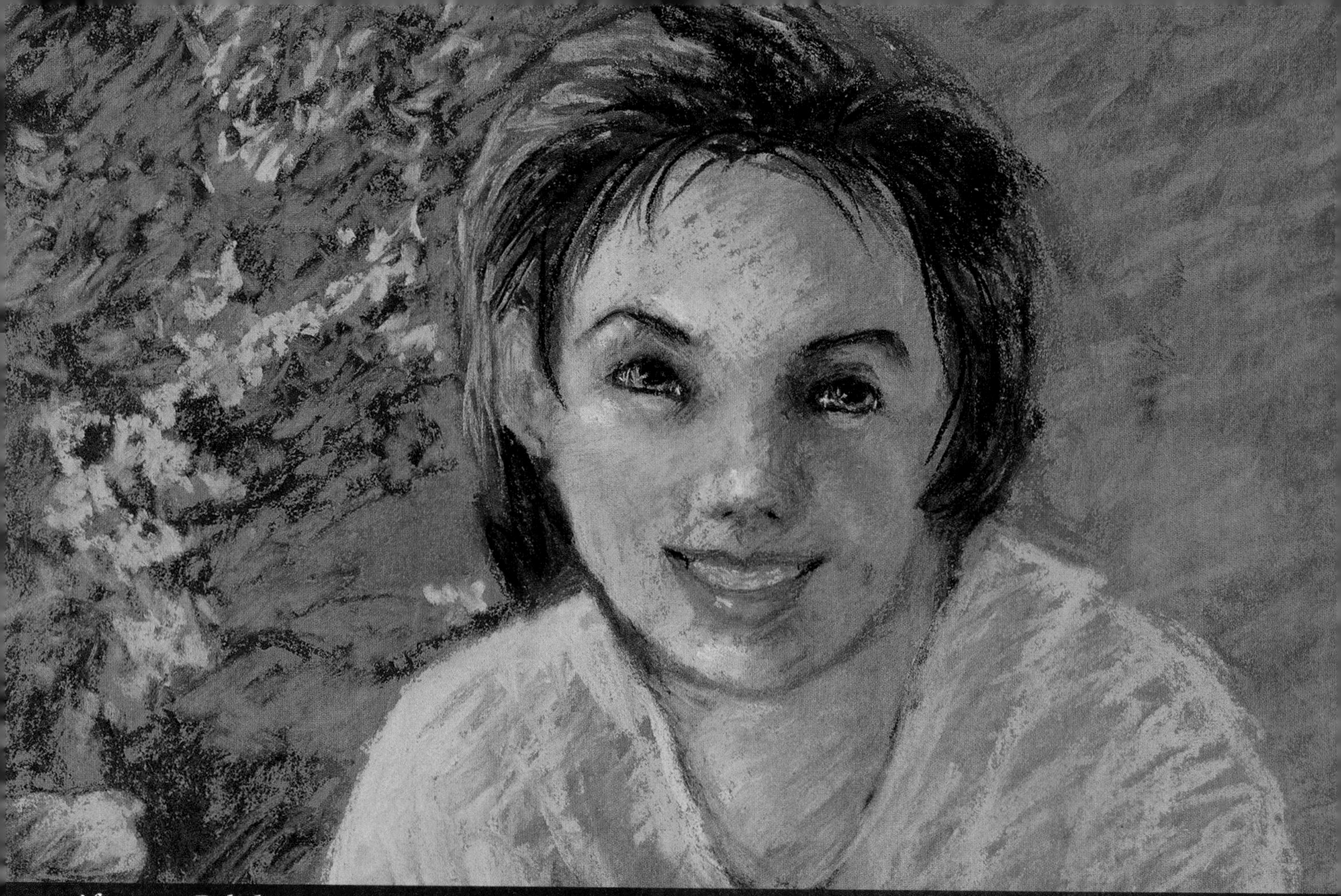

Afternoon Delight

Who Cares for the Caregiver?

Have you ever felt, after a difficult day at school and/or work, that you had nothing left to give? That you were drained? That you were depleted?
Did you ever wish you were learning and experiencing the following:

- *How to balance your life demands.*
- *How to balance and center yourself.*
- *How to find time in the day for quiet and reflection.*
- *How to recognize stressors that are impacting your own health.*
- *How to use techniques of self-care to help you sustain yourself throughout your academic and professional career.*

At first, these questions may appear unusual or perhaps unrelated to psychiatric mental health nursing. As you think about them, you will recognize how caring for your own health and emotional well-being opens a whole new avenue for the further development of your professional life and work. In psychiatric nursing, especially, we are exposed to mental aberrations and severe emotional distresses that can lead to rapid professional burnout. This can be avoided through effective self-care interventions. This chapter focuses on the role of the nurse as self-healer, presenting techniques and tools to support your healthy professional development.

CHAPTER 10

Self-Care for the Nurse

Karilee Halo Shames
Dorothea Hover-Kramer
Noreen Cavan Frisch

CHAPTER OUTLINE

COMPETENCIES

Upon completion of this chapter, the reader should be able to:

1. Explain the occurrences of burnout, emotional fatigue, and emotional exhaustion as occupational risks for nurses.
2. Describe the self-help modalities of meditation, imagery, and self-hypnosis.
3. Describe a few means by which support groups can develop.
4. Identify three ways in which humor promotes healing.
5. Employ the use of relaxation and imagery for self-care.
6. Identify two reasons for centering prior to entering a psychiatric care unit.
7. Use the nursing self-care process to achieve a higher level of personal wellness as a caregiver.

KEY TERMS

Burnout
Circadian Rhythm
Nurse-Self Care
Parasympathetic System Response
Sympathetic System Response

Throughout this text, we are exploring various aspects of psychiatric mental health nursing. We are examining nursing practice, as well as learning about clients, institutions, diagnostic systems, nurse-client relationships, psychiatric disorders, and treatment modalities. We consider how various psychiatric diagnoses are viewed by the people experiencing them. We observe emotional instability, whether it is reflected in a chronic state of low energy, as in depression, or in a fluctuating mood disorder, such as in bipolar illness. In all of these situations, the caregiver is challenged to bring a sense of balance and wholeness to an otherwise unstable situation. We can rightly conclude that providing psychiatric care can be extremely intense for the professional, demanding a vast amount of mental and emotional resourcefulness.

The natural question follows: How does the nurse maintain a sense of balance in the midst of mental chaos? Is it possible to hold on to one's composure, to be centered, while working with emotional instability and tension? How do we, as caregivers, recharge our own supply of energy and health?

In her classic book *Caregiver, Caretaker* (1992), nurse Caryn Summers describes a concept she calls "the chase." She proposes that nurses often gravitate to areas that, somehow, feel comfortable, like our home environments. In other words, as nurses, we might choose specialty areas representative of environments we have endured, and even survived, in our developmental years. Her concept of the chase might lead us to look more closely at our reasons for choosing a specialty. It is possible that many of us are drawn to professional practices in units for reasons outside of our conscious awareness. These areas of subconscious motivation require our full attention lest we succumb to older, less desirable behavior patterns learned in our childhood experiences.

Other authors have written about nurses' involvement with clients' emotional needs, appropriately calling their work *I'm Dying to Take Care of You* (Snow & Willard, 1989). In this book, the authors list the many ways that nurses, because of their caring attributes, become victims of their own dependency needs. The pattern of putting others' requirements ahead of our own is both a gift and a great liability. Nurses may risk losing their sense of boundaries when seeking approval to validate good intentions; nurses may be unduly affected by stress created by those around us. To use a psychological term, nurses may act in a *codependent* fashion, enabling themselves to be abused. The very nature of the organizations within which most of us work may further support this distortion of our healing intentions. The sociologist Anne Wilson Schaef suggested that American organizations, including managed care, hospitals, home care, and health maintenance groups, are addictive in nature (Schaef & Fassel, 1988). The very fabric of our society seems to undervalue the caregiver and emphasize the administrative and financial aspects of organizational structures.

More recently, many writers have drawn attention to the current status of nurses' work, workplace conditions, and workforce demands. There have been trends in all areas of nursing practice that are making it quite difficult for nurses to maintain a life balance and for organizations to sustain a nursing workforce over time. Among these trends are the extended workday and workweek. In 2006, a study of more than 2,000 nurses in the United States documented that 25% of nurses were working over 12 hours per day, nearly 20% of nurses were working two jobs, 17% worked overtime, and nearly 40% were "on call" (Trinkoff, Geiger-Brown, Brady, Lipscomb, & Muntaner, 2006). In addition, reports from this study claim that 27% of nurses had one hour per day or less to relax or to pursue personal activities. Other studies have documented that nurses' worklives are becoming more difficult as patient/client acuity levels increase and nurse to patient ratios decrease (Aiken, Clarke, Sloane, Sochlaski, &

Silber, 2002; Aiken, Clarke, Sloane, Sochlaski, Busse, Clarke, et al., 2001). Nurses working in hospitals find that their professional work is often reduced to a number of discrete tasks that need to be completed each shift. In a time study evaluating nurses' work, Tucker (2002) and Tucker and Spear (2006) describe situations where nurses had to complete 160 tasks in an eight-hour shift, having less than four minutes to attend to each task. Given that, the nurse was still interrupted every 44 minutes. It is not a surprise to read that nurses experience job strain. The work of Aiken et al. (2001) reported that 40% of nurses experienced "burnout," and a later study (Reineck & Furino, 2005) reported that a majority of nurses report job frustration and dissatisfaction. There is little doubt that experiences of frustration, dissatisfaction, and burnout, coupled with extended workdays, homelife demands, and little time for self will certainly lead to emotional exhaustion. Psychiatric mental health nurses, like many of their counterparts in other nursing specialties, work in settings that involve close, intimate, and sustained interactions with clients with the constant demand that the nurse support the client's emotional, spiritual, and physical needs. Psychiatric mental health nurses, as well as other nurses and human service professionals, may be at higher risk for emotional exhaustion as they find themselves in situations where they feel they have been "taken over" by their occupational role as they encounter clients in great need.

This chapter supports the nurse in learning how to care for self and how to find the balance needed to sustain oneself in nursing. When nurses practice self-care, they are in a much better position to be the calm within the storm, to use their hearts and heads to work with people in need. Further, they are in a much better position to prioritize life and work demands and often find it much easier to claim time for self as a legitimate request to others in their lives.

SELF-CARE: A MODALITY FOR PSYCHIATRIC NURSES

Nurses have long been considered the keepers of health, guardians of physical welfare for persons in need. Nursing as a profession has witnessed the phenomenon of **burnout**, whereby caregivers find themselves unable to provide the quality of care that is desirable. A recent search (2008) of the nursing literature through the Cumulative Index to Nursing and Allied Health Literature (CINHAL) indicated 1,474 published articles on the topic of burnout and stress among nursing and only three published articles on the topic of nurse self-care. Clearly, burnout and stress are pervasive and important topics in nursing. Self-care has not yet come to the forefront of nursing awareness. It is important then to start with what we know about burnout. Nurses experiencing burnout may feel a depletion of energy, decreased ability to concentrate, and a sense of hopelessness. They feel pressed and burdened, functioning automatically to meet the demands of an impossible schedule. The constant pressure of the work situation causes many caregivers to become physically, emotionally, or mentally sick. For many, the joy of their work is lost in the chaos, and they need to seek new ways to rejuvenate and redefine their roles.

Nurses who thrive in the workplace have developed attitudes, behaviors, and practices that support their sense of balance and well-being in their work. Early studies of caregivers who maintained high vitality in the workplace (Mabbett, 1989; Hover-Kramer, Mabbett, & Shames, 1996; Wright, 2000) documented that nurses can be empowered to make healthy choices for themselves while they provide effective care. Further, work of holistic nurses has further developed the concept of **nurse-self care** as a guiding principle of nurses' work. As a principle of holistic nursing practice, Quinn wrote that nurses who integrate self-care strategies into their lives are better able to care for their clients (than those who do not) partly because they are then able to model health behaviors that create a sense of harmony and balance for others (2000). In establishing the current Scope and Standards of Holistic Nursing as a Specialty, Mariano writes that "Nurse self-reflection and self assessment, self-care, healing and personal development are necessary for service to others and growth/change in one's own well being" (2007, p. 178). Thus, the following sections will explore how attitudes, behaviors, and practices can assist nurses in making healthy choices.

REFLECTIVE THINKING 10-1

Health Care Trends and Self-Care

The shortage of professional nurses, coupled with financial concerns of institutions, often translate into:

- Shorter stays for clients, meaning nurses have less interaction and relationship-building time with clients and often will see only the acute phase of illness, not the recovery phase
- Downsizing or replacement of trained staff with lesser-skilled workers, which leads nurses to question their job security.

What impact do you think these general trends in health care have on the mental health of nurses? Have you felt the impact of these trends? Have they led you to reflect on the value of being a nurse, or have they underscored for you the importance of caring first for yourself as a means of being an effective caregiver to others?

ATTITUDES

When nurses feel beaten down, they have little left to offer clients. If self-esteem is missing, nurses cannot empower others. If nurses feel unsupported, they may need to examine how nurses as a group helped to create such a situation and work to find remedies together.

Do nurses feel that they have no power? Gordon has written extensively on the issue of nurses' perceived loss of control, loss of voice, and loss of power among nurses (2005). However, exploring the ideas of power and powerlessness, it becomes clear that much power comes from within. Power can be understood as an internally generated strength. From this inner strength comes ability to effect change. Nurses may actually be in a pivotal position, particularly if they agree that responsibility is not a burden, but rather encompasses the full ability to respond and be effectively in charge of their lives. Looking from this vantage point, nurses have the ability to respond in many powerful ways to meet and surpass the demands of daily caregiving.

Nurses must be willing to acknowledge their strengths and limitations and to honor those other health professionals who work alongside nurses as equal partners. Historically, nursing has emphasized caring for others at the expense of self-care, beginning with church-affiliated hospices in the thirteenth century (Donahue, 1985). This attitude certainly requires rethinking today. Nurses know that the maximal benefit to clients is derived from a partnership, one in which physician, nurse, other professionals, and clients work collaboratively, each powerful from his or her own perspective. Nurses, while not the only caregivers, may be in the best position to take time to be deeply connected with clients, to hear the soft words of their hearts, and to articulate a plan of care to the remaining members of the health care team. Physicians have a different, unique, and viable contribution. Nurses' work, as Florence Nightingale stated clearly (in Calabria & Macrae, 1994), is to inspire clients to move beyond their challenges by helping to create an environment for their self-healing.

How can nurses best accomplish this? Martin (2002) indicates that nurses must maintain "personal power" to be healthy and to be in a place to assist clients. She defines *personal power* as one's ability to control one's actions and states that such power is the first step in preventing burnout. One method might well be to embrace an attitude of openness in our own lives, to actualize ourselves as models of physical and emotional health, and to empower these qualities through our living example. This leads to a discussion of the ways in which we might modify our behaviors to bring about healthy changes.

Behaviors

A nurse who is alert and empowered can respond to client requests with new expectations of the best possible outcomes. Nurse behaviors demonstrate an understanding of the interconnectedness between thinking, feeling, and action. Consider, as an example, the following passage written by a nurse who was preparing to work with a hostile client who was dying of acquired immunodeficiency syndrome (AIDS). The nurse exhibits self-caring behaviors that are noteworthy as we move into a deeper understanding of how the word *responsibility* actually becomes her "ability to respond" with creative flexibility.

THE NIGHTINGALE CONSPIRACY

"First, I went into the laundry to take a quiet moment. I did some slow, deep breathing, became aware of any feelings and tension in my body, and consciously released them. I prayed and asked for help and guidance in caring for Mr. Smith. I asked to be granted the perfect words and thoughts to join my soul with him in total harmony, and to be protected from any disease.

Next, I waited until I felt a peaceful calm envelop me, and I had a vision of an angel hovering near, smiling. I emerged back into the hall, feeling eager to be with Mr. Smith.

When I entered, he was belligerent initially. When he felt my calm presence, he quieted immediately, and was soon resting. I sat near his bedside, maintaining loving thoughts and sending peaceful energy into the space we shared. His breathing was labored, and I knew he would be leaving the Earth soon. Suddenly, I felt honored to be with him."

*Jeannette said that at that moment, without the least hesitation, she found herself surrounding him in her arms and cradling him ... He burst out in deep sobs, and she rocked him for a long tender while. Finally, his sobs subsided gradually, and she felt his body relax and go limp. She had helped usher him to another plane. His peaceful smile and energy let her know that he was fine, and she felt humbled and deeply grateful for the opportunity to share in his transition.**

(Shames, 1993, p. 181)

It is evident that Jeannette seized the moment to center, or balance herself, in preparation for her encounter. What she described apparently took a brief amount of time, yet enabled her to be present with her client in a very real and meaningful way.

Nurses today who are rushed and short of time are sometimes unable to make the best decisions on their client's behalf. When they take the time to evaluate the nursing role, nurses can acknowledge that a part of the job is to handle each situation with our full, careful attention.

It may seem that we cannot afford to "waste" time in centering ourselves. Yet, there is much time wasted when one is not fully attentive. For example, when nurses speak improperly or impatiently to coworkers or clients, they find themselves in the uncomfortable position of having to clarify misconceptions and to make amends. Valuable time and energy go into attempts to undo problems that result from hasty actions. From this perspective, it is much more energy efficient to take the time to be well prepared in advance, rather than be burdened later by having to repair damage.

*From *The Nightingale Conspiracy* by K. H. Shames, 1993, Clifton Park, NY: Thomson Delmar Learning.

Understanding that behaviors affect every aspect of our work life, the following section is a discussion of commitment to daily practices that will support optimum self-care and well-being.

Practices

There are a great number of specific practices that can support psychiatric mental health nurses. Beyond preventing occupational burnout, we want to thrive and be vital, effective, and resourceful. The holistic, integrative framework allows us to address our entire energy system—by paying attention to the needs of the *physical* body, by increasing awareness of our *emotional* selves, by developing positive *mental* patterns, and by enhancing our sense of *spiritual* connectedness.

Beginning with the physical dimension, then, nurses want to be attentive to the need for rest as well as for movement. Often, when the body is tired, and we are more prone to accidents and errors, it is because we have exceeded the natural circadian rhythm for optimum attentiveness, which is 90 to 120 minutes in most people. **Circadian rhythm** is a biorhythm that determines human responses to the environment; specifically, it refers to attention span in relation to the presence or absence of daylight (i.e., some people are most alert in the morning, others in the afternoon or evening). Breaks at work, therefore, are not only pleasant but also essential for the physical body to revive itself and for the mind to return to full alertness. In addition, movement that allows the body to stretch to full ranges of motion is a daily requirement for maintenance.

Restful sleep and the need for physical renewal through sleep cannot be overemphasized for nurses. The literature provides evidence of adverse physiological and psychological effects of shift work, including development of sleep disorders, which are associated with cardiovascular disease and digestive tract problems (Admi, Tzischinsky, Epstein, Herer, & Lavie, 2006). A review of existent literature on sleep and the impact of shift rotation for nurses concluded that day-night rotations do impact nurses' health and performance, particularly for those over the age of 40 years (Muecke, 2005). Other research indicated that female nurses had a higher incidence of sleep disorders than did their male counterparts (Admi et al., 2006). Nurses are encouraged to use the sleep hygiene techniques described in Chapter 20 of this text.

Although all nurses know they need to eat regularly, many may not be attentive enough to know which foods truly nourish their bodies. Especially when rushed or under pressure, nurses may eat food as quickly as possible without much thought of its effects. For example, sugar, carbohydrates, and caffeine give a seeming boost in energy levels that is usually short lived and followed by a drop in energy, whereas protein eaten several times during a day sustains the sense of vitality. It is crucial to keep the physical body in shape through proper exercise and diet. Regular cardiovascular exercise coupled with sensible dietary habits allow for a well-oiled machine, one that enables individuals to rise in meeting the demands of everyday life.

Similar to the physical, the emotional body needs nurturing and cycles of activity and rest. Attention to what goes into one's emotional being allows one to sort out the enjoyable feelings from the ones that require releasing. Tension and anger in the workplace as well as in personal life, for example, need quick clearing out in a safe way. When something is amiss, ask who owns the problem. Teamwork issues require resolution at the collegial level; organizational issues belong to management settings; and personal issues or shortcomings require individual attention and willingness to learn from mistakes. Emotional support through friendship circles, specialty groups, and personal counseling allows growth and forward movement.

The mental dimension deserves equal attention as the emotional. Thought patterns can be destructive when they are limiting or excessively negative. For instance, patterns of blaming others and saying we are helpless while waiting for others to take charge significantly limit a nurse's sense of viable choices. Even before considering actions, nurses need to look at the thoughts that precede the action and ask, "Is this the best choice for me? Are there other options? How can I find more resources for myself or for the situation at hand?"

The essentials of energetic self-care require ongoing attentiveness to the quality and state of the personal biofield. One method used by persons recovering from addictions is a personal check-in technique called HALT. HALT is a reminder to ask oneself, right now: Am I Hungry? Am I Angry? Am I Lonely? and Am I Tired? In this way, a simple acronym becomes a means for internal self-assessment that can be prescriptive for relief interventions. In a similar vein, we can use PEMS to assess the Physical, Emotional, Mental, and Spiritual dimensions of the biofield.

The physical body requires nutrition, activity, and rest. If one works with her body proactively and caringly, it lasts longer and self-heals more capably than any man-made device. Self-knowledge is the key to effective physical care since every organism is a unique combination of heredity, life events, and personal mechanisms. Nurses must learn not only to rest, but how often, how long, and how to assess when they are tired. Each nurse must learn the kind of exercise that is optimal for her body type. Likewise, all must learn how much to eat, when to eat, and when to stop.

The emotional body can dominate all other aspects of awareness when it is in disarray. Strong negative emotions require prompt attention and assistance, just as would be required for a physical symptom. Moving toward positive supportive emotions is an integral part of our human journey toward personal fulfillment. Self-understanding requires attention to those "unlovable" parts of ourselves, the parts that constitute the "shadow" (Zweig & Abrams, 1991).

Mental states, as exemplified by our thought patterns, can also overwhelm us if they are destructive, judgmental, or critical. Such patterns can even harm the physical body or cause emotional depression as demonstrated in the vast literature showing mind/body interactions. The practice of creating helpful thought patterns and peaceful images can do much to assist the body and emotions.

Self-assessment in the spiritual dimension may require something as simple as being still and listening to one's inner voice. The practice of centering required in all healing work readily moves us to this new perspective—nothing is quite as demanding, or as immediate, as it seems in the moment. Awareness of one's own spirituality is recognized as a central aspect of nurses' work (Dossey, Keegan, & Guzzetta, 2007).

To assist with our work in psychiatric care settings, the following sections address six specific modalities that are directly helpful in maintaining ourselves as nurse counselors. These are the use of imagery, relaxation skills, self-hypnosis, balancing/centering, humor, and meeting in support groups. Any of these modalities lend themselves to application in a wide variety of settings. It is also helpful to remember that nursing is an art as well as a science: Revitalizing the artist on a daily basis allows for the flow of creativity so that genuine caregiving can occur.

SELF-CARE MODALITIES

Imagery

Imagery is a nursing tool that has been steadily growing in popularity (Reed, 2007; Shames, 1996). It involves the use of internal pictures, sounds, or sensations to evoke our personal healing responses.

As defined in dictionaries, an image is a mental picture, or representation of something, that can be either real or imagined. People experience emotional and physiological responses to images. One might also think of images as a thought with a sensation attached. Not everyone sees visual pictures in the mind's eye, but most people have sensory responses to external symbols.

Consider, for example, the image of a rose. As you read the word *rose,* you may begin to make some mental associations, such as a color, a shape, a smell, or a bush on which a rose grows. To continue, you may recall the last time you held a rose in your hand, the person who gave it to you, or feeling the prick of a rose thorn. Now, if you are asked to imagine a lemon, a very tart, juicy lemon, you may begin to salivate. Your response is not to an actual piece of fruit, but simply to the thought and sensation attached to the word.

Images are extremely powerful and can be used to evoke a wealth of internal experiences, including a sense of health and well-being. When working with clients, nurses can help them feel more relaxed by speaking softly and encouraging them to picture a scene that is peaceful. Clients might envision themselves lounging comfortably in a favorite place, by the ocean, or in a special setting where they would like to be. It does not matter that they are actually in a treatment facility. At that moment, they have actually traveled to a different, more healing place. When a nurse uses such therapeutic imagery, the nurse is helping clients to direct their minds toward a beneficial outcome, rather than repeating patterns of anxiety.

The exercises in Box 10-1 are suggestions for self-care of the nurse using imagery. As you read them, allow yourself to take time to step into each experience as fully as possible and begin to experience the benefits of imagery for well-being.

BOX 10-1
IMAGERY EXERCISES

THE RELEASE BALLOON

Sitting comfortably in a quiet place, allow yourself to release the breath, letting all the stress and tension of the day flow out as you exhale. Do this several times to further unburden yourself. Imagine a pile forming in front of you of specific issues that bother you. Make a symbol of something that is especially annoying to you (e.g., an imposing stack of papers to symbolize paperwork). Let the pile attract many issues like a magnet. Put the pile into the basket of a big, colorful hot air balloon. When the basket is full, gradually untie the lines that hold the balloon. Watch it rise. Drift above the treetops—above the clouds—until it is out of sight. Take several deep breaths and feel lighter and freer.

THE SAFE PLACE

Sitting comfortably in a quiet place, think of the most peaceful place in which you have ever been. It may be a picture that you have seen or a place that you remember. After selecting the site, allow your imagery to develop. See the colors of this safe place. See the surroundings. Hear the sounds associated with this special place. Smell the air of this place. Feel the safety and comfort. If someone is with you, hear the person's soothing words or feel the person's breath. Let your whole body sense the peace of this place. Enjoy the full experience of this safe haven. Gently, come back to full awareness, feeling refreshed and renewed, knowing that you can return to this sensation any time that you choose.

THE IMAGE OF HEALTH AND WHOLENESS

Sitting comfortably in a quiet place, release the breath and note areas of discomfort in your body. Imagine a screen in front of you that shows your body to you with exact detail of the uncomfortable, stressed areas. You may note that the areas that are stressed are tighter and darker, while the healthy areas are warmer and brighter. Gradually, let each area of grayness fill in with a healing color, or sunlight, gently washing away the distress as you breathe into each area. See the whole body filled with light, warmed by your loving breath, filling with health and wholeness. Now, embrace the picture, let it become a part of you. Experience your whole being filling with light and caring. Breathe fully and deeply before moving forward to your next task.

With these understandings, the reader can proceed to a brief exploration of how imagery can be incorporated into work settings. The following excerpt shows how a moment with imagery promoted a priceless experience of healing:

DYING PEACEFULLY

*A nurse was working with an agitated dying client who had always wanted to go to Europe. It was apparent that the wish would never be fulfilled. The nurse took ten minutes of relaxation with the client, mentally escorting him to a quiet place where he felt comfortable and had no pain. The nurse gently guided the client by asking questions such as "Where would you like to go?"; "What would you like to do?"; and "How does that feel?" When she looked over, the client was crying and said he really felt that he had gone to Europe, and that it was wonderful. Within two days, the client died peacefully.**

(Shames, 1996, p. 98)

The imagery was an easily used, effective tool that can be applied any time, any place. It involves the ability of the nurse to assist the client in imagining something more pleasant than the current dilemma. It can allow the client who is upset or in pain an opportunity to escape, perhaps only for a few moments, from his disturbing reality. This brief respite may be all that is needed for the client to become more relaxed or for the person to reconnect to his internal resources, making better decisions for self-healing.

Active use of the imagination, however, may not always be appropriate with psychiatric clients. There are times that using the mind to escape is not appropriate, for instance, when working with psychotic people who cannot distinguish between reality and fantasy. In these instances, the nurse must help the client to relax and "escape" within the parameters of the existing environment, perhaps by focusing on something pleasant in the room, such as a picture or a vase of flowers.

Nurses who use imagery in their daily lives often attest to being more focused, present, and powerful in their interactions. Whereas many other modalities require larger blocks of time, imagery can be amazingly effective in a minute time span. The nurse can go into a laundry room and calm herself by envisioning a peaceful scene, then step out and move into the client environment with a positive outlook. It has often been said that the mind is the builder and the physical a result. If this is so, then it is important for us to use the mind to build healthier, happier surroundings, one thought at a time.

Although imagery may not always be the best tool for psychiatric clients, it is certainly always an appropriate and helpful tool for the psychiatric nurse. Our clients may be emotionally unstable or mentally confused, but we can influence their care through our own focused presence.

Relaxation through Meditation

Throughout human history the concept of quieting the busy mind has been celebrated as the art of the developed, wise person. The word *meditation* simply means to focus one's thoughts, to bring the mind to a state of contemplation and reflection. The effects of setting aside time for contemplation range from calming of the physical body to awareness of our hidden emotions to increased mental clarity and new heights of spiritual enlightenment.

The physical effects of relaxation were described in detail by Hans Selye over 40 years ago (1956) and more recently by Herbert Benson at Harvard Medical School (1987). In Eastern traditions, meditation had been known to have positive physical and emotional benefits, but it was not until the effects were extensively studied in the West that the benefit of a meditative practice was fully appreciated. Consider the physiology of the stress response, which activates a **sympathetic system response** that includes increased heart and breathing rates, increased blood pressure, peripheral blood vessel constriction, muscle tension, gastric hyperacidity, release of adrenaline, and over time the harmful cortisol, to name a few. In short, people have activation of the body's fight-or-flight mechanisms that may be repeated hundreds of times until the body literally goes into overdrive and develops stress-related illness. The effects of calming oneself through meditative practice stimulate the neurons of the autonomic nervous system, which are oppositional to the stress response. **Parasympathetic system response** activation brings about decreases in heart and respiratory rates, dilation of peripheral blood vessels, muscle relaxation, lowered blood pressure, and increased flow of endorphins, the body's own chemicals that increase a sense of well-being. Benson coined the term *relaxation response* to describe these extensive physiological shifts, which can be activated readily through our own willingness to learn ways of relaxing ourselves.

The activation of the relaxation response, then, is one of the most direct benefits of a meditative practice. Other benefits are the deepening of our relationship with our inner selves by connecting with suppressed feelings and thoughts on a regular basis. In working with emotionally disturbed persons, the need to experience one's own center is even more crucial than in more mechanically oriented professions, such as working with computer technologies.

In the *Miracle of Mindfulness*, Thich Nhat Hanh (1987, p. 11) describes mindfulness as "keeping one's consciousness alive to the present reality." If our minds are very cluttered, being present to our inner reality means to experience the clutter and acknowledge it. Mental overloading is well known in the Buddhist tradition, in which it is called the state of the monkey mind. Observing the present state of reality, even one that seems unpleasant at first, opens a path to greater self-understanding.

Box 10-2 provides three examples of meditative practices that build on awareness of the breath, awareness of the body, and awareness of thought patterns. Reading the exercises, allow yourself to take time to recognize an aspect of yourself that may be new to you. Enjoy the discovery of meeting your own best friend!

Any task that is repetitive gives an opportunity for activating the relaxation response. For, example, if you wash dishes, or clean the house, you might do it in a hurry

*From *Creative Imagery in Nursing* by K. H. Shames, 1996, Clifton Park, NY: Delmar Cengage Learning.

BOX 10-2
RELAXATION AND MEDIATION EXERCISES

FOCUSING WITH THE BREATH
Sit or lie comfortably, stretching a few times to release any tension. Exhale fully, letting the breath flow out slowly, as if you are blowing out a candle. Repeat two more times, blowing out even more slowly and deliberately. Note that the inhalations are becoming deeper as well. Now count as you exhale, 1, 2, 3, 4, . . . Wait a moment before inhaling. As you inhale, count slowly, 1, 2, 3, 4, . . . Again, wait a moment as if wondering when the exhale will naturally come. Repeat several times until you get a sense of a natural flow, a cycle of bringing in and releasing—filling and letting go. Just bring your mindful awareness to the breath, aware of the miracle of its flow. In 5 to 10 minutes of this gentle mindfulness practice you will feel calmer and more relaxed.

LEARNING FROM THE BODY
Sitting or lying down comfortably, relax a few times with the breath. Then, follow the path of your body's circulation with your mind's eye. Beginning with the lungs, feel the exchange of air as carbon dioxide is exhaled and fresh oxygen is taken in. Watch the nourished blood from the vessels in the lungs move to the heart pump and through it to the aorta. Watch the flow of nourishing blood to the head, helping the brain to function well. See bright, red blood flowing to the arms and shoulders. Feel the flow in the internal organs, stomach, pancreas, liver, spleen, intestines, kidneys, and bladder. Sense the flow of nourishing blood to the pelvis, thighs, legs, and feet. See the return flow through the tiny capillaries to veins and back to the heart. Feel the continuous flow of support and nourishment in the miracle of your own body. Bring your mindful attention to any part of the body that needs extra nourishment, oxygen, or love. Feel the area fill with the miracle of your mindfulness. Gently, come back to full present awareness so you can move forward, feeling refreshed and replenished.

LEARNING FROM THE MIND
Sitting or lying down comfortably, let your mind wander while you pay attention to its meanderings. As you have a pleasant thought, note to yourself, "This is a pleasant thought." Without any judgment or criticism, just notice how your thoughts roam around—sometimes pleasant, sometimes unpleasant. Maybe you have a tendency to get a little stuck on the unpleasant thoughts, so as soon as you notice one, let yourself move on to a more pleasing thought. Let yourself be both the mind and the observer of the mind—back and forth, just noticing, just bringing the quality of mindfulness to the experience. And, if you wish, imagine that you place the unpleasant thoughts on the back of a little monkey. Let it scamper around, perhaps running up and down a tree, as you feel more quiet and calm. After 10 to 15 minutes, let yourself come back to ordinary awareness, noting what you have learned.

while you are thinking about your next task, or you may take time to be fully present to the moment. Set aside a period of time for self-discovery. Pick up each dish slowly, hold it to the light, feel the water, the soap, and so forth. Experience joy and peace in every moment of this time. Most important, do not get overly ambitious or demanding of yourself:

CREATE AN INNER CALMNESS

*In the first six months, try only to build up your power of concentration, to create an inner calmness and serene joy.... You will be refreshed and gain a broader, clearer view of things, and deepen and strengthen the love in yourself. And you will be able to respond more helpfully to all around you.**

(*Thich Nhat Hanh, 1987, p. 42*)

*From *The Miracle of Mindfulness* by Thich Nhat Hanh, 1987, Boston: Beacon.

Self-Hypnosis

The ability to tap the healing potential of the human mind has been explored for thousands of years. Hypnosis, originally a term related to facilitating sleep or inducing a trance-like state, has come to be understood as a way of using mental suggestions to bring about relaxation and a change in thought patterns. As a tool for personal care, giving ourselves helpful suggestions, through self-hypnosis, is another valuable resource for us as nurse healers. Self-hypnosis further expands and builds on the self-awareness that is developing through our use of imagery and meditative relaxation states.

Using the mind to heal itself is a powerful expansion of the idea of self-healing. Self-hypnosis can be viewed as the creative use of relaxation with mindfulness and specific meaningful imagery. Thus, combining the concepts presented in the previous two sections into integrative exercises (see Box 10-3) can powerfully enhance one's sense of personal identity and emotional health.

Similarly, coming up with one's own problem solutions is no substitute for professional help in problem solving or

BOX 10-3
SELF-HYPNOSIS EXERCISES

THE EQUIVALENT OF AN HOUR OF SLEEP

Since the mind is very flexible, the suggestion of an hour of sleep can actually create the sensation of having experienced an hour of sleep. Needless to say, this is not a replacement for actual sleep, but the exercise can be very helpful when a mental rest is needed.

Set aside at least 10 minutes in an undisturbed place with a timer that will ring after 8 minutes.

Sitting or lying down comfortably, use any of the previous exercises, with imagery or the breath, to relax the body and release emotional tension. Then, let yourself be in the peaceful place that you have selected. Let yourself see, hear, smell, and feel the comfort and safety of the place. Tell yourself, "I will now have the equivalent of an hour of sleep until I hear the wake-up bell." Continue to sense the comfort and peace of your favorite place. Nothing else is important. Experience every aspect of the peaceful place as fully as possible.

When the alarm rings, turn it off and tell yourself, "I have now had the equivalent of an hour of sleep." Allow yourself to stretch as you would on waking and move forward, ready to face the world.

HELPING THE BODY TO HEAL ITSELF

Sitting or lying comfortably, notice a part of the body that hurts or is in need of healing. Surround the body part with your love and bring the light of caring to the area. Take several deep breaths to release tension in the area and to facilitate the flow of blood to the area. Imagine the breath cleansing and nourishing the affected cells. Give yourself the suggestion, "I now bring the light of healing to ________ (name the body part). I now fill __________ with love from the unlimited supply of energy in the universe. With every breath I enhance my healing potential and my desire to heal my _________." Feel the breath steady and surge as you repeat the affirmations. Bring your mindful compassion to the body part in need of your care. After 5 to 10 minutes, complete your work, affirming it is so and returning to ordinary awareness.

LETTING PROBLEM SOLUTIONS COME TO YOU

Sitting or lying down comfortably, set aside at least 15 minutes to speak with your inner friend and resource about a specific problem that seems to be recurring in your life. Increase your relaxation with the breathing release, and then mentally go down a spiral staircase, noting each step carefully and knowing that you will be in a special place for healing resources when you arrive at the bottom of the steps. Count backward slowly: 10, 9, . . ., 1. There is a very comfortable chair for you to sit in and a sophisticated computer at your fingertips. See the details of this "resource place." Now, see or type in the name of the problem you have identified. Let the screen go blank, rest for a moment, taking some more deep breaths. See the possible solutions come on the screen. Some may be funny or unusual; remember not to censor them in any way, just let them pop up in front of you, one by one.

Number them until you have at least three to five possibilities. Thank your inner resources for their time and suggestions. Depart from the room, knowing you can return whenever you wish. Move up the stairs, counting from 1 to 10, feeling lighter and stronger with each step. When you are fully at the top, write down what you received and evaluate the possible solutions for implementation.

NURSINGTIP 10-1

Regarding Self-Hypnosis

When we work with the powerful forces of the mind to heal itself, we must take caution. Just as the suggestion of an hour of sleep is not a substitute for regular sleep, neither is the suggestion of physical healing a substitute for appropriate medical care. As an adjunct or complement to medical treatment, however, self-hypnosis can be exceedingly useful.

psychotherapy when one is dealing with severe issues. In fact, the idea of getting help may be one that comes to nurses as they work with their own inner healer. When one takes stock of the dilemmas our clients are facing because they did not get appropriate help soon enough, nurses can be inspired to receive help as soon as we become aware of issues that exceed our coping skills.

Energy Balancing/Centering

Nurses in psychiatric settings are especially exposed to the effects of mental confusion and emotional anxiety. One might speak of feeling energetically drained by the distress that surrounds self, of being fragmented or scattered, and of feeling pulled in many directions. People often correctly sense that they need to "get it together," to "recharge our batteries," and to gain a sense of one's own center. These descriptions of individuals' energy levels correctly describe conditions in the human energy field. Seeing one's own interactions with others as the movement between human energy fields gives nurses an enhanced way of understanding what really occurs in nurse-client exchanges.

The well-recognized nurse theorist Martha Rogers (see Chapter 3) researched quantum physics extensively. She noted how fields surrounding matter create an effect on surrounding particles. This can be seen readily with a magnet and the path scattered metal pieces will make to align with the invisible energy field of the magnet. The effects of energy fields can also be seen in schools of fish and the ways birds in flight hold together in a pattern as if they were one unit. Rogers expanded the concept of energy fields from physics to conceptualize the interconnectedness of all human interactions with each other and with the environment. Of special relevance to her were nurse-client interrelationships, the foundation of her theory of unitary human beings (Rogers, 1980).

Using Rogers's model, nurses understand that one person, who is an energy field, influences other fields nearby. Focused intent can help to expand and balance one's personal energy field. However, if one is scattered, fragmented, and unaware, the field can become very depleted. Nurses may even unwittingly begin to take on some of the pain that is present in our clients' fields. Thus, it is important that one be centered, especially in the midst of chaos, stress, and confusion.

According to the work of Rogers and related theorists, nurses can calm the disturbed energies around us by effecting change in their own energy fields. It is as if focusing one's own thoughts and intentions creates a vibrational pattern that emanates outward, creating a higher frequency in the client's depleted field through resonance. Conversely, if nurses are not fully focused or intent on creating a sense of calm, their fields can be influenced toward chaos from our challenging surroundings. In psychiatric nursing, then, nurses use their minds as well as their energy fields to restore a sense of balance and wholeness.

Figure 10-1 provides a basic understanding of human energy field interaction, showing how one may assist the client's energy field by allowing energy to flow from the nurse's fuller, more balanced field to the diminished field of the client, in the way water flows from a fuller area in a hose to an emptier one. The image again underscores the importance of engaging in on-going self-care, in order to be sure one's own field is restored before, during, and after each stressful interaction, whether with clients, coworkers, or superiors.

The three exercises in Box 10-4 give beginning steps in working with your own energy field. A number of courses especially designed for nurses and other health care professionals are available to learn energy-oriented healing, such as Transformational Pathways, Therapeutic Touch, and Healing Touch (see Chapter Resources).

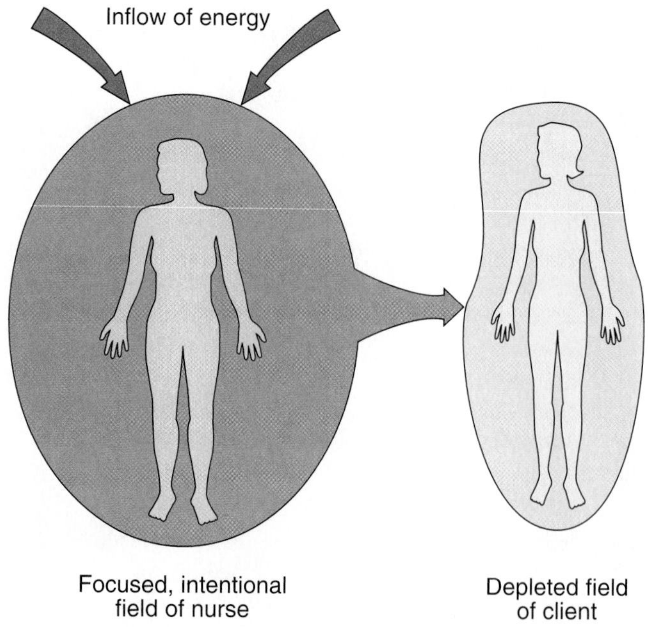

FIGURE 10-1 Flow of energy from nurse to client. (DELMAR/CENGAGE LEARNING.)

HUMOR

Nurse-humorist Patty Wooten (1996) described humor as "a quality of perception that enables us to experience joy even when faced with adversity" (p. 49). She stated that the environments in which nurses function are particularly stress filled and that nurses need to remember to protect themselves to remain balanced and healthy. Laughter seems to be the perfect antidote to stress. For many years, she has been addressing health care providers, offering her own particular, delightful blend of humor and data about the healing effects of laughter. She presents data about the interrelationship between laughter and lowered serum cortisol, activated T lymphocytes, natural killer cells, and T cells with helper/suppressor receptors. She explains how the growing field of psychoneuroimmunology defines communication links between emotional experience and immune response. In other words, there are messages continually sent back and forth between the nervous system and brain and the immune system. When one is distressed, the messages weaken immune response, whereas when one is relaxed and joyful, vitality is enhanced.

Humor enables us to feel better for a variety of reasons. Physiologically, humor and laughter produce changes in blood chemistry. Humor stimulates immune function. Furthermore, human cells are continually changing, occasionally forming cancerous cells. When the immune system is strong, it can mobilize natural killer cells to destroy the abnormal ones. Also, the emotions can trigger release of neurotransmitters from brain neurons, which bond in receptor sites on the surface of the immune cell, altering metabolism positively or negatively.

The groundbreaking work of Norman Cousins (1979) awakened health caregivers to the potential therapeutic effects of laughter. Cousins, suffering from a life-threatening illness, practiced laughing and focusing on positive and

BOX 10-4
ENERGY BALANCING/CENTERING EXERCISES

CENTERING

This practice, once established, should take only 30 to 60 seconds to accomplish, so that you can recenter continuously throughout the workday, especially before approaching a client or doing something new, difficult, or unknown.

Release tension quickly with several deep breaths and full exhalations. Feel the earth under your feet supporting you and enhancing your energy field. Set your intent for the work you are about to do, deciding to be fully present to your client at this time. If needed, review the steps of what you hope to accomplish in the interaction with your client. Ask that whatever occurs be for the highest good of the client, even when you have no idea what the most desirable outcome would be. Affirm that you are fully present with your compassionate intuition and knowledge.

SENSING THE PROTECTIVE LAYERS IN YOUR FIELD

Any time you are feeling vulnerable or unprotected, take a moment to sense your human energy field. The major layers of the field extend out about as far as your arms can comfortably reach in all directions around your body, the sides, the front, and the back.

Use your mind's eye to visualize your energy field as a protective egg of golden light that shines out from your inner center. If you wish, move your arms around you to strengthen the sense of your field, releasing and brushing out any tension. (If it is not appropriate to do this in your work environment, imagine brushing down your arms and releasing tension so your field is unencumbered.) If you are in need of strong boundaries around a difficult individual, let the protective layers build slowly and become thicker to form an invisible shield. If you want to make sure you can receive good messages from the other person, think of the field as a selective semipermeable membrane that lets positive qualities in and bars the harmful vibrations. Reinforce the sense of your confident, protective field throughout the workday.

FILLING WITH ENERGY FROM THE UNIVERSAL ENERGY FIELD

The supply of energy in the universe is literally unlimited. The actual physical nature of the sun, generating the visible light that has nurtured all life on this planet for over 10 billion years, is a good metaphor. Even when we cannot see the sun, its energy is present and we can tap into our internal image of its power.

Sitting or lying down comfortably, release tension with the breath and access the sense of inner peace that may come by being in your favorite place. Let yourself be surrounded by the warmth and nurturing of the sun as well as any other force in nature that is especially meaningful to you. With the breath, bring golden sunlight into your body, let it flow to each major body organ, let it flow with the bloodstream, the immune system, the endocrine system, and so forth. Let each body organ glow with an inner smile as it receives the nurturing warmth. Feel the sunlight accumulating in the energy field's storage area, the solar plexus. Note that this stored energy will be available to you in dark or difficult times. If you wish, place your hands over the solar plexus to feel the continued support of the unlimited supply of energy from the universal energy field. Gently return to full daytime awareness, feeling relaxed and refreshed.

humorous events to inspire joy, hope, and love. He based this idea on the belief that if negative emotions could destructively affect his health, then perhaps positive emotions could beneficially affect his health. His last decade was devoted to researching this relationship at the University of California, Los Angeles Medical School, Department of Behavioral Medicine, where he established the Humor Research Task Force. This project was able to coordinate and support clinical research on humor throughout the world.

Research further indicates that when people engage in humorous activities and responses, they gain a greater sense of mastery. Though people cannot always control events in the external world, they can learn to relax and release positive chemicals such as endorphins and enkephalins, thus having more control over their inner environment.

To have more laughter in one's life, one needs to learn to laugh at self more, seek out people with naturally developed senses of humor, read uplifting and humorous material, and stay in touch with our "inner child," the part that knows intuitively how to laugh at life's events.

However, nurses need also to keep in mind that what often passes for humor is based on making fun of certain people or groups, which can actually be destructive and hurtful. The use of appropriate humor requires a certain level of professional maturity.

There are times when individuals resort to humor to avoid facing painful situations. Humor can be a defense mechanism, covering the deep layers of painful memories or feelings stored beneath the immediate consciousness. Certain individuals develop patterns of injecting humor at tense

NURSING TIP 10-2

Use of Humor

Though humor can be useful in most situations, there are certain times when it would not be helpful or appropriate to attempt to introduce humor. If a person has just received severely distressing news, such as a terminal diagnosis or notification of the death of a loved one, no attempt at humor is appropriate. Similarly, humorous responses can be confusing in serious situations or when important decisions must be made. Humor is inappropriate with individuals who are already challenged to understand, as may occur when communicating with culturally diverse populations, or with individuals who are imbalanced in their psychological orientation. In general, one must be well attuned to the individuals and the situation to inject humor.

moments to avoid feeling the immediate pain of the situation. Some people also laugh when anxious or nervous, confusing those in their presence. This response is often a result of pent-up emotion, but it can result in hurt feelings when others are attempting to deal with the gravity of a dire situation. For these individuals, some stress-relieving maneuvers coupled with opportunities to talk about painful situations can lead to a more appropriate affect over time.

Most nurses can consider humor as a balm to life's constant challenges. Consider a balanced diet between stressful or negative intake and positive, humorous intake. For example, reading the newspapers regularly and watching daily news in graphic detail can be stressful, activating corticosteroid production, which has an immunosuppressive effect. Consider, instead, the health benefits of reading more humorous material and watching less violent, stressful television.

Remember, nurses are constantly receiving and processing information. Be sure that your own energy field has enough laughter and fun to sustain a joyfulness as you undertake a day's work in stress-filled environments. Have you had your laughter fix for the day?

Thus, it is important to relax and remember the lighter side of life, even when life is stressful. For example, consider the following entry written by a breast cancer client:

STANDARD PROCEDURE

Whatever the prognosis is
For better or for worse,
For updating: see the doctor
*For uplifting: see the nurse.**

(Wooten, 1994, p. 37)

*From *Heart, Humor, & Healing* by P. Wooten, 1994, Mt. Shasta, CA: Commune-a-Key.

In another example, written by the mother of a child with cancer, we also see how humor helps people to cope:

HUMOR

*Humor is what got all of us through the clinic visits, the hospital stays, the blood tests, the loss of hair and weight. There is always something on the light side if you can look for it. I'm sure people think "How can he laugh when he has cancer?" Our human nature is such that we can't feel terribly bad all the time.**

(Wooten, 1994, p. 172)

Each of these statements serves to exemplify how people use humor to adapt to the challenges of life. For some, there is more occurring than simply accepting; some people, through maintaining a sense of humor, actually seem to rise above a situation, transforming it for themselves and for everyone around them. This is only one of the many ways in which we can inspire and support each other.

Support Groups

Nurses are making healthy changes, but no one can change a system alone. In addition to personal endeavors to be healthier, nurses need to join forces in order to support each other in making healthy changes in our environments.

Napoleon Hill (1960), in his book *Think and Grow Rich,* left a legacy with his explanation of a "mastermind." He explained that a mastermind group, where many minds join forces in synergistic action or mutual energy exchange, allows people to transcend the limitations of the individual mind and access the largest wisdom, what Jung called the collective unconscious.

When nurses join forces, they are able to give each other exactly what is needed for empowerment. The ingredients needed for true empowerment include skills, tools, information, and support. Nursing has long been rich in the first three, but support has been our weakest link. We can affect our entire profession by recognizing the value of joining forces and supporting each other's goals. *United we thrive.*

Support does not mean nurses have to listen sympathetically to each other's stressful stories or that nurses should help others to the detriment of their own personal or professional well-being. However, support might mean that nurses lend their wisdom and intent, toward creating healthier environments and working conditions.

There are many ways to initiate formal or informal support groups for nurses. One of the simplest is to listen to our colleagues with an open heart. Many nurses, facing challenging situations, find that they need to talk about their experiences, however painful, and to be heard and honored. The act of intentional listening can make all the difference during a difficult time, providing a fair witness to pain and thus

*From *Heart, Humor, & Healing* by P. Wooten, 1994, Mt. Shasta, CA: Commune-a-Key.

releasing previously pent-up emotions that might have been weighing heavily on the soul.

In addition to hearing each other, nurses can also offer suggestions that might empower colleagues. Rather than giving advice, the suggestions might best center around reflective listening, where one reflects on exactly what we are hearing the person say. Sometimes nurses can best hear their own wisdom with this approach. Nurses might realize how they sound, and hearing their own words affirmed can give impetus to healthy changes.

At times, it might be appropriate to offer suggestions. An example of this might be when Chandra, a night nurse, spends a long time complaining about the condition she found a client in after the evening shift. Rather than getting caught up in the politics or personality issues, her colleague might suggest, "Have you spoken to Irma (the evening nurse) about this?" This act can remind Chandra that she needs to go directly to the source for positive action, rather than complain and talk *about* one person to someone else.

A support group can be a meeting between only two nurses, established purely for the purpose of support. Rather than allowing it to turn fully into a griping session, provide some intentional listening; then, at an appropriate point, offer simple suggestions by relating what has worked for you in a similar situation. Consider the following situation:

Wilma spends the first 10 or 15 minutes venting, then catches herself and realizes that she wants some help, rather than to complain. Or, after 20 minutes, Connie decides she needs to intervene to support Wilma's strength in meeting the challenge. Connie suggests, "I had a similar situation last month when working with Dr. Agrwal. Let me tell you how we resolved that. Perhaps you will get some new ideas from this story." In this manner, rather than supporting Wilma's victimized state, Connie is presenting a powerful example of how to handle such a situation.

Many nurses have tried forming support groups only to find that they become gripe sessions with no relief. It might be helpful, in forming a positive group, to elect someone to monitor the energy, perhaps reflecting what has been happening and suggesting a progression toward resolution.

For example, the nurses on Unit C have agreed to meet regularly to discuss their challenges and arrive at policies they all agree with for handling situations. Mary is monopolizing the conversation, groaning about her husband and home problems. Doris, the elected group energy monitor, may step in: "Thank you for sharing what's going on with you, Mary. We will all do whatever we can to support you here. Are there any issues on Unit C we can help you with?"

Hopefully, an intervention like this is all that will be needed to redirect the group's focus. Some groups have found it helpful to limit each person's time to talk so it is even for all members. Each group is a unique composition of individuals and may require special handling. Ultimately, a supportive group will work together to discover ways that work for group members within their beliefs and framework and will learn to eliminate things that do not work well in their experience.

A classic source for information on groups is *Peace and Power: Building Communities for the Future* (Chinn, 1995), which was written by a group of nurses working together for an extended period. The group came up with a framework that supported each individual, allowed each person to feel safe in telling her story, and explored what a true cooperative model might look like. In the beginning of this book, one nurse explains their mission:

SWIMMING UPSTREAM

> *We are tired to death of swimming upstream alone; we want to feel grounded, connected, to be able to touch the earth and put down roots. We are searching for simplicity and balance in our lives, for comradeship and challenge in our work and our relationships. We feel a need for hope, for possibilities in the midst of despair, for integrity and wholeness in the struggle against alienation, for stability in place of rootlessness, for nurturing and closeness based on equality and respect, not on obligation and exploitation. These needs dictate the journey that leads us to community.**
>
> *(Chinn, 1995, p. xv)*

To create community, this group explored its purpose, collective values and beliefs, personal values, expectations, and goals. The depth of their joining is witnessed by the integrity evident in their collective writings. It is a beautiful testament to the power of nurses when they join together. Each group created will differ; some will be loosely structured around the simple purpose of sharing support, while others might be highly organized in terms of structure, purpose, and function.

What is most crucial is that each member be willing to have it be a safe place for every other member, that confidentiality and respect are provided for every member, and that each person be committed to speaking her truth with compassion and clarity. With these guidelines, a support group can be a place of tremendous growth and learning.

NURSING SELF-CARE PROCESS

Through ongoing support, each nurse can create goals for her personal healing journey and can utilize the nursing process to meet those goals. Sherman (2004) believes that appropriate nurse self-care is insulation against stress. We can assess ourselves honestly, with the added positive support from our colleagues, and create a plan of action that is realistic for our complex lifestyles, with change built into the system in small increments. True change takes time, patience, and support, as well as perseverance.

Once nurses establish a proactive plan, they can implement the plan, evaluate its results with supportive feedback, and move accordingly in the direction of a greater and greater sense of well-being. This ongoing process allows us to evolve individually and collectively toward a new model of nurse healer. With healthy support, nursing can redefine its

*From *Peace and Power: Building Communities for the Future* by P. Chinn, 1995, New York: National League for Nursing Press.

purposes, goals, and vision, and each nurse can be an instrumental part of the process. To be effective, however, we need to start with ourselves.

Remember, nurses are all in the process of creating new models for nursing. Nurses do not have to reinvent the wheel, for there have been many who have gone before who have undertaken similar work. Let us commit to learning from them, sharing our heartfelt desires and wisdom, and supporting other nurses with the same loving care and compassion that we would offer to our clients.

KEY CONCEPTS

- Nurses can inspire healing in others through modeling health.
- Nurses are challenged to heal themselves.
- Nurses can provide models of inspiration to those entrusted to their care by allowing themselves to create the support they need.
- Nurses must engage in adequate self-care to remain centered and balanced—the "calm in the storm."
- There are a multitude of pathways to wholeness: imagery, relaxation, meditation, self-hypnosis, centering our energy fields, humor, and support groups.
- Healthy nursing care is a tremendous gift, one that can best be provided by starting with ourselves.

REVIEW QUESTIONS

1. The nurse arrives on the unit after having a very heated argument with her husband. Before entering a client's room, the nurse goes into the medication room and spends a moment deep breathing and chanting. She then resumes her daily assignment. The deep breathing and chanting serves which of the following purposes?
   1. Centering
   2. Avoiding
   3. Reflecting
   4. Transferring

2. A nurse has been working on the same psychiatric unit for 18 years. She dreads going to work each morning and finds she is not as effective with her clients. The nurse is most likely experiencing which of the following?
   1. Burnout
   2. Powerlessness
   3. Depersonalization
   4. Dissociation

3. A nurse must rotate from the day shift to the night shift to be available to her young children during the day. Her husband who previously had this responsibility was forced to work the day shift at his job or be fired. After work, she would rush home to prepare her children's breakfast and send them off to school, and then she would complete her daily chores. Once the children returned home, she would prepare their supper. When she tried to sleep, she found herself staring at the bedroom ceiling. By the second week she was on the night shift, she was so rest broken and exhausted that she could barely function. Which aspect of the nurse's being has most likely been disrupted?
   1. Cardiac functioning
   2. Circadian rhythm
   3. Self-image
   4. Personality structure

4. A client who had experienced anxiety as a response to a phobia related to snakes has been taught relaxation techniques by his nurse. Which of the following would the nurse expect to find if the relaxation techniques have been successful?
   1. Increased heart rate, respiratory rate, and blood pressure with muscle tension
   2. Decreased heart rate, respiratory rate, and blood pressure with relaxed muscles
   3. Increased heart rate, decreased respiratory rate, and blood pressure with relaxed muscles
   4. Decreased blood pressure and heart rate with increased respiratory rate and muscle tension

5. In which of the following situations would it be most appropriate for the nurse to use humor?
   1. A client has just received the diagnosis of a terminal disease
   2. Several members of a client's family were killed in a house fire
   3. A client who is acutely psychotic describes their hallucinations with the nurse
   4. A colleague tells you she is nervous about a presentation she has to give

6. A nurse experiencing burnout is potentially at risk for developing which of the following?
   1. Delirium
   2. Depression
   3. Personality disorder
   4. Psychotic disorder

LEARNING ACTIVITIES

1. Consider the following situation: Lucy is a psychiatric nurse who has been coordinating an inpatient unit in a county facility for 12 years. Lately, she has been feeling exhausted and drained of all enthusiasm while at work. Her staff is similarly depleted, and she would like some new tools for supporting their sense of well-being and empowerment. She would like to feel better, enjoy her work more, and contribute to an elevation in enthusiasm on her unit.
   a. How could you describe the importance of self-care to Lucy?
   b. What would you tell her about the role of attitude and behaviors?
   c. What daily practices could you recommend?
   d. What would you tell her about the use of meditation, self-hypnosis, and imagery?
   e. Could you tell Lucy about the beneficial aspects of humor?
   f. How would you help her to create nurse support groups?
2. What aspects of your professional life would you like to explore to enhance your self-healing endeavors?
3. How might support groups enhance your healing journey?
4. Provide an example of how you might use the nursing self-care process to support your healing goals.

*Study*WARE™ CONNECTION

Using your *Study*WARE™ CD-ROM

1. Complete the Concentration activity for this chapter.
2. Review the audio glossary for key terms in this chapter.
3. Explore the other games and activities that support this chapter.

REFERENCES

Admi, H., Tzischinsky, O., Epstein, R., Herer, P., & Lavie, P. (2006). Shift work in nursing: Is it really a risk factor for nurses' health and patients' safety? *Nursing Economics, 26*(4), 250–257.

Aiken, L., Clarke, S. P., Sloane, D. M., Sochlaski, J., Busse, R., Clarke, H., et al. (2001). Nurses' reports on hospital care in five countries. *Health Affairs, 20*(3), 43–53.

Aiken, L., Clarke, S. P., Sloane, D. M., Sochlaski, J., & Silber, J. (2002). Nursing burnout and patient safety. *JAMA, 295*(5), 549–551.

Benson, H. (1987). *Your maximum mind.* New York: Random House.

Calabria, M., & Macrae, J. (Eds.). (1994). *Suggestions for thought by Florence Nightingale.* Philadelphia: University of Pennsylvania Press.

Chenevert, M. (1994). *STAT: Special techniques in assertiveness training for women in the health professions* (4th ed.). St. Louis: Mosby.

Chinn, P. (1995). *Peace and power: Building communities for the future.* New York: National League for Nursing Press.

Cornell, J. (1994). *Mandala: Luminous symbols for healing.* Wheaton, IL: Quest Books.

Cousins, N. (1979). *Anatomy of an illness.* New York: W. W. Norton.

Donahue, M. P. (1985). *Nursing: The finest art.* St. Louis: Mosby.

Dossey, B., Keegan, L., & Guzzetta, C. (2007). *Holistic nursing: A handbook for practice* (3rd ed.). Gaithersburg, MD: Aspen.

Gordon, S. (2005). *Nursing against the odds.* Ithaca, NY: Cornell University Press.

Grudermeyer, D., & Grudermeyer, R. (1996). *Sensible self-help: The first road map for the healing journey.* Del Mar, CA: Willingness Works Press.

Hill, N. (1960). *Think and grow rich.* New York: Ballantine Books.

Hover-Kramer, D. (1989). Creating a context for self-healing: The transpersonal perspective. *Holistic Nursing Practice, 2,* 3.

Hover-Kramer, D., Mabbett, P., & Shames, K. H. (1996). Vitality for caregivers. *Holistic Nursing Practice, 10,* 2.

Mabbett, P. (1989). *Maintaining vitality.* Unpublished doctoral dissertation, University of Humanistic Studies, Del Mar, CA.

Mariano, C. (2007). Holistic nursing as a specialty: Holistic Nursing—Scope and Standards of Practice. *Nursing Clinics of North American, 42*(2), 165–188.

Martin, B. (2002). Promoting balance between personal health and professional responsibility. *Chart, 99*(5), 4–5.

Muecke, S. (2005). Effects of rotating night shifts: Literature review. *Journal of Advanced Nursing, 50*(4), 433–439.

Quinn, J. A. (2000). Core-Value 3 – Holistic nurse self-care. In N. Frisch, B. Dossey, C. Guzzetta, and J. A. Quinn (Eds.) *AHNA Standards of holistic nursing practice,* pp. 55–72, Gaithersburg, MD: Aspen.

Reed, T. (2007). Imagery in the clinical setting: A tool for nursing. *Nursing Clinics of North America, 42*(2), 261–278.

Reineck, D., & Furino, A. (2005). Nursing career fulfillment: Statistics and statements from registered nurses. *Nursing Economics, 23*(1), 25–30.

Rogers, M. (1980). Nursing: A science of unitary man. In J. Riehl & C. Roy (Eds.), *Conceptual models for nursing practice.* New York: Appleton-Century-Crofts.

Schaef, A. W., & Fassel, D. (1988). *The addictive organization.* San Francisco: Harper & Row.

Selye, H. (1956). *The stress of life.* New York: McGraw-Hill.

Shames, K. H. (1993). *The Nightingale conspiracy.* Montclair, NJ: Enlightenment.

Shames, K. H. (1996). *Creative imagery in nursing.* Clifton Park, NY: Delmar Cengage Learning.
Sherman, D. W. (2004). Nurses' stress & burnout. *American Journal of Nursing, 104*(5), 48–56.
Snow, C., & Willard, D. (1989). *I'm dying to take care of you.* Redmond, CA: Professional Counselor Books.
Summers, C. (1992). *Caregiver, caretaker.* Mt. Shasta, CA: Commune-a Key.
Thich Nhat Hanh. (1987). *The miracle of mindfulness.* Boston: Beacon Press.
Trinkoff, A., Geiger-Brown, J., Brady, B., Lipscomb, J., & Muntaner, C. (2006). How long and how much are nurses now working? *American Journal of Nursing, 106*(4), 60–71.
Tucker, A. (2002). The impact of operational failures on hospital nurses and their patients. *Journal of operations management, 22*(2), 151–169.
Tucker, A., & Spear, S. (2006). Operational failures and interruptions in hospital nursing. *Health Services Research, 41*(3), 643–662.
Wooten, P. (1996). Humor: An antidote to stress. *Holistic Nursing Practice, 10*(2), 49–56.
Wright, S. (2000). Look to the healer inside yourself. *Nursing Standard, 15*(6), 22.
Zweig, C., & Abrams, J. (Eds.). (1991). *Meeting the shadow.* New York: G. P. Putnam's Sons.

LITERARY REFERENCES

Chinn, P. (1995). *Peace and power: Building communities for the future.* New York: National League for Nursing Press.
Shames, K. H. (1993). *The Nightingale conspiracy.* Montclair, NJ: Enlightenment.
Shames, K. H. (1996). *Creative imagery in nursing.* Clifton Park, NY: Thomson Delmar Learning.
Thich Nhat Hanh. (1987). *The miracle of mindfulness.* Boston: Beacon.
Wooten, P. (1994). *Heart, humor, & healing.* Mt. Shasta, CA: Commune-a-Key.

SUGGESTED READING

American Nurses Association, American Holistic Nurses Association. (2007). *Holistic nurses scope and standards of practice.* Washington, D.C.: Author.

RESOURCES: SELF-CARE PROGRAMS FOR NURSES

American Holistic Nurses Association (AHNA) sponsors local networking, and regional and national conferences for nurses. Contact AHNA P.O. Box 2130 Flagstaff, AZ 86003-2130. http://www.ahna.org

Nurses Certificate Program in Interactive Imagery sponsors program in Interactive Imagery in Contact beyond Ordinary Nursing, P.O. Box 8177, Foster City, CA 94467. http://www.integrativeimagery.com

UNIT 2 Clients with Psychiatric Disorders

What are the different mental illnesses that may afflict clients seeking nursing care? How can nurses help heal life's crises? How does anxiety differ from psychosis? How does depression differ from normal grief? How can the nurse help someone who is suicidal? Is there really a difference between dependence on cocaine and dependence on tobacco?

These questions highlight some of the many issues raised in the ten chapters included in this unit on *Clients with Psychiatric Disorders*.

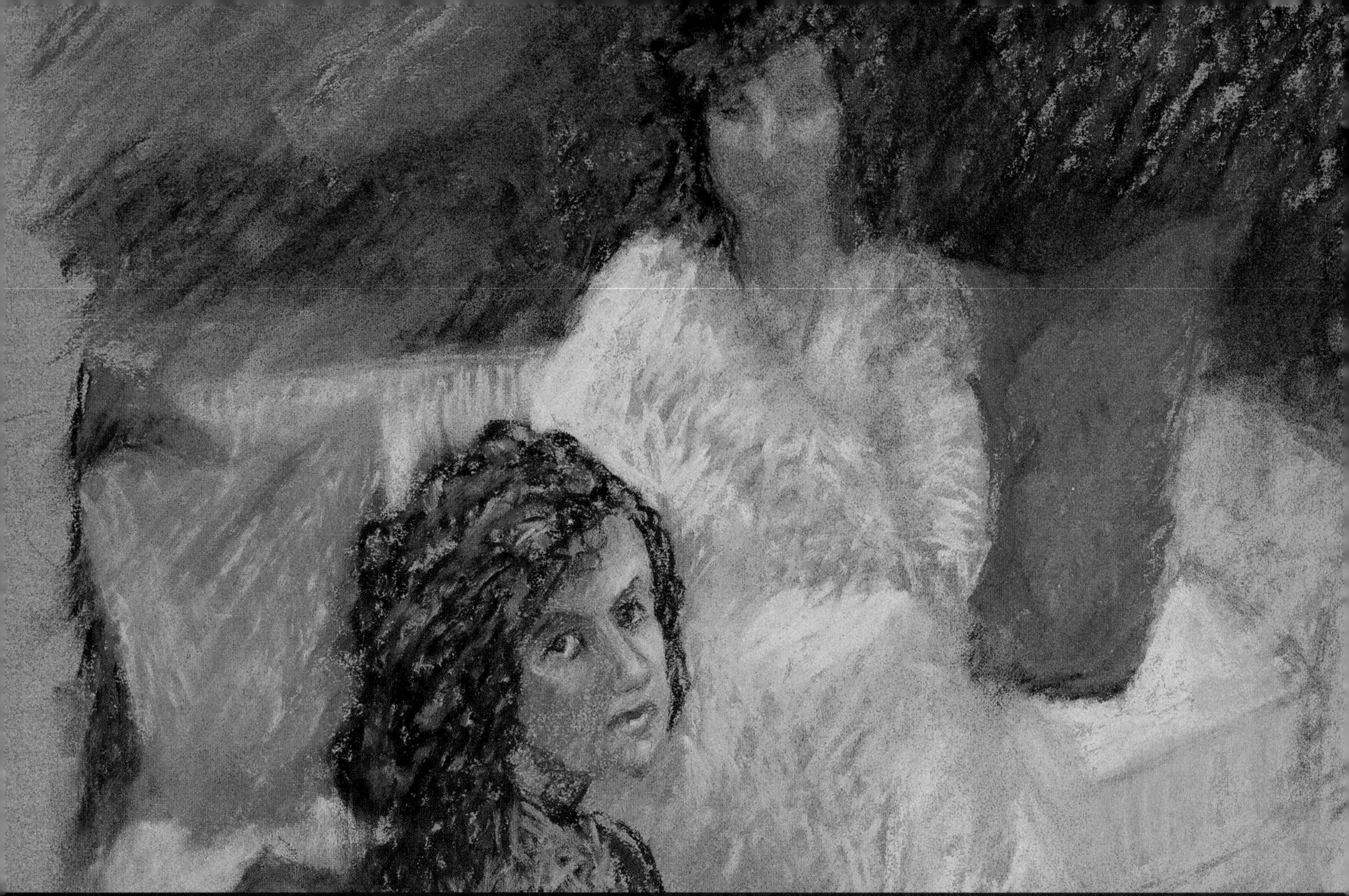

Under Cover

What Have Been the Crises in Your Life?

Consider a time when you had to make a change in your living, for example, graduation, a family move, a death of a family member or loved one, divorce/separation, significant illness, loss of employment, loss of housing, or some other change.

- *Did you believe that you had many choices?*
- *What did you do?*
- *Where did you go for help?*
- *Did you discuss your situation with anyone? If yes, with whom?*
- *What did you do to cope with the emotions?*
- *Can you identify the coping mechanisms that have worked for you?*

Use your answers to these questions to develop an understanding of your personal methods of responding to life's challenging events. As you read through this chapter, continue to examine your own responses to those discussed.

CHAPTER 11

The Client Undergoing Crisis

NOREEN CAVAN FRISCH
LAWRENCE E. FRISCH

CHAPTER OUTLINE

COMPETENCIES

Upon completion of this chapter, the reader should be able to:

1. Identify crises as part of life and describe situations that bring on crisis for many individuals.
2. Describe situational, maturational, cultural, and community crises.
3. Identify four phases of a person's experience of crisis.
4. Use stress theory to interpret an individual's response to crisis.
5. Identify daily stressors in modern life that produce personal stress and require adaptive responses.
6. Use the adaptation nursing theory of Roy and Erickson's Modeling and Role-Modeling theory to evaluate the crisis response, adaptation, and return to an equilibrium state.
7. Use the caring, interpersonal nursing theories of Watson and Peplau to seek to understand the client's subjective experience of the crisis event and provide unconditional, humanistic care.
8. Use cultural care theory to obtain knowledge of the client's culture and to understand the meaning of life's events from within that culture.
9. Apply the nursing process to clients in crisis by:
   - Performing nursing assessments for crisis
   - Analyzing data in terms of nursing and crisis theories
   - Formulating individual nursing diagnoses
   - Deriving a plan of care
   - Evaluating care based on resolution to the precrisis state.

KEY TERMS

Adaptive Energy
Adaptive Potential Assessment Model
Arousal
Community Crisis
Conservative-Withdrawal State
Crisis
Cultural Crisis
Culture Shock
Equilibrium
Fight-Flight Response
General Adaptation Syndrome
Impoverishment
Maturational Crisis
Psychological Development
Situational Crisis
Stress

A **crisis** is one of the many life challenges that call on people to adjust to the unexpected and to adapt to a situation or event that is unpredictable and, more often than not, unwanted. Nurses encounter crises daily in their work. For example, on any given day a nurse may face a crisis in the staffing schedule, a crisis for the client who has just been given a disturbing diagnosis, a crisis for the family victimized by assault, a crisis for a teenager suffering from an accidental injury, or a crisis for a patient contemplating suicide. Nurses themselves face their own individual crises of everyday living, such as failed babysitting arrangements, cars that do not work, health problems, and inability to complete a day's work in a day. Nearly everyone knows something of what it means to live through a crisis. In recent years media attention has made us aware of a seemingly unending succession of serious crises: September 11, 2001, in New York City and Washington, D.C., the southeast Asia tsunami, Hurricane Katrina, cyclones in Burma, and earthquakes in China—to name only a few. Each of these has been responsible for major loss of life and property, and for the destruction of the lives of direct victims and survivors alike. Our understanding of the meaning of crises has been greatly deepened by these events—even though most have taken place far from our own homes.

In many ways, understanding the significance and management of the crises in clients' (and one's own) lives is the essence of learning to be a nurse. While central to all nursing practice, the understanding of crisis is particularly important in psychiatric and mental health nursing. Why is this? A crisis stresses the individual's coping resources, and each person responds differently to seemingly identical situations: Faced with similar adversity, one person may redouble her efforts to achieve success while another may retreat into despondency. Crisis requires that an individual call on all of her personal skills, as well as on the outside social and familial supports that she has built through her life. Each individual has personality strengths, interpersonal networks, and socioeconomic resources that offer some protection against the threat of crisis. When any (or all) of these protections are weak, a person's response to crisis may be dysfunctional, and the result may be one or more symptoms of mental illness. While theories differ in their definitions of crisis and stress, it is generally accepted that most psychiatric problems result from or are strongly influenced by the interaction of stress and overwhelmed coping mechanisms.

The purpose of this chapter is to explore the nature of crisis for individuals, and to a lesser extent, for communities. Later chapters discuss specific forms of mental illness typically encountered by a nurse. While crisis can (and does) occur in every life, mental illness affects only a minority of persons. Even though significant mental illness can occur in the absence of crisis, crisis management skills are very important in psychiatric practice, as they are in all nursing care. Crisis, particularly when trauma is involved, can precipitate long-lasting and debilitating mental illness in some individuals. For many clients, thoughtful nursing intervention early in a crisis may make the difference between mental health and mental illness.

WHAT IS CRISIS?

In psychological terms, a crisis is a stressor that forces an individual to respond and/or adapt in some way. As illustrated in the preceding examples, each nurse faces personal crises of living and comes in daily contact with clients and families undergoing their own crises. Is a crisis always a bad thing? Common usage suggests that it is: No one would wish for a crisis. No one would ask to be out of control, to have an unexpected demand placed on them. But by searching definitions of the word *crisis*, it is clear that crisis itself is neither bad nor good, and the outcome may be positive or negative.

The *Oxford English Dictionary* (1989) defines *crisis* as the turning point in a disease, the decisive stage in the progress of anything, a state of affairs in which change for the better or worse is imminent. The original usage of the term was the turning point in an illness. *Webster's New World Dictionary* (1994) defines a crisis as a turning point, or a decisive or crucial time, stage, or event. In nursing, a crisis is a critical situation, stage, or event in which a person is called on to respond to the unexpected. Thus, a crisis calls for one to face a challenge, to initiate adaptive patterns, and to adjust.

The following example of life-threatening illness as a crisis is presented to illustrate the challenges of crisis and the way in which past coping mechanisms influence responses.

Learning one has a fatal illness would seem to be among the most profound personal crises possible. In the following essay, entitled "Death," the Chinese writer Lu Xun (1881–1936) reflects on his own soon-to-be-fatal illness. Lu Xun died a few weeks after writing this essay.

DEATH

Not till my serious illness this year did I start thinking distinctly about death. At first I treated my illness as in the past, relying on my Japanese doctor, S__________. Though not a specialist in tuberculosis, he is an elderly man with a rich experience who studied medicine before me, is my senior, and knows me very well—hence he talks frankly. Of course, however well a doctor knows his patient, he still speaks with a certain reserve; but at least he warned me two or three times, though I never paid any attention and did not tell anyone. Perhaps because things had dragged on so long and my last attack was so serious, some friends arranged behind my back to invite an American doctor, D__________, to see me. He is the only Western specialist on tuberculosis in Shanghai. After his examination, although he complimented me on my typically Chinese powers of resistance, he also announced that my end was near, adding that [if I had] been a European I would already have been in my grave for five years. This verdict moved my soft-hearted friends to tears. I did not ask him to prescribe for me, feeling that since he had studied in the West he could hardly have learned how to prescribe for a patient five years dead. But Dr. D__________'s diagnosis was in fact extremely accurate. I later had an X-ray photograph made of my chest which very largely bore out his findings.

Though I did not pay much attention to his announcement, it has influenced me a little: I spend all the time on my back, with no energy to talk or read and not enough strength to hold a newspaper. Since my heart is not yet "as tranquil as an old well," I am forced to think, and sometimes I think of death too. But instead of thinking that "twenty years from now I shall be a stout fellow again," or wondering how to prolong my stay in a cedarwood coffin, my mind dwells on certain trifles before death. It is only now that I am finally sure that I do not believe that men turn into ghosts. It occurred to me to write a will, and I thought: If I were a great nobleman with a huge fortune, my sons, sons-in-law, and others would have forced me to write a will long ago; whereas nobody has mentioned it to me....

I remember also how during a fever I recalled that when a European is dying there is usually some sort of ceremony in which he asks pardon of others and pardons them. Now I have a great many enemies, and what should my answer be if some modernized person asked me my views on this? After some thought I decided: Let them go on hating me. I shall not forgive a single one of them either.

Twister

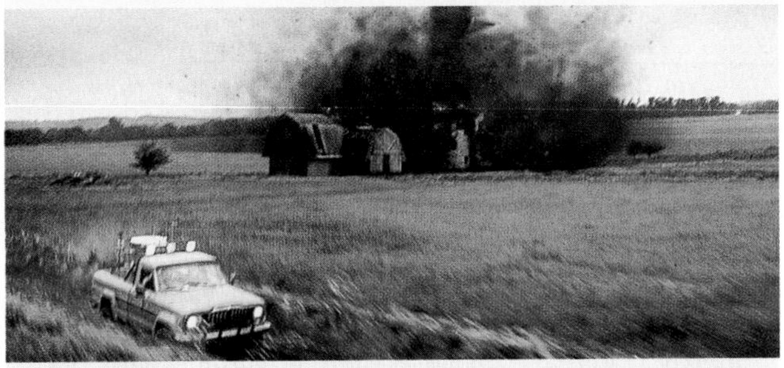

Source: Amblin/Universal/Warners/The Kobal Collection

Natural disasters, such as tornados, floods, and earthquakes, create severe crises in people's lives. Often, individuals and communities require support of mental health professionals to return to their precrisis level of functioning.

*No such ceremony took place, however, and I did not draw up a will. I simply lay there in silence, struck sometimes by a more pressing thought: if this is dying, it isn't really painful. It may not be quite like this at the end, of course; but still, since this happens only once in a lifetime, I can take it.... Later, however there came a change for the better. And now I am wondering whether this was really the state just before dying; a man really dying may not have such ideas. What it will be like, though, I still do not know.**

(Xun, 1994, pp. 192–194)

Lu Xun's crisis comes when his doctors tell him he will soon die from his tuberculosis. He meets this crisis with the ironic humor that was likely also a feature of his healthy life: "I did not ask him to prescribe for me, feeling that since he had studied in the West he could hardly have learned how to prescribe for a patient five years dead." Although he acknowledges that the crisis of his impending death "has influenced me a little," he would have his readers believe that human uncertainty in the face of death is a natural part of life itself. For Lu Xun, the crisis of impending death has no "good or bad" value; it is merely another life challenge to be met with equanimity and ironic curiosity.

Kinds of Crisis

Crises can affect individuals, families, or communities. Crises can be a result of an individual's personal growth and development, including the aging/maturing process. Crises can also be the result of situations external to the individual. Such external situations may affect only one person or may be such that they affect all persons in a community. It is useful to identify and name various kinds of crisis:

- A **situational crisis** is any event that poses a threat or challenge to an individual person. Accidental injury, loss of employment, receiving the diagnosis of a significant illness, and loss of one's possessions through theft or fire are all examples of situational crises.
- A **maturational crisis** is a stage in a person's life where adjustment and adaptation to new responsibilities and life patterns are necessary. Movement from childhood years to young adulthood presents the crisis of adolescence; movement from middle adulthood to old age poses the crises of aging and is often called the time of "midlife crisis."
- A **cultural crisis** is a situation where a person experiences culture shock in the process of adapting/adjusting to a new culture or returning to one's own culture after being assimilated into another.
- A **community crisis** is a crisis of a proportion to affect an entire community of people. Natural disasters, armed conflicts, and significant social ills are community crises.

Nurses deal with all types of crises, and the more information one has in relation to the underlying dynamics of crisis, the better equipped one will be in assessing, diagnosing, and intervening in crisis situations.

Stages of Crisis

Crises have been conceptualized as progressing through four phases (Caplan, 1964). The first phase is a situation or threat to the individual, resulting in anxiety. The individual uses whatever coping mechanisms he has to overcome the anxiety. If anxiety is not reduced, the person enters the second phase, in which anxiety increases and the person's ability to cope decreases. The person feels pressure and is unable to respond. Then, he enters the third phase, in which anxiety continues to escalate. During this third phase, the individual uses every means available to bring his anxiety level and the situation under control. He may use cognitive skills to redefine the crisis so his coping mechanisms can work; he may seek out counseling or support from others as a "last resort." If the person cannot bring his anxiety under control, he enters Caplan's fourth phase of crisis, which presents as a panic state. For some, fourth-phase symptoms may manifest themselves as anxiety or panic; for others, symptoms may include depression or even frank psychosis. How such symptoms manifest is probably determined in large part by an individual's personality, as well as by a range of social support systems important to individual and group coping. Both personality development and social support have been extensively studied and are the subjects of numerous theories. The reader should not assume that the following brief summary is complete, but any understanding of the response to crisis requires some consideration of both personality and social support.

*From *Silent China: Selecting writings of Lu Xun*, 1994, edited and translated by Gladys Yang. Beijing: Foreign Language Press.

Personal Development and Crisis

Nurses are familiar with the process of normal **psychological development**. Each individual's life proceeds through a continuum from infantile dependency to adult autonomy (and then, for many, back through the dependency of old age and chronic illness). Although theories and cultures vary, important psychological milestones include self-differentiation (in which the infant recognizes itself as separate from the mother), basic trust (in which the infant comes to see the animate and inanimate worlds as consistent and trustworthy), and individuation (in which the child and adolescent develops a specific personality and set of aspirations). The psychologically healthy adult has appropriate levels of self-esteem, a sense of personal and social identity that guides interpersonal and vocational choices, and a spiritual identity that provides her with a sense of life-meaning. Crises may severely test any or all of these resources, and an individual's personal history may leave one or more of these resources incompletely established. This, in turn, may lead to vulnerability under crisis.

An individual uses his developmentally determined sense of self-esteem and identity to create a range of social supports and to meet basic life needs. Family ties often require maintenance through a lifetime, but are usually established at birth. In many cultures individuals create extrafamilial networks of meaningful relationships as they mature, pass through schooling, and enter adult and vocational life. In most cultures, marriage is the most common way in which such networks are forged. Basic life needs include at least food, shelter, clothing, health care, and safety from natural and human disasters. Although rarely equitably distributed, financial and social status are of great human importance. There is a strong and consistent empirical relationship between social status and physical well-being. Although possession of wealth rarely single-handedly leads to happiness, few individuals achieve fulfillment while living in abject poverty. Despite the presence of a highly complex relationship between these social factors and an individual's response to crisis, few doubt that those who have strong social supports (including adequate financial resources) can generally weather crises better than those who do not.

Not surprisingly, individuals respond to crises depending on their level of personal development. Nurses providing care to members of a community after a natural disaster have documented the differences in response and needs based on the age group of their clients. Children and adolescents experiencing a natural disaster are left frightened, sad, insecure, and worried about personal safety (Adams, Dolfie, Feren, Love, & Taylor, 1999). Older adolescents are particularly distressed when their interactions with their peer group are disrupted (Grant, Hardin, Pesut, & Hardin 1997). The elderly may have more difficulty coping than younger individuals because of physical infirmities and episodes of disorientation and confusion (Adams, Dolfie, Feren, Love, & Taylor, 1999). The nurse should assess each client to determine each person's focus and needs before establishing interventions.

Stress Theory

Stress, a stimulus that an individual perceives as challenging or harmful, is intimately involved with crisis. While experts may differ on precisely how to define both stress and crisis, that each leads to and/or enhances the other seems nearly certain. There is a well-developed theory of stress, and because of the close relationship between stress and crisis, stress theory is highly relevant to the nurse's understanding of crisis.

Selye, the originator of stress theory, suggested that persons have differing abilities to respond to life's stressors. Each person has resources that he called **adaptive energy**, which allow a response to any stressor. Through physiologic experiments, Selye demonstrated that there is a specific, predictable, physiologic response to stress, which he labeled the **General Adaptation Syndrome** (GAS; Selye, 1974). This response involves an alarm reaction, a stage of resistance, and a stage of exhaustion. The first and third phases were broken down further to include stages of shock and countershock. Table 11-1 provides a summary of the biophysical phenomena of the GAS.

Selye likened the adaptive resources a person has to an inherited fortune. Each individual has adaptive energy; all persons have differing amounts. Once a person uses up whatever adaptive resources he has, there is nothing left from which to draw. The result of a drain of adaptive energy will be illness, disease, or even death. Any crisis can exhaust adaptive resources, but a crisis that is perceived as extremely threatening to life may be most likely to do so.

Other researchers, most notably Engel, observed and recorded psychosocial responses to stress. Engel (1962) observed two major responses to stress: the **fight-flight response**, which is a state of high anxiety and energy, and the **conservative-withdrawal state**, which is one of exhaustion. If you look even casually at Table 11-1, it should not come as a surprise that stress, in addition to causing psychological disturbance in some individuals, can lead to physical health problems. Although scientists still debate whether psychological stress "causes" illness, there is little doubt that it can serve as a trigger for a variety of serious or even fatal physical conditions. Among these are sudden death, heart attack, and even abnormalities in the way that the heart muscle contracts (Dimsdale, 2008).

Stress theory provides a means to understand the following example of an extreme crisis that affected an entire community. In 1972, an ill-constructed dam broke and sent a deluge of floodwater and debris down Buffalo Creek near the town of Man, West Virginia. Over 100 people were killed, and many homes were destroyed. For many, the psychological impact of this flood was life-long and catastrophic. Sociologist Kai Erikson interviewed survivors more than a year later; here is the voice of one survivor:

EVERYTHING IN ITS PATH

For the sake of a little cigarette, I guess, is the reason we're here today. I woke up to get me a cigarette and my

TABLE 11-1 Biophysical Phenomena: General Adaptation Syndrome

ALARM REACTION		STAGE OF RESISTANCE	EXHAUSTIVE STAGE	
SHOCK	COUNTERSHOCK		COUNTERSHOCK	SHOCK
Depressed nervous system	Excretion of epinephrine	Normal range systolic pressure	Excretion of epinephrine	Depressed nervous system
Decreased muscle tone	Elevated systolic blood pressure	Normal range diastolic pressure	Elevated systolic blood pressure	Decreased muscle tone tone
Hypotension	Equal or lower diastolic blood pressure	Normal range pulse	Equal or lower diastolic blood pressure	Hypotension
Leucopenia	Increased pulse pressure	Glyconeogenesis	Increased pulse pressure	Leucopenia
Eosinopenia	Increased pulse rate	Transfer of free fatty acids to triglycerides	Increased pulse rate	Eosinopenia
Hemoconcentration	Glycogenolysis	Protein anabolism	Glycogenolysis	Hemoconcentration
Decreased plasma glucose	Gluconeogenesis	Normal range respiratory rate	Gluconeogenesis	Decreased plasma glucose
Protein catabolism	Mobilization of free fatty acids	Normal range temperature	Mobilization of free fatty acids	Protein catabolism
Hypochloremia	Protein catabolism		Protein catabolism	Hypochloremia
Hypothermia	Increased respiratory rate		Increased respiratory rate	Hypothermia
	Hyperthermia		Hyperthermia	

Source: From *Modeling and Role-Modeling: A Theory and Paradigm for Nursing*, by H. Erickson, E. Tomlin, and M. A. Swain, 2009, Tenth Printing. Printed with permission, EST Company: Cedar Park, TX 78613.

pack was empty. I got up and just put on my trousers and went out of the bedroom—me and my wife was sleeping downstairs with the baby, and the rest of the girls were upstairs. I come through the living room, through the hall, into the kitchen, and got me a pack of cigarettes. For some reason, I opened the inside door and looked up the road—and there it came. Just a big black cloud. It looked like twelve or fifteen foot of water. It was just like looking up Kanawha River and seeing barges coming down four or five abreast.

Well, my neighbor's house was coming right up to where we live, coming down the creek. It was a row of houses, bringing everything as it came. It was coming slow, but my wife was still asleep with the baby—she was about seven years old at the time—and the other kids were still upstairs asleep. I screamed for my wife in a bad tone of voice so I could get her attention real quick—of course I never talk nasty to my wife, but I had to get her attention real quick—and when I screamed at her she knowed something was wrong. She sat up on the side of the bed, pulled the drapes apart, and it was washing cans and tires and everything right over into our yard. I don't know how she got the girls downstairs so fast, but she run up there in her sliptail and she got the children out of bed and downstairs.

Now I had a car parked in back of the house. I looked around. Everything above us was acoming right on down, getting closer and closer, and we didn't have much time nohow. So we all got in that car and I was pulling out going up the valley. There was no way in the world out except going right into it. We had water in the yard all around, but none of the big stuff had got down there yet. We headed up the road. My wife was hollering, "Wilbur, you can't get through there," and my daughter Ann—she was twenty-one at the time—she said, "Yeah Daddy, you can." Well, all the time the water and all those houses was coming right at us in a row.

Well, I don't know what happened. I just turned the key off, left it in the car, and we all rolled out one side, got in the water, run across over to the railroad tracks. And there were cars for the Lundale mines sitting there to put coal in. My wife and some of the children went between the cars; me and my baby went under them because we didn't have much time. My neighbor's house hit the car that we was under while we were still under it and wrecked it, and that turned the big water down through the valley to give us a chance to get up into the woods. We got up into the woods and I looked around and our house was done gone. It didn't wash plumb away. It washed down about four or five house lots from where it was setting, tore all to pieces.

At that time, why, I heard somebody holler at me, and I turned around and saw Mrs. Constable. She lived up there above us. Her husband was a wheelchair patient, got hurt in the Lorado mines, and they had four kids. She had a little baby in her arms and she was hollering, "Hey, Wilbur, come and help me; if you can't help me, come get my baby." Well, there was a railroad car between me and her and I couldn't have got back to her anyway. But I didn't give it a thought to go back and help her. I blame myself a whole lot for that yet. She had her baby in her arms and looked as though she was going to throw it to me. Well I never thought to go help that lady. I was thinking about my own family. They all six got drowned in that house. She was standing in water up to her waist, and they all got drownded....

The first five houses above me, there was about fourteen drowned, and I saw everyone of them in their homes as they floated by where I was at. Well, I looked back on down the valley, and everything had done washed out and gone. I didn't know where my daughter was who lived down below me. And about that time I passed out. I just slumped down. It was around maybe nine o'clock, in that vicinity somewheres.

My house was washed down about five lots from where it had been setting. It had washed up against another big two story house, leaning on about a forty five degree angle, tore all to pieces. The whole back side of it was torn off, the porch was gone, the bathroom was gone, and mud and water and stuff up to the upstairs window. I decided to go over there. I had eight or nine hundred dollars of my money there at the house. I knew where I had it, and I thought maybe I could go in and maybe it wasn't washed away and maybe I'd get some valuable papers and so forth. I got over there and there was a little child had washed up in mine and my wife's bed and it was torn in half. It was laying there in the bed, looked like eight or ten years old by the size of it. There was a truck, a pickup truck, setting in our living room, and it had a dead body in it. There was two dead bodies washed up with the debris that was laying outside of our house, and I had to step over them to get into the house. I just turned and went back....

A fellow by name of Willard Dingess, he asked us was we in the flood and we told him we was. And he asked us where we was going to stay and we said we didn't know. He said, "Well, I've got a little wash house up here, just one room, and you're welcome to it. I've got a little gas heater in it, and you can make your bed down on the floor." So we stayed in that man's wash house, six of us, for nineteen days—a one-room wash house about twelve by twenty....

(Now) I have the feeling that every time it comes a storm it's a natural thing for it to flood. Now that's just my feeling, and I can't get away from it, can't help it. Seems like every time it rains I get that old dirty feeling that it is just a natural thing for it to become another flood.

Why, it don't even have to rain. I listen to the news, and if there's a storm warning out, why I don't go to bed that night. I set up. I tell my wife, "Don't undress our little girls; just let them lay down like they are and go to bed and go to sleep and then if I see anything going to happen, I'll wake you in plenty of time to get you out of the house." I don't go to bed. I stay up.

My nerves is my problem. Every time it rains, every time it storms, I just can't take it. I walk the floor. I get so nervous that I break out in a rash. I'm taking shots for it now.

I live up on a hill now, but that doesn't take away my fear. Every time it rains or goes to come up a storm, I get my flashlight—if it's two o'clock in the morning or if it's three. Now it's approximately five hundred feet from my house to the creek, but I make me a round about every thirty minutes, looking at that creek. And then I come back to the house, light me a cigarette or maybe get me a cup of coffee, and carry my coffee cup with me back down the hill to see if the creek has raised any.

What I went through on Buffalo Creek is the cause of my problem. The whole thing happens over to me even in my dreams, when I retire for the night. In my dreams, I run from water all the time, all the time. The whole thing just happens over and over again in my dreams.

This just puts on me a load I can't carry. It seems like I just got something bulging on my chest. I can't breathe like I should, and it just makes me feel that my chest weighs a hundred pounds. Just a big bulge in there.

I can remember back from 1932 up till 1972 much plainer than I can the past two years. In other words I've got a mental block of some kind. In the past two years, there've been weeks or months went by, and I don't know where they went, what I've done, or what's happened to them.

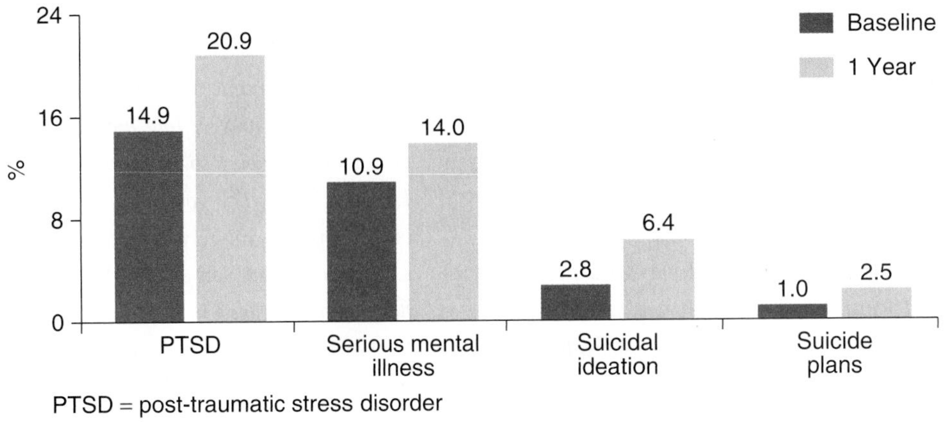

FIGURE 11-1 **Prevalence of Post-Disaster Mental Disorders Increased over Time Following Hurricane Katrina** (CARDIOSOURCE © 2008 BY THE AMERICAN COLLEGE OF CARDIOLOGY FOUNDATION: WWW.CARDIOSOURCE.COM.)

I don't want to get out, see no people ... I didn't even go to the cemetery when my father died. It didn't dawn on me that he was gone forever. And those people that dies around me now, it don't bother me like it did before the disaster.... I don't have the feeling I used to have about something like death. It just don't affect me like it used to....

*Back before this thing happened, you never went up the road or down it but what somebody was ahollering at you. I could walk down the road on a Saturday morning or a Sunday morning and people would holler out their door at me, and maybe I would holler back at them, maybe go sit down and have us a cup of coffee or a cigarette or something. And there'd be half a dozen families would just group up and stand there and talk. But anymore you never see nobody out talking to one another. They're not friendly like they used to be. It's just a whole different life, that's all.**

(Erikson, 1976, pp. 138–147)

Clearly, the catastrophic nature of the flood exhausted the adaptive resources that many of the survivors had. Wilbur, the narrator of the story, describes his own alarm reaction and the fight-flight response during his escape from the water. He further describes his exhaustion immediately following the alarm phase: "I just slumped down." Presumably, he fell into an exhaustive state when all the adaptive energy he could summon had been used up. He goes on to describe less immediate reactions: his recurring guilt of having watched his neighbors die without his own attempts to save them, the devastation of his home, and the horror of the dead bodies that prevented him from rescuing any of his remaining belongings. The crisis caused great stress for him. One year after the flood, he is living with anxiety and fears lasting well beyond the time of the immediate crisis. Further, he describes a change in his whole community, where people no longer talk to one another in quite the same way. Listening to this flood survivor helps the nurse understand the depth of tragedy people experience in severe situations. One of the things that crises of this sort teach us is that individuals vary significantly in their responses to stress. Some people have natural resilience that seemingly allows them to experience trauma and then return fairly quickly to relative normality. Others find themselves "haunted" by memories and flashbacks to varying degrees, sometimes leading to significant disability. When such impairments persist, psychiatric clinicians may make the diagnosis of Post-traumatic Stress Disorder (PTSD). PTSD is classified among the anxiety disorders and is considered in the next chapter. Only a minority of persons who experience overwhelming crisis develop PTSD, and one of the important reasons we still think about the Buffalo Creek dam disaster—despite so many recent catastrophes of equivalent proportions—is that the survivors of that disaster have been studied over many years. Follow-up for more than two decades has shown that about 25% of the Buffalo Creek survivors still have significant PTSD symptoms, but that overall the severity of symptoms has been decreasing for most of the survivor cohort (Green, Lindy, Grace, Gleser, Leonard, Korol, et al., 1990). Follow-up of child Buffalo Creek survivors has found a steady decrease in symptomatology with PTSD diagnosed in 7% of persons up to 17 years after the original event (Green, Grace, Vary, Kramer, Gleser, & Leonard, 1994). Studies of Hurricane Katrina victims have not been so optimistic, though the follow-up interval has been much shorter (see Figure 11-1). PTSD may be increasing in this population over time, along with prevalence of other serious mental health concerns such as depression, suicidality, and actual suicide plan.

The presence of severe psychological symptoms seems to be related to unresolved psychosocial stresses among hurricane survivors—for example, persons whose lives have not yet returned to some semblance of normal following the disaster (Kessler, Galea, Gruber, Sampson, Ursano, & Wessely, 2008). While psychological symptoms continue to be of great concern for Katrina (and some Buffalo Creek) survivors, there are concerns as well about physical effects of

*Reprinted with the permission of Simon & Schuster. From *Everything in its path* by Kai T. Erikson. Copyright © 1976 by Kai T. Erikson.

psychological stress. Post-9/11 there was a significant rise in alcohol and other substance use (Vlahov, Galea, Resnick, Ahern, Boscarino, Bucuvalas, et al., 2002). After a major Japanese earthquake, myocardial infarction mortality increased significantly and remained elevated for at least eight weeks (Ogawa, Tsuji, Shioro, & Hisamichi, 2000).

RESEARCH Highlight 11-1

Family Context of Mental Health Risk in Tsunami-Exposed Adolescents: Findings from a Pilot Study in Sri Lanka

STUDY PROBLEM/PURPOSE

The researchers sought to investigate effects of tsunami exposure on psychosocial losses, depression and PTSD for adolescents in Sri Lanka after the 2004 tsunami.

METHODS

Three-hundred families from two villages (one with ocean exposure and one without) participated in the study. These families agreed to be interviewed by local college-educated women who had been trained to administer research instruments. Participation rate for the families was more than 80% of potential participants. Adolescents and their mothers were asked to respond to questions that included measures of property destruction, social losses (loss of friends, family conflicts, displacements), parent-child relationships, and symptoms of PTSD and depression.

FINDINGS

The prevalence of PTSD was 40.9% for the adolescents and 19% for their mothers. As hypothesized by the researchers, higher levels of tsunami exposure resulted in higher levels of PTSD and depressive symptoms in adolescents. Increased sense of psychosocial loss and displacement also increased symptoms. Positive mother-child relationships helped to mitigate symptoms among their children, while depression in the mother increased symptoms in their children.

IMPLICATIONS

Findings from this study suggest ways to improve recovery and reconstructing programs. Specifically, there is a need for family focused interventions that integrate family and psychiatric therapy with social and economic recovery activities.

Source: "Family context of mental health risk in tsunami-exposed adolescents: Findings from a pilot study in Sri Lanka" by K. A. S. Nickama and V. Kaspur, 2007, *Social Science and Medicine*, *64*, 713–723.

BOX 11-1
MODERN DAY STRESSORS

- Death of a spouse or partner
- Death of a child
- Divorce or separation
- Death of a family member or close friend
- Major illness (self, family)
- Victimization—violence
- Victimization—theft
- Fired at work/laid off at work
- Legal battles/being called to court
- Marriage
- Change in living situation
- Change in eating habits
- Change in social activities
- Gain of a new family member, acquiring stepchildren or stepparents
- Merging two households
- Change in working conditions
- Significant debt
- Chemical abuse, drug dependency (self)
- Chemical abuse, drug dependency (family member/friend)

Less severe than the flood, common life stresses can themselves become crises for many persons. Box 11-1 provides a list of modern-day stresses in American life. These stresses tax individuals daily and create a drain on their coping resources. Ultimately, such stress may result in physical illness or emotional instability. The nurse should remember that these events, unlike the flood or similar disasters, are private stressors. No one necessarily knows that the individual is under stress and coping with impending crises when the problem is personal financial debt. It is always important to allow clients to talk about their lives and to listen to their life challenges.

Critical Incident Stress Management: A Controversial Intervention

Critical incident stress management (CISM) is an intervention commonly incorporated into emergency services. CISM has been thought to assist emergency personnel to deal with the sometimes overwhelming nature of the crises and disasters to which they are called to respond. If emergency personnel are left unsupported, they themselves can be victims of stress-related problems, including burnout, depression, drug or alcohol addiction, and exacerbation of personality disorders (Milstein, Gerstenberger, & Barton, 2002). The technique of CISM is a psychotherapeutic approach of debriefing to help the emergency worker reflect upon the situation, his response, what is particularly troubling for the individual, and how he can handle the stress it produces. It is important to provide supports in such cases, as personnel involved with major disasters have reported continued dealing with the stress even 20 years later (Davis & Stewart, 2000).

While emergency services must address the issues of how best to support emergency workers, one meta-analysis of existing data raises questions about the effectiveness of CISM (Bledsoe, 2003). Not only may debriefing be ineffective, but for some individuals it may actually lead to a worsening of the stress symptoms. The researcher recommends that CISM should never be a mandatory intervention because for some people it may cause harm. Clearly, additional study and evaluation are needed to determine which persons exposed to stressful circumstances will benefit or will be harmed by psychological interventions (Compton, Bahora, Watson, & Oliva, 2008).

NURSING CARE

From emergency departments to community health settings to maternity units, nurses in every area of practice will be called upon to assist those experiencing crisis. Crises are a part of life, and the more tools nurses have to understand and assist clients, the better able our clients will be to respond, cope, and recover. The following sections review nursing theories particularly well-suited to crisis intervention and support, and present examples of nursing interventions and applications of the nursing process to crisis situations.

NURSING THEORY

While psychological and stress theories are important, nursing theories provide further means of understanding behaviors. Of the many nursing models used in current practice, the models addressing adaptation fit best with ideas in general mental health work relating to crisis. Other nursing perspectives, particularly caring theories and cultural care theories, provide important alternative views to crisis. Therefore, each will be addressed in the following discussion.

Adaptation Theories

Nursing theories defining health in terms of successful adaptation and equilibrium are consistent with the general mental health approach to crisis. Roy's adaptation model (Roy & Andrews, 1999) and Erickson's theory of Modeling and Role-Modeling (Erickson, Tomlin, & Swain, 1983) fall into this category. For both of these theories, the person is seen as having component parts. For Roy these parts are biopsychosocial components; for Erickson these parts are biophysical, cognitive, psychological, and social. In both of these theories, health is defined in terms of an equilibrium or balance between the parts that promotes harmony or adjustment. Systems theory has influenced these ideas, such that these nursing theories posit that any event that serves as a stressor on one component of the person will have an effect on the other components.

In light of these theories of adaptation, it is clear that any crisis event serves as a stressor that threatens the balance. The individual undergoing a crisis is in a state of disequilibrium, and any intervention must serve to reestablish balance. The nurse can expect to see symptoms in any of the

BOX 11-2
NEW YORK NURSES RESPOND TO DISASTER

September 11, 2001, plunged the entire country into crisis. The New York State Nurses Association (NYSNA), having its main office in Manhattan, was called upon to react, regroup, and respond to the emergency at its doorstep (Orr, 2002).

These nurses responded first to:

- Arrange transportation for nurses to the disaster area
- Obtain proof of licensure for nurses wanting to gain entry to areas closed to the general public
- Establish communications with emergency services
- Manage volunteers and public relations

The continuing and long-range issues were to:

- Treat survivors admitted to New York City hospitals
- Support rescue workers
- Assist in family support center areas
- Volunteer with the Red Cross triage center
- Provide emergency nursing care

Nurses with two specialties, those who specialize in mental health and counseling and those in burn care, were required most to provide the needed follow-up care. The organization used its Statewide Peer Assistance Network to offer individual and group opportunities to discuss the grief and anger that were common responses among the nurses.

In response to this 9/11 experience, the NYSNA has recommended that ANA:

- Provide leadership to the nursing profession on the need for nurses to volunteer services to assist groups that offer rescue, relief, and disaster services
- Promote workplace initiatives to support nurses volunteering during periods of disaster
- Provide leadership for planning state, regional, and national disaster services

Guernica by Picasso

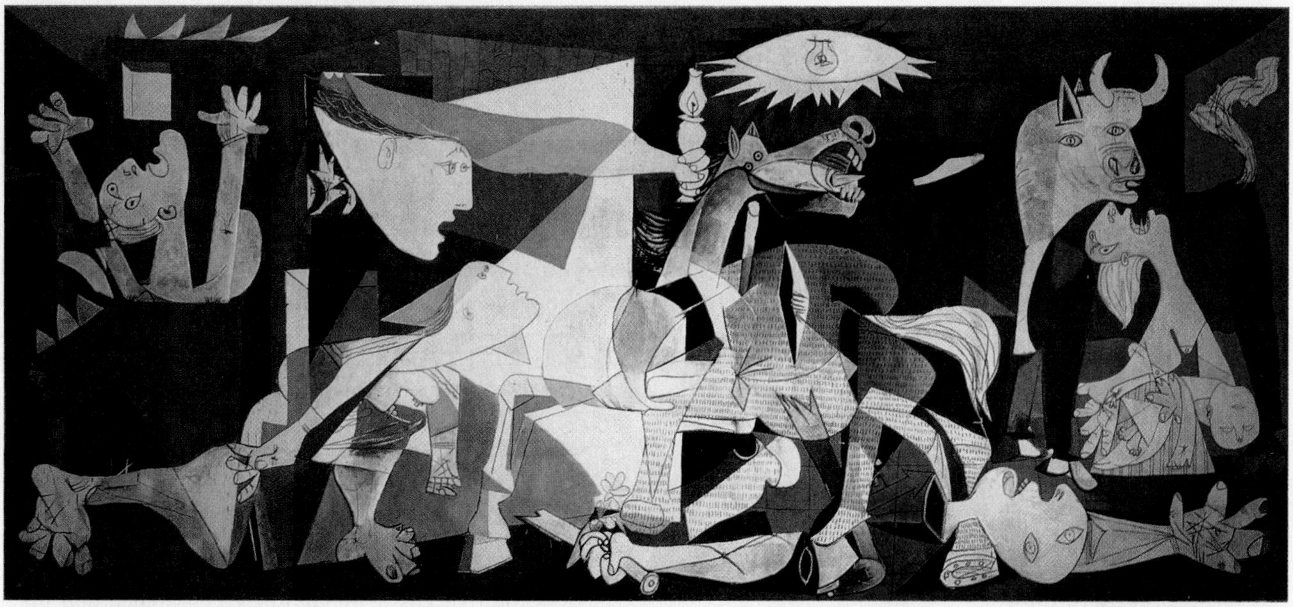

Source: *Archivo fotográphico Museo Nacional Centro de Arte Reina Sofia.* © 2011 Estate of Pablo Picasso/Artists Rights Society (ARS), New York.

An unarmed mountain village is bombed by Fascist airplanes during the Spanish Civil War. Picasso captures in stark black and white the horror and dehumanization of modern warfare. If any of the subjects of this picture, human or animal, survived the war, it would be hard to imagine lives unhaunted by their traumatic experience. Guernica is regarded by many critics and viewers as one of the greatest paintings of the twentieth century. Many viewers have had their perceptions of war—and of painting—forever changed by viewing this monumental canvas.

dimensions of the person; for example, the stress of the crisis may exhibit as an emotional instability, a physical illness, or an inability to concentrate. These reactions to the stress of crisis are highly individual; information from the client about past history and coping will assist the nurse to recognize and interpret the varied symptoms of crisis for an individual.

Erickson's Modeling and Role-Modeling theory provides an integrated view of stress by incorporating ideas of stress theory into a nursing, adaptation framework. Erickson and colleagues introduced the **Adaptive Potential Assessment Model** (APAM) to describe three states of coping potential (Erickson et al., 1983). These states are **arousal**, **equilibrium**, and **impoverishment**. Figure 11-2 depicts the APAM model. Figure 11-3 provides a description of the phenomena specific to each state. Arousal and impoverishment are both stress states. In arousal the person has coping resources, whereas in impoverishment the resources are depleted. A stressful event thrusts a person into a state of arousal. The person will react, attempting to reestablish balance or

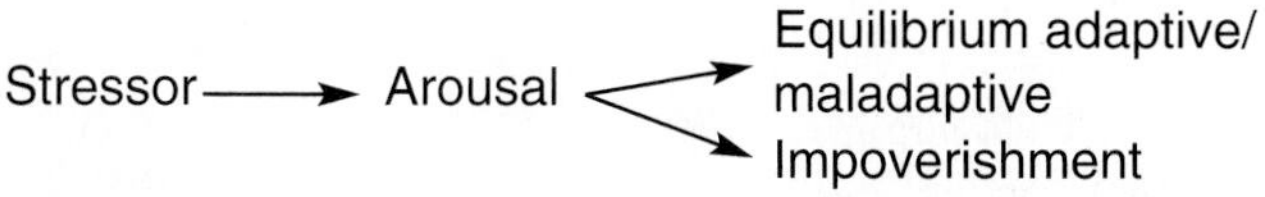

FIGURE 11-2 Adaptive Potential Assessment Model (FROM *MODELING AND ROLE-MODELING: A THEORY AND PARADIGM FOR NURSING,* BY H. ERICKSON, E. TOMLIN, AND M. A. SWAIN. 2009, TENTH PRINTING. PRINTED WITH PERMISSION, EST COMPANY: CEDAR PARK, TX 78613.)

equilibrium. If the reaction is successful, the person will return to an equilibrium state. If the reaction is unsuccessful, the person will drop into a state of impoverishment, as it is not possible to maintain a state of arousal indefinitely.

The theory further states that equilibrium may be either adaptive, that is, a positive state of balance, as in Lu Xun's essay on his impending death from tuberculosis, or maladaptive, that is, a state of balance that provides equilibrium at the expense of one of the individual's dimensions. The flood survivor interviewed by Kai Erikson was in a state of maladaptive equilibrium. One year postcrisis, he was not functioning—he describes being unable to recollect recent events and being unable to tolerate storms and any slight indication of water and flood. He is living in fear and anxiety.

All nursing theories provide suggestions to guide practice. For example, Erickson's Theory of Modeling and Role-Modeling directs the nurse to establish trust, identify strengths, promote positive orientation, promote perceived control, and set mutual goals. Actions directed toward these goals, with an understanding of crisis and the individual client's responses to stress, will form the basis of nursing care.

Caring Theories

Theories that emphasize caring, most notably Watson's Theory of Transperson Caring (2005, 2002, 1988) and Peplau's theory of interpersonal relationship between nurse

Equilibrium (adaptive)
- Normal blood pressure reading
- Normal pulse
- Normal respiration
- Expression of marked hope and positive expectations
- Absent or low feelings of tenseness and anxiousness
- Normal motor-sensory behavior
- Absent or low feelings of fatigue, sadness, and depression

Arousal
- Marked feelings of tenseness and anxiousness without feelings of fatigue, sadness and depression
- Elevated motor-sensory behavior
- Elevated systolic blood pressure
- Elevated pulse
- Elevated respiration
- High score for verbal anxiety

Impoverishment
- Marked feelings of tenseness and anxiousness with feelings of fatigue, sadness, and depression
- Elevated verbal anxiety
- Elevated motor-sensory behavior
- Elevated blood pressure
- Elevated pulse
- Elevated respiration

FIGURE 11-3 Adaptive Potential Assessment Model: phenomena specific to each state. (FROM *MODELING AND ROLE-MODELING: A THEORY AND PARADIGM FOR NURSING*, BY H. ERICKSON, E. TOMLIN, AND M. A. SWAIN, 2009, TENTH PRINTING. PRINTED WITH PERMISSION, EST COMPANY: CEDAR PARK, TX 78613.)

and patient (O'Toole & Welt, 1989), provide a different understanding of crisis and crisis care. If caring and/or relationships are the most important aspects of nursing, a nurse who encounters a person experiencing a crisis will provide unconditional, humanistic care (Figure 11-4). The nurse will be interested in the client's subjective experience of the crisis. Therefore, the theory would direct the nurse to meet the client at the client's level with an attitude of sincere caring, accept the client's view as the important perspective of the event, seek to understand the client's subjective experience of the crisis, and interpret the meaning of the crisis to the client. As the client relates these personal meanings, the nurse will be able to assist the client to make sense of situations that seem random, unfair, and tragic. Nursing care would be planned mutually. Listening is among the most important skills for this type of assistance (Figure 11-5). All too often clients report that their caregivers do not listen to them.

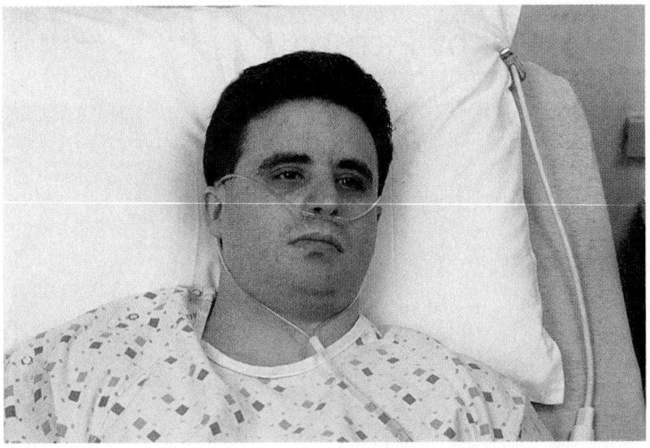

FIGURE 11-4 Clients facing a crisis of physical illness often feel lonely and abandoned. (DELMAR/CENGAGE LEARNING.)

CULTURAL CARE THEORY

Nurses skilled in cultural care understand that there are important cultural perspectives in all life's events. Related to crisis, Cultural Care Theory guides the nurse in two matters: recognizing that crises are culturally determined and understanding that insensitive cross-cultural experiences can produce crisis and culture conflict for the nurse and client.

Leininger's theory (1991) directs the nurse to obtain knowledge of the client's cultural background and to

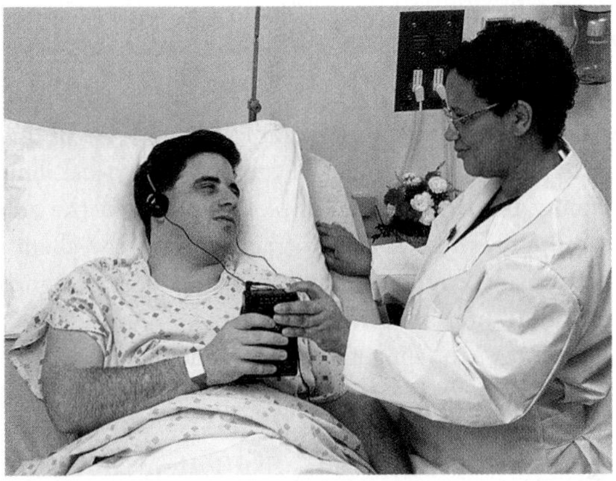

FIGURE 11-5 Listening to clients' feelings and responding to their needs will help you deliver compassionate and effective nursing care. (DELMAR/CENGAGE LEARNING.)

NURSINGALERT 11-1

Crisis and Suicide

The client experiencing crisis who discloses that he is thinking of suicide or implies that he is contemplating self-destructive behaviors of any kind *must be evaluated for suicide risk*. This client needs more than short-term crisis intervention counseling (see Chapter 16).

BOX 11-3
ASSESSMENT QUESTIONS FOR A CLIENT IN CRISIS

- Tell me about the situation that troubled you.
- What was your immediate reaction?
- Were you alone or with others?
- Explain as best you can what you thought and how you felt.
- Have you ever felt like that before? If yes, when?
- Have you discussed this current situation with anyone else?
- Does anyone you know understand what you are going through?
- Are you feeling anxious now?
- Are you able to go to work? To concentrate on other things?
- Are you sleeping at night?
- How do you usually handle stressful events?
- Do you feel you are going out of control?
- Do you feel you are about to harm yourself or others?
- What would be the most supportive thing another person could do for you?
- Do you have anyone to turn to?
- If you were very anxious and afraid in the middle of the night, what would you do?
- Do you have someone you can call on for help?
- How do you usually cope?

REFLECTIVE THINKING 11-1

Selecting a Nursing Theory

There are several nursing conceptual models or theories used in modern practice. Many of these are summarized in Chapter 3, and this chapter on crisis identifies three types of nursing perspectives that are useful in guiding care of the client undergoing a crisis. *How will you choose which to use?*

Begin by selecting one theory or approach that makes sense to you, whether or not it is one of the three the authors have outlined in this chapter. Next, take one of the cases presented in the beginning of the chapter that describes an actual experience of a crisis event. Ask yourself what you need to know and what you need to do as a nurse to assist that person from within your chosen framework. Write down your approach and your rationale for nursing actions.

Next, select a differing perspective, and, taking the same case, answer the same questions.

Compare the nursing actions and the rationale underlying those actions. Were the actions different? Was the rationale for the actions different, depending on the theoretical approach?

Repeat the exercise using yet another perspective.

The ability to examine two or more options for care, with an understanding that both are helpful, will help you develop skills of critical thinking.

understand the meaning of life's events from the client's perspective. It is readily apparent that crisis is highly individual: What is a crisis for one person may not be a crisis for another. The best way to learn of a client's culture and the meaning of events to the individual is to ask the client directly. Questions such as "How does your family interpret this situation?" or "What is the meaning of this loss to you?" help the nurse to understand and help the client to articulate his own response to the crisis situation. It is easy for nurses to believe that all clients can and should be able to handle life's events in the same manner as the nurse or in the same manner as the dominant culture; therefore, talking to the client to gain understanding is extremely important.

To be in a situation where one does not understand the social rules, language, and other aspects of a culture is to be in crisis. Situations where there is a reordering of cultural rules and norms is known as **culture shock**; it could just as easily be called culture crisis. Travel can bring on culture crisis, as can reading to a limited degree.

APPLICATION OF THE NURSING PROCESS 11-1

ASSESSMENT

To provide care, the nurse must be able to assess the individual undergoing crisis and determine the severity of the crisis and the person's responses to it. There are five factors to assess:

1. Determine the event or situation that precipitated the crisis and what caused the individual to seek help.
2. Assess the person's subjective experience of the crisis.
3. Assess the person's level of anxiety.

(*Continues*)

APPLICATION OF THE NURSING PROCESS 11-1 (Continued)

4. Assess the person's coping style and strengths.
5. Assess the supports available to the person.

Figure 11-6 lists a series of questions that could be used in an initial interview when obtaining basic assessment data. In addition to these questions, it is important to determine whether or not the crisis situation has produced feelings of severe despair or anger that could lead to self-destructive, suicidal, or aggressive behavior. If any of these are present, interventions appropriate for such behaviors, such as nursing actions to prevent self-harm, as presented in Chapters 14 and 16, should be instituted immediately. Such a client is not a candidate for crisis intervention, but, rather, must be treated for potentially suicidal and/or violent conditions. Many nurses have found that the APAM (see Figures 11-2 and 11-3) provides a good means of understanding the client's perspective of a crisis event.

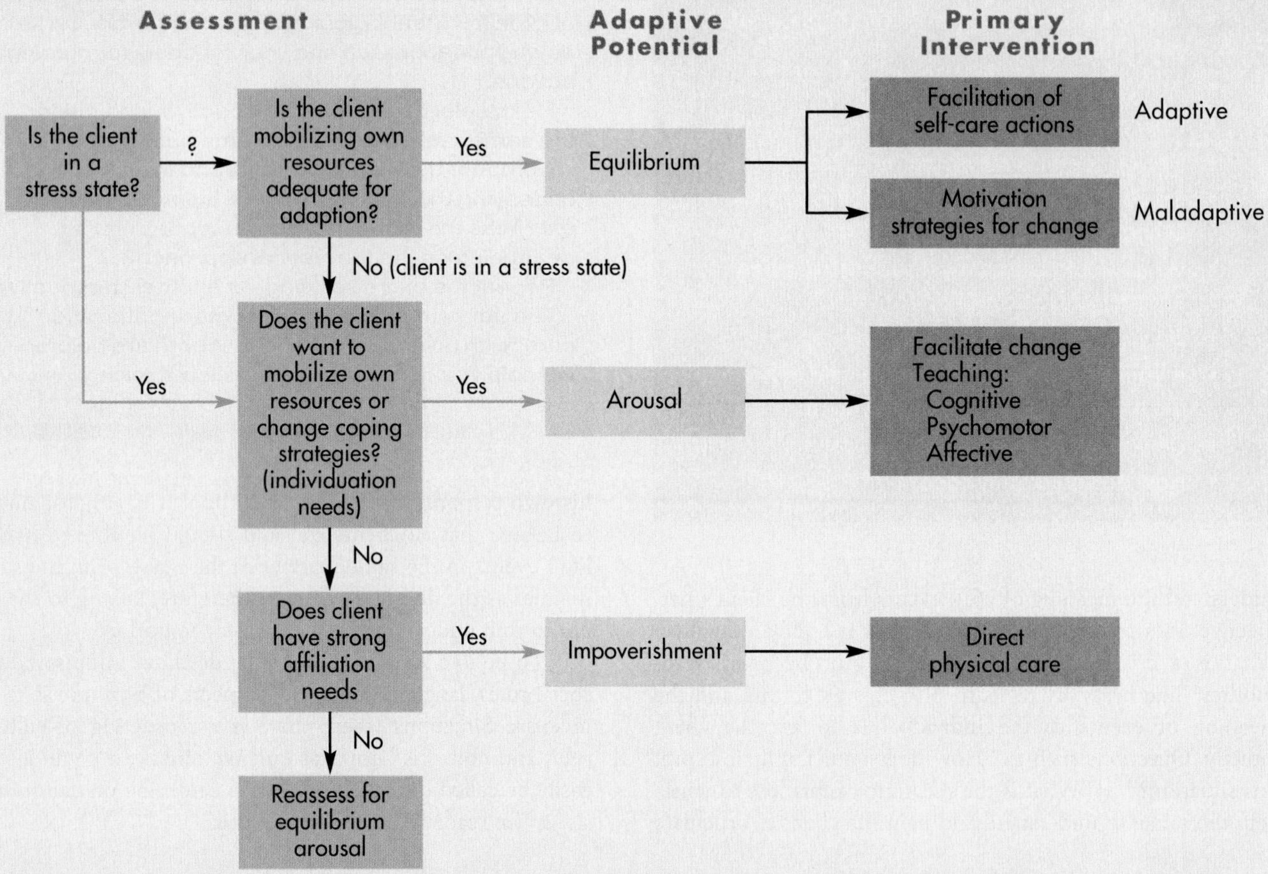

FIGURE 11-6 Adaptive potential as a guide to planning nursing interventions. (FROM S. BOWMAN, HUMBOLDT STATE UNIVERSITY, 1997. REPRINTED WITH PERMISSION.)

NURSING DIAGNOSIS

Bowman (1992) developed a flow chart (see Figure 11-6) that assists both in assessing an individual's adaptive potential and forming appropriate nursing interventions.

Analysis of assessment data should lead to nursing diagnoses and to initiation of a nursing care plan that will guide interventions. In most cases, intervention for crisis is short term and provides support for the here and now, with a goal of restoring equilibrium as soon as possible. Typically, crisis intervention lasts for one month.

(Continues)

APPLICATION OF THE NURSING PROCESS 11-1 (Continued)

Nursing diagnoses (Herdman, 2009) that are common in persons undergoing crisis are:

- *Anxiety* related to the sense of the unknown
- *Fear* related to the precipitating event
- *Ineffective coping* related to the inability to handle the situation
- *Powerlessness* related to the sense of being overwhelmed
- *Hopelessness* related to the sense of inability to recover from the crisis
- *Insomnia* related to the changes in daily patterns and state of excitement or arousal
- *Risk for other-directed violence* related to feelings of anger
- *Complicated grieving* related to the actual or perceived object loss

Anxiety and *fear* are diagnosed when the client reports continued concerns related to his own safety or ability to cope. The difference between the two diagnoses is that *anxiety* is diagnosed when the client experiences a general uneasiness and cannot attribute the feeling to any specific stressor. *Fear* is diagnosed when the client expresses anxiety, uneasiness, or fear directed at some specific object or occurrence. *Ineffective coping* would be diagnosed when the client's coping patterns, or defense mechanisms, do not serve to reestablish an equilibrium or balance in the person's life. Using the Modeling and Role-Modeling theory, any client in impoverishment or in maladaptive equilibrium could be diagnosed as having *ineffective coping*. *Powerlessness* and *hopelessness* are both subjective feelings that express the client's belief that he cannot control the events in his life. The nurse can make these diagnoses only when she has sufficient validation from the client that he, indeed, feels out of control and has given up. *Insomnia* is common post-crisis and for some individuals will be the only clue that they are still feeling stress. Thus, the nurse must ask questions related to sleep even when clients state there are no immediate stressors or crises in their lives. Assessment for *risk for other-directed violence* is always appropriate in situations where the client has experienced a crisis that will seem unfair and unjust. Likewise, *complicated grieving* is to be expected whenever personal loss is involved. It is important for the nurse to remember that clients in crises may not recognize that crisis is at the root of their distress. It is not at all unusual for clients in crisis to present with physical symptoms, either new symptoms, such as shortness of breath, pain, or neurological symptoms (usually with no evident physical explanation for the symptom), or the activation of medical conditions associated with stress, such as headaches or peptic ulcer disease. At times, crises may present as acute psychiatric distress and may receive a DSM-IV-TR diagnosis associated with crisis, such as Acute Stress Disorder. The principles of crisis management do not differ depending on whether the client presents with somatic or psychological symptoms; however, the content of the client's concerns and anxieties will likely be different in each case. It is important to recognize that, by definition, crises cannot last indefinitely—they must either resolve or become diagnosable psychiatric disorders. Depending on its seriousness, an unresolved crisis may lead to any of a variety of adjustment reactions in DSM-IV or even to the anxiety diagnosis Post-traumatic Stress Disorder (the diagnosis that a psychiatrist would likely give Wilbur one year after the Buffalo Creek flood).

OUTCOME IDENTIFICATION

As in all nursing care, the nurse and client must jointly identify expected outcomes of nursing interventions. Dealing with those facing crisis, the nurse will consider both short-term and long-term objectives/goals of care. For example, when the immediate problem is *insomnia,* the nurse may identify the short-term outcome that, within one week, the client will feel safe enough to sleep through the night. When the problem is *grief* related to losses associated with the crisis situation, the expected outcomes will be more long term. For example, a nurse may identify the expected outcome that within two months the client will have resolved the grief and begin to make adjustments/adaptations to "get on with life." It is essential here that the nurse evaluate what can and cannot be accomplished within a predicted time frame and make clear to herself and to her client that crises take time to be resolved and the nurse is willing to assist for the necessary period. Recall that research has indicated that family members/significant others seem to expect the

(*Continues*)

APPLICATION OF THE NURSING PROCESS 11-1 (Continued)

client undergoing crisis to have resolved the emotions long before the client is really able to do so (Stern & Kerry, 1996). Attention to outcomes and time needed to achieve them will help the nurse realistically plan for assisting the client through the duration of the crisis and its aftermath.

PLANNING/INTERVENTIONS

The focus of crisis intervention is to deal with the here and now, to help put the crisis event in perspective of the individual's life, and to allow that life to move on quickly past the crisis. Crisis intervention does not deeply explore a person's past psychological history. Though the individual's personality is formed in large part by the past, and though personality certainly affects response to crisis, crises occur and *are managed* in the present.

A goal of crisis intervention is to reestablish equilibrium or balance. It is imperative that the nurse understand the crisis event from the client's perspective; therefore, the first intervention is that of therapeutic listening. The nurse must establish trust with the client, ensure confidentiality, and seek to develop a good understanding of the client's experiences and feelings. For the client, describing emotions and reactions to the nurse serves to release feelings. The nurse encourages an honest disclosure and does not attempt to avoid emotional reactions such as anger or crying. The Interviewer's voice in the play *The Shadow Box* is abstract and impersonal: Joe can never see the interviewer, who remains offstage, but the voice is at least effective in encouraging Joe to tell some of his story instead of "keeping it all inside." In real life, the voice would likely have been less effective at getting Joe to share his feelings. For example, after Joe admits, "It's not an easy thing" (coping with a fatal illness), the interviewer responds, "You seem fine." But Joe does not really feel (or seem) fine. A more therapeutic response might have been, "No, it never is easy. Can you tell me about some of the things that seem particularly hard *for you*?" Actively listening to clients (and friends and family) is a challenging but very important skill to learn.

If necessary, a change of physical environment may be indicated, as it may serve to alleviate stress and may produce a sense of comfort and/or safety. For example, if the crisis event was the death of a spouse, the client may be more comfortable staying at the home of a family member or close friend rather than returning to the family home on the day of the death.

The nurse should support the client in the use of defense mechanisms that support an adaptive adjustment. All clients will use defenses that they have established as coping mechanisms throughout life. Some will be more adaptive than others. The nurse should never criticize that client's method of coping at a time of crisis, but may gently suggest ways that the client can face the reality of the situation. It is helpful to keep in mind that all defenses serve to maintain self-esteem and that a time of crisis is one when this maintenance is critical for the clients.

There are several means of providing crisis interventions. Individual interactions with the nurse or crisis counselor is one, but groups established for this purpose can be very helpful, particularly if the client can gain support from others who have faced or are facing similar crises. An example would be a support group for survivors of a flood. Nurses should become aware of crisis groups and support groups in their local communities to be able to refer clients as appropriate.

CRISIS INTERVENTION AS MENTAL HEALTH PREVENTION

Data have shown that crisis intervention can prevent the need for psychiatric hospitalization and save money (Hoult, 1986; cited in Sartorius, DeGirdano, Andrews, German, & Eisenberg, 1986, p. 305). Crisis intervention is a very important aspect of primary prevention of more serious mental disorders. Crisis intervention at the primary level refers to the establishment of social, political, and environmental conditions that support health. Community mental health work that provides healthy support for families, schools, and identified community groups (such as the elderly) and helps a community and individuals within it to develop the trust, the skills, and the referral networks needed to cope with unexpected, tragic events is primary mental health at its best.

Many have suggested that the crisis intervention model can be used in treating individuals with severe mental illness. The crisis intervention model was introduced in the 1970s as a method of providing care to

(Continues)

APPLICATION OF THE NURSING PROCESS 11-1 (Continued)

persons with acute phases of mental illness. The intent of the model used in this manner was to provide immediate care, focusing on the present, and helping the client and family to manage the acute condition. A major review of this approach has indicated that most who have studied the model have combined crisis intervention techniques with home care interventions (Joy, Adams, & Rice, 2004). Although review of research indicates crisis intervention with home care interventions may be a viable option for treatment, evidence based on a clinical trial is not available (Joy et al., 2004)

EVALUATION

The nurse must assess the outcomes of the crisis work. The nurse and client together can determine whether there was a successful resolution of the crisis. Does the client feel he can return to a normal life? Does he have the skills and the confidence to return to work? To friends? To family? To carry on?

At times, a crisis opens up new ideas for the affected person and challenges him to examine life from a deeper perspective. For example, many persons who have experienced cancer indicate that receiving the diagnosis of a significant illness created a crisis in their lives. As these persons dealt with the immediate crisis, denial, and shock, they learned to accept the diagnosis and treatment. Because of the experience, they also reexamined their lives, their priorities, and their interactions with others. These persons became different because of having to deal with the crisis, and their personal growth was stimulated by the event. Thus, when a crisis is resolved but the client wishes to pursue continued therapy, group support, and development, the nurse should refer the client to available resources.

REFLECTIVE THINKING 11-2

Crises as a Social Problem

1. What are the factors in your own community that contribute to the community's mental health or lack thereof?
2. Are there supports for identified groups?
   - Children
   - Young families
   - Working parents
   - Handicapped
   - Elderly
   - Poor
   - Victims of abuse
   - Sufferers of addictions
3. If yes, where are these services? Are nurses involved? How does one know where to find them?
4. If no, what is lacking? What would it take to initiate services?
5. To what degree do you believe it is a nurse's role to promote conditions in society that support individuals in their day-to-day lives?
6. Can a nurse be professional without being involved in community issues?

REFLECTIVE THINKING 11-3

Your Own Approach to Significant Illness

Nurses frequently come in contact with others who are facing life-threatening illness. In order to truly empathize with clients, it is helpful for the nurse to reflect on her own experience and feelings about illness. The following questions are a guide:

- Have you ever confronted a significant illness or the threat of a significant illness in yourself? If yes, what were your feelings and your coping mechanisms at the time? If no, can you imagine how you might feel in such a situation?
- Have you ever supported a family member or close friend who was facing significant illness? What was it like for you to be the support person?
- How intense is the threat of disability for you?
- Do you find it difficult to talk with someone who has been diagnosed with a significant illness? If yes, examine what it is that makes this interpersonal contact difficult.

Use your answers to these questions to evaluate areas that are sensitive for you. Get to know your own coping style. Determine how you can best meet clients' needs when clients have issues that overlap with your own sensitive areas.

CARE PLANNING GUIDE 11-1 Client Undergoing Crisis

CLINICAL PICTURE

The client experiencing a crisis event will:

- Describe the crisis event as ''overwhelming''
- Feel a continued threat
- Exhibit symptoms of anxiety, for example: inability to concentrate, agitation, forgetfulness, and social withdrawal

COMMON NURSING DIAGNOSES

Nursing diagnoses commonly employed for the client's undergoing crisis are:

1. Coping: ineffective individual coping OR opportunity to enhance individual coping
2. Powerlessness

The following Care Planning Guides depict suggested interventions, rationales, outcomes, and discharge planning activities for such clients.

NURSING DIAGNOSIS 1: *INEFFECTIVE COPING* RELATED TO RESPONSE TO A CRISIS EVENT

OUTCOMES

1. The client will verbalize a sense of being able to apply coping strategies in the situation.
2. The client will focus on the immediate future, with plans on what to do and how to manage.

NOC: *EFFECTIVE COPING*

INTERVENTIONS (NIC: *COPING ENHANCEMENT*)	RATIONALE
• Assess the client's level of anxiety/stress and the client's past coping patterns.	• Initial assessment provides the nurse with information on where to begin interventions and permits the nurse to capitalize on past strengths.
• Maintain a safe environment.	• Clients undergoing significant crises are threatened; personal safety is required in a therapeutic environment.
• Establish trust through therapeutic presence.	• Presence as a nursing intervention relays concern, undivided attention, and support to clients.
• Focus on the here and now.	• Clients in crisis need to address the immediate situation.
• Mobilize support systems for the client (with the client's permission), if the client is unable to do so for self.	• Many clients in crisis are immobilized or withdrawn and require help to access supports.
• Provide opportunity for the client to talk about precipitating events.	• Talking about the crisis is therapeutic for some individuals.
• Work with the client to develop a realistic plan for self.	• Focus on immediate needs and plans for the client to begin adjusting/coping.

(*Continues*)

CARE PLANNING GUIDE 11-1 Continued

NURSING DIAGNOSIS 2: *POWERLESSNESS* RELATED TO LOSS OF PERSONAL CONTROL OF LIFE EVENTS

OUTCOMES

1. The client will express feelings of control.

NOC: *PERCEIVED CONTROL*

INTERVENTIONS (NIC: GAINING CONTROL)	RATIONALE
Guiding the client in making his or her own decisions about plans of action by:	Feelings of control are achieved when the client has made own decisions about his or her future.
• Assisting the client to explore alternatives of action.	• Exploring alternatives provides a structure for the client to begin to take control of events.
• Assisting the client to evaluate possible consequences of actions.	• Evaluating consequences gives the client a means to make judgments about what to do.
• Allowing the client to talk through his or her ideas and feelings about courses of action.	• Allowing the client to talk gives the client a chance to reason through possible alternatives.
• Supporting the client in making decisions that seem right for the client.	• Provide support for the client in taking control over his or her own actions.
• Assisting the client to formulate a time frame for implementation of the chosen course of action.	• A time frame provides a structure for the client's next steps and supports feelings of direction and control.

LONG-TERM CONSIDERATIONS

1. Resolution of a crisis event is achieved when a client can cope and return to precrisis level of functioning.
2. A significant personal crisis may change an individual's sense of self and of personal vulnerability.

Note: The care planning guides have been adapted from *Plans of Care for Specialty Practice: Psychiatric Mental Health Nursing* by M. Coler, and K. G. Vincent, 1995, Clifton Park, NY: Delmar Cengage Learning.

NURSING CARE PLAN: NURSING PROCESS FORMAT 11-1

Stewart Alsop was a prominent newspaper columnist who developed an unusual form of leukemia. In the following passage from his book *Stay of Execution*, he is in a state of arousal. By his own descriptions, he was sometimes a difficult patient for doctors and nurses alike. He had (and expressed) a strong need for control over an illness and process that constantly denied him that control.

STAY OF EXECUTION

"Is there any chance I have aplastic anemia?" I asked. Aplastic anemia is a serious marrow disease, but it is not malignant.

Dr. Henderson hesitated for a moment. "No," he said.

"Then I do have some form of cancer, leukemia, or something else?"

"Yes," he said quietly.

He left, and. . . . I began, for the first time in about fifty years, to cry. I was utterly astonished, and also dismayed. I was brought up to believe that for a man to weep in public is the ultimate indignity, a proof of unmanliness. Only my elderly roommate was in the room, and he hadn't noticed. I ducked into our tiny shared bathroom, and closed the door, and sat down on the toilet, and turned on the bath water, so that nobody could hear me, and cried my heart out. Then I dried my eyes on the toilet paper and felt a good deal better. . . .

(*Continues*)

NURSING CARE PLAN: NURSING PROCESS FORMAT 11-1 (Continued)

When Dr. Henderson said "no" to my first question and "yes" to my second, a small light went out, a light of hope that I might not have cancer after all. . . .

I spent a lot of time reading—nothing very profound, since I was in a mood for escape, not profundity. I was enjoying. . . . The Day of the Jackal, *the best seller about an attempted assassination of de Gaulle . . . thoroughly when one of the characters told another that his girlfriend had "luke-something." I closed the book hurriedly, sure that the girlfriend would soon die. In fact, I'm told, she didn't, but I've never finished the novel.*

When I wasn't reading for escape, I spent a lot of time trying to remember quotations . . . mostly from school and college days, and I almost always got them wrong. . . . For example, I kept trying to remember T. S. Eliot's eternal Footman. After much brain cudgeling, I scribbled in my notebook:

I have seen the moment of my greatness flicker.
I have seen the eternal Footman hold my coat, and snicker.
In short, I was afraid.

. . . Then there were snatches of nonsense verse, for which I've always had a fondness. From Belloc's Cautionary Tales:

The chief defect of Henry King
Was chewing little bits of string.
At last he swallowed some which tied
Itself in ugly knots inside.
Physicians of the utmost fame
Were called at once; but when they came
They answered, as they took their fees,
"There is no cure for this disease."

*. . . The thrust of these snippets of memory suggests a melancholy frame of mind, but I found it oddly comforting to dig into my small store of remembered quotations. It was a way of papering over misery. I always liked the story about Winston Churchill . . . in the Boer War when he had to spend a couple of days hiding . . . in a dark hole. He passed the time quite happily reciting to himself all the familiar quotations and Latin tags he could recall. This is at least a better way to spend the time than fearing death.**

(Alsop, 1973, p. 68)

Imagine that nurses are actually giving care to the client described here. His expressions of feelings and his behaviors are very similar to those seen by nurses when encountering clients who are life-threatened by illness. This is a fictionalized nursing care plan.

ASSESSMENT

The client is experiencing a crisis of learning that he has a significant illness. He is in a state of arousal—attempting to cope and using his love of books, reading, and quotations as a method of establishing equilibrium. He is mobilizing his resources.

He cries and seeks privacy so that no one will know. His arousal has grown from a sense of denial—a coping mechanism that allows him to believe his tumor is benign. He hears the final declaration from his physician and knows and accepts that he has a malignancy.

NURSING DIAGNOSIS 1 *Fear* related to the unknown course of a life-threatening illness, as evidenced by ability to identify object of fear.

OUTCOMES	NIC	NURSING ACTIONS	EVALUATION
Within 4 weeks, the client will acknowledge and discuss his fear about his illness with his primary care provider and will recognize both adaptive and maladaptive strategies he is using to cope.	• Emotional support • Coping enhancement	• Offer quiet, uninterrupted periods of time for listening and talking. • Assist the client in dealing with his fears. • Encourage the expression of feelings through use of therapeutic communication techniques (active listening, reflecting, restating).	Within 4 weeks, the client was verbalizing his fear. Some of his fears were associated with a lack of information about his illness. The nurse

*Excerpt from page 68 from *Stay of execution*, by Stewart Alsop. © Copyright 1973, J. B. Lippincott. Reprinted with permission of Harper Collins Publishers, Inc.

NURSING CARE PLAN: NURSING PROCESS FORMAT 11-1 (Continued)

OUTCOMES	NIC	NURSING ACTIONS	EVALUATION
NOC: *Fear Control*		• Explore what client sees as coping strategies, identifying which ones he believes are useful and which ones are not.	provided extra information in oral and written form. He was also fearful that he would not be able to control his own emotions and behaviors when undergoing treatment. This fear was expressed.

NURSING DIAGNOSIS 2 *Powerlessness* related to illness treatment regimen, lack of privacy, as evidenced by verbalizations of having no control over situation.

OUTCOMES	NIC	NURSING ACTIONS	EVALUATION
• Within 4 days of hospitalization, client will verbalize feeling in control of treatment choices and his own life activities. • Client will allow himself to express his personal feelings in a variety of ways without self-criticism, particularly during the next 3 months. NOC: *Perceived control over treatment*	• Teaching (individual) • Goal setting • Presence • Patient rights protection • Counseling	• Provide expert assistance to client by answering his questions and allowing him to discuss his various treatment options. • Help client construct an activities schedule that acknowledges his need to read and write. • Identify energy-saving activities that will permit client to both pace himself and do the things that are most important to him. • Encourage expression of feelings by asking open-ended questions and listening actively. • Attempt to limit client's self-critical messages, pointing out his personal strengths and affirming positive aspects of his coping. • Provide for client's need for privacy: procure a private room, knock before entering the room, ask him if this is an acceptable time, arrange activities according to his needs. • Inform client that many persons have the need to reflect and will feel emotional when facing significant illness. Offer to discuss these issues if he wishes.	Client said he particularly appreciated help that allowed him to reflect on the choices he did have. His writing continues to be meaningful to him and should be encouraged. Client began to express his feelings both alone and with others.

(Continues)

NURSING CARE PLAN: NURSING PROCESS FORMAT 11-1 (Continued)

REFLECTIVE QUESTIONS

1. **ASSESSMENT**
   What support mechanisms (family, friends, colleagues) should you include in your assessment?
2. **NURSING DIAGNOSIS**
   What other diagnoses might apply?
3. **OUTCOMES**
   What other mutual goals would be reasonable to explore for this client?
4. **PLANNING/INTERVENTIONS**
   What other strategies might we try with this client? Do you think a support group should be suggested?
5. **EVALUATION**
   What else should we have considered with this client? How could we revise this care plan to better meet his needs?

NURSING CARE PLAN: CONCEPT MAP FORMAT 11-1

BACKGROUND INFORMATION

The Galos family has just been evacuated from their home in the California mountains east of Los Angeles. Burning wildfires have put them in grave danger, as their property is at risk for loss due to fire. While reluctant to leave their home, Mr. and Mrs. Galos and their two children (girls ages 12 and 10 years) recognized the imminent danger and have fled by car to a community 50 miles away. They had some clothing with them, a few important personal possessions, and a small amount of food and water as they left their home. The situation in their neighborhood (a small, friendly subdivision) was relatively calm as they and their neighbors were summoned by emergency service workers and told that evacuation was now mandatory to protect life.

The family arrived at an American Red Cross emergency shelter set up in a school building. Volunteers are assisting to ensure that people's basic needs are met—safety, shelter, food, and clothing. The crisis response nurse notices that Mrs. Galos is particularly distressed. She approaches Mrs. Galos and offers to talk.

Mrs. Galos expresses her feelings. She reports being frightened and extremely anxious. She states that she hasn't slept over the past few nights, being worried about the wildfires burning across an extensive part of the region. She says, "I know we are safe here, but I'm trembling inside. I close my eyes and I see fire!" Mrs. Galos further states, "I don't care about possessions, but I can't deal very well with not knowing what is happening at home."

Mrs. Galos went on to say, "I can usually cope by working at my house—I clean house when I am upset, I exercise by jogging through the neighborhood, I talk to my neighbor. My support system is gone!"

The nurse notices that as Mrs. Galos continues to relate her situation, she appears even more anxious—she is speaking quickly, her breathing is fast, and her color is pale. The nurse further notes that the two Galos children are sitting at a table with other children, drawing pictures and drinking lemonade. The children seem without undue stress at this time. Mr. Galos is talking with one of the Red Cross volunteers about activities needed to move supplies into the building to prepare for housing an estimated 100 evacuees. The nurse also notes that Mrs. Galos is focusing on the present only—she is addressing the "here and now" and

(Continues)

NURSING CARE PLAN: CONCEPT MAP FORMAT 11-1 (Continued)

is not bringing up issues of eventual return to the home and dealing with possible loss of home and all of the related issues such an event would entail.

INITIAL ASSESSMENT AND REFLECTION

The nurse recognizes that Mrs. Galos is facing a significant crisis:

1. She has had to evacuate from her home.
2. She expresses fear of fire.
3. She expresses fear of the unknown.
4. She has lost the context required for her usual coping strategies.
5. She is in a state of fatigue.
6. She is dealing with the present only (is not being future-directed).

INITIAL REVIEW OF NURSING DIAGNOSIS

Knowing that Mrs. Galos is now in a safe environment where she is free from physical harm, the nurse reviews the data and identifies the following nursing diagnoses:

Anxiety, moderate level, related to the unknown outcome of the wildfire
Fear of the wildfire
Ineffective coping, related to loss of the context (house and home) of coping strategies
Insomnia, related to inability to sleep over past few nights

The nurse also identifies the strengths and resources that Mrs. Galos has:

1. Physical safety
2. Provision of basic needs
3. Family members present, safe, and adjusting to the crisis situation

The nurse prepares a concept map, listing the characteristics that contribute to Mrs. Galos's present situation: wildfire spreading near her home, evacuation to a distant town, loss of the setting to implement usual coping strategies, feelings of anxiousness, feelings of fear, and fatigue.

PRIORITIES OF CARE

The concept map for this client in crisis indicates that the immediate crisis event is the focal issue related to virtually all other areas of the client's present situation. The next focal issue is the loss of the home setting, as the home setting is the context required for Mrs. Galos to utilize the coping strategies that have worked for her in the past.

Thus, the nurse chooses *ineffective individual coping* as the primary nursing diagnosis.

The initial and immediate outcome of nursing intervention is for Mrs. Galos to establish effective coping strategies by the end of the day so she can regain/maintain her ability to function with the current crisis. Noting that Mrs. Galos is focusing on the "here and now," the nurse, too, focuses on the present.

NURSING INTERVENTIONS

Nursing interventions are:

- Role enhancement: Assist Mrs. Galos to adopt a role at the crisis shelter that parallels her role at home during a time of anxiety or crisis. The nurse explores the activities needed at the shelter and Mrs. Galos's readiness to take on a volunteer role (cooking, cleaning, and organizing) that would be consistent with her past effective means of coping.
- Self-awareness enhancement: Assist Mrs. Galos to see that she already has important insights into her feelings; for example, she has stated that she is missing her support system. This is very positive and opens up possibilities of identifying other supports in her current environment.

(Continues)

NURSING CARE PLAN: CONCEPT MAP FORMAT 11-1 (Continued)

- Presence: The nurse will be fully present with Mrs. Galos during her time of need. The nurse will allow a certain amount of time to talk with her, maintain positive regard, establish trust by being trustworthy, and provide an attitude of concern and empathy.

OUTCOMES/EVALUATION

Through use of therapeutic communication and presence, the nurse established the trust of Mrs. Galos and provided feedback regarding Mrs. Galos's very positive ability to reflect on the events of the day and conclude that her support system is gone. The nurse explores with Mrs. Galos the kind of activities she would typically do at home to relieve anxiety or stress and attempts to find parallel activities at the shelter. Mrs. Galos related, "I always do better if I have a task and if I am physically busy." The nurse notes that a number of Red Cross volunteers are getting ready to feed about 100 persons at the shelter and could use help in food preparation and organizing people for the meal. Mrs. Galos states, "What else do I have to do anyway?" and permits the nurse to introduce her to the coordinator of the meal so she can get involved in volunteer work herself.

In the early evening, the nurse checks back with Mrs. Galos, who is clearing dishes and assisting with the after-meal cleanup activities. Mrs. Galos states, "It isn't the best day of my life, but we are all managing."

The nurse concludes that the immediate need for assistance has been met, but plans to visit Mrs. Galos tomorrow to evaluate coping, as the events of this crisis will continue for several days and the outcome is still uncertain.

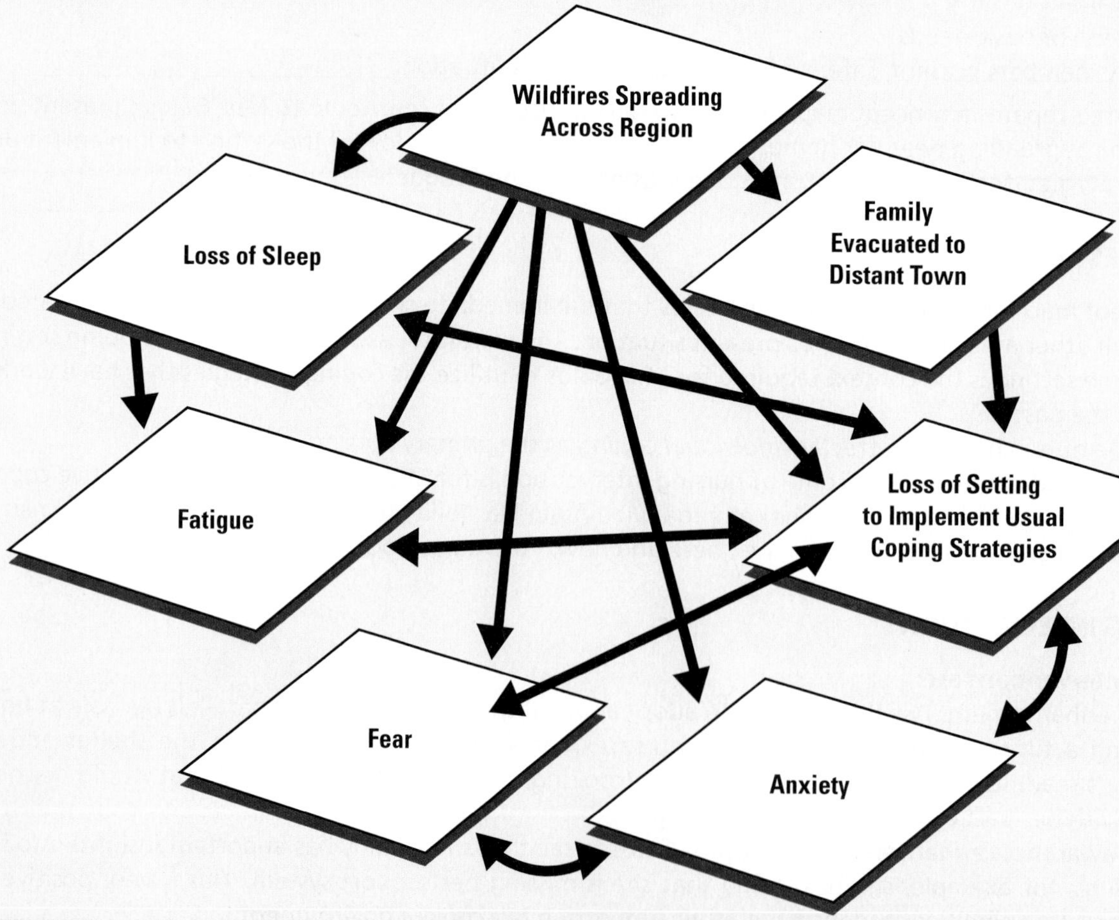

Concept Map of Issues and Problems Mrs. Galos (DELMAR/CENGAGE LEARNING.)

KEY CONCEPTS

- A crisis is one of the many of life's challenges that call on people to adjust to the unexpected and to adapt.
- Crisis stresses each individual's coping resources, and each person responds differently to seemingly identical situations.
- In nursing, a crisis is defined as a critical situation, stage, or life event in which a person is called on to respond and adapt to the unexpected.
- There are several kinds of crisis: situational, an event posing a challenge to an individual; maturational, a stage in a person's growth and development when he must adjust and adapt to new life patterns; cultural, a situation where a person experiences culture shock; and community, a crisis of a proportion to impact an entire community.
- In experiencing crises, persons go through predictable stages in which coping methods used in the past are used to help bring the crisis under control.
- Stress theory provides a means to understand the human experience of crisis. Each person has resources, collectively called adaptive energy, that are used in response to crisis. When all of a person's resources are used up, that person is left in a state of exhaustion.
- Psychosocial responses to stress include the fight-flight response, associated with high energy, and the conservative-withdrawal response, associated with exhaustion.
- The Modeling and Role-Modeling nursing theory includes the Adaptive Potential Assessment Model, which provides the nurse language to describe the client's adaptation to stress.
- Watson's Theory of Transpersonal Caring suggests that listening to the client and understanding the person's subjective experience of the crisis is of the utmost importance.
- Cultural Care Theory points out that a crisis cannot be understood without knowledge of the client's culture.
- Assessment of the crisis and the client's past coping mechanisms and current strengths begin the process.
- Crisis intervention is considered short-term therapy, usually lasting one month.
- The goal of crisis intervention is to return the client to normal life, with adjustment at least at the precrisis level.

REVIEW QUESTIONS

1. A nurse has been planning her retirement for several years. Recently she was informed by her stockbroker that her retirement account had reduced in value by 80% because of the economic recession. The nurse is most likely to develop which type of crisis situation?
1. Maturational crisis
2. Situational crisis
3. Cultural crisis
4. Community crisis

2. A young woman recently graduated from college and moved to a new city to assume employment for a position for which she was hired. While traveling to the new city, her airplane was hijacked and one of the flight attendants was murdered. When rescued, all hostages were taken for debriefing. The nurse's assessment would most likely reveal that the young woman had most likely experienced which types of crisis?
1. Cultural crisis and situational crisis
2. Maturational crisis and situational crisis
3. Situational crisis and community crisis
4. Cultural crisis and maturational crisis

3. A young woman is admitted to the Emergency Room after being attacked and robbed by a mugger. While being examined by the nurse, the client states, "I just want to go home. I'm okay; I just want to go to sleep in my own bed." The nurse assesses the client to be experiencing which stage of crisis as described by Engel?
1. Alarm
2. Fight or flight
3. Reaction formation
4. Conservative-withdrawal

4. A young man is brought to the hospital by his parents who inform the nurse that their son was recently discharged from the army. According to the parents, the young man has been extremely anxious, unable to eat or sleep. He frequently paces the floor during the night, constantly checking the doors and windows to be sure they are locked. A priority nursing diagnosis for this client would be which of the following?
1. Fear of unknown origin
2. Anxiety related to the sense of the unknown
3. Adjustment reaction to living with parents
4. Disturbed sleep pattern related to a state of excitement or arousal

5. A nurse following Watson's Theory of Transpersonal Caring when working while working in a crisis

center recognizes that her approach to the client should demonstrate which of the following?
1. Unconditional, humanistic care
2. Strict adherence to rules and regulations
3. Firm limits and structure
4. Detached conservatism

6. Clients experiencing disturbances in mental health functioning frequently employ ego defense mechanisms. Nurses caring for these clients recognize that the use of defense mechanisms is an attempt to do which of the following?
1. Increase awareness
2. Avoid responsibility
3. Reduce anxiety
4. Delay gratification

7. The nurse is planning to conduct a women's health promotion group. Which of the following approaches to deal with stressful situations would the nurse most likely include in the teaching plan?
1. Avoiding of all stressful situations
2. Indulging in excess food, alcohol, and the use of drugs
3. Referring all stressful situations to a relative to handle
4. Developing positive coping strategies to deal with stressful situations

8. A 65-year-old client recently retired from his place of employment due to health problems. The client is unable to sleep or eat. He frequently returns to his former job site to talk with his former coworkers. The man is most likely experiencing which type of crisis?
1. Cultural crisis
2. Situational crisis
3. Maturational crisis
4. Community crisis

LEARNING ACTIVITIES

1. Identify kinds of crisis (situational, maturational, cultural, and community) and provide an example of each.

2. Describe Caplan's stages of crisis.

3. Explain how personal psychological development influences reaction to crisis.

4. Explain Selye's GAS response to stress.

5. Describe the fight-flight response and the conservative-withdrawal response.

6. Use a nursing adaptation theory to interpret a crisis event.

7. Explain how caring theories and the intervention of listening could be helpful for a person in crisis.

8. Describe how culture influences the perception of and reaction to crisis.

9. Use the flow chart in Figure 11-6 to evaluate whether or not a client is in equilibrium, arousal, or impoverishment.

10. Explain crisis intervention as a form of mental health prevention.

*Study*WARE™ CONNECTION

Using your *Study*WARE™ CD-ROM

1. Complete the Flashcard Activity for this chapter.
2. Review the audio glossary for key terms in this chapter.
3. Explore the other games and activities that support this chapter.

REFERENCES

Adams, S., Dolfie, E., Feren, S. S., Love, R. A., & Taylor, S. W. (1999). Mental health disaster response. *Journal of Psychosocial Nursing, 37*(11), 11–19.

Bledsoe, B. E. (2003). Critical incident stress management (CISM): Benefit or risk for emergency services? *Prehospital Emergency Care, 7*(2), 272–279.

Bowman, S. (1992). *Adaptive potential as a guide to planning nursing interventions.* Paper presented at the Fourth National Modeling and Role-Modeling Conference, Boston, MA.

Caplan, G. (1964). *Principles of preventive psychiatry.* New York: Basic Books.

Coler, M. S., & Hafner, L. P. (1991). An intercultural assessment of the type, intensity and number of crisis precipitating factors in three cultures: United States, Brazil and Taiwan. *International Journal of Nursing Studies, 28*(3), 223–235.

Compton, M. T., Bahora, M., Watson, A. C., & Oliva, J. R. (2008). A comprehensive review of extant research on Crisis Intervention Team (CIT) programs. *Journal of the American Academy of Psychiatry and Law, 36*(1), 47–55.

Davis, J., & Stewart, L. (2000). Air flight disaster, post-traumatic stress, and post-ventive rescue and response; the aftermath of the San Diego PSA 182 plane crash recovery operation, 20 years on. *Accident and Emergency Nursing, 8*(1), 13–19.

Dimsdale, J. E. (2008). Psychological stress and cardiovascular disease. *Journal of the American College of Cardiology, 51*(13), 1237–1246.

Engel, G. (1962). *Psychological development in health and disease.* Philadelphia: W. B. Saunders.

Erickson, H., Tomlin, E., & Swain, M. A. (1983). *Modeling and role-modeling: A theory and paradigm for nursing.* Lexington, SC: Pine Press.

Frohlich, E. D., & Schwartz, R. S. (2007) Stress and cardiovascular disease: Lessons from Katrina. *Medscape Public Health and Prevention.* Retrieved August 10, 2009, from http://www.medscape.com/view article/569342_2.

Grant, S., Hardin, S., Pesut, D., & Hardin, T. (1997). Psychological evaluations, referrals, and follow-up of adolescents after their exposure to Hurricane Hugo. *Journal of Child and Adolescent Psychiatric Nursing, 10*(1), 7–16.

Green, B. L., Grace, M. C., Vary, M. G., Kramer, T. L., Gleser, G. C., & Leonard, A. C. (1994). Children of disaster in the second decade: A 17-year follow-up of Buffalo Creek survivors. *Journal of the American Academy of Child and Adolescent Psychiatry, 33*(1), 71–79.

Green, B. L., Lindy, J. D., Grace, M. C., Gleser, G. C., Leonard, A. C., Korol, M., et al. (1990). Buffalo Creek survivors in the second decade: Stability of stress symptoms. *American Journal of Orthopsychiatry, 60*(1), 43–54.

Herdman, H. (2009). *Nursing diagnosis: Definitions and classification 2009–2011.* Oxford: Wiley Blackwell.

Joy, C., Adams, C., & Rice, K. (2004). Crisis intervention for people with severe mental illnesses. *The Cochrane Library, no 4.*, Oxford, England, ID # CD001087.

Kessler, R. C., Galea, S., Gruber, M. J., Sampson, N. A., Ursano, R. J., & Wessely, S. (2008). Trends in mental illness and suicidality after Hurricane Katrina. *Molecular Psychiatry, 13*(4), 374–384.

Leininger, M. (1991). The theory of culture care diversity and universality. In M. Leininger (Ed.), *Culture care diversity and universality: A theory of nursing* (pp. 55–68). New York: National League for Nursing.

Milstein, J. M., Gerstenberger, A. E, & Barton, S. (2002). Healing the caregiver. *Journal of Alternative and Complementary Medicine, 8*(6), 917–920.

O'Toole, A. W., & Welt, S. R. (Eds.). (1989). *Interpersonal theory in nursing practice: Selected works of Hildegard Peplau.* New York: National League for Nursing.

Ogawa, K., Tsuji, I., Shiono, K., & Hisamichi, S. (2000). Increased acute myocardial infarction mortality following the 1995 Great Hanshin-Awaji earthquake in Japan. *International Journal of Epidemiology, 29*(3), 449–455.

Orr, M. L., (2002, September 30). Ready or not, disasters happen. *Online Journal of Issues in Nursing.* Retrieved November 23, 2003, from http://www.nursingworld.org.ojin/topic19/tpc19_2htm

Oxford English Dictionary. (1989). Oxford, England: Oxford University Press.

Roy, C., & Andrews, H. A. (1999). *The Roy Adaptation Model.* (2nd ed.). Stamford, CT: Appleton & Lange.

Rozanski, A., Blumenthal, J. A., & Kaplan, J. (1999). Impact of psychological factors on the pathogenesis of cardiovascular disease and implications for therapy. *Circulation, 99*(16), 2192–2217.

Sartorious, N., DeGirdano, G., Andrews, G., German, G., & Eisenberg, L. (Eds.). (1986). *Treatment of mental disorders.* Washington, DC: American Psychiatric Press.

Schienle, A., Schafer, A., Hermann, A., Rohrmann, S., & Vaitl, D. (2007). Symptom provocation and reduction in patients suffering from spider phobia: An fMRI study on exposure therapy. *European Archives of Psychiatry Clinical Neurosciences, 257*(8), 486–493.

Selye, H. (1974). *Stress without distress.* Philadelphia: J. B. Lippincott.

Stern, P. N., & Kerry, J. (1996). Restructuring life after home loss by fire. *Image, the Journal of Nursing Scholarship, 28*(1), 11–16.

Vlahov, D., Galea, S., Resnick, H., Ahern, J., Boscarino, J. A., Bucuvalas, M., et al. (2002). Increased use of cigarettes, alcohol, and marijuana among Manhattan, New York, residents after the September 11th terrorist attacks. *American Journal of Epidemiology, 155*(11), 988–996.

Watson, J. (1988). *Nursing: Human science and human care: A theory of nursing.* New York: National League for Nursing.

Watson, J. (2002). Intentionality and caring-healing consciousness: A practice of transpersonal nursing. *Holistic Nursing Practice, 16*(4), 12–19.

Watson, J. (2005). *Caring science as sacred science.* Philadelphia: Davis.

Webster's New World Dictionary (2nd College Ed.). (1994). New York: Simon & Schuster.

LITERARY REFERENCES

Alsop, S. (1973). *Stay of execution.* Philadelphia: J. B. Lippincott.

Erikson, K. (1976). *Everything in its path.* New York: Simon & Schuster.

Xun, L. (1973). *Silent China: Selected writings of Lu Xun,* edited and translated by Gladys Yang. Beijing: Foreign Language Press.

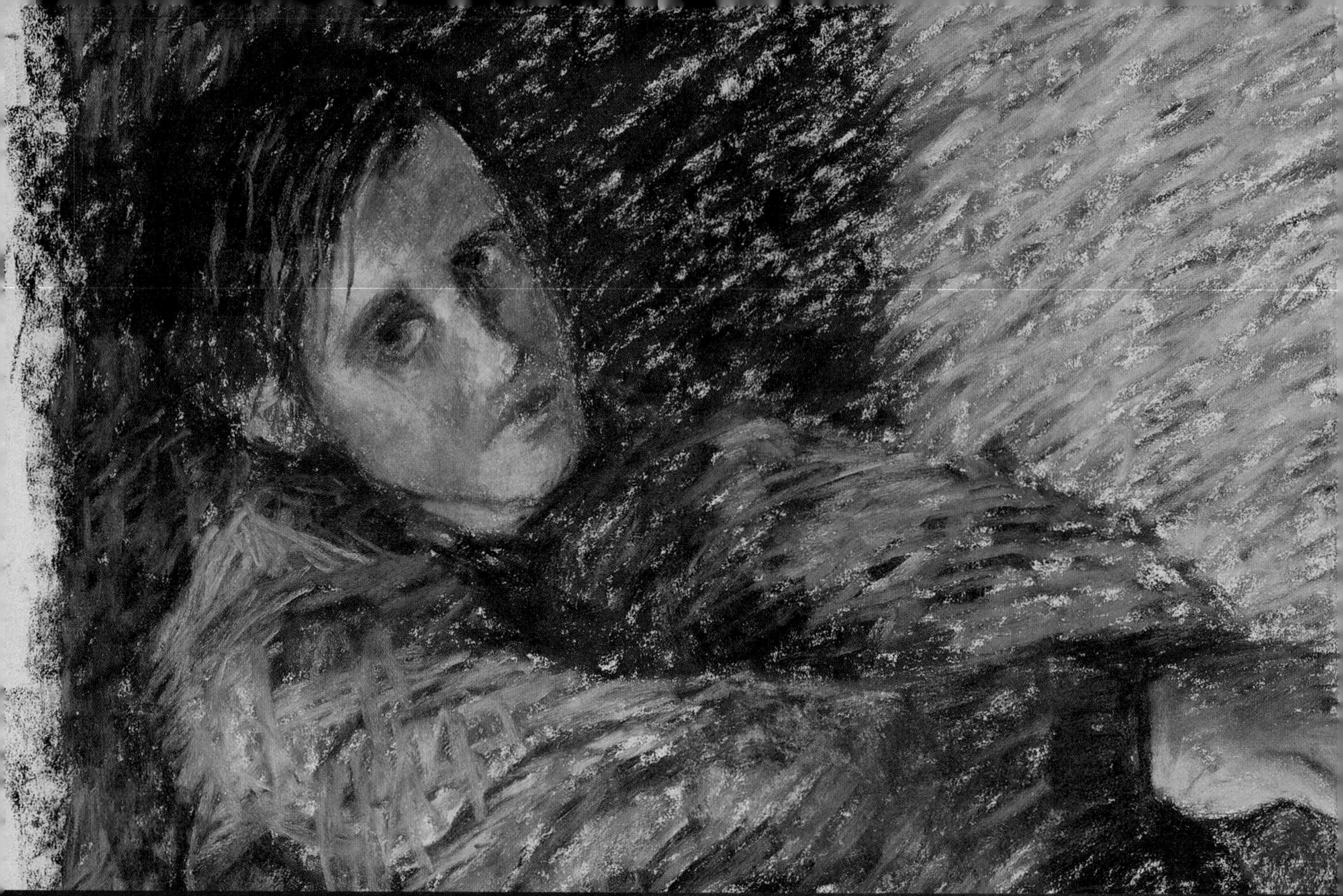

No Way Out

Anxiety in Everyday Life

Modern life is filled with tension and anxieties. Philosophers have stated that anxiety is a part of the human condition, both unavoidable and necessary for persons to seek to understand themselves and define their goals. However, each person tries to find balance within his or her own existence.

Consider the anxieties of your own life:

- ***What are the objects of your worries?***
- ***Are there personal worries stemming from your societal roles and duties?***
- ***Do you have personal fears associated with activities or objects? Are you able to avoid those situations that are anxiety provoking for you?***

How do you find peace?

- ***What does a personal sense of peace mean to you?***
- ***What can you do to find peace in your life?***

As you read this chapter, which focuses on anxiety in illness, remember that all persons, well or ill, experience anxiety. The nurse must understand that anxiety can become an overpowering experience for many persons, and care must focus on a very personal understanding of anxiety, fear, and sense of loss of control.

CHAPTER 12

The Client Experiencing Anxiety

Noreen Cavan Frisch
Lawrence E. Frisch

CHAPTER OUTLINE

COMPETENCIES

Upon completion of this chapter, the reader should be able to:

1. Understand the subjective experience of the emotion of anxiety.
2. Describe the differences between anxiety and fear.
3. Define and describe six major anxiety disorders (Generalized Anxiety Disorder, Panic Disorder, Agoraphobia, Phobias, Obsessive-Compulsive Disorder, Post-Traumatic Stress Disorder).
4. Relate the prevalence of anxiety disorders in the general population.
5. Participate in the major treatments of clients with anxiety disorders, including psychotherapy, medication therapy, and combination treatment.
6. Apply nursing theory and nursing diagnoses in the planning, implementing, and evaluating of nursing care of clients with anxiety disorders.

KEY TERMS

Adversity
Agoraphobia
Cognitive-Behavior Therapy
Compulsions
Generalized Anxiety Disorder
Obsessions
Panic Disorder
Phobia
Positron Emission Tomography
Post-Traumatic Stress Disorder
Trait Anxiety

Anxiety is a nearly universal human experience that has long been of interest to both psychologists and creative writers. As will be seen throughout this chapter, the experience of profound anxiety can be severely disabling. In the short story "He?" by Guy de Maupassant, a young man finds his aversion to marriage overcome by the sudden development of a serious anxiety disorder. In this excerpt, he is talking to a close friend about his upcoming marital plans:

ISN'T IT DREADFUL?

"Isn't it dreadful, to be in this state?"

My dear friend, you are completely baffled by it, aren't you? And I can easily understand why. I suppose you think I have gone mad. Perhaps I am a little insane—but not for the reasons you imagine.

Yes. I'm getting married. It's quite true.

And yet my ideas and convictions on the subject have not changed. I still consider legalized cohabitation to be foolish.... And yet I am getting married.

I might add that I hardly know the girl who will become my wife tomorrow. I have only seen her four or five times. I know that I do not find her displeasing—and that is sufficient for the purpose I have in mind. She is short, fair, and plump. After tomorrow I shall ardently wish for a woman who is tall, dark, and slender....

"Then why on earth do you get married?" you will say.

I hardly dare to tell you the strange, incredible reason which is urging me to commit this senseless action.

I am getting married so I shall not have to be on my own!

I don't know how to tell you about it, how to make myself understood. I am in such a wretched state of mind that you will feel sorry for me, and also despise me.

I cannot bear to be alone any more at night.... I'm afraid of the walls, of the furniture, of familiar objects, which seem to take on a kind of animal life. Above all, I am afraid of the horrible confusion of my thoughts, of the way my reason becomes blurred and elusive, scattered by a mysterious, invisible anguish.

At first I feel a vague uneasiness which enters my soul and sends shivers all over my skin. I look all around me. There's nothing there.... I happen to say something aloud—and I'm frightened by the sound of my own voice! I walk about the room—and I'm afraid there might be something strange behind the door, behind the curtains, in the cupboard, under my bed. And yet I know very well that there is nothing there at all.

Sometimes I suddenly turn round because I'm afraid of what might be behind me—and yet there is nothing there, as I very well know.

I become agitated, feel the nervousness increasing, and so I lock myself in my room, bury myself in my bed and hide myself under the sheets. Then cowering there, all huddled up as round as a ball, I close my eyes in despair and stay like this for a long, long time....

Isn't it dreadful, to be in this state?

I never used to feel in the least like this.... It all started last year in a very curious way ... one damp evening in the autumn....

*Ever since that time I have been afraid when I have been alone at night.... It is ridiculous—but it's horrible. I'm sorry ... I simply can't help it.... But if there were two of us in the place....**

(de Maupassant, 1903/1990, pp. 136–142)

In this excerpt from the short story "He?" the French writer Guy de Maupassant captures the desperate experience of anxiety: "At first I feel a vague uneasiness which enters my soul and sends shivers all over my skin.... I'm afraid of what might be behind me—and yet there is nothing there, as I very well know.... Above all ... I'm afraid of fear, afraid of my panic-stricken mind, afraid of that horrible sensation of incomprehensible terror." Paralyzed by fear, the narrator can only lie curled up in bed and wait until his terror passes. Not only does this excerpt give a vivid sense of what it is like to feel profound anxiety—knowing all along that there is no recognizable reason for fear—but, as will be seen later in this chapter, de Maupassant's story portrays vividly the psychiatric diagnosis of agoraphobia, one of the major categories of anxiety disorders.

Anxiety has a great deal in common with fear, and indeed de Maupassant's narrator freely uses the word *fear* to describe his experience. Still, he is quite careful to separate his anxiety experiences from ordinary fear. Here is another passage from "He?"

Oh, I don't suppose you will understand!

*It's not that I'm afraid of any danger ... if a burglar were to come into the room I would kill him without turning a hair. I'm not afraid of ghosts, and I do not believe in the supernatural. I'm not afraid of the dead.... I am afraid of myself**

(de Maupassant, 1990, p. 137)

It is perfectly natural to fear a stranger entering one's room at night and not at all unusual to be afraid of ghosts, or snakes, or the dead. Humans and chimpanzees both seem to have an innate fear of dead bodies, and baby chickens appear genetically programmed to respond with fear to hawklike shadows (Goodwin, 1986). De Maupassant's agoraphobic narrator denies having these "ordinary" fears. Instead, he is afraid of the creations of his own mind—of fear itself. He is truly a victim of anxiety.

NURSINGTIP 12-1

Difference Between Anxiety and Fear

- **Anxiety** is a state wherein a person feels a strong sense of dread, frequently accompanied by physical symptoms of increased heart rate, respiratory rate, elevated blood pressure (autonomic nervous system responses), without having a specific source or reason for the emotions.
- **Fear** is a state wherein a person feels a strong sense of dread, with autonomic nervous system responses that are focused on a specific object or event—fear of a tornado, fear of surgery, fear of failing in a job.

THE EXPERIENCE OF FEAR AND ANXIETY

Both fear and anxiety are common experiences, and it seems likely that no matter how distressing the experience is, appropriate fear is necessary for individual and species survival. In 1872, Charles Darwin wrote a still-influential book called *The Expression of the Emotions in Man and Animals.* He observed that fear may have two very different functions: to increase ability to fight—"a [frightened] man or animal ... is endowed with wonderful strength, and is notoriously dangerous"; or to flee—"Fear ... soon induces ... the most violent and prolonged attempts to escape from the danger" (p. 81). Darwin also graphically described the degrees of human fear:

EXPRESSIONS OF FEAR

[The] eyes and mouth are widely opened, and the eyebrows raised. The frightened man at first stands like a statue motionless and breathless, or crouches down as if instinctively to escape observation.

The heart beats quickly and violently, so that it palpitates or knocks against the ribs ... the skin instantly becomes pale, as during incipient faintness.... That the skin is much affected under the sense of great fear, we see in the marvelous and inexplicable manner in which perspiration immediately exudes from it. This exudation is all the more remarkable, as the surface is then cold, and hence the term a cold sweat.... The hairs also on the skin stand erect; and the superficial muscles shiver ... the breathing is hurried. The salivary glands act imperfectly; the mouth becomes dry, and is often opened and shut. I have also noticed that under slight fear there is a strong tendency to yawn. One of the best-marked symptoms is the trembling of all the

*From "He?," in *The Dark Side: Tales of Terror and the Supernatural* by Guy de Maupassant, translated by A. Kellet.

muscles of the body; and this is often first seen in the lips. From this cause, and from the dryness of the mouth, the voice becomes husky or indistinct, or may altogether fail....

*As fear increases ... the heart beats wildly or may fail to act and faintness ensue; there is a death-like pallor; the breathing is labored; the wings of the nostrils are wildly dilated; there is a gasping and convulsive motion of the lips, a tremor of the hollow cheek, a gulping and catching of the throat; the uncovered and protruding eyeballs are fixed on the object of terror; or they may roll restlessly from side to side.... The pupils are said to be enormously dilated. All the muscles of the body may become rigid, or may be thrown into convulsive movements.... As fear rises to an extreme pitch, the dreadful scream of terror is heard.**

(Darwin, 1965/1872, pp. 289–292)

Autonomic Nervous System

In this striking description of fearful behavior, Darwin emphasizes the stereotyped patterns of movement and of what would now be termed responses of the autonomic nervous system. Seventy-five years after Darwin's descriptions, Walter Hess won the Nobel Prize for Physiology or Medicine demonstrating in animals that electrical stimulation of the hypothalamus can reproduce complex behavioral patterns closely resembling what animals actually do when they exhibit fear or rage (Kupfermann, 1985). From this and other work, it seems likely that fear behaviors are organized in the limbic system (the subcortical or primitive brain of which the hypothalamus is one part) and are, as Darwin surmised from observation, expressed in patterns common to many higher animals. As Darwin implied in the title of his book, the expression of emotion (which can be observed by others) is not the same as the perception of emotion (which can only be directly studied by human reports). While de Maupassant's anxious narrator must have displayed many of the physical signs of fear, his extreme distress came from his feelings and not their physical expressions.

Neurobiology of Anxiety

Given what is currently known about brain function, it seems nearly certain that the cerebral cortex must be involved in the perception of fear. Studies using **positron emission tomography** (PET scanning—a powerful tool to accurately measure blood flow patterns in the brain) suggest that this hypothesis is likely correct. A PET scanner can identify and precisely localize rapid changes in blood flow that occur as the result of various mental and emotional stimuli. When susceptible persons are made anxious during PET scanning, blood flow increases significantly both in the limbic system and in several specific areas of the cerebral cortex (Rauch, Baer, Breiten, Fischman, Manzo, Moretti, et al., 1995). Functional magnetic resonance imaging (fMRI) scanning has also been used to understand origins of anxiety and their response to treatment. In one study, persons who develop significant anxiety when they see a spider had fMRI done when they looked at pictures of a spider—both before and after a series of cognitive-behavioral treatments. Prior to treatment, and in comparison to persons who did not have spider phobia, the affected individuals had greater fMRI activity in the amygdala (part of the limbic system) and *decreased* activity in parts of the frontal cortex known to modulate or suppress anxiety. After successful treatment the pattern was reversed, leading to much more normal patterns of metabolic activity (Schienle, Schafer, Hermann, Rohrmann, & Vaitl, 2007).

From what is currently known about the neurobiology of anxiety, including the studies reported here, it seems that the anxiety experience has its origins in the limbic system or even deeper in midline brainstem structures. Limbic connections to the autonomic nervous system produce the most striking physical manifestations of anxiety: heart rate changes, pallor, sweating, and hair "standing on end." If Darwin's description is correct and postural changes (crouching, yawning, raising arms) are indeed part of the fear pattern, then they are likely directly patterned by connections from the limbic area to affected muscles. However, simultaneously with this autonomic activation and patterned muscle stimulation, neural messages from the limbic system travel through the nearby temporal lobe and up into the cortical association areas. These association areas are the brain centers in which sensory experiences are linked, joined to memory, and somehow processed as thoughts. Only the involvement of these cortical association centers allows de Maupassant's narrator to feel so vividly his "sensation of incomprehensible terror." When cortical systems act to inhibit the sensation of anxiety, limbic response is lessened, and people perceive less anxiety (Berkowitz, Coplan, Reddy, & Gorman, 2007).

While the sensation of fear has its origin in the limbic system, many of the peripheral manifestations of fear result from the release of hormonal substances (i.e., ACTH) under hypothalamic stimulations, along with activation of the autonomic nervous system via pathways also originating in the hypothalamus. Autonomic activation in turn results in release of cortecholamines (epinephrine and others) by the adrenal glands, with a corresponding rise in heart rate, cardiac contractility, and other signs of autonomic arousal. Recent studies have shown that GABA, a brain neurotransmitter that serves to inhibit the effects of glutamate, is an important factor in anxiety disorders. Many current and evolving treatments for anxiety act on brain receptors for GABA (Lydiard, 2003).

As stated earlier, fear typically occurs in response to a real-life threat or danger. While excessive fear may be self-defeating, fear is commonly an adaptive response allowing an individual to successfully avoid or face danger. In contrast, anxiety is an experience akin to fear but without a realistic source. Although perhaps the majority of anxious people can identify one or more factors that bring on their anxiety responses, most of these persons recognize that their feelings

*From *The Expressions of the Emotions in Man and Animals* by Charles Darwin, in K. Lorenz, 1965/1872, Chicago: University of Chicago Press.

of anxiety are far out of proportion to any real dangers. Both fear and anxiety are common and have likely been part of the human experience for thousands of years. The following passage from the *Book of Job* vividly describes the human experience of fear:

THE HUMAN EXPERIENCE OF FEAR

In thoughts from the visions of the night, when deep sleep falleth on men, fear came upon me, and trembling, which made all my bones to shake. Then a spirit passed before my face; the hair of my flesh stood up. It stood still, but I could not discern the form thereof: an image was before my eyes, there was silence, and I heard a voice, saying, Shall mortal man be more just than God? Shall a man be more pure than his Maker?

(*Job iv. 13*)

Within the last century, anxiety has become a topic of considerable interest to philosophers. The Danish theologian Soren Kierkegaard taught that anxiety was inescapably part of the human condition. In the last decades of the nineteenth century, the stresses of rapidly accelerating social and economic change no doubt contributed to the anxiety felt by many persons. In the first years of the twentieth century, T. S. Eliot wrote a poem that sought to capture the anxiety of a world that had seemingly become caught up in trivial daily concerns to the exclusion of larger spiritual values:

THERE WILL BE TIME

And indeed there will be time
To wonder, "Do I dare?" and, "Do I dare?"
Time to turn back and descend the stair,
With a bald spot in the middle of my hair—
(They will say: "But how his arms and legs are thin!")
Do I dare
Disturb the universe?
In a minute there is time
For decisions and revisions which a minute will reverse. . . .
Should I, after tea and cakes and ices,
Have the strength to force the moment to its crisis?
But though I have wept and fasted, wept and prayed,
Though I have seen my head (grown slightly bald) brought in upon a platter,
I am no prophet—and here's no great matter;
I have seen the moment of my greatness flicker,
And I have seen the eternal Footman hold my coat, and snicker,
And in short, I was afraid. . . .
I grow old . . . I grow old. . . .
I shall wear the bottoms of my trousers rolled.
*Shall I part my hair behind? Do I dare to eat a peach?**

(*Eliot, 1970, pp. 3–4*)

The narrator of Eliot's poem is overwhelmed by anxiety in the course of an uneventful life:

For I have known them all already, known them all—
Have known the evenings, mornings, afternoons,
I have measured out my life with coffee spoons. . . . *

(*Eliot, 1970, p. 6*)

Eating a peach, parting his hair, asking a woman to marry him (the apparent subject of the poem)—these are all decisions that are too complex for the anxious Prufrock, decisions "that lead you to an overwhelming question . . . Do I dare disturb the universe?" And if he did dare propose marriage, and if in response she, "settling a pillow by her head, should say, 'That is not what I meant at all. That is not it, at all: . . . '" Prufrock asks, "Would it have been worth it? . . . " and confesses "in short, I was afraid." (Eliot, 1970). For J. Alfred Prufrock, Job's fear and trembling before God has become anguished indecision over a life measured by nothing larger than coffee spoons.

More than a generation later, in and just after the closing days of World War II, W. H. Auden wrote a much longer poem called "The Age of Anxiety." Anxiety was also a central theme in the philosophy of existentialism, another creation of the years following World War II. Existentialists claimed that a person's major philosophical goal ought to be the choice of a life reflecting authentic personal and social commitment. Imperfect political structures and the fallibility of human nature inevitably made such choices difficult and anxiety-ridden. Seen from the standpoint of more recent history—Hiroshima, political assassinations, wars, refugees, ecological disasters—it is hard to see how any modern life could be lived in awareness and yet without anxiety. Surely the present era is, in Auden's memorable words, an "Age of Anxiety."

Without anxiety, according to Kierkegaard and other modern thinkers, humankind would lose its ability to find both spiritual direction and political freedom. Some psychiatrists disagree strongly, arguing that while mild fear is useful for negotiating truly dangerous situations, virtually any degree of anxiety is self-defeating (Goodwin, 1986). Whatever one's philosophical beliefs about the need for some anxiety in life, few would claim that the crippling anxiety suffered by the narrator of de Maupassant's "He?" or the perhaps milder anxiety affecting Eliot's Prufrock serves any useful human purpose. At least in its extremes, anxiety clearly results in a serious limiting of human potential. Multiple studies document severely impaired quality of life in persons suffering from anxiety (Mendlowicz & Stein, 2000; Olatunji, Cisler, & Tolin, 2007).

*From "The Love Song of J. Alfred Prufrock," *Collected Poems 1919–1962* (pp. 3–7) by T. S. Eliot, 1970, New York: Harcourt Brace & Company.

TABLE 12-1 Stages of Anxiety

Mild	Tension of day-to-day living; individual has an alert perceptual field; can motivate learning. *Example*: anxiety felt when missing the bus.
Moderate	Focus is on immediate concerns; perceptual field is narrowed; individual exhibits selective inattention. *Example*: anxiety felt when taking an exam.
Severe	Focus is on specific detail; perceptual field is greatly reduced. *Example*: anxiety felt when witnessing a car accident.
Panic	Individual experiences a sense of awe, dread, and/or terror; individual loses control; there is a disorganization of the personality. *Example*: anxiety felt when experiencing an earthquake and being unable to cope

STAGES OF ANXIETY

Because anxiety exists as part of each person's everyday existence and also exists as a distinct psychiatric condition, there is general agreement that a continuum of anxiety responses exists ranging from mild anxiety to a panic state. These stages are presented in Table 12-1. In mild anxiety, the person experiences day-to-day tensions and is alert, with an increased perceptual field. In moderate anxiety, the person focuses only on the immediate concerns, with a narrowed perceptual field. In severe anxiety, the person's perceptual field is greatly reduced and the individual focuses on a specific detail. In a panic state, the person has feelings of dread or terror and is unable to control his behaviors.

ANXIETY DISORDERS

The *Diagnostic and Statistical Manual*, third edition (DSM-III), and its successors, DSM-IV (American Psychiatric Association, 1994) and DSM-IV-TR (American Psychiatric Association, 2000), made what was then a radical claim: that it was possible to categorize several varieties of anxiety as psychiatric disorders, distinct both among themselves and from "normal" existential anxiety. It is important for the nurse to be familiar with these disorders. The DSM provides the current definitions for the distinction between anxiety in health and anxiety in illness; that is, it is recognized that all persons experience anxiety, but it is also recognized that some individuals experience such severe anxiety that it interferes with their ability to function in daily life. Thus, there exists anxiety in illness—the anxiety disorders. There is a general category of anxiety disorders, and there are 14 subtypes that have been identified. Six of these are particularly important, distinct, and common. These subtypes of anxiety disorder are summarized in Table 12-2 and are discussed next.

GENERALIZED ANXIETY DISORDER

The primary symptom of **Generalized Anxiety Disorder** is, not surprisingly, excessive anxiety or dread. Clients with Generalized Anxiety Disorder typically recognize that their symptoms are out of proportion to any real threat. According to DSM-IV-TR definitions, anxiety is considered excessive when it is present more days than not for a period of six months or more. Anxiety is "generalized" if it focuses on a variety of life events or activities. The focus of anxiety cannot be solely on certain specific topics, such as gaining weight or fearing illness. Persons anxious only about their weight may have eating disorders, and persons anxious only about their health may have hypochondriasis (one of the somatoform disorders). To meet DSM-IV-TR criteria for a disorder, the anxiety must both be difficult to control and cause significant distress or impairment

The Scream by Munch

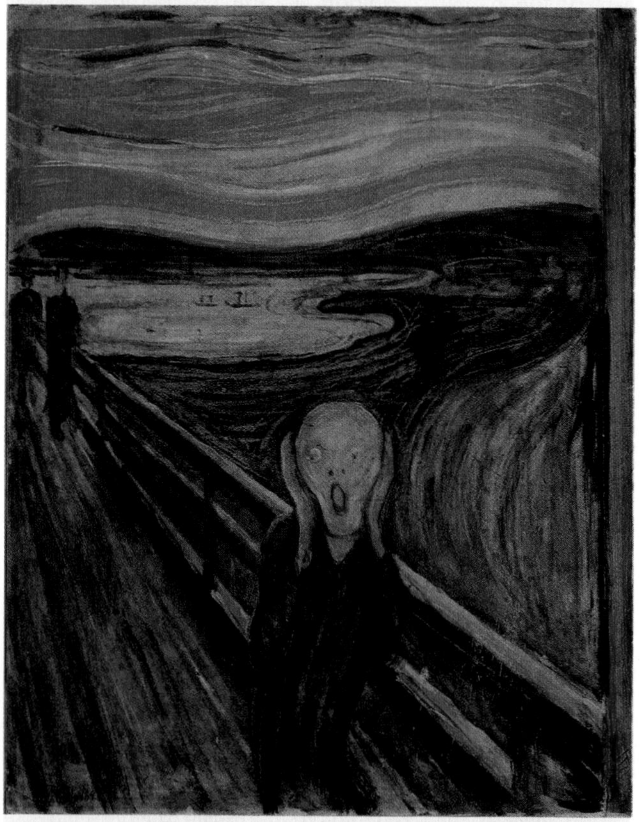

Almost an icon of anxiety, this work reflects the life experiences of a man who was haunted by mental illness—both his own and his sister's. Caught between land and sea, and isolated from the only other humans in sight, the screaming figure occupies a landscape whose unstable shapes and colors are both the source and the expression of unbearable anxiety.

TABLE 12-2 Summary of Major Anxiety Disorders

DISORDER	DEFINITION	SYMPTOMS	PREVALENCE (PERCENTAGE IN ADULT U.S. POPULATION)
Generalized Anxiety Disorder	Anxiety focused on a variety of life events or activities	Restlessness, fatigue, difficulty in concentrating, irritability, muscle tension, sleep disturbances	5
Panic Disorder	Discrete episodes of intense anxiety that begin abruptly and reach a peak within about 10 minutes	Palpitations, sweating, trembling, shortness of breath, sensation of choking, chest pain, nausea, dizziness, fear of losing control, fear of dying, sense of altered reality	6
Agoraphobia	Acute anxiety in crowds; fear of being alone; fear in any physical setting from which the individual may have trouble escaping	Intense feelings of anxiety and/or fear of losing control that results in either refraining from going out or avoiding situations that may bring about anxiety	5
Phobia	Persistent, excessive, or unreasonable fear of a specific object or situation (examples: elevators, airplanes, dogs, spiders, injections, tunnels)	Fears that interfere markedly with life activities	10
Obsessive-Compulsive Disorder	Occurrence of recurrent thoughts, images, and/or impulses that are intrusive and inappropriate, causing anxiety (obsession) and coupled with repetitive actions or behaviors performed to reduce the anxiety (compulsions)	Individual recognizes that his thoughts and/or behaviors are unreasonable; for example, the person who wishes to stop checking and rechecking an alarm clock at night but feels unable to stop the repetitive behavior	2.6
Post-Traumatic Stress Disorder	After exposure to a significant, life-threatening event, the experience of anxiety symptoms in which the event is reexperienced through recollections	Recurrent recollections, dreams, hallucinatory-like flashbacks, impairment of social functioning	3–58 (for person exposed to serious danger)

in functioning. Finally, DSM-IV-TR requires that certain specific symptoms be present and not be caused by medications, drugs, or illness. These symptoms include three or more of the following: restlessness, easy fatigue, difficulty concentrating, irritability, muscle tension, and sleep disturbance. When symptoms are due to another psychiatric illness such as depression, Generalized Anxiety Disorder is usually not diagnosed (American Psychiatric Association, 2000).

Epidemiology

It should be evident from the preceding description that Generalized Anxiety Disorder is very much a "diagnosis of exclusion." Clients are most commonly given this diagnosis when they have disabling symptoms of anxiety that do not fit any other pattern. In the Epidemiological Catchment Area study, 4% to 7% of individuals had met DSM-III criteria for Generalized Anxiety Disorder at some time in their lives (Blazer, Hughes, George, Swartz, & Boyer, 1991). Although the DSM-IV-TR criteria for diagnosis have changed somewhat, 5% may still be the best estimate for the lifetime incidence of generalized anxiety. The more recent European Study of the Epidemiology of Mental Disorders reported that about 2% of men and 4% of women had ever experienced Generalized Anxiety Disorder, based on a sample of about 20,000 in six Western European countries (Alonso,

Angermeyer, Bernert, Bruffaerts, Brugha, Bryson, et al., 2004). Unlike persons with many psychiatric diagnoses (including a number discussed in this chapter), those with generalized anxiety often present in significant distress from their symptoms, which are frequently made harder to tolerate by a variety of social and situational stressors. For example, an individual experiencing daily severe anxiety may find it exceedingly difficult to participate in committee meetings required at work. If so, that person may seek treatment because the anxiety causes difficulty in job performance.

PANIC DISORDER

Panic Disorder is a condition characterized by discrete episodes of intense anxiety that begin abruptly and reach a peak within 10 minutes. They include at least four of a set of specified symptoms. These symptoms include palpitations or rapid heart rate, sweating, trembling, shortness of breath, sensation of choking, chest pain, nausea, dizziness, fear of losing control, fear of dying, numbness or tingling, chills or hot flashes, and some sense of altered reality. There is often a strong wish to run away or otherwise escape from the situation that provoked the attack. Compared to Generalized Anxiety Disorder, the anxiety of Panic Disorder is very much more severe and strikingly episodic. Most persons who experience panic attacks have little or no residual anxiety between attacks. In some individuals, the panic attacks are reproducibly provoked by exposure to certain stimuli (e.g., seeing a snake). In others, they may appear "out of the blue" or be most likely to occur in specific settings (such as the dentist's office).

Many years ago, William Leonard, a professor of English at the University of Wisconsin, described his personal experiences with Panic Disorder. In the following excerpt from his book-length description, he emphasizes both the severity of the anxiety and the rapidity with which symptoms develop (both severity and rapid onset are highly characteristic of Panic Disorder).

LET ME ASSUME

Let me assume that I am walking down University Drive by the Lake. I am a normal man for the first quarter of a mile; for the next hundred yards I am in a mild state of dread, controllable and controlled; for the next twenty yards in an acute state of dread, yet controlled; for the next ten, in an anguish of terror that hasn't reached the crisis of explosion; and in a half-dozen steps more I am in as fierce a panic of isolation from help and home and of immediate death as a man overboard in mid-Atlantic or on his window-ledge far up in a skyscraper with flames lapping his shoulders. The reader who can't understand why I have not whistled or laughed or ordered [the panic attacks] off my psychic premises, or who thinks that I must be grossly exaggerating a mere normal discomfort, like the initial dread in a dentist's chair, is not the reader for whom I am writing one line of this book.... I know that my [panic attacks] at their worst approach any limits of terror that the human mind is capable of in the actual presence of death in its most horrible forms. That I have never fainted away or died under them is due to two factors: first, my physical vitality; and, second, my skill in devising escapes.... The fools say nothing ever happened from one of these [attacks]—so why worry. Nothing ever happened? Well, here is what happens always. First, the [attack] happens—as well say, nothing happens if a

RESEARCH Highlight 12–1

Buddhist Counseling for Symptoms of Anxiety

STUDY PROBLEM/PURPOSE

To describe the effectiveness of a counseling method based on Buddhist principles for Thai clients presenting with symptoms of anxiety.

METHODS

Twenty-one patients presenting with symptoms of anxiety to psychiatric care in Thailand received two sessions of counseling based on Buddhist principles. The clients were part of a culture in which Buddhist beliefs and principles are widely accepted. Anxiety was measured on a standardized scale, and the researchers recorded the amount of antianxiety medication prescribed.

FINDINGS

In a one-month follow-up, those receiving Buddhist "mindfulness" counseling reported less symptoms and required less medication, though there was no formal control group with which to compare outcomes.

IMPLICATIONS

The authors felt that Buddhist counseling had a potential benefit on these individuals' well-being. This study may suggest different paradigms for counseling treatment of anxiety that may be shown effective, especially among persons whose cultural orientation is not Western. The concept of "mindfulness" has found increasing acceptance among Western psychiatric practitioners and may, if further studies are supportive, be usefully incorporated into therapies that are not explicitly Buddhist in content.

Source: "The psychological impact of Buddhist counseling for patients suffering from symptoms of anxiety 2008," S. Rungreangkulkij and W. Wongtakee, *Archives of Psychiatric Nursing*, *22*(3): 127–134. *Journal of the Association of Nurses in AIDS Care*, 14(2), 2–29.

*red-hot iron is run down the throat, even though it should miraculously leave no after-effects. . . . Second, the [attack] leaves me always far more exposed to [panic attacks] for weeks or months [and] increases my fear of the Fear.**

(Leonard, 1927, pp. 66–71)

Leonard's "fear of the Fear" is also a very characteristic aspect of Panic Disorder. Persons who suffer panic attacks often live in severe fear that the attacks will recur, and they often change their lives significantly in an effort to minimize recurrence. Recognizing this feature of panic attacks, DSM-IV-TR defines the diagnosis of Panic Disorder, which in general can be made when panic attacks recur in association with worry about future attacks and/or behavior change related to these attacks. The diagnosis of Panic Disorder also requires that no other physical or psychological condition be present that better explains the panic attacks.

Epidemiology

The Epidemiologic Catchment Area study found that panic attacks occur in about 6% of persons (Robins & Regier, 1991). Multiple studies have demonstrated that between 1.5% and 3.5% of unselected individuals experience Panic Disorder during their lifetimes (American Psychiatric Association, 2000; Alonso et al., 2004). Clearly, only about half of persons with panic attacks have Panic Disorder; most of the rest have other anxiety disorders in which panic attacks may be seen. There is a strong association between Panic Disorder and Major Depressive Disorder (Chapter 16), and over half of persons with Panic Disorder also suffer from significant depression (American Psychiatric Association, 2000). There is also a significant correlation between Panic Disorder and substance abuse. In many cases, the abuse problem may occur because individuals with Panic Disorder treat their symptoms with alcohol or other substances. Panic Disorder tends to occur in relatively young persons, with onset common some time between adolescence and the mid-thirties. There is probably a genetic component to Panic Disorder in that persons are more likely to develop the disorder if their identical twin also has it. There is also a significant increased risk for Panic Disorder in children of individuals with the condition.

Persons with Panic Disorder often do not consult mental health practitioners about their symptoms. Therefore, the diagnosis of Panic Disorder is never made or is made only after many years of suffering. Individuals commonly present to acute health care facilities (often emergency rooms) complaining of physical symptoms: palpitations, chest pain, shortness of breath, faintness, dizziness. Affected individuals are frequently evaluated repeatedly for cardiac, pulmonary, or neurological conditions, and they often undergo complex workups for endocrine problems: thyroid disease or pheochromocytoma. There is almost certainly a link between physical factors and panic attacks, because attacks can often be reproduced by hyperventilation.

The natural history of Panic Disorder is quite variable. However, three stages in the development of Panic Disorder have been described (Kanton, 1989). In the first stage, the panic attack is experienced after a variety of stressors and most often occurs during a routine task (such as driving a car). In the second stage, the individual begins to live in fear that he may have another panic attack, and out of fear, he may avoid an increasing number of events associated with prior panic attacks. Lastly, in the third stage, the person may develop intense avoidant behaviors and refuse to participate in social events. This condition is called **agoraphobia** and refers to a fear of going out in public places. Most individuals with Panic Disorder will improve over long-term follow-up, but about 20% will continue to have the kind of ongoing moderate to severe disability that Leonard reports in the description of his own symptoms. Some studies have indicated that persons with Panic Disorder have a much higher risk of suicide than does the nonaffected population (Weissman, Klerman, Markowitz, & Ouelette, 1989).

> **NURSINGALERT 12-1**
>
> **Panic Disorder and Suicide Risk**
>
> Persons with Panic Disorder have a high risk of suicide; they think about death, feel as though they want to die, and consider or attempt suicide more than do individuals with any other psychiatric condition, including depression. Generalized Anxiety Disorder and Obsessive-Compulsive Disorder also have elevated risks for suicide. The combination of any of these three anxiety disorders with Depression, Schizophrenia, substance misuse, or Post-traumatic Stress Disorder may further increase suicide risk (Hawgood & De Leo, 2008).

AGORAPHOBIA

Only a few years before de Maupassant wrote the story with which this chapter began, the German neurologist Karl Westphal described a group of persons who became acutely anxious both when in crowds and when walking through deserted areas. Westphal called this condition *agoraphobia*, a Greek term meaning "fear of public places." More than 100 years later, this term is still in use for a strikingly common and often severe anxiety disorder. In current usage, Agoraphobia is a description applied to persons who are afraid of crowded public areas. The DSM-IV-TR definition is actually somewhat broader and includes individuals who become fearful in any physical setting from which they might have trouble escaping or getting help in the event of an acute panic attack. Some agoraphobics—like de Maupassant's

*From *The Locomotive-God* by William Leonard, 1927. In L. Y. Rabkin (Ed.), *Psychopathology and Literature* (pp. 66–71), San Francisco: Chandler.

narrator—are afraid of being home alone. More commonly, the opposite situation occurs: Agoraphobic persons are afraid to leave their houses even if, as they leave, they have to walk through deserted (rather than crowded) areas. Since leaving home often results in panic attacks, many agoraphobic individuals are rendered virtually homebound by their fear.

Many agoraphobic persons stay away from public places because of fears they will do something embarrassing (scream uncontrollably, commit a sexual indiscretion) or be dangerous (assault someone). People with Agoraphobia do not actually behave in this way; however, they typically fear each of these consequences with great intensity. Goodwin describes some of the ways that agoraphobics use to mitigate their anxiety to maintain social functioning:

> *Sometimes just carrying an umbrella helps. Other inanimate objects reported to provide relief include canes, shopping baskets on wheels, a bicycle pushed down the street, a folded newspaper carried under the arm.... Agoraphobics almost always are more comfortable in dark places than in sunlight.... If they go to theatres at all, they find an aisle seat near the back to make a fast getaway if necessary ... the most reliable fear-reducer is a trusted companion. Many agoraphobics only venture out of the house when accompanied by someone they know and trust: a husband, friend, child, or even a dog.**
>
> (Goodwin, 1986, pp. 147–148)

NURSINGTIP 12-2

Agoraphobia: Opposing Symptoms, Single Cause

- "Should I ever leave home, which is improbable, I will with much delight, accept your invitation." (Dickinson, 1955)
- "I do not want to be alone any longer at night.... But if there were two of us in the place...." (de Maupassant, 1903/1989)

The various symptoms of Agoraphobia can sometimes seem contradictory. In Agoraphobia, the primary psychological need is to avoid panic; consequently, some persons stay fearfully at home while others experience an inability to remain alone at home. Although these symptoms might seem so opposite to each other that they must have different diagnoses, they do truly have a common root. The similarity comes from underlying motivation rather than behavior, in each case the intense desire to avoid recurrent panic episodes.

Recall that in the opening literary selection, "He?" de Maupassant's narrator plans marriage to a woman he has barely met because any company is preferable to the fear he suffers when home alone. There are some symptoms of Agoraphobia that seem contradictory. The accompanying Nursing Tip helps to explain that differing and even opposite symptoms have a common root.

Many agoraphobics never seek medical or psychiatric treatment for their symptoms and accept a measure of social disability from them. The famous nineteenth-century American poet Emily Dickinson led a remarkably homebound life, which it appears was almost certainly caused by severe Agoraphobia (Garbowsky, 1989). Many of Dickinson's poems seem to describe experiences of intense anxiety, very likely panic attacks. Here, for example, is one poem, "I Felt a Funeral, in my Brain," that might be taken to describe the depersonalization and fear of a typical panic attack:

I FELT A FUNERAL, IN MY BRAIN

I felt a Funeral, in my Brain,
And Mourners to and fro
Kept treading, treading, till it seemed
That Sense was breaking through.
And when they all were seated,
A Service, like a Drum
Kept beating, beating, till I thought
My Mind was going numb.
And then I heard them lift a Box
And Creak across my Soul
With those same Boots of Lead, again,
Then Space began to toll,
As all the Heavens were a Bell,
And Being, but an Ear,
And I, and Silence, some strange Race
Wrecked, solitary, here
And then a Plank in Reason broke,
And I dropped down, and down
And hit a World, at every plunge,
*And Finished knowing—then.**

(Dickinson, 1955, pp. 199–200)

Yet another poem suggests an almost puzzled response to some kind of mental catastrophe, the puzzlement perhaps reflecting Goodwin's (1986) comment that "agoraphobics usually have difficulty explaining why they are afraid" (p. 146):

*From *Anxiety*, by D. W. Goodwin, 1986, New York: Oxford University Press.

*From *The Poems of Emily Dickinson*, edited by T. H. Johnson, 1955, Cambridge: Belknap Press of Harvard University.

I FELT A CLEAVAGE IN MY MIND

I felt a cleavage in my Mind
As if my brain had split;
I tried to match it, seam by seam,
But could not make them fit.
The thought behind I strove to join
Unto the thought before,
But sequence ravelled out of reach
*Like Balls upon a floor.**

(*Dickinson, 1955, p. 358*)

Garbowsky has made a strong case that Dickinson suffered from both Panic Disorder and Agoraphobia, taking the title of her book from a fragment of yet another of Dickinson's poems in which Dickinson seems to describe feeling trapped within a "House without the Door":

Doom is the House without the Door—
'Tis entered from the Sun—
And then the Ladder's thrown away,
*Because Escape—is done.**

(*Dickinson, 1955, p. 358*)

As psychiatrist John Cody writes in a Foreword to Garbowsky's book (Garbowsky, 1989), "The difficult question is not whether there was a diagnosable [psychological] infirmity present—for it is clear that there was—but what was its essential nature." Garbowsky bases her case for Agoraphobia not just on the poetry, but also on the details of Emily Dickinson's unusual life. At age 23, Dickinson wrote to a friend who had invited her to visit, "I thank you Abiah, but I don't go from home, unless emergency leads me by the hand, and then I do it obstinately, and draw back if I can. Should I ever leave home, which is improbable, I will with much delight, accept your invitation" (Garbowsky, 1989, p. 37). In reality, she did make several brief trips in her 20s and 30s, but by the time she reached age 40, she had been completely housebound for five years and wrote to an admirer of her poetry: "I do not cross my Father's ground to any House or town" (Garbowsky, 1989, p. 29). Only after Dickinson died 20 years later did her sister discover the thousands of poems written in her agoraphobic seclusion. All exceedingly brief, some of these are among the most memorable in the English language.

While Agoraphobia likely created for Emily Dickinson the conditions under which she would become one of the nineteenth century's greatest poets, for most persons it creates nothing other than a life of misery. Agoraphobia is among the most disabling and difficult to treat of all the anxiety disorders (Goodwin, 1986). Unfortunately, cases such as Dickinson's, lasting a lifetime and leading to total confinement in the house, still occur with some frequency.

Epidemiology

There is a very strong linkage between Panic Disorder and Agoraphobia. In some studies, 95% of individuals with Agoraphobia also have Panic Disorder, and up to half of all individuals with Panic Disorder also suffer from Agoraphobia. There is considerable variability in estimates of the prevalence of agoraphobia. The U.S. comorbidity study found a lifetime prevalence of nearly 7% (Magee, Eaton, Wittchen, McGonagle, & Kessler. 1996), while the more recent European Study of the Epidemiology of Mental Disorders found that Agoraphobia occurred in about 1% of individuals (Alonso et al., 2004). Symptoms may develop gradually over years or, as in the story told by de Maupassant's narrator, begin suddenly and then persist.

Phobias

A **phobia** is a persistent fear of a specific object or situation. The fear occurs whenever the phobic individual is brought in contact with that object or situation. Phobias are categorized as Social Phobia (e.g., profound fear of public speaking) and Specific Phobia. Social Phobias are also referred to as Social Anxiety Disorders. Social Anxiety Disorder may be the most common phobia, with lifetime incidences up to 14% of the population. It is a phobic disorder where a person experiences severe anxiety when under social stress, such as speaking or performing in public, meeting new people, taking tests, or similar situations. Nursing interventions can include social skills training and exposure to social situations. Psychiatric treatments include medications and cognitive behavioral therapy (Sareen & Stein, 2000). Specific Phobia commonly involves fear of such things as airplane travel, high or exposed places, closed places, animals (often snakes or spiders), or seeing blood. To meet DSM-IV-TR diagnostic criteria for Specific Phobia, the fear must be excessive or unreasonable, must be recognized as excessive or unreasonable by the phobic individual, and must result in significant social, occupational, or academic disruption. As the narrator observes in Erica Jong's novel *Fear of Flying*, multiple phobias are not at all uncommon:

FEAR OF FLYING

*Oh, I have phobias about practically everything you can think of: plane crashes, clap, swallowing ground glass, botulism, Arabs, breast cancer, leukemia, Nazis, melanoma.**

(*Jong, 1973, pp. 253–254*)

*From *The Poems of Emily Dickinson*, edited by T. H. Johnson, 1955, Cambridge: Belknap Press of Harvard University.

*From *Fear of Flying* by Erica Mann Jong.

While most of these phobias get little attention elsewhere in the book, the novel's opening pages vividly describe intense fear of air travel:

> *My husband grabbed my hand therapeutically at the moment of takeoff. "Christ—it's like ice," he said. He ought to know the symptoms by now since he's held my hand on lots of other flights. My fingers (and toes) turn to ice, my stomach leaps upward into my rib cage, the temperature in the tip of my nose drops to the same level as the temperature in my fingers, my nipples stand up and salute the inside of my bra (or in this case, dress—since I'm not wearing a bra), and for one screaming minute my heart and the engines correspond as we attempt to prove again that the laws of aerodynamics are not the flimsy superstitions which, in my heart of hearts, I know they are.... I happen to be convinced that only my own concentration (and that of my mother—who always seems to expect her children to die in a plane crash) keeps this bird aloft. I congratulate myself on every successful takeoff, but not too enthusiastically because it's also part of my personal religion that the minute you grow overconfident and really relax about the flight, the plane crashes instantly.**
>
> *(Jong, 1973, pp. 2–3)*

Terrified as she is, Jong's narrator seems to find herself on airplanes fairly frequently, and not always in her husband's company. By requiring that truly phobic fears interfere markedly with life activities, DSM-IV-TR attempts to distinguish between common fears and true phobias.

NURSING TIP 12-3

Social Anxiety Disorder

Social Anxiety Disorder is a phobic disorder in which a person experiences severe anxiety when under social stress.

- Hospitals, emergency rooms, clinics, and other health care institutions are places that put many people under social stress. Nurses should be cognizant of the fact that many persons are unable to speak up or ask questions in our health care environments.
- Nurses should assess each client's level of anxiety or stress in interactions and assist those who are anxious or intimidated to make their needs known.

*From *Fear of Flying* by Erica Mann Jong.

Epidemiology

While Jong (more accurately, her novel's narrator) may qualify for a DSM-IV-TR diagnosis of Specific Phobia, millions of other individuals do. It is estimated that about 10% of Americans have symptoms of Specific Phobia during any year (American Psychiatric Association, 2000). Available data on one specific phobia, fear of flying among airline passengers, indicate that the incidence may be even higher. Researchers estimate the incidence of fear of flying to be as high as 10–40% of the adult population (VanGerwen & Dieskstra, 2000). Epidemiological studies bear out common stereotypes in showing that women are about twice as likely to have symptoms of Specific Phobia as are men (Eaton, Dyman, & Weissman, 1991). Phobias are notoriously private, and clients with phobic disorders rarely disclose their symptoms, sometimes denying them when asked directly. Goodwin observes:

> *Many people are embarrassed about their phobias and often keep them hidden from even their closest friends. This habit of secrecy may persist even when they see doctors and see them for psychiatric reasons. It is not unusual in psychiatric practice to see a patient for a long period and then have him describe, almost in passing, a phobia that has plagued him for years. In routine questioning of patients, phobias are not even asked about. Many nonpsychiatrists seem unaware even of their existence.*
>
> *(Goodwin, 1986, p. 125)*

Most phobias begin in early adulthood, typically before the age of 30. Animal phobias commonly begin even earlier, often in childhood. While phobic individuals sometimes become adept at avoiding situations that provoke their phobias, in many cases such avoidance is impossible. Elevators, cars, airplanes, dogs, spiders, injections, tunnels—all common foci of phobic anxiety—are remarkably hard to avoid in modern life. In most cases, repeated exposure significantly diminishes the anxiety brought on by the feared situation; in such cases, the phobia may vanish or at least recede to manageable proportions. Follow-up studies suggest that most phobias beginning in adolescence will be cured or much improved within five years (Goodwin, 1986). Phobias that begin later or persist into middle age tend to cause more difficulties with social functioning and may even worsen with time. Many individuals with Specific Phobia can maintain functionality by managing either to cure the disorder via continued exposure or to adapt to their anxiety and avoid the specific object.

OBSESSIVE-COMPULSIVE DISORDER

Persons with Obsessive-Compulsive Disorder suffer from a combination of obsessions and compulsions. "**Obsessions**

Vertigo

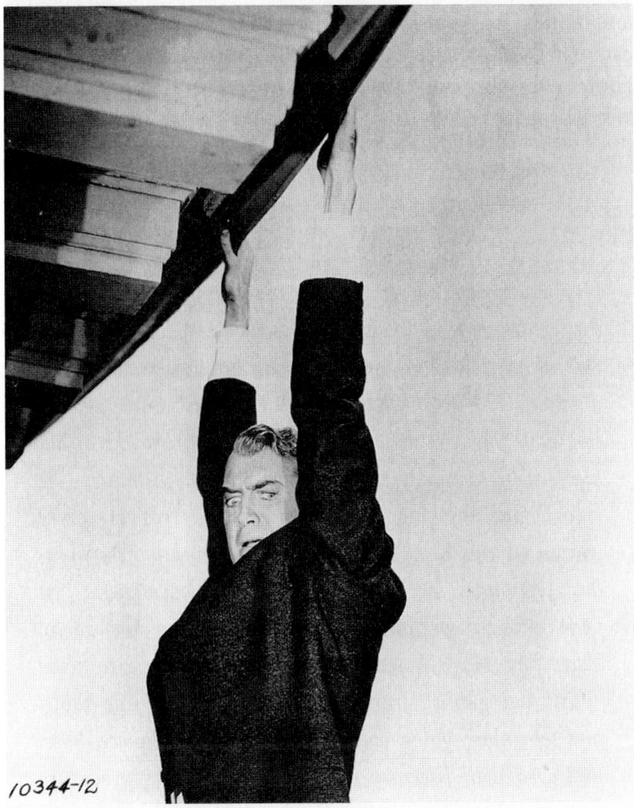

Source: Paramount/The Kobal Collection

In this movie the main character experiences danger in a chase episode involving a friend's fatal fall. He is forced to retire from police work due to his fear of heights—acrophobia.

are recurrent thoughts, images, or impulses that are experienced as intrusive and inappropriate and that cause marked anxiety or distress" (American Psychiatric Association, 2000, p. 457). Common obsessions include fear of self-contamination (becoming infected by touching something or shaking hands), fear that one has forgotten to do something important (such as lock a door or turn off an oven), or a need to have things in one's life (e.g., chairs in a room) in a particular physical arrangement. "**Compulsions** are repetitive behaviors ... or mental acts ... the goal of which is to prevent or reduce anxiety or distress" (American Psychiatric Association, 2000, p. 457). Persons who experience obsessions often find relief from these via repetitive ritualistic actions or compulsions. "For example, individuals with obsessions about being contaminated may reduce their mental distress by washing their hands until their skin is raw; individuals distressed by obsessions about having left a door unlocked may be driven to check the lock every few minutes" (American Psychiatric Association, 2000). While obsessions and compulsions are often experienced by the same individual, Obsessive-Compulsive Disorder refers to individuals who exhibit either obsessions or compulsions or both. In addition, individuals with this diagnosis recognize that their thoughts and/or behaviors are unreasonable.

In a thoughtful discussion of the challenges of practicing obstetrics in areas of the world with very high rates of human immunodeficiency virus (HIV) infection among young women, Douwe Verkuyl observed:

> *Doctors have their own problems and private risks like everybody else and they lose colleagues and acquire extra family responsibilities. Professionally it is difficult to keep up morale when there are tragedies all around and to see the improvements in health indicators of a few years ago wiped out. Needle accidents are more than a 100 times riskier than in most of the first world where they are already cause for serious discussion. Tinkering with your car or even playing sport becomes dangerous because a resulting abrasion might be splashed by blood during the next breech delivery or soaked via a small puncture in a (re-sterilised) glove.*
>
> *Detecting a fungal infection between your toes, an infected mosquito bite, or an aphthous ulcer in your mouth brings on a cold sweat—and empathy with patients who do not want to be tested.**
>
> (Verkuyl, 1995, pp. 293–296)

Although worries of contamination through touching unclean surfaces are common in Obsessive-Compulsive Disorder, it is hard to pass Verkuyl's concerns off as unrealistic anxiety. Practicing obstetrics in Zimbabwe probably is dangerous, and it is likely that any reasonable health care professional would have justifiable anxiety about becoming HIV infected. When concerns are in proportion to risk, the DSM-IV-TR criteria for Obsessive-Compulsive Disorder are not met. Often, however, the fear of contamination greatly exceeds any real risk, a situation well illustrated by the following biographical excerpts from the life and writings of the late Howard Hughes.

NURSING TIP 12-4

- Clients exhibiting compulsions are using the compulsive behaviors to relieve anxiety.
- Do not take away the compulsive rituals (unless they are dangerous) until the client has some other method in place to deal with the anxiety.

*Reprinted with permission from Elsevier (*The Lancet*, Practicing obstetrics and gynecology in areas with a high prevalence of HIV infection by D. A. A. Verkuyl 1995, Vol. 346, pp. 293–296).

Lady Macbeth at the Oregon Shakespeare Festival

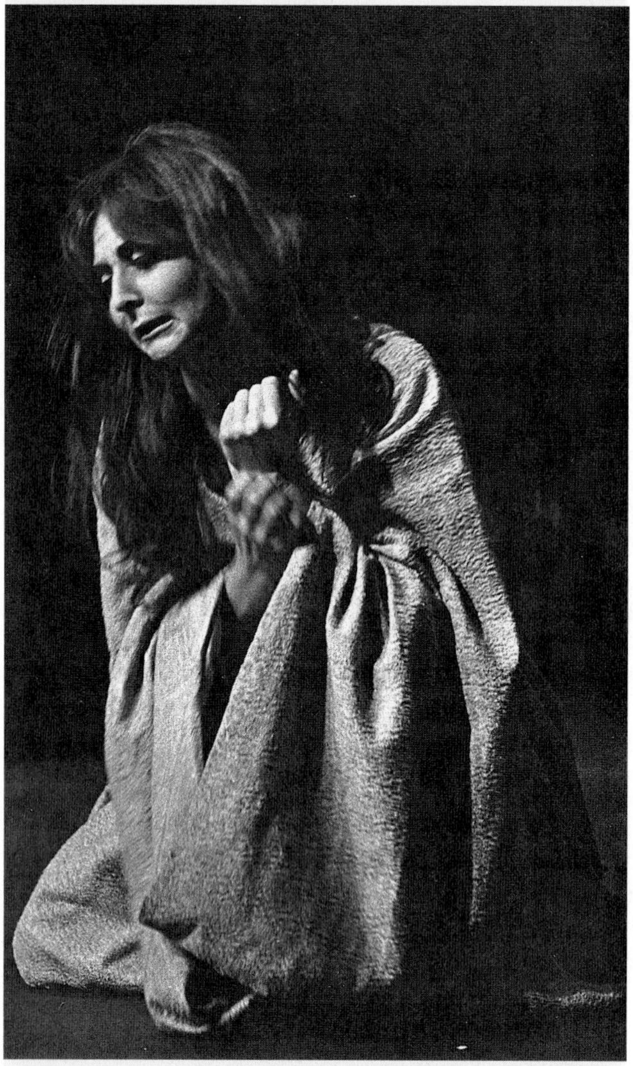

Courtesy of Oregon Shakespeare Festival. Martha J. Tippin as *Lady Macbeth* in the 1971 production of Macbeth at the Oregon Shakespeare Festival. Photographer: Carolyn Mason Jones, Director: Philip Davidson, Costume Designer: Jean Shultz Davidson, Scenic Designer: Richard L. Hay, Lighting Designer: Steven A. Maze.

"Out, damned spot! Out, I say." Lady Macbeth feels guilty for her role in a man's murder. This guilt results in extreme anxiety, and is displayed through Obsessive-Compulsive Behavior. In this scene from Act V, Scene 1, she demonstrates compulsive handwashing—as if to cleanse herself of the deed.

Howard Hughes was one of the most successful and unusual Americans of the twentieth century. Born in 1905, Hughes became a daring airplane pilot, the holder of numerous transcontinental and trans-Atlantic speed records, and, ultimately, the owner of several airlines. He also became a prominent Hollywood director, producer, and movie studio owner. Despite extraordinary wealth and fame (for years he was regarded as the world's richest man), his later life was lived in total isolation and was completely dominated by symptoms of Obsessive-Compulsive Disorder.

HOWARD HUGHES

[By] December 24, 1958, his fifty-third birthday ... Hughes spent almost all his time sitting naked in ... the center of the living room—an area he called the "germ-free zone" ... watching one motion picture after another. The furniture had been pushed back against the walls and the floor was piled high with stacks of old film cans, magazines, and newspapers. Although he rarely read anything, Hughes insisted on receiving every edition of the Los Angeles dailies. As newspapers accumulated, aides stacked them so as to leave aisles just wide enough for one person, criss-crossing the room. Each day Hughes painstakingly used Kleenex to wipe "dust and germs" from his chair, ottoman, side table, and telephone, going over the earpiece, mouthpiece, base, and cord with Kleenex, repeating the cleaning procedure again and again, tossing the used tissues onto a pile behind his chair.

... He dictated a torrent of memoranda aimed at preventing the "backflow" or "back transmission" of germs to him. In one, three pages long and single-spaced, he explained how he wanted a can of fruit opened: "The equipment used in connection with this operation will consist of the following items: 1 unopened newspaper, 1 sterile can opener, 1 large sterile plate, 1 sterile fork, 1 sterile spoon, 2 sterile brushes, 2 bars of soap, sterile paper towels."

Hughes outlined nine steps for opening the can: preparing a table, procuring a fruit can, washing of can, drying the can, processing the hands, opening the can, removing fruit from can, fallout rules while around can, and conclusion of operation. Hughes detailed how each step was to be accomplished. In Step No. 3, "Washing of Can," he wrote:

The man in charge then turns the valve in the bathtub on, using his bare hands to do so. He also adjusts the water temperature so that it is not too hot nor too cold. He then takes one of the brushes, and using one of the bars of soap, creates a good lather, and then scrubs the can from a point two inches below the top of the can. He should first soak and remove the label, and then brush the cylindrical part of the can over and over until all particles

The Aviator

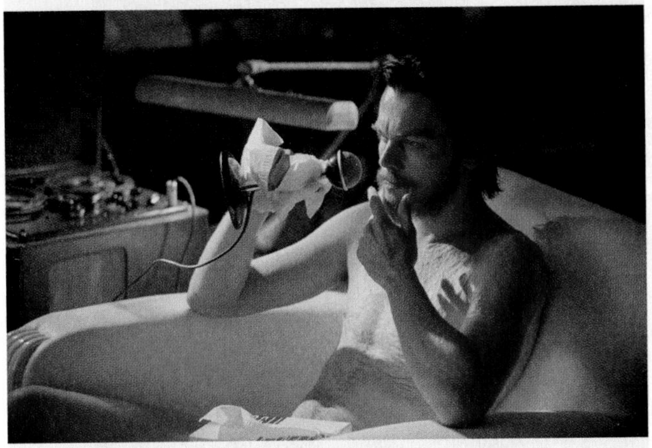

Source: Warner Brothers/The Kobal Collection

A major figure in the history of U.S. aviation, Howard Hughes suffered from severe obsessive-compulsive disorder for much of his life. In this photo from the film *The Aviator*, he holds a microphone with his handkerchief to avoid contaminating himself.

of dust, pieces of paper label, and, in general, all sources of contamination have been removed. Holding the can in the center at all times, he then processes the bottom of the can in the same manner, being very sure that the bristles of the brush have thoroughly cleaned all the small indentations on the perimeter of the bottom of the can. He then rinses the soap from the cylindrical sides and the bottom of the can.

When the fruit was dished onto the plate, Hughes wanted "fallout rules" in effect: "Be sure that no part of the body, including the hands, be directly over the can or the plate at any time. If possible, keep the head, upper part of the body, arms, etc. at least a foot away from the can of fruit and the sterile plate at all times." During the procedure, there must be "absolutely no talking, coughing, clearing of the throat, or any movement whatsoever of the lips."

To make absolutely certain that, with a few authorized exceptions, no one would come in contact with any of the supplies stored in an adjoining bungalow for his use, Hughes issued explicit orders:

No matter how extreme the emergency, no matter how unusual the circumstances may be, no matter what may have arisen, it is extremely important to me that nobody ever goes into any room, closet, cabinet, drawer, bathroom or any other area used to store any of the things which are for me—either food, equipment, magazines, paper supplies, Kleenex—no matter what. It is equally important to me that nobody ever opens any doors or opening to any room, cabinet or closet or anything used to store any of my things, even for one-thousandth of an inch, for one-thousandth of a second. I don't want the possibility of dust or insects or anything of that nature entering.

*... There were even special procedures to be followed in removing his hearing-aid cord from the cabinet where it was stored.**

(Bartlett & Steele, 1979, pp. 232–235)

Unlike Hughes, few sufferers of Obsessive-Compulsive Disorder have the money to hire others to participate with them in the compulsive behavior that "protects" them from fears of contamination. Many persons with this disorder hide their symptoms and rituals from family and friends; others incorporate them into a troubled daily life:

In a fanatic pursuit of cleanliness [one 49-year-old woman] uses up more than 225 bars of soap on herself every month, wears rubber gloves even to switch on a light—and makes her husband sleep alone so she won't be contaminated by him.

(Goodwin, 1986, p. 174)

Epidemiology

While few persons carry their obsessive-compulsive anxieties to the extreme reached by Hughes, the condition that affected this man is far from rare (Nymberg & Van Noppen, 1994). Obsessive-Compulsive Disorder is said to occur about as commonly as diabetes and asthma, and yet clients frequently hide their symptoms from family and health care providers. Figure 12-1 illustrates that anxiety results in physiolgocial change in blood flow to the brain for these clients. Most cases of this disorder begin in quite young individuals, often during young adulthood or before. While most obsessive-compulsive individuals improve with time, some require intensive treatment or hospitalization. As will be discussed later, until recently Obsessive-Compulsive Disorder was very resistant to drug treatment. For persons whose symptoms remain resistant to drugs, recent experience suggests that neurosurgical procedures including reversible deep brain stimulation using implanted electrodes and a pacemaker-like device can be effective (Greenberg, Price, Rauch, Friehs, Noren, Malone, et al., 2005).

*From *Empire: The Life, Legend, and Madness of Howard Hughes* by Donald L. Bartlett and James B. Steele. Copyright © 1979 by Donald L. Bartlett and James B. Steele. Reprinted by permission of W. W. Norton & Company, Inc.

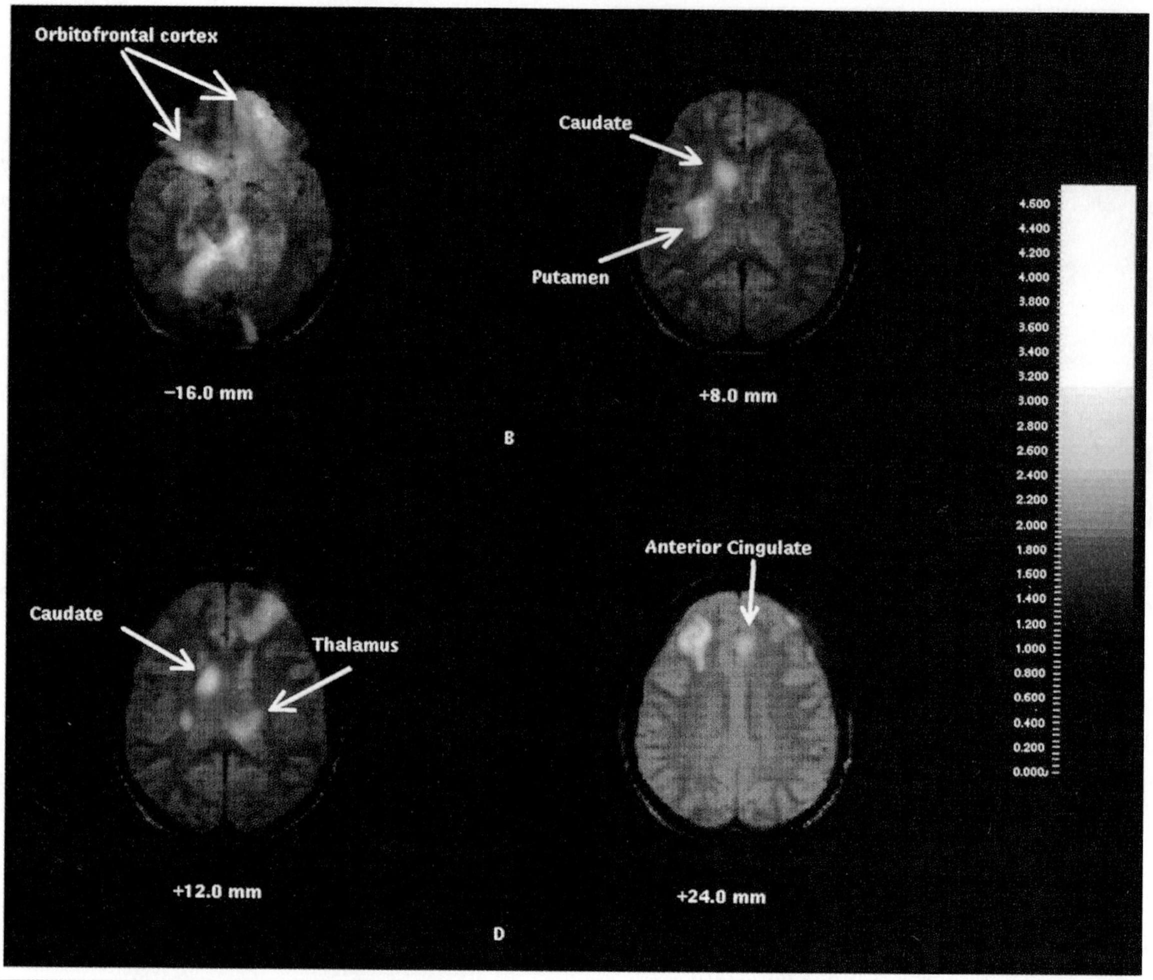

FIGURE 12-1 Obsessive-Compulsive Disorder: PET images. Four persons with Obsessive-Compulsive Disorder were exposed to images or objects that provoked severe anxiety related to obsessive-compulsive symptoms. PET images show increased blood flow (yellow, orange/red) in specific brain areas after exposure compared to exposure to "neutral objects." (FROM "REGIONAL CEREBRAL BLOOD FLOW MEASURED DURING SYMPTOM PROVOCATION IN OBSESSIVE-COMPULSIVE DISORDER USING OXYGEN-15 LABELED CARBON DIOXIDE AND POSITRON EMISSION TOMOGRAPHY" BY S. L. RAUCH, M. A. JENIKE, N. M. ALPERT, L. BAER, H. C. BREITER, C. R. SAVAGE, ET AL., 1994, *ARCHIVES OF GENERAL PSYCHIATRY*, 51, 66. COPYRIGHT © 1994, AMERICAN MEDICAL ASSOCIATION. REPRINTED WITH PERMISSION.)

POST-TRAUMATIC STRESS DISORDER

Post-Traumatic Stress Disorder (PTSD) is an anxiety disorder that typically occurs after a frightening event, most often an accident, crime, or battle. This condition may follow natural disasters, as discussed in Chapter 11. Individuals with this disorder have been exposed to an event that threatened or caused either death or another threat to one's physical integrity, or witnessed an event that involves death, injury, or a threat to the physical integrity of another person (American Psychiatric Association, 2000, p. 463). The response to this exposure must have been one of fear or helplessness, and the event needs to be persistently reexperienced through recurrent recollections, dreams, or hallucinatory-like flashbacks. Additionally, individuals with this diagnosis exhibit impairment of social functioning, the presence of specific anxiety symptoms, and "persistent avoidance of stimuli associated with the trauma and numbing of general responsiveness" (American Psychiatric Association, 2000, p. 463).

It is important to remember that illness and even medical care itself can be profoundly frightening experiences. For some persons, hospital memories can act as stimuli to true Post-Traumatic Stress Disorder. In the 1970s, several cases were reported of surgical patients who awoke out of general anesthesia only to find themselves still mentally undergoing surgery and fully paralyzed. None could remember the actual event, but each suffered marked and sometimes quite prolonged distress, with nightmares and a vague sense of the experience being more than just a dream:

CORONARY BYPASS SURGERY

A 52 year old man was extremely anxious and irritable following coronary bypass.... He had repetitive dreams of being tied down and unable to move. He related his anxiety to a recollection of being sewn up at the end of surgery.

EXAMINER: Are you sure it wasn't a dream?

PATIENT: I'm positive!

EXAMINER: Are you sure?
PATIENT: I'm absolutely sure!
EXAMINER: I think you're right. You were awake at the end of surgery.
*PATIENT: (With amazement) I was?**

(Blacher, 1975, pp. 67–68)

Each of the surgical patients described in this report had a remarkably rapid cure after recognizing that their symptoms originated from awakening paralyzed during surgery.

HYSTERECTOMY

A 25 year old hospital secretary underwent a hysterectomy.... [Later] she ... disclosed that she had been plagued by a nightly nightmare of hearing voices and then seeing people floating over her. She would fight their taking her somewhere, and felt she was choking and couldn't defend herself. The prominent feeling was that she was dead or dying and she would awaken in terror and be unable to go back to sleep. She was constantly preoccupied with death.

*She had not told of her symptoms in the hospital for fear she would be considered insane, but now she felt overwhelmed by them. When it was suggested that she must have been awake during surgery, she began to connect the dream with specific people. She recalled her surgeon giving orders; she related the choking to the endotracheal tube.... The night after this discussion, she had the dream again but instead of experiencing the usual terror, she rolled over and went back to sleep. The nightmare never recurred, her irritability disappeared, and she felt normal by the next day.**

(Blacher, 1975 p. 67)

In none of the cases described by Blacher was there any independent corroboration that anesthesia had lightened. And while the explanations seemed to relieve all clients' symptoms, and midsurgical awakenings have previously been documented by anesthesiologists, there can be no absolute certainty that each client truly suffered paralysis while awake. Establishing the reality of a post-traumatic stress episode may not be critically important when surgery is the cause and reassurance brings about a rapid cure. However, in recent years there has been great interest in adult post-traumatic stress due to unrecalled childhood trauma, most commonly sexual abuse. In several highly publicized cases, individuals "remembered" sexual assaults that occurred many years before and brought criminal charges against alleged perpetrators (Crews, 1994). Psychologists are strongly divided as to where the truth lies in these complex stories, but there is little doubt that individuals can vividly remember events that did not happen and confess to crimes they did not commit. In fact, there is reason to believe that under some circumstances, a person who confesses to a crime may be more likely to be innocent than one who denies involvement (Cohen & Stewart, 1995). The psychological dynamics of Post-Traumatic Stress Disorder are exceedingly complex and interesting; truth is sometimes difficult or impossible to determine. While some apparently repressed memories may involve events that never truly happened, many, if not most, of the events giving rise to post-traumatic stress are well documented, violent, and all too real. A particularly famous example of Post-Traumatic Stress Disorder due to a disastrous flood is discussed in detail in Chapter 11.

Epidemiology

Post-Traumatic Stress Disorder is quite commonly seen in military situations. The conditions of war are exceedingly frightening to civilians and soldiers alike. The more violence experienced, the more likely it is that post-traumatic stress will occur. In civilian life, experiencing or witnessing violent crime or trauma are common antecedents of Post-Traumatic Stress Disorder. The degree of personal involvement or threat influences the likelihood of subsequent development of symptoms. For example, persons who are very close witnesses to violence may be more likely to be affected than those who observe violence at a distance. In recent years it has been suggested that Post-Traumatic Stress Disorder may occur after stressful, but not explicitly violent, events such as unexpected pregnancy loss. Children who witness violence (including domestic violence perpetrated by a parent or other caretaker) are also at significant risk of long-term sequelae. Not surprisingly, there was a significant increase in persons reporting symptoms of post-traumatic stress in New York following the September 11, 2001, terrorist attack. Interestingly, a substantial number of persons who were not directly affected by the attack also met diagnostic criteria for probable post-traumatic stress. Data seem to show that the consequences of such large-scale trauma may extend into the general population and not be limited to those directly affected by the trauma (Galea, Vlahov, Resnick, Ahern, Susser, Gold, et al., 2003).

In Post-Traumatic Stress Disorder, the degree of anxiety and the duration of symptoms may be highly variable from person to person (Goodwin, 1986) and may depend importantly on pretraumatic mental health and subsequent social support. There is an exceedingly wide prevalence range reported for this condition. In surveys of persons exposed to serious danger, Post-Traumatic Stress Disorder has been found in as few as 3% and as many as 58% of individuals (American Psychiatric Association, 2000). Although persons with pretraumatic psychiatric symptoms may be more likely to develop serious Post-Traumatic Stress Disorder, given a severe enough psychological stressor, virtually anyone seems likely to be susceptible. Half of individuals are completely

*From "On Awakening Paralyzed during Surgery" by R. S. Blacher, 1975, *Journal of the American Medical Association, 234*, pp. 67–68. Copyright 1975, American Medical Association. Reprinted with permission.

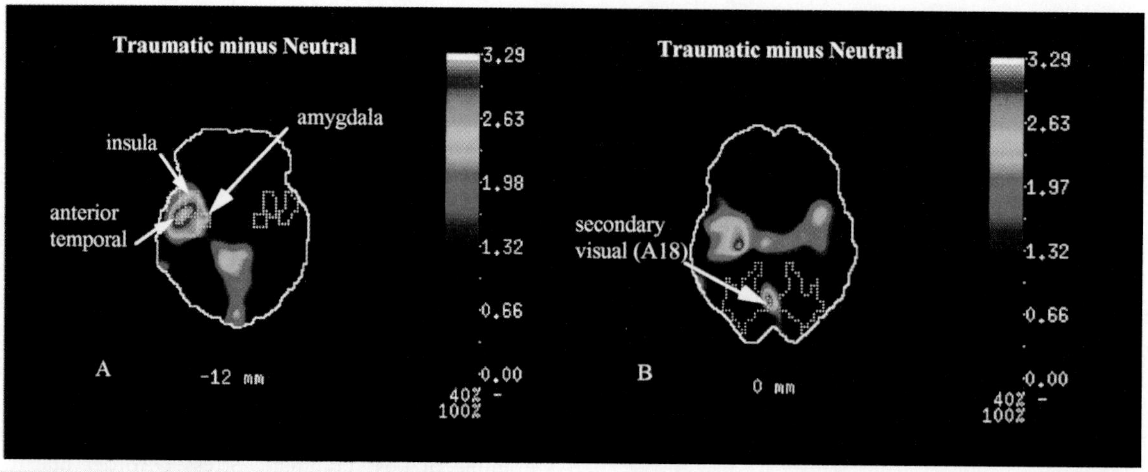

FIGURE 12-2 **Post-Traumatic Stress Disorder: PET image. These PET scans depict brain blood flow changes in two clients with Post-Traumatic Stress Disorder who were asked to listen to a recorded "neutral voice" describing an episode of trauma similar to one they had previously experienced. Listening to this script greatly increased heart rate and fear (as reported on a standardized scale). The PET results show marked increases in brain blood flow to specific areas.** (FROM "A SYMPTOM PROVOCATION STUDY OF POST-TRAUMATIC STRESS DISORDERS USING POSITRON EMISSION TOMOGRAPHY AND SIGHT-DRIVEN IMAGERY" BY S. L. RAUCH, B. A. VANDERKOLK, R. E. FISHER, N. M. ALPERT, S. P. ORR, C. R. SAVAGE, ET AL., 1996, *ARCHIVES OF GENERAL PSYCHIATRY, 53,* 385. COPYRIGHT © 1996, AMERICAN MEDICAL ASSOCIATION. REPRINTED WITH PERMISSION.)

recovered by three months, but the remainder may continue to be affected for a year or more (American Psychiatric Association, 2000). As with many other anxiety disorders, PET scanning suggests specific localized areas of brain dysfunction in Post-Traumatic Stress Disorder (see Figure 12-2; Bremner, 1999). Functional magnetic resonance imaging (fMRI) shows findings similar to those reported for some other anxiety disorders; compared to controls, individuals with PTSD exposed to provoking stimuli have greater activation of the amygdala and *decreased* activation of cortical brain centers that normally suppress amygdala activity (Shin, Wright, Cannistraro, Wedig, McMullin, Martis, et al., 2005). These findings are consistent with the current views that 1) the amygdala is a major source of emotions related to anxiety, and 2) in persons with anxiety disorders the amygdala's response is not as effectively inhibited by "emotional control" areas in the medial prefrontal cortex.

CAUSES OF ANXIETY DISORDERS

While the symptoms of anxiety have their biological origins in the amygdala or adjacent limbic system of the brain, many forms of anxiety occur in response to environmental stimuli. Psychologists have developed a wide range of theories to explain anxiety. While psychoanalysis offers somewhat different explanations for each person's symptoms, psychoanalytic theories typically postulate the origin of anxiety as being infantile conflicts involving sexual development. The essence of psychoanalytic theory is that mental processes are unconscious and, as a result, only dimly accessible to personal understanding, most often through dreams. Anxiety, according to psychoanalysis, comes from unconscious processes that originate in early childhood experiences. Such psychoanalytic explanations are virtually impossible to validate, given how subjective and private an individual's unconscious experience really is. As one sympathetic critic has observed:

> *The question is not whether Freud got it exactly right, or whether strong criticisms cannot be made of some of his case histories, but whether the types of explanation he introduced substantially amplify the understanding of ourselves and others that common-sense psychology provides.**
>
> *(Nagel, 1994a, p. 34)*

Recently, such "commonsense" theories have seemed more attractive to many psychologists than psychoanalysis. One such theory postulates two highly individual factors: adversity and trait anxiety. **Adversity** is a measure of how strong a given stimulus for anxiety is: A large earthquake or explosion is likely to make almost anyone anxious, whereas a small spider is unlikely to bother most individuals very much. **Trait anxiety** is an abstract but measurable personality characteristic based on the everyday observation that some quite normal individuals appear to experience more anxiety than do others. Persons who admit to feeling more anxious than others are said to have high levels of trait anxiety. A model for perceived anxiety based on these two concepts is illustrated in Figure 12-3.

In this model of perceived anxiety, the individual appraises an event based on its actual adversity and on inherent patterns of trait anxiety. The result is a degree of arousal that may or may not lead to symptoms. Arousal often also results in efforts to reduce anxiety. These can take the form of symptom-reducing activities such as deep breathing or stimulus-reducing activities such as getting out of a closet that has a spider in it. This

*From "Freud's Permanent Revolution" by T. Nagel, 1994, *New York Review of Books, 41,* pp. 34–38.

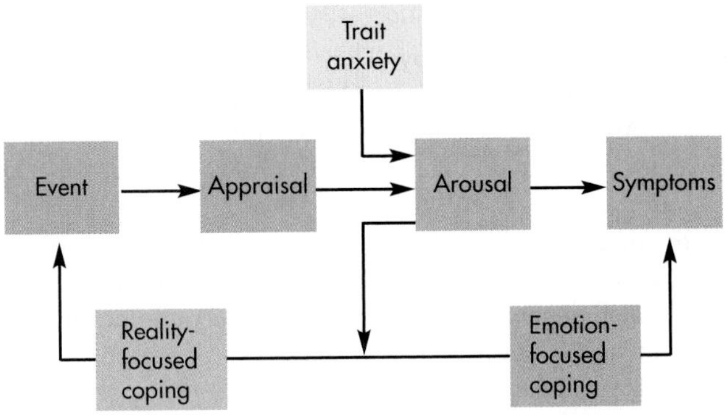

FIGURE 12-3 Model for Anxiety (FROM *TREATMENT OF ANXIETY DISORDERS:A CLINICIAN'S GUIDE AND PATIENT MANUALS* BY ANDREWS, CREAMER, CRINO, HUNT, LAMPE, & PAGE, 1994, NEW YORK: CAMBRIDGE UNIVERSITY PRESS. REPRINTED WITH PERMISSION OF CAMBRIDGE UNIVERSITY PRESS.)

model refers to these two coping methods as "emotion-focused coping" and "reality-focused coping," respectively.

This kind of commonsense model can be useful in understanding anxiety and in helping clients to improve their abilities to cope with anxiety symptoms. However, many psychologists are uncomfortable with ideas like trait anxiety, which do not seem to offer any deep explanation of why some people are more anxious than others. Some have sought biological explanations in neurotransmitters, brain blood flow, and brain receptors for tranquilizer-like substances. While much research has been reported, to date, none of these biological explanations has provided a complete explanation for the mystery of anxiety. It has been shown that many different neurotransmitter systems are altered in anxiety disorders, and scientists have yet to identify either the most important of these or a characteristic pattern (Mathew, Price, & Charney, 2008). Fortunately, effective treatment for anxiety disorders seems not to require a full understanding of the causes of human anxiety, though it is almost certain that improved understanding will lead to better treatment options as well.

TREATMENT OF ANXIETY DISORDERS

PSYCHOTHERAPY

Psychotherapy continues to be widely used in the treatment of anxiety disorders. Psychotherapy can be viewed as falling into two general categories: those therapies based on helping individuals achieve insight into *why* they feel anxiety and those that emphasize behavioral means of controlling the anxiety.

Insight-Based Treatments

Psychotherapy based on insight into symptoms may sometimes be valuable, especially for highly motivated individuals whose symptoms are not disabling. Psychoanalysis is among the best known of the insight therapies and has been widely employed to assist persons with anxiety. Although there is now evidence that some forms of psychotherapy significantly improve anxiety (Smits & Hofmann, 2008), and a small randomized trial does suggest that psychoanalysis is effective in panic disorder (Milrod, Leon, Busch, Rudden, Schwalberg, Clarkin, et al., 2007), the benefits claimed for psychoanalysis in anxiety are largely anecdotal:

> *While I don't know whether psychoanalysis is more or less effective in eliminating unwanted symptoms than medication or behavior therapy, for example, I am quite sure that it has a different kind of effect on patients from more "external" forms of treatment. My observation is that psychoanalysis can confer a valuable form of self-knowledge which is deep though essentially perceptual and not theoretical, and that this self-understanding, whether or not it cures [anxiety] directly, can be used by those who have it to anticipate, identify and manage forms of irrationality that would otherwise victimize or even disable them. It also permits a subtler response to [anxiety] in others, through the enhancement of psychological imagination. For this reason I believe it will survive the development of simpler symptomatic cures.**
>
> (Nagel, 1994b, p. 56)

Behaviorally Based Treatments

In contrast, there is strong empirical evidence that behaviorally based treatments are effective in treating at least some anxiety disorders (Hunot, Churchill, Silva de Lima, & Teixeira, 2007). For example, studies consistently show that cognitive-behavior therapy results in significant benefit for persons suffering from panic attacks (Goldfried, Greenberg, & Marmar, 1990). **Cognitive-behavior therapy** assumes that clients can learn to identify the common stimuli that give rise to their anxiety, develop plans to respond to those stimuli with non-anxious responses, and problem solve when unanticipated anxiety-provoking situations arise. Although insight is very much involved in this process, it is not insight into deep psychological causes, as in psychoanalysis, but, rather, practical commonsense problem solving. Data show that cognitive-behavior therapy is better than placebo in treating phobic disorders, Obsessive-Compulsive Disorder, and Generalized Anxiety Disorder (Andrews, 1993). Treatment appears both to be effective during the relatively brief course of therapy and to remain effective for some months after therapy finishes. It is still unclear, however, how long benefit from cognitive-behavior therapy truly lasts (Andrews, 1993). As a result, there may be an important need for medical and psychological follow-up to ensure satisfactory improvement. Since part of cognitive behavioral therapy is educational, there has been interest in using computer programs to enhance learning and reduce costs (Nakagawa, Marks, Park, Bachofen, Baer, Dottl, et al., 2000). Further information about cognitive-behavior therapy is found in Chapter 28.

*From "Letter to the Editor" by T. Nagel, 1994, *New York Review of Books, 41*, p. 56.

Techniques for enhancing relaxation might seem to be of use in controlling acute symptoms of anxiety, but studies suggest relaxation alone may be no more beneficial than placebo in affecting long-term symptoms of Generalized Anxiety Disorder (Andrews, 1993; Conrad, Isaac, & Roth, 2008).

Programs to treat flying phobia are widely available both in this country and abroad. These programs include two basic elements: an educational component and a test flight (VanGerwen & Diekstra, 2000). For simple phobias the evidence strongly supports the effectiveness of "exposure therapy" in which the person experiencing phobia is exposed to the inciting factor under supervised conditions (Wolitzky-Taylor, Horowitz, Powers, & Telch, 2008).

Emergency Treatments for Acute Stress

Victims of traumatic events (floods, earthquakes, bombings, etc.) often seek treatment in emergency departments for psychological as well as physical injuries. The aim of emergency treatment is to help persons cope and prevent post-traumatic stress. Treatment for trauma victims aims to reframe their cognitive appraisal so they no longer feel helpless. Acute intervention should restore psychological safety, provide information, restore and support coping, and ensure social support (Osterman & Chemtob, 1999). Experience in England after a bombing incident indicates that when support to victims included education regarding post-traumatic stress, simple advice about managing stress, advice about seeking treatment if symptoms continued, and the number for a telephone help line, individual counseling of each victim was not needed (Guthrie, Wells, Pilgrim, Mackway-Jones, Minshull, Pattinson, et al., 1999). Systematic review of numerous similar studies has, however, concluded that single-session "debriefing" after a traumatic event is not helpful and may result in paradoxically higher incidence of post-traumatic symptoms.

PHARMACOLOGY

Humans have known for centuries that certain drugs (alcohol, in particular, but also opiates) are effective in reducing anxiety under some circumstances. In recent years, safer and more effective pharmacological treatments have been developed. Antidepressants are effective in many forms of anxiety disorders, including Obsessive-Compulsive Disorder, generalized anxiety, social phobia, and Panic Disorder. Symptoms of Post-Traumatic Stress Disorder may also respond to antidepressants. Table 12-3 lists antidepressant medications commonly employed in the management of these conditions. Buspirone, neither a tranquilizer nor an antidepressant, may also be effective for anxiety and appears to have very few side effects. Beta blockers (propranolol and other drugs) are an effective treatment for acute symptoms of performance anxiety such as shaking hands or loss of voice control that an individual experiences during public presentations.

Benzodiazepines have established short-term effectiveness in the control of anxiety symptoms. They are clearly the treatment of choice for acute episodes of anxiety, such as occur during crises. They are widely used to reduce anxiety responses to uncomfortable or frightening medical procedures such as colonoscopy. Their long-term effectiveness is more uncertain. In one study, 61% of 31 persons with Generalized Anxiety treated for 6 to 12 months with diazepam (Valium) sought additional psychological counseling (Power, Simpson, Swanson, & Wallace, 1990). One might conclude from these findings that benzodiazepines only partially relieve the symptoms of anxiety. What benefit these drugs do bring is often achieved at the expense of significant physical dependence. In one 40-month study, 65% of persons put on benzodiazepine medication were still taking the drug after the 40 months (Rickelsk & Schweizer, 1990). Withdrawal from benzodiazepines frequently produces moderate to severe symptoms of insomnia, anxiety, and even seizures. Benzodiazepines are controlled substances and should probably be used with more discretion than is currently the case. As Saraceno and colleagues observed in a World Health Organization review of psychiatric treatment:

> *The recent literature concerning [benzodiazepines] has focused almost exclusively on their potential to produce dependence.... Their prescription is widespread in general practice, and an important fraction of long-term consumers start off with symptomatic treatment irrespective of formal diagnoses of mental disorder and eventually become "cases" of formal psychiatric interest precisely on the grounds of their developing dependence.*
>
> *Because of such concerns, most persons needing drug treatment for anxiety should probably receive antidepressants.**
>
> *(Saraceno, Tognoni, & Garattini, 1993, p. 63)*

Benzodiazepines are not effective in the treatment of Obsessive-Compulsive Disorder, however, in many cases this condition responds quite well to antidepressants. Commonly used drugs include clomipramine and a variety of SSRI medications (paroxetine, fluoxetine, sertraline, and others). Fluvoxamine, an SSRI drug *not* typically used as an antidepressant, was one of the first drugs found effective for OCD, but may offer little benefit over other choices.

COMBINATION THERAPY

In many cases, it would appear that the ideal treatment for anxiety disorders is a combination of medication and psychotherapy. For Generalized Anxiety Disorder, psychotherapy, particularly cognitive-behavior therapy, should likely be the main treatment, with benzodiazepines used as needed to control acute episodes not responding to learned cognitive skills. Post-Traumatic Stress Disorder is often treated with a combination of antidepressants and psychotherapy, although the effectiveness of antidepressant treatment has not been consistently shown (Andrews, 1993). This disorder often proves particularly difficult to treat, and clients frequently

*From "Critical Questions in Clinical Psychopharmacology" by B. Saraceno, G. Tognoni, & S. Garattini, 1993. In N. Sartorius, G. Girolamo, G. Andrews, G. A. German, & L. Eisenberg (Eds.), *Treatment of Mental Disorders* (pp. 63–87), Washington, DC: American Psychiatric Press.

TABLE 12-3 Representative Antidepressants and Other Drugs Used in Long-Term Treatment of Anxiety Disorders

DRUG CLASS AND SPECIFIC AGENT	DISORDERS COMMONLY TREATED	TYPICAL DOSAGE (mg)	SIDE EFFECTS
Tricyclics	GAD, PD	(300 mg typically maximum)	Dry mouth Low blood pressure Urinary obstruction Sedation
Amitryptiline		10–150	
Desipramine		10–150	
Imipramine		10–150	
Nortryptiline		10–150	
Clomipramine	(Primarily OCD)	25–250	
SSRIs	GAD, PD, OCD, SP		Weight change Sexual dysfunction Arousal, akisthesia
Fluoxetine		10–80	
Fluvoxamine		50–300	
Paroxetine		20–50	
Sertraline		25–200	
Escitalopram		10	
Citalopram		20–60	
Newer Antidepressants			
Mirtazapine	(Indications still uncertain)	15–45	Drowsiness, dry mouth, weight gain
Venlafaxine (extended release)	GAD, OCD	75–225	Drowsiness, dizziness, nausea
Desvenlafaxine	(Indications still uncertain)	50–400	Dry mouth, constipation dizziness, insomnia
Duloxetine	GAD	60–120	Nausea
Other Drugs			
Buspirone	GAD	15–60 (divided dosage)	
Anticonvulsant/mood stabilizers	GABA-modulating agents still largely under study		
Monoamine oxidase inhibitors (Phenelzine)	SP	45–90	Drug-drug and drug-diet interactions
Beta blockers	PA	Dosage varies	Fatigue, low bp
Pregabalin	GAD	200–600	dizziness, drowsiness

GAD (Generalized Anxiety Disorder); OCD (Obsessive-Compulsive Disorder); PA (Performance Anxiety); PD (Panic Disorder); SP (Social Phobia); GABA (gamma amino butyric acid—an inhibitory neurotransmitter in the brain).

remain seriously impaired by their symptoms despite the best of current treatment efforts.

Panic Disorder without Agoraphobia usually responds effectively to drugs, but side effects (antidepressants) and dependence (alprazolam) often limit long-term use. Cognitive-behavior therapy has been shown to be at least as effective as drug therapy, though some evidence favors using both (Barlow, Gorman, Shear, & Woods, 2000). With or without associated Panic Disorder, Agoraphobia is often very difficult to treat. Antidepressants are of value in some persons and may be combined with behavior therapy. One effective behavior therapy for Agoraphobia may be "exposure therapy," in which clients are exposed for two hours or more to the stimuli that bring on their symptoms. Studies using nurses trained as behavior therapists show high levels of effectiveness (Marks, 1987). Exposure therapy is successful in reducing symptoms, but few clients experience full relief from their anxiety.

The best treatment for Specific Phobia is almost certainly some form of behavioral therapy, probably controlled exposure therapy (Cottraux, 1993). There is some evidence that adding benzodiazepines may increase effectiveness, but this has not been confirmed. In the absence of associated depression, tricyclic antidepressants have little benefit in this disorder.

RESEARCH Highlight 12–2

Comparing Telephone and Face-to-Face Interviews in Assessing Social Anxiety

STUDY PROBLEM/PURPOSE

To determine how effectively telephone interviews could be used to identify one anxiety disorder.

METHODS

One hundred undergraduate student subjects were interviewed twice, once by telephone, and the second time in person using standardized survey instruments.

FINDINGS

Fifty-two percent of the students interviewed met the study's criteria for social anxiety disorder. There was strong agreement between the ratings done in person and those done by telephone. The kappa statistic, a measure of agreement beyond chance, was 84, indicating significant agreement between observers.

IMPLICATIONS

The authors' hypothesis, that telephone interviews could be useful in screening for social anxiety, was borne out by this study. However, basing the diagnosis on a questionnaire—even one that has been standardized as in this case—may risk over-identifying psychiatric disorders. While the questionnaire clearly performed comparably in person and over the telephone, the very high rate of anxiety disorder seems unlikely to accurately reflect the health of an unselected population of student volunteers. This study was done in Brazil, and could reflect local differences in diagnostic criteria or anxiety prevalence.

Source: "Comparability between telephone and structured face-to-face clinical interview for DSM-IV in assessing social anxiety disorder" by J. A. S. Crippa, et al., 2008, *Perspectives in Psychiatric Care*, *44*(4), 241–47.

As noted previously, Obsessive-Compulsive Disorder often responds well to selective serotonin reuptake inhibitor (SSRI) antidepressants such as fluvoxamine and clomipramine, but relapse is very common after medication is stopped. It is thought by some that combining cognitive-behavior psychotherapy and medication may be particularly effective (Mavissakalian & Jones, 1989), but there is no strong evidence that such combination treatment is better than either treatment alone. When Obsessive-Compulsive Disorder is extremely severe, as in the description of Howard Hughes earlier in this chapter, neurosurgical procedures may occasionally be the only effective treatment (Griest, 1990). This surgery involves making lesions to interrupt efferent tracts from the frontal cortex to the limbic and basal ganglia structures thought to be involved in Obsessive-Compulsive Disorder. Less than 0.5% of clients with Obsessive-Compulsive Disorder become surgical candidates, but for those that do, outcomes are particularly positive. In one study, 65% were symptom free without additional treatment; others were much improved (Griest, 1990).

NURSING CARE FOR CLIENTS EXPERIENCING ANXIETY

From a perspective of nursing care, two major ideas are relevant to caring for clients with anxiety disorders. First, providing such care requires great patience, trust, and intuition, and, second, the nurse must fully understand the nature of the client's anxiety and sense of being overpowered by the emotion.

Nursing Theory

The Modeling and Role-Modeling theory gives clear direction in providing care to any client with anxiety disorders. Modeling and Role-Modeling suggests two nursing interventions critical to initiating care: building trust and modeling the client's world. Both of these interventions are effective, but, for many nurses, difficult to accomplish when working with clients experiencing anxiety.

Building trust requires that the nurse accept the client as he is, without demands or judgments. The nurse must show the client that the nurse comes to the relationship in an atmosphere of caring. Supportive presence, then, is the first step in establishing trust. Modeling the client's world means entering into the client's perceptions, seeing the world from the client's perspective, and basing interactions on the nurse's understanding of the client's subjective experiences.

Building trust with a person overcome by anxiety will take patience. The nurse must have a true understanding that the client's emotions are real, overpowering, and not within the client's conscious control. It is easy for a nurse to assume that the client is exaggerating her emotions, because of the fact that the emotions themselves are an exaggeration of the situation. In anxiety disorders, the client knows that her emotions are extreme for the context; however, these emotions are still a very real part of her existence. Before trust can be established, the client needs assurance that the nurse is accepting and will not simply expect that the client can "snap out of it."

The best way for the nurse to show acceptance is to model the client's world—to understand the client's subjective experience, to consider what the outside world is like from the client's perspective, and to enter figuratively into the client's personal world. If the nurse understands the client's emotions, feelings, and needs, the nurse will be able to assist the client to use whatever resources are available to reestablish balance.

APPLICATION OF THE NURSING PROCESS 12-1

ASSESSMENT

Since all persons experience anxiety in everyday living and all persons seeking health care express at least some anxiety related to their need for care, it is essential that the nurse have the ability to make an assessment of anxiety and determine if the anxiety being expressed is healthy or not. One author states, "Recognizing anxiety and assessing its cause are as essential [to nursing care] as monitoring vital signs" (Spear, 1996, p. 41). Another author cautions that nurses in home care settings will see clients with anxiety, and the nurses must be in a position to make careful assessment of that anxiety (Busch, 1996). In such an assessment, the nurse must be able to determine if the client's anxiety is a symptom of one of the anxiety disorders presented in this chapter or if the anxiety is a temporary response to a current stressor.

In making the assessment, the nurse should begin with the observable, physical signs of anxiety—increased pulse, blood pressure, and respiratory rate; a heightened startle response; and "gut symptoms" such as urinary

BOX 12-1
ASKING CLIENTS ABOUT SYMPTOMS OF ANXIETY DISORDERS

Here are questions that have been useful in asking clients about symptoms of anxiety disorders. You may find that you prefer to word these questions somewhat differently, but the important thing is to ask them. Many clients experience anxiety symptoms for years before a doctor, nurse, or psychologist takes the time to ask about these symptoms.

Generalized Anxiety Disorder	Do you find yourself worrying frequently about a number of different things, such as the way things are going for you at home, work, or school? Do you find yourself feeling anxious or tense much of the time without any obvious reason?
Panic Disorder	Have you ever experienced sudden, intense fear for no reason? Have you found yourself experiencing intense physical symptoms of chest pain, shortness of breath, dizziness, or sweating, along with a sense that something terrible or life-threatening was happening to you?
Agoraphobia	Do you find yourself uncomfortable in places where you can't get help or escape, such as walking alone, or on a bridge, or in a crowded area? Are you uncomfortable leaving your home or going traveling without a friend or companion?
Specific Phobia	Are there certain things, places, or activities that you usually or always find fearful—such as spiders, high places, or flying in an airplane? If you do have fears about specific things, places, or activities, do these fears affect any of your activities at work, home, or school?
Obsessive-Compulsive Disorder	Do you find yourself troubled by persistent or recurrent thoughts that you can't easily get out of your mind—such as thoughts of death, illness, or doing something socially embarrassing (for example, saying something inappropriate, rude, or indecent)? Do you find yourself unable to easily stop doing certain activities over and over again: activities such as checking that doors are locked, washing your hands, or counting objects?
Post-Traumatic Stress Disorder	Have you ever had a particularly traumatic experience such as witnessing or experiencing violence or a catastrophic event (such as a flood or fire)? Have you ever found yourself reexperiencing a violent or catastrophic event through dreams or waking "flashbacks"?

(Continues)

APPLICATION OF THE NURSING PROCESS 12-1 (Continued)

frequency or abdominal distress. Then, the nurse should inquire about the client's cognitive responses—sense of disorientation, difficulty concentrating, and/or fear of losing control. When anxiety level rises, the client may become confused and/or distressed, may have difficulty thinking, and may not be able to cope.

The nurse may find that both the client and his family members can provide information on how he usually copes and what degree of stress he has been experiencing. Knowledge of the client's support system will also assist in determining to what degree the client's environment is able to support his own ability to cope. Box 12-1 lists 12 questions that are an excellent tool for use in screening for anxiety disorders. By asking them, the nurse has a measure to assess if an anxiety disorder may exist.

Once data are collected and screening is completed, the nurse may assess that the client has anxiety to the level that psychiatric care need be initiated.

NURSING DIAGNOSIS

Several nursing diagnoses are relevant to any of the anxiety disorders, and some are likely to be relevant to one of the specific disorders. Box 12-2 lists diagnoses and related factors commonly assigned to clients with anxiety disorders. These diagnoses address not the anxiety disorder itself, but the *human response* to the disorder.

BOX 12-2

NURSING DIAGNOSES AND RELATED FACTORS COMMON IN CLIENTS WITH ANXIETY DISORDERS

- *Anxiety* related to unconscious conflicts
- *Fear* related to a phobic stimulus, for example, a phobic fear of heights
- *Insomnia* related to anxiety of being alone, fear of the dark, or flashbacks associated with post-traumatic stress
- *Social isolation* related to restriction of travel away from home or places felt to be "safe"
- *Interrupted family processes* related to adjustments family members must make to accommodate compulsive and/or phobic behaviors of one of their members
- *Powerlessness* related to feeling out of control of one's own thoughts and behaviors
- *Post-trauma syndrome* related to anxiety felt following a significant, life-threatening event
- *Complicated grieving* related to inability to cope with grief following significant losses associated with a significant, life-threatening event.

From H. Herdman, (Ed). *Nursing Diagnoses and Classification, 2009–2011*. Copyright © 2009, Wiley Blackwell.

OUTCOME IDENTIFICATION

Nursing care for any of the anxiety disorders must be based on achieving realistic outcomes of care. The nurse will set outcome goals in collaboration with the client and will recognize that it may take weeks for the client to feel a sense of control of his life, or months to achieve a day-to-day perception of decreased anxiety. Realistic outcomes might be that the client's anxiety is decreased so that he may drive a car on the freeway without fear of a panic attack or that he may leave the house in the morning at least two days without excessive anxiety regarding being out in public.

PLANNING/INTERVENTIONS

The nurse's independent role in treating anxiety disorders is to plan interventions aimed at assisting the client to cope with subjective, human responses to the anxiety experienced. The nurse's collaborative role is to work with a psychiatric team to carry out a multidisciplinary treatment plan. Thus, the following interventions will include both the nurse's independent and collaborative roles.

(Continues)

APPLICATION OF THE NURSING PROCESS 12-1 (Continued)

As described in the section related to nursing theory, the nursing interventions of therapeutic listening, building trust, and establishing a positive nurse-client relationship are essential to providing care. The nurse must let the client know that he understands and accepts her symptoms of anxiety as real and important; the nurse knows the client feels she is about to lose control and does not make demands that the client is unable to meet. Nursing interventions for specific nursing diagnoses are directed toward alleviating symptoms, for example, identifying symptoms of an impending panic attack and administering medication. The nurse can use his understanding of the client's typical response to anxiety to help the client enhance her coping skills and social supports. The nurse may be able to help the client redirect activities so there is less time and focus on the symptoms and more time and focus on present, constructive activities. For example, the nurse may help a client with Obsessive-Compulsive Disorder to engage in satisfying activities—walking with others, going to movies, doing volunteer work—instead of directing attention to the client's particular symptoms. The nurse may frequently fill the role of coordinating various community resources, such as visits to mental health clinics, participation in support groups, and follow-up home visiting services evaluating the effects of medication.

Nurses can be involved in a collaborative role in all treatments previously described, including cognitive-behavioral training, supportive group therapy, insight-based psychotherapy, and use of medications. One author points out that the nurse is in a good position to support cognitive-behavioral therapy by assisting the client to identify thought patterns contributing to anxious feeling and to help the client become more realistic about her worries (Thobaben, 2005). Further, the nurse will frequently be in a position to provide support and guidance to family members who are attempting to live their own lives while accommodating the special needs of the client. Family members will need information, suggestions for reasonable accommodation of family processes, and emotional support.

EVALUATION

Nursing care should be evaluated in terms of whether or not the expected outcomes were achieved. In anxiety disorders, one cannot expect the client to experience a complete "cure" or remission of the disorder. However, the therapeutic goal should be that the client achieve a level of control over his anxieties and be able to experience life in a personally satisfying manner. There is obviously a need for the nurse and client to discuss realistic expectations and to determine the client's needs and wants in relation to his own illness.

The following three case studies illustrate the application of the nursing process to clients having different anxiety disorders.

CARE PLANNING GUIDE 12-1 Client Experiencing Anxiety: Generalized Anxiety Disorder

CLINICAL PICTURE

The clinical picture of a client with generalized anxiety is:

- Unrealistic or excessive worry
- Motor tension (restlessness, muscle tension)
- Wariness, vigilance (difficulty concentrating, jumpy, edgy)

COMMON NURSING DIAGNOSES

The nursing diagnosis most commonly used is:

1. *Anxiety*

(Continues)

CARE PLANNING GUIDE 12-1 Continued

NURSING DIAGNOSIS: *ANXIETY*

OUTCOMES

1. The client will demonstrate decreased anxiety.
2. The client will use effective coping strategies when faced with anxiety-producing stimuli.

NOC: *ANXIETY LEVEL; ANXIETY SELF-CONTROL; COPING*

INTERVENTIONS (NIC: *ANXIETY REDUCTION; COGNITIVE RESTRUCTURING; COUNSELING*)	RATIONALE
• Appraise the anxiety level and degree of interference with normal activities.	• Initial assessment provides baseline data. Ongoing appraisal permits early identification of changes.
• Encourage the client to notice stimuli (both internal and external) that increase sense of anxiety.	• Reflection provides insight as of the probable causes of anxious feelings.
• Initiate supportive therapy.	• Therapy must be directed at building trust, self-esteem, and personal sense of control.
• Teach skills of cognitive restructuring.	• Client can learn to control anxious feelings rather than be controlled by them.
• Provide information regarding medications, if prescribed.	• Information on medications is needed for management of the therapeutic regimen.

LONG-TERM CONSIDERATIONS FOR THE CLIENT WITH GENERALIZED ANXIETY

1. Monitor management of the therapeutic regimen.
2. Provide for continued follow-up. This client will have a fear of being abandoned and will require a sense of continued support.
3. Group therapy may be helpful to control symptoms over the long term.

CARE PLANNING GUIDE 12-2 Client With Obsessive-Compulsive Disorder

CLINICAL PICTURE

The clinical picture of the client with Obsessive-Compulsive Disorder is:

- Obsessions or compulsions, or both, cause serious distress and take up more than one hour per day or interfere with functioning.
- Depression and substance abuse may complicate the disease.

COMMON NURSING DIAGNOSES

Nursing diagnoses most frequently used for this client are:

1. *Anxiety*
2. *Ineffective coping*

(Continues)

CARE PLANNING GUIDE 12-2 Continued

NURSING DIAGNOSIS 1: *ANXIETY*

OUTCOMES

1. The client will understand the need to reduce time in performing rituals.
2. The client will substitute positive anxiety reduction practices.
3. The client will learn to express thoughts and feelings.
4. The client will schedule time to include normal and recreational activities.

NOC: *ANXIETY LEVEL; ANXIETY SELF-CONTROL*

INTERVENTIONS (NIC: *ANXIETY REDUCTION; COUNSELING*)	RATIONALE
• Direct the client to record the duration of rituals.	• Recording of rituals helps in understanding the context of the behavior and in planning for change.
• Teach and practice inhibiting/delaying rituals, substituting other activities.	• Prevention of anxiety escalation reduces tension and interrupts ritualistic behaviors.
• Encourage expression of thoughts and feelings.	• Opportunity for safe expression of feelings sets a context of acceptance.
• Teach and assist to schedule time for normal/recreational activities.	• Enlisting the client to plan time for other activities promotes problem solving and adherence to the plan.
• Educate about medications prescribed.	• Knowledge of medication and realistic expectations enhances adherence to the treatment.

NURSING DIAGNOSIS 2: *INEFFECTIVE COPING*

OUTCOMES

1. Client will verbalize the need for behavioral change.
2. Client will identify maladaptive behaviors.
3. Client will identify strengths.
4. Client will identify goals and need for changes.
5. Client will seek follow-up care.

NOC: *COPING*

INTERVENTIONS (NIC: *ANXIETY REDUCTION, COPING ENHANCEMENT; COUNSELING*)	RATIONALE
• Complete a thorough history—both physical and psychosocial.	• Baseline data assist to understand the client's life situation and the effects of coping patterns on roles and relationships.
• Use a calm, reassuring presence; provide an atmosphere of acceptance.	• Begin working with the client by gaining the client's trust.
• Assist the client in developing an objective appraisal of his behaviors.	• Use the client's cognitive skills to reflect on behaviors and consequences.

(*Continues*)

CARE PLANNING GUIDE 12-2 Continued

INTERVENTIONS (NIC: *ANXIETY REDUCTION, COPING ENHANCEMENT; COUNSELING*)	RATIONALE
• Assist the client to identify behavior patterns he wishes to change.	• Develop mutually agreed-upon goals.
• Assist the client to identify his own strengths.	• Use the client strengths in planning for change.
• Teach problem-solving techniques.	• Assist the client to sort through alternatives, choose actions, and determine his own goals/solutions.
• Encourage socialization.	• Activities can decrease anxiety and increase subjective feelings of connectedness with others.

LONG-TERM CONSIDERATIONS FOR THE CLIENT WITH OBSESSIVE-COMPULSIVE DISORDERS

1. Behavioral and pharmacologic treatments require long-term adherence to the treatment plan.

Note: The care planning guides have been adapted from *Plans of Care for Specialty Practice: Psychiatric Mental Health Nursing* by M. Coler, and K. G. Vincent, 1995, Clifton Park, NY: Delmar Cengage Learning.)

NURSING CARE PLAN: NURSING PROCESS FORMAT 12-1

Client Experiencing Panic Attacks

MENTAL HEALTH CLINIC

Earlier in the chapter, Professor Leonard explained his own experience with Panic Disorder. He made it clear that he was writing for the reader who understood his "fear of Fear," not for the reader who minimalized his overpowering emotions. The nurse will understand that, even though there is no rational basis for the panic, the panic is real and that one attack will leave the professor vulnerable to repeated attacks.

When a client comes to a mental health clinic seeking help for her panic attacks, the psychiatric nurse could assist her, providing support and assurance that others have presented with the same symptoms. One fear of many clients with panic attacks is that they are alone in their symptoms. It is reassuring to the client if the nurse can relay that he has seen others in similar situations and understands both the severity of and the inability to control the symptoms. The nurse would support the treatment plan offered by mental health workers as a team and accepted by the client. Behaviorally based treatment for the purpose of helping the client identify stimuli that precipitate panic would be helpful. Further, since some clients find comfort through the use of transitional objects (for example, carrying an umbrella), this approach could be explored with him.

Imagine that nurses are giving care to Professor Jones, a college professor who experiences panic attacks. The nurses encounter Professor Jones in two settings, an emergency department where he comes for treatment of symptoms, and in the mental health clinic, where he has been referred for follow-up care. A fictionalized nursing care plan follows.

EMERGENCY ROOM

It is highly likely that Professor Jones would, at some point in his illness, appear in an emergency room in the midst of one of his panic attacks. At this point, he would present with symptoms of palpitations,

(*Continues*)

NURSING CARE PLAN: NURSING PROCESS FORMAT 12-1 (Continued)

sweating, trembling, shortness of breath, a sensation of choking, chest pain, nausea, and dizziness. Emergency room staff would immediately initiate treatment to rule out physical causes for his symptoms (cardiac arrhythmias). By the time such assessments had been completed, the panic attack would be subsiding, and the professor would have diminished symptoms.

Nursing care in this situation first requires an immediate assessment of the potential dangerous physical causes of the symptoms, so treatment can be provided. Second, the nurse must have a professional understanding of the condition of Panic Disorder to provide compassionate and appropriate care to a client with a psychiatric condition. Because many clients with panic attacks do not seek help for their condition but, rather, live in fear and distress, it is those times when the client is brought into emergency settings that the nurse can provide support and make appropriate referral.

ASSESSMENT

Professor Jones's panic attacks are unpredictable and intense. He has the classic symptoms of breathing abnormalities, chest pain, and a paralyzing fear that led to more frequent attacks over time. He is becoming increasingly debilitated by these attacks and is seeking professional assistance.

NURSING DIAGNOSIS 1 *Anxiety* related to perceived threat of death secondary to increasing frequency of panic attacks and previous experience of panic attacks, as evidenced by tension, apprehension, and uncertainty.

OUTCOMES	NIC	NURSING ACTIONS	EVALUATION
• Within 1 month Professor Jones will develop an awareness of his own anxiety by becoming aware of the antecedents to his panic attacks • Within 1 month, the client will practice anxiety control techniques: use of medication; use of transitional objects; and use of support system.	• Counseling • Presence • Anxiety reduction • Support system enhancement • Emotional support	• Establish a therapeutic client • Offer reassurance and support • Engage the client in self-reflective discussions • Assist the client to identify life-style and stress patterns while encouraging the client to monitor anxiety levels and the number of attacks. • Educate client about prescribed medications and their uses in controlling anxiety • Explore other approaches, such as use of transitional objects (umbrella), that symbolize safeness and which some find make them feel more secure • Provide assistance over the phone. Professor Jones may call if he is afraid he may be developing an attack. He can then talk to someone rather than feel alone.	Professor Jones found that he had many stressors in his life: high work demands, large number of students, and poor time management. He discovered through self-reflection that his number of panic attacks increased when he felt too much was going on. Professor Jones took prescribed medications and reported feeling less "worried" He disclosed that carrying books made him "feel better." He thought this was silly, but, given that the nurse explained that others with his condition sometimes felt less anxious with an object, he decided he would carry his books when

(Continues)

NURSING CARE PLAN: NURSING PROCESS FORMAT 12-1 (Continued)

OUTCOMES	NIC	NURSING ACTIONS	EVALUATION
			walking to and from work. Professor Jones did call into the clinic—2 or 3 times the first few weeks. The nurse is now helping him to establish and use a support system.

NURSING DIAGNOSIS 2 *Social isolation* related to alterations in mental status, as evidenced by insecurity in public

OUTCOMES	NIC	NURSING ACTIONS	EVALUATION
• Professor Jones will maintain social contact with at least one personal friend over the next 2 months	• Socialization enhancement	• Assist Professor Jones to reflect on the purpose and role social withdrawal served for him right now. • Help Professor Jones to establish social contacts lost during his recent experiences with increased panic attacks; encourage him to invite a colleague to lunch, write a note to a friend, and use the phone to talk to others. • Invite Professor Jones to attend supportive group therapy/ social therapy meetings.	Within 2 weeks, Professor Jones reestablished contact with a trusted friend. Professor Jones attended two campus social events and interacted with other faculty there. Professor Jones declined the groups at this time, wishing to try other approaches.

NURSING DIAGNOSIS 3 *Risk for suicide* related to psychological alterations secondary to a diagnosis of Panic Disorder

OUTCOMES	NIC	NURSING ACTIONS	EVALUATION
• Professor Jones will make a plan to obtain immediate help should he feel he is going out of control	• Suicide prevention	• Discuss the risks with him • Identify supports available in his community: emergency department, 911 for ambulance	Professor Jones never attempted to injure himself. He did not use either the emergency room or the 911 emergency number during the time of treatment.

(*Continues*)

NURSING CARE PLAN: NURSING PROCESS FORMAT 12-1 (Continued)

REFLECTIVE QUESTIONS

1. **ASSESSMENT**
   What other aspects of Professor Jones's life should be evaluated as possibly influencing his mental health?
2. **NURSING DIAGNOSIS**
   What other diagnoses might apply with this client? Could he be having a heart attack? How do we discriminate between extreme anxiety and a physiological emergency?
3. **OUTCOMES**
   What other mutual goals would be reasonable? How would goals change if Professor Jones had always been reclusive?
4. **NURSING ACTIONS**
   What other strategies might we try? If we found out that he was an academic genius who relied on scientific reports for personal and professional decision making, how might we modify our interventions?
5. **EVALUATION**
   If Professor Jones had more panic attacks rather than fewer, what then?

NURSING CARE PLAN: NURSING PROCESS FORMAT 12-2

Client Experiencing Obsessive-Compulsive Disorder

Obsessive-Compulsive Disorder is relatively common, and the average person experiencing the disorder is unable to make the world adjust to the obsessions and compulsions in the manner used by Howard Hughes, described earlier in the chapter. Few have the resources to demand so much of others, and accommodation of the individual and his family will require much patience, understanding, and professional support. Consider the following example of Mrs. Vail, who was diagnosed with the same condition:

Mrs. Vail is a 47-year-old woman who lives with her husband, Fred, in a three-bedroom home in a small city. Fred is employed as an accountant.

The Vails have a number of longtime friends in their community, and they frequently enjoy playing bridge, going to the movies, and participating in social events at their church. The Vails have two children, both grown—a 23-year-old son, working in an urban center 50 miles away, and a 20-year-old daughter, who is newly married and living in the same community as her parents. Mrs. Vail has always been a homemaker and takes pride in her ability to organize a household and provide service to community and church groups. For the past two years, Mrs. Vail has become increasingly nervous and has become progressively more concerned about the cleanliness of her home.

Over the past three months, she has become excessively concerned with contamination of her household by germs from the outside. She has insisted that family members and guests remove their shoes before entering the house. She washes the floors every day and sometimes two or three times a day. She is uncomfortable with anyone bringing things into the house from outside; for example, she does not want her husband to bring papers home from work. She will wear only one coat when going outside, and she will leave the coat and her shoes on her back porch, never bringing them in. She has become overly concerned with her food as well, and over the past few days, she will not eat food anyone else has purchased or prepared. She has established elaborate rituals of washing vegetables, boiling meat, and preparing food in a manner that releases her from anxiety over eating contaminated food.

Her husband has attempted to understand her concerns and is willing to "humor" her by removing his shoes and eating foods she has prepared in her "new way." But, he is losing his patience; he wants to go out to eat with friends, and she will go, but refuses to eat. Their daughter thinks her mother is "weird" and finally convinced her

(*Continues*)

NURSING CARE PLAN: NURSING PROCESS FORMAT 12-2 (Continued)

mother to discuss her feelings with the family doctor. Mrs. Vail readily agreed that her feelings and behaviors are different and changed and describes herself as increasingly lonely, anxious, and afraid of others.

The physician has diagnosed Mrs. Vail as having Obsessive-Compulsive Disorder, prescribed clomipramine, and recommended follow-up care and treatment through the county mental health clinic.

ASSESSMENT

Mrs. Vail is a 47-year-old homemaker who has had difficulty with increasing anxiety over the past two years. During the past two months, she has become completely focused on the cleanliness of her home and the purity of her food. She has developed and uses to excess elaborate systems for "keeping the germs away," systems that have interrupted and changed every aspect of daily living for the Vail family. Mr. Vail does not understand his wife's unusual behaviors; Mrs. Vail realizes she has a serious problem and is very unhappy.

NURSING DIAGNOSIS 1 *Anxiety* related to unconscious conflicts as evidenced by unexplained fears of contamination in the home and excessive cleaning rituals.

OUTCOMES	NIC	NURSING ACTIONS	EVALUATION
• The client will acknowledge and discuss her anxiety and preoccupation with home cleanliness, she will recognize her inflexibility and rigidity in her current day-to-day living processes, and she will identify the need for behavioral change. • Mrs. Vail will demonstrate a decrease in repetitive cleaning behaviors in the home within 8 weeks. • Mrs. Vail will demonstrate at least one problem-solving skill that can be used to decrease her feelings of anxiety.	• Anxiety reduction • Complex relationship building • Coping enhancement • Mutual goal setting	• Assist the client in recognizing her fears and behaviors. • Communicate to Mrs. Vail unconditional acceptance of her and her problems. • Use active and empathetic listening techniques. Recognize Mrs. Vail's strengths in these situations: her clear role with the family, her protection of the family, and her concern for her family. • Collect data with Mrs. Vail and set mutual goals for decreasing redundant cleaning behaviors over the next 8 weeks (i.e., wash floor six times rather than eight times a day the first week; clean vegetables three times rather than four). • Encourage Mrs. Vail to become involved in other activities, to redirect her focus to other events.	Within 8 weeks, Mrs. Vail was able to discuss her anxieties and behaviors. She identified the behaviors she most wanted to change—the redundant cleaning behaviors involved with food preparation. Mrs. Vail was able to see her desire to change the behavior as a strength. The data collection was useful. Mrs. Vail was unaware of how many times she had performed the same activities. Mrs. Vail explored different activities she could pursue when she thought she was becoming anxious, like taking a walk. Medication also decreased both her anxiety and her repetitive actions in the home

NURSING DIAGNOSIS 2 *Powerlessness* related to her lifestyle and feeling of helplessness, as evidenced by inability to control her repetitive cleaning behaviors.

(Continues)

NURSING CARE PLAN: NURSING PROCESS FORMAT 12-2 (Continued)

OUTCOMES	NIC	NURSING ACTIONS	EVALUATION
• Mrs. Vail will verbalize feeling in control of her actions in the home within 8 weeks.	• Cognitive restructuring	• Provide expert assistance to Mrs. Vail by encouraging her to discuss and learn about Obsessive-Compulsive Disorder. • Help Mrs. Vail construct a reasonable work schedule at home that builds in time for cleaning, food preparation, and other home activities not currently part of the obsessive-compulsive behaviors.	Mrs. Vail maintained schedule.

NURSING DIAGNOSIS 3 *Social isolation* related to inability to engage in satisfying personal relationships, as evidenced by preoccupation with thoughts of contamination, repetitive acts (cleansing rituals), and inability to meet expectations of family and friends.

OUTCOMES	NIC	NURSING ACTIONS	EVALUATION
• Mrs. Vail will identify previous social activities that she enjoyed before becoming so anxious. • Mrs. Vail will leave the home at least twice a week for activities unrelated to homemaking activities.	• Support system enhancement • Socialization enhancement	• Discuss with the family unit Mrs. Vail's need for support in making gradual changes. • Identify social activities and networks Mrs. Vail had before her Obsessive-Compulsive Disorder became problematic.	Mrs. Vail began to identify social activities. She left the home once during the past 2 weeks.

NURSING DIAGNOSIS 4 *Interrupted family processes* related to situation transition (the need of the family to accommodate Mrs. Vail's behaviors), as evidenced by inability to accept Mrs. Vail's behavior.

OUTCOMES	NIC	NURSING ACTIONS	EVALUATION
• The family will gain knowledge about Obsessive-Compulsive Disorder. • The family will express concern about Mrs. Vail's condition and support her in obtaining professional help. • The family will distinguish between supportive and nonsupportive	• Teaching • Family support • Family integrity promotion	• Educate and provide materials to the family about Obsessive-Compulsive Disorder, its course, and its treatment. • Supervise Mrs. Vail's medication regimen. • Support Mr. Vail by encouraging his questions, concerns, and expressions of feeling.	Within 6 weeks, the Vail family had a better understanding of the behaviors Mrs. Vail has been demonstrating. They were relieved to have a supportive nurse of whom they could ask a myriad of questions. They had initially thought that Mrs. Vail was "beyond help" and were encouraged to see early progress. Mr. Vail was

(*Continues*)

NURSING CARE PLAN: NURSING PROCESS FORMAT 12-2 (Continued)

OUTCOMES	NIC	NURSING ACTIONS	EVALUATION
behaviors for both Mrs. Vail and each other.		• Encourage Mrs. Vail's children to become more involved in Mrs. Vail's progress and to provide respite to Mr. Vail.	especially glad to have help with his wife's problems; he said, "You know I love her. I just didn't know what to do."

REFLECTIVE QUESTIONS

1. **ASSESSMENT**
   What other environmental factors should be considered concerning Mrs. Vail and her family?
2. **NURSING DIAGNOSIS**
   What other diagnoses might apply to this client's situation?
3. **OUTCOMES**
   Were mutual goals with Mrs. Vail possible during the initial phases of contact? How might those goals change once Mrs. Vail was beginning to improve?
4. **NURSING ACTIONS**
   What nursing interventions were used to engender trust with Mrs. Vail? How could you move beyond her anxiety without adding to that anxiety?
5. **EVALUATION**
   In what other ways might this scenario have gone? If Mrs. Vail's behaviors had actually escalated with this plan?

NURSING CARE PLAN: NURSING PROCESS FORMAT 12-3

Client Experiencing Post-Traumatic Stress Disorder

Returning to the literary excerpt presented in Chapter 11—the story of Wilbur, the man who experienced the crisis of the West Virginia flood—one can recognize the tragedy of significant disaster. Wilbur is experiencing Post-Traumatic Stress Disorder. One year after the flood experience, he describes guilt, anxiety, sleeplessness, and fear of water/rain. A nurse involved in his care recognizes that the anxiety is recurrent and, after one year, becoming a pattern that Wilbur cannot control. Upon evaluation of those losses in his life that are associated with the flood, the nurse uncovers that the grief is prolonged—that is, he has not worked through the grief he is holding.

Imagine that nurses are giving care to Wilbur, who has come to the facility for treatment. A fictionalized nursing care plan follows.

NURSING DIAGNOSIS 1 *Post-trauma syndrome* related to disaster (flood), as evidenced by flashbacks and nightmares and verbalization of guilt.

OUTCOMES	NIC	NURSING ACTIONS	EVALUATION
• Wilbur will verbalize an understanding of Post-	• Teaching: Disease process	• Provide information to Wilbur regarding post-traumatic response: the	Within 1 month, Wilbur had a good understanding of PTSD and

(Continues)

NURSING CARE PLAN: NURSING PROCESS FORMAT 12-3 (Continued)

OUTCOMES	NIC	NURSING ACTIONS	EVALUATION
Traumatic Stress Disorder (PTSD). • Wilbur will begin to be more involved with his family and community; his anxiety will decrease over the next 6 months as his interest in others increases.	• Anxiety reduction • Support system enhancement	relationship among his fear of rain, sleeplessness, and anxiety. • Assist Wilbur to identify activities he might enjoy to redirect his attention to the present. • Identify support groups that might be available in Wilbur's local area.	could relate the information to his own experience. Wilbur began to enjoy and engage in outdoor activities with old friends, for example, hiking.

NURSING DIAGNOSIS 2 *Complicated grieving* related to actual losses, as evidenced by reliving of past experiences.

OUTCOMES	NIC	NURSING ACTIONS	EVALUATION
Wilbur will begin the grieving process to identify his losses and work through the emotions of anger and depression.	• Presence • Active listening • Grief work facilitation	• Encourage Wilbur to slowly and gradually discuss his experiences in a safe and secure setting. • Assess Wilbur for depression, anxiety, and the potential for self-harm or neglect. • Support Wilbur through the grieving process. • Facilitate creating an environment that would most enable Wilbur to heal based on his perspective. • Provide positive feedback for Wilbur's growth and improvement.	Over time, Wilbur dealt with the severe losses from the flood. He realized the normalcy of grieving and how one "sometimes cannot make sense of these things." He kept thinking that he and his whole family would have died had he not gotten up to smoke. When the most intense grieving period had passed, he grinned and commented that everybody thinks smoking is so bad. He believes it saved his life.

REFLECTIVE QUESTIONS

1. **ASSESSMENT**
   How could you assess the impact of Wilbur's relationship with his family members over the past year on his current state of mental health?
2. **NURSING DIAGNOSIS**
   Are there other diagnoses that might better manage Wilbur's issues?
3. **OUTCOMES**
   What do you think Wilbur thought about these goals? Would they have to be mutual to work?
4. **NURSING ACTIONS**
   Could the same strategies used with Wilbur work for other flood victims? Where does care need to be personalized?
5. **EVALUATION**
   Do plans always work? How would we know with Wilbur? With other clients?

NURSING CARE PLAN: CONCEPT MAP FORMAT 12-1

Anxiety

BACKGROUND INFORMATION

Marsha is a 19-year-old freshman student attending a liberal arts college where she intends to major in biology. She moved into a rather nicely decorated dorm where she shares a pod with three other students. She has her own sleeping room, and a study room/living room, kitchenette, and bathroom are shared with her roommates. She has moved away from her parents' home for the first time to go to college. She is the oldest of three siblings, and her two younger brothers are in high school.

Marsha believes that she has made a reasonably good adjustment to college life. She does miss her family because she and her brothers and parents are close. She has made new friends—mostly other students from her classes. She did well in her classes during the first term. It is now February in her second semester. She will soon be facing midterm tests, dealing with upcoming due dates for writing assignments, and functioning in her student work job as a secretary/helper in the college's alumni office. She finds she cannot sleep well at night, lying awake until at least 3:00 A.M., and she feels an uncomfortable state of worry over forgetting to do something she was supposed to do. She does not concentrate well in her classes, and worries that she is missing something in her reading assignments. She is invited to activities with her friends, but feels badly about going because of her worries about school work. However, when she turns down invitations to go out, she worries that her friends will not like her and will not understand.

She goes to the College Health Office and discusses her feelings with the nurse. She tells the nurse she is most worried about not sleeping, and that the more she tries to sleep, the more anxious and uncomfortable she feels. She is feeling isolated from others and wants more social interactions, but now believes that her friends think she is "weird" because her behavior has changed over the past few months. She is afraid of not performing well in school. The nurse has performed a very basic physical assessment, and notes that her vital signs and blood pressure are within normal range, and that she has lost 10 pounds since the beginning of the academic year.

INITIAL ASSESSMENT AND REFLECTION

Ms. Shennan, the nurse, reflects on Marsha's situation and is concerned that Marsha is exhibiting some of the characteristics of Generalized Anxiety Disorder. While the nurse cannot document that Marsha has had symptoms over a six-month period, her symptoms have persisted and have become more severe over the course of the academic year. She is also concerned about Marsha's inability to sleep, loss of weight, and her stated need for more social interaction. She is concerned that Marsha has lost her self-confidence and wonders if Marsha could be developing a self-image problem.

INITIAL REVIEW OF NURSING DIAGNOSES

The nurse believes that there are several nursing diagnoses that might be applicable for Marsha's situation:

1. *Disturbed sleep pattern* related to negative thoughts of poor performance
2. *Fear* of school failure to recurrent thoughts of poor performance
3. *Anxiety:* generalized, mild to moderate level persisting for several months
4. *Impaired social interaction* related to inability to make commitments to spend time with friends
5. *Risk for self-image disturbance* related to thought of poor performance
6. *Imbalanced nutrition: less than body requirements*, related to 10-lb weight loss.

The nurse prepares a concept map, taking into account the various issues that Marsha faces to assist in determining priorities.

(Continues)

NURSING CARE PLAN: CONCEPT MAP FORMAT 12-1 (Continued)

PRIORITIES OF CARE

Fear of school failure emerged as a focal point on the concept map because it is impacting on several other issues, including state of worry, decreased social contacts, inability to sleep, and loss of self-confidence. Mapping the issues has assisted the nurse to conclude that the focal issue is the priority issue, and she speaks to Marsha about this. Marsha agrees that much of her worry is related to this fear. Ms. Shennan and Marsha begin to look at goals and projected outcomes of their work together.

The priority issue is stated as a nursing diagnosis:

Fear of school failure related to recurrent thoughts of not being able to perform on assignments/tests and inability to concentrate on assigned tasks.

Other nursing diagnoses exist; however, the plan of care is to address one initially. Continual evaluation of outcomes will determine if issues related to the other diagnoses continue over time. It is expected that once the issue of fear of school failure is addressed, there will be improvement in related issues and the priorities of care will change.

NURSING INTERVENTIONS

Ms. Shennan and Marsha develop the following goals of care:

Marsha will perform adequately on school work (defined as obtaining a "B" or better on tests and assignments) by the semester's end.

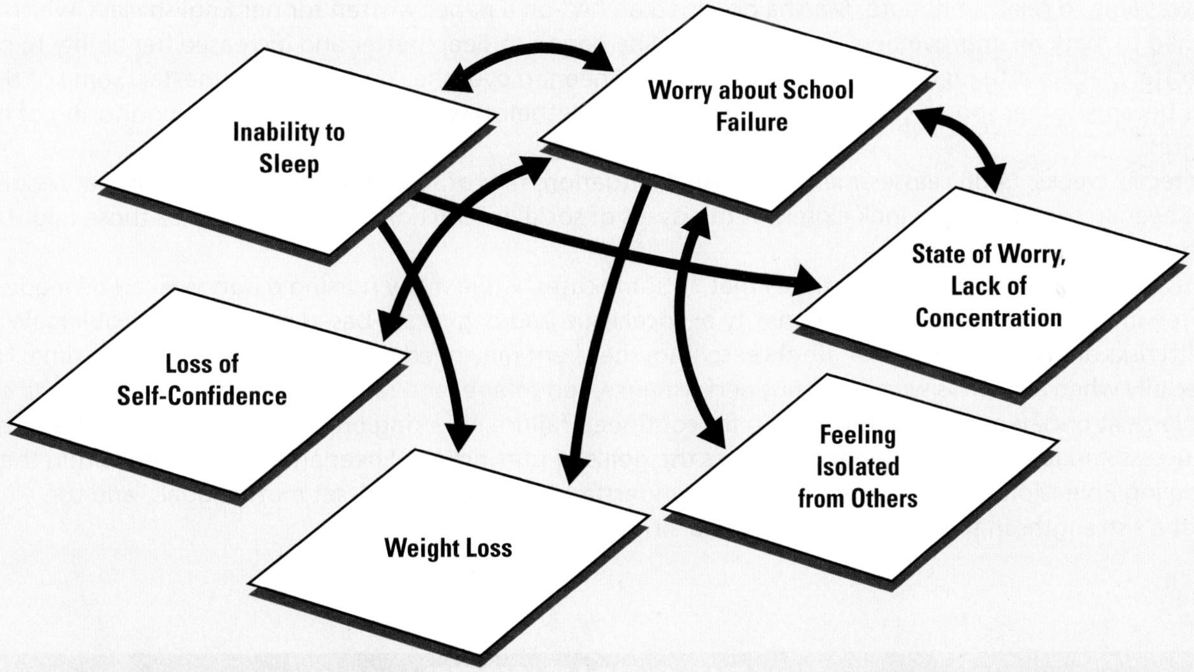

CONCEPT MAP OF ISSUES AND PROBLEMS Issues Related to Worry about School Failure (DELMAR/CENGAGE LEARNING.)

NURSING INTERVENTIONS

Nursing interventions are:

- Marsha will attend sessions of preparing for tests and test-taking at her college. She will also go to the campus Writing Center for tutoring and feedback on her written work.

(Continues)

NURSING CARE PLAN: CONCEPT MAP FORMAT 12-1 (Continued)

- Marsha will keep an appointment that Ms. Shennan has made with the medical doctor regarding assessment of her possible need for antidepressants and to evaluate her physical health status (including weight loss).
- Marsha will meet with Ms. Sheenan weekly to discuss her work and her feelings.

Rationale for this plan of care is that Marsha must have a realistic goal and objective for herself. Agreeing that adequate school performance can be defined as a "B" or better relieves Marsha of the demands on her self that she must be perfect and obtain "A's." Second, Ms. Sheenan realized that Marsha had several supports for her college work (test preparation session, writing help) that she was not using. Third, the evaluation for use of medication is an appropriate collaborative intervention as the level of anxiety Marsha describes may be assisted by antidepressant use. Lastly, Ms. Sheenan intends to build trust, set mutual goals, and emphasize Marsha's strengths to provide the nurturing support that Ms. Sheenan believes are needed for Marsha to succeed. Ms. Sheenan is operating under the Modeling Role-Modeling theory here, as she is beginning with the five aims of intervention and using her understanding of Marsha's situation to build a therapeutic relationship.

OUTCOMES EVALUATION

Marsha did focus on her school performance and attended the study sessions and the other services available to her. The medical doctor evaluated Marsha and prescribed antidepressants, which she took for the duration of the semester. Marsha found that as she felt better prepared for school tests and assignments, she was able to relax a bit more. Marsha obtained an "A" on a paper written for her English class, which seemed to mark an improvement in her feelings. She began to sleep better and increased her ability to concentrate. Marsha attended weekly sessions with Ms. Sheenan over the course of the semester. Some of these visits became rather short—just a "checking in," but nonetheless were important for the monitoring of her progress.

After six weeks, upon reassessment of Marsha's situation, fear of school failure was not a primary issue. Ms. Sheenan then began to look closely at the issues of social interaction and weight loss as those might pose continued health risks.

This exemplar from practice illustrates that, in some cases, while many nursing diagnoses can be made, it is often important to determine the priority or focal issue and begin care based on only one problem. When health risks are not immediate or life-threatening, the client may need to focus on one thing at a time. Here especially when a client is worried about performance, self-image, and failure, attempting to deal with six problems at once would be setting her up for continued failure. Working on one issue for which there can be success impacts on the others and achieves the goals of nursing. Ms. Sheenan worked from within the Modeling Role-Modeling theory to attempt to understand Marsha's world, set mutual goals, and use Marsha's strengths in the application of the nursing process.

KEY CONCEPTS

- Anxiety is a subjective feeling of uneasiness associated with the autonomic nervous system.
- Anxiety and fear have much in common; however, anxiety is a generalized response, and fear is a response to a specific, identified object or situation.
- While there is some disagreement among psychiatrists, most believe that anxiety is a part of the human condition. In its extremes, however, anxiety results in serious limitations.
- Stages of anxiety have been described to identify the emotions and responses on a continuum of severity.
- There are six major anxiety disorders (summarized in Table 12-2).
- Treatment for anxiety disorders includes psychotherapy, which can be insight based or behaviorally based, as well as medication. Therapy and drugs are frequently used in combination.

- Nursing theory, particularly the Modeling and Role-Modeling theory, provides direction for nursing care, beginning with the need to establish trust and understand the client's subjective experience of emotion.

REVIEW QUESTIONS

1. A client is admitted to the psychiatric unit with a diagnosis of severe anxiety. After the admission interview, which nursing action would be most helpful?
   1. Provide the client with a tour of the unit
   2. Contact the attending physician for standing orders
   3. Introduce the client to the staff and other patients on the unit
   4. Take the client to his room and assist him with putting up his belongings

2. When interviewing a new admission, the client states to the nurse, "I know something horrible will happen to my family while I am in this hospital." The most appropriate response by the nurse would be which of the following?
   1. "What do you think will happen to your family?"
   2. "That's silly; your family will be fine without you."
   3. "Why do you think something will happen to your family?"
   4. "Your family will be fine. You need to worry about yourself now."

3. A 40-year-old woman arrives at the emergency room with her husband. The nursing assessment reveals that the woman is diaphoretic and uncoordinated. She expresses a concern that she is loosing control and the nurse believes she has misperceptions of the environment. The client is most likely experiencing which level of Anxiety?
   1. Mild
   2. Moderate
   3. Severe
   4. Panic

4. A client scheduled for several laboratory tests calls the nurse screaming, "I think I am having a heart attack. My heart feels like it is racing." The first action by the nurse is to do which of the following?
   1. Contact the physician on call
   2. Check the client's vital signs
   3. Tell the client to calm down
   4. Administer the client's PRN medication

5. A young man recently discharged from the military after serving in Afghanistan for two years is brought to the hospital by his father. His father states, "My son is rest broken. He is unable to sleep at night because of recurring dreams about the atrocities he has witnessed." Which of the following explanations, provided by the nurse, regarding Post-Traumatic Stress Disorder is correct?
   1. "Post-Traumatic Stress Disorder is a life-long disorder that cannot be treated."
   2. "Post-Traumatic Stress Disorder is an example of dissociative personality."
   3. "Post-Traumatic Stress Disorder is an anxiety disorder that typically occurs after a frightening event."
   4. "Post-Traumatic Stress Disorder is a psychotic disorder characteristic of men in their twenties."

6. A client is given a prescription for Valium to treat her anxiety. The nurse would evaluate that further teaching is needed, if the client makes which of the following remarks?
   1. "I should not drive when taking this medication."
   2. "I should take my medication according to the physician's orders."
   3. "I should not stop taking my medication without medical supervision."
   4. "I should not have any more than two drinks of alcohol while taking Valium."

7. A client diagnosed with Obsessive-Compulsive Disorder washes her hands every 15 minutes. When developing the plan of care for the client, the nurse would include which of the following nursing diagnosis?
   1. Risk for infection
   2. Altered body image
   3. Poor personal hygiene
   4. Nutritional deficit—less than body requirement

8. A client is admitted with obsessive-compulsive personality. While conducting morning rounds, the nurse finds the client performing her ritual. Which action by the nurse is a priority at this time?
   1. Allow the client to complete the ritual
   2. Interrupt the ritual and tell the client to report to the nurse's station
   3. Tell the client she is showing how weak she is because she can not control her behavior.
   4. Place the client in seclusion because her behavior is inappropriate

9. The nurse caring for a client experiencing a panic attack would hypothesize that if the panic attack continues without treatment, the client would be at risk for which of the following?
   1. Renal failure
   2. Generalized anxiety
   3. Mitral valve prolapse
   4. Development of a mood disorder

LEARNING ACTIVITIES

1. Define anxiety and fear and differentiate between the two.
2. Describe what is meant by calling modern times the "age of anxiety." Describe when anxiety becomes a psychiatric concern.
3. List the six major anxiety disorders and describe their symptoms.
4. Select one client you have cared for in the general hospital who exhibited anxiety. Describe the presenting symptoms of the anxiety, the client's need for support, and the response of the nursing staff.
5. Select one client you have cared for in the psychiatric setting who exhibited a phobia. Describe the presenting symptoms of the anxiety, the client's need for support, and the response of the nursing staff.
6. Plan out an information session you would have with a family who had a son with Obsessive-Compulsive Disorder. What does this family need to know and how will you teach it?
7. Do the same exercise in question #6 for a woman who has a husband with Post-Traumatic Stress Disorder.

*Study*WARE™ CONNECTION

Using your *Study*WARE™ CD-ROM

1. Complete the Crossword activity for this chapter.
2. Complete the Quiz for this chapter in Test Mode.
3. Explore the other games and activities that support this chapter.

VIDEO LINK

Obsessive-Compulsive Disorder

Read and contemplate the questions below about Chuck, the client experiencing Obsessive-Compulsive Disorder. Then watch the video "Obsessive-Compulsive Disorder" on your StudyWARE CD-ROM to observe Chuck's interview with a psychiatrist. Consider these questions prior to listening to the psychiatrist's analysis.

1. Define Obsessive-Compulsive Disorder.
2. What is the prevalence in the adult population?
3. Which did Chuck determine were the most difficult of his symptoms?
4. Does Chuck recognize that his thoughts and actions are unreasonable?
5. Does his compulsive behavior reduce his anxiety?
6. At what age did Chuck first notice his symptoms?
7. What are some of the ideas about the cause of Anxiety Disorders?
8. What are the treatments for Obsessive-Compulsive Disorder?
9. What are the pharmacological treatments for Obsessive-Compulsive Disorder?
10. Which of the movement disorders do you feel Chuck exhibited?
11. Depression many times co-exists with Obsessive-Compulsive Disorder. Which type of depression do you think Chuck suffered from?
12. From a nursing perspective what are the two major ideas that are relevant to caring for clients experiencing Anxiety Disorders?
13. What questions would be therapeutic in assessing the symptoms of Obsessive-Compulsive Disorder?
14. Develop a care plan for Chuck.

Panic Disorder

Read and contemplate the questions below about Steve, the client experiencing Panic Disorder. Then watch the video "Panic Disorder" on your StudyWARE CD-ROM to observe Steve's interview with a psychiatrist. Consider these questions prior to listening to the psychiatrist's analysis.

1. Describe how Panic Disorder is characterized?
2. How does it differ from Generalized Anxiety Disorder?
3. What is the prevalence and age of onset?
4. At what age did Steve's panic start?
5. Describe Steve's symptoms?
6. At which time did Steve not notice his symptoms?
7. Which medical assessments did Steve undergo in order to determine his diagnosis?
8. Were these assessments necessary?
9. Did you feel that Steve was at risk for suicide at the most acute point in his illness?
10. Which other anxiety disorder did Steve have?
11. What are some of the ideas about the cause of Anxiety Disorders?
12. Explore the treatments for Panic Disorder?
13. Which pharmacological treatments are considered?
14. Give examples of questions that would be helpful in the assessment of this disorder.
15. Which other mental illness did Steve suffer from?
16. Is there a significant correlation between this mental health challenge and Panic Disorder?
17. How was Steve's family affected?

REFERENCES

Alonso, J., Angermeyer, M. C., Bernert, S., Bruffaerts, R., Brugha, T. S., Bryson, H., et al. (2004). Prevalence of mental disorders in Europe: Results from the European Study of the Epidemiology of Mental Disorders (ESEMeD) project. *Acta Psychiatrica Scandinavica Supplement, 109* (Suppl. 420), 21–27.

American Psychiatric Association. (1994). *Diagnostic and statistical manual of mental disorders* (DSM-IV). Washington, DC: Author.

American Psychiatric Association. (2000). *Diagnostic and statistical manual of mental disorders* (4th Ed.-TR.). Washington, DC: Author.

Andrews, G. (1993). The benefits of psychotherapy. In N. Sartorius, G. Girolamo, G. Andrews, G. A. German, & L. Eisenberg (Eds.), *Treatment of mental disorders* (pp. 235–247). Washington, DC: American Psychiatric Press.

Andrews, G., Creamer, M., Crino, R., Hunt, C., Lampe, L., & Page, A. (1994). *Treatment of anxiety disorders: A clinician's guide and patient manuals.* New York: Cambridge University Press.

Barlow, D. H., Gorman, J. M., Shear, M. K., & Woods, S. W. (2000). Cognitive-behavioral therapy, imipramine, or their combination for panic disorder: A randomized controlled trial. *Journal of the American Medical Association, 283*(19), 2529–2536.

Berkowitz, R. L., Coplan, J. D., Reddy, D. P., & Gorman, J. M. (2007). The human dimension: How the prefrontal cortex modulates the subcortical fear response. *Review of Neurosciences, 18*(3–4), 191–207.

Blazer, B. G., Hughes, D., George, L. K., Swartz, M., & Boyer, R. (1991). Generalized anxiety disorder. In L. Robins & D. Regier (Eds.), *Psychiatric disorders in America* (p. 192). New York: Free Press.

Bremner, J. D. (1999). Alterations in brain structure and function associated with post-traumatic stress disorder. *Seminars in Clinical Neuropsychiatry, 4*(4), 249–255.

Busch, P. E. (1996). Panic disorder. *Home Healthcare Nurse,* 14, 111–116.

Cohen, J., & Stewart, I. (1995). Beyond all reasonable DNA. *Lancet, 345,* 1586–1587.

Coler, M., & Vincent, K. G. (1995). *Plans of care for speciality practice: Psychiatric mental health nursing.* Clifton Park, NY: Thomson Delmar Learning.

Conrad, A., Isaac, L., & Roth, W. T. (2008). The psychophysiology of generalized anxiety disorder: 2. Effects of applied relaxation. *Psychophysiology, 45*(3), 377–388.

Cottraux, J. (1993). Behavior therapy. In N. Sartorius, G. Girolamo, G. Andrews, G. A. German, & L. Eisenberg (Eds.), *Treatment of mental disorders* (pp. 199–233). Washington, DC: American Psychiatric Press.

Crews, F. (1994). The revenge of the repressed. *New York Review of Books, 41,* 54–60.

Davis, T., Rocc, C., & MacDonald, G. (2002). Screening and assessing adult asthmatics for anxiety disorders. *Clinical Research in Nursing, 11*(2), 173–189.

Eaton, W., Dyman, A., & Weissman, W. W. (1991). Panic and phobia. In L. N. Robins & D. A. Regier (Eds.), *Psychiatric disorders in America: The epidemiologic catchment area study.* New York: Free Press.

Galea, S., Vlahov, D., Resnick, H., Ahern, J., Susser, E., Gold, J., et al. (2003). Trends of probable post-traumatic stress disorder in New York City after the September 11 terrorist attack. *American Journal of Epidemiology, 158*(6), 514–524.

Garbowsky, M. (1989). *The house without the door: A study of Emily Dickinson and the illness of agoraphobia.* Cranbury, NJ: Associated University Presses.

Goldfried, M. R., Greenberg, L. S., & Marmar, C. (1990). Individual psychotherapy: Process and outcome. *Annual Review of Psychology, 41,* 659–688.

Goodwin, D. W. (1986). *Anxiety.* New York: Oxford University Press.

Greenberg, B. D., Price, L. H., Rauch, S. L., Friehs, G., Noren, G., Malone, D., et al. (2003). Neurosurgery for intractable obsessive-compulsive disorder and depression: Critical issues. *Neurosurgical Clinics of North America, 14*(2), 199–212.

Griest, J. H. (1990). Treatment of obsessive compulsive disorder: Psychotherapies, drugs and other somatic treatments. *Journal of Clinical Psychiatry, 51*(8, Suppl.), 44–50.

Guthrie, E., Wells, A., Pilgrim, H., Mackway-Jones, K., Minshull, P., Pattinson, S., et al. (1999). The Manchester bombing: Providing a rational response. *Journal of Mental Health, 8* (2), 149–158,

Hawgood, J., & De Leo, D. (2008). Anxiety disorders and suicidal behaviour: An update. *Current Opinions in Psychiatry, 21*(1), 51–64.

Herdman, H. (Ed). (2009). *Nursing diagnoses: Definitions and classification 2009–2011.* Oxford: Wiley Blackwell.

Hunot, V., Churchill, R., Silva de Lima,, M., & Teixeira, V. (2007). Psychological therapies for generalised anxiety disorder. *Cochrane Database of Systematic Reviews,* (*1*).

Kanton, W. (1989). *Panic disorder in the medical setting* (DHHS Pub. No. ADM 89-1629). Washington, DC: U.S. Government Printing Office.

Kemppainen, J., Holzemer, W., Nokes, K., Eller, L., Corless, I., Bunch, E., et al. (2003). Self-care management of anxiety and fear in HIV disease. *Journal of the Association of Nurses in AIDS Care, 14*(2), 21–29.

Kupfermann, I. (1985). Hypothalamus and limbic system I: Peptidergic neurons, homeostasis, and emotional behavior. In E. R. Kandel & J. H. Schwartz (Eds.), *Principles of neural science* (2nd ed., pp. 623–624). New York: Elsevier.

Lydiard, R. B. (2003). The role of GABA in anxiety disorders. *Journal of Clinical Psychiatry, 64*(Suppl. 3), 21–27,

Magee, W.J., Eaton, W.W., Wittchen, H.U., McGonagle, K.A., & Kessler, R.C. (1996). Agoraphobia, simple phobia, and social phobia in the National Comorbidity Survey. *Archives of General Psychiatry, 53*(2), 159–168.

Marks, I. (1987). *Fears, phobias, and rituals: Panic, anxiety, and their disorders.* New York: Oxford University Press.

Mathew, S. J., Price, R. B., & Charney, D. S. (2008). Recent advances in the neurobiology of anxiety disorders: Implications for novel therapeutics. *American Journal of Medical Genetics Part C Seminars in Medical Genetics, 148*(2), 89–98.

Mavissakalian, M. R., & Jones, B. A. (1989). Antidepressant drugs plus exposure treatment of agoraphobia/panic and OCD. *International Review of Psychiatry, 1,* 275–282.

Mendlowicz, M. V., & Stein, M. B. (2000). Quality of life in individuals with anxiety disorders. *American Journal of Psychiatry, 157*(5), 669–682.

Milrod, B., Leon, A. C., Busch, F., Rudden, M., Schwalberg, M., Clarkin, J., et al. (2007). A randomized controlled clinical trial of psychoanalytic psychotherapy for panic disorder. *American Journal of Psychiatry, 164*(2), 265–272.

Nakagawa, A., Marks, I. M., Park, J. M., Bachofen, M., Baer, L., Dottl, S. L., et al. (2000). *Journal of Telemedicine and Telecare, 6*(1), 22–26.

Nymberg, J. H., & Van Noppen, B. (1994). Obsessive-compulsive disorder: A concealed diagnosis. *American Family Physician, 49,* 1129–1137.

Olatunji, B. O., Cisler, J. M., & Tolin, D. F. (2007). Quality of life in the anxiety disorders: A meta-analytic review. *Clinical Psychology Review, 27*(5), 572–581.
Osterman, J. E., & Chemtob, C. M. (1999). Emergency intervention for acute traumatic stress. *Psychiatric Services, 50*(6), 739–740.
Power, K. G., Simpson, R. J., Swanson, V., & Wallace, L. A. (1990). A controlled comparison of cognitive-behavior therapy, diazepam, and placebo, alone and in combination, for the treatment of generalized anxiety disorder. *Journal of Anxiety Disorders, 4,* 267–292.
Rauch, S. L., Baer, L., Breiten, H. C., Fischman, A. J., Manzo, P. A., Moretti, C., et al. (1995). A positron emission tomographic study of simple phobic symptom provocation. *Archives of General Psychiatry, 52,* 20–28.
Rickelsk, P., & Schweizer, E. (1990). The clinical course and long term management of generalized anxiety disorder. *Journal of Clinical Psychopharmacology, 10*(Suppl.), 101S–110S.
Robins, L. N., & Regier, D. A. (1991). Psychiatric disorders in America: The epidemiologic catchment area study. New York: Free Press.
Saraceno, B., Tognoni, G., & Garattini, S. (1993). Critical questions in clinical psychopharmacology. In N. Sartorius, G. Girolamo, G. Andrews, G. A. German, & L. Eisenberg (Eds.), *Treatment of mental disorders* (pp. 63–87). Washington, DC: American Psychiatric Press.
Sareen, L., & Stein, M. (2000). A review of the epidemiology and approaches to the treatment of social anxiety disorder. *Drugs, 59*(3), 497–509.
Schienle, A., Schafer, A., Hermann, A., Rohrmann, S., & Vaitl, D. (2007). Symptom provocation and reduction in patients suffering from spider phobia: An fMRI study on exposure therapy. *European Archives of Psychiatry and Clinical Neurosciences, 257*(8), 486–493.
Shin, L. M., Wright, C. I., Cannistraro, P. A., Wedig, M. M., McMullin, K., Martis, B., et al. (2005). A functional magnetic resonance imaging study of amygdala and medial prefrontal cortex responses to overtly presented fearful faces in posttraumatic stress disorder. *Archives of General Psychiatry, 62*(3), 273–281.
Smits, J. A., & Hofmann, S. G. (2008). A meta-analytic review of the effects of psychotherapy control conditions for anxiety disorders. *Psychological Medicine, 38,* 1–11.
Spear, H. L. (1996). Anxiety: When to worry, what to do. *RN, 59*(7), 40–45.
Thobaben, M. (2005). Psychological perspectives: Generalized Anxiety Disorder (GAD). *Home Health Care Management and Practice, 17*(2), 140–142.
VanGerwen, L. J., & Dieskstra, R. F. (2000). Fear of flying treatment programs for passengers: An international review. *Aviation Space Environmental Medicine, 71*(4), 430–437.
Weissman, M., Klerman, G., Markowitz, J., & Ouelette, R. (1989). Suicidal ideation and suicide attempts in panic disorder and attacks. *New England Journal of Medicine, 321,* 1209–1214.
Wolitzky-Taylor, K. B., Horowitz, J. D., Powers, M. B., & Telch, M. J. (2008). Psychological approaches in the treatment of specific phobias: A meta-analysis. *Clinical Psychology Review. 28*(6), 1021–1037.

LITERARY REFERENCES

Auden, W. H. (1948). *Age of anxiety*. London: Faber and Faber.
Bartlett, D. L., & Steele, J. B. (1979). *Empire: The life, legend, and madness of Howard Hughes*. New York: W. W. Norton.
Blacher, R. S. (1975). On awakening paralyzed during surgery. *Journal of the American Medical Association, 234,* 67–68.
Darwin, C. (1965/1872). In K. Lorenz, *The expression of the emotions in man and animals*. Chicago: University of Chicago Press.
de Maupassant, G. (1989). He? In *The dark side: Tales of terror and the supernatural* (A. Kellett, Trans.). New York: Carol & Graf.
Dickinson, E. (1955). In T. H. Johnson (Ed.), *The poems of Emily Dickinson*. Cambridge: Belknap Press of Harvard University.
Eliot, T. S. (1970). The love song of J. Alfred Prufrock. In *Collected poems 1919–1962*. New York: Harcourt, Brace, and World.
Jong, E. (1973). *Fear of flying*. New York: Holt Rinehart and Winston.
Leonard, W. (1927). *The locomotive-god*. New York: Century. As quoted in L. Y. Rabkin (Eds.), *Psychopathology and literature* (pp. 66–71). San Francisco: Chandler.
Nagel, T. (1994a). Freud's permanent revolution. *New York Review of Books, 41,* 34–38.
Nagel, T. (1994b). Letter to editor. *New York Review of Books, 41,* 56.
Verkuyl, D. A. A. (1995). Practising obstetrics and gynecology in areas with a high prevalence of HIV infection. *Lancet, 346,* 293–296.

SUGGESTED READINGS

Bemis, J., & Barrada, A. (2000). *Embracing the fear: Learning to manage anxiety and panic attacks*. Minneapolis, MN: Hazelden Education Information.
Dozois, D. A., & Dobson, K. S. (2004). *The prevention of anxiety and depression: Theory, research, and practice*. Washington, DC: American Psychological Association.
Flynn, C. A., & Chen, V. C. (2003). Antidepressants for generalized anxiety disorder. *American Family Physician, 68*(9), 1757–1758.
Fryer, A. (1992). *National anxiety disorders screening day screening questionnaire*. New York: Anxiety Disorders Clinic, New York State Psychiatric Institute.
Rauch, S. L., Jenike, M. A., Alpert, N. M., Baer, L., Breiten, H. C., Savage, C. R., et al. (1994). Regional cerebral blood flow measured during symptom provocation in obsessive compulsive disorder using oxygen-15 labeled carbon dioxide and positron emission tomography. *Archives of General Psychiatry, 51,* 66.
Rauch, S. L., Vanderkolk, B. A., Fisher, R. E., Alpert, N. M., Orr, S. P., Savage, C. R., et al. (1996). Symptom provocation study of posttraumatic stress disorders using positron emission tomography and sight-driven imagery. *Archives of General Psychiatry, 53,* 385.
Westenberg, H., Boer, J., & Murphy, D. (1997). *Advances in neurobiology of anxiety disorders*. New York: John Wiley.

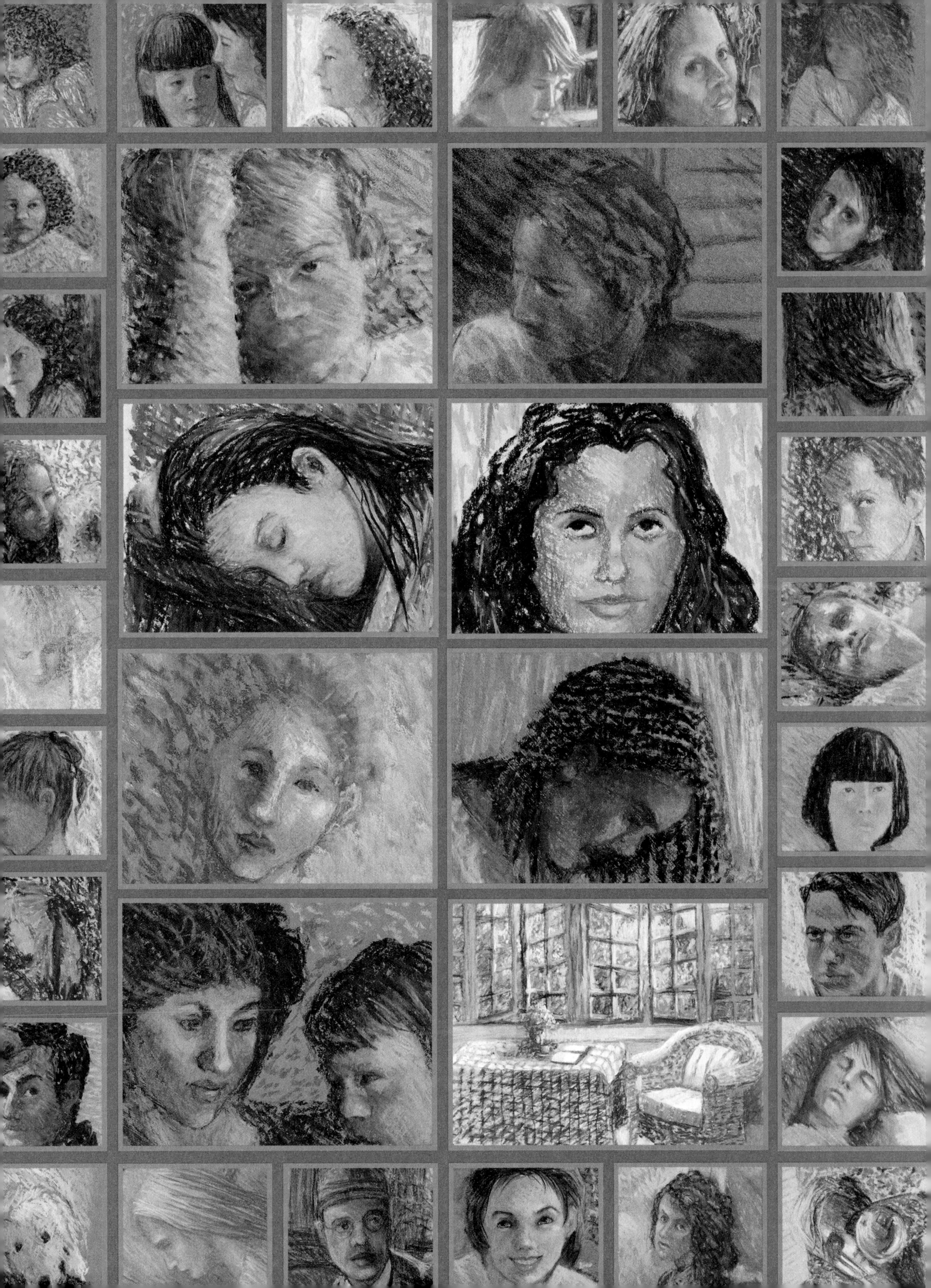

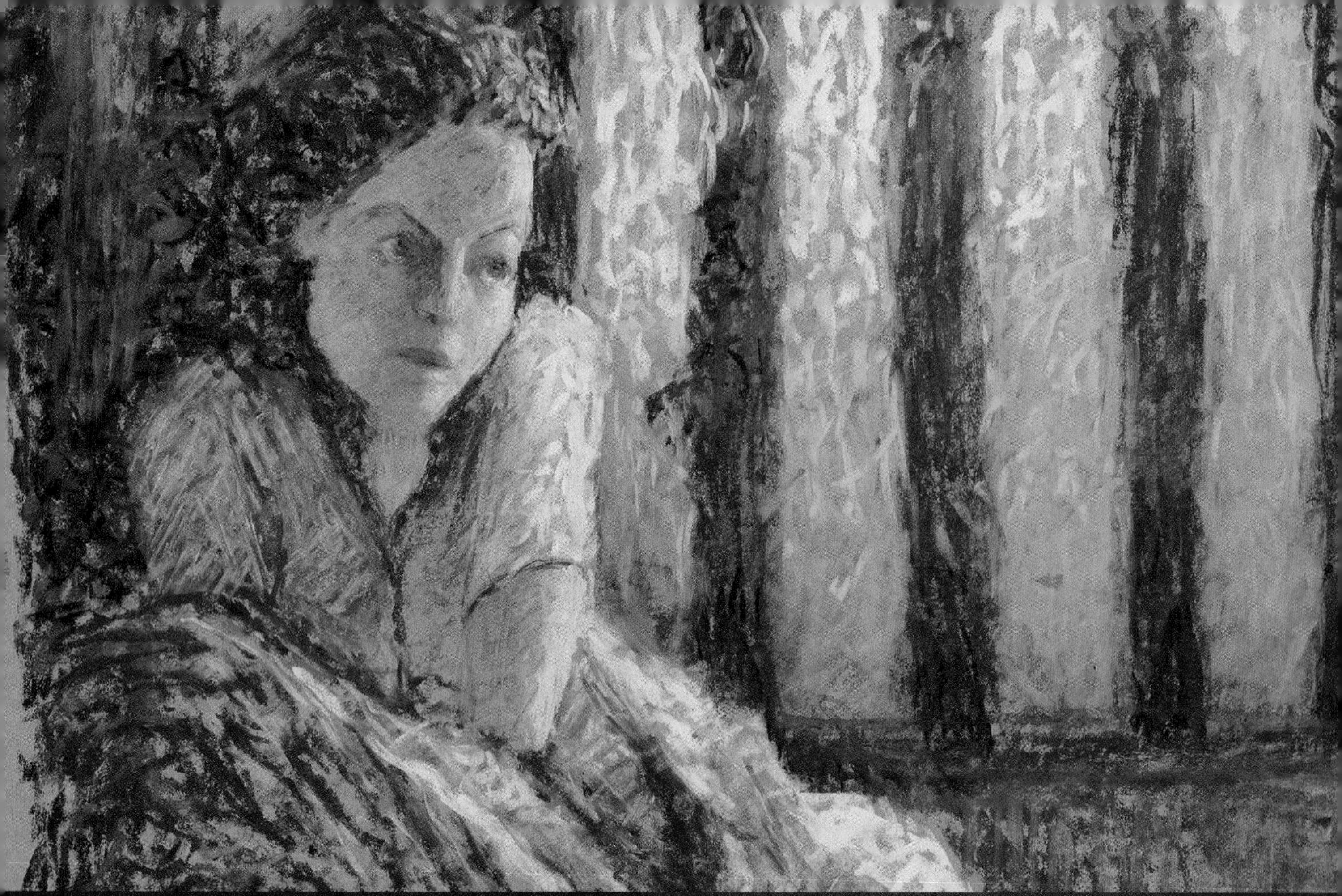

Mind's Prison

In Touch with Reality

Nurses may become apprehensive when they begin working with clients who are out of touch with reality. Consider the following:

- *Think of the last time you tried to talk to someone who, no matter how hard you tried to explain, just could not understand you or your perspective?*
- *When falling asleep at night in a darkened room, have you ever thought someone was present, only to see that there was just a pile of clothes on a chair that gave the illusion that a person was in the room?*
- *Have you ever been certain you heard something (the doorbell, for example) when no one else in the room heard the sound?*
- *Have you ever experienced a life event that seemed overwhelming and incomprehensible and learned you still had to go on with life even if you couldn't explain all that had happened to you?*

Most persons have experienced at least one of the above. These represent relatively common and completely normal experiences. As you begin to study those conditions that cause altered thought processes, remember that altered thought processes and the other accompanying human responses are part of the human condition. What one sees in mental illness is an exaggeration of the normal human response, not something totally different but, rather, something different only in degree. It is the degree that makes the condition a mental illness.

CHAPTER 13

The Client Experiencing Schizophrenia

NOREEN CAVAN FRISCH
LAWRENCE E. FRISCH

CHAPTER OUTLINE

COMPETENCIES

Upon completion of this chapter, the reader should be able to:

1. Contrast disturbed thought processes as normal human responses with the psychiatric conditions schizophrenia and psychosis.
2. Empathize with the lived experiences of those who have schizophrenia and those who have a family member with the condition.
3. Recognize the presenting symptoms of schizophrenia.
4. Discuss the epidemiology of schizophrenia.
5. Explain the etiology of schizophrenia as an organic disease.
6. Discuss the genetic factors known with regard to the transition of schizophrenia.
7. Engage in psychosocial therapeutic treatments for individuals and their families.
8. Explain the role of neuroleptic drugs in the management of schizophrenia.
9. Provide nursing care to persons suffering from schizophrenia, based on nursing theory and the nursing process.
10. Develop a personal perspective on the social policies that guide treatment and care of chronically mentally ill persons in the United States.

KEY TERMS

Akathisia	Derailment	Persecutory Delusions
Akinesia	Dystonia	Psychotic
Alogia	Flattened Affect	Referential Delusions
Anhedonia	Grandiose Delusions	Schizophrenia
Avolition	Hallucinations	Tangentiality
Catatonia	Incoherence	Tardive Dyskinesia
Delusion	Neologistic Word	Word Salad

The *Diagnostic and Statistical Manual*, 4th ed., text revision (DSM-IV-TR), describes psychotic symptoms as the defining feature of several disorders, schizophrenia being the one most commonly seen by nurses. While the term **psychotic** has had many interpretations, all include the loss of rational thought and/or loss of ability to accurately interpret the environment. **Schizophrenia** is defined as a mental disorder characterized by disordered thoughts, hallucinations, and delusions.

Many persons have heard a lot about the word "schizophrenia," and many believe that the term means "split" or "dual personality"; this, however, is not the case. Another common misconception is that schizophrenia is caused by factors such as family dysfunction or drug and alcohol abuse. Box 13-1 lists these and other myths about the disease.

The reader needs to leave behind the myths and preconceptions and consider the following excerpt as the actual, real-life experience of one person:

ANONYMOUS AUTOBIOGRAPHY

On my first day of externship at a hospital I was waiting for the pharmacy to open since I was early by an hour. I was sitting in a lobby wearing a white lab coat and required name tag and catching a catnap. A young male patient approached me.

"Excuse me, miss. Do you know that every morning when I get out of bed I feel there is danger everywhere?"

Because I had a white coat he assumed I had an answer to this problem, or at least that I was not in his situation and could offer some assistance. I was taken off guard by this psychiatric patient but said, "You sound very frightened." He said, "Yes. Are you sad or just resting?" I felt he was seeing right through me. "No," I replied, "I'm not sad; I'm just very tired." "Oh," he said, "then I'll leave you alone," and he walked away.

My white coat and name tag offered me no immunity from schizophrenia. Pharmacy students are vulnerable just as everyone else is, in spite of the fact that we are taught about all diseases as if we were an immune group.

Inside, while I spoke to this patient I wanted to say: "Yes, I too sense danger everywhere, each morning and all day. It's hard for me to get out of bed, to go out of the house, to talk to people; it's hard just to get dressed and

BOX 13-1
DISPELLING COMMON MYTHS ABOUT SCHIZOPHRENIA

- Schizophrenia does not mean split personality, as in Dr. Jekyll and Mr. Hyde. There are psychiatric disorders of multiple personalities, but they are very different from schizophrenia. The word "schizophrenia" does mean "splitting of the mind," but this name was chosen to reflect the effects of schizophrenia on thought and language, not personality.
- Schizophrenic individuals are *not* unusually prone to violence. While schizophrenic persons do commit crimes and some are very dangerous, the majority of schizophrenic individuals are not violent. Although schizophrenic persons are rarely dangerous to others, their risk of suicide is very high, approaching 10%.
- Schizophrenia is not caused by family dysfunction. Psychological factors influence the way individuals and families cope with schizophrenia, but families do not cause schizophrenia any more than they cause multiple sclerosis or cancer. While the biological factors leading to schizophrenia remain unknown, schizophrenia is clearly a disease of the brain, not a primary psychological disorder.

get outside and function. I'm afraid of people, of change. I'm sensitive to sunlight and noise. I never watch the news or read a newspaper because it frightens me."

Talking to this patient had made the conflict within me very obvious. This young man and I are related in a way I cannot share with him, with my fellow students, or with faculty. Yes, I am a pharmacy student. But yes, I have been diagnosed as schizophrenic and have been hospitalized on three occasions when I could not function. Yes, I am on neuroleptics and must see a psychologist at least once a week, and sometimes more often, in order to function.

I wanted to tell him, "Yes, I know how it feels, and isn't it terrible?" ... Even now ... in a professional pharmacy school, it would probably shock many people to know a schizophrenic was in their class, would be a pharmacist, and could do a good job.... So even now I must write this article anonymously. But I want people to know I have schizophrenia, that I need medicine and psychotherapy, and at some times I have required hospitalization. But I also want them to know that I have been on the dean's list, and have friends, and expect to receive my pharmacy degree from a major university.

*When you think about schizophrenia next time, try to remember me; there are more people like me out there trying to overcome a poorly understood disease and doing the best they can with what medicine and psychotherapy have to offer them. And some of them are making it.**

(*Anonymous, 1983, pp. 152–155*)

Disordered thought is a major characteristic of schizophrenia, and while all persons with this diagnosis have had disordered thought at some time in their lives, they do not have disordered thoughts all of the time, as the excerpt from a pharmacy student makes clear. However, disordered thoughts occur in schizophrenia and often present along with hallucinations and delusions. These three phenomena—disordered thoughts, delusions, and hallucinations—are the characteristics of psychosis. While not all three are present in every psychotic client, most schizophrenic individuals manifest a complex mixture of all three. Along with manic-depressive disorder, schizophrenia is the major cause of prolonged psychosis seen in psychiatric practice. Distinguishing between psychosis caused by schizophrenia and by manic-depressive illness may sometimes be difficult, and reflecting this difficulty, some clients who manifest characteristics of both manic-depressive disorder and schizophrenia are given the DSM-IV-TR diagnosis of "schizoaffective disorder." Schizoaffective disorder is discussed briefly in Chapter 18; this chapter focuses on schizophrenia alone.

THE EXPERIENCE OF SCHIZOPHRENIA

A nursing perspective on disordered thought requires consideration of the subjective human experience of the disease. Because rational cognitive ability is so important for functioning, there are human responses that pervade every aspect of a person's living when one is unable to think. Several nursing diagnoses apply when caring for such a person. These will be discussed as the reader examines the presenting symptoms and current definitions of schizophrenia.

Disordered Thoughts

Disturbed, or disordered, thoughts are a major characteristic of schizophrenia. When schizophrenic individuals talk, they demonstrate a flow of thought that can be described as "loose," that is, topics and ideas follow one another with far less order than one expects in everyday speech. Often one idea or thought is followed by a seemingly unrelated one; either topic might make good conversational sense, but when put together, the ideas do not quite seem to mesh. Here is an example of fairly disordered thinking from a published study of schizophrenic language:

*From *Schizophrenic Bulletin*, 9, by Anonymous, 1983, 152–155.

*You ask me to define contentment? Well uh, contentment, well the word contentment, having a book perhaps, perhaps your having a subject, perhaps you have a chapter of reading, but when you come to the word "men" you wonder if you should be content with men in your life and then you get to the letter "I" and you wonder if you should be content having tea by yourself or be content with having it with a group and so forth.**

(Lorenz, 1961, p. 604)

In this passage, the speaker at times seems to make quite good sense (it is perfectly reasonable to wonder if it is better to have tea by oneself or in a group), but the rapid shift of ideas (here, around the focus of a single word—"contentment") is characteristic of disordered thought. The confusion is not in speech alone, but in the thinking process itself. One schizophrenic individual reported, "I try to read even a paragraph in a book, but it takes me ages because each bit I read starts me thinking in ten different directions at once" (Sass, 1992, p. 178). More extreme examples of schizophrenic thought may be completely devoid of any obvious sense:

*Chirps in a box. If you abstract yourself far enough from a given context you seem somehow to create a new kind of concretion.... You explode like when stars explode. In the sky a plate which burned bright. Symbol of all light and energy with me contracted into this plate.**

(Lorenz, 1961, p. 604)

Schizophrenia often evolves slowly over years. In the early stages of schizophrenia, formal thought disorder may be very subtle and hard to recognize (Harrow & Quinlan, 1985). As the condition evolves, language becomes even more bizarre than the examples preceding and may lead to a loss of any ability to communicate.

Incomprehensible Language

The following example illustrates a further degree of disordered communication in schizophrenia:

*That's wish-bell double vision. Like walking across a person's eye and reflecting personality. It works on you like dying and going into the spiritual world but landing in the vella world.***

(Harrow & Quinlan, 1985, p. 423)

In this last passage, the word "vella" is an invented or **neologistic word**. Schizophrenic individuals frequently invent their own vocabularies and may sometimes offer definitions so that others can better understand their worlds:

Snortie—to talk through walls.

Trominoes—tiny people who live in one's body.

Split-kippered—to be simultaneously alive in Lancashire and dead in Yorkshire.†

(McKenna, 1994, p. 14)

There have been a number of studies of schizophrenic language, and many aspects of thought disorder have been formally categorized (Andreasen, 1979). There are specific terms used to describe schizophrenic speech: **derailment**, going off the point or subject; **tangentiality**, failure to reach a goal or stick to the original point; **incoherence**, speech that is not logically connected; and **word salad**, a group of disconnected words. These characteristics of speech are part of DSM-IV-TR diagnostic criteria for schizophrenia (American Psychiatric Association, 2000). As long as students understand that thought and speech can be disrupted in a variety of ways, the actual distinctions among these categories may not be of great importance for nursing practice. Remember, of course, that all of us lose our train of thought, drift from the main topic, and lapse from logic at some times; persons with schizophrenia exhibit these characteristics commonly and persistently—though sometimes with varying degrees of severity.

Without coherent language, the individual loses the ability to communicate verbally. When trying to communicate, it becomes very difficult for the client and his family and friends and others because, as hard as they try, they cannot connect with and understand each other. The client sometimes recognizes his communication deficits, but is unable to express needs, ideas, and intentions to others. Not surprisingly, the progressive loss of language often leads to social failure.

Loss of Function

A person without ability to think and communicate cannot maintain behavior that conforms to accepted social norms. In addition to disruptions in language and thought, behavior in schizophrenia is often disordered. Appearance and dress may range from sloppy to eccentric or even bizarre, and behavior may be equally affected:

The person may appear markedly disheveled, may dress in an unusual manner (e.g., wearing multiple overcoats, scarves, and gloves on a hot day), or may display clearly inappropriate sexual behavior (e.g., public masturbation) or unpredictable and untriggered agitation (e.g., shouting or swearing).‡

(American Psychiatric Association, 2000, p. 300)

*From "Problems Posed by Schizophrenic Language," by M. Lorenz, 1961, *Archives of General Psychiatry, 4*, 603–610.

**From *Discarded Thinking and Schizophrenic Psychopathology*, by M. Harrow and D. M. Quinlan, 1985, New York: Gardner.

†From *Schizophrenia and Related Syndromes*, by P. J. McKenna, 1994, New York: Oxford University Press. Reprinted with permission from Oxford University Press.

‡From *Diagnostic and Statistical Manual of Mental Disorders*, 4th ed., text rev., 2000, Washington, DC: Author.

The extreme of disordered behavior is **catatonia**: "a marked decrease in reactivity to the environment, sometimes reaching an extreme degree of complete unawareness ... maintaining a rigid posture and resisting efforts to be moved ... the assumption of bizarre postures." Catatonia is among the most striking psychotic manifestations. The following reflections of one psychotic young woman, edited and published by her therapist, may give some insight into the perceived world that holds a catatonic individual in such rigidity:

AUTOBIOGRAPHY

*For me, madness was definitely not a condition of illness; I did not believe that I was ill. It was rather a country, opposed to Reality, where reigned an implacable light, blinding, leaving no place for shadow; an immense space without boundary, limitless, flat; a mineral, lunar country, cold as the wastes of the North Pole. In this stretching emptiness, all is unchangeable, immobile, congealed, crystallized. Objects are stage trappings, placed here and there, geometric cubes without meaning.**

(Anonymous, 1955, pp. 677–689)

Catatonia may be seen in psychiatric diagnoses other than schizophrenia and may manifest itself as mutism alone (inability to talk) without the other symptoms of body rigidity. Since loss of speech may also occur in conversion disorders (Chapter 19) in which disordered thought is absent, the Bush-Francis Catatonia Screening Instrument (readily available on the Internet) has been shown valuable in screening for catatonia. This is important since treatment with benzodiazepines (Chapter 12) and, in severe instances, electroconvulsive therapy (Chapter 32) can be effective in restoring more normal functioning.

DELUSIONS

Many schizophrenic persons express **delusions**, false beliefs that misrepresent either perceptions or experiences. Delusions are a major defining characteristic of psychosis. Delusions are commonly characterized as grandiose, persecutory, or referential. **Grandiose delusions** involve perceptions of importance; delusional persons often believe themselves to have special powers and may claim to be religious messiahs. Persons with **persecutory delusions** are paranoid; they believe that others intend to do them harm. Persons with **referential delusions** believe that common events—such as passages in songs, patterns of clouds in the sky, or comments of passersby—refer specifically to them. In the following passage, written about himself in the third person, a young schizophrenic man describes grandiose delusions and multiple ideas of reference developing after he presented a paper at a psychology conference:

GRANDIOSE DELUSIONS

David's paper was viewed as a monumental contribution to the conference and potentially to psychology in general. If scientifically verified, his concept of telepathy, universally present at birth and measurable, might have as much influence as the basic ideas of Darwin and Freud.

Each speaker focused on David. By using allusions and nonverbal communications that included pointing and glancing, each illuminated different aspects of David's contribution. Although his name was never mentioned, the speakers enticed David into feeling that he had accomplished something supernatural in writing the paper....

David was described as having a halo around his head, and the Second Coming was announced as forthcoming. Messianic feelings took hold of him. His mission would be to aid the poor and needy....

David's sensitivity to nonverbal communication was extreme; he was adept at reading people's minds. His perceptual powers were so developed that he could not discriminate between telepathic reception and spoken language by others. He was distracted by others in a way that he had never been before.... Several hundred people at the conference were talking about David. He was the subject of enormous mystery, profound in his silence. Criticism, though, was often expressed by skeptics of the anticipated Second Coming. David felt the intense communication about him as torturous. He wished the talking, nonverbal behavior, and pervasive train of thoughts about him would stop....

*Everyday, David studied the patterns in the sky formed from clouds of airplane exhaust. These patterns, always vivid, typically expressed a favorable view of David.**

(Zelt, 1981, pp. 527–531)

Delusions are described as bizarre if they bear no understandable relationship to ordinary life experiences. David's paranoid and grandiose delusions are relatively nonbizarre: People could be talking about him, and it is in accord with accepted Christian belief that the Second Coming could be imminent. His referential delusions vary from personal hypersensitivity to bizarre delusions of personal messages seen in airplane vapor trails. Particularly bizarre schizophrenic delusions involve the perception that one's body has been physically changed:

OUT OF THE DEPTHS

I was told [by a hallucinatory voice] to feel on the back of my neck and I would find there a sign of my new mission. I therefore examined and found a shuttle-like affair about three-fourths of an inch long.†

(Boisen, 1960, p. 91)

*From "An Autobiography of a Schizophrenic Experience," by Anonymous, 1995, *Journal of Abnormal and Social Psychology, 51*, 677–689.

*From "Grandiose Delusions," by D. Zelt, 1981, *Schizophrenic Bulletin, 7*, 527–531.

†From *Out of the Depths*, by A. Boisen, 1960, New York: HarperCollins. Reprinted with permission from HarperCollins Publishers.

Bizarre delusions may be much more severe, as when a client believes "a stranger has removed his or her internal organs and has replaced them with someone else's organs without leaving any wounds or scars."

Delusions of persecution are among those most commonly seen in schizophrenia. David Zelt, in the article previously quoted, goes on to describe elaborate persecutory delusions involving the CIA and thought control. Another first-person account of schizophrenic experience describes vaguely persecutory delusions about the nursing staff of a mental hospital:

PERSECUTORY DELUSIONS

My feelings about the nursing staff during the first episode were rather complicated. I tried to get as much as I could out of contact with the young student nurses in the ward, but I felt that none of them was in a position to take care of me. On the contrary, they were much younger than myself, and I felt protective of them at times when I did not regard them as making active attempts to harm me. In such instances, I was on the defensive and felt some antagonism. It seemed to me that most of the nurses were like marionettes on a string, with no personalities of their own, being manipulated by powerful forces outside themselves. I saw them as under the influence of hypnotic suggestion. They were, I thought, in the control of others whose minds were more powerful than theirs....

*Ordinary simple people like these nurses were, I had felt, being educated to hateful, intolerant, and prejudiced attitudes toward others by the dominant forces in the society around them ... [I] developed a strong attachment to one of the nurses—a head nurse—who seemed to me particularly kind, understanding, and sensitive. There were times when only her presence could reassure me. In spite of this I began to develop the idea that it would be dangerous for her to have too much to do with me. She could not really help me because she too was subject to influence from my enemies even though her intentions were good.**

(Anonymous, 1955, pp. 678–679)

Hallucinations

Hallucinations are another major part of the psychotic experience and are also very common in schizophrenia (see Figure 13-1). **Hallucinations** are sensory experiences not perceptible to other nonpsychotic individuals. While hallucinations can involve virtually any sensory modality, they are most commonly auditory. Psychotic individuals typically describe "hearing voices," and these voices are perceived as quite distinct from the individual's own thoughts. The voices generally have specific content, and this is most frequently of a threatening or negative nature: "The voices schizophrenics hear tend to emanate not from any particular person or object in external space but from inside the body or from the sky, as if permeating the entire universe" (Sass, 1992, p. 233). Schizophrenic hallucinations occur while the individual is fully awake, and are thought not to be different from experiences considered normal in some cultures (American Psychiatric Association, 2000). It is not unusual for schizophrenic persons to hear two or more voices talking with each other or actually commenting on the individual's stream of thought. This type of multivoice auditory hallucination is highly characteristic of schizophrenia:

*A twenty-four year old man repeatedly heard a couple of voices discussing him. A deep, rough voice would say, "G.T. is a bloody paradox"; then a higher-pitched one would chime in, "He is that, he should be locked up"; and a female voice would occasionally interrupt, saying, "He is not, he is a lovely man."**

(Mellor, 1970, p. 16)

While voices heard by hallucinating individuals may not always be this distinct, persons experiencing auditory hallucinations often describe them as actually quite loud. Dr. Ralph Hoffman's group at the Yale Psychiatric Institute has played human voice recordings to persons with schizophrenia in order to estimate that the perceived sound level of many hallucinations is 60–70 dB, about the level of normal conversation at arm's-length distance (www.webmd.com/schizophrenia/news/20000323/schizophrenia-voices-in-head-relief). More recent work by Hoffman (Hoffman, Varanko, Gillmore, & Mishara, 2007) suggests that persons with schizophrenia report they can distinguish voices from their own "thinking out loud" by analyzing the verbal content, their own sense of being in control of the thought, and whether or not they perceived the voice as being their own.

Symptoms

These features of schizophrenia—disordered thoughts and behavior, delusions, and hallucinations—are often referred to as "positive symptoms." Positive symptoms typically manifest themselves as behaviors that seem clearly bizarre even to persons with no special training in psychology, such as schizophrenic persons displaying eccentricities of language, appearance, and behavior that cause them to seem highly unusual. In fact, some writers and psychiatrists have portrayed persons with schizophrenia as individualistic heroes in a society that celebrates conformity and materialistic values:

*From "An Autobiography of a Schizophrenic Experience," by Anonymous, 1995, *Journal of Abnormal and Social Psychology, 51*, 677–689.

*From "Firsthand Symptoms in Schizohrenia," by C. S. Mellor, 1970, *British Journal of Psychiatry, 117*, 16–18.

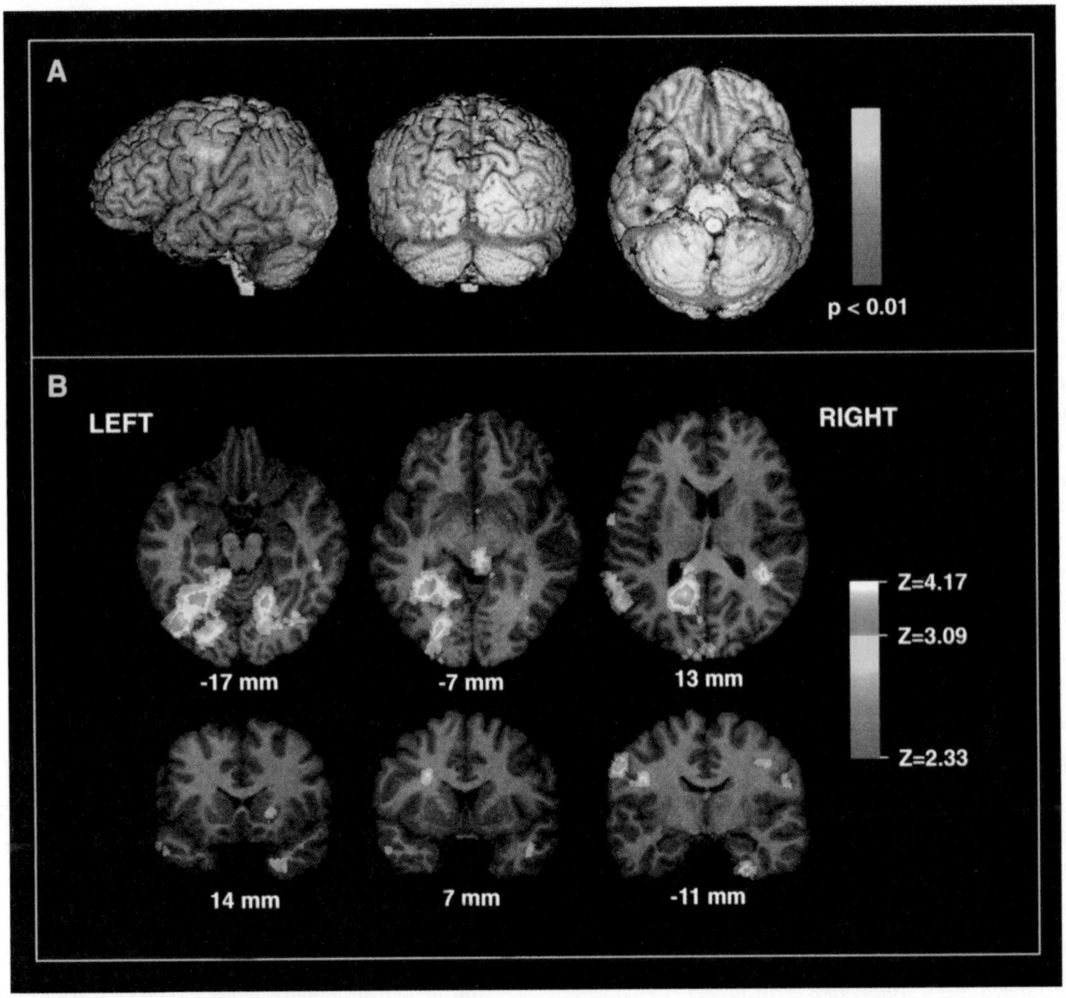

FIGURE 13-1 **Surface and slice images of the brain of a client with schizophrenia, showing areas of increased activity (in color) while he was having hallucinations—hearing voices and seeing visions that weren't there. These activated brain regions, detected with specifically designed positron-emission tomography (PET)–imaging techniques, are involved in complex auditory-linguistic, visual, and emotional processing.** (COURTESY OF D. SILBERSWEIG, M.D., AND E. STERN, M.D., THE NEW YORK HOSPITAL–CORNELL MEDICAL CENTER FUNCTIONAL NEUROIMAGING LABORATORY,. FROM "A FUNCTIONAL NEUROANATOMY OF HALLUCINATIONS IN SCHIZOPHRENIA," BY D. SILBERSWEIG, E. STERN, ET AL. 1995. *NATURE,* 378, 176–179.)

> *In* The Politics of Experience, *R. D. Laing describes madness as a release from constraint and a return to "primal man" that may even have the power to heal "our own appalling state of alienation called normality."**
>
> (*Sass, 1992, p. 22*)

This romantic view of madness has little practical relevance to the very real difficulties that most schizophrenic individuals encounter in finding a satisfactory way to live in modern society. The more modern echo of Sass's (1992) viewpoint comes from geneticists who believe that the susceptibility to schizophrenia may derive from genes that actually enhance our cognitive abilities. In this view, the very processes that give us the ability to remember better and think faster also result in susceptibility to schizophrenia. While much of this remains speculation, we will discuss some of these ideas in more detail below. For most schizophrenic individuals, the greatest impediments to social integration come not from their madness—the delusions, hallucinations, and disordered thought—but from what are commonly termed "negative symptoms."

Negative symptoms of schizophrenia are both more difficult to describe and, in their subtlest forms, more difficult to detect than are the positive symptoms. In many ways, however, the negative symptoms—flattened affect, alogia, avolition, and anhedonia—are far more debilitating.

- **Flattened affect** describes the loss of expressiveness that most schizophrenic persons develop during their illness. While schizophrenic individuals may sometimes smile or seem to develop some human warmth, the overall impression of schizophrenia is that of extreme emotional distance and lack of human response.
- **Alogia** refers to the tendency of schizophrenic individuals to speak very little and, even when speaking openly, to use brief and often seemingly empty phrases.
- **Avolition** is the tendency for those with schizophrenia to lack motivation for work or other goal-directed activities.

*From *Madness and Modernism*, by L. Sass, 1992, New York: Basic Books.

- **Anhedonia** is the seeming inability to find enjoyment in activities that would be pleasurable to unaffected individuals. While by no means unique to schizophrenia—indeed, anhedonia is a major part of the experience of depression—most schizophrenic individuals do display a significant degree of loss of pleasure in daily activities.

While the positive symptoms of schizophrenia (disordered language, hallucinations) are rarely seen among normal persons, many nonschizophrenic persons display negative symptoms at times—either as part of normal life or as a symptom of another disorder such as depression. In comparison to their occurrence in others, negative symptoms are more common and more severe in persons with schizophrenia and are especially striking when a schizophrenic individual is contrasted with the person she was before the illness began. The following passage is a description of one family's experience of schizophrenia with an emphasis on the debilitating effects of negative symptoms.

MOURNING WITHOUT END

[Gary's] childhood up to his teenage years was, as we say in medicine, "unremarkable." There was, however, something remarkable for us: Gary was a terrific kid, the kind of appealing child that parents feel lucky to have. If you had been gathering data about him during his senior year of high school, this is what you would have learned: academically, he was ranked first in his class, with a combined score of 1500 on his SATs, and had been accepted to Harvard early decision; he had a close relationship with a girlfriend for 2 years; he was the leader of a jazz group and acknowledged as an outstanding jazz drummer. It is no wonder, then, that he did not go to the 10th reunion of his high school class, because his life has not been the same since his senior year.

I have often been asked, "when did Gary's illness begin?" If I were his psychiatrist writing up the case history, I would say, "when he dropped out of Harvard during his sophomore year" or "at the time of his first hospitalization 2 years later." But when the onset of the illness is so insidious, as it was in Gary's case, and as it is in so many of these young people, it is an impossible question to answer. In retrospect, we have reason to believe that his illness started much earlier ... During high school Gary quit the tennis team, saying that he wanted to concentrate on his drumming and band work. At the time it seemed reasonable, but in retrospect it was the beginning of a tendency toward isolation....

Since that time there have been three relatively short hospitalizations, the first of which was necessary because he was suicidal ... What has it been like for us these past 10 years? I will begin with what has always been most painful for me ... feelings of loss, grief, and mourning ... I feel the loss of the son that I once had because in many ways he is quite different. Struggling as he does with many of what we now call the "negative symptoms," he has lost that gleam in his eye, that joyous good humor, that zest for life which he once showed. Today, it is hard for him to feel things strongly, or to enjoy his music, sports, or being with the family.

For a long time, when I looked into his eyes I felt that there was no one there. This is one of those manifestations that are difficult for the observer, let alone the person with the illness, to put into words. Some of the expressions that came into my mind were these: "He has become a shell of a person, there is no one there, he has lost his self, he looks different, his face has changed, he's a lost soul" ... These symptoms and the cognitive impairment disturb me much more than they do my wife, who gets more distressed over his delusional thinking. For me, the delusional thinking, as upsetting as it is, is still a sign of lively mental activity ... I am more hopeful that the delusions can be altered by medication: I worry that the cognitive impairment cannot be reversed....

I know that I should be most proud of Gary, and I can often feel that. The problem is that it is not easy to see that he is displaying great courage in coping with what has happened to him. The symptoms of the illness make him appear lacking in motivation, initiative, and will, and even he accuses himself of not trying hard enough. It is hard for

Spider

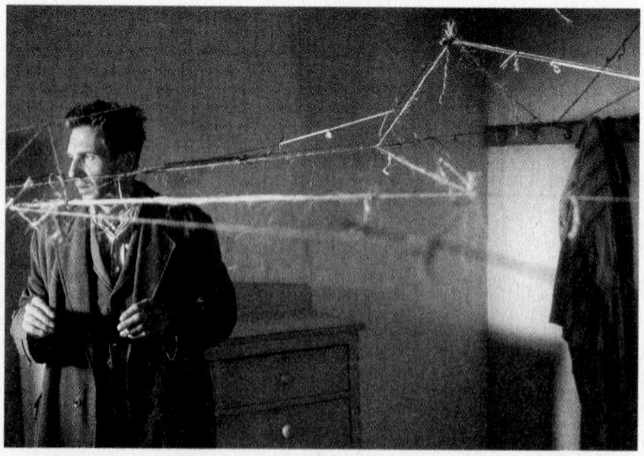

Courtesy: Sony Pictures/The Kobal Collection/Seida, Takashi

Here, Ralph Fiennes is cast in *Spider* as Dennis Clegg, whose schizophrenic thoughts become a tangled web as he struggles to understand a violent episode at the onset of his illness.

*an observer to see how difficult it must be for him to get up every day, hoping to feel different, only to awake with the same feeling of anhedonia.**

(*Willick, 1994, pp. 5–19*)

As Gary's father observes, cognitive impairment is yet another aspect of schizophrenia, in some ways the most disabling. While not part of the diagnostic criteria for schizophrenia, cognitive impairment has a major influence on functional outcome.

The diagnosis of schizophrenia in DSM-IV-TR (American Psychiatric Association, 2000) requires the presence of two positive or negative symptoms for a significant portion of time during a one-month period, with some associated social or occupational dysfunction. Even in the absence of symptoms, there must also be a six-month period of some detectable prodromal or residual symptoms.

CLINICAL COURSE

As in Gary's case, schizophrenia most commonly manifests itself in the early to mid-twenties in men. The disorder often begins somewhat later in women, typically in the late twenties. Gary's case was once again typical in that he had at least two years of steadily progressing symptoms before hospitalization was required, and, in retrospect, mild symptoms could be traced back to early adolescence. There is increasing evidence that a preschizophrenic state can be fairly reliably identified among adolescents with a set of symptoms including substance abuse, social withdrawal, and peculiar, often persecutory, thinking. Whether treatment (antidepressants may be the best current choice) can delay or prevent progression to psychosis remains uncertain (McGorry, Yung, Bechdolf, & Amminger, 2008).

The long-term course of schizophrenia is somewhat different in men and women (Tamminga, 1997). Overall, women tend to have a somewhat more benign course with fewer negative symptoms and less long-term cognitive impairment. This may be a function of the later onset of the disorder, since the same relatively more benign course is also seen in men whose symptoms start later in life. Other factors associated with relatively better prognosis include a psychologically sound personality prior to developing schizophrenia; good functioning between relatively short episodes of decompensation; the presence of significant depressive symptoms, especially in association with a family history of mood disorder; no family history of schizophrenia; and normal neurological status with no signs of structural brain damage on computed tomography (CT) or magnetic resonance imaging (MRI) (American Psychiatric Association, 2000).

Much of the current understanding about the natural course of schizophrenia comes from a landmark 20-year study done by Manfred Bleuler (1974). Bleuler found that schizophrenia most commonly evolved over approximately five years, after which time it tended to stabilize with little subsequent deterioration and, in about a third of clients, showed a tendency for some improvement. Unfortunately, another third of clients continued to worsen after five years, and a significant proportion of these clients tended to develop very severe intellectual and functional deficits. While negative symptoms surely compounded difficulties of social adjustment, severe cognitive deficits were associated with the worst outcomes.

Numerous other studies have examined cohorts of schizophrenic persons in a variety of settings and countries. Overall, the outcome for schizophrenia seems to have improved somewhat in the past 20 years, presumably as a result of treatment. Second, despite such improvement, schizophrenia is still a socially devastating disorder: In one study, less than 20% of clients were fully employed, and less than 50% were fully independent (Johnstone, 1991). Some clients may be free of positive symptoms and therefore be considered to have a "good outcome," but a good functional outcome may not follow directly from the relative absence of positive symptoms.

Studies of prognosis may be biased by who is included and excluded from the study. Some experts feel that many follow-up studies have systematically omitted clients with unusually high functioning (such as the pharmacy student whose story opens this chapter) as well as those whose outcomes are very poor. One of the important unanswered questions is whether outcome in schizophrenia is improved by early treatment (McGlashan & Johannessen, 1996). Since early symptoms may be subtle, several years often have elapsed by the time treatment begins. If medication and psychotherapy do act to preserve brain function and reduce the severity of negative symptoms, then early detection, even by population screening, may have importance. This question has become particularly relevant with the advent of newer "atypical" medications that some experts feel may actually modify the course of disease if administered early. Many experts feel that early diagnosis and treatment of psychotic disease (including that due to schizophrenia) offer the best chance for good social and clinical outcomes (Reed, 2008). But evidence so far is inconclusive on whether such interventions truly make a difference (Marshall & Rathbone, 2006). The U.S. CATIE (Clinical Antipsychotic Trials of Intervention Effectiveness) Study seems to suggest that treatment with medication (either older or newer medications) may improve functioning to some degree; however, many individuals require social and vocational rehabilitation services to improve (Swartz et al., 2007).

No discussion of outcome in schizophrenia would be complete without some discussion of the risk of suicide in this disorder. Suicide is discussed in more detail in Chapter 18, but it is worth emphasizing here that schizophrenia carries a very high suicide risk, possibly the highest of any psychiatric diagnosis (including major depressive disorder). Overall, at least 10% of schizophrenic individuals eventually commit suicide (Gottesman, 1991). Suicide may occur at

*From "A Parent's Perspective: Mourning without End," by Martin Willick, 1994. Reprinted with permission from *Schizophrenia: From Mind to Molecule* (pp. 5–19), © Copyright 1994, Washington, D.C.: American Psychiatric Press.

any time in the course of the disorder and occurs with equal frequency in men and women, in contrast to suicide in the general population, which is much more common in men. Retrospective studies have not been able to identify unusual risk factors in individuals who have killed themselves (Allenbeck, 1989), and the pervasive negative symptoms of schizophrenia make any prediction based on assessing degree of depression exceedingly difficult.

EPIDEMIOLOGY

The major challenge in much of psychiatric epidemiology is case definition: determining who actually has a given diagnosis. While this is of great importance in virtually all psychiatric conditions, nowhere is it more important or difficult than with schizophrenia, for which widely accepted definitions have emerged only recently. Mentally ill individuals frequently tend to have several seemingly different overlapping diagnoses, the border between diagnoses is often obscure, and social and economic factors may play a major role both in cause and in outcome of psychiatric disorders. The *Diagnostic and Statistical Manual* has been of value in standardizing case definitions, but as the DSM evolves through DSM-III, III-R, IV, and IV-TR criteria continue to change, potentially affecting conclusions of earlier studies.

Despite these limitations, there is actually much known about the epidemiology of schizophrenia (Gottesman, 1991). One highly regarded study using a cross-sectional methodology was a Swedish door-to-door survey of all 2,550 individuals in a rural community. Careful psychiatric interviews were conducted, and to these were added data from hospital and other community health records. There is reason to believe that the case definitions used for schizophrenia were similar to those in use today. Twenty-one schizophrenic persons were found, for a prevalence of 8.2 per 1,000 persons in the community. It is important to recognize that a number of the schizophrenic community members interviewed in this study had neither been previously diagnosed with schizophrenia nor received any mental health treatment (in several cases despite obvious psychosis). Based on a set of plausible assumptions, the lifetime risk for schizophrenia in this part of Sweden was estimated to be 1.39%. This study established that at any point in time, 8.2 persons with schizophrenia would likely be found for every 1,000 residents of a particular community. If the entire population were followed for a lifetime, it is probable that 1.39% would develop sufficient symptoms to result in a diagnosis of schizophrenia.

An even more ambitious Danish study followed a cohort of persons born during a four-year period on a small Danish island. Those who lived to age 11 years ($N = 4{,}130$) were entered in the study and followed for the next 55 years. Over this period, 38 developed schizophrenia, for a lifetime risk of just under 1%, reasonably close to the 1.39% figure in the Swedish cross-sectional study.

Yet other studies report an incidence rate of one new case per 10,000 individuals yearly (American Psychiatric Association, 2000).

SOCIAL COSTS

Epidemiological studies can help understand how common schizophrenia is, but a broader viewpoint is required to understand the very high social and financial costs of this relatively uncommon disorder (Flynn, 1994). In one year, it was estimated that mental illness cost Americans $129.7 billion. About half this amount was attributed to lost productivity, and the other half to actual medical care. While schizophrenic persons represent only 10% of the outpatient mental health caseload in the United States and only 15% of the overall inpatient caseload (36% in state and county mental hospitals), their care accounts for 75% of all mental health direct costs and 90% of all costs due to loss of productivity (Flynn, 1994). While it would appear that by far the majority of U.S. mental health care expenditures have been devoted to persons with schizophrenia, these expenditures by no means benefit all schizophrenic individuals. Many, if not most, schizophrenic persons may be living without any ongoing contact with the formal mental health system:

> *A rising tide of schizophrenic and other severely disordered individuals are now being seen in American jails.... Jails have, in fact[,] become the new asylums as many police departments feel that it is more humane to arrest severely mentally ill people than to leave them outdoors where they risk freezing to death under bridges or in city parks. Today, we have more seriously mentally ill individuals in the Los Angeles County Jail than in all five California mental hospitals combined. In fact, the Los Angeles County Jail has more mentally ill individuals than the nation's largest state hospital.**
>
> *(Flynn, 1994, p. 21)*

While the above quote was written in 1994, there is current evidence that little has changed. It is believed that in the United States, more than a million inmates of the prison system have severe mental illness (Kinsler & Saxman, 2007), and data also indicate that the severely mentally ill represent approximately 11% of the homeless population as well (Folsom & Jeste, 2002).

Evaluating the issue from a different perspective, a group of researchers in Ohio documented that 7.9% of severely ill individuals known to the county mental health system had at least one incarceration during the study year (Munetz, Grande, & Chambers, 2001). Many authors have raised concerns that severely mentally ill persons come to the attention of law enforcement and receive care (if at all) in jails rather than in hospitals or mental health clinics (Kinsler & Saxman, 2007; Lamb & Weinberger, 2005). Concerns are raised further that individuals can be "recriminalized" in the prison system. Severe mental illness has been shown to be

*From "Schizophrenia from a Family Point of View," by L. Flynn, 1994. Reprinted with permission from *Schizophrenia: From Mind to Molecule* (pp. 21–30), © Copyright 1994, Washington, DC: American Psychiatric Press.

associated with homelessness and substance abuse, creating conditions where jails have come to be the institutions primarily responsible for the care of these individuals (McNeil, Binder, & Robinson, 2005). The social costs of severe mental illness are great, and these costs compound when there is no comprehensive and sustainable treatment system (see Chapter 22 for further discussion on this topic).

ETIOLOGY

The nineteenth-century search for etiology was based on the widely held conviction that schizophrenia is a disorder of the brain and not primarily a psychological condition. This view that organic or biological factors are more important than psychological factors in causing schizophrenia has emerged more clearly in recent years. When schizophrenia made its appearance at the end of the eighteenth century, there were several theories about its cause. Given that its discovery coincided with the European Industrial Revolution, schizophrenia was initially thought to be a direct consequence of stress and urbanization (Gottesman, 1991).

Psychoanalytic Theory

While Freud did not believe that psychotherapy could cure psychosis, he did offer a range of potential psychoanalytic explanations for the symptoms of schizophrenia. Spurred by some apparent therapeutic successes, some of his followers eventually proposed psychoanalytical theories of the etiology of schizophrenia. These included a view that childhood temper tantrums and other unneutralized aggressions might ultimately lead to psychosis. At about the same time, a psychoanalytic theory emerged that portrayed schizophrenia as arising out of inadequate maternal nurturance in early infancy (Fine, 1979). Irving Gottesman, a psychologist, makes the following observations about psychological theories of schizophrenia:

> *It must be said that much of Freud's doctrine has been overly generalized by his disciples and followers beyond the conditions for which it may be of use. This has confused the study and understanding of schizophrenia by delaying biological and genetic research, and we have lived with that confusion for much of the twentieth century. Mental health professionals believe that environmental, interpersonal, and intrapsychic stressors are contributing factors; we do not believe, however, that a bad mother or father, bad mothering, or any other environmental factor alone can cause someone to become schizophrenic.**
>
> (*Gottesman, 1991, p. 15*)

In addition, multiple research studies have evaluated a wide range of developmental, environmental, and psychological factors and have failed to find any suggestion that such factors are in any way direct causes of schizophrenia (McKenna, 1994).

*Adapted from *Schizophrenia genesis,* by Irving I. Gottesman, 1991. Reprinted with permission from W. H. Freeman and Company.

Genetics

For individuals of certain genetic background, the incidence of schizophrenia may be very much higher than average. For example, while the overall risk of schizophrenia developing in a lifetime is about 1%, an individual with two schizophrenic parents has nearly a 50% chance of becoming schizophrenic. Schizophrenia is clearly a disorder with a major genetic component. This component has been investigated most dramatically through studies of twins. These studies are summarized in Research Highlight 13-1, and the results of

RESEARCH Highlight 13-1

Twin Studies in Schizophrenia

Several twin studies have been conducted, and the major findings are the following:

1. Studies have examined hospitalized clients and compared the frequency of similarly affected twins for both identical (monozygotic) and fraternal (dizygotic) twins. In four studies, 60–70% of hospitalized identical twins had a twin who also had the disease; for fraternal twins, only 0–15% had a twin with the disease (McKenna, 1994*).
2. Other studies have focused on cross-sectional population samples rather than on hospitalized individuals. For identical twins, if one twin had schizophrenia, his co-twin was 2–3 times more likely to have schizophrenia than were nonidentical co-twins of affected individuals (Gottesman, 1991**).
3. Studies that evaluate twins reared apart (in different families, often because of adoption or other family disruptions) are useful for separating genetic and environmental effects. Most twins, of course, share both similar genetics and a similar developmental environment. When identical twins are reared apart (that is, when they share the same genetics, but different environments), if one twin has schizophrenia, the co-twin also had schizophrenia in 64% of pairs (Reveley, 1994***). While it is difficult to find a large number of such twin pairs, and so in consequence results may remain somewhat speculative, these data further emphasize the importance of genetics in schizophrenia.

Source: "The inheritance of neuropsychological dysfunction in twins discordant for schizophrenia" by T. D. Cannon, M. O. Huttunen, J. Lonnqvist, A. Tuulio-Henriksson, T. Pirkola, D. Glahn, et al. (2000). *American Journal of Human Genetics*, 67(2), 369–382.

**Schizophrenia and related syndromes* by P. J. McKenna. New York: Oxford University Press 1994.

***Schizophrenia genesis* by I. I. Gottesman. New York: Freeman (1991).

****"Phenomenology, environmental risk, and genetics: Twin studies of schizophrenia" by A. M. Reveley, in N. C. Andreasen (Ed.), Schizophrenia: From Mind to Molecule* (pp. 105–118). Washington, DC: American Psychiatric Press, 1994.

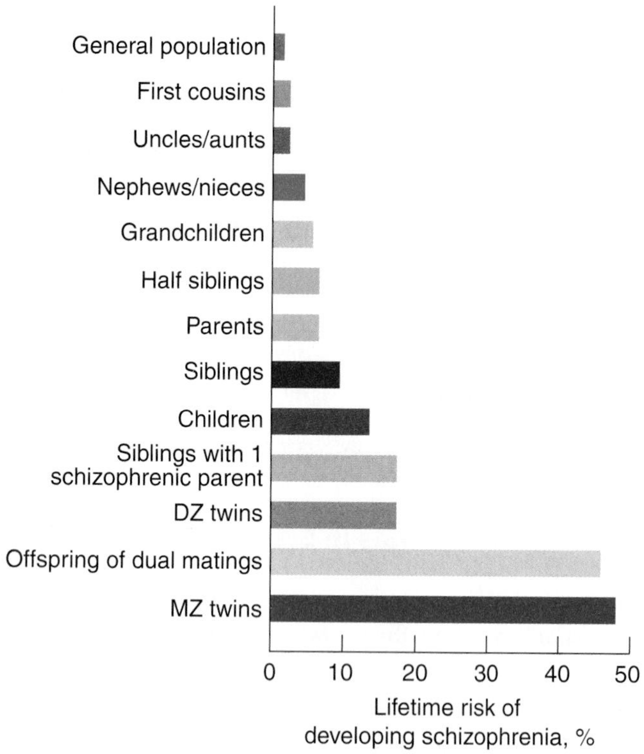

FIGURE 13-2 **Genetic risk for developing schizophrenia.**
(ADAPTED FROM *SCHIZOPHRENIA GENESIS* BY IRVING I. GOTTESMAN, 1991. REPRINTED WITH PERMISSION FROM W. H. FREEMAN AND COMPANY.)

twin studies argue convincingly that there is a genetic component to the disease (Gottesman, 1991; McKenna, 1994; Reveley, 1994).

The inheritance of schizophrenia, however, is very complex and still incompletely understood (DeLisi, 2000). As can be seen from Figure 13-2, there is a clear genetic risk for developing schizophrenia, with the highest risk occurring for identical twins (50%) and for children whose parents both have schizophrenia (45%). Intermediate (10–15%) risk occurs for nonidentical-twin siblings of schizophrenic individuals and for children of schizophrenics. Risks for other genetic relationships, although higher than the general population's baseline of 1%, are under 10%.

The current belief is that genetic factors account for about 70% of the risk of developing schizophrenia, although the majority of schizophrenics (63%) have no family history of the disease. Furthermore, many identical twins with schizophrenic siblings never develop schizophrenia despite having virtually all of their genes in common. While genetics clearly plays a role, other as yet unidentified environmental factors must also be involved in the development of schizophrenia (Dawson, 1998; Tsuang, 2000).

REFLECTIVE THINKING 13-1

Schizophrenia and Genetic Tendency

If a family had one child with schizophrenia and asked you about the genetic tendencies of the disease, what would you tell them?

CURRENT VIEWS

If psychological factors are not fundamental causes and genetic factors only play a partial role, what *does* cause schizophrenia? By the end of the nineteenth century, some leading psychiatrists felt strongly that schizophrenia was due to "organic causes"; that is, there was something physically and structurally wrong with the brains of schizophrenic individuals. The trouble with this theory was that no one could find any structural abnormalities in brains examined at autopsy. Dr. Alois Alzheimer (who was able to show a definitive link between senile dementia and brain structure) was able to show only mild generalized cell loss and scarring (gliosis) in schizophrenia, findings too nonspecific to offer clues to causation (Johnstone, 1991).

There was little progress in the search for organic causes of schizophrenia until the mid-1970s, when the newly developed CT scanner was used to evaluate brain structure in schizophrenic individuals. This powerful tool was able to show that schizophrenic males (but not females) have larger lateral ventricles than do nonschizophrenic persons. It appears that this finding has been established beyond any reasonable doubt, but its meaning is unclear (Figure 13-3). No one knows if the ventricular enlargement is a cause or a consequence of schizophrenia, and the degree of enlargement seems to have no consistent relationship to the degree or nature of illness. There is, however, some evidence that ventricular enlargement may progress during the course of schizophrenia and be associated with subtle shrinking of brain substance (cerebral atrophy). These observations remain speculative but do suggest that schizophrenia may come to be viewed as a progressive degenerative neurologic disease (DeLisi, 2000).

Soon after the development of CT scanning, various techniques became available to study regional brain blood flow and metabolic activity, and these techniques were soon used to study clients with schizophrenia. Despite early suggestions of regional blood flow abnormalities, two decades of research have produced many interesting findings in different forms of schizophrenia (Liddle et al., 1992) but little definitive insight into the cause of the disorder (Soares & Innes, 1999).

Dopamine Hypothesis

Although the cause of schizophrenia remains unknown, the brain in this disorder has been examined in remarkable detail. It seems extraordinary that such profound disruption of function can result with such little anatomic change. Many scientists feel that the pathological explanation for such profound but as yet invisible abnormalities can only be found at the molecular level: in specific enzymes and neurotransmitters. This view has given rise since the 1960s to what is termed the "dopamine hypothesis" (McKenna, 1994). This hypothesis states that the functional abnormalities in schizophrenia are due to excessive activity of brain dopamine. Dopamine is normally produced in the brain,

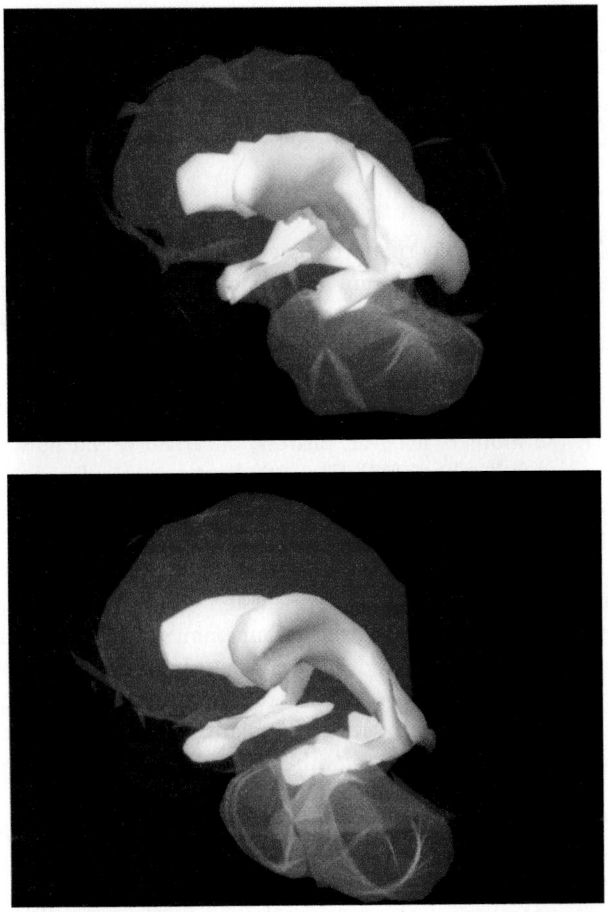

FIGURE 13-3 **MRI images in schizophrenia. These two MRI images depict a person with schizophrenia (top) and a normal control (bottom). The brain is seen from the side. The most striking difference is in the hippocampus (yellow), which is much smaller in the schizophrenic individual. The ventricles (gray) are larger in the person with schizophrenia.** (REPRINTED WITH PERMISSION FROM NANCY C. ANDREASON, UNIVERSITY OF IOWA, IOWA CITY, IA.)

and it serves as a signaling molecule or neurotransmitter. Dopamine seems to have its most important effects in the basal ganglia of the brain; reduction of dopamine in these structures leads to Parkinson's disease (a movement disorder most commonly seen in the elderly). Several pieces of evidence provide support for the hypothesis that dopamine is also involved in the causation of schizophrenia. First, drugs effective in the control of positive symptoms of schizophrenia all seem to have significant dopamine receptor–blocking activity; that is, these drugs seem to work because they reduce the effect of an individual's own dopamine on his or her brain. Secondly, drugs like amphetamines, which have the ability to cause strikingly schizophrenic-like psychoses, act by increasing brain dopamine concentrations (McKenna, 1994; Svenningsson et al., 2003).

Finally, of all the neuropathological findings from multiple autopsies of persons dying with schizophrenia, the most reproducible is an increase in dopamine receptors in the brain's basal ganglia. If receptors are increased in number, then any given amount of brain dopamine can exert a stronger biological effect (Clardy, Hyde, & Kleinman, 1994). Quite recent work adds to the likelihood that dopamine receptors play a role in the genesis of schizophrenia. The dopamine-related brain-signaling protein called DARPP-32 has been known for some time to affect brain functioning. Persons whose genetic makeup gives them adequate quantities of DARPP-32 (about 75% of us) seem to have better memory function and more flexible thought processes. However, these cognitive advantages seem also to put them at higher risk for schizophrenia if, in addition to the commonest genetic form of DARPP-32, they also have exposure to as-yet-unknown genetic or environmental causative factors (Meyer-Lindenberg et al., 2007).

Other Neurotransmitters

Despite the intriguing evidence supporting the finding of increased dopamine and dopamine receptors in schizophrenia, there is also some evidence against the hypothesis, which remains at best incomplete. While dopamine levels and receptor numbers are clearly correlated with schizophrenic symptoms, they may themselves be affected by other brain processes, particularly those in the prefrontal and cortical areas shown to be abnormal by imaging studies (Moore, West, & Grace, 1999).

The reader will recall from Chapter 4 of this text that brain synapses may be either excitatory or inhibitory. Recent research shows that in schizophrenia, there is a decrease in the number of inhibitory neurons, particularly those in which gamma-aminobutyric acid (GABA) is the predominant neurotransmitter. Expression of the signaling neuropeptides cholecystokinin and somatostatin is also decreased in schizophrenia. Loss of inhibitory function may account for the increased brain activity seen in some specific brain sites, notably the hippocampus and parts of the prefrontal cortex (Freedman, 2003). While inhibitory pathways are prominently affected, there is also evidence that effects of the excitatory neurotransmitter glutamine are potentiated by the actions of dopamine. In other research, a genetically determined relative deficiency of brain receptors for nicotine has been implicated in the pathogenesis of schizophrenia, perhaps not a surprise in a condition associated with such a very high prevalence of tobacco usage. In many ways, however, the most interesting link between inhibitory pathways and schizophrenia comes from epidemiological work linking adolescent and young adult marijuana use to the onset of schizophrenia. In Chapter 4 we discussed briefly how scientists have recently discovered brain endocannabinoid receptors that affect the way that inhibitory neurotransmitters are released. Cannabinoids in marijuana bind to these receptors, producing an experience of intoxication that in some individuals may involve paranoia or manic-like experiences. In susceptible individuals (and the nature of that susceptibility has not yet been defined), regular marijuana usage is associated with the onset of schizophrenia with a dose response relationship (i.e., more usage increases risk; Leweke & Koethe, 2008). Regular marijuana users are several times more likely to develop schizophrenia (odds ratio 2–9) than nonusers (Semple, McIntosh, & Lawrie, 2005). Whether these individuals would have eventually become schizophrenic in the absence of marijuana usage remains uncertain. Clearly, the neurochemical pathways involved in schizophrenia are complex and still incompletely understood. However, what is known at least allows a better understanding of how drug treatments affect this disorder.

Other Considerations: The Role of Viruses

While it has become increasingly clear that a variety of biochemical changes in the brain, almost certainly inherited in some way, make it more likely that someone will develop schizophrenia, the actual "cause" of this disease—why, for example, one identical twin will succumb and the other will not—remains a mystery. One theory has been that virus infection either in postnatal life or during pregnancy may cause a genetically susceptible individual to subsequently develop schizophrenia—perhaps many years after that exposure. Many viruses and the parasite toxoplasma have been implicated—though none as yet convincingly. One case control study implicated adult toxoplasma infection in the onset of schizophrenia among military recruits (all of whom had had blood drawn and stored before the development of schizophrenia) (Niebuhr et al., 2008). Some researchers have speculated that it is not the virus or parasite that causes schizophrenia in susceptible individuals, but the individual's (or, when infection is acquired prenatally, his or her mother's) immune response to that infection.

TREATMENT

There are two main approaches to the treatment of schizophrenia: the psychosocial approach and the pharmacological approach. The nurse has a role in each (Gournay, 1995). There is an autonomous nursing role in directing and managing the psychosocial treatment as well as an obvious collaborative role in working with other professionals to provide for the psychosocial therapies and to monitor the pharmacological treatment. Each will be discussed next, with specific attention paid to nursing perspectives on care in the section that follows.

Psychosocial Treatment

The goals of psychosocial treatment interventions can be conceived in a number of different ways, but one useful approach has been to divide interventions into three categories: clinical and family support services, rehabilitative services, and humanitarian aid/public safety (Hargreaves & Shumway, 1989). The goal of clinical interventions is to reduce both positive and negative symptoms and to maximize functional outcome. Clinical support involves outpatient management and family/community services. Rehabilitation involves increasing clients' capacities, both for social interactions and for productive activity (including gainful employment when feasible). Humanitarian interventions are those efforts that maximize an individual's independence and quality of life within the bounds of his or her mental disability. Public safety involves balancing personal liberty with the recognition that some social control may be needed to prevent harm, both to the individual and to society.

Clinical and Family Support Services

Clinical and family support services include educating family members about the nature and meaning of schizophrenia as well as providing specific skills training in stress management and functional coping for both client and family.

Assisting family members is a priority of nursing care. One study of mothers of schizophrenic young men revealed that the mothers felt fear, distress, uncertainty, and powerlessness (Wheeler, 1994). These findings echo similar observations among parents who care for mentally ill children (Eakes, 1995). Families can be supported through education, group activities, and community involvement/advocacy. Internet bulletin boards and discussion groups provide new methods of linking individuals and family members with others around the world in electronic support groups. For example, over a three-month period, one discussion group on the general topic of schizophrenia had 54 named participants from ten countries with over 1,000 entries (Schizophrenia Discussion Groups, 2004).

In addition, nurses and others can help families to better understand the purpose and side effects of medication in an effort to ensure compliance with treatment. Multiple studies have shown that adding these kinds of psychosocial interventions to drug treatment significantly reduces the frequency of relapses (Huxley, Rendall, & Sederer, 2000; McGlashan, 1994). The CATIE study showed that good compliance with treatment is one of the major determinants of psychosocial outcomes in schizophrenia (Swartz et al., 2007).

Rehabilitation

Rehabilitation efforts for persons with schizophrenia may be directed toward vocational goals for some individuals, but for a majority, the presence of negative symptoms makes any kind of social functioning so problematic that the primary focus has to be on enhancing social skills. Training in social functioning can potentially increase clients' knowledge and skill levels; it may also sometimes reduce rates of psychotic relapse (Hogarty et al., 1986). Programs can address emotional insight and family problem-solving skills and both verbal and nonverbal communication, including the importance of eye contact and facial expressions. As two authorities observe,

> *The most effective psychosocial treatment—whether provided in individual, group, or family therapy, inpatient ward or community program—contains elements of practicality, problem-solving of everyday challenges, socialization and vocational activities, and specific goal orientation ... It is likely that future research will establish the benefit of indefinite psychosocial support and training in the long-term*

NURSINGTIP 13-1

Family Management of Members with Schizophrenia

Three underlying concepts of programs directed to families have been summarized as follows (Barrowclough & Tarrier, 1992):

1. Living with a person who suffers from schizophrenia can be very difficult; most relatives feel stressed and upset, at least some of the time.
2. When the client with schizophrenia lives with his family, a lot of the day-to-day help and rehabilitation are carried out by family members. Thus, if they are to effectively help the client, family members must have help in managing their stress and coping with difficult situations.
3. Additionally, people who suffer from schizophrenia are unusually sensitive to stress in others, so by feeling more in control of oneself, a family member may indirectly help the client.

*management of schizophrenia. Just as neuroleptic drugs are most effective in maintaining symptomatic improvement when continued indefinitely, it is not surprising that psychosocial treatments are similarly optimized by continuity.**

(Vaccaro & Roberts, 1992, p. 114)

Individual and family stress is clearly associated with both onset and exacerbation of schizophrenic symptoms. Failure to take medication is a major cause of symptoms worsening. Enhancing family functioning, decreasing measures of interpersonal stress, and maximizing medication compliance are among the important areas for psychosocial intervention. This intervention may be effected by a nurse, a social worker, a psychologist, or a multidisciplinary team involving all three professions. Special programs have been developed to assist schizophrenic persons with activities of daily living, and one of these is summarized in Research Highlight 13-2 (Heinssen, Liberman, & Kopelowicz, 2000).

Humanitarian Aid/Public Safety

In recent years, mental health workers have used the term "challenging behavior" to describe the most difficult positive symptoms of schizophrenia: bizarre, socially disruptive, and perhaps potentially dangerous behavior. Prior to deinstitutionalization, many such clients would have been hospitalized in an effort to enhance their own safety as well as that of the public. Today the options for managing and treating such challenging behavior are probably more limited.

*From *Teaching Social and Coping Skills*, by J. V. Vacarro & L. Roberts. In M. Birchwood and N. Tarrier (Eds.), 1992. *Innovations in the Psychological Management of Schizophrenia*. Reprinted with permission from John Wiley & Sons.

RESEARCH Highlight 13-2

Living among Strangers: The Needs and Functions of Persons with Schizophrenia Residing in Assisted Living Facilities

PURPOSE

The purpose of the research was to investigate the levels of functioning, the needs, and the medication knowledge of persons with schizophrenia in assisted living facilities.

METHODS

The researcher used a descriptive, correlational design to evaluate relationships among the variables of needs, symptoms, medication knowledge, and demographics. There were 58 persons in the study sample.

RESULTS

The findings suggest that the average person with schizophrenia living in assisted living facilities is a 43-year-old Caucasian male who dropped out of high school and suffered from a psychiatric illness for 21 years. This average resident had five inpatient psychiatric hospital admissions in his life and was prescribed four different psychiatric medications at the time of the study. A majority received treatment at a community mental health center. The two most commonly identified needs of these residents were for social activity and to learn domestic skills, followed by work-related needs and transportations needs. Level of functioning was positively correlated with the global assessment of functioning (GAF) score and medication knowledge.

IMPLICATIONS

Better understanding of the level of functioning and the needs of schizophrenic individuals permits facilities to develop standards designed to assist in meeting such needs.

Source: "Living among Strangers: The Needs and Function of Persons with Schizophrenia Residing in an Assisted Living Facility," by S. V. Cadena, 2006, *Issues in Mental HealthNnursing*, *27*, 25–41.

Beginning in the mid-1960s, the United States embarked on an extraordinary program to remove the severely mentally ill from mental hospitals. Many hospitals were indeed uncaring, filthy, and brutal; from a human perspective, "deinstitutionalized" care seemed to offer the severely mentally ill potential for far more normal lives. As a result, between 1965 and 1975 the population of U.S. mental institutions was purposefully reduced by 60%; and it had actually declined even more dramatically between 1955 and 1965. Experts have

REFLECTIVE THINKING 13-2

Schizophrenia and the Homeless

Clinicians who examine the homeless consistently conclude that about a third of them have severe mental disorders, and in direct surveys of the homeless, the homeless themselves report clear symptoms of psychosis.

In the 1950s and 1960s, most of these persons would have been placed in hospitals on the basis of their mental illnesses. Deinstitutionalization moved these persons to the least restrictive environment, and in the 1980s and 1990s, social policies were such that these persons had the right to be on their own but with little support and no money with which to manage other than on the street. Courts have ruled that mental illness is not sufficient justification for involuntary commitment to a hospital, and hospitals are not allowed (or, at least, are not reimbursed) for keeping clients longer than a specified number of days.

- How would you create social policy to maintain the individual rights of mentally ill persons and at the same time provide them with care and treatment?
- Who would agree with your position, and who would not? How can the nurse best implement this role?

observed that the results were not quite as intended: "With help from improvements in antipsychotic drugs, many schizophrenics have returned to the community. Some are in supervised public settings, and we are still able to count those, but some are in jails and prisons, others are lost among the hordes of homeless, and a few are in private treatment" (Gottesman, 1991, p. 64).

While this revolutionary program of deinstitutionalization is not fully responsible for the current American epidemic of homelessness, many feel it has contributed significantly. About a third of the homeless are estimated to be seriously mentally ill, as are up to 20% of the nearly 1 million individuals in U.S. jails and prisons (Gottesman, 1991).

While numerous problems were documented and care in some hospitals was inappropriate, the best psychiatric facilities of the 1960s provided clients with a protective and supportive environment that cannot be duplicated today. As distinguished Yale University psychiatrist Thomas McGlashan observes,

> *We must tell the accountants that the alternatives to institutionalization are equally if not more expensive ... We have thrust the severely mentally ill out of the institutions [and onto the sidewalks] only to forget that ... they are disabled and they need asylum, in the sense of support and protection from stress ... I am not sure what will be our next great leap forward, but I do know one thing—we sure are ready for something because it sure is bad out there.**
>
> (McGlashan, 1994, p. 213)

Many mental health workers define humane care as the least restrictive care needed to provide psychosocial and rehabilitative services to the client. Although deinstitutionalization ensured that persons live in environments with fewer restrictions, one knows from a social perspective that the settings in which many schizophrenic persons currently live are neither caring nor therapeutic. The individual's right to the least restrictive environment has all too often meant the right to be homeless, starving, and without treatment.

Pharmacological and Physical Treatments

Antipsychotic Medications

For centuries, rauwolfia root had been used in India to sedate persons with severe psychiatric disorders. In 1952, the active ingredient of rauwolfia, reserpine, was found to have useful properties in the management of schizophrenia (though for a variety of reasons it is no longer used). At virtually the same time, two newly synthesized antihistamine-like drugs, promethazine and chlorpromazine, were found to have very similar effects in clients. By the mid-1960s, multiple placebo-controlled double-blind trials had established beyond any doubt the effectiveness of chlorpromazine in controlling both negative and positive symptoms of schizophrenia, although the effect on negative symptoms was far less than that on positive symptoms. Not only was the effectiveness of chlorpromazine proven by these careful studies, but also the improvement—especially in positive symptoms of paranoia, hallucinations, and agitation—was quite remarkable for some clients. Numerous "antipsychotic" medications have become available over the past 40 years; collectively, these drugs have been called "antipsychotics" or "neuroleptics."

Antipsychotics are now thought of as falling into two categories: first- and second- generation medications. Several decades of antipsychotic use have led clinicians to a variety of conclusions about these medications, which are summarized in Box 13-2. These medications are helpful, but they do not cure schizophrenia, and they have some significant adverse side effects, which are discussed in the following paragraphs.

Side Effects of Antipsychotics

Most antipsychotics share similar therapeutic properties and side effects. Sudden death has occasionally been reported after neuroleptic administration, especially by injection, but experts are not yet sure whether medication has caused these deaths (Editors, 1995). Other than this still-unresolved concern, the most serious antipsychotic side effects involve the

*From "Psychosocial Treatments" of Schizophrenia, by T. H. McGlashan, 1994. Reprinted with permission from *Schizophrenia: From Mind to Molecule* (p. 213), Copyright © 1994, Washington, DC: American Psychiatric Association.

nervous system and appear to result from the very dopamine receptor blockade that makes these drugs so useful.

The most readily treated side effect is called **dystonia**. Dystonic reactions usually manifest as painful muscle spasms lasting anywhere from a few seconds to days. These may involve any muscle group and are most often localized to just a few muscles at a time. Contractions of the neck, known as torticollis, and of the facial muscles are probably most common. Clients may present with the head drawn forcefully to one side, with spasms of the mouth muscles, or with fixed tongue protrusion. These spasms are rarely dangerous unless the laryngeal muscles are involved, in which case the airway is at risk of obstruction. Dystonic reactions typically occur within a few hours or days of starting an antipsychotic, stop fairly quickly when medication is discontinued, and respond almost instantaneously to intravenous diphenhydramine (benadryl) or to other anticholinergic medications. Benzodiazepines (diazepam or clonazepam) are also effective. Acute dystonia is fairly rare but occurs in 2–3% of clients given chlorpromazine and rather more commonly in clients given haloperidol (Haldol) and a long-acting injectable neuroleptic such as fluphenazine.

Akathisia is a somewhat more common side effect that affects both motor function and behavior. Clients with akathisia become physically restless and unable to sit still: they pace, shift their weight from foot to foot, and tap their feet. The upper extremities and face are rarely involved, but many clients develop emotional changes: at times, they show decreased ability to concentrate along with euphoria but sometimes malaise, depression, and worsening psychosis. Compared to acute dystonia, akathisia begins somewhat later in the course of treatment, but rarely after six months. It sometimes diminishes or disappears without stopping treatment, but virtually always goes away when the antipsychotic medication is stopped.

Symptoms of Parkinsonism may be induced by antipsychotic drugs and occur in up to 40% of clients treated with these medications. Older clients are affected more than younger, and, like akathisia, Parkinsonism tends to occur within the first months of treatment. The primary finding is **akinesia**, or poverty of movement. This is different from the usual avolition of schizophrenia; clients with Parkinsonian akinesia initiate very slowly any movement (seen commonly in getting out of a chair) and show reduced arm swinging when walking. In most cases, symptoms resolve even without stopping medication, but about 1% of individuals continue to have Parkinsonism despite drug withdrawal. It is felt by many that these individuals had underlying "idiopathic" Parkinsonism that was unmasked by neuroleptic treatment. Clients with drug-induced Parkinsonism are thought to respond particularly well to anticholinergic medication treatment.

Tardive dyskinesia is a troublesome movement disorder that is commonly found in schizophrenic clients maintained on antipsychotics for long periods of time. The incidence is said to be up to 4% per year but is clearly highest in older clients, especially women. The movements of tardive dyskinesia are typically repetitive and most commonly involve the face. Common findings are repetitive smacking, chewing, grimacing, cheek puffing, and tongue protrusion. Similar movements can involve the hands, and on occasion, ticlike movements occur, including grunts or other vocal utterances.

Curiously, increasing the dose of medication sometimes significantly suppresses tardive dyskinesia. However, tardive dyskinesia is often very resistant to any treatment and permanently stigmatizes clients who have the misfortune to develop symptoms that are unresponsive to treatment. Early diagnosis and treatment, including drug holidays and decreased dosages, are the best courses of action.

Neuroleptic malignant syndrome. The most serious antipsychotic side effect, neuroleptic malignant syndrome, is also the rarest, but nurses must be familiar with it because if left untreated, it may rapidly lead to death. Most clients develop this syndrome only when on high or increasing doses of medication and often after a dosage increase. The most striking features are confusion or decreased level of consciousness

BOX 13-2
ANTIPSYCHOTIC MEDICATIONS

- Antipsychotics are valuable medications, but they do not cure schizophrenia.
- Twenty percent of clients have complete remission when treated with first-generation antipsychotics.
- In about a quarter of clients, even positive symptoms remain highly resistant to antipsychotic medications.
- While the antipsychotic medications do have an effect on negative symptoms, these symptoms frequently remain socially incapacitating.
- These medications have a range of significant adverse side effects.
- With the exception of clozapine, there is little evidence that any one neuroleptic is more effective than the others.
- All the antipsychotics seem to share the ability to block dopamine from interacting with brain dopamine receptors.
- Newer neuroleptics increase the risk of heart disease and must be used cautiously when long-term treatment is contemplated.

NURSINGALERT 13-2
Tardive Dyskinesia

Unlike the other neuroleptic-induced movement disorders, tardive dyskinesia frequently cannot be reversed by withdrawing medication.

and high fever. Clients also acutely develop Parkinsonian symptoms of rigidity and akinesia, but the significance of these is sometimes overlooked in the erroneous search for an infectious cause of fever. Fever is most often very high in neuroleptic malignant syndrome, not infrequently rising to dangerous levels (above 106°F); but in rare cases, it may be absent, and high fever is not required to make the diagnosis. Serum creatine kinase (CK) is the definitive diagnostic test; because of muscle damage, presumably due to extreme rigidity, CK reaches very high levels, often associated with myoglobinuria. Treatment is largely symptomatic, and both vigorous hydration and cooling are often required to ensure survival. Antipsychotic medication is stopped, and various medications to increase central nervous system (CNS) dopamine levels may be given.

First- and Second-Generation Antipsychotics

Thioridizine and clozapine are regarded as atypical antipsychotics partly because they do not seem to cause movement disorders. Whereas thioridizine is clearly *less* effective than the other antipsychotics, clozapine has been shown in controlled trials to be more effective and often to produce improvement in clients resistant to other antipsychotics. Unfortunately, this improvement sometimes comes at a price: Clozapine occasionally and unpredictably causes severe agranulocytosis (reduction in numbers of white blood cells). This complication has proven fatal for some clients, and in some states, mental health client advocacy groups have forced tight regulation in the use of clozapine. With careful monitoring of white blood cell counts, clozapine can be used with relative safety, but this requirement for monitoring makes it very difficult to employ in community outpatient settings unless compliance can be ensured. There is currently much interest in developing new drugs that have clozapine's effectiveness without its effect on white blood cells.

In addition to clozapine (Clozaril), currently available second-generation drugs include quetiapine (Seroquel), olanzapine (Zyprexa), ziprasidone (Geodon), aripipraazole (Abilify), and risperidone (Risperdal). A combination medication with olanzapine and fluoxetine (Prozac) is also marketed under the name of Symbyax. Each of these medications has a significantly decreased risk of tardive dyskinesia compared to classical agents such as haloperidol. Clozapine, despite the risk associated with its use, still seems to be more effective than the others and is the treatment of choice for symptoms resistant to other drugs. Many psychiatrists have chosen to use atypical drugs as "first-line" treatments because they are less likely to cause tardive dyskinesia and because initial evidence suggested that these drugs might prove effective in relieving negative as well as positive symptoms (Worrel, Marken, Beckman, & Ruehter, 2000). Subsequent studies have not shown newer agents to be more effective, especially in reducing negative symptoms, and their metabolic side effects have raised concerns about long-term safety (Tandon et al., 2008).

Weight gain is common with most second-generation drugs, and gains of 40 pounds are not unusual. It is perhaps because of this weight gain that diabetes sometimes accompanies long-term use of the second-generation medications, and diabetic ketoacidosis has been reported in some patients (Freedman, 2003). There appears to be increased risk of coronary heart disease in persons who take second-generation antipsychotics for prolonged periods, and with the exception of clozapine (whose clinical effectiveness seems paradoxically linked to its ability to cause weight gain and increased cardiac risk), these drugs may afford no added efficacy over first-generation antipsychotics (Bai et al., 2006). Whether cardiac risk associated with second-generation neuroleptics can be reduced by control of conventional coronary risk factors (and how effective that control might prove among individuals with schizophrenia) remains to be seen. Studies are currently underway to determine if ziprasidone may have additional mortality risk because of its tendency to slightly prolong the cardiac QT interval (thereby possibly increasing susceptibility to dangerous arrhythmias). Because of evidence that mortality is also increased among elderly patients who are given atypical antipsychotics to control behavior associated with dementia, the U.S. Food and Drug Administration (FDA) has placed a black box warning on these drugs when used in the elderly. No treatment program is uniformly successful or unequivocally alters the course of the disease (Schultz & Andreasen, 1999). Further reports from CATIE and other similar long-term studies will be necessary to determine the best and safest drug treatments for schizophrenia.

While current practice is generally to start treatment with a second-generation medication other than clozapine, those clients who do not improve may be switched either to a first-generation medicine or to clozapine. In clients with the highest levels of functioning, clozapine may be used preferentially (and with close hematological monitoring) despite its risk of life-threatening bone marrow suppression. Clients who respond to antipsychotics but relapse because of failure to adhere to prescribed medication regimens are candidates for injectable medicines or perhaps for long-acting oral preparations that are currently being evaluated. Injectable first-generation medicines do risk producing tardive dyskinesia, but they allow better compliance with therapy and can lead to improved neuropsychological outcomes in many clients. A large prospective trial called PROACTIVE is currently evaluating whether injection treatment leads to better outcomes than does conventional oral administration of antipsychotics. It will be a number of years before the results of PROACTIVE become known.

Risk of Suicide

Suicide is a major risk among clients with schizophrenia. While depression not infrequently accompanies schizophrenia (often leading to a diagnosis of schizoaffective disorder), suicide may take place in the absence of recognized depression. Suicide is more likely to occur when positive symptoms are improving, but overall suicidal risk may be decreased in clients taking clozapine (Freedman, 2003). A large Finnish observational study showed that suicide risk was lower among schizophrenic patients treated with antipsychotics in combination with antidepressants, but it remains unclear

RESEARCH Highlight 13-3

Student Nurses and Severe Mental Illness

One of the goals of instruction in psychiatric mental health illness is to increase students' empathy with mentally ill persons and to help students feel more comfortable in working with people whose mental experiences are very different than their own.

STUDY PROBLEM PURPOSE

Nurse researchers conducted a before-and-after study involving third-year university nursing students who were exposed to a four-week clerkship in mental health nursing. The goal of this study was to see if the students' exposure to mental illness altered their professional attitudes toward severely ill clients.

METHODS

One hundred twenty-six students were given a paper-based exercise involving four separate vignettes of persons with schizophrenia. The students were asked questions about the cases in these vignettes both before and following their four-week clerkship.

FINDINGS

Based on the students' pre- and postclerkship responses, instructors felt students had become more compassionate, more willing to care for patients with significant mental illness, and more accepting of community—rather than institutional—care for these individuals.

IMPLICATIONS

While the lack of a control group and the evaluation of the questionnaires by instructors who might wish to find the results reported risk bias in this study, the results support the subjective experience of many who teach courses in psychiatric mental health nursing. Spending a period of concentrated time among persons with schizophrenia and other serious mental illnesses under the tutelage of sensitive and committed instructors can have lasting effects on students' personal growth and on their willingness to provide care to people whose lives and thoughts are very different than their own.

Source: "Reshaping Students' Attitudes toward Individuals with Mental Illness through a Clinical Nursing Clerkship," by P. Romem et al., 2008, *Journal of Nursing Education*, *47*(9), 396–402.

whether this treatment actually reduced suicide or identified more compliant patients at lower risk of self-injury. It remains uncertain whether adding psychological treatments, such as cognitive-behavioral therapy, to drug and supportive treatment of schizophrenia reduces the risk of suicide. While there is enthusiasm for cognitive therapy based on limited evidence (Tandon, 2005), other studies do not suggest that it has major benefits in reducing suicide risk (Tarrier et al., 2006).

Other Physical Treatments

Medication is not the only treatment employed for schizophrenia. Electroconvulsive therapy (shock therapy) has been used, especially for individuals in catatonic states, and, while there may be only short-term benefit, evidence suggests electroconvulsive therapy to be valuable in selected patients when used in association with antipsychotic medications (Tharyan & Adams, 2005; see Chapter 32 for further discussion of electroconvulsive therapy).

NURSING CARE

The nurse is a major participant in the care of schizophrenic persons.

Nurses will work with other mental health care workers and be part of a collaborative team providing service to and advocacy for clients. A nursing perspective, however, is unique because the nursing focus is on the human response to the condition. As demonstrated in the discussions preceding, the human responses to living with schizophrenia are directly related to the individual's experience and symptoms. Applicable nursing diagnoses parallel these symptoms, as illustrated in Table 13-1.

What approach to care should the nurse use? There are basic guidelines for each nursing diagnosis. To address the diagnosis of *disturbed thought processes*, the nurse must first recognize that the client is unable to easily follow verbal speech. The nurse must speak clearly, making only one point at a time or giving clear and simple directions. When a client is delusional, the nurse should not enter into the delusion, that is, should not ask the client to "Tell me more" or engage the client in conversation about the delusional ideas. Rather, the nurse should attempt to learn the meaning of the delusion to the client. Also, the nurse can and should express doubt over the reality of delusional thoughts; for example, the nurse could say, "I don't see how you can be receiving

TABLE 13-1 Symptoms Experienced with Schizophrenia and Associated Nursing Diagnoses

SYMPTOMS	NURSING DIAGNOSES
Disordered thought	*Disturbed thought processes*
Incomprehensible language	*Impaired verbal communication*
Loss of function	*Ineffective role performance*
Delusions	*Disturbed thought processes*
Hallucinations	*Disturbed sensory perception*

Art of Healing by Edward Adamson and John Timlin

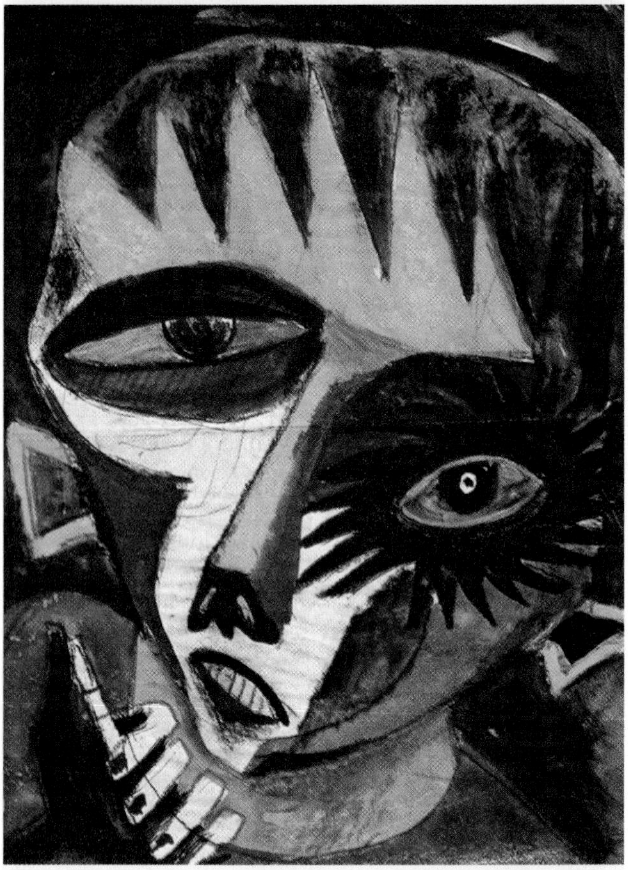

Courtesy: Reprinted with permission of Adamson Collection Charity.

While the influences of Cubism may be apparent, this painting is not by a follower of Pablo Picasso or Georges Braque but was painted by an individual suffering from schizophrenia. The intensity of schizophrenic experiences is evident in the frenzied shapes and colors.

messages from outer space," but must avoid entering into an argument with the client over the validity of his thoughts. The nurse should redirect the conversation away from the delusions and back to reality by introducing another topic. When a client has been diagnosed with *impaired verbal communication* because of disordered speech, the nurse can assist by taking time to understand the client's needs, maintaining a calm and peaceful environment to help the client center and express himself, and communicating to the client in clear, short phrases. Interventions aimed at developing and maintaining social skills (to be discussed later) will also apply.

The diagnosis of *ineffective role performance* will cause great difficulty for the client in society. Loss of job, friends, and support may be results of the client's inability to perform in socially acceptable ways. The client may lose the ability to care for himself. Such situations lead to dependence on others to the degree where hospital care or care through structured settings such as board-and-care homes is necessary. The community nurse will frequently have a role in evaluating the living and care environments for clients and assisting in procuring appropriate and safe arrangements. Further, the nurse should assist the client in activities that foster socially acceptable interactions with others.

The diagnosis of *disturbed sensory perceptions* due to hallucinations can be frightening to the client, his family and friends, other clients on a hospital unit, and the nurse herself. The nurse must understand that the hallucinations are very real to the client and that clients will respond to their hallucinatory experiences. In an acute setting, the nurse should provide a quiet and nonstimulating environment and talk to the client, letting him know that she is present and will maintain safety for the client. It is appropriate for the nurse to tell the client that she does not see or hear the client's hallucination. For example, the nurse might say, "I know it is very real to you, but I do not hear the voice." Because medications can control hallucinations, the nurse can administer medication as prescribed by the physician. The nurse must remember that clients may respond to hallucinations in unpredictable ways and that there is always a potential for violent outbursts. For example, a client may hear voices telling him to harm someone else. The goals of the nursing interventions are to establish safety and to help attune the client to reality.

Impaired social interactions result from the negative symptoms of the disease. Social support and social training groups can be important interventions. The nurse must begin by establishing a one-on-one, supportive, therapeutic relationship and build from that relationship to assist the client to interact with others. On an interdisciplinary team, recreational and occupational therapists can make important contributions to meeting the client's needs for socialization through planned therapeutic activities.

NURSING THEORY

The overriding need of a long-term schizophrenic client is to be supported so that he can maintain ability to function as independently as possible. Frequently, the client's inability to interact with others and meet expected social norms prevents independent functioning. Nursing theories grounded in establishing a trusting nurse-client relationship help provide the framework to serve as a basis for all therapeutic interaction.

The Modeling and Role-Modeling Theory (Erickson, Tomlin, & Swain, 1983; Frisch & Bowman, 2008) assists by providing the nurse with the five aims of intervention that can become the foundation for all work with the schizophrenic client:

1. Build trust.
2. Promote positive orientation.
3. Promote perceived control.
4. Promote strengths.
5. Set mutual goals that are health directed.

The nurse can begin with building trust and work from an established nurse-client relationship to design care aimed at realistic and appropriate goals.

APPLICATION OF THE NURSING PROCESS 13-1

ASSESSMENT

An important consideration in assessing a client with schizophrenia is the degree to which symptoms of the disease are currently affecting the client's functioning. Box 13-3 lists important parameters of assessment. The nurse will need to obtain information from the client and, often, from other sources. For example, a person with schizophrenia may not be able to communicate regarding negative symptoms, such as lack of motivation or poverty of speech, and will not be able to tell the nurse if current behavior is a change from previous functioning. Such information is appropriately obtained from family members or others who may relate observations over a period of time.

In assessment, the nurse is not just looking for evidence that symptoms of schizophrenia exist, but also looking for clues as to the immediate concerns of and the kind of assistance desired by the client or family members/caretakers.

BOX 13-3
ASSESSMENT PARAMETERS FOR SCHIZOPHRENIC CLIENTS

Observe for:

1. Presence of delusions
   - Does the client have ideas or beliefs that others say are untrue?
   - Does the client have the belief that neutral cues in the environment refer to him?
   - Does the client believe he has special talents and extraordinary powers?
2. Presence of hallucinations
   - Does the client see, hear, or smell things others do not?
3. Disorganized speech
   - Can the client communicate logically and rationally?
4. Problems in basic grooming
5. Negative symptoms of schizophrenia, including:
   - Flat affect (dampening of emotions)
   - Poverty of speech
   - Lack of motivation
   - Symptoms of depression
6. Level of independence and functioning

NURSING DIAGNOSIS

Nursing diagnoses are made based on priority needs. For example, in an acute episode where the client is being admitted to hospital for symptoms of disordered thoughts, hallucinations, delusions, and loss of function, control and management of the symptoms are the highest priority. Once symptoms are brought under control, the concerns of loss of function, social isolation, and role performance can be addressed over a rehabilitative plan of care.

Nursing diagnoses made during the acute episode may be:

- *Disturbed thought processes* related to physical and psychological stressors
- *Disturbed sensory perceptions—auditory hallucinations* related to biochemical imbalance and/or psychological stress

APPLICATION OF THE NURSING PROCESS 13-1 (Continued)

- *Self-care deficit (specify)* related to disturbed thought processes
- *Insomnia* related to fear of falling asleep

In contrast, in a rehabilitative phase of treatment, the nursing diagnoses may be:

- *Ineffective role performance* related to change in self-perception of role
- *Social isolation*, related to absence of or inability to engage in satisfying personal relationships
- *Ineffective therapeutic regimen management* related to knowledge deficit and complexity of therapeutic regimen

OUTCOME IDENTIFICATION

For each diagnosis, the nurse must establish appropriate and expected outcomes and goals. Again, the expected outcomes will be different depending on whether the client is being treated in an acute or rehabilitative phase.

ACUTE PHASE

In the acute phase, the immediate goal of treatment is to bring symptoms under control. For example, for the diagnosis of *disturbed thought processes*, a stated outcome might be "within 3 days of initiating treatment, the client will be able to answer simple direct questions." For the diagnosis of *disturbed sensory perception—auditory hallucinations*, the outcome might be "within 3 days of initiating medication, the client will experience a decline in number of hallucinations." For the diagnosis of *insomnia*, the stated outcome might be "within 3 days of hospital admission, the client will sleep through the night."

REHABILITATIVE PHASE

Clearly, the nurse providing care in the rehabilitative phase will establish goals aimed at helping the client and his family to make the best adjustment possible to a chronic illness and will take any measures possible to maintain the client's independence to whatever degree possible. Outcomes should be identified for every nursing diagnosis. Examples are (1) for the diagnosis of *ineffective role performance*, related to inability to keep a job, the nurse and client together might determine that the problem is getting up to go to work and might establish a goal that the client will attend work regularly by going to work with his neighbor; and (2) for the diagnosis of *ineffective therapeutic regimen management*, related to forgetting to take needed medications, the nurse and client might come up with an outcome that the client will take medications regularly and that his sister will visit daily to inquire about medication.

PLANNING/INTERVENTIONS

ACUTE PHASE

In the acute phase of schizophrenia, the assessment, plan, and outcomes are all based on alleviating acute symptoms. Thus, much of the nursing care will be collaborative and involve use of medications to bring symptoms under control. Independent nursing care—for example, care directed at assisting a client to sleep—will be done through interventions that establish a safe and trusting environment and provide an acutely ill client a space for sleep without interference from others.

REHABILITATIVE PHASE

In the rehabilitative phase, the interventions must be planned by the nurse and client together, not by the nurse alone. The most successful interventions will be creative, as the nurse and client attempt to identify

(Continues)

APPLICATION OF THE NURSING PROCESS 13-1 (Continued)

BOX 13-4
PRINCIPLES FOR CARING FOR SCHIZOPHRENIC CLIENTS: ACUTE PHASE

The following principles are helpful in planning interventions for schizophrenic clients in the acute phase:

- The symptoms of disordered thoughts, hallucinations, and loss of function are often frightening to the client. Nursing actions to promote a calm, peaceful, trusting atmosphere are essential in alleviating fear and establishing a nurse-client relationship.
- The nurse should express reality regarding client reports of hallucinations and delusions but should not enter into arguments regarding whether or not the delusions are true or the hallucinations are real. For example, the nurse should say, "I don't understand how you could be getting secret messages from the president of Poland while you are here in our hospital," and then should redirect the conversation to another topic. Regarding hallucinations, the nurse should say, "I don't hear the voices you are talking about, but I understand they are real to you."
- The nurse should work collaboratively with the treatment team to initiate a plan to control the acute symptoms and move the client into rehabilitative care.

the reasons that impede successful meeting of client goals and to come up with plans that work for the client. For example, the nurse helps her client find volunteer work in his community, assists the client to interact with others, and helps him maintain a socially acceptable role within the community. The nurse also works with her client and his family members to monitor daily medication intake and assists the client to keep acute symptoms under control.

EVALUATION

Evaluation of nursing care is always based on whether or not the identified outcomes have been met. When the outcomes are written in behavioral and measurable terms, the nurse can readily evaluate if the outcome has been met.

BOX 13-5
PRINCIPLES FOR CARING FOR SCHIZOPHRENIC CLIENTS: REHABILITATIVE PHASE

The following principles are helpful in planning interventions for clients with schizophrenia in the rehabilitative phase:

- Clients tend to do better with a structured daily schedule and a daily plan of activities. Therefore, it is helpful for the client to have a written schedule to follow.
- Social isolation is common, and activities that promote supportive contacts with others help to meet social needs and to boost self-esteem.
- *Risk for ineffective therapeutic regimen management* is high, such that frequent home visits from the nurse coupled with assistance from family or significant others may be essential for success.
- Factors such as lack of transportation to follow-up visits, lack of supportive and affordable housing, and difficulty in obtaining health care insurance or social assistance usually require that the nurse work closely with social workers and community agencies to meet client needs.
- Family members and/or significant others are frequently involved in client care; the nurse's care to the caregiver and the elimination of caregiver role strain are always important considerations.

CARE PLANNING GUIDE 13-1 Client with Schizophrenia (Acute Phase)

CLINICAL PICTURE

The clinical picture of a client with acute presentation of schizophrenia includes both the positive and negative symptoms of the disease:

- Delusions, hallucinations, and disorganized speech
- Flat affect, avolition, alogia, and anhedonia
- Decreased level of functioning

COMMON NURSING DIAGNOSES

The nursing diagnoses commonly used are:

1. *Disturbed thought processes*
2. *Disturbed sensory perceptions: hallucinations*
3. *Self-care deficit (specify)*
4. *Impaired social interaction*

NURSING DIAGNOSIS 1: *DISTURBED THOUGHT PROCESSES*

OUTCOMES

1. Verbalize decreased distress related to delusions or cognitive distortions.
2. Be oriented to person, time, and place.
3. Be able to participate in therapeutic activities.

NOC: *DISTORTED THOUGHT SELF-CONTROL*

INTERVENTIONS (NIC: *DELUSION MANAGEMENT; REALITY ORIENTATION*)	**RATIONALE**
• Monitor for changes in orientation, cognitive, and behavioral functioning, and document.	• Allows for early recognition of change from baseline data, allowing for individualized care.
• Provide reality orientation—express doubt, and do not enter into the delusion.	• Helps to correct distortions and misperceptions of the environment.
• Address the themes that may express the client's underlying concerns and feelings.	• Themes may indicate fears or concerns (e.g., safety or need to escape).
• Redirect toward therapeutic, reality-oriented activities.	• Brings the client into reality, provides distractions from delusions, and provides means to cope.
• Provide education and support for taking antipsychotic medications.	• Client needs to be accepting of the role medications have in controlling symptoms.

NURSING DIAGNOSIS 2: *DISTURBED SENSORY PERCEPTIONS: HALLUCINATIONS*

OUTCOMES

1. Client will verbalize one method of coping with hallucinations.

NOC: *DISORDERED THOUGHT SELF-CONTROL*

INTERVENTIONS (NIC: *HALLUCINATION MANAGEMENT*)	**RATIONALE**
• Monitor for signs of hallucinations, and document.	• Allows for early identification and treatment and documentation of treatment response.
• Be attentive to themes that may express the client's underlying concerns and feelings.	• Themes may express fears, distortions, or possible danger to self/others.

(*Continues*)

CARE PLANNING GUIDE 13-1 Continued

INTERVENTIONS (NIC: *HALLUCINATION MANAGEMENT*)	RATIONALE
• Teach client how to cope with distressing hallucinations: humming, using a radio, and telling the voices to "go away."	• Distraction techniques can be used for symptom relief.
• Provide education and support for taking antipsychotic medications.	• Assist the client to understand the role of medication in controlling symptoms.

NURSING DIAGNOSIS 3: *SELF-CARE DEFICIT*

OUTCOMES

1. Client will manage day-to-day activities, beginning with appropriate dressing, grooming, and nutrition.

NOC: *SELF-CARE: ACTIVITIES OF DAILY LIVING (ADL)*

INTERVENTIONS (NIC: *SELF-CARE ASSISTANCE*)	RATIONALE
• Monitor client's ability for independent self-care, and document.	• Allows for early identification of changes and individualized care.
• Ensure easy access to clothing and grooming materials.	• Clients with thought disorders can easily be overwhelmed if preparatory activities are too complicated.
• Provide a schedule of daily activities that includes a consistent routine for dressing, bathing, meals, and exercise/activity.	• Clients with disordered thoughts respond well to having their time structured and are unable to structure their time themselves.

NURSING DIAGNOSIS 4: *IMPAIRED SOCIAL INTERACTION*

OUTCOMES

1. Client will exhibit less discomfort in social situations.
2. Client will pick up on social cues when interacting with others.

NOC: *SOCIAL INTERACTION SKILLS; SOCIAL INVOLVEMENT*

INTERVENTIONS (NIC: *SOCIALIZATION ENHANCEMENT; BEHAVIOR MODIFICATION, SOCIAL SKILLS*)	RATIONALE
• Monitor patterns of social activity, including areas of strengths and weaknesses.	• Care can be individualized based on the client's specific patterns.
• Identify client goals for interaction.	• Set mutual goals for interaction.
• Support and reinforce efforts at social interaction.	• Client will need encouragement; reinforcement of new behaviors is important when the client is trying to master new patterns.
• Provide a supportive group to enhance and to practice social skills.	• Gives the client a safe place to try out new skills and new interactive patterns.
• Teach essential components of social interactions: making eye contact, how to have productive patterns of speech, how to relate a message, and how to enter into a conversation.	• Address gaps in knowledge about social skills.

(*Continues*)

CARE PLANNING GUIDE 13-1 Continued

LONG-TERM CONSIDERATIONS FOR THE CLIENT WITH SCHIZOPHRENIA

1. Symptom management will become a key issue for living with the disease in the long term. The role of antipsychotic medications must be understood.
2. Social interactions, social skills, and structured activities will be needed for management of negative symptoms.

Note: The care-planning guides have been adapted from *Plans of Care for Specialty Practice: Psychiatric Mental Health Nursing*, by M. Coler and K. G. Vincent, 1995, Clifton Park, NY: Thomson Delmar Learning.

NURSING CARE PLAN: NURSING PROCESS FORMAT 13-1

Refer to the literary excerpt "Mourning without End." Imagine that nurses are giving care to Gary as if he were coming to the hospital for an acute admission. His symptoms and behaviors are expected to be similar to those of other clients with schizophrenia. This is a fictionalized nursing care plan.

ASSESSMENT

Gary is a highly intelligent college student who has firsthand experience with schizophrenia. He is currently in school, and until recently has adequately managed his academic work. Gary has been hospitalized three times in the past for acute schizophrenic episodes that included delusions and suicidal ideation. He has been well maintained for several months on medications and weekly psychotherapy. Gary has noticed an increase in problems over the past three weeks. He is having difficulty concentrating, is increasingly afraid of people, and senses danger is everywhere. Gary has cut the cable of his television because he believes it has the power to hurt him and refuses to deal with answering the phone or checking his messages. He recognizes he is increasingly isolating himself from his friends, his peers, his family, and his work. It is very hard to even get up in the morning. He forgets to take his prescribed medications. Gary is very close to his father, who has stood by him since his illness began. Gary decides to drive to his father's private office to talk to him about getting help. He is very fearful.

Gary and his father decide that he needs some intensive intervention. The psychotherapist is called, and Gary is admitted to a private mental health clinic. Gary's father arranges for a short-term leave of absence from the college for Gary.

NURSING DIAGNOSIS 1 *Ineffective coping* related to situational crises, as evidenced by inability to cope, meet role expectations, or meet basic needs

OUTCOMES	NIC	NURSING ACTIONS	EVALUATION
• Within 4 days, Gary will identify those factors he believes may have precipitated the need for this hospitalization.	• Coping enhancement	• Assist Gary in verbally exploring the source of his stress over the past 3 weeks by asking about life events prior to hospitalization.	Gary's stress was primarily in response to his classes, where he has had stress related to performance.

(Continues)

NURSING CARE PLAN: NURSING PROCESS FORMAT 13-1 (Continued)

OUTCOMES	NIC	NURSING ACTIONS	EVALUATION
• Within 4 days, Gary will reestablish the effective coping strategies he has used in the past (physical exercise in the form of two 30-minute walks a day). • Within 7 days, Gary will demonstrate an ability to manage his medications and daily activities in a supervised home setting. • Within 2 weeks, Gary will return to his apartment, demonstrating prehospital behavior, as evidenced by preillness stable eating, sleeping, and activity patterns.	• Medication management	• Encourage Gary to use strategies that have worked well in the past, such as taking supervised walks or setting up a structured daily schedule. • Work with Gary to achieve understanding of the importance of establishing a schedule as a means of maintaining control of his life and a link to reality. • Help Gary to reestablish normal perspectives about his behavior, his medications, his stress level, and his environment.	Gary's greatest fear was of slipping back into a delusional state and "losing all the progress I had made." Gary did not initially make the connection, but as his fear escalated, he stopped walking each day, missed two appointments with his therapist, and forgot to take his medications. His symptoms increased. Once hospitalized, he realized he was perfectly capable of staying well enough to manage his daily affairs.

NURSING DIAGNOSIS 2 *Impaired social interaction* related to social withdrawal, as evidenced by verbalization of discomfort in social situations and dysfunctional interactions with peers

OUTCOMES	NIC	NURSING ACTIONS	EVALUATION
• Within 24 hours of hospitalization, Gary will establish a beginning relationship with a nurse. • Within 4 days, Gary will attend a small inpatient group session. • Within 2 weeks, Gary will attend an outpatient group meeting (with his father, if he so chooses). • Within 1 month, Gary will reconnect with at least two friends and regularly attend his therapy sessions.	• Counseling • Socialization enhancement • Support group • Support system enhancement • Discharge planning	• Assist Gary in his socialization, starting with one-on-one interactions. • Encourage Gary to expand his world by initiating conversation with one staff person and one client per day. • Attend a small inpatient counseling session with Gary. • Include outpatient meetings in the discharge plan for Gary. • Help Gary locate and reestablish contact with one or two friends of his choice. • Follow up with telephone calls first to Gary's dad	In the hospital, Gary was open to discussing his problems. He felt particularly comfortable with Ben, a nurse who expressed how much he respected Gary for working toward a college degree. Ben liked to walk and talk, so he and Gary were able to do a lot of reflection about what had gone on the past few weeks. With Ben's encouragement, Gary did get involved in inpatient and outpatient counseling sessions. Gary also asked his psychotherapist to let Ben

(Continues)

NURSING CARE PLAN: NURSING PROCESS FORMAT 13-1 (Continued)

OUTCOMES	NIC	NURSING ACTIONS	EVALUATION
		(with Gary's permission) and then to Gary to encourage his continued participation in group and other interactions.	know he was "back on track with school."

REFLECTIVE QUESTIONS

1. **ASSESSMENT**
   What additional personal or environmental factors should be evaluated as possible stressors for Gary?
2. **NURSING DIAGNOSIS**
   What is the role of family in mental health problems such as Gary's? What additional nursing diagnoses, including family-oriented diagnoses, might be appropriate in Gary's case?
3. **OUTCOMES**
   Where do regular life challenges fit in the lives of persons with schizophrenia? Do you think the outcomes identified for Gary would be typical or expected for other individuals with schizophrenia?
4. **NURSING ACTIONS**
   What are the best ways to instill "hope" in the lives of clients? Where did hope fit for Gary?
   What additional interventions would you recommend to get Gary back to his prehospital level of functioning?
5. **EVALUATION**
   Does successful management of acute mental illnesses engender success in future potential episodes? Why or why not? Do you think that Gary's initial progress promises continued improvement?

NURSING CARE PLAN: CONCEPT MAP FORMAT 13-1

Client with Schizophrenia

BACKGROUND INFORMATION

Jack is a 22-year-old man diagnosed with schizophrenia for 5 years. He is a college graduate with a degree in accounting and maintains a job at a local bank. He is on maintenance doses of medication (Clozaril) and has been functioning on his own, living in an apartment by himself, with support from his family over the past year.

Nurse Lea comes to the psychiatric unit this morning and learns that Jack was admitted last night. He was brought to the hospital by his father, who was increasingly concerned that Jack was not managing his own affairs and that something was wrong. The immediate history is that Jack has missed work for one week, he has been withdrawn, and he has been spending much of his time alone in a darkened room. While not able to describe his feeling/experiences to his father or to his doctor, Jack did relate that he is hearing voices, he has been unable to sleep, and he feels anxious. When his father decided to seek help, Jack's appearance was disheveled, there was no evidence of food in his apartment, he had been smoking, and his father noted cigarette butts randomly strewn about the floor. Jack was in agreement with his father to seek care.

(Continues)

NURSING CARE PLAN: CONCEPT MAP FORMAT 13-1 (Continued)

The night nurse reported that Jack did not sleep last night. He sat in his room quietly. Lea is assigned to care for Jack today. She notes that he is sitting in the day room. He is looking at others from a distance, he is not asking questions, and he is not interacting with others. Lea approaches, and Jack does not respond to her. Lea introduces herself as his nurse. Jack acknowledges the introduction with a nod but does not speak. Lea then indicates to Jack that there is a breakfast meal for him, and Jack responds by sitting to eat alone, without saying anything.

INITIAL ASSESSMENT AND REFLECTION IN BUILDING A CARE MAP

While there are many needs one could identify for Jack on the morning after his hospital admission, Lea recognizes that the hospitalization itself is an intervention aimed at controlling what could be unpredictable behaviors and ensuring a safe environment for Jack. Jack is experiencing a self-care deficit. He is unable to meet his own needs for safety, for food, and for security. There are obvious concerns that his symptoms are a result of nonadherence to his medication program. Through structured hospital care, his medications will be reinstituted. The fact that Jack has withdrawn and maintained a state of isolation over the past week is not unexpected, because many schizophrenic clients who experience psychiatric symptoms in the community withdraw, staying alone and away from stimuli as a means of coping with hallucinations.

INITIAL REVIEW OF NURSING DIAGNOSES

Issues that Lea raises in Jack's plan of care are the following:

1. Self-care deficit: hygiene, activities of daily living
2. Insomnia
3. Disturbed sensory perception: hallucinations (reports of hearing voices)

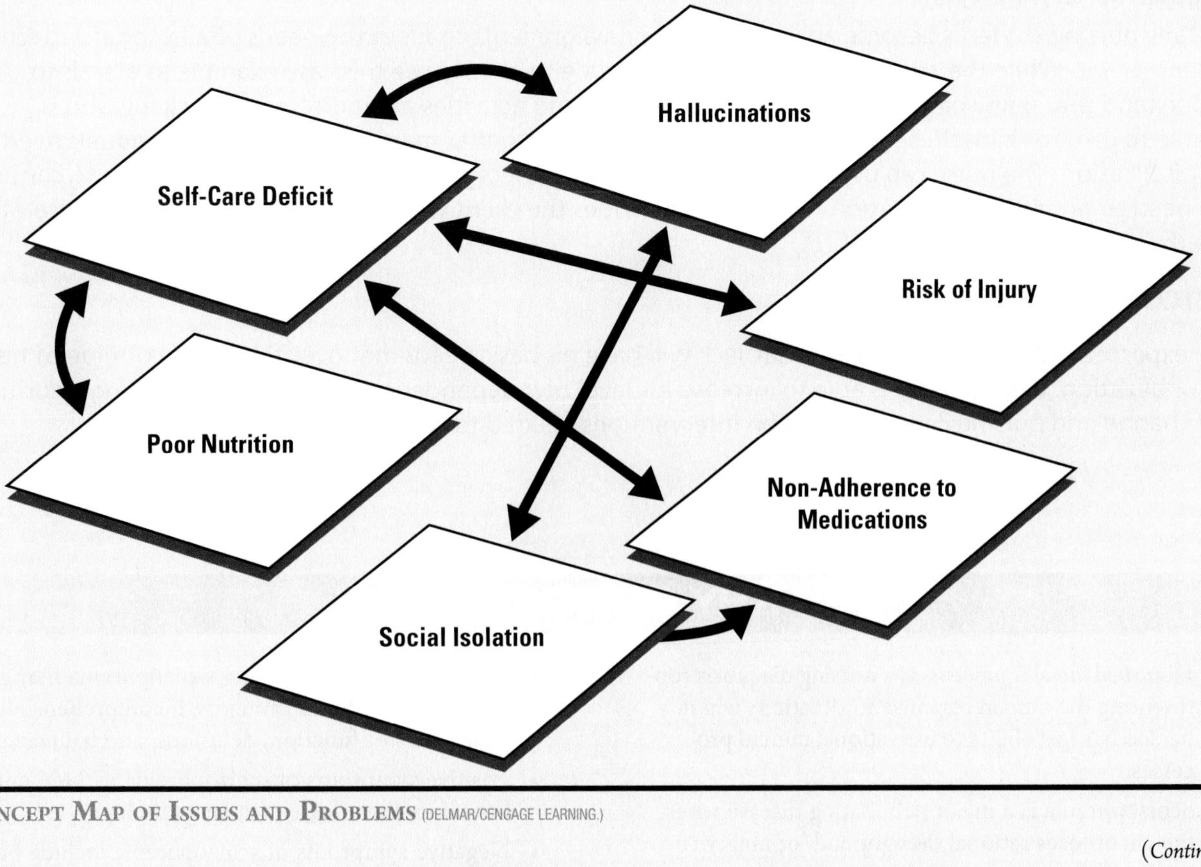

Concept Map of Issues and Problems (DELMAR/CENGAGE LEARNING.)

(*Continues*)

NURSING CARE PLAN: CONCEPT MAP FORMAT 13-1 (Continued)

4. Risk for injury (to self and others) related to cognitive and affective changes and to inattention to safety needs at home (cigarettes)
5. Imbalanced nutrition: less than body requirements
6. Ineffective management of the therapeutic regimen
7. Social isolation

PRIORITIES OF CARE

Lea's immediate care is designed to meet Jack's immediate needs: Lea will focus on self-care activities and assist Jack to maintain a daily schedule that permits a routine of meals, activities, free time, and one-on-one interaction. Lea will also monitor medication compliance. Her goals are to meet basic self-care needs/requirements, and to establish a trusting relationship. Longer term goals for the hospitalization are to reestablish medication compliance in preparation for hospital discharge and to promote social behaviors.

The immediate nursing diagnosis is:

Self-care deficit related to cognitive and perceptual impairments as evidenced by inability to meet self-care requirement of safety and security, hygiene, nutrition.

NURSING INTERVENTIONS

- Lea will monitor and control Jack's environment, ensuring that he is physically and psychologically safe. Specifically, Jack will remain in the hospital; he will have basic needs met and he will be supported to behave as he wishes.
- Lea will provide Jack with a schedule, indicating times for meals, activities, medications, and so forth to structure his day.

Rationale for this diagnosis and plan of care is that Jack's immediate needs are related to his inability to maintain in the community.

Many nursing students become anxious over their assignments to meet the needs of a hospitalized schizophrenic client. While the anxiety is understandable, students should use this case example as a basis to understand that many basic, fundamental nursing skills and activities are indicated for a client who is unable to care for himself. Self-care deficits may be the reason that many schizophrenic individuals need hospitalization. The nurse can use Orem's Self-Care Deficit Theory of Nursing or related theories to consider the need to provide compensation for self-care activities the client would do on his own, given a state of health.

OUTCOME/EVALUATION

The expected outcome of this care is that Jack will have his basic needs met over the period of time of his hospitalization. Clearly, as he is able to increase his level of independence/autonomy, the nursing priorities will change and nursing care will focus on interventions needed to return Jack to his home.

KEY CONCEPTS

- *Disturbed thought processes* is a nursing diagnosis representing the human response to situations where a person has lost ability to use rational mental processes.
- Schizophrenia is a major debilitating disease where the client loses rational thought and/or ability to interpret the environment.
- An individual experiencing schizophrenia may present with disordered thoughts, incomprehensible language, loss of function, delusions, and hallucinations.
- Positive symptoms of schizophrenia include outward behaviors that clearly display pathology.
- Negative symptoms of schizophrenia include behaviors that represent a change from the individual's

prior personality and lead to social isolation and anhedonia.

- There is no predictable clinical course for any individual person diagnosed with schizophrenia.
- With about one new case of schizophrenia per 10,000 persons, the social costs are exceedingly high.
- Schizophrenia is an organic disease with a strong genetic component.
- Psychosocial treatment includes individual and family support services as well as socially directed rehabilitation.
- Pharmacological treatment is primarily through antipsychotic medications.
- Nursing theory focusing on the nurse-client interactions is most helpful.
- The five aims of intervention provide a framework for nursing care.

REVIEW QUESTIONS

1. A nurse admitting a client experiencing an acute schizophrenic episode, would most likely assess which of the following?
1. Open and outgoing personality
2. Loss of contact with reality
3. Feelings of guilt and worthlessness
4. Logical and precise thinking

2. The client is prescribed a first-generation neuroleptic for his schizophrenia. Discharge teaching by the nurse should include contacting the health provider if which of the following occurs?
1. Elevated temperature
2. Blurred vision
3. Difficulty concentrating
4. Inability to remain seated for long periods of time

3. The client has been on Haldol since admission four days earlier. Which assessment by the nurse would best determine the effectiveness of a client's antipsychotic medication?
1. The client no longer has hallucinations
2. The client is no longer depressed
3. The client has made a friend on the unit
4. The client requests discharge

4. A client has developed neuroleptic malignant syndrome. A priority nursing intervention would be which of the following?
1. Provide comfort and rest
2. Measure intake and output
3. Encourage client to remain active
4. Monitor vital signs and blood pressure

5. A client is admitted to the emergency room with complaints of sore throat and fever. The client's mother informs the nurse that the client has been taking Clozaril. Which of the following laboratory tests is a priority at this time?
1. Fasting blood sugar
2. Cholesterol level
3. Blood urea nitrogen
4. White blood cell count

6. A client is prescribed Haldol 5mg three times a day and questions the nurse about the dose. The best response by the nurse is which of the following?
1. That is an appropriate dose for an adult of your size.
2. If that is the dose your physician ordered, it must be right.
3. The dose does seem very high; I will contact your physician to verify the dose.
4. The dose seems very low for your condition; I will contact your physician to verify the dose.

7. A new graduate has been assigned four patients whom she must perform an assessment on. Her assessment reveals several client complaints. Which client complaint should receive priority?
1. A client receiving Cogentin who states, "I can't read my book, everything seems blurred."
2. The client receiving clozapine who states, "I think I might be getting the flu, my throat is sore and I feel very tired."
3. A client who was admitted for alcoholism and states, "I took my Valium but I still feel nervous.
4. A client receiving Prozac who states "This medicine makes me sleepy. Is that normal?"

8. During a one-to-one session with a client, the nurse notes that the client is unable to stop moving. He frequently stands-up and begins pacing while answering the nurse's questions. The nurse assesses the client's need to be in constant motion as which of the following?
1. Akathesia
2. Flight-of-ideas
3. Echopraxia
4. Neuroleptic syndrome

9. During morning rounds, a client complains to the nurse that he has been constipated since beginning his medication. The nurse teaches the client about the types of foods which help with constipation. Which of the following menus, if selected by the client, would indicate to the nurse that the client understood the health teaching?
1. Bacon and cheese sandwich on white bread with a glass of whole milk
2. Sausage and two fried eggs, two pieces of white bread toast and coffee

3. Orange juice, bran flakes with milk, and a honey-bran muffin
4. Egg and cheese omelet with salsa and a glass of chocolate milk

10. Following a client's admission to a psychiatric unit, the nurse's initial action would be to do which of the following?

1. Provide safety and security for the client
2. Obtain a complete health history
3. Interview the relative who accompanied the client
4. Place the client in seclusion from other clients

LEARNING ACTIVITIES

1. How would you identify that a client brought to your emergency room had had an altered thought process?
2. How would you tell the difference between a drug-induced condition and schizophrenia?
3. Describe the clinical course of schizophrenia.
4. Explain the difference between positive and negative symptoms of the disease.
5. How would you design social supports for schizophrenic persons in your community?
6. What is your opinion of the current supports and services in your community?
7. Explain the major antipsychotic medications and their side effects.
8. How does the nurse-client relationship impact care of the schizophrenic person?
9. Explain how the five aims of intervention assist in planning nursing care.

*Study*WARE™ CONNECTION

Using your *Study*WARE™ CD-ROM

1. Complete the Concentration activity for this chapter.
2. Complete the Quiz for this chapter in Test Mode.
3. Explore the other games and activities that support this chapter.

VIDEO LINK

Read and contemplate the questions below about Etta, the client experiencing schizophrenia. Then watch the video "Schizophrenia" on your *Study*WARE™ CD-ROM to observe Etta's interview with a psychiatrist. Consider these questions prior to listening to the psychiatrist's analysis.

1. Identify the positive symptoms of schizophrenia that Etta is experiencing.
2. What are the negative symptoms that she displays?
3. When Etta speaks, there is disorder in her ideas and topics. Are there specific terms to describe schizophrenic speech? Give examples of this language.
4. What types of delusions is Etta experiencing?
5. Are these the most common types of delusions that clients with schizophrenia experience?
6. Why do you suppose that she now has relief from some of her delusions?
7. How might you respond to a client who reports such delusions to you? What therapeutic strategies would you use to respond?
8. Do you think Etta experiences hallucinations?
9. What was the classification of medication prescribed for Etta at the onset of her schizophrenia?
10. Did you notice any medication side effects that she is experiencing? Is there treatment for such side effects?
11. What are the two major treatment approaches to schizophrenia?
12. Is the onset of Etta's schizophrenia in keeping with the general statistics? What is the downside to an earlier onset (e.g., between ages 16 and 18)?
13. What is the incidence of schizophrenia for a child if one parent has the disease?
14. Etta identified stressors that affect her illness? What are they?
15. What challenges has Etta's family faced?
16. What therapeutic programs and community supports would be valuable for them?
17. If we were engaged in discharge planning with this individual, what would we need to consider?

REFERENCES

Allenbeck, P. (1989). Schizophrenia: A life-shortening disease. *Schizophrenia Bulletin, 15,* 81–89.

American Psychiatric Association. (2000). *Diagnostic and statistical manual of mental disorders* (4th ed., text rev.). Washington, DC: Author.

Andreasen, N. C. (1979). Thought, language and communication disorders: Clinical assessment, definition of terms and evaluation of their reliability. *Archives of General Psychiatry, 36,* 1315–1321.

Anonymous. (1955). An autobiography of a schizophrenic experience. *Journal of Abnormal and Social Psychology, 51,* 677–689.

Anonymous. (1983). [Anonymous autobiography]. *Schizophrenic Bulletin, 9,* 152–155.

Bai, Y. M., Lin, C. C., Chen, J. Y., Lin, C. Y., Su, T. P., & Chou, P. (2006). Association of initial antipsychotic response to clozapine and long-term weight gain. *American Journal of Psychiatry, 163*(7), 1276–1279.

Barrowclough, C. B., & Tarrier, N. T. (1992). Interventions with families. In M. Birchwood & N. Tarrier (Eds.), *Innovations in the psychological management of schizophrenia.* Chichester, UK: Wiley.

Bleuler, M. (1974). The long term course of the schizophrenic psychoses. *Psychological Medicine, 4,* 244–254.

Cannon, T. D., Huttunen, M. O., Lonnqvist, J., Tuulio-Henriksson, A., Pirkola, T., Glahn, D., et al. (2000). The inheritance of neuropsychological dysfunction in twins discordant for schizophrenia. *American Journal of Human Genetics, 67*(2), 369–382.

Clardy, J. C., Hyde, T. M., & Kleinman, J. E. (1994). Postmortem neurochemical and neuropathological studies in schizophrenia. In N. C. Andreasen (Ed.), *Schizophrenia: From Mind to Molecule.* Washington, DC: American Psychiatric Press.

Dawson, P. J. (1998). Schizophrenia and genetics: A review and critique for the psychiatric nurse. *Psychiatric Mental Health Nursing, 5*(4), 299–301.

DeLisi, L. E. (2000). Critical overview of current approaches to genetic mechanisms in schizophrenia research. *Brain Research Review, 31*(2–3), 187–192.

Eakes, G. G. (1995). Chronic sorrow: The lived experience of parents of chronically mentally ill individuals. *Archives of Psychiatric Nursing, 9,* 77–84.

Editors. (1995). Anti-drug counterblast in mental health [Editorial]. *Lancet, 346,* 323.

Erickson, H., Tomlin, E., & Swain, M. A. (1983). *Modeling and role-modeling: A theory and paradigm for nursing.* Lexington, KY: Pine.

Fine, R. (1979). *A history of psychoanalysis.* New York: Columbia University Press.

Flynn, L. (1994). Schizophrenia from a family point of view. In N. C. Andreasen (Ed.), *Schizophrenia: From Mind to Molecule* (pp. 21–30). Washington, DC: American Psychiatric Press.

Folsom, D., & Jeste, D. V. (2002). Schizophrenia in homeless persons: A systematic review of the literature. *Acta Psychiatrica Scandinavica, 105*(6), 404–413.

Freedman, R. (2003). Schizophrenia. *New England Journal of Medicine, 349,* 1738–1745

Frisch, N., & Bowman, S. (2008). The modeling and role-modeling theory. In J. George (Ed.), *Nursing theories: The base for professional practice* (6th ed.). Upper Saddle River, NJ: Prentice Hall.

Gottesman, I. I. (1991). *Schizophrenia genesis.* New York: Freeman.

Gournay, K. (1995). New facts on schizophrenia. *Nursing Times, 91*(25), 32–33.

Hargreaves, W. A., & Shumway, M. (1989). Effectiveness of mental health services for the severely mental ill. In C. A. Taube & A. Hohmann (Eds.), *The future of mental health services research.* Washington, DC: NIMH, U.S. Government Printing Office.

Harrow, M., & Quinlan, D. M. (1985). *Disordered thinking and schizophrenic psychopathology.* New York: Gardner.

Heinssen, R. K., Liberman, R. P., & Kopelowicz, A. (2000). Psychosocial skills training for schizophrenia: Lessons from the laboratory. *Schizophrenia Bulletin, 26*(1), 21–46.

Hoffman, R. E., Varanko, M., Gillmore, J., & Mishara, A. L. (2007, November). Experiential features used by patients, with schizophrenia to differentiate "voices" from ordinary verbal thought. *Psychological Medicine,* 1–10.

Hogarty, G. E., Anderson, C. M., Reiss, D. J., Kornblith, S. J., Greenwald, D. P., Javna, C. D., et al. (1986). Family psychoeducation, social skills training and maintenance chemotherapy. *Archives of General Psychiatry, 43,* 633–642.

Huxley, N. A., Rendall, M., & Sederer, L. (2000). Psychological treatments in schizophrenia: A review of the last 20 years. *Journal of Nervous and Mental Disorders, 188*(4), 187–201.

Johnstone, E. C. (1991). Disabilities and circumstances of schizophrenic patients: A follow-up study. *British Journal of Psychiatry, 159*(Suppl.), 4–46.

Kinsler, P. J., & Saxman, A. (2007). Traumatized offenders: Don't look now, but your jail's also your mental health center. *Journal of Trauma and Dissociation, 8*(2), 81–92.

Lamb, H. R., & Weinberger, L. E. (2005). The shift of psychiatric inpatient care from hospitals to jails and prisons. *Journal of the American Academy of Psychiatry and the Law, 33*(4), 529–534.

Leweke, F. M., & Koethe, D. (2008). Cannabis and psychiatric disorders: It is not only addiction. *Addiction Biology, 13*(2), 264–275.

Liddle, P. F., Friston, K. J., Frith, C. D., Hirsch, S. R., Jones, T., & Frackowisk, R. S. J. (1992). Patterns of cerebral blood flow in schizophrenia. *British Journal of Psychiatry, 160,* 179–186.

Lorenz, M. (1961). Problems posed by schizophrenic language. *Archives of General Psychiatry, 4,* 603–610.

Marshall, M., & Rathbone, J. (2006). Early intervention for psychosis. *Cochrane Database of Systematic Reviews,* (18):CD004718.

McGlashan, T. H. (1994). Psychosocial treatments of schizophrenia. In N. C. Andreasen (Ed.), *Schizophrenia: From Mind to Molecule* (pp. 189–215). Washington, DC: American Psychiatric Press.

McGlashan, T., & Johannessen, J. (1996). Early detection and intervention with schizophrenia: Rationale. *Schizophrenia Bulletin, 22*(2), 201–222.

McGorry, P. D., Yung, A. R., Bechdolf, A., & Amminger, P. (2008). Back to the future: Predicting and reshaping the course of psychotic disorder. *Archives of General Psychiatry, 65*(1), 25–27.

McKenna, P. J. (1994). *Schizophrenia and related syndromes.* New York: Oxford University Press.

McNeil, D. E., Binder, R. L., & Robinson, J. C. (2005). Incarceration associated with homelessness, mental disorder, and co-occurring substance abuse. *Psychiatric Services, 56*(7), 840–846.

Mellor, C. S. (1970). Firsthand symptoms in schizophrenia. *British Journal of Psychiatry, 117,* 16–18.

Meyer-Lindenberg, A., Straub, R. E., Lipska, B. K., Verchinski, B. A., Goldberg, T., Callicott, J. H., et al. (2007). Genetic evidence implicating cDARPP-32 in human frontostriatal structure, function, and cognition. *Journal of Clinical Investigation, 117,* 672–682.

Moore, H., West, A. R., & Grace, A. A. (1999). The regulation of forebrain dopamine transmission. *Biological Psychiatry, 46*(1), 40–55.

Munetz, M. R., Grande, Y. P., & Chambers, M. R. (2001). The incarceration of individuals with severe mental disorders. *Community Mental Health Journal, 37*(4), 361–372.

Niebuhr, D. W., Millikan, A. M., Cowan, D. N., Yolken, R., Li, Y., & Weber, N. S. (2008). Selected infectious agents and risk of schizophrenia among U.S. military personnel. *American Journal of Psychiatry, 165,* 99–106.

Reed, S. I. (2008). First-episode psychosis: A literature review. *International Journal of Mental Health Nursing, 17,* 85–91.

Reveley, A. M. (1994). Phenomenology, environmental risk, and genetics: Twin studies of schizophrenia. In N. C. Andreasen (Ed.), *Schizophrenia: From Mind to Molecule* (pp. 105–118). Washington, DC: American Psychiatric Press.

Sass, L. (1992). *Madness and modernism.* New York: Basic Books

Schizophrenia Discussion Groups. (2004). *The Schizophrenia homepage.* Retrieved December 11, 2004, from http://www.schizophrenia.com/contact/html

Schultz, S. K., & Andreasen, N. (1999). Schizophrenia. *Lancet, 353*(9162), 1425–1430.

Semple, D. M., McIntosh, A. M., & Lawrie, S. M. (2005). Cannabis as a risk factor for psychosis: Systematic review. *Journal of Psychopharmacology, 19*(2), 187–194.

Soares, J. C., & Innes, R. B. (1999). Neurochemical brain imaging investigations in schizophrenia. *Biological Psychiatry, 46*(5), 600–615.

Svenningsson, P., Tzavara, E. T., Carruthers, R., Rachleff, I., Wattler, S., Nehls, M., et al. (2003). Diverse psychotomimetics act through a common signaling pathway. *Science, 302*(5649), 1412–1415.

Swartz, M. S., Perkins, D. O., Stroup, T. S., Davis, S. M., Capuano, G., Rosenheck, R. A., et al. (2007). Effects of antipsychotic medications on psychosocial functioning in patients with chronic schizophrenia: Findings from the NIMH CATIE Study. *American Journal of Psychiatry, 164,* 428–436.

Tamminga, C. A. (1997). Gender and schizophrenia. *Journal of Clinical Psychiatry, 58*(Suppl. 15), 33–37.

Tandon, R. (2005). Suicidal behavior in schizophrenia. *Expert Review of Neurotherapeutics, 5*(1), 95–99.

Tandon, R., Belmaker, R. H., Gattaz, W. F., Lopez-Ibor, J. J., Jr, Okasha, A., Singh, B., et al. (2008). [For the Section of Pharmacopsychiatry, World Psychiatric Association. Pharmacopsychiatry Section statement on comparative effectiveness of antipsychotics in the treatment of schizophrenia]. *Schizophrenia Research, 100*(1–3), 20–38.

Tarrier, N., Haddock, G., Lewis, S., Drake, R., & Gregg, L.: SoCRATES Trial Group. (2006). Suicide behaviour over 18 months in recent onset schizophrenic patients: The effects of CBT. *Schizophrenia Research, 83*(1), 15–27.

Tharyan, P., & Adams, C. E. (2005, April 18). Electroconvulsive therapy for schizophrenia. *Cochrane Database of Systematic Reviews,* (2):CD000076.

Tsuang, M. (2000). Schizophrenia: Genes and environment. *Biological Psychiatry, 47,* 212–220.

Vaccaro, J. V., & Roberts, L. (1992). Teaching social coping skills. In M. Birchwood & N. Tarrier (Eds.), *Innovations in the psychological management of schizophrenia.* Chichester, UK: John Wiley.

Wheeler, C. (1994). The diagnosis of schizophrenia and its impact on the primary caregiver. *Nursing Practice in New Zealand, 9,* 15–23.

Worrel, J. A., Marken, P. A., Beckman, S. E., & Ruehter, V. L. (2000). Atypical antipsychotic agents: A critical review. *American Journal of Health Systems Pharmacology, 57*(3), 238–255.

LITERARY REFERENCES

Anonymous. (1955). An autobiography of a schizophrenic experience. *Journal of Abnormal and Social Psychology, 51,* 677–689.

Anonymous. (1983). *Schizophrenic Bulletin, 9,* 152–155.

Boisen, A. (1960). *Out of the depths.* New York: HarperCollins.

Sechehaye, M. (Ed.). (1970). *Autobiography of a schizophrenic girl.* New York: New American Library.

Willick, M. S. (1994). A parent's perspective: Mourning without end. In N. C. Andreasen (Ed.), *Schizophrenia: From Mind to Molecule* (pp. 5–19). Washington, DC: American Psychiatric Press.

Zelt, D. (pseudonym). (1981). Grandiose delusions. *Schizophrenic Bulletin, 7,* 527–531.

SUGGESTED READINGS

Harman, C. E. (2003). *The diagnosis and stigma of schizophrenia stigma.* Brookings, OR: Old Court Press.

Loudon, M. (2006). *Relative stranger: A life after death.* Edinburgh: Cannongate.

Murray, R. (2003). *The epidemiology of schizophrenia.* Oxford: Oxford University Press.

Saks, E. R. (2007). *The center cannot hold: My journey through madness.* New York: Hyperion.

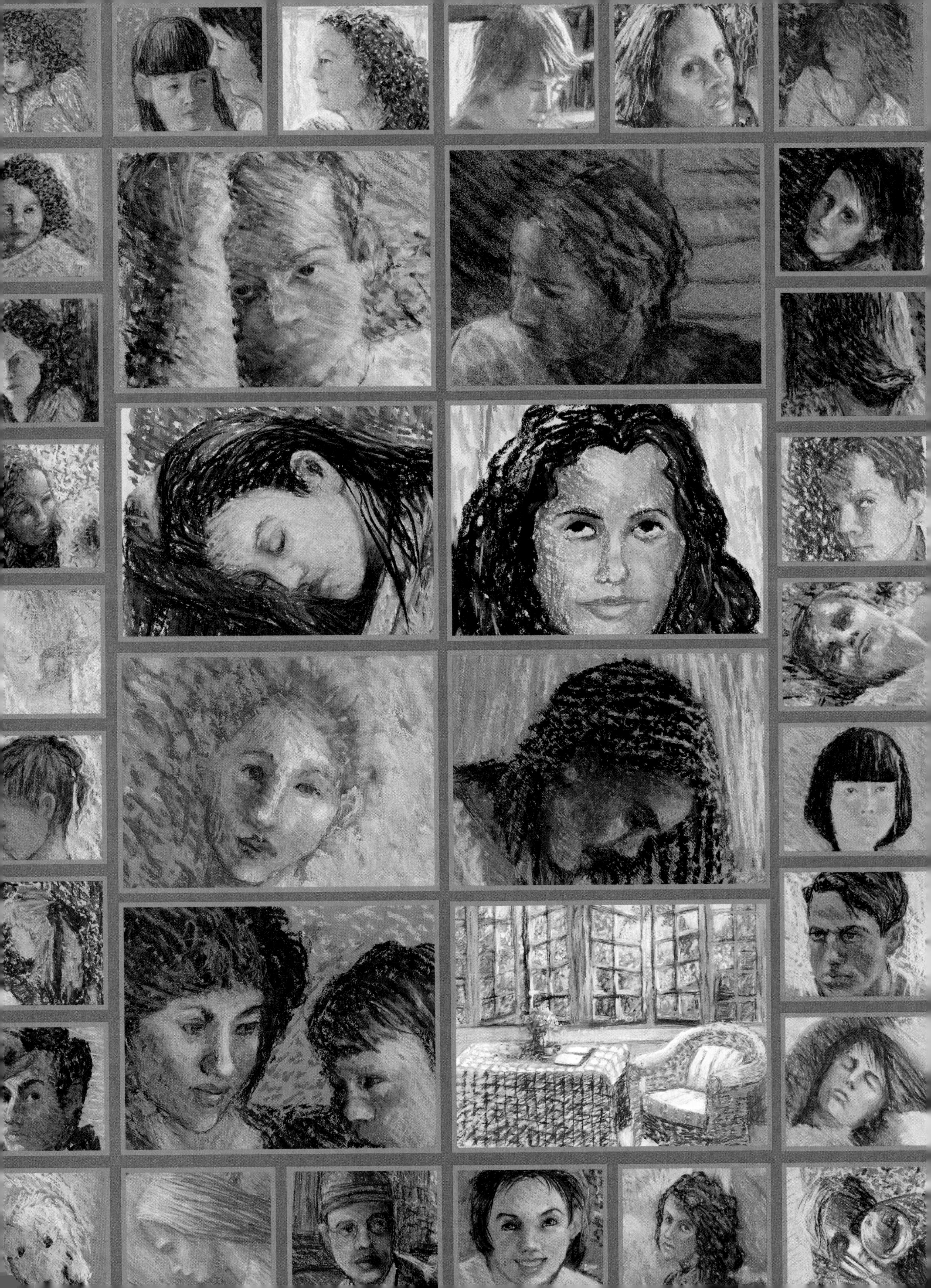

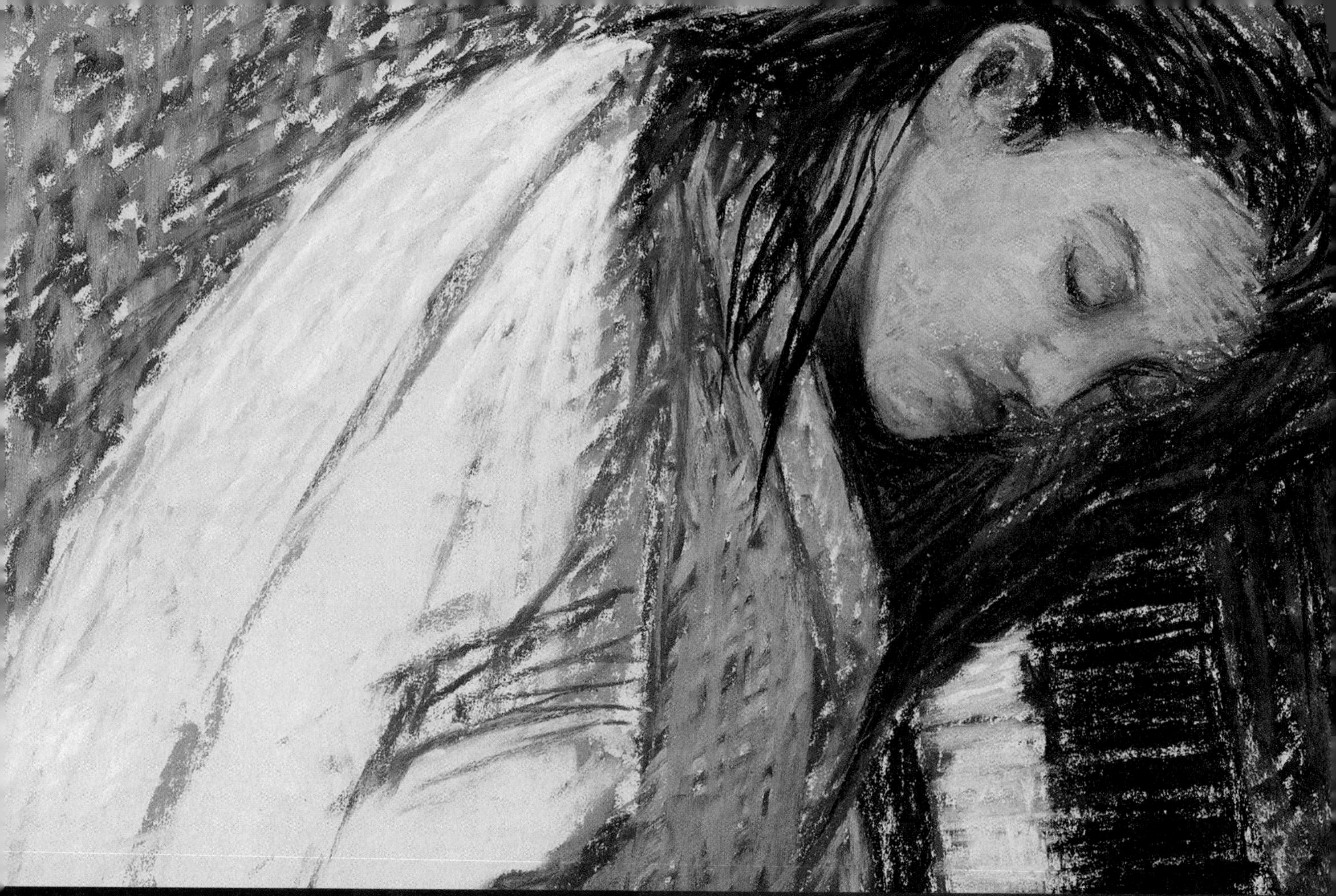

Mood Swings and You

Consider your life over the past few months:

- ***What were the "ups" and "downs" for you?***
- ***Do you notice changes in emotions or energy over time?***
- ***Are there days (or times) when you feel closer to people around you and other times when you feel isolated?***
- ***Can you identify patterns in the moods of your life?***
- ***Do you notice patterns in mood in persons close to you?***

Everyone has mood swings. Life events affect each of us such that some days are happier ("better") than others. In this chapter, we begin to explore the range of moods that people experience.

CHAPTER 14

The Client Experiencing Depression

NOREEN CAVAN FRISCH
LAWRENCE E. FRISCH

CHAPTER OUTLINE

COMPETENCIES

Upon completion of this chapter, the reader should be able to:

1. Identify mood swings as a normal part of the human emotional experience.
2. Employ empathy to understand one's own experience of depression and to understand the depressive feelings of others.
3. Define *depression* and differentiate between major and minor depressive disorders.
4. Describe the concepts of grief and bereavement.
5. Analyze predisposing factors to grief and depression.
6. Identify major psychological theories that explain depression.
7. Integrate a nursing theory base into care for depressed clients.
8. Apply the nursing process to clients who are depressed by:
    - Performing nursing assessments for depression
    - Analyzing data in terms of nursing and psychological theories
    - Formulating individualized nursing diagnoses
    - Suggesting appropriate outcomes
    - Deriving a plan of care
    - Evaluating nursing care based on outcomes

KEY TERMS

Bipolar Depression
Chronic Grief
Cognitive Therapy
Delayed Grief
Depression
Ego
Emotion-Focused Therapy
Exaggerated Grief
Grief
Marital Therapy
Masked Grief
Mood Disorder
Mood Episode
Nurse Agency
Self-Care Agency
Superego
Supportive-Educative Role
Unipolar Depression

Mood swings are a part of everyone's life. There are days when each of us feels up, and days when we feel down. However, when one's mood is significantly "down," usually for several days or more, depression may be diagnosed. The longer a downswing lasts and the more severe it is, the more likely it is that an individual is suffering from depression. Although clinical depression is a common human experience and the cause of a "depressed mood," the inevitable human experience of loss also has a potent effect on mood. Understanding how people feel when confronted with loss can give a better understanding of the experience of depression.

WRITTEN ON SEEING THE FLOWERS, AND REMEMBERING MY DAUGHTER

I grieve for my second daughter.
Six years I carried her about,
Held her against my breast and helped her eat,
Taught her rhymes as she sat on my knee.
She would arise early and copy her elder sister's dress,
Struggling to see herself in the dressing table mirror.
She had begun to delight in pretty silks and lace
But in a poor family she could have none of these.
I would sigh over my own recurring frustrations,
Treading the byways through the rain and snow.
But evenings when I returned to receive her greeting
My sad cares could be transformed into contentment.
What were we to do, that day when illness struck?
The worse because it was during the crisis of war;
Frightened by the alarming sounds, she sank quickly into death.
There was no time even to fix medicines for her.
Distraught, I prepared her poor little coffin;
Weeping, accompanied it to that distant hillside.
It is already lost in the vast void.
Disconsolate, I still grieve deeply for her.

I think how last year, in the spring,
When the flowers bloomed by the pond in our old garden
She led me by the hand along under the trees
And asked me to break off a pretty branch for her.
This year again the flowers bloom;
Now I live far from home, here by this river's edge.
All the household are here, only she is gone.
I look at the flowers, and my tears fall in vain.
A cup of wine brings me no comfort.
*The wind makes desolate sounds in the night curtains.**

(Ch'i, in Weir, 1980, p. 156)

The loss of a child is such an overwhelming experience that even this beautiful poem can only hint at a mother's grief. What would we think if, instead of telling us that "I still grieve deeply for her," Kao Ch'i described how cheerful and happy she was? When the French writer Camus opens his famous novel *The Stranger* with the lines "Mother died today, or maybe yesterday. I can't be sure," the reader knows something is profoundly wrong. Death and loss call for grief and sadness. These are the *normal* human responses; anything less is a sign of poor mental health, of blocked emotions, of crisis.

So, it is clear that feelings of sadness are normal for each of us at some times. Losses and stresses far less profound than death can make us sad, but the feelings are usually fleeting, perhaps lasting a few hours or days. These fluctuations in mood are so much a part of life that the thought of life with all ups and no downs seems to be completely outside of normal human experience. And yet, there are people for whom the ups or the downs become too extreme and last too long. Because of their moods, these people may find it hard or impossible to function in their families, in their work, or in social affairs. They may behave bizarrely, hold unreasonable beliefs, and in their extremes of mood, bring harm to themselves or to others. These people have what we term a **mood disorder**. In his book *As a Man Grows Older*, the Italian novelist Italo Svevo describes an extreme example of such a mood disorder:

AMALIA

He had just shut the door of his flat behind him and was standing hat in hand in the dining room, uncertain what to do next, and wondering whether he could after all face an hour of boredom in his sister's mute society. Suddenly there came from Amalia's room the sound of two or three unintelligible words, and finally a whole phrase: "Get away, you ugly brute!" He shuddered. Her voice was so changed by fatigue or emotion that it resembled his sister's only as an inarticulate shout proceeding from the throat can resemble the modulated speaking voice. Was she asleep at this hour and dreaming by day?

He opened the door noiselessly, and a sight presented itself to his eyes which till his dying day he could never forget. For ever afterwards one or other of the details of that scene had only to strike his senses for him to recall the whole of it immediately and to feel again the appalling horror of it....

Amalia's clothes lay scattered all over the floor and a skirt prevented him from opening the door completely; there were a few garments under the bed ... her boots had been arranged with evident care in the middle of the table.

Amalia was sitting on the edge of the bed, clothed only in a short chemise. She had not noticed her brother's entry, and continued gently to pass her hands up and down her legs, which were as thin as spindles. Emilio was surprised and shocked to see that her naked body resembled that of an ill-nourished child....

"Amalia! What are you doing?" he said reprovingly. She did not hear him, though she seemed to be conscious....

"Amalia!" he repeated in a faint voice, overwhelmed by this obvious proof that she was delirious. He put his hand on her shoulder. Then she turned. She looked first at the hand whose touch she had felt, then she looked him in the face.... It was a slight relief to him to notice that she had heard him. She looked at him again, thoughtfully, as if she were trying to understand the meaning of those cries and of the repeated pressure on her shoulder. She touched her chest as if she had suddenly become conscious of the weight upon it which tormented her. Then forgetting Emilio and her own exhaustion, she shouted again: "Oh, still those horrible creatures!" and there was a break in her voice as if she were going to burst out crying. She rubbed her legs vigorously with both her hands; then bent down with a swift movement as if she were about to surprise an animal in the act of escaping. She seized one of her toes in her right hand and covered it over with her left, then carefully raised both her closed hands as if she were holding something in them. When she saw they were empty she examined them several times, then returned to her foot, ready to stoop down again and renew her strange chase.

A shivering attack reminded Emilio that he ought to induce her to get into bed. He approached her.... His task was however quite easy, for she obeyed the first firm pressure of his hand; she lifted one leg after the other on to the bed, without any shame, and allowed him to pull the bedclothes over her. But she showed an inexplicable reluctance to lie down altogether, and remained leaning on one elbow.

*From "Written on Seeing the Flowers, and Remembering My Daughter" by Ch'i K., from *Anthology of Chinese Literature: Volume II*, edited by Cyril Birch. Copyright 1972 by Grove Press, Inc. In Weir, R. F. (1980) *Death in Literature*. New York: Columbia University Press. Reprinted with permission.

Very soon, however, she could no longer hold out in that position, and abandoned herself on the pillow, uttering for the first time an intelligible sound of grief. "Oh, my God! my God!"

"But what has happened to you?" asked Emilio who, at the sound of that one sensible cry, thought that he could talk to her like a reasonable person. She made no reply, for she was intent on discovering what it was that still went on tormenting her.... She hunched herself all up together, sought out her legs with her hands, and in the deep plot she was evidently meditating against the things or creatures which tormented her, she even contrived to make her breathing less noisy. Then she drew up her hands again and gazed at them in incredulous surprise when she found them empty. She lay for a while beneath the sheets in a state of such distress that she seemed even to forget her terrible bodily fatigue.

"Are you better?" Emilio asked, in a tone of entreaty. He wanted to console himself by the sound of his own voice.... He bent over her, so that she might hear him better.

She lay looking at him for a long time, while her quick feeble breath rose towards him. She recognised him; the warmth of the bed seemed to have revived her senses. However far she wandered afterwards in her delirium, he never forgot that she had recognised him....

Amalia listened to all he had to say, but she seemed also to be listening inwardly to other words beside his; then she said "If you want it I must do it. We will stay here then, but ... so much dirt...." Two tears flowed down her cheeks which had been dry till that moment; they rolled like two pearls down her flaming cheeks....

Soon after she forgot that grievance, but her delirium soon produced another source of distress. She had been out fishing and could not catch any fish: "I can't understand! What is the good of going out fishing if there are not any fish? One has to go such a long, long way and it is so cold." The others had taken all the fish and there were none left for them. All her grief and fatigue now seemed to be due to that fact. Her fevered words, to which her exhaustion gave a kind of tired rhythm, were continually interrupted by some sound of distress.

*He had ceased to pay any attention to her; he must find some way out of the situation, he must devise some means of fetching a doctor.... He had not made up his mind yet what he should do, but he must make haste and get some help for his unfortunate sister.**

(Svevo, 1949, pp. 193–199)

*From Edited by Italo Svevo, translated Beryl De Zoete, from AS A MAN GROWS OLDER, copyright © 1949 by Italo Svovo and Beryl De Zoete. Reprinted by permission of New Directions Publishing Corp.

Amalia's mood disorder of **depression**, the state wherein an individual experiences a profound sadness, has become so severe that she has become psychotic; she has almost completely lost touch with reality. She very likely needs psychiatric hospitalization to recover. Depression varies from a mild downturn in mood to a severe disorder (such as Amalia's) that may threaten life either from suicide or from failure to provide for basic needs such as nutrition and personal safety. This chapter discusses depressive disorders, those mood disorders in which mood swings are always down (or **unipolar depression**). The next chapter discusses mood disorders in which, at least some of the time, persons experience upswings to a manic or hypomanic level (referred to as **bipolar depression**, even in those rare instances where the swings are only up). The reader cannot tell from the preceding excerpt whether Amalia's depression is unipolar or bipolar: The symptoms and severity of depression may be identical in both conditions.

WHAT IS DEPRESSION?

Sadness and loss are universal, but symptoms severe enough or long-lasting enough to justify a diagnosis of depression are much rarer. Epidemiological studies suggest that 7% to 12% of men and 20% to 25% of women are likely to become significantly depressed at some time in their lives. The definition of "significantly depressed" is clearly arbitrary, but the *Diagnostic and Statistical Manual, Fourth Edition-Text Revision* (DSM-IV-TR) is currently the best guide to definition. DSM-IV-TR presents definitions and criteria for mood disorders so there can be definitional consistency in mental health care.

DSM-IV-TR makes a fundamental distinction between a mood episode and a mood disorder. A **mood episode** is the experience of a strong emotion of depression, mania, or a mixture of both for a period of at least two weeks. To be diagnosed as an episode, the symptom must be newly present or have clearly worsened over the preepisode state and must be present nearly every day for most of the day for two consecutive weeks. A mood disorder is diagnosed based on the pattern of mood episodes.

Depression is the intense feeling of a depressed, down mood. However, not everyone who feels depressed meets DSM-IV-TR criteria for depression, and it is *possible* (but *unusual*) to meet those criteria *without feeling depressed.* DSM-IV-TR defines a range of depressive mood disorders, the most important of which are Major Depressive Disorder, Minor Depressive Disorder, Dysthymic Disorder, and Bereavement. These are common and important clinical conditions with which the nurse should be thoroughly familiar.

MAJOR DEPRESSIVE DISORDER

To qualify for this diagnosis, DSM-IV-TR requires the presence of at least one major depressive episode. This episode must: (1) last at least two weeks, (2) represent a change from previous functioning, and (3) cause some impairment in a person's social or occupational functioning. During an

Old Man in Sorrow by Vincent Van Gogh

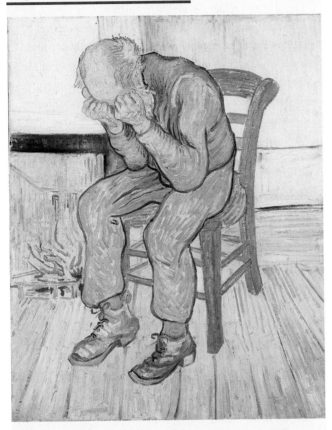

Courtesy: Collection Kröller-Müller Museum, Otterlo, The Netherlands.

Van Gogh painted this relatively unknown picture not long before he killed himself, a few months after his release from the asylum at Arles (see Van Gogh painting in Chapter 2). Although the chair recalls several famous paintings from somewhat happier days (*The Rocking Chair, Gauguin's Armchair*), the figure is an extraordinary evocation of despair.

episode, it is also required that five or more symptoms be present. One of these symptoms *must* be either depressed mood or loss of interest in previously enjoyable activities. The individual must also experience at least four additional symptoms, which may include changes in appetite or weight; sleep disturbance (usually trouble staying asleep); fatigue or loss of energy; feelings of worthlessness or guilt; difficulty concentrating, thinking, or making decisions; or recurrent thoughts of death or suicide.

A person experiencing a depressive episode may express feelings of sadness and hopelessness, or may express the sense of feeling empty or having no feelings. Some persons express somatic symptoms such as bodily aches and pains rather than sadness. Also, some individuals, particularly adolescents, will exhibit irritability or crankiness rather than sadness. Family members or close friends will notice a change in the individual, most commonly a social withdrawal and a neglect of activities that previously brought the person pleasure. Nearly 100 years ago, the great Russian writer Leo Tolstoy eloquently described the onset of his own recurrent major depressive episodes:

MY CONFESSIONS

But five years ago something very strange began to happen to me. At first I experienced moments of perplexity and arrest of life, as though I did not know how to live or what to do; and I felt lost and became dejected. But this passed, and I went on living as before. Then these moments of perplexity began to recur oftener and oftener, and always in the same form. They were always expressed by the questions: What's it for? What does it lead to? ...

My life had come to a standstill. I could breathe, eat, drink, and sleep, and I could not help doing these things; but there was no life, for there were no wishes the fulfillment of which I could consider reasonable. If I desired anything, I knew in advance that whether I satisfied my desire or not, nothing would come of it. Had a fairy come and offered to fulfill my desires I should not have known what to ask. If in moments of intoxication I felt something which, though not a wish, was a habit left by former wishes, in sober moments I knew this to be a delusion, and that there was really nothing to wish for. I could not even wish to know the truth, for I guessed of what it consisted. The truth was that life is meaningless. I had, as it were, lived, lived and walked, walked, till I had come to a precipice and saw clearly that there was nothing ahead of me but destruction....

It had come to this, that I, a healthy, fortunate man, felt I could no longer live; some irresistible power impelled me to rid myself one way or other of life. I cannot say I wished to kill myself. The power which drew me away from life was stronger, fuller, and more widespread than any mere wish. It was a force similar to the former striving to live, only in the opposite direction....

And all this befell me at a time when all around me I had what is considered complete good fortune. I was not yet fifty; I had a good wife who loved me and whom I loved, good children, and a large estate which without much effort on my part improved and increased. I was respected by my relations and acquaintances more than at any previous time. I was praised by others, and without much self-deception could consider that my name was famous. And far from being insane or mentally diseased, I enjoyed on the contrary a strength of mind and body such as I have seldom met with among men of my kind; physically, I could keep up with the peasants at mowing, and mentally I could work for eight and ten hours at a stretch without experiencing any ill results from such exertion....

But life had lost its attraction for me; so how could I attract others? ... I was like one lost in a wood who, horrified at having lost his way, rushes about, wishing to find the road. He knows that each step he takes confuses him more and more; but still he cannot help rushing about.

*... The horror of darkness was too great.... That was the feeling which drew me most strongly towards suicide.**

(Tolstoy, 1932, pp. 201–207)

Major depressive episodes frequently develop over a few days or weeks, and without treatment they may last longer than six months. Up to 10% of persons with Major Depressive Disorder have, as did Tolstoy, symptoms that persist for two or more years. Major Depressive Disorder is quite common in clients visiting general medical outpatient facilities; it appears to occur in up to 9% or 10% of clients (Löwe, Spitzer, Williams, Mussell, Schellberg, & Kroenke, 2008; APA, 2000).

Minor Depressive Disorder

An additional 10% of clients may suffer from less severe symptoms that may interfere with their functioning but may not qualify for a diagnosis of Major Depressive Disorder. The diagnosis Minor Depressive Disorder has been proposed for these individuals, but this diagnosis has yet to be validated for formal inclusion in DSM. In the Epidemiologic Catchment Area (ECA) study (see Chapter 8), minor depression was strongly associated with other psychiatric comorbidity, especially alcohol dependence and anxiety disorders. "Minor" depression can be brief or associated with fewer than the five symptoms required for diagnosis of major disorder. It need not feel minor to the person who experiences it. The American novelist F. Scott Fitzgerald described his own struggles with depression in an essay that he called *The Crack-Up*:

THE CRACK-UP

Of course all life is a process of breaking down, but the blows that do the dramatic side of the work—the big sudden blows that come, or seem to come, from outside—the ones you remember and blame things on and, in moments of weakness, tell your friends about, don't show their effect all at once. There is another sort of blow that comes from within—that you don't feel until it's too late to do anything about it, until you realize with finality that in some regard you will never be as good a man again. The first sort of breakage seems to happen quick—the second kind happens almost without your knowing it but is realized suddenly indeed.

Before I go on with this short history, let me make a general observation—the test of a first-rate intelligence is the ability to hold two opposed ideas in the mind at the same time and still retain the ability to function. One should, for example, be able to see that things are hopeless and yet be determined to make them otherwise. This philosophy fitted on to my early adult life, when I saw the improbable, the implausible, often the "impossible," come true....

For seventeen years, with a year of deliberate loafing and resting out in the center—things went on like that, with a new chore only a nice prospect for the next day. I was living hard, too, but: "Up to forty-nine it'll be all right," I said. "I can count on that. For a man who's lived as I have, that's all you could ask."

—And then, ten years this side of forty-nine, I suddenly realized that I had prematurely cracked.

Now a man can crack in many ways—can crack in the head—in which case the power of decision is taken from you by others! or in the body, when one can but submit to the white hospital world; or (like the present writer) in the nerves ... too much anger and too many tears....

Suffice it to say that after about an hour of solitary pillow-hugging, I began to realize that for two years my life had been a drawing on resources that I did not possess, that I had been mortgaging myself physically and spiritually up to the hilt....

I realized that in those two years, in order to preserve something—an inner hush maybe, maybe not—I had weaned myself from all the things I used to love—that every act of life from the morning tooth-brush to the friend at dinner had become an effort. I saw that for a long time I had not liked people and things, but only followed the rickety old pretense of liking. I saw that even my love for those closest to me has become only an attempt to love, that my casual relations—with an editor, a tobacco seller, the child of a friend, were only what I remembered I should do, from other days. All in the same month I became bitter about such things as the sound of the radio, the advertisements in the magazines, the screech of tracks, the dead silence of the country—contemptuous at human softness, immediately (if secretively) quarrelsome toward hardness—hating the night when I couldn't sleep and hating the day because it went toward night. I slept on the heart side now because I knew that the sooner I could tire that out, even a little, the sooner would come that blessed hour of nightmare which, like a catharsis, would enable me to better meet the new day....

Trying to cling to something, I liked doctors and girl children up to the age of about thirteen and well-brought-up boy children from about eight years old on. I could

*From *A Confession and What I Believe* by L. Tolstoy, translated by A. Maude, 1932, Oxford, England: Oxford University Press. Reprinted with permission.

have peace and happiness with these few categories of people. I forgot to add that I liked older men—men over seventy, sometimes over sixty if their faces looked seasoned. I liked Katharine Hepburn's face on the screen, no matter what was said about her pretentiousness, and Miriam Hopkins' face, and old friends if I only saw them once a year and could remember their ghosts.

All rather inhuman and undernourished, isn't it? Well, that, children, is the true sign of cracking up.

It is not a pretty picture. Inevitably it was carted here and there within its frame and exposed to various critics.

"Instead of being so sorry for yourself, listen—(one of the critics) said. (She always says "Listen," because she thinks while she talks—really thinks.) So she said: "Listen. Suppose this wasn't a crack in you—suppose it was a crack in the Grand Canyon."

"The crack's in me," I said heroically.

"Listen! The world only exists in your eyes—your conception of it. You can make it as big or as small as you want to. And you're trying to be a little puny individual. By God, if I ever cracked, I'd try to make the world crack with me. Listen! The world only exists through your apprehension of it, and so it's much better to say that it's not you that's cracked—it's the Grand Canyon."

... She spoke, then, of old woes of her own, that seemed, in the telling, to have been more dolorous than mine, and how she had met them, over-ridden them, beaten them.

*I felt a certain reaction to what she said, but I am a slow-thinking man, and it occurred to me simultaneously that of all the natural forces, vitality is the incommunicable one ... You have it or you haven't it, like health or brown eyes or honor or a baritone voice. I might have asked some of it from her ... but I could never have got it—not even if I'd waited around for a thousand hours with the tin cup of self-pity. I could walk from her door, holding myself very carefully like cracked crockery, and go away into the world of bitterness, where I was making a home.**

(Fitzgerald, 1945, pp. 520–524)

Fitzgerald describes sadness ("too many tears"), insomnia, and loss of pleasure in some activities and relationships. He is able to take pleasure in some people and activities (for example, watching Katherine Hepburn movies). From his essay, we can be confident that he was severely troubled by depression, but he probably does not describe sufficiently numerous or severe symptoms to allow a diagnosis of major depression.

Dysthymic Disorder

Whereas the essence of Major Depressive Disorder is discrete episodes of depression, persons with Dysthymic Disorder feel depressed nearly all of the time. DSM-IV-TR criteria for Dysthymic Disorder include "depressed mood for most of the day, for more days than not ... for at least 2 years" (American Psychiatric Association, 2000, p. 376). A person with Dysthymic Disorder must also have at least two of the following symptoms: appetite disturbance, sleep disturbance, fatigue, low self-esteem, poor concentration or difficulty making decisions, and feelings of hopelessness. As with Major Depressive Disorder, the symptoms must cause clinically significant distress or impairment in social or occupational functioning. Dysthymic Disorder is somewhat rarer than Major Depressive Disorder, occurring during a lifetime in about 6% of persons. At any time, between 2% and 4% of persons visiting outpatient medical facilities have Dysthymic Disorder (APA, 2000), and up to 36% of persons in outpatient mental health facilities have Dysthymic Disorder (Klein, Shankman, & Rose, 2006). Like Major Depressive Disorder, Dysthymic Disorder often begins in childhood or adolescence. Researchers presenting results of a 10-year longitudinal study of the course of Dysthymic Disorder report that while more than 70% of persons recovered with treatment, individuals with Dysthymic Disorder carry a significant risk of developing another period of chronic depression at some time in their lives. Seventy-five percent of persons with this disorder will experience major depression (Klein et al., 2006). In his play *Uncle Vanya*, the great writer Anton Chekhov would seem to be convincingly describing Dysthymic Disorder. Here, the middle-aged country doctor Astrov is visiting in the home of Sonia, a young woman who is in love with him:

UNCLE VANYA

SONIA: You're dissatisfied with life then?

ASTROV: I love life as such—but our life, our everyday provincial life in Russia, I just can't endure. I despise it with all my soul. As for my own life, God knows I can find nothing good in it at all. You know, when you walk through a forest on a dark night and you see a small light gleaming in the distance, you don't notice your tiredness, not the darkness, nor the prickly branches lashing you in the face.... I work harder than anyone in the district—you know that—fate batters me continuously, at times I suffer unbearably—but there's no small light in the distance. I'm not expecting anything for myself any longer, I don't love human beings ... I haven't cared for anyone for years.

SONIA: Not for anyone?

ASTROV: No one. I feel a sort of fondness for your old nurse—for the sake of old times. The peasants are all too much alike, undeveloped, living in squalor. As for the educated people—it's hard to get on with them. They tire me so. All of them, all our good friends here are shallow in thought, shallow in feeling, unable to see further than their noses—or to put it quite bluntly, stupid. And the ones who are a bit more intelligent, of a higher mental calibre, are hysterical, positively rotten with introspection and futile cerebration. They whine, they are full of hatreds and morbidly malicious, they sidle up to a man, look at him out of the corner of their eyes, and pronounce their judgement: "Oh, he's a psychopath!," or "Just a phrase-monger." And when they don't know how to label me, they say: "He's a queer fellow, very queer!" I love forests—that's queer, I don't eat meat—that's queer too. There isn't any direct objective, unprejudiced attitude to people or nature left.... No, there isn't! [About to drink.]

SONIA: [Prevents him.] No, I beg you, I implore you, don't drink any more.

ASTROV: Why not?

SONIA: It's so unlike you! You have such poise, your voice is so soft.... More than that, you are beautiful as no one else I know is beautiful. So why do you want to be like ordinary men, the kind who drink and play cards? Don't do it, I implore you. You always say that people don't create anything, but merely destroy what has been given them from above. Then why, why are you destroying yourself? You mustn't, you mustn't, I beseech you, I implore you!

ASTROV: [Holds out his hand to her.] I won't drink any more!

SONIA: Give me your word.

ASTROV: My word of honour.

SONIA: [Presses his hand warmly.] Thank you!

ASTROV: Enough! My head's clear now. You see I'm quite sober—and I'll stay sober to the end of my days. [Looks at his watch.] Well, to continue. As I said, my time's over, it's too late for me now ... I've aged too much, I've worked myself to a standstill, I've grown coarse and insensitive ... I believe I could never really become fond of another human being. I don't love anybody and never shall now. What still does affect me is beauty. I can't remain indifferent to that. I believe that if Yeliena Andryeevna wanted to, for instance, she could turn my head in a day.... But that's not love, of course, that's not affection.... [Covers his eyes with his hands and shudders.]

SONIA: What is it?

ASTROV: Nothing.... In Lent one of my patients died under chloroform.

SONIA: It's time to forget about that. [A pause.] Tell me, Mihail Lvovich.... If I had a girl friend, or a young sister and if you got to know that she ... well, suppose that she loved you, what would you do?

*ASTROV: [Shrugging his shoulders.] I don't know. Probably nothing. I should let her know that I couldn't love her.... besides I've got too many other things on my mind. However, if I'm going, I'd better start now. I'll say goodbye, my dear girl, or we'll not finish till morning. [Shakes hands with her.]**

(Chekhov, 1954, pp. 210–212)

Nurses must be aware of the fact that nearly 15% of hospitalized clients may meet criteria for Major Depressive Disorder. This is a complex issue, however, because DSM-IV-TR criteria do not permit a diagnosis of either Dysthymic Disorder or Major Depressive Disorder to be made when depressive symptoms are thought to be due to physical illness. Some additional material on depressive illness in persons with physical illness is found in Chapter 21 (on care of the physically ill) and in Chapter 25 (on care of the elderly client). Although the presence of chronic physical illness may influence the precise diagnosis given to persons with physical illness, it does not change the importance of providing effective treatment. Physical illness and its treatments may alter the side effects of drug therapy, especially of psychiatric medications that interact with drugs used for other conditions. It has been known that depression can increase mortality in patients with chronic illness, especially the elderly (Schultz, Beach, Ives, Martire, Ariyo, & Kop, 2000) and those with coronary artery disease (Busell & Stuart, 1999). The Whitehall II study in the United Kingdom showed that persons with mild depression had the kinds of abnormalities in small arteries that are often associated with the development of coronary disease and similar cardiovascular disorders (Hemingway, Shipley, Mullen, Kumari, Brunner, Taylor, et al., 2003). More recent studies continue to document a significant association between depression and cardiac disorders (Fan, Strine, Jiles, & Mokdad, 2008), and depression and diabetes and hypertension (Kagee, 2008; Swenson, Rose, Vittighoff, Stewart, & Schellinger, 2008).

Postpartum Depression

One setting in which depression frequently manifests itself is after the birth of a baby. Zauderer presents a useful case study and review of the literature on this important condition (Zauderer, 2008). Beck, in turn, provides a review of international nursing research contributions to our understanding of postpartum depression (Beck, 2008a, Beck 2008b). According to the DSM criteria for depressive episodes and mood disorders, the symptoms of postpartum depression do not differ from the symptoms of non-postpartum mood disorders (APA, 2000, p. 422). The postpartum presentation is a qualifier from the diagnosis, signifying that the depression occurs within four weeks after childbirth. Postpartum depression may have a variety of serious consequences for the health and well-being of both mother and infant. Depression

*From "Uncle Vanya," in *Plays*, by Anton Chekhov (pp. 210–212), translated by Elisaveta Fen, 1954. Reproduced with permission from Rosemary Davidson.

occurs following approximately 10% to 15% of births, but ranges greatly in seriousness. The risk appears higher among younger mothers, those from lower socioeconomic groups births (CDC, 2008), and perhaps smokers (Whitaker, Orzol, & Kahn, 2007). Many suggestions have been made about causes of postprartum depression, most focusing on changes in hormonal levels following delivery. A variety of hormones have been implicated in the causation of postpartum depression; these include estrogen, progesterone, thyroxine, melatonin, cortisol, and prolactin.

Whatever role hormones may eventually be found to play, personal risk factors have been consistently shown to be important in predicting postpartum symptoms. Among the most important predictors are prior depression (especially following a previous birth) and low levels of social support. Pregnancy loss may contribute to depression, but premature birth or other neonatal complications do not seem to play a role (Bernazzani & Bifulco, 2003). Studies show that many obstetric providers fail to ask mothers explicitly about symptoms of depression, and may not schedule visits until six weeks after delivery—when symptoms may already have led to adverse consequences. The Edinburgh Postnatal Depression Scale (EPDS) is a commonly used short screening instrument (Cox, Holden, & Sagovsky, 1987) that has been shown to perform well in detecting this disorder (Morris-Rush, Freda, & Bernstein, 2003). Undetected postpartum depression may lead to serious disturbances in mother-infant bonding, breastfeeding effectiveness, and family functioning. In rare circumstances, postpartum depression may result in psychosis or infanticide, or both (Meier, 2002). While the majority of attention has been given to female postpartum depression, postpartum depression has also been reported in men (Schumacher, Zubaran, & White, 2008) and seems to predict adverse later psychological problems among their children (Ramchandani, Stein, O'Connor, Heron, Murray, & Evans, 2008).

Bereavement versus Depressive Disease

It is important that the nurse understand and recognize the difference between bereavement or **grief**, a normal and healthy condition, and depressive disease. While DSM-IV-TR recognizes the diagnosis of Bereavement (loss), no diagnostic criteria are given because this is assumed to be a normal human condition. However, the nurse will recognize Grieving—*anticipatory or dysfunctional* as nursing diagnoses described by NANDA (2005) and calling for a nursing response. A person experiencing grief will have many of the same symptoms as one who is depressed—that is, a grieving person will feel sad and hopeless and express feelings of depression. A grieving person may also exhibit loss of appetite, weight loss, sleep disturbances, and inability to concentrate, make decisions, and carry out daily activities. The difference is that the grieving person has experienced a recent loss, acknowledges that loss, and experiences great pain in giving up attachment to that which was lost. Bereavement may last for days or months, depending on the degree of attachment involved. The level of severity can only be determined by the individual grieving, not the particular circumstances that provoked the grief. A person will respond to the emotions of grief using the same coping strategies that he has used to deal with other, powerful emotions in the past. One learns how to grieve by learning how to understand and accept emotions, how to feel emotions, and how to use supportive persons to talk about feelings. Successful resolution of normal grief requires that a person accept, understand, and deal with painful emotions.

NURSINGALERT 14-1

Risk Factors for Depression

- Family history of depression
- Having experienced recent negative stressors
- Having childhood experiences in a negative home environment
- Lacking a social support system
- Having significant, physical disease

Three stages of the normal grieving process have been accepted as a pattern that is followed by most individuals suffering loss (Manning, 1984); these are discussed following.

Stage 1: The Period of Shock

The person describes feeling "numb." This stage lasts from days to a month or more. The *Old Testament* story of David and Jonathan's friendship and Jonathan's death in a battle on Mount Gilboa is told primarily in 1 *Samuel.* The following lament was written by Peter Abelard (best known for his own tragic love affair with Heloise). In Abelard's version, David is in shock after learning of Jonathan's death.

PLANCTUS VI — KING DAVID'S LAMENT ON THE DEATH OF SAUL AND JONATHAN

Overcome with sorrow, I play my harp.
What else to do when mourning is everywhere: Saul is dead
And Jonathan too.

Oh Jonathan. We were more than brothers.
Our hearts and souls were joined as one
What was our sin, what was our crime, to be so parted?

Ye daughters of Zion, begin your lamentation for the death of Saul
But I alone will mourn Jonathan
Never again will dew or rain fall on Gilboa, but my tears will flow unending.

Oh why, oh why, did I listen to them? Why did I let you fight apart from me?
Had we died together there would be no lasting pain in my heart.
United in death, not parted as now.

How many times did you save my life in battle! But where was I in your need?
Half a soul is not enough to live
When surviving means to die each day.

What joy is there in victory over the enemy?
Yes, I rejoiced, until the messenger came
And when he told me of your death — I had him killed —
Death to the messenger of sorrow.

My voice is hoarse from lamenting
My hand bleeds from striking the strings
*Overcome with sorrow, I put my harp to rest.**

(Peter Abelard, 1079-1142)

Stage 2: The Reality Stage

Most of the painful experience begins here, when the individual consciously realizes the meaning of the loss to her life. Reactions may include anger, guilt, hurt, frustration, helplessness, or fear. The following selection is from Julian Barnes's novel *Flaubert's Parrot*. The narrator is an English doctor, Geoffrey, whose wife has recently committed suicide. Geoffrey is obsessed by the life and writings of Gustave Flaubert, who wrote *Madame Bovary*, a nineteenth-century novel about the adultery and suicide of a country doctor's wife.

FLAUBERT'S PARROT

This is a pure story, whatever you may think. When she dies, you are not at first surprised. Part of love is preparing for death. You feel confirmed in your love when she dies. You got it right. This is part of it all.

Afterwards comes the madness. And then the loneliness: not the spectacular solitude you had anticipated, not the interesting martyrdom of widowhood, but just loneliness. You expect something almost geological—vertigo in a shelving canyon—but it's not like that; it's just misery as regular as a job. What do we doctors say? I'm deeply sorry, Mrs Blank ... rest assured you will come out of it; ... I would suggest; perhaps a new interest, Mrs Blank; car maintenance, formation dancing?; don't worry, six months will see you back on the roundabout; come and see me again any time; oh nurse, when she calls, just give her this repeat prescription will you, no I don't need to see her, well it's not her that's dead is it, look on the bright side. What did she say her name was?

And then it happens to you. There's no glory in it. Mourning is full of time; nothing but time ... I've tried drink, but what does that do? Drink makes you drunk, that's all it's ever been able to do. Work, they say, cures everything. It doesn't; often, it doesn't even induce tiredness; the nearest you get to it is a neurotic lethargy. And there is always extra time. Have some more time. Take your time. Extra time. Time on your hands.

Other people think you want to talk. "Do you want to talk about Ellen?" they ask, hinting that they won't be embarrassed if you break down. Sometimes you talk, sometimes you don't; it makes little difference. The words aren't the right ones; or rather, the right words don't exist. "Language is like the cracked kettle on which we beat out tunes for bears to dance to, while all the time we long to move the stars to pity." You talk, and you find the language of bereavement foolishly inadequate. You seem to be talking about other people's griefs. I loved her; we were unhappy; I miss her.... There is a limited choice of prayers on offer: gabble the syllables.

"It may seem bad, Geoffrey, but you'll come out of it. I'm not taking your grief lightly; it's just that I've seen enough of life to know that you'll come out of it." The words you've said yourself while scribbling a prescription.... And you do come out of it, that's true. After a year, after five. But you don't come out of it like a train coming out of a tunnel, bursting through the Downs into sunshine and that swift, rattling descent to the Channel; you come out of it as a gull comes out of an oil slick. You are tarred and feathered for life.

And still you think about her every day ...

*I sometimes feel embarrassed by people's sympathy.**

(Barnes, 1985, p. 190)

Stage 3: The Recovery Stage

During the final, recovery phase, the person integrates the loss into the reality of her life and begins to live again. From Flaubert's *Madame Bovary*, a friend tries to console Dr. Bovary after his wife's suicide:

*Translation by Lawrence Frisch from the Latin as given by Lorenz Weinrich. Weinrich L. (Translation by Marshall R.) (1969) Peter Abaelard as Musician—II, *The Musical Quarterly.* 55:464-486.

MADAME BOVARY

*I know what it's like, he said, slapping him on the shoulder. I was like you, I was! After I lost my poor departed wife, I used to go off into the fields, to be on my own. I'd drop down at the foot of a tree, crying, calling on the good Lord, telling him off. I wanted to be like the moles, hung up on the branches, their bellies crawling with maggots—dead, I mean. And when I thought of the others, at that very moment, hugging their bonny little wives close to them, I'd strike the ground with my stick, hard. I was crazy, like, didn't even eat, the thought of going to the inn sickened me, you wouldn't believe it. Ah well, slowly but surely, one day chasing another, spring on top of winter, autumn on top of summer, it leaked away, drop by drop, little by little; it left, it went away—it sank down, I should say, because there's always something that stays, at the bottom, so to speak ... a weight there, on the chest! But it's the same for all of us, we mustn't let ourselves go, and want to die just because others are dead.... You must pull yourself together Monsieur Bovary—it will pass! Come and see us. My daughter thinks of you from time to time, you know, and you are forgetting her, so she says. It'll be spring soon; we'll get you to shoot a rabbit in the woods, to help take your mind off things.**

(Flaubert, 1983, pp. 113–114)

Grief experienced after the death of a loved one was once thought to take about one year to reach resolution. Now it is clear that normal grieving may take two or even three years, depending on many factors surrounding the attachment and loss (Bower, 1987). During normal grieving, however, the person is progressing though the stages described previously, often adaptive behaviors in relatively uniform patterns (Steeves, 2002).

Even when depressive symptoms are severe, unless a grieving individual is suicidal, Major Depressive Disorder is not diagnosed within the first two months after the loss of a loved one. Abnormal grief reactions do occur, particularly in situations where the individual had ambivalent feelings toward the person lost or unresolved emotional work within that relationship.

In abnormal grieving, the individual experiences grief as overwhelming and resorts to maladaptive behaviors. The literature describes four types of abnormal grief reactions (Worden, 1991): **chronic grief**, in which the grief never reaches conclusions; **delayed grief**, in which the grief work is not accomplished at the time of loss and remains with the individual; **exaggerated grief**, in which the grief is experienced as overwhelming; and **masked grief**, in which the grief is masked by either a physical symptom or a maladaptive behavior and the person is unaware of the connections to grief and loss.

A nurse will need to support and care for persons undergoing grief, and some of the nursing interventions will be similar to those used when caring for one who is depressed. It is important, though, that the nurse have basic underlying knowledge of the course and dynamics of both grief and depression so that specialist care can be sought when grieving becomes complicated by a mood disorder (Kendler, Hettema, Butera, Gardner, & Prescott, 2003).

> **NURSING TIP 14-1**
>
> **Identifying Successful Grieving**
>
> A person moving successfully through normal grieving will:
>
> - Consciously recognize she has experienced a significant loss
> - Progress through the stages of shock (emotional numbness), reality (deep pain), and recovery (beginning to live again)
> - Use adaptive coping behaviors such as action strategies (keeping busy), cognitive coping ("can do" attitude), and interpersonal coping (talking with others, joining a support group)

THEORIES OF DEPRESSION

Depression is such a profound and devastating human experience that it seems to demand an explanation. As in the story of Amalia, depression can rapidly transform a person from relatively normal functioning to psychosis. F. Scott Fitzgerald describes his own "cracking up" as occurring both more slowly and less profoundly, but neither he nor his friend have a clear understanding of why this has happened to him. There are numerous psychological theories that try to explain the cause of mood disorders. The nurse should have at least some acquaintance with a few of the major theories of depression.

PSYCHOANALYSIS

Psychoanalysis derives from Sigmund Freud's studies of dreaming as a window into the unconscious mind (Fine,

*From *Madame Bovary* by G. Flaubert, 1983. In D. J. Enright (Ed.), *The Oxford Book of Death* (pp. 113–114), Oxford: Oxford University Press.

Tarnation

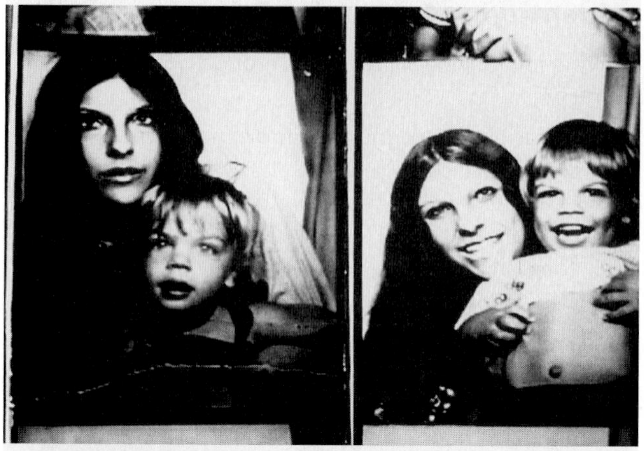

Courtesy: Wellspring Media/The Kobal Collection/The Picture Desk

In this set of stills from the film *Tarnation* we see two views from the family album of a mother who suffers from a psychotic depression, an illness that causes immense grief for all around her family. Only her son, Jonathan, manages to extricate himself from the catastrophe that Renee's illness brings upon everyone involved.

1979). Since there are currently many schools of psychoanalysis, not all strictly adhering to Freud's theories, it is not possible to define a single psychoanalytic perspective on depression. In fact, although Freud himself suffered from symptoms of depression, neither the diagnosis nor the explanation of depressive symptoms plays a large part in his work. In 1917, Freud published "Mourning and Melancholia," a paper that described mourning as the "psychically prolonged ... existence of the lost object (of love)." By this he meant that the mourner feels as if somehow the lost person is still emotionally present until "the work of mourning is completed." In this paper, Freud described depression (melancholia) as loss of an *internal* quality such as self-esteem during the crisis deriving from a child's discovery of his inability to assume the social and sexual role of the same-sex parent. Freud later viewed depression as a conflict between the **ego** (the conscious self) and the **superego** (an inner voice, something like an internalized parent). In depression, the superego punishes the ego for having forbidden wishes or for not living up to the superego's expectations (usually similar to those of one's actual parents). The result of that conflict was guilt, self-hate, and anger turned inward; these processes, in turn, led to depression.

Although perhaps somewhat out of favor presently, psychoanalysis offers at least two important insights into the understanding of depression. First, the concept that depression may derive from the superego allows the nurse or other therapist to explore with a client how childhood experiences and parental expectations may influence present feelings. Second, since psychoanalysis traces the roots of depression into childhood, it supports the understanding that children may be significantly depressed. Depression *does* occur in children, and the nurse who works with children and their families should be alert to its detection and treatment.

Object Loss Theory

Object loss theory is also based in psychoanalysis, but derives from a specific historical event. After World War II, millions of children were orphaned and left homeless and grew up in abject poverty. John Bowlby's psychoanalytic study of these children concluded that adult mental health required a young child to experience a close and loving relationship with its mother (or an appropriate mother substitute; Fine, 1979). Two ideas are important in the theory that derived from Bowlby's observations: (1) a traumatic loss early in life may predispose one to depression, and (2) a subsequent loss or separation in adulthood may serve as a stimulus to depression. These ideas have been strongly attacked by other psychoanalysts, particularly Freud's daughter, Anna. Anna Freud believed that many factors other than maternal separation influence the development of a child's personality (more precisely, *ego*) and that a strong ego can resist the crisis of maternal loss. This disagreement over the role that object loss plays in depression was once known as the Bowlby controversy. Object loss theory may be important in understanding the personal histories of depressed individuals whose childhoods were particularly traumatic and loss filled.

Learned Helplessness Theory

The learned helplessness theory of depression is based on the work of Seligman (1974). He defines helplessness as the sense that one has no control over life events and defines hopelessness as the sense that no one can do anything about life's events. This theory suggests that it is not any specific situation that causes depression, but, rather, it is the individual's belief that there is nothing either he or anyone else can do to make things better. Learned helplessness is caused by a series of reinforcers in one's environment that serve to take control away from the individual, thus producing a personality trait of "giving up." A person who has learned helplessness in growing up has no sense of herself as master of her own destiny and will lack the skills and incentive to try.

Cognitive Theory

Cognitive theory emerged in contrast to psychoanalysis. Psychoanalysis emphasizes the unconscious childhood origins of adult emotional experiences. Psychoanalysts Albert Ellis and Aaron Beck initiated something of a revolution when they came to believe that how clients *think about their feelings* may be more important for their recovery than *deep understanding of the origins of those feelings*. Beck views depression as a condition in which the individual has come to accept faulty thoughts and to hold dysfunctional assumptions. Ellis termed these thoughts "irrational beliefs" (Beck, 1967). According to cognitive theory, the client is depressed because he accepts a view of himself and the world that allows for dysfunctional thoughts, painful emotions, and maladaptive behaviors (Perris & Herlofson, 1993). By learning to see the world differently, the client can come to adopt a healthier and more functional self-image. Cognitive therapy derives from cognitive theory and relies on individual learning and teaching from a skilled therapist. Psychologists refer to the recent developments leading to cognitive therapy as the "cognitive revolution," in part because supporters of cognitive approaches have consistently demanded that their theories be judged on whether they make clients better. Cognitive treatments *do* work, and it has been difficult to demonstrate such consistent effectiveness for any other type of psychotherapy. In this successful insistence on demonstrable effectiveness, cognitive therapy truly *is* revolutionary.

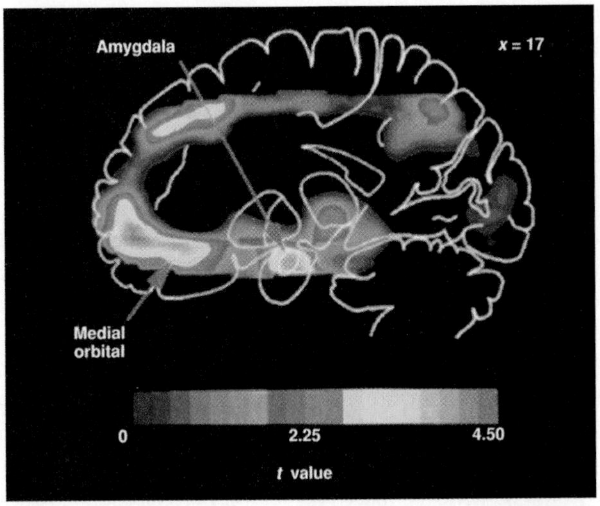

FIGURE 14-1 **PET Scanning in Depression. This PET image shows that depressed persons commonly have increased blood flow in specific brain areas as compared to nondepressed persons. This image depicts a parasagittal "slice" as if the image were seen from the left side of a transparent head. Areas depicted in yellow, orange, or red have more blood flow than do comparable anatomic areas in persons without depression. This scan provides evidence for increased metabolic activity in the amygdala (and other brain areas) in persons with familial major depression.** (FROM "LINKING MIND AND BRAIN IN THE STUDY OF MENTAL ILLNESSES: A PROJECT FOR A SCIENTIFIC PSYCHOPATHOLOGY" BY NANCY C. ANDREASEN. *SCIENCE 275*: 1586–93 (1997). USED WITH PERMISSION OF THE AMERICAN ASSOCIATION FOR THE ADVANCEMENT OF SCIENCE.)

Physical/Biological Models

With recent advances in biochemical studies, explicitly biological and biochemical models of depression have been proposed. It has long been known that some drugs make depression worse, whereas others clearly improve depressive symptoms. Although their effects may be different, such drugs seem to have in common that they affect concentrations of monoamines (especially norepinephrine and serotonin) in the brain. This effect on monoamines has been of interest to physiologists because norepinephrine and serotonin are produced in only very localized areas of the brainstem. This localized production might imply that depression is a disease that could be shown to have its origins in a very specific area of the brain.

Recently, the very powerful tools of functional magnetic resonance imaging (fMRI), single-photon emission computed tomography (SPECT), and positron emission tomography (PET) have allowed measurements to be made of metabolism and blood flow in different parts of the brain in depressed and nondepressed persons (see Figure 14-1; George, Ketter, & Post, 1993). These scanning techniques can measure both blood flow and glucose utilization in different, very highly localized brain areas. Emerging studies seem to show that depression is associated with consistent changes in the temporal and especially the frontal lobes: Depressed persons do not metabolize glucose well in these areas, but when their depression resolves, metabolism returns to normal (Videbech, 2000). There is increased metabolic activity within the amygdala in persons with familial major depression as compared to a control group.

These findings are both interesting and important, and they suggest that depression is truly, at some level, a disease of the brain. The findings do not explain *why* glucose uptake is abnormal, and they do not explain how (or whether) psychological factors such as grieving can affect brain function measured by PET scanning. As a result, it still remains unknown whether the observed PET findings are a *cause* or an *effect* of depression. While PET and SPECT findings do not yet hold clinical importance for the nurse, it is likely that evolving highly technical studies will cast new light and understanding on both the causes and treatments of depression.

As mentioned previously and discussed in Chapter 4, the amygdala has recently been recognized to be the major brain structure associated with feelings and expressing emotions such as fear, apprehension, and perhaps sadness. It is then not surprising that neuroimaging studies have linked the amygdala to the emotions of depression. Recent work has shown a strong link between the amygdala (where "primitive" emotions seem to originate), and the *left* prefrontal cortex (apparently involved in the suppression of negative emotions). When persons without depressive disorder are shown images (automobile crashes, threatening animals) likely to provoke strong adverse feelings and then are asked to consciously suppress those feelings, fMRI demonstrates that activation of their left prefrontal cortex suppresses activity in the amygdala. In contrast, persons with depression develop strong activation of both left and right prefrontal areas—a response that results in activation of the amygdala and associated limbic structures (Johnstone, van Reekum, Urry, Kalin, & Davidson, 2007). These data suggest a biophysiological explanation for one of the most important findings in depression: that persons with depression are less able to suppress negative thoughts than are normal individuals. Research suggests that both providers and patients view imaging as valuable in understanding, treating, and destigmatizing depressive disorders (Illes, Lombera, Rosenberg, & Arnow, 2008).

While studies attempting to localize abnormal functioning within the brain of depressed individuals have led to dramatic new insights about the nature of affective disorders, in recent years scientists have also explored the way that substances produced *outside* the brain can have an effect on feelings and emotions. Interferon, a substance synthesized naturally by human cells, usually in response to viral infections, has found a role in treating several cancers, a number of viral infections, and some other disorders. Depression has proved to be one of the major side effects of interferon treatment, and this side effect has been linked to changes in brain concentrations of serotonin (Sakai, Hasegawa, Okura, Morikawa, Ueyama, Shirai, et al., 2003). However, researchers have recently recognized that interferon and certain related "cytokines" are frequently produced by the body in response to some cancers and chronic inflammatory illnesses (such as rheumatoid arthritis). These substances appear to have a direct effect on the brain and may be responsible, at least in part, for the depression that often accompanies malignancies and chronic illnesses (Raison & Miller, 2003).

TREATMENT

In the following section, a variety of treatments that have proved effective in managing depression are discussed. Data suggest, however, that barely half of persons with depression receive treatment, and that less than half of that treatment is judged adequate based on number and timing of follow-up visits (Kessler, Berglund, Demier, Jin, Koretz, Merikangas, et al., 2003). While many factors contribute to failures in treating depression, currently clients with depression are more likely to be diagnosed and offered treatment than in the 1980s. Significant progress has been made in managing depression, but much more remains to be done. Current treatments that are discussed include psychotherapy, somatic or physical therapies, and medications.

PSYCHOTHERAPY

Psychotherapy refers to any of more than 250 types of largely verbal techniques designed to help individuals surmount psychological stresses including depression. Psychotherapy based on psychoanalytic interventions emphasizes helping clients gain insight into the causes of their depression. This approach is long term and requires much motivation on the part of the client to invest considerable time, effort, and money. Although psychoanalytic interventions have long been used in treating depression, there is little evidence establishing effectiveness, and several newer approaches have gained favor in recent years as evidence has accumulated in their favor. The discussion that follows covers three types of short-term psychotherapy: emotion-focused therapy, marital therapy, and cognitive therapy. Nurses will have many clients who receive other types of therapeutic interventions, but these three therapies are among the most carefully studied in mood disorders.

Emotion-focused therapy recognizes the importance of emotional responses in depression and encourages the recognition and conscious control of these responses (Greenberg & Bolger, 2001). Emotions involved in depression include sadness, guilt, and shame. Greenberg distinguishes between "constructive" and "unconstructive" emotions. "Most therapists," he claims, "are skilled at helping patients **swiftly eliminate** unpleasant emotions. Most therapists have been trained in some approach to emotion regulation. The methods differ … but the goal is generally the same: the prompt reduction of unpleasant emotion…. After years of enthusiasm for emotion control therapies, practitioners around the world are awakening to realize they've missed half the picture. In mistakenly suppressing our patients' **constructive** unpleasant emotions, we've inadvertently stunted their growth and jeopardized their adaptation" (Greenberg, 2009). Emotion-focused therapy helps people to become aware of feelings and needs and then to communicate these to others in ways that lead to personal support and growth. "Anxiety, anger, sorrows and regret are useful or they would not exist. Unpleasant feelings draw people's attention to matters important to their well-being. However when unpleasant emotions endure even when the circumstances that evoked them have changed, or are so intense that they overwhelm, or evoke past loss or trauma they can become dysfunctional. Healthy adaptation thus necessitates learning to be aware of, to tolerate, and to regulate negative emotionality" (Greenberg & Pascual-Leone, 2006) In this form of therapy, the therapist works as an "emotions coach" to help people be aware of their emotional responses, to accept these (when constructive), and then to make sense of these experiences.

Greenberg and his colleagues have provided evidence that suggests emotion-focused therapy may have relatively prolonged benefit in moderate depression when compared with short-term client centered therapy (Ellison, Greenberg, Goldman, & Angus, 2009). Emotion-based therapy contrasts with other brief dynamic approaches where the therapist takes an active role to direct sessions toward resolution of emotionally charged conflicts. In more traditional dynamic therapy, techniques of confrontation and interpretation of behaviors and events are frequently used. As with emotion-focused therapy, conflicts, their meanings, and individuals' choices are emphasized—though perhaps with less particular emphasis on explicitly emotional content. Unlike emotion-focused work, which more commonly involves either individuals or couples, brief dynamic therapy can be done in a group format.

Marital therapy attempts to resolve problems that occur within a marriage. Marital therapy is relevant to the treatment of depression because marital distress is common and often includes at least one depressed spouse. Studies suggest that relapses of depression are often preceded by marital discord. Behavioral marital therapy focuses on enhancing behaviors that are supportive of healthy marital relationships. Through therapy sessions, each partner comes to understand the feelings and experiences of the other. Building a stronger marital bond helps to ward off future depressive episodes. The therapist here takes an active role as well and uses techniques similar to those in brief dynamic therapy. A systematic review of a small number of studies of marital therapy suggests that this therapy is as effective as antidepressant medications, but no more effective than individual psychotherapy (Barbato & D'Avanzo, 2006). Emotion-focused therapy has been used with couples (Denton, Burleson, Clark, Rodriguez & Hobbs 2000), but its effectiveness has not been compared directly with marital therapy.

Cognitive therapy focuses on removing symptoms by identifying and correcting perceptual biases in clients' thinking and correcting unrecognized assumptions. The therapy concentrates on changing negative thoughts and behaviors into alternatives that do not sustain depression (Abraham, Neese, & Westerman, 1991). Cognitive behavioral therapy has been among the best-studied nonpharmacological treatments for depression and there is evidence for its effectiveness in depression overall, but not as clearly among the depressed elderly (Wilson, Mottram, & Vassilas, 2008). In recent years, researchers at Duke University have shown that "self-system therapy" (SST) is more effective than cognitive behavior therapy for the identifiable minority of persons with depression who have difficulty improving self-esteem and motivation despite successfully reducing negative symptoms through cognitive techniques (Strauman, Vieth, Merrill, Kolden, Woods, Klein, et al., 2006).

Most psychotherapists currently endorse brief treatment approaches. Significant improvement should be seen by 6 to 12 weeks. In contrast to long-term psychotherapy, which may extend over years, brief treatment does not generally exceed 40 sessions (see Chapter 28).

Effect of Psychotherapy

Studies of psychotherapy have shown fairly consistent benefit for depression. Brief dynamic psychotherapy has not been compared to placebo, but overall efficacy in six studies appeared to be about 35%. Marital therapy has been shown to effectively alleviate depressive symptoms especially and, not surprisingly, in clients who report marital discord. Cognitive therapy has been extensively studied and compared to both placebo and drug treatment. No studies show conclusively that cognitive therapy differs in effectiveness from any other psychotherapeutic technique *or* that medication treatment is more effective than cognitive therapy. In some studies, cognitive therapy seems to be more effective than medication, but a large study of chronically depressed individuals treated with either drugs or cognitive-behavioral therapy showed that a combination of the two was significantly more effective than either alone (Keller, McCullough, Klein, Arnow, Dunner, Gelenberg, et al., 2000), though these finding have not been confirmed in subsequent studies. Cognitive therapy may be effective in preventing relapse once remission has occurred (Lau, 2008). Several studies have now shown the effectiveness of computer-assisted cognitive therapy (Wagner, Knaevelsrud, & Maercker, 2007; Spek, Nyklicek, Smits, Cuijpers, Riper, Keyzer, et al., 2007). This may be an important advance since one of the strongest criticisms of psychotherapy is its cost in comparison to treatment with medications (Kaltenthaler, Shackley, Stevens, Beverley, Parry, & Chilcott, 2002).

Physical Therapies

Although many physical therapies have been in use for depressed clients, this discussion will be limited to three: electroconvulsive therapy, light therapy, and deep brain electrical stimulation.

Electroconvulsive Therapy

Electroconvulsive therapy (ECT) is a procedure in which clients are treated with pulses of electrical energy sufficient to cause a brief convulsion or seizure (Bolwig, 1993). Electroconvulsive therapy is carried out under anesthesia. Muscle-depolarizing agents are also given so that no actual convulsive movements occur; the primary effect of ECT is on the brain itself. Studies show that clients do not find the actual ECT treatment frightening, painful, or unpleasant. Although deaths have occurred from ECT, particularly in elderly clients or those with heart disease, the risk is quite low. Side effects depend on the specific technique used, but are mostly limited to memory deficits. These are typically mild, but may be permanent (see also Chapter 32).

Effect of ECT Electroconvulsive therapy is utilized in depression because multiple studies have shown it to be highly effective in helping severe depression resistant to all other treatments. Many studies on ECT and depression produce response rates as high as 90%. In comparison to medications (tricyclic antidepressants and monoamine oxidase [MAO] inhibitors), ECT has been clearly shown to be the superior treatment (Abraham et al., 1991). Studies using "sham ECT" have demonstrated that ECT effectiveness is not solely due to a placebo effect. A recent report indicates that ECT can improve the quality of life for adults with major depression and that this change can be maintained for at least six months (Rosenquist, Brenes, Arnold, Kimball,

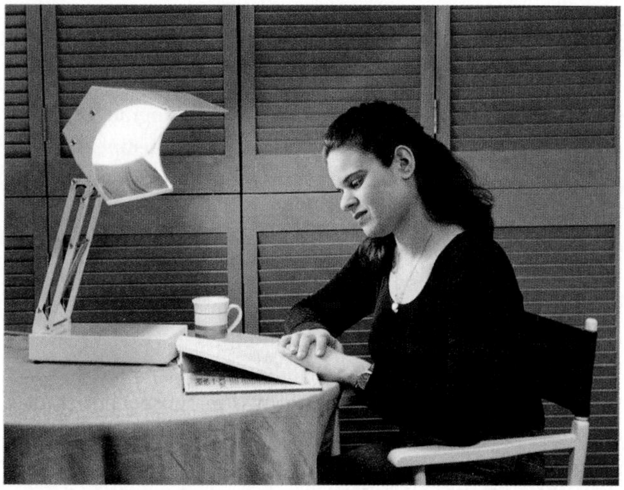

FIGURE 14-2 **Many clients with seasonal affective disorder will find their spirits lifted when using light therapy.** (COURTESY NORTHERN LIGHT, MONTREAL, CANADA.)

& McCall, 2006). Other data suggest that ECT is particularly effective for depression in the elderly (Tew, Mulsant, Haskett, Prudic, Tase, Crowe, et al., 1999).

Light Therapy

Light therapy is a form of treatment most commonly indicated for clients who have Seasonal Affective Disorder (SAD), a nonpsychotic depression that occurs repeatedly during the winter months and is usually seen in areas of high latitude where daylight time during the winter is limited (Birtwhistle & Martin, 1999). By exposing clients to bright lights for a period of time each day, light therapy simulates summer light conditions (Figure 14-2).

EFFECT OF LIGHT THERAPY When used for SAD, light therapy relieves symptoms in about 75% of persons. Response should occur within two weeks, and neither safety nor efficacy has been established for treatment lasting longer than this (see also Chapter 32). Other researchers evaluated the use of light therapy in a small population of women with nonseasonal depression and reported significant improvements, indicating that light therapy may have use in treating depression outside of SAD (McEnany & Lee, 2005).

BRAIN STIMULATION

Brain stimulation using powerful localized magnetic fields has recently become an area of intense research interest. Repetitive transcranial magnetic stimulation (rTMS) has had some effectiveness in a variety of neurological and psychiatric disorders (George, 2003), although its usefulness in depression has yet to be firmly established (Martin, Barbanoj, Schlaepfer, Thompson, Perez, & Kulisevshy, 2003). The technique involves placement of a small magnetic coil over specific areas of the brain. A powerful magnetic field is induced within the brain, and if treatments are repeated over time, improvement in mood may result, at least in some individuals. Whether such improvement is lasting, and whether it can be obtained less expensively with other psychiatric treatments, remains to be seen. In recent years neurosurgeons have developed techniques to implant stimulating electrodes in the brain. These electrodes are attached to a pacemaker-like device that provides ongoing stimulation (Howland, 2008). While evidence for effectiveness of deep brain stimulation in depression is still accumulating, preliminary studies suggest it may be effective for persons who have failed all other kinds of treatment (Larson, 2008).

MEDICATIONS

Four types of medications are commonly used to treat depression. Lithium and some anticonvulsants (especially valproate) are most commonly, but not exclusively, used for clients with bipolar disorder. They are discussed in Chapter 15. The other three categories are tricyclic and related antidepressants, selective serotonin reuptake inhibitors (SSRIs), and MAO inhibitors.

Drugs are chosen based on client characteristics, prior response to medications, family history of response to medication, concurrent illnesses and medications, and the provider's preferences. Since most medications take a month or more to be effective, dose increases or changes in medication should generally be made only after several weeks. Some clinicians begin tricyclic antidepressants at low doses and increase at one- to three-day intervals in an effort to accommodate clients to medication side effects.

Antidepressant medications are generally prescribed for four to nine months and may then be discontinued. Many clients, however, should remain on antidepressants indefinitely. Indications for continuing antidepressant treatment include three or more episodes of Major Depressive Disorder, history of recurrence within one year of discontinuing previous antidepressants, family history of recurrent depression or bipolar depression, onset of depression before age 20, and sudden onset of past depressions.

Psychotically depressed clients like Amalia are likely to receive antipsychotic medications such as phenothiazines or atypical neuroleptics. Since psychosis is such an important part of the psychiatric disorder schizophrenia, these medications are discussed at length in Chapters 13 and 27. When indicated by psychotic symptoms, they are used comparably in depressed and schizophrenic clients.

Because symptoms of anxiety are typically prominent in depressed clients seen in primary care, these clients are often wrongly treated with antianxiety medications, sometimes instead of effective antidepressant medications. The excerpt "The Crack-Up," presented earlier, offers a good example of depression in which anxiety is a major symptom—the very idea of "cracking" is an anxiety-related symptom. Although it may seem logical to use antianxiety medications when treating individuals such as the narrator in Fitzgerald's essay, experts strongly oppose such treatment except in highly unusual cases (Wells, Katon, Rogers, & Camp, 1994). Anxiolytics (antianxiety medications) should be avoided for at least four reasons: (1) symptoms of anxiety in depressed clients almost always respond to antidepressant medications; (2) controlled studies show no benefit from adding anxiolytics to antidepressants; (3) most anxiolytic medications have a strong tendency to produce dependency, and (4) studies show that antidepressant medications are among the most effective antianxiety agents.

The following is a discussion of the commonly used medications.

Tricyclic and Related Antidepressants

Tricyclics and related antidepressants were the first medications to prove effective in the management of depression. They are still the standard against which newer drugs are measured. Although called *antidepressants,* these medications do have other uses in client care. For example, they are used to treat enuresis (bed wetting in children), chronic pain, Panic Disorder, Obsessive-Compulsive Disorder, migraine headaches, and bulimia as well as depression. Table 14-1 lists tricyclic and related antidepressants, daily dosage ranges, and common side effects. Clients with sleep disturbances are often given a drug with high to moderate sedative effects. Anticholinergic effects (dry mouth, constipation, inability to pass urine) are often the side effects that clients find most unacceptable and lead to discontinuation of medication. Orthostatic effects result in dizziness or fainting on changing position and are especially troublesome for elderly clients and those with relatively low blood pressure. Moderate weight gain is another common side effect of many of these medications, and most can cause sexual dysfunction in both men and women. Many of the medications in Table 14-1 are very dangerous and often fatal if taken in overdose. For this reason, great caution is used in prescribing these medications to potentially suicidal clients. The medications in Tables 14-2 and 14-3 (SSRIs and others) may be much safer and rarely result in death, even if taken in large quantities.

Tricyclic antidepressants are usually given as a single dose at bedtime. Sleep may improve almost immediately (though some clients are troubled by vivid dreams), but any improvement in depressive symptoms takes at least two to three weeks. Full response typically requires four to six weeks. Blood testing to determine plasma levels of antidepressant drugs is often used for amitryptiline (Elavil), imipramine (Tofranil), desipramine (Norpramin), and nortriptyline (Pamelor). If medication is stopped, it should be tapered rather than withdrawn abruptly. Recent studies have suggested that lower dosages of tricyclics than those given in Table 14-1 may be equally effective with fewer side effects (Furukawa, McGuire, & Barbui, 2003).

NURSING ALERT 14-2

Bupropion and Maprotiline

Bupropion may cause seizures, especially in doses above 300 mg daily. Seizures are also seen with Marpotiline—even at usual therapeutic dosages.

NURSING ALERT 14-3

Antidepressant "Black Box" Warning

Antidepressants now carry an FDA "black box warning" about an increased risk of suicide in medication-treated depressed children and adolescents/young adults through the age of 24. There is no evidence of increased suicidal risk in older adults. For a useful review of the risks and benefits of antidepressants and this FDA decision, see Friedman and Leon's article on "Expanding the Black Box" (Friedman & Leon, 2007)

Selective Serotonin Reuptake Inhibitors

The SSRIs have become increasingly popular in recent years. They have not yet been clearly demonstrated to be as effective as tricyclic medication in treating severely depressed

TABLE 14-1 Tricyclic Antidepressants

GENERIC NAME	PROPRIETARY NAME	DOSE RANGE (mg)	SEDATION	ANTICHOLINERGIC EFFECTS	ORTHOSTATIC EFFECTS
Amitriptyline	Elavil	150–200	High	High	High
Amoxapine	Asendin	150–200	Low	Low	Moderate
Clomipramine	Anafranil	150–200	High	High	High
Desipramine	Norpramin	150–200	Low	Low	Moderate
Doxepin	Sinequan/Adapin	150–200	High	Moderate	Moderate
Imipramine	Tofranil	150–200	Moderate	Moderate	High
Maprotiline	Ludiomil	150–200	Moderate	Low	Moderate
Nortriptyline	Pamelor	75–100	Low	Low	Lowest
Protriptyline	Vivactil	30	Low	High	Low
Trimipramine	Surmontil	150–200	High	Moderate	Moderate

NURSING ALERT 14-4

Tricyclic Antidepressants

Tricyclic antidepressants are very dangerous in overdose; administration must be carefully monitored, especially in clients at risk for suicide.

individuals but are widely used among outpatients (Parker, 2002). The influential "STAR*D" trial found that 70% of clients treated with SSRIs did not achieve complete remission from depression (Sussman, 2007). There are currently five SSRIs available: fluoxetine (Prozac), sertraline (Zoloft), paroxetine (Paxil), citalopram (Celexa), and fluvoxamine (Luvox; Table 14-2). They differ in recommended dose, but otherwise seem to have relatively few differences between them (Kroenke, West, Swindle, Gilsenan, Eckert, Dolo, et al., 2001). Fluoxetine (Prozac) seems to have the highest incidence of interactions with other drugs, and paroxetine (Paxil) is excreted at high levels in breast milk, making it perhaps less desirable for treating women of reproductive age.

The SSRIs work by inhibiting the reuptake of serotonin at brain synapses and hence increasing the available serotonin at serotonin-sensitive receptors. Some newer SSRIs under development also stimulate the serotonin receptors. Like tricyclics, the SSRIs take several weeks to have an effect and may not achieve maximum effectiveness for four to six weeks.

These medications have achieved their current popularity not because they are more effective than tricyclic antidepressants, but, in large part, because their side effects are less troublesome. The SSRIs lack the anticholinergic and orthostatic side effects of tricyclic antidepressants. The SSRI side effects may include agitation, restlessness, insomnia, weight loss, headache, nausea, and diarrhea. Sexual dysfunction may also occur, especially in men. The SSRIs are generally safe if taken in overdose, a major advantage for treating potentially suicidal clients. Although SSRIs still cost a great deal more than generic tricyclic drugs, many clients prefer more expensive SSRI treatment because of fewer significant side effects. A generic form of fluoxetine has reduced treatment costs modestly.

Monoamine Oxidase Inhibitors

Monoamine oxidase (MAO) inhibitors increase the availability of brain neurotransmitters by interfering with their metabolism. These drugs act to increase the concentrations of serotonin, epinephrine, and norepinephrine in brain tissue. This metabolic effect seems to be responsible for their usefulness as antidepressants. The traditional MAO inhibitors (now referred to as MAO-A drugs) are not used frequently because they require clients to use great care in choosing foods and over-the-counter medications. Since these inhibitors act both on the brain and in the gut, they also prevent the gastrointestinal tract from breaking down ingested catecholamines, which are found in large quantities in some foods and medications. Clients taking MAO inhibitors who consume certain foods or drugs may experience a dangerous rise in blood pressure. This may result in stroke or other cardiovascular catastrophe. Among the substances and foods that should not be taken while consuming MAO-A inhibitors are fermented foods including some cheeses and alcoholic beverages, and a variety of drugs including many over-the-counter cold remedies, certain street substances, and a number of prescription drugs. The amino acid tryptophan, freely available in pharmacies and health food stores, may also cause significant reactions. Anyone taking MAO inhibitors should receive clear written instructions from his or her pharmacist and physician about what foods and drugs must be avoided. Box 14-1 lists many of these foods and drugs.

New MAO inhibitors with fewer interactions and/or effects that can be rapidly reversed have recently been marketed. These drugs may increase the safety and popularity of

TABLE 14-2 Selective Serotonin Reuptake Inhibitor (SSRI) Antidepressants

GENERIC NAME	PROPRIETARY NAME	DOSE RANGE (mg)	SEDATION	ANTICHOLINERGIC EFFECTS	ORTHOSTATIC EFFECTS
Citalopram	Celexa	20–40	Low	Very low	Very low
Escitalopram	Lexapro	10–20	Low	Very low	Very low
Fluoxetine*	Prozac (also generic)	20–80 (A once-weekly dosage form is also available.)	Very low	Very low	Very low
Fluvoxamine	Luvox	50–300 (divided dose if >100/day)	Moderate	Very low	Very low
Paroxetine	Paxil	20–50 (controlled release: 25–62.5)	Low-moderate	Very low	Very low
Sertraline	Zoloft	50–200	Low-moderate	Very low	Very low

*Available in a long-acting oral formulation—dosage may differ from short-acting form.

the MAO group of medications. Drugs that have no gut effects and are active only in the brain are also being developed and may prove less susceptible to drug and food interactions. Whether safer MAO inhibitors will have therapeutic advantages over SSRIs remains to be seen. Currently available MAO-A inhibitors include tranylcypromine (Parnate), phenelzine (Nardil), isocarboxazid (Marplan) and the reversible MAO-A inhibitor moclobemide which has a shorter half-life and "washout" time than other MAOs. Moclobemide is available in Canada as Manerix and Aurorix, but it is not FDA-approved for prescription in the United States At the time of this writing selegiline in a skin patch preparation is the only MAO-B drug available on the North American market (see also Chapter 27).

Miscellaneous Antidepressants

The agents in Table 14-3 are often regarded as new non-SSRI antidepressants. They have been effectively promoted to physicians by their manufacturers, and collectively they account for approximately one-fourth of antidepressant prescriptions given by primary care providers (Pirraglia, Stafford, & Singer, 2003). While each is effective for depression, these medications differ significantly in their side-effect profiles. Bupropion has effectiveness and side effects similar to the SSRIs, but it does not cause sexual dysfunction. Trazadone may be somewhat less effective than other antidepressants, and it is very sedating. For this reason, relatively low dosage nighttime trazadone is often given in combination with other antidepressants for use in clients who suffer from insomnia. Nefazadone is very similar to trazodone, but may be more effective with less sedation. Venlafaxine, an agent that has an effect on both serotonin and norepinephrine brain pathways, is similar in side effects to SSRIs, however it may elevate blood pressure in some persons. There is some evidence that venlafaxine (and the similar drug duloxetine) may be more effective than SSRIs in the management of depression—especially when associated with physical pain

BOX 14-1
FOOD AND MEDICATIONS THAT MUST BE AVOIDED BY CLIENTS TAKING MAO INHIBITORS

FOODS TO BE COMPLETELY AVOIDED

- Cheese: except for cottage and cream cheese
- Smoked, dried, pickled, cured, or preserved meats and fishes
- Caviar
- Fava beans
- Avocados (probably only if overripe)
- Yeast extracts
- Chianti wine
- Beer containing yeast

FOODS WITH SOME RISK UNLESS USED IN MODERATION

- Chocolate
- Coffee

MEDICATIONS TO BE AVOIDED

- Prescription medications: tricyclic antidepressants, Prozac, Demerol, amphetamines and amphetamine-like medications including all sympathomimetics
- Nonprescription medications: cold or allergy medications, nasal decongestants and inhalers, cough medications except for plain guaifenesin, stimulants and diet pills, pain medications except for aspirin, acetaminophen, and ibuprofen

TABLE 14-3 Miscellaneous Antidepressants (Some generic preparations have brand names that differ from those given here)

GENERIC NAME	PROPRIETARY NAME	DOSE RANGE (mg)	SEDATION	ANTICHOLINERGIC EFFECTS	ORTHOSTATIC EFFECTS
Bupropion*	Wellbutrin	300	Low	Very Low	Very low
Trazodone	Desyrel	150–400	High	Very low	High
Nefazadone	Serazone	300–600	Low	Very low	Moderate
Mirtazapine	Remeron	15–45	Low-Moderate	Very low	Low
Maprotiline	Ludiomil	100–225	Low-Moderate	Moderate	Moderate
Venlafaxine*	Effexor	75–375	Low	Low	Low
Duloxetine	Cymbalta	20–60	Low-Moderate	Moderate	Low

Note: Bupropion and trazodone are pharmacologically not tricyclic antidepressants. Bupropion and maprotiline may cause seizures, especially in doses of bupropion above 300 mg daily. Venlafaxine and Duloxetine are selective serotonin-norepinphrine reuptake inhibitors (SNRIs).

*Available in a long-acting oral formulation—dosage may differ from short-acting form.

(Sussman, 2003). Mertazapine does not interfere with sexual functioning, but it may cause weight gain and it is sedating.

Effect of Medications

Multiple studies have shown that antidepressant medications are more effective than placebo in resolving symptoms of depression. Few studies suggest any major difference in effectiveness among any of the available drugs. In general, if clients can tolerate medication side effects, a response occurs in 60% to 70% of both inpatients and outpatients. Most studies show a placebo improvement in depression of about 18% to 30%. While many other studies used symptom improvement as their therapeutic endpoint, the STAR*D study was designed on the premise that complete resolution of depressive symptoms was the desired outcome for treatment. Using this criterion, only 30% of enrolled patients achieved remission in the study's "Level 1" in which citralopram was utilized. In this study, clients not responding at Level 1 were enrolled in Level 2, where they were given the choice of several treatment options: medication change to bupropion sustained release, sertraline, or venlafaxine extended release, or addition of a second medication (bupripion SR or buspirone) to the citralopram, or to add (or switch to) cognitive behavioral therapy. About 20% of the "switch group" had resolution of their depression, whereas this outcome occurred in 30% of those who received addition of a second medication. Results from the cognitive behavioral part of the study, in which the fewest clients chose to enroll, showed benefits comparable to adding additional antidepressants but with more delayed effectiveness (Thase, Friedman, Biggs, Wisniewski, Trivedi, Luther, et al., 2007). STAR*D reached the following five conclusions that many experts feel are important:

1. Response in depression treatment should be carefully monitored and based on the assumption that normal mental functioning is the appropriate endpoint.
2. Treatment responses may take up to six weeks so that changes in therapy, once appropriate dosage levels have been achieved, should be delayed until sufficient time has lapsed to assure an effect.
3. Either drug substitution or augmentation with addition of a second drug is likely to enhance response if there is treatment failure to an initial SSRI given in adequate dose for an adequate time.
4. For those who do not respond to substitution or addition (Level 2), two additional levels were defined, but neither produced a large treatment effect.
5. Primary care doctors were able to achieve desired treatment responses as often as were psychiatric specialists (Gaynes, Rush, Trivedi, Wisniewski, Balasubramani, McGrath, et al., 2008).

STAR*D is not the "final word" in depression treatment, but it has taught us that the effectiveness of SSRIs is quite limited. This message was emphasized in a British meta-analysis that suggested that antidepressants may only have proven efficacy among the most seriously depressed clients (Kirsch, Deacon, Huedo-Medina, Scoboria, Moore, & Johnson, 2008). This study was widely publicized, and has led to the recognition (already implicit in the STAR*D study) that much remains to be learned about the best clinical approach to this common and often debilitating condition (Turner and Rosenthal, 2008).

One of the important recognitions in recent years has been that depression is not just a disorder of "feelings." The symptoms of depression produce as much disability and interference with daily functioning as do more "physical" disorders such as rheumatoid arthritis or multiple sclerosis. Workers with depression lose an average of 5.6 hours of work weekly because of their disorder, a loss that accounts for much of the estimated $44 billion cost of this disorder just in lost productivity (Stewart, Ricci, Chee, Hahn, & Morganstein, 2003). Perhaps more striking, depression has been shown to be a significant risk factor for myocardial infarction. It remains unclear exactly how depression influences the heart, and—perhaps more important—we are still unsure whether treatment for depression reduces the risk of heart attacks (Frasure-Smith & Lesperance, 2003). Nursing research suggests that women who suffered a heart attack report that in the weeks before their attack they had felt unusually fatigued, anxious, and had difficulty sleeping (McSweeney, Cody, & Crane, 2001). Whether these depressive-like symptoms were the cause of their heart attacks or came about as a result of some metabolic or inflammatory process that itself led to the heart attack will require further study. In older individuals, depression is also linked to the development of stroke, diabetes, and

NURSING TIP 14-2

What You Need to Know about St. John's Wort (*Hypericum*)

There is much popular interest in the use of St. John's Wort as a treatment for depression. What do nurses need to know?

What It Is

A biological extract from a plant.

Advantages

- Available without prescription.
- More acceptable to some patients than standard antidepressants.
- Evidence for effectiveness in mild to moderate depression.

Disadvantages

- Preparations are nonstandard; amount of *hypericum* may vary in lots and among manufacturers.
- May be less effective than drug or cognitive therapy.
- Drug interactions occur and may be significant (Hammerness, Basch, Ulbricht, Barrette, Foppa, Basch, et al., 2003)
- May cause "switch" to mania in patients with unrecognized Manic-Depressive Disease.

From "St. John's Wort for Depression: A Systemic Review" by B. Gaster and J. Holroyd, 2000, *Archives of Internal Medicine*, *160*(2), 153–156.

osteoporosis (Krishnan, Delong, Kraemer, Carney, Spiegel, & Gordon, 2002). The relationship between depression and overall health will remain a fertile area for nursing and medical scholarship in the years to come.

NURSING CARE

Nursing theories assist nurses in planning care for a client who is depressed, but the particular theory a nurse selects will depend on many factors. Although the authors believe that caring theories and self-care deficit theory are especially helpful in approaching and planning nursing care for depressed clients, other practitioners may choose different theories with equally good results. The principles of theory application highlighted in the following discussion should be applicable to many alternative theoretical frameworks.

Caring Theories

Isolation and loneliness are among the most prominent personal characteristics of persons who are depressed. For example, earlier in this chapter, Tolstoy describes his depression as a *force* drawing him away from life, work, and family. Comparable feelings of detachment are expressed in many of the other excerpts quoted and by almost all depressed persons. In some cases social isolation is a major *cause* of an individual's depression—a person who has no important others in his life may become depressed as a consequence of isolation. This is often the case for the elderly. In contrast, other depressed people have opportunities for social interaction that they actively reject—their depression results in social isolation. For example, Tolstoy was a father, a world-famous author, and a large landowner at the time of his depression. He had friends, family, colleagues, and numerous admirers; for him, social isolation was entirely self-imposed. Whether the client chooses isolation or has it thrust on him by depression, an interpersonal, caring approach will provide the basis for a helping relationship. Although Wiedenbach (1964) and Leininger (1978) have also developed important theories based on caring, this discussion will focus on Watson's (2008) theory of caring science.

Watson's theory calls for each individual to be valued, cared about, and cared for. For a depressed person, the theory dictates that the nurse would value the individual, seek to understand him, and provide respect, nurturing, and support. The nurse will initiate a nurse-client relationship that is based on mutuality and affirmation. The nurse should approach the depressed client with an attitude of sincere caring and strive to build a relationship with the client that demonstrates the nurse's respect for the person.

Watson (2008) believes that nursing is a transpersonal value. She suggests that the process of nursing requires engagement such that two persons (nurse and client) connect in meaningful ways that are transpersonal and unpredictable. The human caring process may create a bridge for the depressed person to reach out, to feel and experience human interaction once again (Kelley & Johnson, 2002).

A caring approach could serve to provide the client with a sense of belonging as well as a sense that he is "likeable." The nurse would strive to understand the world from the client's perspective and be willing to listen to the client's subjective experiences. Through a positive nurse-client relationship, the nurse could aid the client in experiencing a positive view of self and a positive sense of future hope.

It is important to recognize that Watson's theory requires mutuality, that is, that the client respond with some kind of involvement in the therapeutic relationship. The withdrawn, angry, suspicious, and depressed person may be very slow to enter into this kind of mutuality. Despite the strong therapeutic potential of nursing intervention based on caring, some depressed individuals may respond slowly or not at all. The nurse faced with such a client must be willing to persevere, to consult with colleagues and mentors who have extensive experience in reaching the depressed, to carefully examine her own feelings and responses, and perhaps at some point to consider a switch in theory and approach.

Self-Care Deficit Theory

Although diagnosis often focuses on how a depressed person feels, for many depressed individuals the biggest problems are not those of affect (feeling) but of self-care. For example, weight loss is a cardinal symptom of depression, and it frequently results from failure to eat. The depressed may lose interest in their appearance, in hygiene, and in their surroundings. In the excerpt from Italo Svevo's writing quoted earlier, both Amalia's personal appearance (especially her weight loss) and the dishevelment of her dressing and room emphasize her profound self-care deficit.

Orem's (2001) self-care deficit theory views nurses' work to be doing for the client that which he cannot do for himself. In this theory, the concept of **nurse agency** refers to nursing activities required to compensate for the client's inability to meet his own self-care needs. Since a depressed client is often neglectful of basic health and personal requirements, the nurse should direct the client's activities toward correcting any apparent care deficit. The nurse may do this both by directly assisting the client to meet health needs and by demonstrating to the client that the nurse believes he is sufficiently important and worthy of his needs being met.

In using this approach with a depressed client, the nurse must take care not to do for the client anything he is truly capable of doing for himself. In Orem's theory, the concept of **self-care agency** refers to the client's ability to provide for his own needs. Whenever possible, the nurse should encourage the client to meet his own health requirements, thus increasing self-care agency. The nurse will approach the client with an attitude of kindness and understanding and demonstrate via behaviors that the client is valued as a person. When the client begins to be able to care for his basic physical and personal needs, the nurse will move to a **supportive-educative role**, which focuses on enhancing the client's ability both to carry on effectively without nursing support and to rise above the feelings of depression that brought on the initial deficit in self-care.

Theory of Transitions

A "theory of transitions" was proposed by Meleis et al. (Meleis, Sawyer, Im, Hilfinger Messias, & Schumacher 2000) as a middle range theory that examined the change individuals experience when confronted with life's transitional events. Meleis noted that changes in health status can provide opportunities for enhanced well-being. Among other factors, successful resolution of transitions requires awareness, engagement, and change. A research group in Sweden reported use of this theory in a population of adults with major depression (Skärsäter & Willman, 2006). The concept of transitions (moving through, moving on) was used as a framework to understand client's recognition of depression in self and to describe the recovery process. The researchers report that the experience of major depression served as a "trigger" for life changes. They proposed a set of nursing interventions to assist the client through recovery based on the transition process that includes: awareness of the condition, engagement with others, change in one's life, taking time needed for resolution, and management of critical events. Nursing interventions supportive of these processes follow under discussion of nursing interventions.

APPLICATION OF THE NURSING PROCESS 14-1

ASSESSMENT

The majority of depressed persons are seen in general medical settings, not in psychiatric clinics and wards. The nurse will come in contact with depressed persons in all areas of practice and on virtually every working day. Thus, all nurses should have basic skills in the assessment and management of depression. While for many nurses that management may be referral to a mental health professional, initial assessment is a fundamental nursing skill. The recognition of depression is an important collaborative issue as well—the Medical Outcomes Study clearly showed that primary care practitioners do not do a good job of recognizing or treating depression (Wells, Stewart, Hays, Burnam, Rogers, Daniels, et al., 1989). This failure is important because depression itself, far from being a minor problem, causes more functional impairment than do many chronic medical disorders, such as diabetes. Recognizing and treating depression are not only of critical importance in primary care, but also equally necessary for hospitalized medical clients, the elderly, new mothers, children, and adolescents.

How, then, does one know that an individual is depressed? The answer is simple: by observing and talking to him. However, even if the answer is simple, the process of discovering depression is often far from easy. Relatively few individuals present to the nurse with a ready-made diagnosis of depression, and even fewer seek care complaining primarily of depression. From past experience, persons may feel that doctors and nurses want to hear only about physical symptoms; so depressed persons are far more likely to volunteer information about their physical symptoms than about their feelings. In addition, many people just do not talk well about feelings, or they may come from a culture in which admitting depression results in loss of face or status. Even a person who knows his symptoms are due to depression is likely to share information about his feelings only with an interviewer he feels to be sympathetic and unhurried. Open-ended questions are best for eliciting feelings, questions such as "So how would you say your life has been going?" or "How does this illness make you feel?" More direct questioning may also be helpful and sometimes necessary: "Do you ever feel down-in-the-dumps or sad?"

The nurse should ask most, if not all, clients about their feelings. However, certain individuals should be interviewed more intensively. These include persons with prior episodes of depression or suicide

(Continues)

NURSINGTIP 14-3

Recognizing Depression

Persons who are depressed often have the following characteristics:

- Find that previously enjoyable activities no longer produce joy
- Loss of interest in friends; isolation from others
- Difficulty concentrating
- A history of significant loss or trauma
- A sense of powerlessness and hopelessness
- Loss of appetite and weight
- Sleep disturbances, particularly early morning awakening with inability to fall back asleep
- Make few demands on nursing staff

APPLICATION OF THE NURSING PROCESS 14-1 (Continued)

attempts, persons under age 40 or over 70, postpartum mothers, persons with significant medical illness, persons who have limited social support or stressful life circumstances, and persons who abuse alcohol or other substances. Each of these groups is at higher-than-average risk for significant depression (Depression Guideline Panel, 1993). Women seem to suffer more commonly from depression than do men, so some experts recommend that women be interviewed about depressive symptoms somewhat more intensively than men. A family history of depression should probably also prompt more detailed questioning, although unipolar Major Depressive Disorder only sometimes runs in families. People who present with or admit to problems with sleep, appetite, sexual functioning, chronic pain, or weight change may have depression even if they deny depressed mood. They may instead have fatigue, trouble concentrating, anxiety, or guilt as important alternate symptoms of depression (Depression Guideline Panel, 1993).

The effectiveness of a nurse's interview can be enhanced by questionnaires designed to assist in the detection of depression. These are of two general types: those intended to be completed by the client (self-rating scales) and those intended to be completed by the nurse during an interview. Common depression scales are the Beck Depression Inventory, Zung Self-Rating Depression Scale, and the Edinburgh Postnatal Depression Scale (EPDS). These scales are valuable instruments for nursing practice because they rarely miss persons who are significantly depressed. While these scales do not diagnose depression, they do indicate when further assessment is needed. A recent report of the use of the EPDS with prenatal (rather than postpartum) women indicated that use of this scale resulted in referrals to liaison psychiatry where nearly a third (31%) of the women had diagnosable depression, another third had significant adjustment disorders, and a remaining 4% had other diagnosable conditions (such as PTSD and Borderline Personality Disorder; Harvey & Pun, 2007). A skilled interviewer familiar with DSM-IV-TR should evaluate any client who has an abnormal result on any of the depression questionnaires; although only 60% to 75% of these people will have a final diagnosis of depression, many of the remainder who score "falsely positive" for depression can benefit from supportive nursing interventions.

The nurse should also remember that intuition can be one of the most powerful tools for detecting depression. The appearance of a depressed person can often be a strong clue to feelings and diagnosis. In

(Continues)

BOX 14-3
CULTURAL ASPECTS OF DEPRESSION: REPORT OF A KOREAN IMMIGRANT POPULATION LIVING IN THE UNITED STATES

In reviewing available literature on the topic, the authors remind the reader that for much of the world's population, psychobiological affect is presented through physical complaints. In Asian traditions, there is emphasis on inhibiting emotions. Emotions are understood as pathogenic factors that can cause bodily disturbances. Therefore, emotions will frequently be expressed through somatic metaphors.

Investigators studied a Korean immigrant population in the United States and have documented that these individuals will present with somatic complaints, intermixed with affective complaints. Common presentations of depression will be insomnia, indigestion, palpitations, along with general aches and pains. The Korean culture leads individuals to view health in general and mental health as a balance between mind, body, and nature. Illness then, is an imbalance of the body's natural components. Mental illness holds stigma within this culture, thus the presentation and the description of the condition is often in terms of being "out-of-balance." Korean Americans tend to be reluctant to seek out mental health services and when they do accept treatment, they are likely to prefer structured, problem-solving techniques to relieve specific symptoms. Nurses must seek to interpret symptoms and behaviors from within their client's worldview and to understand the client's presenting complaints as reflective of specific cultural ideals and adaptations.

Nurses are cautioned that depression in any client cannot be fully understood without entering into the client's culture. These issues are thoroughly discussed in Chapter 7.

From: Park, S.Y., & Bernstein, K.S., 2008. Depression and Korean American Immigrants. *Archives of Psychiatric Nursing*, *22*(1), 12–19.

APPLICATION OF THE NURSING PROCESS 14-1 (Continued)

REFLECTIVE THINKING 14-1

How Do You Feel When Interviewing a Depressed Client?

Think about a depressed individual you have worked with and reflect on the following:

- Do depressed clients raise feelings of depression or grief in you? If yes, how do you know this has happened?
- Do you believe that depression is justified in some persons and situations and not in others? If yes, what is the difference?
- Is it hard to empathize with one who is depressed, particularly if you do not believe he has the "right" to feel so down?
- Do some clients leave you feeling drained and fatigued? Which ones? In what settings?
- Do some clients leave you feeling angry? Which ones? In what settings?

general, a depressed person presents with little affect or (even if they deny feeling sad) with visible sadness. The individual may look tired, appear withdrawn, and have less facial and bodily expression than is normal. Of course, many medical conditions (hypothyroidism is an excellent example) can produce such an appearance, but the person's appearance is often an important clue for recognition of depression. Another very important diagnostic clue is much harder to describe and learn: Many skilled nurses report that depressed people make them (the nurses) feel a certain way. After talking for a few minutes to a depressed client, many sensitive persons find themselves fatigued and a little depressed. By listening to her own feelings, the nurse can greatly enhance her ability to recognize depression and so provide caring help to clients in need. Many nurses are attracted to psychiatric care precisely because it gives them an opportunity to develop and use their highest intuitive skills.

NURSING DIAGNOSIS

By listening and hearing the experience of a depressed person, the nurse will be able to assess that individual's response to the emotion. Some persons will feel lonely, and others guilty. Some will describe not having feelings. Some will lose all connection to others and to a meaning and purpose in their lives. Some, as in F. Scott Fitzgerald's writing, will be personally and spiritually bankrupt. The following is a list of nursing diagnoses (Herdman, 2009) that are common in depressed persons:

- *Hopelessness,* related to long-term stress; abandonment; lost belief in transcendent values
- *Powerlessness*, related to lack of ability to exert control
- *Spiritual distress*, related to challenged belief and value system
- *Low self-esteem (may be situational or chronic)*, related to lack of positive reinforcement of one's value and worth
- *Social isolation*, related to inability to engage in satisfying personal relationships
- *Self-care deficit (may be in several areas)*, related to lack of concern or regard toward self
- *Insomnia*, related to internal stress

The first five of these diagnoses can be made only when the nurse has sufficient interactions with the client to be able to validate that the defining characteristics of the diagnosis are present. The definition of the diagnosis of hopelessness states that it is a "subjective state," and the major defining characteristics include both physical observations and verbal cues (Herdman, 2009). A nurse must validate that the client's subjective feelings are those of seeing limited or no alternatives or choice, and having no energy to mobilize resources, in order to make the diagnosis of *hopelessness*. *Powerlessness* is diagnosed when an individual feels that his own action cannot affect an outcome; the person has a perceived lack of control over his current situation. *Spiritual distress* is used as a nursing diagnosis when there is a disruption in a person's life principles such that he questions the meaning of life and of his own existence and lacks a sense of future and of belonging. *Low self-esteem* refers to negative evaluations of self or of self-capabilities. *Social isolation* is diagnosed when a client expresses the desire to be more involved with others than he is currently able to be. Clearly, formulating and validating these diagnoses require considerable nursing skill and effort toward establishing therapeutic communication and rapport with the client.

(Continues)

APPLICATION OF THE NURSING PROCESS 14-1 (Continued)

The diagnoses of *self-care deficit* and *insomnia* can be made through objective observation and the client's subjective feelings. *Self-care deficit* is diagnosed when the client is unable to perform basic activities of daily living and hygiene. *Insomnia* can be used as a diagnosis when the client's sleep cycle causes discomfort. For many depressed individuals, early morning awakening with inability to fall back asleep and feelings of never being rested would lead to this diagnosis. Accuracy in diagnoses is important in guiding nursing staff to individualize care. In each case, nursing staff will address the client's human response to the depression.

OUTCOME IDENTIFICATION

Expected outcomes of nursing care will be as varied as the individual clients and the circumstances surrounding their needs for care. For a client hospitalized with psychotic depression, the nurse may focus on risk for injury related to loss of touch with reality. A reasonable expected outcome would be that the client remain free of injury during the hospitalization. When the focus of care is self-care deficit, an expected outcome could be that within one week the client will initiate activities of grooming and daily living. In contrast, when the client is being followed as an outpatient and the depression is of long-term duration, the expected

BOX 14-4
NURSING LITERATURE ON DEPRESSION: FINDINGS AND REPORTS

- Researchers examined the impact of insurance coverage and co-payment costs for antidepressant medications for older adults. A population of elders was studied throughout a western Canadian province tracking the impact of policies that provided full coverage, co-payments of $10–$25, and income-based deductibles. The researchers reported that the co-pay policy was associated with a significant drop in frequency of antidepressant initiation. Alternate forms of medication cost sharing may have important influences on treatment and health of elders. Clinical consequences of payment policies need to be addressed (Wang, Patrick, Dormuth, Avorn, Maclure, Canning, & Schneeweiss, 2008).
- There is a considerable number of women who develop depressive symptoms during their childbearing years. A study of pregnant women documented that over 10% had some risk factors for depression and screening scores indicating possible depression. These women also identified that several barriers existed that could inhibit them from receiving treatment. These barriers were: cost, lack of insurance, lack of transportation, long waits for treatment, previous bad experience with mental health care, and not knowing where to receive treatment. Such financial and logistical barriers need to be addressed (Kopelman, Moel, Mertens, Stuart, Arndt, & O'Hara, 2008).
- Using a qualitative research approach, researchers interviewed 30 elderly women about their experiences and views of depression. The women considered depression to be severe and indicated that medication was their preferred treatment. Causes of depression included loss of health, family, and roles. The informants in this study emphasized fatigue and weakness as the major components of depression, in contrast to DSM-IV, which emphasizes feelings of guilt, worthlessness, weight loss, and suicidal ideation (Ugarriza, 2002).
- The psychological effects of exercise training have been thought to reduce depressive symptoms. To study the effects of an aerobic exercise training program on the feelings of depression in an HIV-positive population, researchers used a randomized controlled trial of a supervised, 12-week aerobic training program. At the end of the 12-week exercise intervention, the experimental group showed reductions in depressive symptoms (Neidig, Smith, & Brashers, 2003).
- Researchers found that adults who were diagnosed for the first time with major depression had a lowered sense of coherence and low perception of social supports. During recovery, their sense of coherence improved as did their perception of social supports. Researchers concluded that these clients have a need for interventions involving social and family supports (Huggstrom & Denkar, 2005).
- Researchers that set up a home care, community-based service for depressed adults reported that homecare supports decreased length of hospital stay and provided cost-effective care (Blacock, 2006).

(Continues)

APPLICATION OF THE NURSING PROCESS 14-1 (Continued)

outcomes of care will take longer to achieve. For example, for a client experiencing social isolation and feelings of loneliness, the expected outcome of therapy combined with a socialization group could be that within one month the client will initiate a social contact with one person. The three care plans presented at this chapter's end illustrate differing care situations and a range of expected outcomes of care.

PLANNING/INTERVENTIONS

There are several interventions for the depressed client. These include: (1) independent nursing actions based on nursing diagnoses, and (2) collaborative interventions associated with treatment plans made by a multidisciplinary psychiatric team. Major approaches are discussed in the following section.

The nurse would identify the priority diagnoses for each client and establish a plan of care directed toward the circumstances that contributed to the condition. A depressed person will not take initiative to solve problems and find solutions to uncomfortable conditions. A nurse must take care to use a nursing perspective/theory to build a relationship with the client and suggest options for care that serve to keep the client in control of his own treatment and that move the client and nurse to mutually agreed-on interventions.

Nursing interventions include establishing a one-on-one relationship to provide human contact and relief from the loneliness often described by clients who are depressed; providing positive regard and unconditional acceptance to enhance client self-esteem and feelings of worthiness; engaging the client in activities, often beginning with activities of daily living and moving to social activities, to provide a pattern of functional living and recreation; listening to the client, providing time to understand the client's subjective experience of depression and pain; educating the client (and client's family/significant others) about the prevalence of depression and the use of antidepressive medications; assisting the client to establish a true sense of his own strengths and weaknesses; and addressing the feelings of hopelessness and lack of future by permitting the client to talk through his feelings. Box 14-5 discusses other techniques found useful, including group therapy (see Chapter 30), movement therapy, and exercise (see Chapter 32; Figure 14-3). In addition, Box 14-6 presents nursing interventions for depression derived from Skarsater and Willman's research documenting the recovery process based on Meleis' theory of transitions.

BOX 14-5
NURSING INTERVENTIONS AND THERAPIES FROM THE NIC USEFUL TO CONSIDER WHEN WORKING WITH DEPRESSED CLIENTS

Interventions	Therapies
Active listening	Animal Assisted Therapy
Assertiveness training	Art Therapy
Body image enhancement	Group Therapy
Cognitive restructuring	Guided Imagery
Coping enhancement	Recreation Therapy
Counseling	Relaxation Therapy
Emotional support	
Mood management	
Presence	
Self-esteem enhancement	
Sleep enhancement	
Socialization enhancement	
Support group	
Teaching: Disease process and prescribed medications	

From *Nursing Interventions Classification* (5th Ed.) by G. Bulechek, H. Butcher, and J. Dochterman 2008, St. Louis: Mosby.

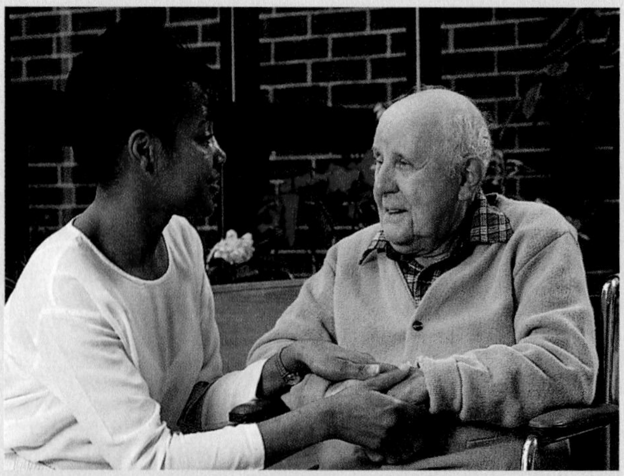

FIGURE 14-3 Supportive nursing care for depressed clients can include one-to-one interactions, caring touch, listening with empathy, and helping the client to identify personal strengths. (DELMAR/CENGAGE LEARNING.)

(Continues)

APPLICATION OF THE NURSING PROCESS 14-1 (Continued)

BOX 14-6
NURSING INTERVENTIONS THAT SUPPORT PROPERTIES OF THE TRANSITION PROCESS FOR PERSONS RECOVERING FROM MAJOR DEPRESSION

AWARENESS

- Meet and understand the individual as a whole person within the framework of family and work, needs and wishes.
- Illuminate the individual situation; carefully explore resources and plan together for individualized care during the acute phase.

ENGAGEMENT

- Provide information on where to contact former patients, or support groups, who can share experiences, in order to provide informational and appraisal support.
- Develop and use information methods that strengthen the individuals to participate in and make appropriate decisions.
- The encounter should make the individual feel welcome to participate in a caring relationship.

CHANGE AND DIFFERENCE

- Encourage the person to set boundaries and prepare them, especially female patients, for the possibility that they may not obtain the support they need as such changes can be inconvenient for other persons.
- Discuss with parents how they talk to their children about the changed family situation, and carefully explore the needs of all family members.
- Discuss the meaning of the changed internal values/mode of life and how comfortable the individual is about this change.

TIME SPAN

- Support the individual to establish structure in terms of time and care.

CRITICAL POINTS AND EVENTS

- Support individuals to take charge of their life and initiate necessary changes.
- Recommend women to take sick leave for as long as necessary, in order to fulfill their own needs and make use of their own space.
- Support males to return to work, or similar, on a part-time basis.

From Skärsäter, I., & Willman, A., 2006, The Recovery Process in Major Depression, *Advances in Nursing Science*, *29*(3), p. 250 used with permission.

EVALUATION

When evaluating a client's progress in managing depression, the nurse should first ask the client's view of changes that have occurred since therapy began. Specific indicators such as stronger sleep patterns, return of appetite, renewed or increasing sense of control and self-worth, and renewed interest in previous or new activities are all good signs of progress. Depressed individuals may experience progress in some areas (return to normal weight) but not in others (continued lack of ability to concentrate). The nurse needs to keep in mind and to remind the client that managing depression often requires significant energy and a conscious effort on the client's part to balance emotions and maintain perspective. It is also important to remember that depression resulting from a significant loss, such as loss of a loved one, may take many weeks or months to overcome and that the client will need sensitive nursing care to adapt to the new situations and roles that accompany such a loss.

CARE PLANNING GUIDE 14-1 Client with Depression (Major Depression Episode)

CLINICAL PICTURE

The clinical picture of a client with depression includes:

- Depressed mood
- Anhedonia
- Fatigue
- Weight loss or gain
- Feelings of worthlessness or guilt
- Poor concentration

COMMON NURSING DIAGNOSES

Nursing diagnoses most commonly employed include:

1. *Low self-esteem* (may be situational or chronic)
2. *Hopelessness*

(See also the care planning guide in Chapter 16 for the client who is suicidal.)

NURSING DIAGNOSIS 1: *CHRONIC LOW SELF-ESTEEM*

OUTCOMES

1. Decrease the number of self-negating comments.
2. Verbalize own area(s) of strengths/abilities.
3. Verbalize a positive view of self.

NOC: *SELF-ESTEEM*

INTERVENTIONS (NIC: *SELF-ESTEEM ENHANCEMENT; TEACHING: DISEASE PROCESS*)	RATIONALE
• Monitor negative thought patterns for logic, validity, and frequency; reality test with the client.	• Allows for early identification of changes associated with rumination on negative thoughts of self that are out of proportion to one's own weaknesses.
• Assist to set realistic self-expectations.	• Setting realistic self-expectations provides a goal for treatment.
• Encourage to attend activities as a break in the pattern of self-criticism.	• Attention directed outside of self assists in breaking the pattern of self-criticism and provides activities to balance the sense of fatigue.
• Teach that negative ruminations about self are part of depression and can be treated with therapy and medications.	• Education can provide a sense of relief that treatment is available and helpful.

NURSING DIAGNOSIS 2: *HOPELESSNESS*

OUTCOMES

1. The client will verbalize at least one positive expectation for the future.

NOC: *HOPE*

(*Continues*)

CARE PLANNING GUIDE 14-1 Continued

INTERVENTIONS (NIC: *HOPE INSPIRATION*)	RATIONALE
• Monitor for level of hope and plans for the future.	• Allows for early identification of changes in level of hope and presence of future plans and contributes to individualized care.
• Assist in identification of areas of hope in life	• Provides a basis for understanding and mutual goal setting.
• Recognize the client's intrinsic worth, viewing illness as only one facet of the individual.	• Attention to one's self-worth from external sources demonstrates hope for the individual's future.
• Provide an open, trusting therapeutic relationship.	• The client needs to begin to trust another and enter into a therapeutic relationship that encourages discussion of feelings.
• Encourage participation in activities.	• Activities provide stimulation and opportunities for expressing feelings.
• Encourage visits/support from family/significant others.	• Others who are important in the client's life break the self-imposed isolation and validate the client's worth.

LONG-TERM CONSIDERATIONS FOR CLIENTS WITH MAJOR DEPRESSION

1. Treatment, including therapy and medication, makes a real difference in individuals' recovery, but takes time.
2. Group or family therapy may provide ongoing support.
3. There is always a need to assess for potential of suicide.

Note: The care planning guides have been adapted from *Plans of Care for Speciality Practice: Psychiatric Mental Health Nursing* by M. Coler and K. G. Vincent, 1995, Clifton Park, NY: Thomson Delmar Learning.

NURSING CARE PLAN: NURSING PROCESS FORMAT 14-1

The description of Amalia is presented in the introductory section of this chapter.

Amalia is experiencing a major depressive disorder. She has lost touch with reality; she does not respond to her brother as he enters her room and calls to her; she is uttering words that are unintelligible; she responds to unknown images as she talks about horrible creatures; she cries; and she is in obvious distress and fatigue. While her brother refers to her condition as *delirium*, it is really *psychosis*, the difference being that a person in a psychotic state can be brought back to reality and can acknowledge others in the real world, whereas the person in a delirious state cannot recognize reality. Amalia can recognize and interact with her brother, and she does so when he puts his hand on her shoulder and speaks to her firmly; thus she is psychotic. Imagine that nurses are giving care to Amalia. A fictionalized nursing care plan follows.

ASSESSMENT

Amalia's psychotic depression has incapacitated her. She is nonverbal, minimally responsive, fearful of unknown images, and unable to meet the most basic of needs. She is admitted to an inpatient unit by her brother, who is absolutely shocked by what he has seen.

(*Continues*)

NURSING CARE PLAN: NURSING PROCESS FORMAT 14-1 (Continued)

NURSING DIAGNOSIS 1 *Risk for injury,* related to loss of touch with reality

OUTCOMES	NIC	NURSING ACTIONS	EVALUATION
• Amalia will remain free of injury during the inpatient period	• Surveillance: Safety	• Monitor Amalia's condition and location frequently to ensure her safety. • Assign a one-to-one nurse-client ratio. • Provide the least restrictive environment that allows for the level of observation, a private room, and remove any object that could potentially be used for self-harm.	Amalia was admitted without any sense of reality. She was tormented by creatures and was extremely fearful. She was put into a protected environment with frequent monitoring. She remained free of injury during the inpatient period.

NURSING DIAGNOSIS 2 *Disturbed thought processes,* related to loss of touch with reality and lack of sleep, as evidenced by inaccurate interpretation of environment and distractibility

OUTCOMES	NIC	NURSING ACTIONS	EVALUATION
• Amalia will experience fewer psychotic symptoms within 48 hours and remain oriented to person, time, and place.	• Reality orientation	• Engage Amalia in brief conversations using simple sentences. • Reorient Amalia as necessary. • Provide for adequate rest and sleep. • Monitor sleep, food consumption, and affect, closely watching for psychotic tendencies and depression.	Amalia was gradually oriented to person, time, and place. Within 72 hours, Amalia was calmer, was able to interact with her primary caregiver, and finally slept.

NURSING DIAGNOSIS 3 *Self-care deficit,* related to perceptual and cognitive impairment

OUTCOMES	NIC	NURSING ACTIONS	EVALUATION
• Amalia will demonstrate functional behaviors with activities of daily living within 48 hours.	• Self-care assistance: IADL	• Gently guide Amalia through self-care activities, gradually shifting responsibilities for activities of daily living (ADL) to Amalia. • Initially focus on safety, dressing, and eating.	Initially, Amalia was minimally responsive, required complete physical care and protection, and was fed. As her condition improved, however, she was able to assume increasing responsibility for her physical care. She remained extremely

(*Continues*)

NURSING CARE PLAN: NURSING PROCESS FORMAT 14-1 (Continued)

	• Give progressive activities associated with ADL. • Provide positive feedback for Amalia's increasing assumption of ADL.	fatigued and lethargic, so activities were clustered. Rest periods were built into Amalia's day. By day 4, she was able to bathe and dress herself and began to discuss her problems with the nurse.

REFLECTIVE QUESTIONS

1. **ASSESSMENT**
   Would it be valuable to also interview Amalia's brother and/or friends?
2. **NURSING DIAGNOSIS**
   What other diagnoses are especially important with Amalia?
3. **OUTCOMES**
   How dependent can the nurse allow Amalia to be? Is it necessary to get Amalia focused on self-care?
4. **NURSING ACTIONS**
   What differences in Amalia's care would there be if she were in an active-destructive state rather than a neglectful one?
5. **EVALUATION**
   Do plans always work? How does the nurse maintain her own positive attitude?

NURSING CARE PLAN: NURSING PROCESS FORMAT 14-2

The description of F. Scott Fitzgerald's feelings of depression are presented within the discussion of Minor Depressive Disorder earlier in this chapter.

Fitzgerald is describing depression in terms of emptiness (drawing on resources he did not possess), being physically and spiritually drained, and feeling anger and annoyance at the world going on around him (being bitter at the sound of the radio). His life has become an extreme effort, and he is worried about his own ability to cope any longer.

Based on this brief description, one could assume that Fitzgerald has a level of depression that could benefit from treatment, medication, and therapy.

Imagine that nurses are giving care to Mr. Curpin, a man expressing his depression in a manner similar to Fitzgerald.

ASSESSMENT

Mr. Curpin is depressed to the point of admitting, "I have no real life in me." He has isolated himself from family and friends, sees no purpose in his life, and forces himself to "appear normal." He is reliant on old patterns of behavior to get him through the long days and longer nights. He is restless, fatigued, unhappy, and discouraged.

(Continues)

NURSING CARE PLAN: NURSING PROCESS FORMAT 14-2 (Continued)

NURSING DIAGNOSIS 1 *Ineffective coping,* related to depression, as evidenced by verbalization of inability to cope and expression of discouragement

OUTCOMES	NIC	NURSING ACTIONS	EVALUATION
• Within 6 weeks, Mr. Curpin will demonstrate an increased use of coping mechanisms. • Within 1 month, Mr. Curpin will reconnect with family or friends. • Within 2 months, Mr. Curpin will verbalize feeling a greater sense of control over his life.	• Coping enhancement • Counseling • Emotional support	• Encourage Mr. Curpin to discuss the loss of life's purpose through use of communication techniques and open-ended questions and by spending time with Mr. Curpin. • Establish a relationship with Mr. Curpin based on trust: set aside time to talk with him; keep promises; initiate interactions; and keep an atmosphere of positive regard. • Explore the coping mechanisms Mr. Curpin used before to manage difficult times. • Assess the personal meaning of his social isolation; explore means to reach out to others. • Facilitate discussion about his illness, treatment plan, and personal goals. • Emphasize Mr. Curpin's strengths and progress in gaining control over his life. • Clarify Mr. Curpin's understanding of his treatment.	Mr. Curpin revealed that part of his life's concerns related to a sense of fatigue and depression over "getting older" and "not feeling well." His coping mechanism was to withdraw and become uninvolved, yet he felt lonely and isolated. He was willing to try to reach out to others; he willingly agreed to enter therapy and to explore his means of coping.

(Continues)

NURSING CARE PLAN: NURSING PROCESS FORMAT 14-2 (Continued)

NURSING DIAGNOSIS 2 *Spiritual distress*, related to intense suffering, as evidenced by apathy and questioning own existence

OUTCOMES	NIC	NURSING ACTIONS	EVALUATION
• Within 4 weeks, Mr. Curpin will verbalize a mood change consistent with hope.	• Spiritual support	• Use therapeutic communications with Mr. Curpin to establish trust and empathic caring. • Be open to Mr. Curpin's expressions of concern. • Encourage Mr. Curpin to discuss views about meaning and purpose of life and relationships that provided spiritual strength and support.	Mr. Curpin began to explore his life and what a positive future would mean to him. Over time, he was able to identify future-oriented goals.

REFLECTIVE QUESTIONS

1. **ASSESSMENT**
   What physical clues might you look for when interviewing someone whom you suspect is suffering from depression?
2. **NURSING DIAGNOSIS**
   What means do you really have to help someone adopt new coping patterns?
3. **OUTCOMES**
   How can you predict outcomes for another's feelings?
4. **NURSING ACTIONS**
   What does it mean when someone has truly lost the meaning and purpose of life? What do you think is a nurse's role in relieving the distress of the human spirit?
5. **EVALUATION**
   Have you accomplished your goal as a nurse when this client sees a future and describes a sense of hope? What other role would you have?

NURSING CARE PLAN: NURSING PROCESS FORMAT 14-3

The description of Geoffrey is presented within the discussion of bereavement earlier in this chapter.

Geoffrey is undergoing acute grieving due to the death of his wife through suicide. He is describing the reality stage of grieving, coming to terms with the pain, the emptiness, and the extreme sadness that he feels. He relates that others offer themselves to him should he want to talk, but that talking about his grief makes little difference. He implies that others who are concerned for him enter his world, talk, take him out, let him know that he will "get over it," and finally leave him to himself, where he can feel his grief once again.

(Continues)

NURSING CARE PLAN: NURSING PROCESS FORMAT 14-3 (Continued)

Normal grieving is one of the most painful events in a person's life. The nurse recognizes that this is so and also is aware of the fact that the pain is a healthy human response to loss. The nurse cannot make the pain go away. Persons who undergo grief do not always want distractions, medications, and the like. They need to feel their sorrow.

Imagine that nurses are caring for Harold, a man who has experienced similar circumstances to Geoffrey.

ASSESSMENT

Harold's wife committed suicide three weeks ago. He knew she was depressed, but had no idea she would take her own life. He feels detached, lost, depressed, and overwhelmed. He does not feel like eating, has nightmares when he sleeps, and is unable to respond to the many friends and family offering support. He is secluded and withdrawn.

NURSING DIAGNOSIS *Grieving*, related to death of spouse, as evidenced by self-care deficits, social seclusion, withdrawal, and sense of depression and emotional pain

OUTCOMES	NIC	NURSING ACTIONS	EVALUATION
• Within 2 weeks, Harold will begin to express his feelings associated with his wife's death. • Within 2 months, Harold will establish an adequate balance of sleep, rest, activity, and eating. • Within 3 months, Harold will show evidence of reengaging in life's activities, including work and social interactions.	• Grief work facilitation • Support system enhancement	• Facilitate Harold's involvement with a therapist or group so he can explore the loss of his wife to suicide. • Monitor Harold's grief reactions, watching for statements of hopelessness, self-blame, agitation, or threats of suicide. • Encourage and support Harold in completing normal daily activities and contacts by helping him to plan a schedule and carry through with plans. • Monitor Harold's physical condition. • Teach about grief work, normal responses, and strategies for dealing with grief reactions. • Underscore that grieving is real, it is painful, and it takes time to resolve.	Harold went to one bereavement group meeting, but found it too painful to return. Harold did agree to meet with a counselor. He needed time to talk, to cry, and to feel the pain of grief. He did so with the counselor. Within 6 weeks, Harold was able to function adequately in the world. He went back to work and continued therapy. Harold understands grief and grief work intellectually. Harold is beginning to see a future for himself. Harold continues in counseling.

(*Continues*)

NURSING CARE PLAN: NURSING PROCESS FORMAT 14-3 (Continued)

REFLECTIVE QUESTIONS

1. **ASSESSMENT**
   What characteristics would you look for to distinguish normal grief from dysfunctional grief or depression?
2. **NURSING DIAGNOSIS**
   How do you think grief is complicated by death through suicide? How can you differentiate normal grief from depression?
3. **OUTCOMES**
   The time frame of grief resolution is highly individualized. How does a nurse establish outcomes? What do you do when your outcomes prove unrealistic?
4. **NURSING ACTIONS**
   What nursing theory or theories do you think support your work in bereavement? Why?
5. **EVALUATION**
   How would you know if Harold's grief became a dysfunctional grief reaction? What would you look for?

NURSING CARE PLAN: CONCEPT MAP FORMAT 14-1

Depression

BACKGROUND INFORMATION

Sarah is a young professional woman in her late 20s. She is a single woman with significant positive ties to her family and has many close friends. She dates somewhat infrequently and is highly selective in her decisions to go out with male friends. She has had one serious relationship with a male friend that lasted three years. About one year ago, she and her friend separated based on mutual agreement that neither was ready or able to make a long-term commitment to one another. Sarah believes that her need for autonomy, professional enhancement, and independence are primary in her life at the moment.

Sarah has recently been transferred from her position in the South, where she has spent her entire life, to a large urban city in the Midwest. Her successes at work have earned her two promotions in the past five years, and she eagerly pursued the changes that relocation would bring her. Once in her location, now for five months, she realizes she can meet her basic needs, but feels that something is really lacking in her life. She no longer enjoys photography and reading (her main interests outside of work). She has been invited to join a book club by one of her new colleagues at work and she has declined. She increasingly is unable to sleep well, awakening at 4 A.M. and not able to return to sleep. When awake, she is worried that she is not performing at her optimal level at work, and she is having trouble concentrating. She does not eat well anymore and thinks she has lost some weight. She is seeking help at her employee assistance center. She tells the nurse there that she cannot sleep, that she feels tired all of the time, and that she is turning down social activities because she does not have the energy to go anywhere. She tells the nurse she believes her major problem is fatigue and an overarching feeling that she is unable to change any aspects of her current situation to make her life better.

(Continues)

NURSING CARE PLAN: CONCEPT MAP FORMAT 14-1 (Continued)

INITIAL ASSESSMENT AND REFLECTION

The nurse recognizes that Sarah has several characteristics of depression:

1. Recent move that triggered a loss
2. No pleasure in previously enjoyable activities
3. Increasing sense of isolation from others
4. Sleep disturbances
5. Lack of ability to concentrate

INITIAL REVIEW OF NURSING DIAGNOSES

The nurse's first concern is to assess if Sarah has any issues related to safety or critical illness requiring immediate attention and intervention. The nurse assesses that there are no such issues. Next, the nurse proceeds to review the nursing diagnoses that could be present and recognizes that there are several that need to be considered, based on the history and interview with Sarah:

- *Insomnia*, related to early morning awakening
- *Social isolation*, related to lack of social contacts and refusal to participate in social activities
- *Low self-esteem*, related to questioning professional role
- *Imbalanced nutrition: less than body requirements*, related to failure to eat regular meals/healthy food
- *Powerlessness*, related to expressed feelings of not being able to change aspects of her life
- *Fatigue*, expressed by statements of not having enough energy

The nurse prepares a concept map, listing the following characteristics as important to Sarah's health in her current situation: move to a new city, social isolation with continued withdrawal from others, feelings of sadness, fatigue, insomnia, worry about work performance, powerlessness to change her situation, and nutritional imbalance. The nurse then uses the concept map to connect the characteristics/factors that were related.

PRIORITIES OF CARE

The concept relationships indicate that two issues that are related to most of the others (the focal issues) have emerged and are the priorities for the nurse's attention and care plan:

1. Sleep disturbances
2. Social interaction

Rationale for beginning interventions on these two nursing diagnoses:

- Failure to sleep exacerbates feelings of fatigue, sadness, powerlessness, and social isolation. Taking care of sleep is the first step in dealing with all of these other issues.
- Sarah is concerned about her sleep patterns, and in efforts to set mutual goals for a care plan, the nurse knows she should begin where the client wished to begin.
- Sleep patterns are an objective and treatable condition, and the nurse and Sarah can set goals and see progress toward outcomes with sleep issues.
- Social interaction also emerges as a focal diagnosis. Socialization is viewed by Sarah as an important, and now unfulfilled, aspect of her life.
- Social interactions can be pursued, again in an objective manner with clearly identified mutual goals.

(Continues)

NURSING CARE PLAN: CONCEPT MAP FORMAT 14-1 (Continued)

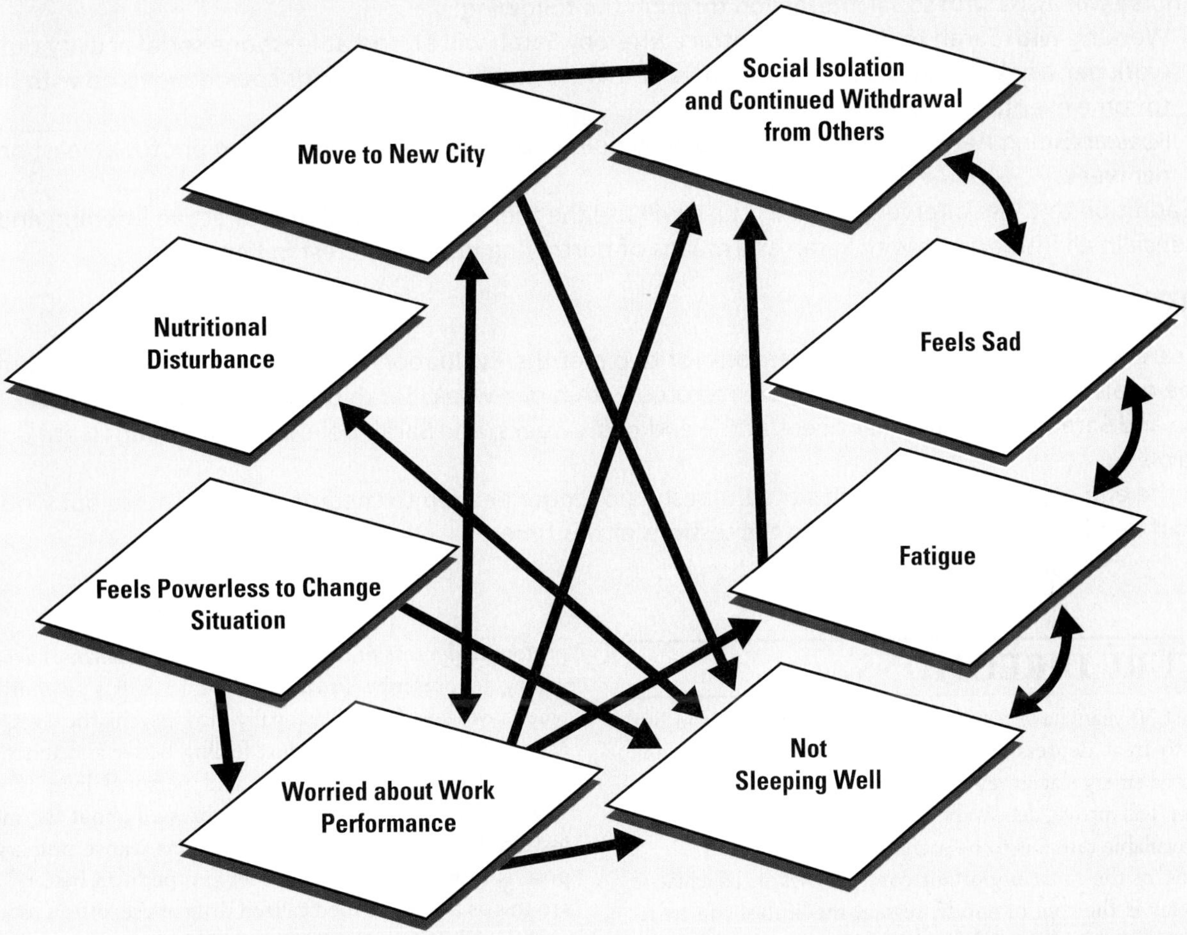

Concept Map of Issues and Problems (DELMAR/CENGAGE LEARNING.)

Thus, the concept map permits the nurse to begin interventions with Sarah that are focused and mutually important, with the expectation that with short-term interventions, other aspects of Sarah's life will also improve.

NURSING INTERVENTIONS

- Setting mutually agreed-upon goals:
  By the end of one week, Sarah will sleep through the night and will awaken feeling rested.
  By the end of the month, Sarah will be able to reestablish previous sleep patterns.
  By the end of the month, Sarah will reestablish regular weekly social interactions with friends outside of work.
- Planning interventions based on the assessment and the goals, the nurse will assist with a sleep regimen through sleep enhancement activities such as:
  Assisting Sarah to adjust the environment to promote sleep (light, noise, temperature)
  Encouraging Sarah to establish a bedtime routine (use of bed for sleeping and not for reading, watching TV, eating, or drinking); eliminating bedtime food or drinks that could interfere with sleep
  Maintaining a predictable pattern of time to go sleep
  Evaluating of use of Trazadone with Sarah's primary care provider, because the medication will assist with sleep and at the same time assist in treating depression.

(Continues)

NURSING CARE PLAN: CONCEPT MAP FORMAT 14-1 (Continued)

The nurse will assist with social interaction through the following:

Working with Sarah to develop a contract whereby Sarah will attend at least one social activity out of work per week. Sarah will attend activities or invite one of her new friends/coworkers to go with her to some event.

Reestablishing her interest in photography by going out of the house and taking photos at least once per week.

In addition to these interventions, the nurse will use the therapeutic techniques of active listening and presence in all interactions with Sarah as a means of portraying honest interest in her.

OUTCOMES/EVALUATION

The care was continued with weekly sessions for two months. Evaluation was based first on accomplishment of the goals set. Once sleep patterns were restored within one week, Sarah began her socializing again. The nurse and Sarah reevaluated her needs at the end of six weeks, and Sarah believed that "things were under control."

At the end of eight weeks, Sarah stated that she no longer needed to check in with the nurse but would do so if needed. The nurse terminated the sessions at this time.

FUTURE DIRECTIONS

The past 30 years have resulted in important advances in our ability to treat depression. New antidepressant medications will likely emerge at an ever-accelerating rate. Whether any of these will prove decisively superior to medications currently available remains to be seen.

One of the most important controversies in psychiatric care today is the role of antidepressant medications in treating persons who do not have Major Depressive Disorder. While the concept of Minor Depressive Disorder remains invalidated, studies suggest that antidepressants and cognitive and marital therapies may benefit persons with less profound depression. In recent years, clinicians have been willing to prescribe Prozac and other SSRIs to individuals who have few (or occasionally no) psychiatric symptoms. Many of these persons report feeling better and functioning more effectively in their jobs and personal lives (Kramer, 1993). Much concern has been expressed about the medical justification for prescribing medications whose primary purpose is to make individuals "feel and perform better." Some see this as a form of medicalized drug abuse, others as a legitimate medical practice (Nuland, 1994). Surely, these issues will continue to be major social and even political concerns in the coming years.

KEY CONCEPTS

- Mood swings are part of everyone's life; however, there are people for whom typical ups and downs become too extreme and too long.
- Depression is the intense feeling of a depressed, down mood.
- DSM-IV-TR lists specific criteria for the depressive conditions of Major Depressive Disorder, Dysthymic Disorder, and Bereavement. Minor Depressive Disorder has not been validated by DSM, but exists as a category for many who do not meet the exact criteria of other depressive disorders.
- A depressed person loses interest in activities that were previously enjoyable and often experiences loss of appetite or weight, sleep disturbance, fatigue, feelings of worthlessness, trouble with concentration, and recurrent thoughts of death or suicide.
- Persons who are grieving experience the same feelings as those who are depressed.
- Grief is a normal, albeit painful, human experience.
- Major theories that explain depression include psychoanalytic theory, object loss theory, learned helplessness theory, cognitive theory, and physical/biological theories.
- The nursing theories of Watson and Orem are particularly helpful in working with depressed clients.
- Caring nursing theories emphasize the need for the nurse to establish a trusting relationship with the client.

- The self-care deficit nursing theory addresses the need for the nurse to provide care to meet the client's needs that he is not able to meet on his own.
- Medications are frequently used in alleviating depressive symptoms. Tricyclic and related antidepressants, SSRIs, and MAO inhibitors are the most frequently used.

REVIEW QUESTIONS

1. A nurse is developing a care plan for a client being admitted for depression. A priority nursing diagnosis would be which of the following?
   1. Risk for injury
   2. Ineffective coping
   3. Chronic low self-esteem
   4. Disturbed sensory perception

2. Which assessment by the nurse would best indicate that the client's prescribed antidepressant has been effective?
   1. The client eats only small portions at meal time each day
   2. Staff members comment that the client is more cooperative
   3. The physician decides to increase the medication dose
   4. The client seldom participates in all unit activities

3. Prior to administering a tricyclic agent, the nurse should do which of the following?
   1. Check the chart to see if the results of the chest x-ray and complete blood work are available
   2. Determine that the client has not taken an MAO inhibitor in the last two weeks
   3. Determine that the client has not taken an SSRI in the last three weeks
   4. Check the chart to determine if the client has completed a living will

4. The physician writes several orders for a client admitted with a diagnosis of major depression. Which of the following orders should the nurse question?
   1. General diet
   2. Activities as tolerated
   3. Referral for occupational therapy
   4. Discontinue Parnate (tranylcypromine) and immediately begin Anafranil (clomipramine) 50 mg four times per day.

5. A depressed client tells the nurse that nothing will help and he still plans to kill himself. Which of the following statements by the client indicates that he is still suicidal?
   1. The client states that he is unable to enjoy eating anymore.
   2. The client states that he is unable to get a good night's sleep.
   3. The client states that no one cares about him.
   4. The client states he will purchase a gun once he is discharged.

6. A client has been admitted to the psychiatric unit with depression. Which of the following statements by the nurse would be most therapeutic?
   1. "What is your daily routine?"
   2. "When was your last doctor's visit?"
   3. "Tell me what brought you to the hospital today."
   4. "Have you been taking your prescribed medications?"

7. A client who has been prescribed Elavil (amytriptyline) for her depression asks the nurse which side effects she should be watching for. The nurse's best response would be:
   1. "Generally there are no side effects from Elavil."
   2. "The most common side effects of Elavil include: hypertension, drowsiness, fatigue, and tremors."
   3. "Dehydration is a common complaint, so you should drink at least eight glasses of water each day."
   4. "You should avoid foods high in tyramine such as smoked salmon, luncheon meats, aged cheeses and wines."

8. A client receiving an MAOI is attending a session with the hospital nutritionist. Which group of foods should the client plan to avoid when preparing meals?
   1. Foods high in sodium
   2. Foods high in fat content
   3. Foods containing tyramine
   4. The client will need to be on a general diet

LEARNING ACTIVITIES

1. Differentiate between unipolar and bipolar depression.

2. Identify those who are at risk for developing depression.

3. Describe the characteristics of major depression, minor depression, and dysthymia.

4. Describe bereavement or grief; identify the stages of normal grieving.

5. Consider a client diagnosed with major depression. Explain the depression from the perspective of each of the following theories: psychoanalytic, object loss, learned helplessness, cognitive, and physical/biological.
6. Watson's nursing theory guides practice with depressed persons. How would her theory suggest you initiate interaction with a client?
7. What nursing interventions for a depressed person are consistent with Orem's theory?
8. List assessment parameters for nursing care of one who is at risk for depression.
9. What are the cultural considerations related to nursing care of one who is depressed?
10. Suggest the process needed to validate nursing diagnoses associated with depression.
11. Describe independent nursing interventions for depression. How are these interventions evaluated in practice?
12. Describe the nurse's role in monitoring clients on tricyclic antidepressants and other drugs.

*Study*WARE™ CONNECTION

Using your *Study*WARE™ CD-ROM

1. Complete the Crossword Puzzle for this chapter.
2. Complete the Quiz for this chapter in Test Mode.
3. Explore the other games and activities that support this chapter.

VIDEO LINK

Read and contemplate the following questions about Barbara, the client experiencing a Major Depressive Disorder. Then watch the video "Major Depressive Disorder" on your *Study*WARE™ CD-ROM to observe Barbara's interview with a psychiatrist. Consider these questions prior to listening to the psychiatrist's analysis:

1. Does Barbara display all the symptoms of a Major Depressive Disorder?
2. At what age did Barbara feel she became depressed? How did this depression present?
3. What health risks do you feel Barbara may be predisposed to as a result of her long-term depression?
4. Do you feel that there is a possibility of another underlying depressive disorder?
5. Does Barbara suffer from seasonal affective disorder?
6. Given Barbara's history, do you feel that she was at risk for a postpartum depression?
7. Reflect back on Barbara's life; how do you think her depression has impacted on her happiness and productivity?
8. Consider the impact of her illness on her children.
9. What unrealistic expectation did she place on them?
10. What community resources and therapeutic programs are available for families of depressed persons?
11. What do epidemiological studies reveal about the incidence of depression in the general population? What is the predicted incidence for Barbara's children?
12. Discuss the classifications of medications that are used to treat depression. What are the major associated side effects?
13. Given the longevity of Barbara's illness, which classification of medication do you think she may have been initially prescribed? Which medications are currently realizing the greatest benefit?
14. Which medications would be given with caution considering her history of suicide?
15. How long does it take for the majority of antidepressants to reach a therapeutic level?
16. Which other therapeutic regimes should be incorporated into a treatment plan in order to gain a holistic approach to treating depression?
17. Is Barbara a high suicide risk right now? What assessments did you make to draw this conclusion?

REFERENCES

Abraham, I. L., Neese, J. B., & Westerman, P. S. (1991). Depression: Nursing implications of a clinical and social problem. *Nursing Clinics of North America, 26*(3), 527–544.

American Psychiatric Association. (2000). *Diagnostic and statistical manual of mental disorders* (Fourth Ed.–Text Rev.). Washington, DC: Author.

Barbato, A., & D'Avanzo, B. (2006). Marital therapy for depression. *Cochrane Database of Systematic Reviews* (2).

Beck, A. (1967). *Depression: Causes and treatment.* Philadelphia: University of Pennsylvania Press.

Beck, C. T. (2008a). State of the science on postpartum depression: What nurse researchers have contributed—Part 1. *MCN American Journal of Maternal and Child Nursing, 33*(3), 151–156.

Beck, C. T. (2008b). State of the science on postpartum depression: What nurse researchers have contributed—Part 2. *MCN American Journal of Maternal and Child Nursing, 33*(2), 121–126.

Bernazzani, O., & Bifulco, A. (2003). Motherhood as a vulnerability factor in major depression: The role of negative pregnancy experiences. *Social Science Medicine, 56*(6), 1249–1260.

Birtwhistle, J., & Martin, N. (1999). Seasonal affective disorder: Its recognition and treatment. *British Journal of Nursing, 8*(15), 1004–1009.

Blacock, E. (2006). Home clinic programme: An alternative model for private mental health facilities and sufferers of major depression. *International Journal of Mental Health Nursing, 15,* 3–9.

Bolwig, T. (1993). Biological treatment other than drugs. In N. Sartorius, G. DeGirdano, G. Andrews, G. A. German, & L. Eisenberg (Eds.), *Treatment of mental disorders* (pp. 92–111). Washington, DC: American Psychiatric Press.

Bower, B. (1987). Bereavement: Reeling in the years. *Science News, 131*(6), 84.

Bulecheck, G., Butcher, H., & Dochterman, J. (2008). *Nursing interventions classification* (5th ed.). St. Louis: Mosby.

Busell, E. F., & Stuart, E. M. (1999). Influences of psychosocial factors and biopsychosocial interventions on outcomes after myocardial infarction. *Journal of Cardiovascular Nursing, 13*(3), 60–72.

CDC. (2008) Prevalence of self-reported postpartum depressive symptoms—17 states. 2004–2005. *Morbidity and Mortality Weekly Report.* 57(14)361–366.

Cox, J. L, Holden, J. M., & Sagovsky. R. (1987). Detection of postnatal depression. Development of the 10-item Edinburgh Postnatal Depression Scale. *British Journal of Psychiatry, 150,* 782–786.

Denton, W. H., Burleson, B. R., Clark, T. E., Rodriguez, C. P., & Hobbs, B. V. (2000). A randomized trial of emotion-focused therapy for couples in a training clinic. *Journal of Marital and Family Therapy. 26,* 65–78.

Depression Guideline Panel. (1993). *Depression in primary care: Detection and diagnosis.* Rockville, MD: Agency of Health Care Policy and Research.

Ellison, J. A., Greenberg, L. S., Goldman, R. N., & Angus, L. (2009) Maintenance of gains following experiential therapies for depression. *Journal of Consulting and Clinical Psychology 77,* 103–112.

Fan, A. Z., Strine, T. W., Jiles, R., & Mokdad, A. H. (2008). Depression and anxiety associated with cardiovascular disease among persons aged 45 years and older in 38 states of the United States, 2006. *Preventive Medicine, 46*(5), 445–450.

Fine, R. (1979). *A history of psychoanalysis.* New York: Columbia University Press.

Ford, K. (1992). Seasonal depression: Management of seasonal affective disorder. *Professional Nurse, 8,* 94–98.

Frasure-Smith, N., & Lesperance, F. (2003). Depression: A cardiac risk factor in search of treatment. *Journal of the American Medical Association,* 289, 3171–3173.

Friedman, R. A., & Leon, A. C. (2007). Expanding the black box—depression, antidepressants, and the risk of suicide. *New England Journal of Medicine, 356*(23), 2343–2346.

Furukawa, T., McGuire, M., & Barbui, C. (2003). Low dosage tricyclic antidepressants for depression. *Cochrane Database Systematic Review,* (3), CD003197.

Gaster, B., & Holroyd, J. (2000). St. John's Wort for depression: A systematic review. *Archives of Internal Medicine, 160*(2), 153–156.

Gaynes, B. N., Rush, A. J., Trivedi, M. H., Wisniewski, S. R., Balasubramani, G. K., McGrath, P. J., et al. (2008). Primary versus specialty care outcomes for depressed outpatients managed with measurement-based care: Results from STAR*D. *Journal of General Internal Medicine, 23*(5), 551–560.

George, M. S. (2003). Stimulating the brain. *Scientific American, 289*(3), 66–73.

George, M. S., Ketter, T. A., & Post, R. M. (1993). SPECT and PET imaging in mood disorders. *Journal of Clinical Psychiatry, 54,* 6–13.

Greenberg, B. D., Price, L. H., Rauch, S. L., Friehs, G., Noren, G., Malone, D., et al. (2003). Neurosurgery for intractable obsessive-compulsive disorder and depression: Critical issues. *Neurosurgery Clinics of North America, 14*(2), 199–212.

Greenberg, L. S. (2009). Overview. Retrieved August 12, 2009 from http://www.emotionfocusedtherapy.org/Overview.htm.

Greenberg L.S., & Pascual-Leone, A. (2006) Emotion in psychotherapy: a practice-friendly research review. *Journal of Clinical Psychology, 62,* 611–630.

Greenberg, L.S., & Bolger, E. (2001) An emotion-focused approach to the overregulation of emotion and emotional pain. *Journal of Clinical Psychology, 57,* (197–211).

Hammerness, P., Basch, E., Ulbricht, C., Barrette, E. P., Foppa, I., Basch, S., et al. (2003). St. John's Wort: A systematic review of adverse effects and drug interactions for the consultation psychiatrist. *Psychosomatics, 44*(4), 271–282.

Harvey, S. T., & Pun, P. K. (2007). Analysis of positive Edinburgh depression scale referrals to a consultation liaison psychiatry service in a two-year period. *International Journal of Mental Health Nursing, 16,* 1161–1167.

Hemingway, H., Shipley, M., Mullen, M. J., Kumari, M., Brunner, E., Taylor, M., et al. (2003). Social and psychosocial influences on inflammatory markers and vascular function in civil servants (the Whitehall II study). *American Journal of Cardiology, 92*(8), 984–987.

Herdman, H. (Ed). (2009). *Nursing diagnoses: Definitions and classifications 2009–2011.* Oxford: Wiley Blackwell.

Howland, R. H. (2008). Neurosurgical approaches to therapeutic brain stimulation for treatment-resistant depression. *Journal of Psychosocial Nursing and Mental Health Services, 46,* 15–19.

Huggstrom, L., & Denker, K. (2005). Sense of coherence and social support in relation to recovery in first episode patients with major depression. *International Journal of Mental Health Nursing, 14,* 258–264.

Illes, J., Lombera, S., Rosenberg, J., & Arnow, B. (2008). In the mind's eye: Provider and patient attitudes on functional brain imaging. *Journal of Psychiatric Research,* 43, 107–114.

Johnstone, T., van Reekum, C. M., Urry, H. L., Kalin, N. H., & Davidson, R. J. (2007). Failure to regulate: Counterproductive recruitment of top-down prefrontal-subcortical circuitry in major depression. *Journal of Neuroscience, 27*(33), 8877–8884.

Kagee, A. (2008). Depression and anxiety in South African patients. *Journal of Health Psychology, 13*(4), 547–555.

Kaltenthaler, E., Shackley, P., Stevens, K., Beverley, C., Parry, G., & Chilcott, J. (2002). A systematic review and economic evaluation of computerized cognitive behaviour therapy for depression and anxiety. *Healthy Technology Assessment, 6*(22), 1–89.

Keller, M. B., McCullough, J. P., Klein, D. N., Arnow, B., Dunner, D. L., Gelenberg, A. J., et al. (2000). A comparison of nefazodone, the cognitive behavioral-analysis system of psychotherapy, and their combination for the treatment of chronic depression. *New England Journal of Medicine, 342*(20), 1462–1470.

Kelley, J., & Johnson, B. (2002). Theory of transpersonal caring. In J. George (Ed.), *Nursing theories: The base for professional practice* (pp. 405–426). Upper Saddle River, NJ: Prentice Hall.

Kendler, K. S., Hettema, J. M., Butera, F., Gardner, C. O., & Prescott, C. (2003). Life event dimensions of loss, humiliation, entrapment and danger in the prediction of onsets of major depression and generalized anxiety. *Archives of General Psychiatry, 60*(8), 789–796.

Kessler, R. C., Berglund, P., Demier, O., Jin, R., Koretz, D., Merikangas, K. R., et al. (2003). The epidemiology of major depressive disorder: Results from the National Comorbidity Survey Replication (NCS-R). *Journal of the American Medical Association, 289*, 3095–3105.

Kirsch, I., Deacon, B. J., Huedo-Medina, T. B., Scoboria, A., Moore, T. J., & Johnson, B. T. (2008). Initial severity and antidepressant benefits: A meta-analysis of data submitted to the Food and Drug Administration. *PLoS Medicine, 5*(2).

Klein, D., Shankman, S., & Rose, S. (2006). Ten-year prospective follow-up study of the naturalistic course of Dysthymic Disorder and Double Depression. *American Journal of Psychiatry, 163*, 872–880.

Kopelman, R. C., Moel, J., Mertens, C., Stuart, S., Arndt, S., & O'Hara, M. W. (2008). Barriers to care for antenatal depression. *Psychiatric Services, 59*(4), 429–432.

Kramer, P. D. (1993). *Listening to Prozac.* New York: Viking Press.

Krishnan, K. R., Delong, M., Kraemer, H., Carney, R., Spiegel, D., & Gordon, C. (2002). Comorbidity of depression with other medical diseases in the elderly. *Biological Psychiatry, 52*(6), 559–588.

Kroenke, K., West, S. L., Swindle, R., Gilsenan, A., Eckert, G. J., Dolo, R., et al. (2001). Similar effectiveness of paroxetine, fluoxctine, and sertraline in primary care: A randomized trial. *Journal of the American Medical Association, 286*(23), 2947–2955.

Kurlowicz, L. H. (1993). Social factors and depression in late life. *Archives of Psychiatric Nursing, 7*(1), 30–36.

Larson, P. S. (2008). Deep brain stimulation for psychiatric disorders. *Neurotherapeutics, 5*, 50–58.

Lau, M. A. (2008). New developments in psychosocial interventions for adults with unipolar depression. *Current Opinions in Psychiatry, 21*(1), 30–36.

Leininger, M. M. (1978). *Transcultural nursing: Concepts, theories, and practices.* New York: John Wiley and Sons, Inc.

Löwe, B., Spitzer, R. L., Williams, J. B., Mussell, M., Schellberg, D., & Kroenke, K. (2008). Depression, anxiety and somatization in primary care: Syndrome overlap and functional impairment. *General Hospital Psychiatry, 30*(3), 191–197.

Manning, D. (1984). *Don't take my grief away.* San Francisco: Harper & Row.

Martin, J. L., Barbanoj, M. J., Schlaepfer, T. E., Thompson, E., Perez, P., & Kulisevshy, J. (2003). Repetitive transcranial magnetic stimulation for the treatment of depression: Systematic review and meta-analysis. *British Journal of Psychiatry, 182*, 480–491.

McEnany, G. W., & Lee, K. A. (2005). Effects of ECT on sleep, mood, and temperature in women with nonseasonal depression. *Issues in Mental Health Nursing, 26*, 81–794.

McSweeney, J. C., Cody, M., & Crane, P. B. (2001). Do you know them when you see them? Women's prodromal and acute symptoms of myocardial infarction. *Journal of Cardiovascular Nursing, 15*(3), 26–38.

Meier, E. (2002). Andrea Yates: Where did we go wrong? *Pediatric Nursing, 28*(3), 296–297, 299.

Meleis, A. I., Sawyer, L. M., Im, E. O., Hilfinger Messias, D.K., Schumacher, K. (2000). Experiencing transitions: A middle range theory. *Advances in Nursing Science, 23(1)*, 12–28,

Morris-Rush, J. K., Freda, M. C., & Bernstein, P. S. (2003). Screening for postpartum depression in an inner-city population. *American Journal of Obstetrics and Gynecology, 188*(5), 1217–1219.

Neidig, J. L., Smith, B. A., & Brashers, D. E. (2003). Aerobic exercise training for depressive symptom management in adults living with HIV infection. *Journal of the Association of Nurses in AIDS Care, 14*(2), 30–40.

Nuland, S. B. (1994). The pill of pills. *New York Review of Books, 41*(11), 48.

Orem, D. E. (2001). *Nursing: Concepts of practice* (6th ed.). St. Louis: Mosby.

Parker, G. (2002). Differential effectiveness of newer and older antidepressants appears mediated by an age effect on the phenotypic expression of depression. *Acta Psychiatrica Scandinavica, 106*(3), 168–170.

Perris, C., & Herlofson, J. (1993). Cognitive therapy. In G. Andrews, G. A. German, & L. Eisenberg (Eds.), *Treatment of mental disorders* (pp. 151–153). Washington, DC: American Psychiatric Press.

Pirraglia, P. A., Stafford, R. S., & Singer, D. (2003). Trends in prescribing of selective serotonin reuptake inhibitors and other newer antidepressant agents in adult primary care. *The Primary Care Companion to the Journal of Clinical Psychiatry, 5*(4), 153–157.

Prevention, C. F. (2008). Prevalence of self-reported postpartum depressive symptoms—17 states, 2004–2005. *MMWR Morbidity and Mortality Weekly Reports, 57*(14), 361–366.

Raison, C. L., & Miller, A. H. (2003). Depression in cancer: New developments regarding diagnosis and treatment. *Biological Psychiatry, 54*(3), 283–294.

Ramchandani, P. G., Stein, A., O'Connor, T. G., Heron, J., Murray, L., & Evans, J. (2008). Depression in men in the postnatal period and later child psychopathology: A population cohort study. *Journal of the American Academy of Child and Adolescent Psychiatry, 47*(4), 390–398.

Rosenquist, P. B., Brenes, G. B., Arnold, E. M., Kimball, J., & McCall, V. (2006). *Journal of ECT, 22*(1), 18–24.

Sakai, K., Hasegawa, D., Okura, M., Morikawa, O., Ueyama, T., Shirai, Y., et al. (2003). Novel variants of murine serotonin transporter mRNA and the promoter activity of its upstream site. *Neuroscience Letter, 342*(3), 175–178.

Schultz, R., Beach, S. R., Ives, D. G., Martire, L. M., Ariyo, A. A., & Kop, W. J. (2000). Association between depression and mortality in older clients. *Archives of Internal Medicine, 160*, 1761–1768.

Schumacher, M., Zubaran, C., & White, G. (2008). Bringing birth-related paternal depression to the fore. *Women and Birth, 21*(2), 65–70.

Seligman, M. (1974). Depression and learned helplessness. In R. Friedman & M. Katz (Eds.), *The psychology of depression: Contemporary research and theory.* Washington, DC: Winston & Sons.

Skärsäter, I., & Willman, A. (2006). The recovery process in major depression. *Advances in Nursing Science, 29*(3), 245–259.

Spek, V., Nyklicek, I., Smits, N., Cuijpers, P., Riper, H., Keyzer, J., et al. (2007). Internet-based cognitive behavioural therapy for subthreshold depression in people over 50 years old: A randomized controlled clinical trial. *Psychological Medicine, 37*(12), 1797–1806.

Steeves. R. H. (2002). The rhythms of bereavement. *Family and Community Health, 25*(1), 1–10.

Stewart, W. F., Ricci, J. A., Chee, E., Hahn, S., & Morganstein, D. (2003). Cost of lost productive work time among U.S. workers with depression. *Journal of the American Medical Association, 289*, 3135–3144.

Strauman, T. J., Vieth, A. Z., Merrill, K. A., Kolden, G. G., Woods, T. E., Klein, M. H., et al. (2006). Self-system therapy as an intervention for self-regulatory dysfunction in depression: A randomized comparison with cognitive therapy. *Journal of Consulting and Clinical Psychology, 74*(2), 367–376.

Sussman, N. (2003). SNRIs versus SSRIs: Mechanisms of action in treating depression and painful physical symptoms. *Journal of Clinical Psychiatry, 5*(Suppl. 7), 19–26.

Sussman, N. (2007). Translating science into service: Lessons learned from the Sequenced Treatment Alternatives to Relieve Depression (STAR*D) Study. *Primary Care Companion to the Journal of Clinical Psychiatry, 9*(5), 331–337.

Swenson, S. L., Rose, M., Vittighoff, E., Stewart, A., & Schellinger, D. (2008). The influence of depressive symptoms on clinician-patient communication among patients with type 2 diabetes. *Medical Care, 46*(3), 257–265.

Tew, J. D., Jr., Mulsant, B. H., Haskett, R. F., Prudic, J., Tase, M. E., Crowe, R. R., et al. (1999). Acute efficacy of ECT in the treatment of major depression in the old-old. *American Journal of Psychiatry, 156*(12), 1865–1870.

Thase, M. E., Friedman, E. S., Biggs, M. M., Wisniewski, S. R., Trivedi, M. H., Luther, J. F., et al. (2007). Cognitive therapy versus medication in augmentation and switch strategies as second-step treatments: A STAR*D report. *American Journal of Psychiatry, 164*(5), 739–752.

Turner, E. H., & Rosenthal, R. (2008). Efficacy of antidepressants. *British Medical Journal, 336*(7643), 516–517.

Ugarriza, D. N. (2002). Elderly women's explanation of depression. *Journal of Gerontological Nursing, 28*(5), 54–55.

Videbech, P. (2000). PET measurements of brain glucose metabolism and blood flow in major depressive disorder: A critical review. *Acta Psychiatrica Scandanavica, 101*(1), 11–20.

Wagner, B., Knaevelsrud, C., & Maercker, A. (2007). Internet-based cognitive-behavioral therapy for complicated grief: A randomized controlled trial. *Death Studies, 30*(5), 429–453.

Wang, P. S., Patrick, A. R., Dormuth, C. R., Avorn, J., Maclure, M., Canning, C. F., & Schneeweiss, S. (2008). The impact of cost sharing on antidepressant use among older adults in British Columbia. *Psychiatric Services, 59*(4), 377–383.

Watson, J. (2008). *Nursing: Philosophy and science of caring (revised and updated* edition). Boulder: University of Colorado Press.

Wells, K. B., Katon, W., Rogers, B., & Camp, P. (1994). Use of minor tranquilizers and antidepressant medications by depressed outpatients: Results from the medical outcomes study. *American Journal of Psychiatry, 151*, 694–700.

Wells, K. B., Stewart, A., Hays, R. D., Burnam, M. A., Rogers, W., Daniels, M., et al. (1989). The functioning and well-being of depressed patients: Results from the medical outcomes study. *Journal of the American Medical Association, 272*(7), 914–919.

Whitaker, R. C., Orzol, S. M., & Kahn, R. S. (2007). The co-occurrence of smoking and a major depressive episode among mothers 15 months after delivery. *Preventive Medicine, 45*(6), 476–480.

Wiedenbach, E. (1964). *Clinical nursing: A helping art.* New York: Springer.

Wilson, K. C., Mottram, P. G., & Vassilas, C. A. (2008). Psychotherapeutic treatments for older depressed people. *Cochrane Database of Systematic Reviews*(1).

Worden, J. W. (1991). *Grief counseling and grief therapy* (2nd ed.). New York: Springer.

Zauderer, C. R. (2008). A case study of postpartum depression & altered maternal-newborn attachment. *MCN American Journal of Maternal Child Nursing, 33*(3), 173–178.

LITERARY REFERENCES

Barnes, J. (1985). *Flaubert's parrot.* New York: Knopf.

Chekhov, A. (1954). Uncle Vanya. In *Plays* (E. Fen, Trans., pp. 185–247). New York: Viking.

Ch'i, K. (1980). Written on seeing the flowers and remembering my daughter. In R. F. Weir (Ed.), *Death in literature.* New York: Columbia University Press.

Fitzgerald, F. S. (1945). *The crack-up.* New York: New Directions.

Flaubert, G. (1983). Madame Bovary. In D. J. Enright (Ed.), *The Oxford book of death* (pp. 113–114). Oxford: Oxford University Press.

Svevo, I. (1949). *As a man grows older.* New York: New Directions.

Tolstoy, L. (1932/1882). *A confession and what I believe* (A. Maude, Trans.). Oxford, England: Oxford University Press.

Weinrich L. (Translation by Marshall R.) (1969) Peter Abaelard as Musician—II, *The Musical Quarterly.* 55:464–486.

SUGGESTED READINGS

Cohen, D. B. (1994). *Out of the blue: Depression and human nature.* New York: Norton.

Goodwin, F., & Redfield, K. (2007). *Manic-depressive illness.* New York: Oxford University Press.

Horwitz, A. V., & Wakefield, J. C. (2007). *The loss of sadness: How psychiatry transformed normal sadness into depressive disorder.* New York: Oxford University Press.

Jamison, K. R. (1993). *Touched with fire.* New York: Free Press.

Kramer, P. D. (2005). *Against depression.* New York: Viking.

Williams, J. M. G. (1995). *The psychological treatment of depression: A guide to the theory and practice of cognitive behavioral therapy.* New York: Routledge.

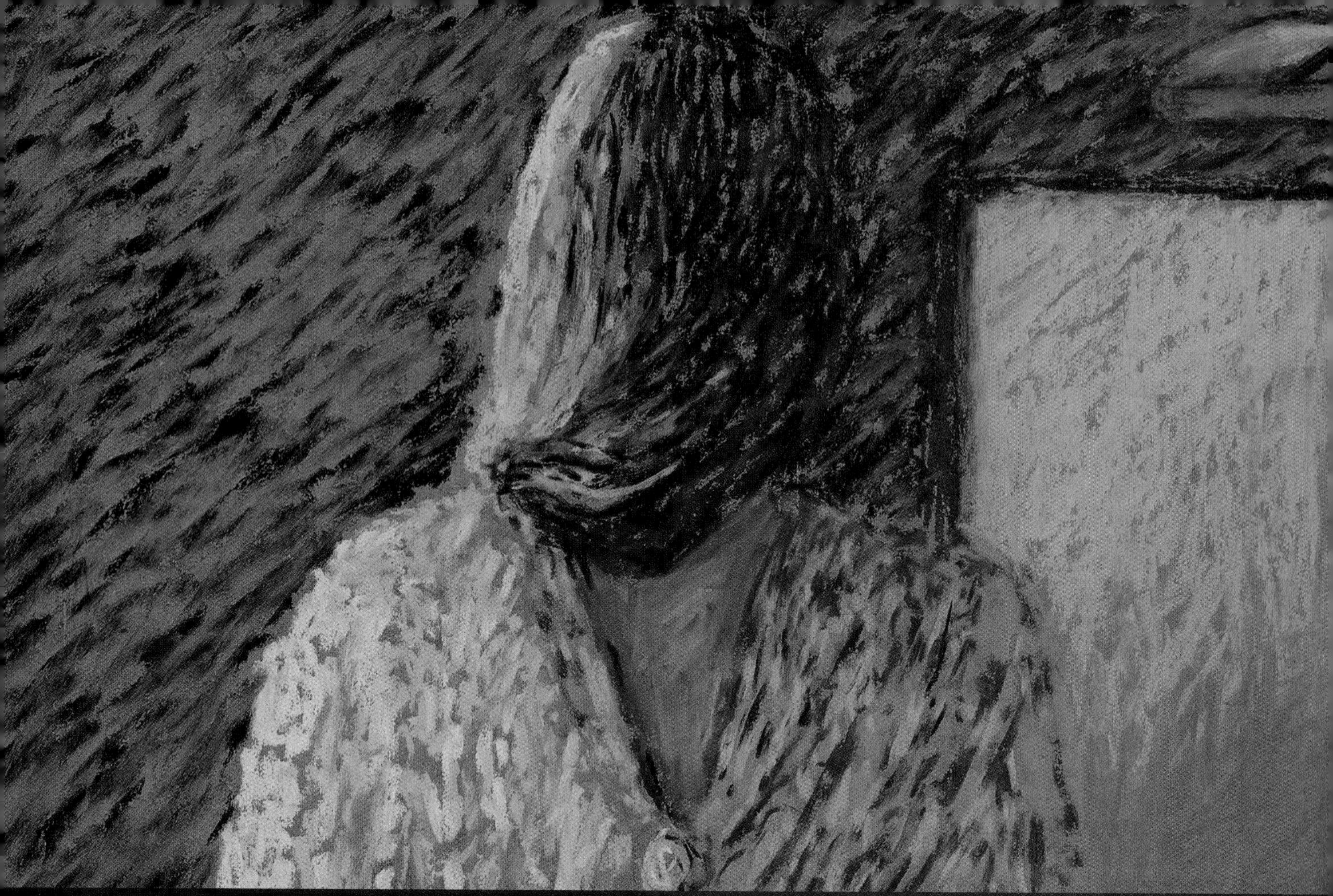

Going Up?

Life in the Fast Lane

Have you ever done any of the following?

- ***Neglected your physiological need for sleep because you were just too busy to rest?***
- ***Found yourself driving on a freeway late at night with the radio on and the windows open to keep yourself awake when you knew you should be in bed rather than driving?***
- ***Missed meals because work took precedence? Or eaten meals standing up, on the run, or in your car?***
- ***Been completely involved in your own projects, such that you could not really explain to other people what you were doing and why?***
- ***Neglected medical or dental appointments because you were just too busy?***
- ***Became upset with others who told you they just could not understand what you were up to?***

If you have experienced any of these situations, you have some notion of that part of life called "the fast lane." As you begin to learn about the mood disorder called mania, think of the disorder as an extension and exaggeration of the situations in which many of us find ourselves.

CHAPTER 15

The Client Experiencing Mania

NOREEN CAVAN FRISCH
LAWRENCE E. FRISCH

CHAPTER OUTLINE

COMPETENCIES

Upon completion of this chapter, the reader should be able to:

1. Define *mania* and state the behaviors associated with the condition.
2. Describe the cyclical relationship of mania and depression.
3. Explain the genetic and inherited nature of manic disease.
4. Describe the clinical course of mania.
5. Safely administer drugs in the treatment of mania.
6. Integrate nursing theory in assessing and understanding clients with mania.
7. Employ empathy in interactions with manic persons.
8. Use the nursing process and nursing diagnoses to plan and evaluate nursing care.

KEY TERMS

Bipolar Disorder (BPD)	Grandiosity	Rapid Cycling
Borderline Personality	Hypomania	Schizoaffective Disorder
Continuous Cycling	Mania	Switch Process
Cyclothymic Patterns	Manic Episode	

Mania is a term used to describe a common disorder associated with an elevated, expansive, or irritable mood. Although many individuals suffer from both mania and depression at times in their lives, mania is in many ways the exact opposite of depression. For example, individuals with depression have a depressed and slowed mood, whereas individuals experiencing mania generally have a markedly elevated mood. Manic individuals are talkative, excitable, and energetic, and their words and ideas often move rapidly from topic to topic. Self-esteem and libido are usually decreased in depression. By contrast, in mania, self-esteem is inflated, often to the point of **grandiosity**, and sexual behavior may be indiscriminately impulsive. Manic individuals often go for days without sleep, and they may indulge in buying sprees and other impulsive activities with potentially destructive consequences. Many manic individuals lose touch with reality and become psychotic. They may be paranoid, agitated, or delusional, and they may suffer from hallucinations. Manic clients may span the spectrum from fascinating, creative company to violent, out-of-control individuals, highly dangerous to themselves and others. For the manic client, "life is 'effortless,' 'charged with intensity,' and 'filled with special meaning.' [The person] is 'racing,' 'speeded up,' 'wired,' 'hyper,' 'high as a kite,' 'moving in the fast lane,' 'ecstatic,' 'full of energy,' 'flying.' Other people are described as 'too slow' and 'can't keep up'" (Goodwin & Jamison, 1990, p. 16).

Some psychiatrists have suggested that there are stages of mania, as illustrated in Table 15-1. As an individual moves between these stages, his mood, thinking, and behavior may all change. Like depression, mania is typically a cyclical disorder—affected individuals go into and out of episodes of mania that may last a few days to many weeks. In between manic episodes, most of these individuals are unaffected and may lead highly productive lives. In fact, as will be discussed later in this chapter, many individuals who suffer from mania seem to be unusually creative, and when well, they may be successful professionals and leaders.

In the early stages of mania, an individual may recognize that his behavior is manic, as in this writing of the poet Theodore Roethke about his own manic episode:

FOR NO REASON

*For no reason I started to feel very good. Suddenly I knew how to enter into the life of everything around me. I knew how it felt to be a tree, a blade of grass, even a rabbit. I didn't sleep much. I just walked around with this wonderful feeling. One day I was passing a diner and all of a sudden I knew what it felt like to be a lion. I went into the diner and said to the counter-man, "Bring me a steak. Don't cook it. Just bring it." So he brought me this raw steak and I started eating it. The other customers made like they were revolted, watching me. And I began to see that maybe it was a little strange.**

(Seager, 1991, p. 101)

In an excerpt from *Outside the Dog Museum*, the novelist Jonathan Carroll also captures some of the strange behavior seen in Stage I mania:

*From *The Glass House: The Life of Theodore Roethke* by Allan Seager, 1992, Ann Arbor: University of Michigan Press.

TABLE 15-1 Stages of Mania

	STAGE I	STAGE II	STAGE III
Mood	Liability of affect; euphoria predominates; irritability if demands not satisfied	Increased dysphoria and depression, open hostility and anger	Clearly dysphoric; panic stricken; hopeless
Cognition	Expansivity, grandiosity, over-confidence; thoughts coherent but occasionally tangential; sexual and religious preoccupation; racing thoughts	Flight of ideas; disorganization of cognitive state; delusions	Incoherent, definite loosening of associations; bizarre and idiosyncratic delusions; hallucinations in one-third of patients; disorientation to time and place; occasional ideas of reference
Behavior	Increased psychomotor activity; increased initiation and rate of speech; increased spending, smoking, telephone use	Continued increased psychomotor acceleration; increased pressured speech; occasional assaultive behavior	Frenzied and frequently bizarre psychomotor activity

Source: "The Stages of Mania: A Longitudinal Analysis of the Manic Episode" by G. A. Carlson and F. K. Goodwin, 1973, *Archives of General Psychiatry*, *28*, 221–228.

GOING INSANE

There was no screech of tires, screams, or thunderous crash when my mind went flying over the cliff into madness, as I gather is true in many cases. Besides, we've all seen too many bad movies where characters scratch their faces or make hyena sounds to indicate they've gone nuts.

Not me. One minute I was famous, successful, self-assured Harry Radcliffe in the trick store, looking for inspiration in a favorite spot. The next, I was quietly but very seriously mad, walking out of that shop with two hundred and fifty yellow pencil sharpeners. I don't know how other people go insane, but my way was at least novel.

Melrose Avenue is not a good place to lose your mind. The stores on the street are full of lunatic desires and are only too happy to let you have them if you can pay. I could.

*Anyone want an African gray parrot named Noodle Koofty? I named him in the ride back to Santa Barbara. He sat silently in a giant black cage in the back of my Mercedes station wagon, surrounded by objects I can only cringe at when I think of them now: three colorful garden dwarves about three feet high, each holding a gold hitching ring; five Conway Twitty albums that cost twenty dollars each because they were "classics"; three identical Sam the Sham and the Pharaohs albums, "classics" as well, twenty-five dollars a piece; a box of bathroom tiles with a revolting peach motif; a wall-size poster of a chacma baboon in the same pose as Rodin's The Thinker ... other things too, but you get the drift.**

(Carroll, 1992, pp. 16–17)

Although this last excerpt is from a novel, an almost identical story comes from the real-life descriptions of a manic individual:

MANIA

*Unfortunately, for manics anyway, mania is a natural (if unnatural) extension of the economy. What with credit cards and bank accounts there is little beyond reach. So, I bought twelve snake bite kits, with a sense of urgency and importance. I bought precious stones, elegant and unnecessary furniture, three watches within an hour of one another (in the Rolex rather than Timex class) ... and totally inappropriate siren-like clothes. During one spree I spent several hundreds on books having titles or covers that somehow caught my fancy: ... twenty sundry Penguin books because I thought it could be nice if the penguins could form a colony, five Puffin books for a similar reason ... I imagine I must have spent far more than $30,000 during my two manic episodes.**

(Goodwin & Jamison, 1990, p. 29)

Although the experience of Stage I mania is often described as highly pleasant with "great joy and elation" (Goodwin & Jamison, 1990, p. 26), as mania persists and progresses, it takes on more frightening, or ego-dystonic, aspects:

THE FIRST TIME I WAS MANIC

In fact, the most awful I have ever felt in my entire life ... was the first time I was manic. I had been high many

*From *Outside the Dog Museum* by J. Carroll, 1992, New York: Doubleday. Reprinted with permission.

*Excerpted from *Manic Depressive Illness* by Frederick K. Goodwin and Kay Redfield Jamison, 1990. Oxford, England: Oxford University Press, Inc. Reprinted with permission.

*times before, but they had never been frightening experiences—ecstatic at best, confusing at worst. In fact, I had learned to accommodate quite well to them. I developed mechanisms of self-control to keep down the peals of otherwise singularly inappropriate laughter, and rigid limits on my irritability. I learned to avoid situations that might otherwise trip or jangle my hypersensitive wiring, and I learned to pretend I was paying attention or following a logical point when my mind was off chasing rabbits in a thousand directions. My work and professional life flowed. But nowhere did this, or my upbringing, or my intellect, or my character, prepare me for insanity. Although I had been building up to this for weeks, and certainly knew something was seriously wrong, there still was a definite point when I knew I was insane. My thoughts were so fast that I couldn't remember the beginning of a sentence halfway through. Fragments of ideas, images, sentences raced around and around.... Finally ... they became meaningless melted pools. Nothing once familiar to me was familiar. I wanted desperately to slow down but could not. Nothing helped—not running around a parking lot for hours on end or swimming for miles. My energy level was untouched by anything I did.**

(Goodwin & Jamison, 1990, p. 27)

BOX 15-1
MANIC BEHAVIORS

- Inflated self-esteem or grandiosity
- Decreased need for sleep (e.g., feels rested after only three hours of sleep)
- More talkative than usual or pressure to keep talking
- Flight of ideas or subjective experience that thoughts are racing
- Distractibility (i.e., attention too easily drawn to unimportant or irrelevant external stimuli)
- Increase in goal-directed activity (either socially, at work or school, or sexually) or psychomotor agitation
- Excessive involvement in pleasurable activities that have a high potential for painful consequences (e.g., engaging in unrestrained buying sprees, sexual indiscretions, or foolish business investments)

From *Diagnostic and Statistical Manual of Mental Disorders, Fourth Edition-Text Revision*, 2000, Washington, D.C. American Psychiatric Association. Reprinted with permission.

MANIA

Although the excerpts provide an intuitive idea of which behaviors are considered manic, there are specific definitions of mania. These are divided into categories, based on the severity of the symptoms.

Manic Episode

A **manic episode** is defined as follows:

- A distinct period of abnormally and persistently elevated, expansive, or irritable mood lasting at least one week (or any duration if hospitalization is necessary).
- During the period of mood disturbance, three (or more) of the specific symptoms listed in Box 15-1 have persisted to a significant degree.

For a diagnosis of a manic episode, symptoms causing marked impairment in job or personal functioning that are not due to illness, drugs, or medications must be present.

Hypomania

Although extreme mania is clearly abnormal, some experts believe that there is no fine line dividing normal happiness and mild mania—indeed most of us probably have some maniclike experiences at times in our lives (Klerman, 1981). Mild manic states may become abnormal when they are recurrent, lengthy, and associated with change in functioning, uncharacteristic of the person when not symptomatic (American Psychiatric Association, 2000). In an effort to capture this difference between normal happiness and mild mania, the fourth edition, text revision of the *Diagnostic and Statistical Manual* (DSM-IV-TR) also defines **hypomania**. The defining characteristics of hypomania include the same seven criteria for mania, but to diagnose hypomania, only three symptoms need be present, and these need only have lasted four days. In contrast to mania, hypomanic symptoms need not cause any disturbance in functioning, but must be observable by others.

*Excerpted from *Manic Depressive Illness* by Frederick K. Goodwin and Kay Redfield Jamison, 1990. Oxford, England: Oxford University Press, Inc. Reprinted with permission.

Bipolar Disorders

Whereas mania is an important psychiatric condition and requires unique nursing and medical interventions, it is most commonly seen along with Major Depressive Disorder (MDD). The combination of mania and depression is typically referred to as **Bipolar Disorder (BPD)**. Although clients may be depressed and manic at the same time, the two conditions most commonly occur sequentially—most often the mania comes first, followed soon after by depression. Psychiatrists refer to the mood change from mania to depression or depression to mania as the **switch process**. The

The Devil and Daniel Johnston

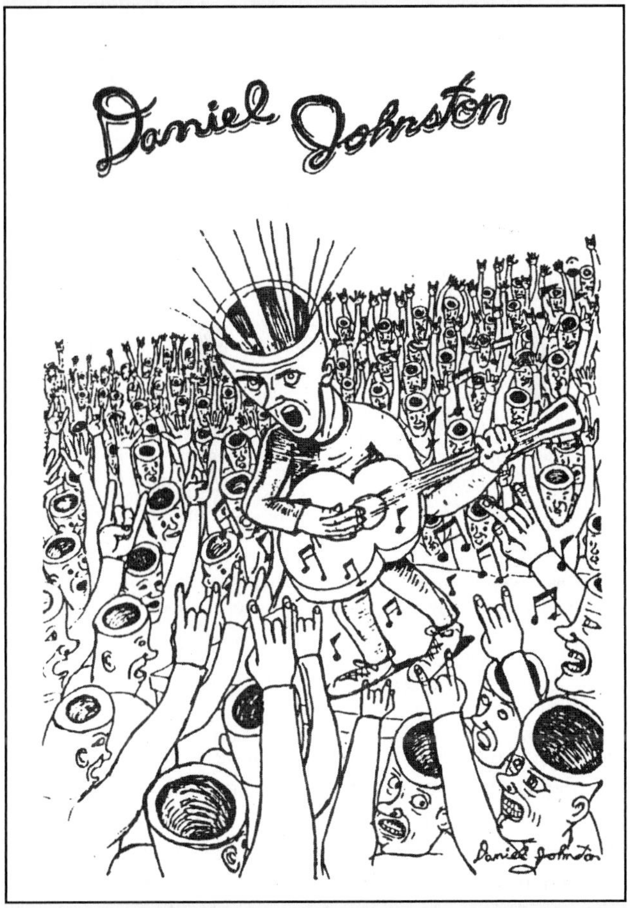

Courtesy: Sony Pictures/The Kobal Collection

The Devil and Daniel Johnston portrays musician/cartoonist Johnston's struggles with Bipolar Disorder—here powerfully portrayed through one of Johnston's drawings.

association between depression and mania has been recognized for more than 2,000 years:

ARETAEUS

*According to Aretaeus (100 AD), the classical form of mania was the bipolar one: the patient who previously was gay, euphoric, and hyperactive suddenly "has a tendency to melancholy; he becomes, at the end of the attack, languid, sad, taciturn, he complains that he is worried about his future, he feels ashamed." "Melancholia is without any doubt the beginning and even part of the disorder called mania."**

(Roccataggliata, 1986, pp. 230–231)

This linkage between mania and depression had not been forgotten when in 1679, Brouchier wrote about a client:

"There are twin symptoms, which are her constant companions, Mania and Melancholy, and they succeed each other in a double and alternate act" (Goodwin & Jamison, 1990, p. 45). While the association between these disorders has been long and consistently recognized, modern clinicians now regard mania and depression (when they occur together in the same client) as a single disorder with two manifestations. This synthesis into the term bipolar or manic-depressive illness was most decisively made in the early years of this century by the German psychiatrist Kraepelin. In 1988, Post and coworkers at the National Institute of Mental Health summarized Bipolar Disorder graphically. Figure 15-1 presents a summary of the clinical course of 82 bipolar persons (Post, Roy-Bryne, & Uhde, 1988). From this representation, it can be seen that depression and mania may occur either separately or in close proximity to each other. These early studies on the course of Bipolar Disorder have been recently augmented by a system of symptom recording using a home computer (Bauer, Grof, Gyulai, Rasgon, Glenn, & Whybrow, 2004). This technique can potentially provide researchers with more accurate and comprehensive data on the course of symptoms in Bipolar Disorder. Joffe, MacQueen, Marriott, and Trevor-Young (2004) have used more traditional life-charting data to track the course of symptoms in nearly 200 clients with Bipolar Disorder followed for a mean duration of three years. These authors have shown that, in contrast to the data in Figure 15-1, which implies that clients have relatively long periods free of symptoms, individuals with Bipolar Disorder spend a significant proportion of their lives confronting the symptoms of mania or depression, or both. With treatment these symptoms are usually not severe enough to meet diagnostic criteria for mental illness, but they may greatly influence quality of life. The work of Joffe and colleagues emphasizes that studies of the efficacy of treatment may need to focus on the client's perception of benefit, not on DSM-based diagnostic criteria. Except when due to organic causes, mania almost never occurs without depression—nearly all persons with mania have a form of Bipolar Disorder (Suppes, Dennehy, & Gibbons, 2000).

DSM-IV-TR defines two types of bipolar major depressive disorders: Bipolar I and Bipolar II. Bipolar I is classic manic-depressive disease, with the combination of depression and at least one episode of mania. Bipolar II is diagnosed when one hypomanic episode has accompanied major depression but there has been no mania. DSM-IV-TR also describes **cyclothymic patterns** in which individuals cycle between hypomanic and melancholic states but do not qualify for a diagnosis of Major Depressive Disorder (and hence Bipolar II).

EPIDEMIOLOGY

Epidemiological surveys are consistent in showing that neither mania nor Bipolar Disorder are particularly common in the population as a whole. Leff, Fischer, and Bertelson (1976) found that only 2.6 persons per 100,000 were newly hospitalized for mania each year. Others have suggested that

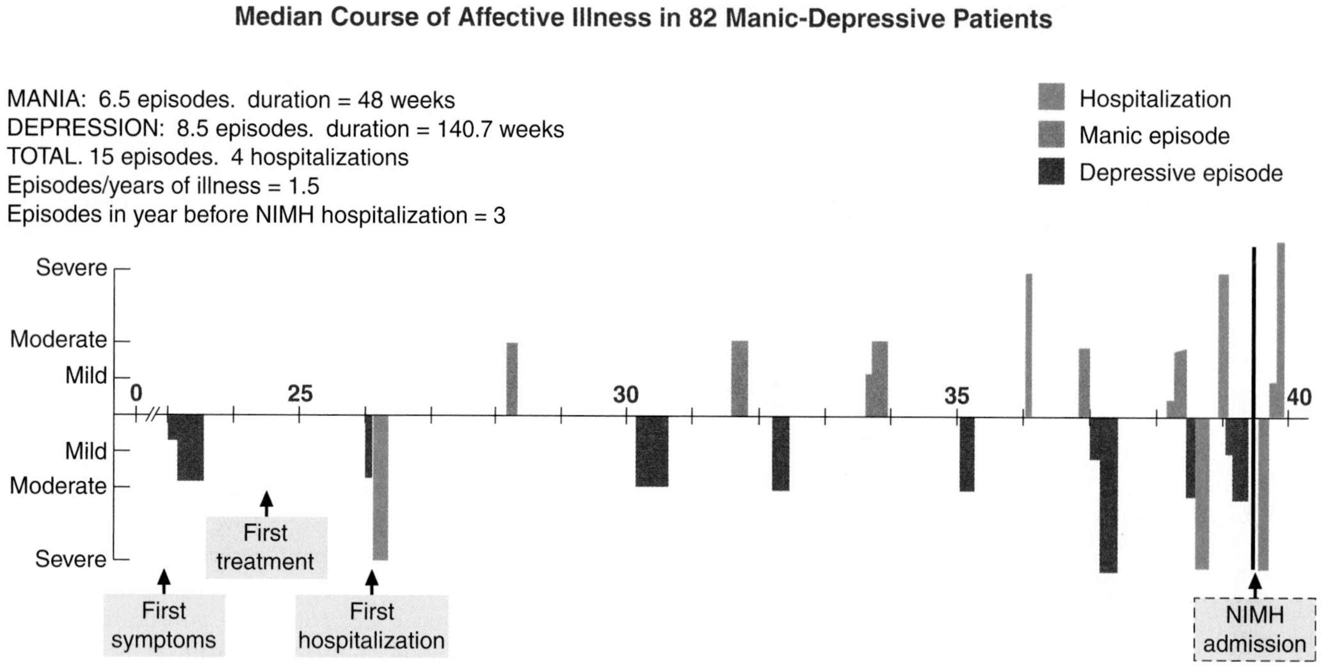

FIGURE 15-1 Clinical course of mania (FROM GRAPHIC REPRESENTATION OF THE LIFE COURSE OF ILLNESS IN PATIENTS WITH AFFECTIVE DISORDER, 145, 847, 1988. AVAILABLE AT HTTP://AJP.PSYCHIATRYONLINE.ORG. REPRINTED WITH PERMISSION FROM THE AMERICAN PSYCHIATRIC ASSOCIATION.)

mania (of a degree requiring hospitalization) is the rarest of all the major psychoses (Krauthammer & Klerman, 1979). While severe mania may be relatively rare, the nurse working at a community mental health facility is certain to see this condition regularly, in part because individuals with severe mania often experience recurrent manic episodes. For example, in a random community-based household survey, Fogarty, Russell, Newman, and Bland (1994) found a lifetime prevalence of mania of 0.6%, but in those who reported mania, the mean number of manic episodes was 23. A Danish study evaluating over 2 million individuals found that 2,299 of these persons received a diagnosis of Bipolar Disorder during the collective follow-up of over 30 million "person years" (Mortensen, Pedersen, Melbye, Mors, & Ewald, 2003). This is a significantly lower incidence than in some of the other studies noted previously. The authors noted several factors that increased an individual's likelihood of being diagnosed with Bipolar Disorder. These included having a first-degree relative (parent, sibling) with Bipolar Disorder or experiencing the loss of a parent prior to age five. The same Danish group has also reported that suicide of a mother or sibling greatly increases the risk of hospitalization for mania (Kessing, Agerbo, & Mortensen 2004). Other stressful life events that the authors found moderately associated with mania included recent unemployment, divorce, or marriage.

Although severe mania is relatively rare, the milder forms, for which clients may often not seek hospitalization—or even treatment—are not uncommon. The Epidemiologic Catchment Area Study (discussed in more detail in Chapter 8) found lifetime prevalence rates for Bipolar I Disorder of 4.4% (Weissman, Bruce, Leaf, Florio, & Holzer, 1991). This means that over a lifetime, about 4% of individuals are likely to experience at least one manic episode. Unipolar depressive disorder is about two to four times more common than is bipolar disease, but the difference in rate of occurrence is obscured somewhat by the way in which the two conditions affect men and women differently. Since women are about twice as likely to be affected by unipolar depression as are men, but women are no more likely than are men to have Bipolar Disorder, some of the difference in rate between the two conditions is due to the increased frequency of Unipolar Disorder in women. Depressive disease in men is about evenly divided between unipolar and Bipolar Disorder (Shivakumar, Bernstein, & Suppes, 2008). The course of Bipolar Disorder differs significantly between sexes as well (Arnold, 2003). Bipolar II, predominant depression, and (as noted next) rapid cycling are more common in women. Women with Bipolar Disorder have more associated medical and psychiatric disorders (perhaps in part because the onset of bipolar illness is later in women than in men).

While women may not have a higher overall incidence of bipolar depression than do men, the length of their symptom cycles can be different in important ways from those of men. One of the major characteristics of Bipolar Disorder is cycle length: the time between episodes. While cycle length may vary from weeks to years and may gradually accelerate over time (with episodes eventually coming more frequently; see Figure 15-1), psychiatric epidemiologists have arbitrarily divided persons with manic-depressive disorder into those with long and those with short cycle lengths, the latter being called *rapid cyclers*. Rapid cyclers are defined as individuals who have four or more episodes in a year. Although the overall incidence of Bipolar Disorder does not differ much between men and women, nearly all rapid cyclers are women

(Kupka, Luckenbauth, Post, et al., 2005; Pariser, 1993). Rapid cyclers may be particularly difficult to treat, so that while rapid cyclers constitute only 13% to 20% of persons with manic-depressive disorder (Calabrese & Woyshville, 1994), these persons may seek care more frequently than would be predicted from their absolute numbers.

Although the onset of bipolar disease can occur from childhood to old age, on average persons with Bipolar Disorder tend to become ill in their thirties or before, a decade earlier than do those with unipolar disease (Goodwin & Jamison, 1990). In recent years, Bipolar Disorder has been increasingly diagnosed in adolescents and children. Because symptoms of mania may differ in young children from those in adults, this disorder is discussed at greater length in Chapter 23. There also has been increased recognition of the importance of Bipolar Disorder among the elderly (Sajatovic, 2002). While Sajotovic reports that up to 19% of depression in the elderly is due to Bipolar Disorder, there is still much to be learned about the degree to which this disorder contributes to illness among elders. Bipolar Disorder seems to occur with fairly comparable incidence among persons of widely differing ethnicity and race. Carefully controlled studies in China have suggested few differences from manic-depressive disorder seen in the United States (Dunner, Jie, Ping, & Dunner, 1984). Although most mental illness seems to disproportionately affect the poor, at least some forms of bipolar disease occur more often among the well-off, particularly affecting men with professional or managerial jobs (Coryell, Endicott, Keller, Anderson, Growe, Hirschfield, et al., 1989).

Most of the previous observations apply largely to Bipolar I disorder. The frequency of Bipolar II disorder is less well understood. One study suggested a community prevalence of between 8% and 12% percent (double that for Bipolar I; Goodwin & Jamison, 1990), but subsequent studies suggest that about 5% of persons will develop Bipolar II symptoms sometime in their life (Benazzi, 2007).

ETIOLOGY

MOLECULAR BASIS

A very striking finding about bipolar depressive disorder is its tendency to be inherited. Some of the best data on the inheritance of manic-depressive illness come from studies of twins (Goodwin & Jamison, 1990). If one of two identical twins is manic-depressive, the other is almost certain to develop the disease. For fraternal twins (who share much less of their genetic makeup), the risk is much lower, about 20%. Although social and environmental factors surely play a role in how (and perhaps whether) some mental illness develops, genetics seems to be the strongest influence for manic-depressive disorder. Even when identical twins are separated early in life and brought up in completely different adoptive families, when one has manic-depressive disorder, the risk for the second twin seems to be at least 70%. Manic-depressive disorder is not only shared between twins, it is also often passed from parents to their children.

MARIANA

With blackest moss the flower-plots
Were thickly crusted, one and all:
The rusted nails fell from the knots
That held the pear to the gable-wall.
The broken sheds looked sad and strange:
Unlifted was the clinking latch;
Weeded and worn the ancient thatch
Upon the lonely moated grange.
She only said, "My life is dreary,
He cometh not," she said;
She said, "I am aweary, aweary,
*I would that I were dead!"**

(Tennyson, 1830)

Here is Tennyson at his poetic gloomiest and seemingly a match for the tragic story told by Jamison's psychological genealogy of the Tennyson family (Figure 15-2). While the Tennyson family tree illustrates a remarkable inheritance of mental illness, including manic-depressive disease, it also illustrates the inheritance of both unipolar and bipolar depression within manic-depressive families. The finding that unipolar depression is common in relatives of clients with Bipolar Disorder has been shown in more formal studies as well—clients with manic-depressive disorder are two to three times more likely to have relatives with Unipolar or Bipolar Disorder than are controls (Gershon, Hamovil, Guroff, Dibble, Leckman, & Banney, 1982). Children of parents with Bipolar Disorder are about ten times more likely to develop bipolar symptoms than are children of unaffected parents (Craddock & Jones, 1999). Further, diagnosis of early onset bipolar disease is higher for children whose first-degree relatives have Bipolar 1 Disorder than for those whose relatives do not have such a diagnosis (Wozniak, 2007).

Although twin studies and case-control studies provide strong evidence that manic-depressive disorder is often inherited, in recent years, geneticists have sought stronger confirmation of the way in which Bipolar Disorder is transmitted. There are potentially two approaches to obtaining this confirmation. The first is to define a defective gene product (typically a protein) thought to cause manic-depressive illness and then look for its presence in affected persons and their relatives. This approach has not yet proved possible. The second approach is to seek other well-defined genetic conditions that are inherited along with Bipolar Disorder. Often, the conditions sought produce no symptoms but are only detected by chemical analysis of protein or DNA. These kinds of studies, known as linkage studies, can be powerful genetic tools and have been remarkably productive in studying other psychiatric/neurological conditions (Gusella, Wexler, Conneally, Naylor, Anderson, Tanzi, et al., 1983). Multiple linkages have been found and experts in psychiatric

*From *Poems & Plays* by A. Tennyson, 1968, Oxford, England: Oxford University Press. Reprinted with permission.

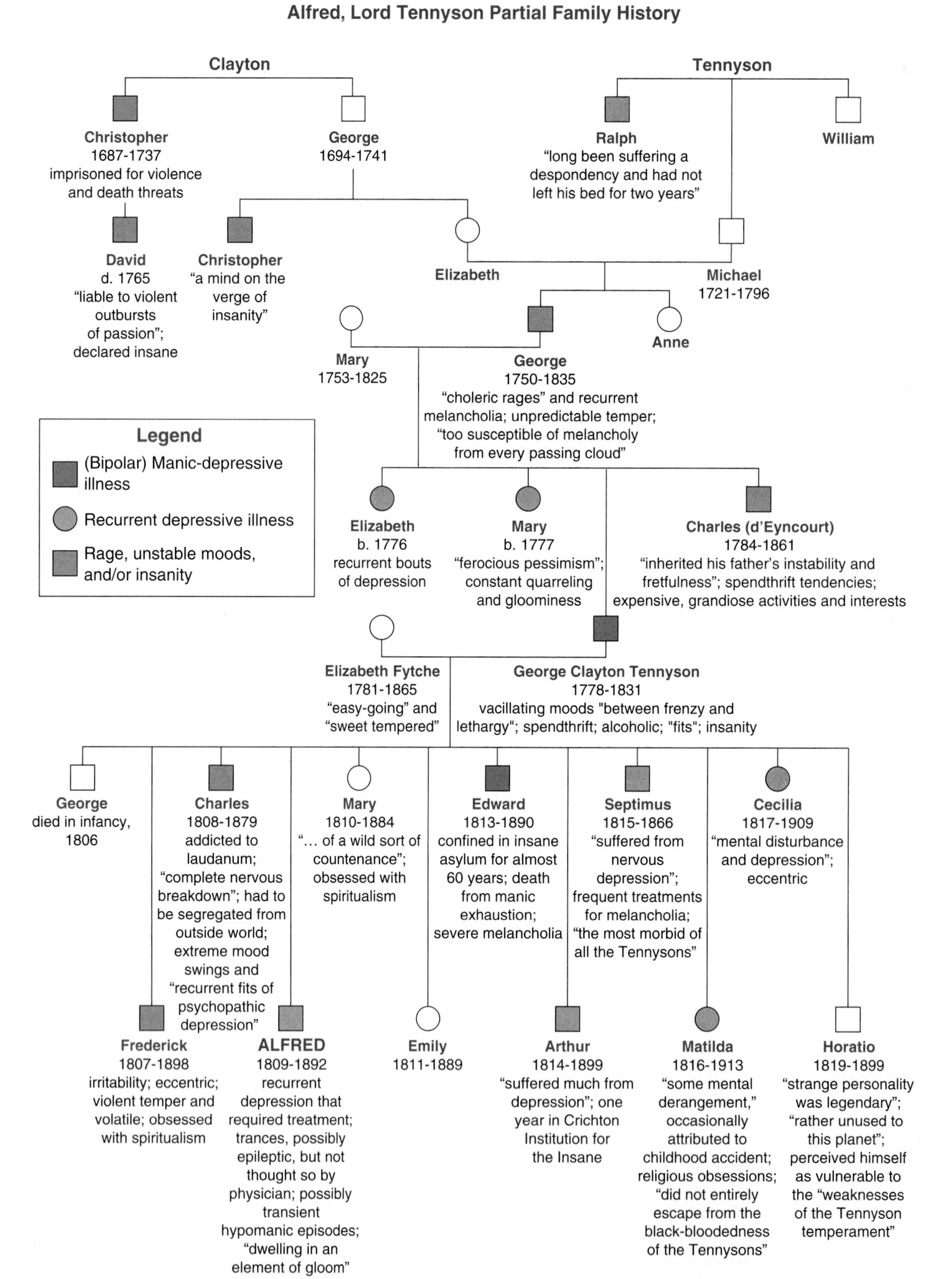

FIGURE 15-2 **Psychologic genealogy: Family with bipolar and depressive disease** (FROM *TOUCHED WITH FIRE: MANIC DEPRESSIVE ILLNESS AND THE ARTISTIC TEMPERAMENT* BY KAY REDFIELD JAMISON, 1993, ALL RIGHTS RESERVED. REPRINTED WITH PERMISSION OF THE FREE PRESS, A DIVISION OF SIMON & SCHUSTER ADULT PUBLISHING GROUP.)

genetics predict that the next decade should see major advances in the understanding of how genetics and environment affect the development of bipolar symptoms (Craddock & Jones, 1999). Some, if not all, investigators have reported links between Bipolar Disorder and genes for an enzyme that metabolizes serotonin in the brain. Such studies eventually could lead to a better understanding of Bipolar Disorder or even to new forms of treatment (Preisig, Bellivier, Fenton, Baud, Berney, Courtet, et al., 2000). Genetic studies, however, have so far failed to offer a comprehensive explanation for Bipolar Disorder (Kennedy, Farrer, Andreasen, Mayeux, & St. George-Hyslop, 2003). One of the most interesting ideas to emerge from genetic studies is a possible linkage between bipolar psychosis and schizophrenia. Both chromosomes 8p and 13q are associated with psychosis in both conditions—suggesting that there may be shared predispositions between these two conditions that are usually considered distinct (Goes, Sanders, & Potash, 2008). Further study on this connection may eventually break down long-lived distinctions between the two major psychotic disorders (Craddock, O'Donovan, & Owen, 2006).

The cause of manic-depressive illness is not known. There have been numerous theories about the factors causing the disorder, but none yet seems remotely adequate to explain the clinical findings. It is widely believed that manic-depressive disease is due to some genetically determined biochemical abnormality of the brain. Support for this view comes from the technique of positron emission tomography (PET) scanning. The PET scan is somewhat similar to the computed tomography (CT) scan, but instead of viewing brain structure, it detects areas of metabolic activity. While the significance of findings remains unknown, there do appear to be recognizable differences between brain metabolism in normal persons and in persons suffering from mania (Blumberg, Stern, Ricketts, Martinez, de Asis, White, et al., 1999). As noted in Chapter 14 on depression, many experts believe that abnormalities of brain neurotransmitters such as serotonin and dopamine play a major role in affective disorder. Bipolar clients have different patterns of urinary and plasma catecholamines than do unipolar depressed clients. Although these findings are interesting and fairly consistent (Goodwin & Jamison, 1990), they do not yet offer any clear causal information about bipolar depression. Studies focusing on brain signaling pathways have suggested that Bipolar Disorder may involve abnormalities in these brain functions (Bezchlibnyk & Young, 2002). The ERK-MAPK (extracellular signal regulated kinase/mitogen activated protein kinase) pathway has been a prime suspect, largely because of its association with apparent mania in a mouse model (Einat, Manji, Gould, Du, & Chen, 2003). Lithium, a drug highly effective in treating mania, appears to act on ERK-MAPK pathways in the brain. Because this pathway is highly complex (http://www.emdbiosciences.com) and because it plays a role in many process—not just those involving mania—it is unlikely that a final view of the cause of bipolar depression will emerge soon. Other complex pathways may also be involved in the production and treatment of mania (Gould & Manji, 2002). One emerging challenge is identifying individuals with depression who have latent Bipolar Disorder—and consequently may benefit from mood stabilization in addition to treatment for depression. There is some evidence that neuroimaging techniques may allow this distinction to be made early in the course of depressive symptoms (Keener & Phillips, 2007).

One of the interesting goals of research on Bipolar Disorder has been to define the molecular basis for the switch process—the change, often very sudden, between depressive and manic states. Work on switching has been limited by the great difficulty in distinguishing between cause and effect. Although a given measurement—typically an increase in a chemical substance in blood, urine, or spinal fluid—may cause switching, it may also be, like the observed change in mood, merely the result of switch.

Switching from depression to mania may often be provoked by antidepressant medication, especially tricyclics (Compton & Nemeroff, 2000). St. John's wort, a preparation currently unregulated by the FDA and available without prescription, has been reported to provoke switching in some individuals who use it to treat depressive episodes (Nierenberg, Burt, Matthews, & Weiss, 1999). There is some evidence that selective serotonin reuptake inhibitors (SSRIs) have a decreased risk of provoking switching (Parker & Parker, 2003). *Discontinuation* of antidepressants may also lead to mania in some individuals (Ali & Milev, 2003). Some neurophysiologists have evoked the concept of "kindling" to explain aspects of the course of Bipolar Disorder, especially the switch process from depression to mania. Further research will be required to assess the importance of current observations to clinical treatment (Barley, 1999).

Other Causes

Drugs

A diagnosis of a manic episode can be made only when symptoms have no definable organic cause. Some illnesses and many drugs can precipitate mania. It is important that these factors be considered before a client is labeled with a psychiatric diagnosis or potentially treated inappropriately. Although persons of any age may have organic causes of mania, since most manic episodes present for the first time before the age of 40, organic causes should always be sought in older adults presenting with a first episode of mania (Young & Klerman, 1992).

Alcohol and drug withdrawal (particularly from benzodiazepines) are among the most common extrinsic factors leading to agitated states and may be particularly hard to diagnose if, as is often the case, clients do not admit to drug use. The elderly are particularly sensitive to drug effects and may develop either mania or delirium in response either to single drugs or to polypharmacy (the administration of multiple drugs, often for multiple medical indications). Common drugs that may induce mania in clients of any age include oral corticosteroids and levodopa. Clients taking anabolic steroids may be at particular risk for mania and may not admit to steroid use even if asked (Pope & Katz, 1994). Other medications that may occasionally cause mania include baclofen, bromocriptine, captopril, chloroquine, and thyroxine (Peet & Peters, 1995). Intoxicated persons (particularly with stimulant drugs such as cocaine, PCP, or amphetamines) frequently present with mania.

Physical Disease

A wide range of diseases can also produce mania. Among infectious diseases, syphilis, human immunodeficiency virus (HIV), and Lyme disease should always be considered (Fallon, Nields, Parsons, Liebowitz, & Klein, 1993; Baillargeon, Ducate, Pulvino, Bradshaw, Murray, & Olivera, 2003). Thyroid and other endocrine abnormalities (particularly Cushing's disease or syndrome) can cause manic symptoms. Many neurological conditions, including brain tumors and the aftermath of brain injury from trauma or stroke, can precipitate mania (Strakowski, McElroy, Keck, & West, 1994). Wilson's disease, an uncommon treatable inherited disorder of copper metabolism, may rarely present with mania (Machado, Deguti, Caixeta, Spitz, Lucato, & Barbosa, 2008).

CLINICAL COURSE

As emphasized in Figure 15-1, the spectrum of Bipolar I Disorder includes recurrent episodes of both mania and depression. Episodes may last several months to a year or more and are often shortened by effective treatment. For any given person, the length of episodes is fairly constant, with manic episodes typically somewhat shorter than depressive episodes (Goodwin & Jamison, 1990). The following excerpt relates how suddenly manic episodes can appear:

IN THE SUMMER OF 1955

*In the summer of 1955 when I was 33, the thousand unacknowledged human ... pressures in my being exploded. I ran barefooted in the streets, spat at members of my own family, exposed myself, was almost bodily thrown out of the house of a Nobel Prize-winning author, and believed God had ordained me to act out every conceivable human impulse without an ounce of hypocritical caution.**

(*Krim, 1961, p. 64*)

Depressive symptoms are generally thought more likely to develop over days or weeks, although, as in the following personal description by the famous psychologist William James, they can also occur with striking rapidity:

SUDDENLY

*Suddenly there fell upon me without any warning, just as if it came out of the darkness, a horrible fear of my own existence. Simultaneously there arose in my mind the image of an epileptic patient whom I had seen in the asylum, a black-haired youth with greenish skin, entirely idiotic, who used to sit all day on one of the benches ... with his knees drawn up against his chin.... This image and my fear entered into a species of combination with the other.... It was as if something hitherto solid within my breast gave way entirely, and I became a mass of quivering fear. After this the universe was changed for me altogether.... (My fear) gradually faded, but for months I was unable to go out into the dark alone.**

(*James, 1961, pp. 160–161*)

Individual episodes in clients with manic-depressive disease may be either manic or depressive. Manic and depressive phases may follow each other rapidly (Winokur, Clayton, & Reich, 1969), or clients may have only a single episode of either mania or depression. About half of persons with Bipolar Disorder begin their illnesses each with a single depressive episode and no history of mania. Individuals differ widely in cycle length, with more than four episodes per year defined as **rapid cycling**; occasional clients exhibit **continuous cycling**, which is defined as recurrent movement from mania to depression without an intervening normal period.

Social Prognosis

Although continuous cyclers do not have normal intercycle periods, the remainder of bipolar individuals seem quite unaffected between episodes. On recovery, many return successfully to their families and jobs; however, the social prognosis of Bipolar Disorder is not uniformly good. In one study where clients were followed up six months after hospital admission for mania, 80% were free of symptoms, but only 21% were fully employed (Dion, Tohen, Anthony, & Watermaux, 1988). In a longer follow-up study, significant psychosocial and occupational impairments were documented in clients, despite remissions of up to two years (Coryell, Scheftner, Keller, Endicott, Maser, & Klerman, 1993). A more current study reports that those with Bipolar Disorder lose approximately 65 workdays per year as a result of severe and persistent depressive episodes (Kessler Akiskal, Ames, Birnbaum Greenberg, Hirshfeld, et al, 2006). This study concluded that lost workdays are associated more often with the depressive than the manic phases of the disease.

Clients with manic-depressive disorder not only have psychosocial difficulties as a result of their illness, they are also at risk of dying from it. All-cause mortality is approximately twice as high for manic-depressive clients as for age-matched controls, but coexisting medical conditions seem to account for most natural causes of death (Black, Winokur, & Nasrallah, 1987). Suicide, discussed at more length in

*From *Views of a Nearsighted Cannoneer* by S. Krim, 1961, New York: Excelsior. Reprinted with permission.

*From *Varieties of Religious Experience* by William James. Copyright © 1961 by Macmillian Publishing Group. Reprinted with the permission of Scribner, an imprint of Simon and Schuster Adult Publishing Group.

> **NURSINGALERT 15-1**
>
> **Risk for Suicide in Mania**
>
> The risk of successful suicide in persons with mania increases in the presence of substance abuse or prior suicide attempt (Goodwin & Jamison, 1990).

Chapter 16, is a major risk for clients with Bipolar Disorder. Although one older study suggested that 46% of all suicides occur in persons with manic-depressive illness, this finding has not been corroborated by other studies. More consistently, researchers have found a high suicide rate among persons with Bipolar Disorder—as high as 60% in some studies, but with a mean of 19% (Goodwin & Jamison, 1990). One or more suicide attempts occur in 25% to 50% of persons diagnosed with Bipolar Disorder (Jamison, 2000).

There is some evidence that persons who are appropriately treated and intensively followed have diminished likelihood of suicide. Nonetheless, a retrospective review of 92 suicides by manic-depressive individuals found that 70% of these occurred despite high-quality medical and psychiatric care (Schou & Weeke, 1988). Treatment of Bipolar Disorder with lithium (see the treatment section) has been associated with a decreased risk of suicide compared to the use of divalproax, another common medication (Goodwin, Fireman, Simon, Hunkeler, Lee, & Revicki, 2003). The atypical psychotic medication clozapine may also reduce suicide risk (Muller-Oerlinghausen, Berghofer, & Ahrens, 2003).

Life Stress

Life stresses may precipitate manic-depressive illness, particularly the first-ever episode, but the majority of recurrent episodes seem to occur without external stimuli (Goodwin & Jamison, 1990). Sleep deprivation may sometimes trigger mania, and in some persons, symptoms seem to respond to restorative sleep (Nowlin-Finch, Altshuler, Szuba, & Mintz, 1994).

One of the curious, and not absolutely consistent, aspects of mania is its seasonal tendency. Numerous studies suggest that mania is more likely to present in the summer than at other times of the year (Takei, O'Callaghan, Sham, Glover, Tamura, & Murray, 1992).

ASSOCIATED DISORDERS/DUAL DIAGNOSES

Substance Abuse

One of the factors that complicates both the understanding and treatment of manic-depressive disorder is that many persons with this diagnosis have other complicating psychiatric diagnoses. Among such dual diagnoses, alcohol abuse plays a particularly important role since there are strong associations between Bipolar Disorder and alcohol abuse, especially in men. Although there are problems with consistent definition of alcohol abuse among different studies, about 35% of persons with manic-depressive disorder are said to abuse alcohol. The corresponding rate for the population as a whole is probably one-third to one-half of this (Goodwin & Jamison, 1990). At least one study suggested a much stronger relationship between alcoholism and mania than between alcohol and depression (Helzer & Prybeck, 1988). Although studies have not consistently shown higher alcohol intake during manic as compared to depressive phases, some observers have suggested steady and frequent drinking during mania contrasted with more binge drinking during depressive phases. There have been few studies comparing individuals with Bipolar I and Bipolar II Disorders, but where this question has been examined, alcohol abuse does seem to be associated with both diagnoses (Goodwin & Jamison, 1990). Nonalcoholic-substance abuse is similarly associated with Bipolar Disorder (Ringen, Melle, Birkenaes, Engh, Faerden, Jonsdottir, et al., 2008; Ostacher & Sachs, 2006), cocaine being a particularly commonly used substance during manic episodes. Whether the high frequency of cocaine use reflects specific efforts to replicate or prolong manic euphoria or merely reflects community drug use patterns is unknown. Persons with Bipolar Disorders are also said to engage in excessive use of narcotics, marijuana, and hallucinogens. Tobacco abuse is extremely common among persons with Bipolar Disorder and is among the most dangerous associations, leading to loss of life and increased morbidity (Ziedonis, Williams, & Smelson, 2003). There are only limited data on the frequency with which persons with Bipolar Disorder are offered smoking cessation counseling and treatment. In a study of psychiatric practice utilizing the National Ambulatory Medical Care Survey, Himelhoch and Daumit (2003) report that clients with Bipolar Disorder were more likely to receive smoking-related counseling than were those with some other disorders. However, overall, only 13.4% of smokers in the study received any intervention for this addiction from psychiatric caregivers. This failure to prioritize smoking cessation is important because many patients with Bipolar Disorder are at high risk for cardiovascular disease—often related to the use of antipsychotic medications that lead to weight gain, diabetes, and metabolic syndrome (van Winkel, De Hert, Van Eyck, Hanssens, Wampers, Scheen, et al., 2008). The combination of any of these risks with smoking substantially increases the risk of heart attack or stroke. Varenicline (an effective medication to reduce nicotine craving) has limited usefulness in psychiatric clients as it may lead to mania in susceptible individuals with Bipolar Disorder (Kohen & Kremen, 2007). Bupropion—another useful adjunct to smoking cessation—is much less likely to cause manic switch, though this has been reported with high dosages (Goren & Levin, 2000) and it may be contraindicated in Bipolar Disorder (West, 2003).

Schizoaffective Disorder

A second very important dual diagnosis is **Schizoaffective Disorder**, bipolar type, a condition in which elements of schizophrenia combine with manic-depressive disorder. Schizoaffective persons have prolonged delusions and/or hallucinations, typically at times when their mood disorders (either mania or depression or both) are in remission. It is often difficult to determine whether persons have pure manic-depressive illness or are schizoaffective, but long-term prognosis may be worse for individuals in the latter category (Goodwin & Jamison, 1990). Since they are by definition psychotic, schizoaffective clients are more difficult to treat successfully than are purely manic-depressive individuals, and, like schizophrenics whom they resemble, they often have major difficulties holding jobs and maintaining personal relationships.

Borderline Personality

Clients with **borderline personality** often overlap diagnostically with Bipolar II disorder (Berrocal, Ruiz Moreno, Rando, Benvenuti, & Cassano, 2008). As discussed in Chapter 18, these individuals have very rapid mood swings that tend to react much more to their environment than do the moods of purely hypomanic clients. Recognizing subtle bipolar features is important in the assessment of borderline personality. If Bipolar II is present and not diagnosed, a manic attack may occasionally result from administering antidepressant medication to one who is bipolar but thought to be borderline—though the risk in Bipolar II Disorder is likely lower than in Bipolar I.

BIPOLAR DISORDER AND CREATIVITY

MADNESS

*The greatest of goods comes to us through madness.... The prophetess at Delphi and the priestesses at Dodona achieve much that is good for Greece when mad, both on a private and on a public level, whereas when sane they achieve little or nothing;.... Among the ancients too those who gave things their names did not regard madness as shameful or a matter of reproach; otherwise they would not have connected the very word with the finest of the sciences, that by which the future is judged, and named it "manic." No, they gave it the name thinking madness a fine thing.... The man who arrives at the doors of poetry without madness from the muses, persuaded that expertise will make him a good poet, both he and his poetry, the poetry of the sane, are eclipsed by that of the mad.**

(Plato in Rowe, 1974)

Thus, the ancient Greeks appreciated that madness and mania could form the basis for poetic inspiration. A remarkable number of modern poets, writers, artists, and musicians have suffered from manic-depressive disorder, and many psychologists and artistic critics have felt that this illness contributed significantly to their artistic greatness. Experts may not agree that the manic state truly facilitates artistic creativity—surely few individuals in Stage 2 or 3 mania are sufficiently in touch with reality to produce creatively—but there is little doubt that the unusual psychic energy and decreased needs for sleep associated with hypomania make for enhanced productivity. Perhaps the willingness to take risks seen in mania also has a counterpart in productive creative work, where risk taking may lead to unanticipated accomplishment.

Not only is manic-depressive illness frequently seen among creative artists, but striking mood swings also appear with some frequency among political and military leaders. When writing of historical figures or creative artists, it is of course highly risky to try to make psychological diagnoses from fragmentary sources. Despite this problem, Goodwin and Jamison (1990) suggest after careful consideration that a surprising array of famous historical figures may have suffered from elements of manic-depressive illness. Individuals considered by Goodwin and Jamison to have been influenced by cyclothymia or hypomania include Oliver Cromwell, Alexander Hamilton, Napoleon Bonaparte, Robert E. Lee, Theodore Roosevelt, Winston Churchill, and Benito Mussolini. Goodwin and Jamison note that biographies of notable poets, composers, and artists document a prevalence of extremes in mood; however, it is important to recognize that many creative persons have no psychopathology: "that the illness and its related temperaments are associated with creativity seems clear. The clinical, ethical, and social implications of this association are less so" (p. 367).

TREATMENT AND CLINICAL MANAGEMENT

Pharmacological Treatment

Acute Mania

The acute condition is most effectively treated with either mood stabilizers (lithium or divalproex) or neuroleptic (antipsychotic) agents (see also Chapter 27). Benzodiazepines (clonazepam [Klonopin] is frequently used) may occasionally be helpful in controlling nonpsychotic symptoms of pressured speech, hyperactivity, agitation, and anxiety, but there is no evidence that these agents add to the effectiveness of mood stabilizers or antipsychotics. The effectiveness of atypical neuroleptics such as olanzapine in the management of acute mania has been clearly shown through a series of randomized controlled trials (Rendell, Gijsmann, Keck, Goodwin, & Geddes, 2003). Valproic acid (divalproex) has a direct mood-stabilizing effect, and it may begin to work within 24 to 72 hours. Consequently, it is sometimes administered as part of the initial pharmacological treatment of

*From *Phaedrus and the Seventh and Eighth Letters* (2nd ed.) by Plato, translated by C. J. Rowe, 1988, 1986, Warminster, Wiltshire, England: Aris & Philips.

Tasso in the Asylum by Eugene Delacroix

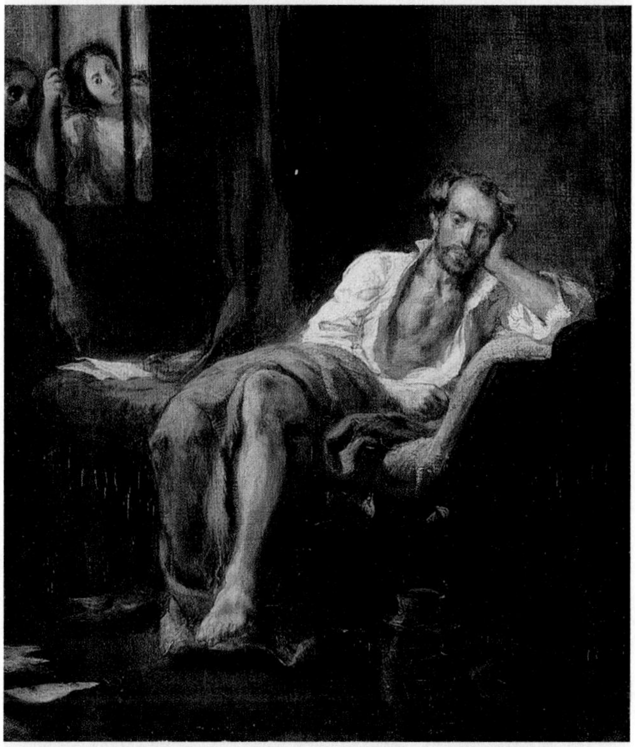

Courtesy: Oskar Reinhart Collection, "Am Romerholz," Winterthur

The English Romantic poet Lord Byron was one of the nineteenth century's best documented manic-depressives. Not surprisingly, he wrote a number of long poems whose narrators or subjects were either frankly manic or had manic characteristics. His widely read "Lament of Tasso" romanticized the life of sixteenth-century Italian poet Torquato Tasso, who was confined seven years for what seems to have been a combination of psychosis (probably manic) and political imprudence. The painting (by another great Romantic artist) contrasts the poet's repose with the manic intensity of the arm forced between the bars of his cell. The woman at the bars is also striking, perhaps an inmate, perhaps a lover or wife.

THE LAMENT OF TASSO

*When the impatient thirst of light and air Parches the heart: and abhorred grate, Marring the sunbeams with its hideous shade, Works through the throbbing eyeball to the brain With a hot sense of heaviness and pain.**

(Byron, 1905)

acute mania, it or may be used alone. Lithium has long been used for control of acute mania but may have higher potential toxicity than either olanzepine or valproate. Combination therapy with an atypical antipsychotic (olanzepine) and either lithium or valproate has proven most effective in controlled studies but needs to be shown valuable in everyday clinical practice (Keck, 2003).

One report documents the effectiveness of a lengthy first night of sleep in some clients presenting with acute mania to an inpatient facility (Nowlin-Finch, Altshuler, Szuba, & Mintz, 1994). While such sleep therapy may be potentially dangerous if it is achieved only with high doses of medication, it certainly has much to commend it for simplicity and the client's need for rest.

Maintenance Treatment

The 1993 Agency for Health Care Policy and Research (AHCPR) Clinical Practice Guidelines for depression do not treat bipolar depression separately from unipolar depression. These guidelines recommend maintenance pharmacological treatment for all persons who have had three or more episodes of major depressive disorder or for those with two episodes of major depression and one of the following:

1. Family history of Bipolar Disorder or recurrent major depression (parent or sibling)
2. History of recurrence within one year after medication being discontinued
3. First episode occurring before age 20
4. Both episodes that were severe, sudden, or life-threatening and occurred within three years.

Analysis of published data suggests that for Bipolar Disorder, only two relapses might justify maintenance without any of the additional preceding criteria. Goodwin and Jamison (1990) suggest that even a single episode justifies long-term prophylaxis if the first episode is manic, the client is male, onset is sudden or later than age 30, the episode is severe or suicidal, no external precipitants were involved, and/or the client is an adolescent.

"Mood stabilizers" are the primary treatment for Bipolar Disorder, and recent work suggests that lithium remains an important drug in the management of this condition despite a variety of challenges in its effective usage (Bauer & Mitchner, 2004).

Lithium

Discovered to be effective in 1949 and used in this country since the late 1960s, lithium has been shown to have beneficial effects in the great majority of people treated. Lithium is used both to treat individual episodes of mania and to prevent recurrences of both mania and depression. Multiple studies have established the efficacy of lithium in both treatment and prevention of symptom recurrence. Lithium is most effective in persons whose symptoms began after puberty (Goodwin & Jamison, 1990) and who are not short cyclers (have fewer than four episodes yearly). Other than a therapeutic trial, there is no satisfactory way to predict which individuals will or will not respond to lithium.

Lithium is given orally in one to three 300-mg doses. Lithium affects all parts of the body; however, three organs

*From the *Complete Poetical Works of Lord Byron* by Lord Byron, 1905, Boston: Houghton Mifflin Company.

are most important to evaluate for potential adverse effects: the thyroid gland, for possible hypothyroidism, which occurs in 5% to 35% of cases; the kidneys (Shuster, 1999), since lithium is excreted through the kidneys and it has been established that lithium decreases renal concentrating ability; and the nervous system, since tremor and decreased motor coordination occur in some individuals. Before initiating treatment, blood counts, electrolyte and other chemistry determinations, urinalysis and creatinine clearance, and thyroid studies should be done; these should be repeated at six-month to yearly intervals during maintenance treatment. After an acute episode of mania, lithium is typically continued for at least 6 to 12 months (Goodwin & Jamison, 1990) and then consideration is given to long-term maintenance treatment. Lithium levels must be carefully monitored to prevent toxicity associated with overdose. Potentially interfering drugs must be avoided. These include certain antibiotics, many antihypertensive drugs, and anticonvulsants. Lithium takes up to two weeks to have any effect on mood. Side effects include increased thirst and appetite, weight gain, memory problems, and impaired motor coordination. Although lithium may cause cardiac arrhythmias, this is an unusual complication that may be related to unrecognized thyroid dysfunction (Namuta, Abe, Tarao, & Nakashima, 1999). Thyroid replacement treatment is occasionally required in clients on long-term lithium treatment. Lithium is embryotoxic, particularly in the first trimester, but the absolute risk of fetal damage is very low and may not justify any change in medication during pregnancy (Warner, 2000).

NURSINGALERT 15-2

Lithium Toxicity

WARNING SIGNS OF LITHIUM TOXICITY

- Anorexia
- Nausea and vomiting
- Hand tremor
- Muscle twitching
- Hyperactive deep tendon reflexes
- Ataxia
- Tinnitus
- Vertigo
- Weakness, drowsiness

SIGNS OF LITHIUM INTOXICATION

- Fever
- Decreased urine output
- Decreased blood pressure
- Irregular pulse
- Electrocardiographic changes
- Altered level of consciousness
- Seizures
- Coma
- Death

NURSINGTIP 15-1

Managing Lithium Toxicity

- Obtain history.
- Discontinue lithium doses.
- Evaluate vital signs.
- Obtain blood lithium level.
- Obtain other blood work: electrolytes, blood urea nitrogen, creatinine, urinalysis, and complete blood count.
- Evaluate cardiac status through electrocardiography.
- If acute overdose, provide emetic.
- Provide hydration.
- In severe cases, implement osmotic diuresis (with urea or mannitol), increase lithium clearance (with aminophylline), provide intake of sodium chloride (NaCl) to promote lithium excretion, and implement dialysis.

Lithium's major side effects concern neurological and cognitive functioning. Although some psychiatrists believe that these effects may be lessened by keeping lithium blood levels at the lowest consistent with effectiveness, there is little scientific data to support this view. Clients may need to accept slowed mental functioning in trade for the "leveling off" of emotions that typically results from lithium use. This is not a trade-off that will be acceptable to all clients.

Compliance is a problem for many clients. Kate Millett, author and painter, has described her own ambivalence about restarting lithium in the face of recurrent symptoms of mania:

LITHIUM

I maintain that ... the issue is my own freedom: to take lithium or not to as I choose. It's a voluntary program I was in. Even my shrink doesn't capture people and put them away; he has given me his word on this a number of times. I am free to go off lithium, then if I so choose, though the results of doing so are in his opinion dire. And the experience of my friend Martha Ravich is dire too ... a professional photographer. She was manic as a monkey, they say. I'd like to know what she says. But I know she's back on lithium. Humiliation, capitulation, cure? That was her attempt to throw the drug; the shaky hands (lithium's side effect), which she hated just as I do, needing steady hands for the camera as I do for the brush. The fear in the trembling hands that hold a 16mm movie camera. I always thought her hands were unsteady because they had scared her, broken her confidence. Thereafter you are *afraid, unsound; they have said so, proved it with incarceration with the parole of medication, the continual and eternal doses of lithium—without which you will always be crazy, will lapse into it again in weeks. Look at me—it is six weeks, and I do not feel crazy even though now they say I am. Because I stopped lithium? ... If I had never told would they know?**

(*Millett, 1990, pp. 65–66*)

The use of lithium by writers and creative artists has been studied, and there is a suggestion that lithium does have negative effects on some aspects of creativity (Shaw, Mann, Stokes, & Manevitz, 1987). In studies reported by Goodwin and Jamison (1990), 4 of 24 artists and writers refused to continue taking lithium because of side effects of loss of work effectiveness. Two other subjects reported that their productivity was decreased but agreed to continue medication at least for the study's duration.

One client with manic-depressive illness came to terms with the meaning of lithium in his life. He wrote the "Rules for the Gracious Acceptance of Lithium into Your Life," presented in Box 15-2, as a guide for all.

With a medication that has so many actual and potential physical and psychological side effects, it is important for clients to clearly understand the risks and benefits of taking lithium, particularly when it is given for long-term prophylaxis of mood symptoms. The nurse has a major role in assisting clients to understand the known effects of lithium and the reasons why it is recommended. Unfortunately, because of the variable and highly individual course of Bipolar Disorder and difficulty of monitoring and assuring treatment adherence, it is hard to assess any individual's outcome with certainty. Still, studies do show long-term benefit with the use of lithium, including reduction in suicide risk (Tondo & Baldessarini, 2000).

BOX 15-2
RULES FOR THE GRACIOUS ACCEPTANCE OF LITHIUM INTO YOUR LIFE

1. Clear out the medicine cabinet before guests arrive for dinner or new lovers stay the night.
2. Remember to put the lithium back into the cabinet the next day.
3. Don't be too embarrassed by your lack of coordination or your inability to do well the sports you once did with ease.
4. Learn to laugh about spilling coffee, having the palsied signature of an 80 year old, and being unable to put on cufflinks in less than 10 minutes.
5. Smile when people joke about how they think they "need to be on lithium."
6. Nod intelligently, and with conviction, when your physician explains to you the many advantages of lithium in leveling out the chaos in your life.
7. Be patient when waiting for this leveling off. Very patient. Re-read the Book of Job. Continue being patient. Contemplate the similarity between the phrases "being patient" and "being a patient."
8. Try not to let the fact that you can't read without effort annoy you. Be philosophical. Even if you could read, you probably wouldn't remember most of it anyway.
9. Accommodate to a certain lack of enthusiasm and bounce which you once had. Try not to think about all the wild nights you once had. Probably best not to have had those nights anyway.
10. Always keep in perspective how much better you are. Everyone else certainly points it out often enough and, annoyingly enough, it's probably true.
11. Be appreciative. Don't even consider stopping your lithium.
12. When you do stop, get manic, or get depressed, expect to hear two basic themes from your family, friends, and healers:
    - But you were doing so much better, I just don't understand it.
    - I told you this would happen.
13. Restock your medicine cabinet.

Anticonvulsants

Anticonvulsants, particularly carbamazepine (Tegretol) and valproic acid, have been used with some frequency in treating manic-depressive disorder. Their quicker action may make them of value in acute mania, and their different profile of side effects may offer advantages when, for example, renal dysfunction makes the use of lithium difficult or dangerous. These medications, particularly carbamazepine, seem to have their most important use in clients who do not respond to a therapeutic trial of lithium. Because of the high incidence of nonresponse among rapid-cycling bipolar clients, some psychiatrists will begin them directly on an anticonvulsant. The indications for acute and maintenance use of anticonvulsants are probably the same as those for lithium. Carbamazepine is begun at low dose (typically 100 mg in a single dose) and increased as tolerated, usually to 600 to 1,000 mg/day in divided doses, until blood levels reach a therapeutic level of 6 to 10 mg/mL. Valproic acid (most commonly, Depakene) is typically given in a dose of 500 to 1,000 mg daily with blood levels of 50 to 100 mg/mL.

Lithium and carbamazepine can be used together, particularly for rapid cyclers or for those who have dose-dependent lithium side effects such as excessive urination or memory difficulties. Although the antimanic effectiveness of carbamazepine has been well established, there is somewhat less evidence demonstrating its antidepressant effect in Bipolar Disorder.

Side effects of carbamazepine include drowsiness, ataxia, dizziness, visual difficulties, tremor, nausea, rash, liver test abnormalities, and changes in white blood count. Carbamazepine is related to tricyclic antidepressants, so persons sensitive to these drugs should not use carbamazepine. Periodic blood testing and serum levels are required for safe and effective use. Valproic acid side effects are usually minimal but include sedation, tremor, headache, and visual disturbance. A small percentage of clients develop massive liver damage while on valproic acid. Such damage typically occurs without warning, is independent of dosage, and rarely affects persons over 12 years of age.

Fatal adult liver failure due to valproate has occasionally been reported, mostly in patients treated for seizure disorders (Konig, Schenck, Sick, Holm, Heubner, Weiss, et al., 1999). Patients who begin on valproate are often advised to have liver function tests, at least for the first 6 to 12 months of treatment. The first signs of liver failure may include malaise, weakness, lethargy, or vomiting. Patients may be advised to discontinue treatment and seek diagnostic medical care if they develop any of these symptoms. A variety of newer anticonvulsants (lamotrigine, topiramate, tiagabine, and others) have recently come into use for the treatment of Bipolar Disorder. There are data showing the *ineffectiveness* of gabapentin, but the relative usefulness of these other medications remains largely unproven (Evins, 2003).

One of the major current challenges in treating Bipolar Disorder is the risk of metabolic syndrome. This is a condition related to abdominal obesity in which insulin resistance gives rise to significant risk for cardiovascular disease. There is a significant association between Bipolar Disorder and metabolic syndrome (Birkenaes, Opjordsmoen, Brunborg, Engh, Jonsdottir, Ringen, et al., 2007), which likely translates into substantial risk for heart attack and stroke. As nurses come to recognize the importance of this risk, it is likely there will be more emphasis on using mood stabilizers that do not lead to weight gain—perhaps primarily lamotrigine (Ketter et al., 2008) and cambamazepine (Torrent, Amann, Sanchez-Moreno, Colom, Reinares, Comes, et al., 2008).

RESEARCH Highlight 15–1

Coping Styles of Outpatients with a Bipolar Disorder

STUDY PROBLEM PURPOSE

The researchers wanted to gain insights regarding the coping styles used by persons with Bipolar Disorder when those individuals were confronted with problems or unpleasant events.

METHODS

A sample of 157 community dwelling patients with Bipolar Disorder agreed to participate in the study. They were interviewed at the clinic where they received treatment by the researcher or a trained research assistant. The patients completed two self-assessment questionnaires and provided demographic data to the researchers.

FINDINGS

More women than men participated in the study (65% women). A good majority (75%) lived with others, about 45% had completed high school or college. Most had a euthymic [elevated] mood state at the time of the study. Almost all were using mood stabilizers.

Based on the questionnaire responses, these bipolar patients used less-active coping styles than the general population. They also reported a more passive and avoidant coping style than their counterparts in the general population.

IMPLICATIONS

Nurses may be able to assess coping styles of bipolar clients and work with them to develop action plans around dealing with unpleasant life events. Clearly, further research is needed to understand if action plans devoted to coping can impact the quality of life and daily mood of such individuals.

Source: "Coping styles of outpatients with a bipolar disorder" by P. J. J. Goossens, E. A. M. Knoppert-van der Klein, and T. van Achterberg. (2008). *Archives of Psychiatric Nursing*, *22*(5), 245–253.

Antipsychotics

Traditional antipsychotic medications (neuroleptics) such as thioridazine, haloperidol, and others have not been shown to be generally effective in the long-term management of Bipolar Disorder. Newer neuroleptics, the second-generation antipsychotics such as olanzapine, clozapine, quetiapine, risperidone, and ziprasidone do appear to have usefulness in chronic management of Bipolar Disorder and may have some safety advantages over lithium, carbamazepine, and divalproex (Yatham, 2003). These drugs may be used by themselves ("monotherapy") or may be combined with other agents to increase effectiveness (Goodwin, 2003). As noted previously, these medications are associated with significant weight gain and may increase risk for cardiovascular disease unless careful attention is paid to both weight and the consequences of metabolic syndrome (blood pressure, cholesterol and other lipids, and blood sugar). Ziprasidone and aripiprazole are atypical antipsychotics that are unlikely to be associated with weight gain and as a result may not increase cardiovascular risk (Baptista, De Mendoza, Beaulieu, Bermudez, & Martinez, 2004).

Antidepressants and Bipolar Disorder

Since Bipolar Disorder is associated with depression in nearly all cases, it may seem self-evident that antidepressants would be useful in therapy. However, antidepressant therapy may stimulate the development of mania (switching) or rapid cycling. These complications occur in up to 84% of clients not treated with mood stabilizers, and the addition of antidepressants does not appear to improve the effectiveness of treatment (Ghaemi, Rosenquist, Ko, Baldassano, Kontos, & Baldessarini, 2004). The authors report that SSRIs and other "modern antidepressants" did not have a more favorable effect on depression. While the 2000 Expert Consensus Guidelines for the Treatment of Bipolar Disorder (http://www.psychguides.com) endorse the use of antidepressants if lithium or other mood stabilizers fail to prevent breakthrough depression, the guidelines emphasize the importance of mood stabilization as the primary approach to Bipolar Disorder. Antidepressants are only advised as one of several options (including lamotrigine) that can be used when depressive symptoms make it necessary to supplement lithium.

Mood Stabilization and Weight Gain

As noted before, lithium and especially divalproex and the atypical antipsychotics are associated with significant weight gain in the majority of clients to whom they are prescribed. This weight gain may lead to serious health problems, including the development of diabetes and metabolic syndrome (Aronne & Segal, 2003). Risk factors for developing obesity seem to include the type of mood stabilizer prescribed, binge eating, depressive symptoms, excess carbohydrate intake, and low exercise (Keck & McElroy, 2003; Fagiolini, Frank, Houck, Mallinger, Swartz, Buysse, et al., 2002). Studies involving clients taking atypical antipsychotics (not all of whom had Bipolar Disorder) show benefit from active interventions to prevent weight gain (Vreeland, Minsky, Menza, Rigassio Radler, Roemheld-Hamm, & Stern, 2003). Divalproex (valproic acid) may also be associated with polycystic ovarian syndrome in women—a relatively common condition nearly always associated with obesity (Joffe, Hall, Cohen, Taylor, & Baldessarini, 2003).

Psychotherapy

It is uniformly accepted that the primary treatment for Bipolar Disorder is medication. Treating bipolar clients with psychotherapy alone is thought by some to be at least ethically dubious (Goodwin & Jamison, 1990), if not negligent. Nonetheless, there is much support in the literature for the combined use of medication and psychotherapy in the management of manic-depressive illness (Lam, Watkins, Hayward, Bright, Wright, Kerr, et al., 2003; Zaretsky, 2003). There have been few, if any, good clinical trials showing that psychotherapy adds to the effectiveness of treatment, and it is likely that not all clients require psychotherapeutic interventions. Studies suggest better outcomes for clients receiving individual and family psychotherapy. One of the major goals in psychotherapy is to increase compliance in taking lithium, and there is evidence that psychotherapy does enhance that compliance (Paykel, 1995). From a nursing perspective, Cutler (2001) has conducted self-management groups for clients with Bipolar Disorder (see Research Highlight). In addition to compliance, issues addressed by nurse-led psychotherapy can include dealing with vocational and interpersonal issues, helping clients come to terms with their feelings about past manic and depressive episodes, and assisting clients in dealing with fear about the potential recurrence of symptoms. Similar results have been reported from studies based on the concept of "psychoeducation" (Colom, Vieta, Reinares, Martinex-Aran, Torrent, Goikolea, et al., 2003). For some clients, there is real concern about the risk of passing manic-depressive disorder on to children, and this concern can be addressed in a group setting. For many clients, group therapy can be guided to help persons deal with common problems affecting those with Bipolar Disorder (Rothbaym & Astin, 2000).

Other Treatments

There are some situations where treatments other than medications and psychotherapy will be used, and the following merit mention. Although rarely used, electroconvulsive therapy is effective in treating mania (Small, Milstein, & Small, 1991; see Chapter 32). It may have a role in situations where lithium is contraindicated, particularly during early pregnancy. Some evidence supports the usefulness of calcium channel blockers in mania unresponsive to either lithium or anticonvulsants (Cook & Winokur, 1990).

There has been recent interest in the use of low-field magnetic stimulation of the brain in the management of affective conditions, including Bipolar Disorder (Rohan, Parrow, Stoll, Demopulos, Friedman, Dages, et al., 2004). Preliminary data suggest some evidence for improvement in depressive symptoms.

Treatment Effectiveness under Study

While there is evidence supporting many of the individual steps that psychiatric providers use in treating Bipolar Disorder, guidelines for practice remain more based on consensus than on hard evidence. The disorder is highly variable between clients, and it has proven very difficult to design studies to assess general recommendations. The multicenter STEP-BD (systematic treatment enhancement program for Bipolar Disorder) study was begun in 2002 to attempt to gather data about which combinations of treatments work best in the management of this complex condition. STEP-BD has confirmed earlier reports that adding antidepressants to mood stabilizers does not improve outcomes (Goldberg, Perlis, Ghaemi, Calabrese, Bowden, Wisniewski, et al., 2007). The STEP-BD study has also shown that long-term intensive psychotherapy does improve functioning in many persons with Bipolar Disorder (Miklowitz, Otto, Frank, Reilly-Harrington, Kogan, Sachs, et al., 2007).

NURSING CARE

The nurse caring for a manic client must begin with an understanding of the disorder and a recognition that the experiences of the condition are unique to each individual. To be effective, the nurse will need to handle three major components of care:

1. Use nursing theory to assess how to best assist the client in dealing with a chronic condition.
2. Determine how to support the client's family in adapting to having a family member with Bipolar Disorder.
3. In cases where the nurse works on an inpatient unit, establish a supportive ward milieu for the manic client and the other clients on the unit.

Each of these is addressed in the following discussion.

NURSING THEORY

It often is difficult for nurses to understand the experiences and the point of view of a manic client. In a manic state, the client appears out of control or on the verge of being so. The client does not have the time or interest to sit and talk with the nurse and frequently does not see any way that a nurse can assist him or does not understand why others view him as confused. In between manic episodes, the client must come to terms with the knowledge that he has a chronic illness and that professionals are recommending a continuous dose of medications for management of the condition. Further, the client experiences a range of emotions—ecstasy, joy, fear, depression, embarrassment, guilt—when going through life and reflecting on his past behaviors.

NURSINGALERT 15-3

Women and Bipolar Disorder

Women frequently develop symptoms of bipolar disease during childbearing years. Many of the drugs used for treatment of Bipolar Disorder, however, may be harmful during pregnancy. For example, divalproex can cause significant fetal abnormalities if given early in pregnancy. Further, several of the medications used to treat bipolar disease can reduce the effectiveness of birth control pills and possibly of the hormones used to relieve the symptoms of menopause (Burt & Rasgon, 2004).

Recent epidemiological data suggest a strong link between Bipolar Disorder and postpartum psychosis (Chaudron & Pies, 2003). Women with depression occurring either before pregnancy or during the course of gestation must be followed closely during and after pregnancy to anticipate the potential for postpartum depression or psychosis.

The special needs of women with Bipolar Disorder have only recently come to be appreciated. Care for these women should be provided by nurses and others who can coordinate the range of services needed to ensure effective and safe management of Bipolar Disorder.

THEORY OF HUMAN BECOMING

Parse's theory (Fawcett, 2001; Hickman, 1995; Parse, 1992) is a very useful perspective in a situation where the nurse must build rapport and a beginning level of trust with a client too busy to be bothered with establishing a nurse-client relationship and in a situation where the client seeks ongoing support in coming to terms with illness. The theory suggests that individuals find personal meaning in the process of living. Further, the theory states that each person establishes his own value priorities, making sense out of his existence. Thus, the nurse does not need to focus on the nurse's reality or bring control to her interactions with the client (neither of which the client would easily accept). Rather, the nurse brings presence and unconditional support. The nurse seeks to understand the client's interpretation of his lived experiences. Nursing interventions begin with being fully present for the person and making no demands. Next, in the context of caring and support, the nurse will tease out multiple complex realities of the client's experiences. Understanding the client's world will form the basis for nursing care. Nursing interventions must be planned, then, within the context of the client's meaning in life, his goals, and his illness. Consider the exercise in Reflective Thinking 15-1 from the perspective of Parse's theory.

REFLECTIVE THINKING 15-1

The Decision to Use Lithium

Consider Kate Millet's discussion on her own, very personal decision to use or not to use lithium. (Excerpt can be found in lithium discussion earlier in this chapter.)

Understanding that each individual makes personal choices and understands his condition based on his own interpretation of life, his own values, and his own lived experiences, consider the following:

- Can a nurse or psychiatrist ever really know what is best for another?
- Under what conditions can mental health professionals force an individual to receive treatments or medications he does not choose to take?
- Describe a collaborative (rather than paternalistic) model of psychiatric care.

Self-Care Deficit Theory

When a client is clearly out of control and unable to meet even his own basic needs, the nurse may use Orem's Self-Care Deficit theory to guide the nursing role. According to Orem's theory, in situations where client agency is limited and the client is unable to care for his own health needs, the nurse must ensure that those needs are met. Thus, in situations where the client is potentially dangerous to self or others, the nurse has a role to intervene and provide for safety. For example, when a manic client is on the verge of physical exhaustion and yet does not see the need to stop physical exercise, the nurse may have to establish her ability and authority to see that the client stops, rests, and takes fluids as the nurse cares for the client's physical needs.

In other situations, particularly when the nurse and client have an ongoing therapeutic relationship, the client may ask the nurse to intervene in his manic behaviors before he engages in behaviors that will be hurtful and/or embarrassing to him later. In such cases, the client will tell the nurse or his psychiatrist or mental health workers that he wants to be stopped if he stops sleeping, becomes agitated, spends large sums of money, and the like. In such a case, the client tells the nurse in advance which behaviors he believes indicate he has lost ability to care for himself, and the nurse knows when interventions (such as hospital admission) are indicated.

SUPPORT FOR THE CLIENT'S FAMILY

Family members and close friends/significant others are often involved in the client's care and frequently seek support and education from nurses. Because of the inherited nature of the disorder, family members may request genetic counseling and may report others in the family who are either depressed or manic. These family members may seek education about the disease, and most will benefit from having someone listen to their feelings and responses to the information that a family member has bipolar disease. Worry of becoming ill, fear of not being able to handle the client, and guilt over the genetic aspects of passing a disease on to offspring are common themes expressed by families. The nurse's role is one of both support and listening, as well as one of educating the family and friends about the disease and what to expect. Because manic individuals may rapidly cycle into depression, the risk of self-injury and suicide must be discussed with family and friends.

THE WARD MILIEU AND THE MANIC CLIENT

One aspect of caring for the manic individual that challenges every psychiatric nurse is the overall management of a hospital inpatient unit when one (or two or three) manic individual(s) arrive on the floor. Taking a perspective from systems theory, consider that a ward may be in equilibrium. Clients and staff have their personalities, activity levels, patterns for day-to-day activities, and unwritten rules of how interactions take place. Once an individual arrives in a state of mania, the equilibrium is upset, and all of the old, predictable patterns of activity and interactions change. The manic client is hospitalized because he is unable to control racing thoughts, feels full of energy, and knows that his life is filled with special meaning. Feelings of grandiosity are a common part of the presenting symptoms, as are feelings of paranoia. Thus, the manic client has more energy and stamina than anyone else present, more ideas of what should be done on the unit, and more confidence than others in his abilities to fix any perceived problem. In addition, the manic client has less ability to use social conventions when approaching others and will not pick up on other's nonverbal indicators that they want to be alone. Experienced nurses offer the following suggestions for coping with this situation:

1. Take a deep breath and relax.
2. Remember that just as anxiety is contagious, so are feelings of calm and peace.
3. Work together with all unit staff to project an image of patience and confidence.
4. Treat all persons with respect and dignity.
5. Provide the manic client with enough personal space so he does not disturb others with behaviors he cannot control. Often a private room is indicated.

Take these suggestions and ask other psychiatric nurses for additional ideas.

APPLICATION OF THE NURSING PROCESS 15-1

ASSESSMENT

Nursing assessment should begin with presenting symptoms, past history of manic and depressive cycles, evaluation of compliance with prescribed medications, and supporting data. Assessment for a newly hospitalized client should include the current status of the client, including information on the following:

- How long has this manic episode lasted?
- When was the last time the client slept or ate?

(*Continues*)

APPLICATION OF THE NURSING PROCESS 15-1 (Continued)

BOX 15-3
SUPPORTING ASSESSMENT DATA FOR THE CLIENT WITH MANIA

Evaluate for the presence of the following:

- Euphoric, expansive, or irritable mood
- Excessive use of makeup, jewelry, and brightly colored clothing, which the person may change several times a day
- Hyperverbal speech, including slurred speech, flight of ideas, loose associations, and racing thoughts
- Irritability when ideas and plans are thwarted
- Intrusiveness and poor sense of boundaries
- Inability to sit still or join an activity that requires participation
- Expansiveness, with indiscriminate enthusiasm for interpersonal, sexual, or occupational interests
- Inflated self-esteem or grandiosity

Adapted from *Instant Nursing Assessment: Mental Health* by P. D. Mabbett, 1996, Clifton Park, NY: Thomson Delmar Learning.

BOX 15-4
SEVEN QUESTIONS TO ASK WHEN ASSESSING A MANIC CLIENT

1. Do you experience ups and downs in your moods?
2. Do you have difficulty focusing your thoughts or conversation?
3. Have you spent more money than usual recently?
4. When is the last time you slept, and how long did you sleep?
5. Have you noticed a change in your sexual interest or sexual activity recently?
6. Do you feel irritated when other people tell you to slow down or when they do not seem to follow your thoughts?
7. Do you believe you have extraordinary abilities or powers?

Adapted from *Instant Nursing Assessment: Mental Health* by P. D. Mabbett, 1996, Clifton Park, NY .

- What is the degree of irritability?
- What is the potential for violent outbursts?
- Is the client oriented and in touch with reality?
- Is the client exhibiting delusions?
- What event precipitated the client's coming in for care?

Further, assessment should include observations for data that support the diagnosis of mania. Boxes 15-3 and 15-4 present such supporting data and questions the nurse might ask when completing the initial assessment interview.

NURSING DIAGNOSIS

Nursing diagnoses most commonly assigned manic individuals are listed in Table 15-2. These nursing diagnoses are grouped into categories: safety needs, physical needs, social needs, cognitive needs, and family needs.

OUTCOME IDENTIFICATION

First, outcomes will be based on meeting immediate needs of safety and physical supports. The nursing care plan should reflect these as priorities and establish that these basic needs must be met. Second, the nurse

(*Continues*)

APPLICATION OF THE NURSING PROCESS 15-1 (Continued)

TABLE 15-2 Common Nursing Diagnoses for a Manic Client

AREA OF NEED	NURSING DIAGNOSIS
Safety needs	*Risk for violence (self or other directed)*
	Risk for suicide
Physical needs	*Insomnia or Sleep Deprivation*
	Imbalanced nutrition: less than body requirements
	Fatigue
Social needs	*Impaired social interaction*
Cognitive needs	*Disturbed thought processes*
	Ineffective coping
	Ineffective self-health management
Family needs	*Interrupted family processes*
	Risk for caregiver role strain

will initiate care directed at meeting the client's needs and desires for appropriate social contacts with others; the expected outcome will be that client will interact within socially acceptable boundaries. Lastly, the nurse will provide care related to cognitive aspects of the disease, with a focus on assisting the client to manage his illness.

PLANNING/INTERVENTIONS

Outcomes such as "the client will recognize own behaviors that place him at risk for manic episodes" or "the client will seek help to prevent the exacerbation of symptoms" are examples of outcome statements that may be appropriate.

Interventions include providing a safe and structured environment for the manic client, free of objects that could be used to harm self or others and free of extraneous noise or stimulation. All verbal communication from the nurse should be short, concise, and clear. With regard to client socialization, the nurse should provide an environment with minimal social contacts until the client is able to interact and must always ensure that the client is redirected away from situations that could be embarrassing on recovery. Nursing interventions focus on the client's need to learn to manage his own condition. It is important to provide information about the disease, its treatment and progression, and sources of help. Lastly, assistance to the client's family/significant others is almost always required, as these persons need to become partners in the management of the condition.

EVALUATION

When evaluating client progress, the nurse can first look at the client's surrounding environment to see that potential hazards have been removed and that excessive stimuli have been reduced or eliminated. Once immediate dangers to the client's physical well-being have been controlled, the nurse should consider the client's level of functioning and social interactions as compared to those at the beginning of treatment. The level of social interaction, for example, must take into account the client's cognitive abilities, desires, and initial level of functioning. The nurse must be careful to view progress in terms of degree and to view the actions of a client who has not inflicted physical harm to self or others during treatment as the first positive steps in a potentially long road to recovery.

CARE PLANNING GUIDE 15-1 Client With Mania

CLINICAL PICTURE

The clinical picture of the client with mania generally includes:

- Positive family history of manic disease in a first-generation relative
- Inability to attend to questions, irritability, and psychomotor agitation in the acute phase
- Bipolar depression

COMMON NURSING DIAGNOSES

Nursing diagnoses most commonly employed for the manic client are:

1. *Risk for injury*
2. *Impaired social interaction*
3. *Noncompliance to the treatment regimen*
4. *Insomnia*
5. *Imbalanced nutrition: Less than body requirements*
6. *Disturbed thought processes*

NURSING DIAGNOSIS 1: *RISK FOR INJURY,* RELATED TO IMPAIRED JUDGEMENT, GRANDIOSITY, POOR CONCENTRATION

OUTCOMES

1. The client will be free of injury during the acute phase.
2. The client will recognize behaviors that place self in potentially dangerous situations.

NOC: *RISK CONTROL*

INTERVENTIONS (NIC: *SURVEILLANCE: SAFETY; TEACHING: DISEASE PROCESS*)	RATIONALE
• Monitor judgment regarding potentially dangerous activities.	• Poor judgment and decision-making skills put the client at risk for injury.
• Monitor for physical or cognitive (attention span, ability to concentrate, feelings of grandiosity) function alterations that might lead to unsafe behaviors.	• Risk taking, hypersexuality, and decreased ability to concentrate due to racing thoughts place the client at risk for injury. Hospitalization may be required for the client's safety.
• Assess for suicidal ideation.	• Depression can be associated with suicidal ideation.
• Provide a safe, structured environment (ward management).	• The nurse controls the environment, preventing injury by controlling the client's behaviors/movements.
• Speak in short, simple sentences.	• Communicate so that the client understands within his or her attention span.
• Teach about high-risk behaviors that could be harmful.	• Interventions beyond the acute phase address lifestyle management with an illness that alters judgment.
• Monitor behaviors and responses to environmental stimuli that may be harmful in the inpatient and community setting.	• Assess and reassess with the client as part of helping him or her deal with a life-long illness.

(*Continues*)

CARE PLANNING GUIDE 15-1 Continued

NURSING DIAGNOSIS 2: *IMPAIRED SOCIAL INTERACTION,* RELATED TO INTRUSIVE BEHAVIOR, PRESSURED SPEECH, AGITATION, OR GRANDIOSITY

OUTCOMES

1. The client will interact with others appropriately.

NOC: *SOCIAL INVOLVEMENT*

INTERVENTIONS (NIC: *BEHAVIOR MODIFICATION: SOCIAL SKILLS*)	RATIONALE
• Monitor the quality of social interactions with peers, family, staff, etc.	• Allows for identification of changes from baseline data regarding behaviors.
• Monitor others' reactions to interactions with the client.	• Use these observations for feedback to the client, providing information of the impact of the client's behaviors on others.
• Assist the client to gain insight into the appropriateness of interactions with others.	• Poor judgment and manic behaviors cloud insights.
• Provide a safe environment where the client will not be embarrassed by his or her own behavior upon recovery.	• Uncontrolled interactions may lead to anger in others; socially inappropriate behaviors cannot be controlled by the client.
• Redirect to activities with minimal socialization, until the client is ready to interact appropriately.	• Keep the client in a quiet, nonstimulating environment.
• Encourage the client to verbalize feelings about the manic episode during the recovery phase.	• Provide support and acceptance of the client's behavior as part of an illness.

NURSING DIAGNOSIS 3: *NONCOMPLIANCE TO THE TREATMENT REGIMEN,* RELATED TO DENIAL OF NEED FOR MEDICATION; INCREASED ENERGY, ELATION, SENSE OF INFALLIBILITY

OUTCOMES

1. The client will perform treatment regimen as prescribed.
2. The client will state the need for medication.
3. The client will participate in designing the discharge plan.

NOC: *COMPLIANCE BEHAVIORS*

INTERVENTIONS (NIC: *MEDICATION MANAGEMENT*)	RATIONALE
• Monitor adherence to the treatment plan.	• Establishes baseline behaviors and past consequences of not following regimen.
• Monitor insight regarding the need for medications.	• Provides information about acceptance and knowledge base about the client's own disease.
• Involve the family/significant others in education and follow-through, if appropriate, and only with the client's permission.	• If the family/significant others are involved, they can be a continuing support to the client.
• Tailor medication times to the client's lifestyle.	• Promotes feelings of control over the treatment and increases chances of adherence.
• Reality-test the pros and cons of manic highs vs. stable moods.	• Education re-treatment plan must include the impact of uncontrolled, manic episodes on one's person life.

(*Continues*)

CARE PLANNING GUIDE 15-1 Continued

NURSING DIAGNOSIS 4: *INSOMNIA,* RELATED TO IRRITABILITY, AGITATION, SENSE OF URGENCY TO ACCOMPLISH TASKS

OUTCOMES

1. The client will maintain sufficient sleep/rest for bodily needs.

NOC: *SLEEP*

INTERVENTIONS (NIC: *SLEEP ENHANCEMENT*)	RATIONALE
• Provide a private room and limit stimuli, especially at night.	• A quiet and private space is conducive to rest and sleep.
• Keep conversation to a minimum.	• Avoids verbal stimuli.
• Make observations about sleep/rest needs and provide reassurance that the nurse is nearby.	• Expresses the client's need for sleep and the nurse's willingness to provide support/protection.

NURSING DIAGNOSIS 5: *IMBALANCED NUTRITION: LESS THAN BODY REQUIREMENTS,* RELATED TO NOT TAKING TIME TO EAT

OUTCOMES

1. The client will maintain sufficient food intake to avoid losing weight.

NOC: *ADEQUATE NUTRITION AND HYDRATION*

INTERVENTIONS (NIC: *NUTRITION MANAGEMENT*)	RATIONALE
• Provide "finger foods" (sandwiches, fruits, foods that can be eaten while moving along).	• A manic client will not sit down at a table to eat with others.
• Provide fluids in containers that can be handed to the client.	• The client is at risk for dehydration, particularly if physically active and not replacing fluids.
• Remind the client to eat/drink frequently.	• The client may not eat if not reminded.

NURSING DIAGNOSIS 6: *DISTURBED THOUGHT PROCESSES,* RELATED TO BIOLOGICAL AND PSYCHOLOGICAL STRESSORS

OUTCOMES

1. The client will begin to concentrate and increase attention span.
2. The client will begin to gain insight over realistic sense of what he can and cannot do.

NOC: *DISTORTED THOUGHT SELF-CONTROL*

INTERVENTIONS (NIC: *BEHAVIOR MANAGEMENT, DELUSION MANAGEMENT*)	RATIONALE
• Keep interactions short; focus attention on one thing at a time.	• Directs the client's attention to activities around him, bringing him back to the reality of his situation.
• As the client moves to the recovery phase, discuss the differences between his manic and nonmanic phases and appraisals of self.	• Builds insight into the challenges of living with this chronic illness as the client begins to think realistically about his behaviors.

(*Continues*)

CARE PLANNING GUIDE 15-1 Continued

LONG-TERM CONSIDERATIONS FOR THE MANIC CLIENT

1. Individual therapy to provide support and to monitor symptoms
2. Inpatient hospitalization as required for safety
3. Group/family support
4. Community-based support groups

Note: The care planning guides have been adapted from *Plans of Care for Speciality Practice: Psychiatric Mental Health Nursing* by M. Coler and K. G. Vincent, 1995, Clifton Park, NY: Delmar, Cengage Learning.

NURSING CARE PLAN: NURSING PROCESS FORMAT 15-1

Refer to the excerpt "The First Time I Was Manic," found in the introductory section of this chapter. Consider a client, whom we shall call Joe, who is describing his feelings that he knew he was going insane. He states, "My thoughts were so fast that I couldn't remember the beginning of a sentence halfway through." Further, he relates, "I wanted desperately to slow down but could not. Nothing helped—not running around a parking lot for hours on end or swimming for miles."

Imagine that Joe is our client.

ASSESSMENT

Joe, 34 years old, has been admitted to the psychiatric hospital in an acute manic episode, referred from the emergency department. His three friends brought him to the hospital; they know him well and know that he has had two manic episodes before. His friend Tom states that Joe has been prescribed lithium, but that no one really knows if Joe has been taking it. Tom says that Joe has not slept in days and that he has been out running today for approximately three hours. No one knows the last time Joe had anything to eat. Joe agreed to come to the hospital with his friends, evidently willing to accept that he "needed a rest." On admission, Joe could not communicate well and exhibited flight of ideas. Although he was oriented to person and place, Joe did not know the date. Joe has agreed to get a rest; however, he is pacing the floor when the psychiatric nurse arrives and states he is "ready to rest, but there are a lot of things that need help around this place, and it took forever to get the doc to bring me here, and I ran across the marsh today and saw the gulls, and it's time for spring and when will school be out?"

ACUTE PHASE

NURSING DIAGNOSIS 1 *Insomnia*, related to sensory alterations (psychological stress), as evidenced by verbal report of difficulty sleeping.

OUTCOMES	NIC	NURSING ACTIONS	EVALUATION
• Within the first 24 hours on the unit, Joe will sleep 4 hours and obtain rest.	• Sleep enhancement	• Provide Joe a private room. • Keep stimulation to a minimum.	Joe says he isn't tired at all; he wants to know what is going on around the unit.

(Continues)

NURSING CARE PLAN: NURSING PROCESS FORMAT 15-1 (Continued)

OUTCOMES	NIC	NURSING ACTIONS	EVALUATION
		• Orient Joe to his room, letting him know that you are present and willing to assist him. • Keep all conversation to a minimum. • Establish trust by letting Joe know you are there to help meet his needs. Speak clearly, letting him know that you agree he does need rest. • Administer medications as prescribed (divalproex/ valproic acid). • Talk with Joe about the need for rest.	Joe decides to take a shower; only after the shower does he agree to try to sleep; he goes to bed at 1:00 A.M. and does sleep until 7:00 A.M.

NURSING DIAGNOSIS 2 *Imbalanced nutrition: less than body requirements related to disturbed thought processes secondary to manias,* as evidenced by reported inadequate food intake.

OUTCOMES	NIC	NURSING ACTIONS	EVALUATION
• Within 2 hours after admission, Joe will be adequately hydrated and will have eaten some food.	• Nutrition management	• Bring water, juice, cold beverages to Joe's room. • Arrange for "finger foods" (sandwiches, crackers, and fruit) to be brought to Joe's room. For the first hour on the unit, offer food every 15 minutes.	At the nurse's direction, Joe consumed four glasses of water and two glasses of juice during the first 2 hours in the hospital. He also consumed one sandwich and three pieces of fruit over the next 24 hours.

NURSING DIAGNOSIS 3 *Disturbed thought processes,* related to biological and psychological stressors secondary to mania as evidenced by distractibility, racing thoughts, and inability to concentrate.

OUTCOMES	NIC	NURSING ACTIONS	EVALUATION
• Within 48 hours of admission, Joe will be able to concentrate on the immediate task at hand; he will be able to complete a sentence and carry on a simple conversation.	• Behavior management: overactivity	• Administer medications as prescribed; talk to Joe in simple, clear language; direct Joe to unit activities. • Invite Joe to participate in a volleyball game.	Joe takes his medications; he states that the unit needs help in decorating and in making the environment "fun." He asks why there isn't more going on.

(*Continues*)

NURSING CARE PLAN: NURSING PROCESS FORMAT 15-1 (Continued)

OUTCOMES	NIC	NURSING ACTIONS	EVALUATION
		• By late afternoon, communicate with Joe regarding his feelings of "things moving too fast."	Joe played the volleyball game, although he did not follow the rules of keeping score. Joe states he understands he can't keep up with his thoughts; he has felt this way before.

RECOVERY PHASE

After three days in the hospital, Joe enters the recovery phase. He has slept well for two nights; he describes a basic understanding that he has missed medications and has entered a manic state again. The nursing care is now focused on helping Joe recognize risks for exacerbation of his symptoms and learn how to manage his own care at home. His friends have come to visit and have all told him he is doing much better. He is able to communicate with his friends.

NURSING DIAGNOSIS 4 *Ineffective self-health management*, related to perceived excessive demands and denial as evidenced by inability to report or recall prior compliance to medication regimen.

OUTCOMES	NIC	NURSING ACTIONS	EVALUATION
• By the time of hospital discharge, Joe will have a plan for compliance with his prescribed medication regimen and will understand the reasons for taking his medication.	• Case management • Medication management • Case management	• Refer Joe to a cognitive-therapy group for persons with Bipolar Disorder who have similar challenges and needs to Joe's. • Instruct Joe about medications, diet, and side effects and provide information in writing. • Arrange for the community mental health nurse to visit Joe's home for follow-up.	Joe attends the first group meeting his fourth day in the hospital (other clients in the group are outpatients); Joe indicates an understanding of his medications. Joe is willing to have the community nurse visit; the hospital nurse arranges for Joe to meet this nurse before discharge.

REFLECTIVE QUESTIONS

1. **ASSESSMENT**
   How would you assess the safety of Joe's environment? What other questions could you ask Joe's friends to gain insight into the course of his illness?
2. **NURSING DIAGNOSIS**
   What other nursing diagnoses would you develop for Joe? How do you assess for his safety? Do you have a concern regarding self-esteem and socialization?

(Continues)

NURSING CARE PLAN: NURSING PROCESS FORMAT 15-1 (Continued)

3. **OUTCOMES**
What outcomes are realistic for Joe? Can he return home to his own care? How will you know what is safe for him?

4. **NURSING ACTIONS**
Are there other approaches to the care plan? Why does the nurse ask him to participate in a volleyball game? What activities are appropriate for a manic client on the unit where you work?

5. **EVALUATION**
The nurse did not encounter escalating mania or violence with Joe. Have you seen risk for violence in a manic client? What did the nurse do? What are your feelings regarding the role of medication in the treatment of Bipolar Disorder?

NURSING CARE PLAN: CONCEPT MAP FORMAT 15-1

BACKGROUND INFORMATION

For this Nursing Care Plan we will assume that Mr. Jones, from a movie of he same name (see Chapter 33), has just been admitted. He has Bipolar Disorder and his symptoms have been escalating over the past few days, and he had just created a civil disturbance—at a concert, he leapt up on stage and took over from the conductor because he felt the music wasn't being played fast enough. He is agitated, pacing, and talking very fast, believing that there has been some mistake with bringing him into the hospital. He begins talking very loudly; he wants to tell the nurse what went wrong. He begins "conducting" at the nurses' station, letting everyone know that he should be in charge of the unit and that he will be leaving the unit as soon as someone figures out that he doesn't need to be there. Another client confronts him by saying he is as "crazy as the rest of us." At this point, Mr. Jones takes on an aggressive stance—his face is red, and he clinches his right fist.

INITIAL ASSESSMENT AND REFLECTION

Nurse Jeff is on the unit and he has observed Mr. Jones's behaviors described here. He recognizes that Mr. Jones is in the hospital for his own safety and for stabilization of his condition. Jeff moves over to talk with Mr. Jones. Mr. Jones moves away and begins to speak loudly, but his words do not make sense. Jeff offers Mr. Jones his medication, and Mr. Jones says, "Not now, I'm too busy, catch me later."

Jeff is concerned about many issues/problems during this first night of hospitalization. Jeff recognizes the need to establish trust with Mr. Jones and to begin interaction with his client that is positive and supportive and that will form the basis of a therapeutic nurse-client relationship. He also sees immediately that he must be in control of Mr. Jones's behaviors. Jeff knows that there is a real risk for violence if the anger escalates in a manic client who is unable to control his behavior and who may be feeling invincible.

The initial nursing problems written as nursing diagnoses follow:

- *Risk for injury*, related to lack of judgment regarding activities and consequences of behaviors
- *Risk for violence: other directed*, related to lack to tolerance of other's criticisms
- *Insomnia*, related to increasing agitation
- *Noncompliance*, related to unwillingness to take ordered medications at this time

Jeff uses the concept map as a tool to evaluate the situation.

PRIORITIES OF CARE

The concept map draws attention to two focal issues: the need for external control of the client's behavior and, of course, the nonadherence to the therapeutic regimen that is the probable cause of the relapse. It is clear that the need for Jeff to control Mr. Jones's behavior is the immediate and very pressing issue and

(Continues)

NURSING CARE PLAN: CONCEPT MAP FORMAT 15-1 (Continued)

must take first priority. The concept map, however also demonstrates another interesting relationship. The need for external control of Mr. Jones's behavior is related to the need for the nurse to build trust with the client and will be affected by how well Jeff can accomplish this basic client care goal.

NURSING INTERVENTIONS

Jeff takes two immediate actions. First, he separates Mr. Jones from the other clients on the unit. Jeff directs other staff to redirect other clients to an activity room, and Jeff maintains a presence with Mr. Jones in the hallway. He directs Mr. Jones (who is pacing) to walk with him in the direction of Mr. Jones's room. This is an important (and often unrecognized) nursing intervention of "ward management' needed in many settings where the nurse must maintain the safety (physical and emotional) of all on the unit. Second, Jeff speaks to Mr. Jones in short, simple sentences and directs his attention to the immediate activity of walking toward the room that will be his. Jeff's interaction is kind and yet firm.

Jeff says, "I'll be thé nurse with you over the night tonight. I'd guess we can get a lot of things straightened out in the morning." Jeff is careful to not move into Mr. Jones's personal space, remaining about two to three feet away, and he speaks softly and slowly. Jeff says, "we'll walk to your room." As they come to the room, Mr. Jones enters and looks around. Jeff inquires about sleep patterns and learns that Mr. Jones "hasn't slept in days." Jeff ensures that Mr. Jones has a private room, and maintains the environment as one with little stimulation. He asks Mr. Jones if there is anything he can do to assist him to prepare for sleep tonight. As he leaves Mr. Jones so his client can prepare for sleep, Jeff says, "I'll be right back with your medicine." Jeff leaves the room, returns, and Mr. Jones takes it, saying, "More of this stuff again!" Jeff will maintain a careful watch over Mr. Jones's behavior over the night.

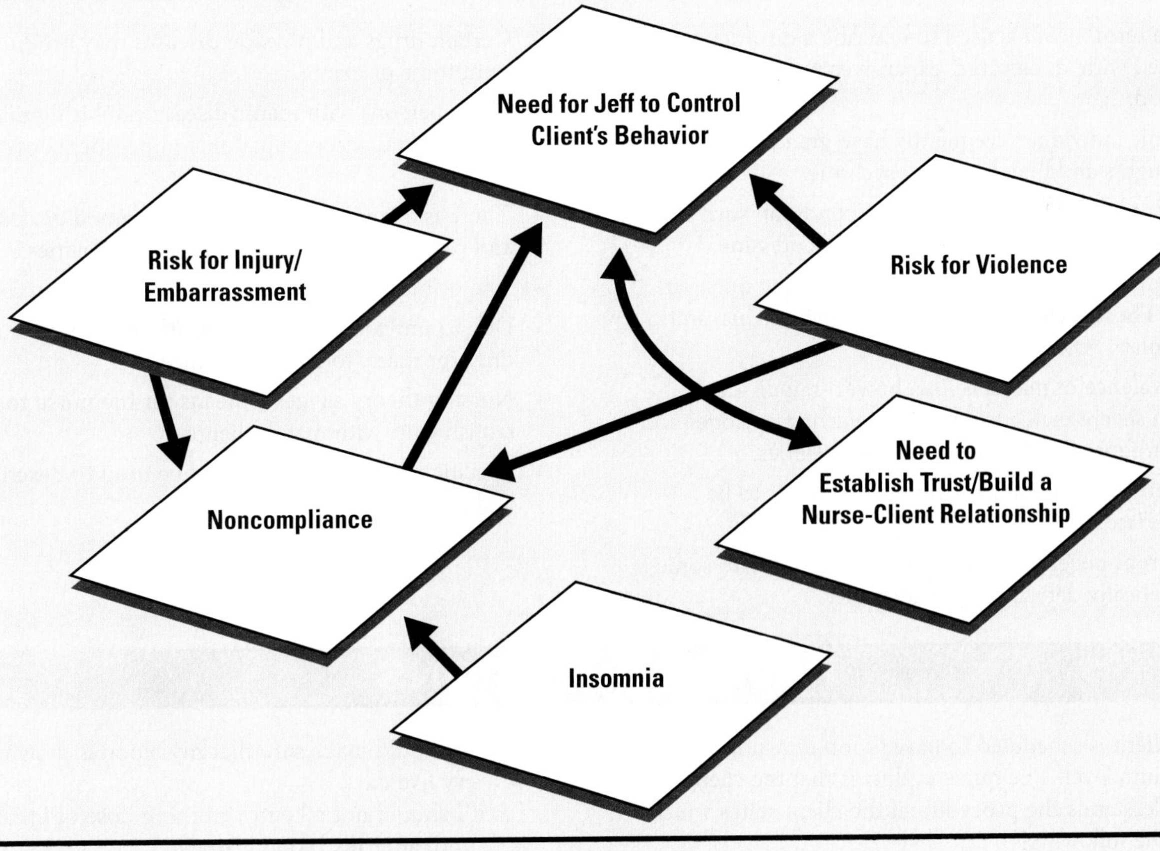

Concept Map of Issues and Problems (DELMAR/CENGAGE LEARNING.)

(Continues)

NURSING CARE PLAN: CONCEPT MAP FORMAT 15-1 (Continued)

OUTCOMES/EVALUATION

The immediate need to address the risk for violence was met. At the same time, Jeff uses skills in communication to interact with Mr. Jones and begin a nurse-client relationship. He controls the environment and his interactions with the client. Jeff takes every effort to prevent escalation of violence—separating Mr. Jones from others, providing a private room with little stimulation, maintaining a physical distance from the client so as not to move into personal space, and directing attention to the room, to sleep, thus avoiding confrontations.

The psychiatric mental health nurse often uses the intervention of "ward management" to meet client needs. This concept map illustrates the relationship of ward management to both risk for violence and the need to develop a therapeutic relationship with clients. When the nurse can successfully maintain a calm environment on the unit, then he or she can more easily develop a positive and, ultimately, trusting relationship with the clients.

The other issues that clearly must be addressed in this hospitalization include Mr. Jones's nonadherence to the treatment regimen. This will need to be addressed once the acute phase of mania has subsided and it becomes possible to work with the client and other members of the health care team to establish a treatment plan preparing for discharge.

KEY CONCEPTS

- The term *mania* is used to describe a disorder associated with an elevated, expansive, and/or irritable mood.
- Manic individuals frequently have grandiose thoughts and may become psychotic.
- There is a cyclical nature to the condition such that persons move between mania and depression.
- There are categories of mania, depending on severity. These include manic episode, hypomania, and Bipolar Disorder.
- Prevalence of mania is low; however, individuals with severe mania experience recurrent episodes and are frequently seen in psychiatric facilities.
- There is a tendency for Bipolar Disorder to be inherited.
- Current belief is that bipolar disease is due to some genetically determined abnormality.
- Certain drugs and physical diseases may produce symptoms of mania.
- Many persons with manic disease exhibit significant psychosocial and occupational impairments over time.
- There is a link between mania and mood disorders and persons with artistic and creative abilities.
- The primary treatment for mania is pharmacological.
- Due to unwanted side effects, lithium is a difficult drug for many to take over time.
- Nursing theory suggests means for the nurse to establish trust with manic clients.
- Specific nursing diagnoses can be used to describe and plan nursing care.

REVIEW QUESTIONS

1. A client is scheduled to have blood drawn for her lithium level. The nurse evaluates that the client understands the procedure if the client states which of the following?
   1. "I should eat a large breakfast before having my blood drawn."
   2. "I should make sure that my blood is drawn every five days."
   3. "I should not take my morning dose of lithium until after my blood is drawn."
   4. "I should not wear any metal jewelry to the hospital when I come for my test."

2. The physician writes several orders for a client admitted with a diagnosis of Bipolar Disorder. Which of the following orders should the nurse question?
   1. Begin lithium after blood work
   2. Low sodium diet
   3. Activities as tolerated
   4. Referral for occupational therapy

3. During your session with a client admitted with a diagnosis of Bipolar Disorder, you assess that the client is having flight of ideas. Your most therapeutic response would be to say which of the following?
   1. "Tell me what you are feeling right now."
   2. "I will come back when you are feeling better."
   3. "You are talking too fast. Can you slow down a little?"
   4. "What you are saying does not make any sense to me, does it make sense to you?"

4. A client newly admitted to the psychiatric unit introduces herself to each of the staff and states, "I'm the minster of health for the president of the United States." The nurse would chart this behavior as the client experiencing which of the following?
   1. Delusions of grandeur
   2. Auditory hallucinations
   3. Delusions of persecution
   4. Ideas of reference

5. An outcome for a client with mania, who was experiencing hallucinations and delusions, would be which of the following?
   1. Client will sleep at least eight hours each day
   2. Client will interact with others in group meetings
   3. Client will be oriented to time, place, and person
   4. Client will act more appropriately

6. Prior to administering a client's daily dose of lithium, the nurse reviews the laboratory report, which indicates the blood lithium level is 2.0. Which of the following is the priority action by the nurse?
   1. Administer the lithium as ordered
   2. Administer only half of the ordered amount
   3. Hold the medication and contact the physician
   4. Hold the medication and contact the nursing supervisor

7. A man contacts the police because his wife and five-year-old daughter have been missing for 24 hours. He tells the police, "My wife has bipolar disease and she hasn't been taking her medications and I'm worried that something has happened to them." Later that evening, the police find the wife and child wandering the streets in the snow without being properly clothed. The police take them to the local emergency department. Which action by the nurse would take priority?
   1. Schedule a family conference
   2. Assess the child's physical condition
   3. Assess the mother's psychological state
   4. Refer the mother and child to the psychiatrist

LEARNING ACTIVITIES

Consider the following case: Mari, a 20-year-old college student, has been up for five nights in a row working on a project for her design class. She has not had time to sleep, eat, or bathe. She has plans to win a prize at an international exhibit, although this is her first attempt at design. She is enthusiastic and seems capable. When her roommates suggest that she take a break, she becomes angry and verbally abusive to them, stating she has to continue with her work. Her closest friend has just discovered that Mari has spent over $5,000 on this project and has neglected all of her other classes for the past week. Because you are a nursing student, her roommates come to you for advice.

1. What evidence do you have that Mari is exhibiting mania?
2. Does Mari fit into a risk category? How would you know?
3. What else would you want to know about Mari?
4. How could you tell if there were a potential for violence?
5. Where on your campus could you refer Mari for help?
6. At what point would you notify an authority on your campus about Mari's condition?

*Study*WARE™ CONNECTION

Using your *Study*WARE™ CD-ROM

1. Complete the Crossword activity for this chapter.
2. Complete the Quiz for this chapter in Test Mode.
3. Explore the other games and activities that support this chapter.

VIDEO LINK

Read and contemplate the following questions about Mary, the client experiencing Bipolar Disorder. Then watch the video "Bi-Polar Disorder" on your *Study*WARE™ CD-ROM to observe Mary's interview with a psychiatrist. Consider these questions prior to listening to the psychiatrist's analysis.

1. In this interview you see Mary first in her depressive state and then switching into mania. Describe this change in her behavior.
2. What psychotic symptoms does Mary exhibit? Does she experience these in both her depressive and manic state?
3. How do they affect her behavior?
4. How would you chart Mary's mood—in the depressive state; in the manic state?
5. What terms would you use to describe her ability to communicate?
6. Does Mary recognize the triggers to her illness?
7. Mary self-medicated while experiencing one of her most profound depressions. What was she using? Do you feel that this self-medication regime was beneficial?
8. Mary states that she has a disease of the brain. What does the latest research finding reveal on the brains of people with Bipolar Disorder?
9. Which symptoms of mania bothered Mary the most?
10. What particular actions did she engage in that might cause her to lose her friends and family?
11. Mary was combative toward her husband while he was visiting her in hospital. What therapeutic interventions do you believe were necessary?
12. How do we create a therapeutic milieu for someone in a manic state?
13. What medications are used to treat Bipolar Disorder?
14. How do we monitor these medications for the therapeutic dosage? What are the general side effects?
15. What other therapies have proven to be beneficial for persons experiencing Bipolar Disorder?
16. Create a care plan that could be used for the duration of Mary's hospital stay.
17. Which community resources would you want to recommend to Mary and her family in preparation for her discharge?

REFERENCES

Ali, S., & Milev, R. (2003). Switch to mania upon discontinuation of antidepressants in patients with mood disorders: A review of the literature. *Canadian Journal of Psychiatry, 48*(4), 258–264.

American Psychiatric Association. (2000). *Diagnostic and Statistical Manual of Mental Disorders*, Fourth Edition-Text Revision. Washington, DC: Author.

Arnold, L. M. (2003). Gender differences in bipolar disorder. *Psychiatric Clinics of North America, 26*(3), 595–620.

Aronne, L. J., & Segal, K. R. (2003). Weight gain in the treatment of mood disorders. *Journal of Clinical Psychiatry, 64*(Suppl. 8), 22–29.

Baillargeon, J., Ducate, S., Pulvino, J., Bradshaw, P., Murray, O., & Olivera, R. (2003). The association of psychiatric disorders and HIV infection in the correctional setting. *Annals of Epidemiology, 13*(9), 606–612.

Baptista, T., De Mendoza, S., Beaulieu, S., Bermudez, A., & Martinez, M. (2004). The metabolic syndrome during atypical antipsychotic drug treatment: Mechanisms and management. *Metabolic Syndrome and Related Disorders, 2*(4), 290–307.

Barley, K. P. (1999). Electrophysiologic kindling and behavioral sensitization as model for bipolar illness: Implications for nursing practice. *Journal of the American Psychiatric Nurses Association, 5*(2), 62–66.

Bauer, M., Grof, P., Gyulai, L., Rasgon, N., Glenn, T., & Whybrow, P. C. (2004). Using technology to improve longitudinal studies: Self-reporting with ChronoRecord in bipolar disorder. *Bipolar Disorders, 6*(1), 67–74.

Bauer, M. S., & Mitchner, L. (2004). What is a "mood stabilizer"? An evidence-based response. *American Journal of Psychiatry, 161*(1), 2–18.

Benazzi, F. (2007). Bipolar II disorder: Epidemiology, diagnosis and management. *CNS Drugs, 21*(9), 727–740.

Berrocal, C., Ruiz Moreno, M. A., Rando, M. A., Benvenuti, A., & Cassano, G. B. (2008). Borderline personality disorder and mood spectrum. *Psychiatry Research, 159*(3), 300–307.

Bezchlibnyk, Y., & Young L. T. (2002). The neurobiology of bipolar disorder: Focus on signal transduction pathways and the regulation of gene expression. *Canadian Journal of Psychiatry, 47*(2), 135–148.

Birkenaes, A. B., Opjordsmoen, S., Brunborg, C., Engh, J. A., Jonsdottir, H., Ringen, P. A., et al. (2007). The level of cardiovascular risk factors in bipolar disorder equals that of schizophrenia: A comparative study. *Journal of Clinical Psychiatry, 68*(6), 917–923.

Black, D. W., Winokur, G., & Nasrallah, A. (1987). Is death from natural causes still excessive in psychiatric patients? A follow-up of 1593 patients with major affective disorder. *Journal of Nervous and Mental Diseases, 175*, 674–680.

Blumberg, H. P., Stern, E., Ricketts, S., Martinez, D., de Asis, J., White, T., et al. (1999). Rostral and orbital prefrontal cortex dysfunction in the manic state of bipolar disorder. *American Journal of Psychiatry, 156*(12), 1986–1988.

Burt, V. K., & Rasgon, N. (2004). Special considerations in treating bipolar disorder in women. *Bipolar Disorders, 6*(1), 2–13.

Calabrese, J. R., & Woyshville, M. J. (1994). A medication algorithm for bipolar rapid cycling. *Journal of Clinical Psychiatry, 56* (Suppl. 3), 11–18.

Carlson, G. A., & Goodwin, F. K. (1973). The stages of mania: A longitudinal analysis of the manic episode. *Archives of General Psychiatry, 28*, 221–228.

Chaudron, L. H., & Pies, R. W. (2003). The relationship between postpartum psychosis and bipolar disorder: A review. *Journal of Clinical Psychiatry, 64*(11), 1284–1292.

Colom, F., Vieta, E., Reinares, M., Martinex-Aran, A., Torrent, C., Goikolea, J., et al. (2003). Psychoeducation efficacy in bipolar disorders: Beyond compliance enhancement. *Journal of Clinical Psychiatry, 64*(9), 1101–1105.

Compton, M. T., & Nemeroff, C. B. (2000). The treatment of bipolar depression. *Journal of Clinical Psychiatry, 61*(Suppl. 9), 57–67.

Cook, B. L., & Winokur, G. (1990). Perspective on bipolar illness. *Comprehensive Therapy, 16*, 18–23.

Coryell, W., Endicott, J., Keller, M., Anderson, M., Growe, W., Hirschfield, R. M. A., et al. (1989). Bipolar affective disorder and high achievement: A familial association. *American Journal of Psychiatry, 146*, 983–988.

Coryell, W., Scheftner, W., Keller, M., Endicott, J., Maser, J., & Klerman, G. L. (1993). The enduring psychosocial consequences of mania and depression. *American Journal of Psychiatry, 150*, 720–727.

Craddock, N., & Jones, I. (1999). Genetics of bipolar disorder. *Journal of Medical Genetics, 36*(8), 585–594.

Craddock, N., O'Donovan, M. C., & Owen, M. J. (2006). Genes for schizophrenia and bipolar disorder? Implications for psychiatric nosology. *Schizophrenia Bulletin, 32*(1), 9–16.

Cutler, C. G. (2001). Self-care agency and symptom management in patients treated for mood disorder. *Archives of Psychiatric Nursing, 15*(1), 24–31.

Depression Guideline Panel. (1993). *Depression in primary care: Detection and diagnosis.* Rockville, MD: Agency of Health Care Policy and Research.

Dion, G. L., Tohen, M., Anthony, W. A., & Watermaux, C. S. (1988). Symptoms and functioning of patients with bipolar disorder six months after hospitalization. *Hospital and Community Psychiatry, 39*, 652–657.

Dunner, D. L., Jie, S. Q., Ping, Z. Y., & Dunner, P. Z. (1984). A study of primary affective disorder in the People's Republic of China. *Biological Psychiatry, 19*, 353–359.

Einat, H., Manji, H. K., Gould, T. D., Du, J., & Chen, G. (2003). Possible involvement of the ERK signaling cascade in bipolar disorder: Behavioral leads from the study of mutant mice. *Drug News Perspectives, 16*(7), 453–463.

Evins, A. E. (2003). Efficacy of newer anticonvulsant medications in bipolar spectrum mood disorders. *Journal of Clinical Psychiatry, 64* (Suppl. 8), 9–14.

Fagiolini, A., Frank, E., Houck, P. R., Mallinger, A. G., Swartz, H. A., Buysse, D. J., et al. (2002). Prevalence of obesity and weight change during treatment in patients with bipolar I disorder. *Journal of Clinical Psychiatry, 63*(6), 528–533.

Fallon, B. N., Nields, J. A., Parsons, B., Liebowitz, M. R., & Klein, D. F. (1993). Psychiatric manifestations of lyme borreliosis. *Journal of Clinical Psychiatry, 54*, 263–268.

Fawcett, J. (2001). The nurse theorists: 21st Century update: Rosemarie Rizzo Parse. *Nursing Science Quarterly, 14*(2), 126–131.

Fogarty, F., Russell, T. M., Newman, S. C., & Bland, R. C. (1994). Mania. *Acta Psychiatrica Scandinavica, 376*(Suppl.), 16–23.

Gershon, E. S., Hamovil, J., Guroff, J. J., Dibble, E., Leckman, L. R., & Banney, W. E., Jr. (1982). A family study of schizoaffective, bipolar I, bipolar II, unipolar, and normal control probans. *Archives of General Psychiatry, 39*, 1157–1167.

Ghaemi, S. N., Rosenquist, K. J., Ko, J. Y., Baldassano, C. F., Kontos, N. J., & Baldessarini, R. J. (2004). Antidepressant treatment in bipolar versus unipolar depression. *American Journal of Psychiatry, 161*(1), 163–165.

Goes, F. S., Sanders, L. L., & Potash, J. B. (2008). The genetics of psychotic bipolar disorder. *Current Psychiatry Reports, 10*(2), 178–189.

Goldberg, J. F., Perlis, R. H., Ghaemi, S. N., Calabrese, J. R., Bowden, C. L., Wisniewski, S., et al. (2007). Adjunctive antidepressant use and symptomatic recovery among bipolar depressed patients with concomitant manic symptoms: Findings from the STEP-BD. *American Journal of Psychiatry, 164*(9), 1348–1355.

Goodwin, F. K. (2003). Rationale for using lithium in combination with other mood stabilizers in the management of bipolar depression. *Journal of Clinical Psychiatry, 64*(Suppl. 5), 18–24.

Goodwin, F. K., & Jamison, K. R. (1990). *Manic-depressive illness.* Oxford, England: Oxford University Press.

Goodwin, F. K., Fireman, B., Simon, G. E., Hunkeler, E. M., Lee, J., & Revicki, D. (2003). Suicide risk in bipolar disorder during treatment with lithium and divalproex. *Journal of the American Medical Association, 290*(11), 1467–1473.

Goren, J. L., & Levin, G. M. (2000). Mania with bupropion: A dose-related phenomenon? *Annals of Pharmacotherapy, 34*(5), 619–621.

Gould, T. D., & Manji, H. K. (2002). The Wnt signaling pathway in bipolar disease. *Neuroscientist, 8*(5), 497–511.

Gusella, J. F., Wexler, N. S., Conneally, P. M., Naylor, S. L., Anderson, M., Tanzi, R. E., et al. (1983). A polymorphic DNA marker genetically linked to Huntington's disease. *Nature, 306*, 234–238.

Helzer, J. E., & Prybeck, T. R. (1988). The co-occurrence of alcoholism with other psychiatric disorders in the general population and its impact on treatment. *Journal on Studies of Alcohol, 49*, 219–224.

Hickman, J. S. (1995). Rosemarie Rizzo Parse. In J. George (Ed.), *Nursing theories: The base for professional nursing practice* (4th ed.; pp. 335–354). Norwalk, CT: Appleton & Lange.

Himelhoch, S., & Daumit, G. (2003). To whom do psychiatrists offer smoking-cessation counseling? *American Journal of Psychiatry, 160*(12), 2228–2230.

Jamison, K. R., (2000). Suicide and bipolar disorder. *Journal of Clinical Psychiatry, 61*(Suppl. 9), 47–51.

Joffe, H., Hall, J. E., Cohen, L. S., Taylor, A. E., & Baldessarini, R. J. (2003). A putative relationship between valproic acid and polycystic ovarian syndrome: Implications for the treatment of women with seizure and bipolar disorders. *Harvard Review of Psychiatry, 1*(2), 99–108.

Joffe, R. T., MacQueen, G. M., Marriott, M., Trevor-Young, L. (2004). A prospective, longitudinal study of percentage of time spent ill, patients with bipolar I or bipolar II disorders. *Bipolar Disorders, 6*(1), 62–66.

Keck, P. E., & McElroy, S. L. (2003). Bipolar disorder, obesity, and pharmacotherapy-associated weight gain. *Journal of Clinical Psychiatry, 64*(12), 4126–1435.

Keck, P. E., Jr. (2003). The management of acute mania. *British Medical Journal, 327*(7422), 1002–1003.

Keener, M. T., & Phillips, M. L. (2007). Neuroimaging in bipolar disorder: A critical review of current findings. *Current Psychiatry Reports, 9*(6), 512–520.

Kennedy, J. L., Farrer, L. A., Andreasen, N. C., Mayeux, R., & St. George-Hyslop, F. (2003). The genetics of adult-onset neuropsychiatric disease. *Science, (302-5646)*, 822–826.

Kessing, L. V., Agerbo, E., & Mortensen, P. B. (2004). Major stressful life events and other risk factors for first admission with mania. *Bipolar Disorders, 4*(6), 122–129.

Kessler, R. C., Akiskal, H. S., Ames, M., Birnbaum, H. Greenberg, P., Hirshfeld, R., Jin, R., Merikangas, K. R., Simon, G. E., & Wang, P. S. (2006). Prevalence and effects of mood disorders on work performance in a nationally representative sample of U.S. workers. *American Journal of Psychiatry, 169*(9), 1561–1568.

Ketter, T. A., Brooks, J. O., Hoblyn, J. C., Champion, L. M., Nam, J. Y., Culver, J. L., Marsh, W. K., Bonner, J. C. (2008). Effectiveness of lamotrigine in bipolar disorder in a clinical setting. *Journal of Psychatric Research, 43*(1), 13–23.

Klerman, G. L. (1981). The spectrum of mania. *Comprehensive Psychiatry, 22,* 11–20.

Kohen, I., & Kremen, N. (2007). Varenicline-induced manic episode in a patient with bipolar disorder. *American Journal of Psychiatry, 164*(8), 1269–1270.

Konig, S. A., Schenck, M., Sick, C., Holm, E., Heubner, C., Weiss, A., et al. (1999). Fatal liver failure associated with valproate therapy in a patient with Friedreich's disease: Review of valproate hepatotoxicity in adults. *Epilepsia, 40*(7), 1036–1040.

Krauthammer, C., & Klerman, G. L. (1979). The epidemiology of mania. In B. Shopsin (Ed.), *Manic illness* (pp. 11–28). New York: Raven.

Kupka, R., Luckenbauth, D. A., Post, R. M., et al. (2005). Comparison of rapid-cycling and non-rapid-cycling bipolar disorder based on prospective mood ratings in 539 outpatients. *American Journal of Psychiatry, 162,* 1273.

Lam, D. H., Watkins, E. R., Hayward, P., Bright, J., Wright, K., Kerr, N., et al. (2003). A randomized controlled study of cognitive therapy for relapse prevention for bipolar affective disorder: Outcome of the first year. *Archives of General Psychiatry, 60*(2), 45–52.

Leff, J. P., Fischer, M., & Bertelson, A. C. (1976). A cross-rebreak national study of mania. *British Journal of Psychiatry, 129,* 428–442.

Leibenluft, E. (1997). Issues in the treatment of women with bipolar illness. *Journal of Clinical Psychiatry, 58*(Suppl 15), 5.

Mabbett, P. D. (1996). *Instant nursing assessment: Mental health.* Clifton Park, NY: Thomson Delmar Learning.

Machado, A. C., Deguti, M. M., Caixeta, L., Spitz, M., Lucato, L. T., & Barbosa, E. R. (2008). Mania as the first manifestation of Wilson's disease. *Bipolar Disorders, 10*(3), 447–450.

Miklowitz, D. J., Otto, M. W., Frank, E., Reilly-Harrington, N. A., Kogan, J. N., Sachs, G. S., et al. (2007). Intensive psychosocial intervention enhances functioning in patients with bipolar depression: Results from a 9-month randomized controlled trial. *American Journal of Psychiatry, 164*(9), 1340–1347.

Mortensen, P. B., Pedersen, C. B., Melbye, M., Mors, O., & Ewald, H. (2003). Individual and familial risk factors for bipolar affective disorder in Denmark. *Archives of General Psychiatry, 60,* 1209–1215.

Muller-Oerlinghausem, B., Berghofer, A., & Ahrens, B. (2003). The antisuicidal and morality-reducing effect of lithium prophylaxis. Consequences for guidelines in clinical psychiatry. *Canadian Journal of Psychiatry, 48*(7), 433–439.

Namuta, T., Abe, H., Tarao, T., & Nakashima, V. (1999). Possible involvement of hypothyroidism as a case of lithium-induced sinus mode dysfunction. *Pacing Clinical Electrophysiology, 22*(6), 954–957.

Nierenberg, A. A., Burt, T., Matthews, J., & Weiss, A. P. (1999). Mania associated with St. John's wort. *Biological Psychiatry, 46*(12), 1707–1708.

Nowlin-Finch, N. L., Altshuler, L. L., Szuba, M. P., & Mintz, J. (1994). Rapid resolution of first episodes of mania: Sleep related? *Journal of Clinical Psychiatry, 55,* 26–29.

Ostacher, M. J., & Sachs, G. S. (2006). Update on bipolar disorder and substance abuse: Recent findings and treatment strategies. *Journal of Clinical Psychiatry, 67*(9).

Pariser, S. F. (1993). Women and mood disorders: Menarche to menopause. *Annals of Clinical Psychiatry, 5,* 249–254.

Parker, G., & Parker, K. (2003). Which antidepressants flick the switch? *Australian and New Zealand Journal of Psychiatry, 37*(4), 464–468.

Parse, R. R., (1992). Human becoming: Parse's theory of nursing. *Nursing Science Quarterly, 5,* 35–42.

Paykel, E. S. (1995). Psychotherapy, medication combinations, and compliance. *Journal of Clinical Psychiatry, 56*(Suppl. 1), 24–30.

Peet, M., & Peters, S. (1995). Drug induced mania. *Drug Safety, 12,* 146–153.

Pope, H. G., Jr., & Katz, D. L. (1994). Psychiatric and medical effects of anabolic-androgenic steroid use: A controlled study of 160 athletes. *Archives of General Psychiatry, 51,* 375–382.

Post, R. M., Roy-Byrne, P. P., & Uhde, T. W. (1988). Graphic representation of the life course of illness in patients with affective disorder. *American Journal of Psychiatry, 145,* 844–848.

Preisig, M., Bellivier, F., Fenton, B. T., Baud, P., Berney, A., Courtet, P., et al. (2000). Association between bipolar disorder and monoamine oxidase A gene polymorphisms: Results of a multicenter study. *American Journal of Psychiatry, 157*(6), 948–955.

Rendell, J. M., Gijsmann, H. J., Keck, P., Goodwin, G. M., & Geddes, J. R. (2003). Olanzapine alone or in combination for acute mania. *Cochrane Database Systematic Review,* (4), CD004040.

Ringen, P. A., Melle, I., Birkenaes, A. B., Engh, J. A., Faerden, A., Jonsdottir, H., et al. (2008). Illicit drug use in patients with psychotic disorders compared with that in the general population: A cross-sectional study. *Acta Psychiatrica Scandinavica, 117*(2), 133–138.

Rohan, M., Parrow, A. Stoll, A. L., Demopulos, C., Friedman, S., Dages, S., et al. (2004). Low-field magnetic stimulation in bipolar depression using an MRI-based simulator. *American Journal of Psychiatry, 161*(1), 93–98.

Rothbaym, B. D., & Astin, M. C. (2000). Integration of pharmacotherapy and psychotherapy for bipolar disorder. *Journal of Clinical Psychiatry, 61*(Suppl. 9), 68–75.

Sajatovic, M. (2002). Aging-related issues in bipolar disorder: A health services perspective. *Journal of Geriatric Psychiatry and Neurology, 15,* 128–133.

Schou, M., & Weeke, A. (1988). Did manic-depressive patients who committed suicide receive prophylactic or continuation treatment at the time? *British Journal of Psychiatry, 153,* 324–327.

Shaw, E. D., Mann, J. J., Stokes, P. E., & Manevitz, A. Z. A. (1987). Effects of lithium carbonate on associative productivity and idiosyncrasy in bipolar outpatients. *American Journal of Psychiatry, 143,* 1166–1169.

Shivakumar, G., Bernstein, I., Suppes, T., & the Stanley Foundation Bipolar Network. (2008). *Journal of Women's Health, 17*(3), 473–478.

Shuster, J. (1999). Adverse drug reaction: Lithium and sodium depletion. *Nursing, 28*(9), 29.

Small, J. G., Milstein, J., & Small, I. F. (1991). Electroconvulsive therapy for mania. *Psychiatric Clinics of North America, 14,* 887–903.

Strakowski, S. M., McElroy, S. L., Keck, P. W., Jr., & West, S. A. (1994). The co-occurrence of mania with medical and other psychiatric disorders. *International Journal of Psychiatry, 24,* 305–328.

Suppes, T., Dennehy, E. B., & Gibbons, E. W. (2000). The longitudinal course of bipolar disorder. *Journal of Clinical Psychiatry, 61*(Suppl. 9), 23–30.

Takei, N., O'Callaghan, E., Sham, P., Glover, G., Tamura, A., & Murry, R. (1992). Seasonality of admission in the psychoses: Effect of diagnosis, sex, and age at onset. *British Journal of Psychiatry, 161,* 506–511.

Tondo, L., & Baldessarini, R. J. (2000). Reduced suicide risk during lithium maintenance treatment. *Journal of Clinical Psychiatry, 61*(Suppl. 9), 97–104.

Torrent, C., Amann, B., Sanchez-Moreno, J., Colom, F., Reinares, M., Comes, M., et al. (2008). Weight gain in bipolar disorder: Pharmacological treatment as a contributing factor. *Acta Psychiatrica Scandinavica, 118*(1), 4–18.

van Winkel, R., De Hert, M., Van Eyck, D., Hanssens, L., Wampers, M., Scheen, A., et al. (2008). Prevalence of diabetes and the metabolic syndrome in a sample of patients with bipolar disorder. *Bipolar Disorders, 10*(2), 342–348.

Vreeland, B., Minsky, S., Menza, M., Rigassio Radler, D., Roemheld-Hamm, D., & Stern, R. (2003). A program for managing weight gain associated with atypical antipsychotics. *Psychiatric Services, 54*(8), 1155–1157.

Warner, J. P. (2000). Evidence based psychopharmacology 3, assessing the evidence of harm: What are the teratogenic effects of lithium carbonate? *Journal of Psychopharmacology, 14*(1), 77–80.

Weissman, M. M., Bruce, M. L., Leaf, P. J., Florio, L. P., & Holzer, C., III. (1991). Affective disorders. In L. N. Robins & D. A. Regier (Eds.), *Psychiatric disorders in America: The epidemiologic catchment area study* (pp. 53–80). New York: Free Press.

West, R. (2003). Bupropion SR for smoking cessation. *Expert Opinion in Pharmacotherapy, 4*(4), 533–540.

Winokur, G., Clayton, P. J., & Reich, T. (1969). *Manic depressive illness.* St. Louis: Mosby.

Wozniak, J., (2007). Bipolar disorder is common in first degree relatives of children with prepubertal and early adolescent bipolar 1 disorder. *Evidenced Based Mental Health, 10*(2), 63.

Yatham, L. N. (2003). Acute and maintenance treatment of bipolar mania: The role of atypical antipsychotics. *Bipolar Disorders, 5*(Suppl. 2), 7–19.

Young, R. C., & Klerman, G. N. (1992). Mania in late life: Focus on age at onset. *American Journal of Psychiatry, 149,* 867–875.

Zaretsky, A. (2003). Targeted psychosocial interventions for bipolar disorder. *Bipolar Disorders, 5*(Suppl. 2), 80–87.

Ziedonis, D., Williams, J. M., & Smelson, D. (2003). Serious mental illness and tobacco addition: A model program to address this common but neglected issue *American Journal of Medical Science, 6*(4), 223–230.

LITERARY REFERENCES

Byron, Lord. (1905). *The complete poetical works of Lord Byron.* Boston: Houghton Mifflin Company.

Carroll, J. (1992). *Outside the dog museum.* New York: Doubleday.

James, W. (1961). *The varieties of religious experience.* New York: Macmillan.

Krim, S. (1961). *Views of a nearsighted cannoneer.* New York: Excelsior.

Millett, K. (1990). *The looney-bin trip.* New York: Simon & Schuster.

Plato. (1988, c1986). *Phaedrus and the seventh and eighth letters* (2nd ed.; C. J. Rowe, Trans). Warminster, Wiltshire, England: Aris & Phillips.

Roccataggliata, G. (1986). *A history of ancient psychiatry.* Westport, CT: Greenwood Press.

Seager, A. (1991). *The glass house: The life of Theodore Roethke.* Ann Arbor: University of Michigan Press.

SUGGESTED READINGS

Martin, E. R. (2007). *Bipolar expeditions: Mania and depression in American culture.* Princeton: Princeton University Press.

Noel, K. (2006). *Halfway house.* New York: Atlantic Monthly Press.

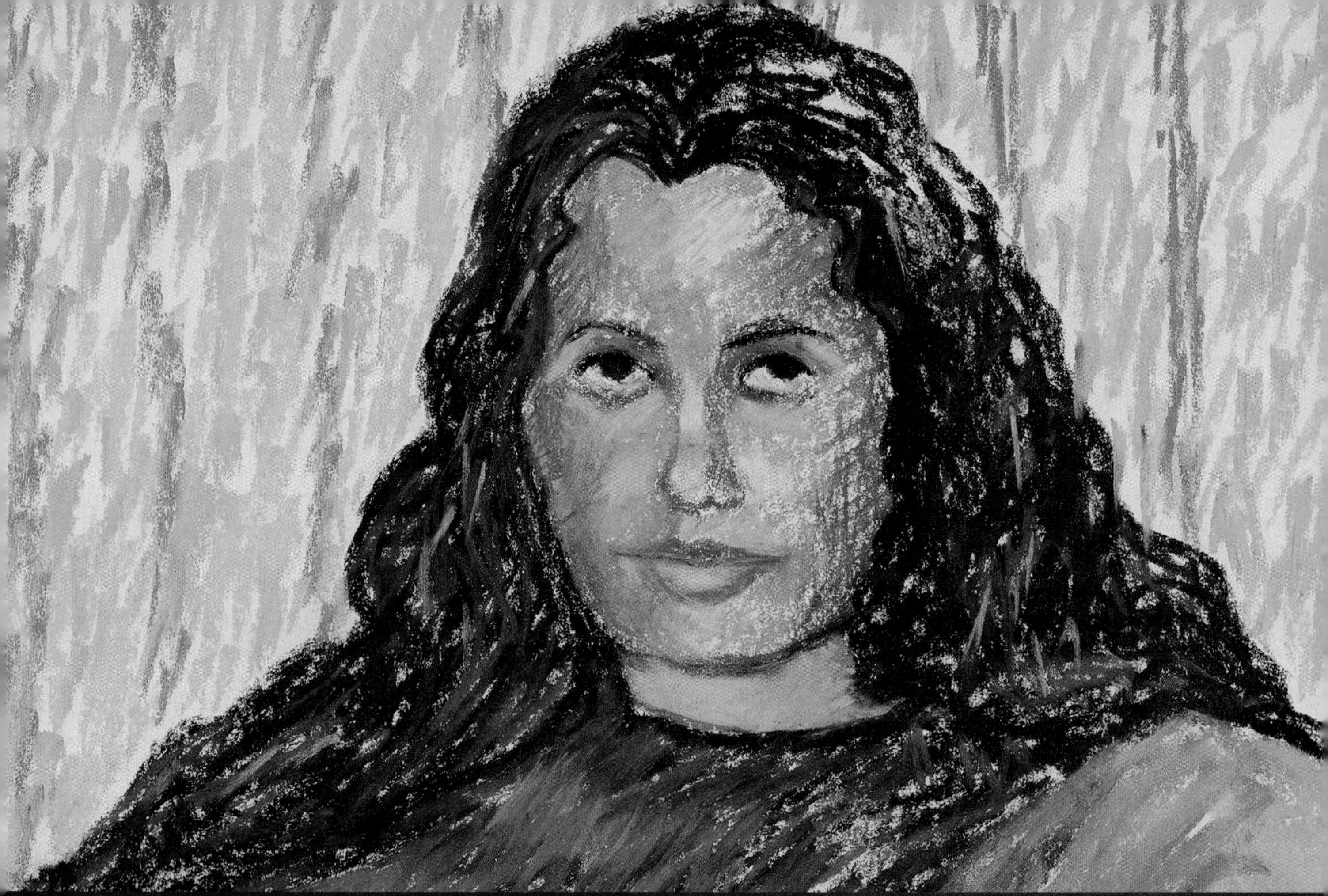

Exploration of Hope and Hopelessness

- *What does it mean to you to have meaning and purpose in life?*
- *What is your source of inner strength?*
- *What in your life helps to make you feel connected to others?*
- *Do you believe that those around you can support your needs?*
- *Do you have a sense of your own future?*

Consider your own very personal answers to these questions. Recognize that hopelessness is a human emotion stemming from a distress of the human spirit.

CHAPTER 16

The Client Who Is Suicidal

NOREEN CAVAN FRISCH
LAWRENCE E. FRISCH

CHAPTER OUTLINE

COMPETENCIES

Upon completion of this chapter, the reader should be able to:

1. Explore the significance of hopelessness and loss of meaning and purpose in life.
2. Identify the conditions and circumstances that make an individual at high risk for suicide.
3. Describe a means of assessing suicide potential in a client.
4. Know the means of providing a safe environment for the suicidal client.
5. State the psychiatric and medical conditions that significantly increase a client's risk of suicide.
6. Use theory to understand and interpret suicidal behaviors.
7. Use the nursing assessment to evaluate one's sense of meaning and purpose in life.
8. Use nursing theory to develop a therapeutic nurse-client relationship and as a framework to provide care.
9. Apply the nursing process when providing care to individuals at risk for suicide.
10. Administer care to family members who have experienced the loss of a loved one to suicide.

KEY TERMS

Euthanasia
Suicidal Ideations
Suicide
Suicide Potential
Suicide Survivors

Purposefully taking one's own life, or **suicide**, is the ultimate form of self-destruction. Clients who are suicidal often feel overwhelmed by life events and decide that the only relief will come from ending their own lives. Intense feelings of fear, loss, anger, or despair can drive individuals to commit suicide, and the effects of an attempted or completed suicide can be devastating and long lasting. Nurses must learn how to recognize the danger signs of clients at risk for suicide and know the appropriate interventions to help clients preserve their health and dignity.

ON DEATH

I am a student nurse. I am dying. I write this to you who are, and will become, nurses in the hope that by my sharing my feelings with you, you may someday be better able to help those who share my experience.

I'm out of the hospital now—perhaps for a month, for six months, perhaps for a year—but no one likes to talk about such things. In fact, no one likes to talk about much at all. Nursing must be advancing, but I wish it would hurry. We're taught not to be overly cheery now, to omit the "Everything's fine" routine, and we have done pretty well. But now one is left in a lonely silent void. With the protective "fine, fine" gone, the staff is left with only their own vulnerability and fear. The dying patient is not yet seen as a person and thus cannot be communicated with as such. He is a symbol of what every human fears and what we each know, at least academically, that we too must someday face. What did they say in psychiatric nursing about meeting pathology with pathology to the detriment of both patient and nurse? And there was a lot about knowing one's own feelings before you could help another with his. How true.

But for me, fear is today and dying is now. You slip in and out of my room, give me medications and check my blood pressure. Is it because I am a student nurse, myself, or just a human being, that I sense your fright? And your fears enhance mine. Why are you afraid? I am the one who is dying!

I know you feel insecure, don't know what to say, don't know what to do. But please believe me, if you care, you can't go wrong. Just admit that you care. That is really for what we search. We may ask for why's and wherefore's, but we don't really expect answers. Don't run away—wait—all I want to know is that there will be someone to hold my hand when I need it. I am afraid. Death may get to be a routine to you, but it is new to me. You may not see me as unique, but I've never died before. To me, once is pretty unique!

You whisper about my youth, but when one is dying, is he really so young anymore? I have lots I wish we could talk about. It really would not take much more of your time because you are in here quite a bit anyway.

*If only we could be honest, both admit of our fears, touch one another. If you really care, would you lose so much of your valuable professionalism if you even cried with me? Just person to person? Then it might not be so hard to die—in a hospital—with friends close by.**

(*Anonymous, 1970, p. 336*)

Death of the young and suicide have much in common—each seems particularly tragic, somehow avoidable, in some way incomprehensible. It is rare that the dying can call so eloquently for understanding, comfort, simple touch, and friendship as does this anonymous student nurse. Much is both said and unsaid in this moving essay. As readers, we sense remarkable self-awareness, a resignation coupled with defiance, a strong expression of fear, and anger: "Why are *you* afraid? I am the one who is dying! ... I write this ... in the hopes ... you may someday be *better able* to help.... Then, it might not be so hard to die" (italics added). Today it may not be so hard for some to die. The years since 1970 have seen many changes in our understanding of the process of death, in the way we can reach out to the dying of all ages, and in the tools we can offer to ease the pain and fear that so often accompany death. But the mixture of fear, anger, despair (veiled but seemingly just under the surface of this remarkable essay), and the loss both of human touch and of any control over life and death are present, and these experiences are the stuff of which suicide is made.

The purpose of this chapter is to address the topic of suicide from the perspective of psychiatric mental health nursing. Suicide is not inherently a psychiatric problem. By no means do all persons who commit suicide have a psychiatric illness. Indeed, there is growing pressure for medical and nursing involvement in legally assisted suicide of persons thought to be fully mentally competent who decide to end their lives. Nonetheless, suicide currently takes place primarily among the psychiatrically disturbed and in an atmosphere of alienation, disconnectedness, and despair. Most who kill themselves are no less in need of solace, touch, and listening than was the student nurse who wrote so eloquently about impending death. Many reach out prior to acting and, like the student nurse, find there is no human response.

PREVALENCE OF SUICIDE AND RELATED STATISTICS

In the United States, suicide accounts for approximately 11 deaths yearly per 100,000 persons: 1.4% of all U.S deaths in 2005 (just over 32,000 deaths; Centers for Disease Control and Prevention [CDC], 2007). Suicide is the second leading cause of death among persons aged 25–34. Before 1978, the suicide rate was highest for persons older than 24 years, but between 1955 and 1978, a steady rise in adolescent and young adult suicide brought the rates for this age range from 5 per 100,000 to over 13 per 100,000. In 1987, there were 4,924 suicidal deaths among persons aged 15 to 24, making suicide the third leading cause of death among young persons (Berman & Jobes, 1991) a ranking that it still holds (CDC, 2007) despite a decrease in suicide rate for this age grouping that began about 1995 (McKeown, Cuffe, & Schulz, 2006).

While suicide occurs at all ages, males over age 75 have a suicide rate nearly three times the national average (CDC, 2007). The overall suicide rate for Americans 65 and older had been increasing steadily into the 1990s (Saluatore, 2000), but it then declined through 2005 to a rate that is still about 40% higher than the comparable rate for those under 65 (McKeown et al., 2006). Suicide is more common among divorced and separated men (Kposawa, 2000). Suicide rates rose in nearly all countries during the Great Depression of the 1930s, and studies for several countries support a significant correlation between unemployment and risk of suicide (Lewis & Sloggett, 1998). Among the employed, neither occupation nor income correlate consistently with suicide rates, but high rates have been reported for U.S. physicians (notably women and psychiatrists), and to a lesser extent for nurses (Hawton & Vislisel, 1999). Students interested in further data on suicide (as well as other causes of injury) should consult the National Center for Injury Prevention and Control's "WISQARS" interactive data site (available at: http://webappa.cdc.gov/sasweb/ncipc/mortrate10_sy.html).

Completed suicide rates have dropped significantly in a number of countries over the past decade, especially for children and adolescents. One of the hypotheses explaining this decline in suicide rate has been the greater use of antidepressant medication in young persons during this time. There is good correlation between increasing use of SSRIs and other "new generation" antidepressants and decreased suicide rate (Gibbons, Hur, Bhaumik, & Mann, 2005). This correlation does not prove that the increased antidepressant usage causes suicide rates to fall, but it does suggest the possibility of a causal connection. Since 2003, when authorities in the United States and the Netherlands placed "black box" warnings on antidepressants prescribed for children and adolescents (the United Kingdom went further and prohibited the use of most medications to treat depression in children), antidepressant prescription rates declined by 22% in the United States and the Netherlands. Between 2003 and 2004, suicide in children and adolescents increased by 14% in the United States and 49% in the Netherlands (Gibbons, Brown, Hur, Marcus, Bhaumik, Erkens, et al., 2007). Experts do not yet know if these increases are directly attributable to the drop in antidepressant usage, but this remains a very likely possibility. During the same period, the percentage of adults—for whom there was no evidence of increased suicide risk related to antidepressant prescription—who received no antidepressant medication after a diagnosis of depression increased from 20% to 30% (Valuck, Libby, Orton, Morrato, Allen, & Baldessarini, 2007). There is as yet no indication that this decreased use of medication resulted in higher suicide rates.

*From "On Death—I Am a Student Nurse" by Anonymous, 1970, *American Journal of Nursing, 70*, p. 336. Reprinted with permission.

Suicide Potential

The nurse must be able to assess for **suicide potential** and know when a client's risk is severe and a chance of completing suicide is imminent. Prevalence data assist in establishing those instances where the risk is high. In general, a client who is rational, has a suicidal plan, and has the means to carry out the plan is at very high risk. For example, a client who expresses suicidal thoughts, has a plan to shoot himself, and has a loaded gun in the closet is at very high risk for completing suicide. Table 16-1 presents a tool for assessing suicide potential. The reader should examine each aspect to become familiar with high-risk behaviors.

Suicide or Accident

Although it may sometimes not be possible to identify suicidal intent in accidents, one study found that nearly 15% of actual suicides were misclassified as nonsuicidal in official death reports (Phillips & Ruth, 1993). The World Health Organization (WHO) reports that suicide rates may be significantly underreported, depending on the processes used by each reporting country (Bertolote & Fleischmann, 2002). Clearly, efforts to understand the phenomenon of suicide are potentially made more complicated by the difficulties of ensuring accurate recording of events.

Suicide Attempts

Suicide attempts appear to be strikingly more common than are completed suicides. Unfortunately, though, it is much more difficult to measure suicide attempts than to measure suicides, and accurate statistics are quite a challenge to obtain. The World Health Organization reports that no country in the world provides official statistics on attempted suicides (Bertolote & Fleishmann, 2002). The community surveys and the epidemiological studies from the 1980s remain as the best set of available estimates of suicide attempts. In these studies persons were asked retrospectively if they had ever contemplated suicide or attempted it. These reports indicated that up to 10% of people in Canada reported having made a suicide attempt sometime in their lives (Bagley, 1985), and in the United States, estimates for suicide attempts were 2.9% in the U.S. Epidemiologic Catchment Area Study (Moscicki, O'Carrol, Rae, Locke, Roy, & Regier, 1988), and in Israel estimates were as high as 7.9% (Levav, Magnes, Aisenberg, & Rosenblum, 1988). As mentioned in Chapter 8 (Epidemiology) there have been no other major community studies, and it is unlikely that current governments will fund such major undertakings again. However, in addition to those community studies, one set of researchers surveyed adolescents anonymously and reported that in the 1990s, 7% to 10% of adolescents reported one or more prior suicide attempts (Safer, 1997). More recently, trends reported by the U.S. National Hospital Medical Care Survey suggest that emergency room visits for suicide attempts and self-injury have been rising over the last decade and now account for 1.5 visits per 1,000 in U.S. emergency rooms (Larkin, Smith, & Beautrais, 2008). Data over the years has consistently shown that suicide attempts are more common in women, whereas successful suicide is more common in men (Bertolote & Fleishman, 2002; Lester, 1992). Factors such as childhood sexual abuse also seem to serve as predictors for both suicidal attempts and ideation (Brezo, Paris, Tremblay, Vitaro, Hebert, & Turecki, 2008).

Suicidal Ideation

Suicidal thoughts, called **suicidal ideations**, are even more common than suicidal attempts for persons in all age groups. The Epidemiologic Catchment Area Study referred to previously reported a history of suicidal ideation (ever having thought seriously about suicide) in 10.7% of persons surveyed (Robins & Regier, 1991). More recently, in a study of cancer patients, 17.7% were found to have suicidal ideation, and this ideation was reported as not necessarily a manifestation of depression as being related to poor physical health that also influences individuals' thinking about suicide and death (Schneider & Shenassa, 2008). In a National College Health Assessment Survey, 9.5% of college students exhibited suicidal ideation in the year preceding the study (Schwartz, 2006). Undetected suicidal ideation clearly remains a grave concern as reports suggest that for every one completed suicide, there are 100–200 attempts (National Institutes of Mental Health, 2008).

Methods

There is an extensive literature on methods chosen by persons attempting and successfully completing suicide (Lester, 1992). Firearms are used by the majority of persons, particularly younger individuals. Medication overdose is another commonly chosen method, and most dangerous overdoses involve psychotropic prescription medications, especially older tricyclic antidepressants. In areas where tricyclics are more widely used, suicide rates are higher—suggesting that access to more lethal means may increase the risk of suicide or that the use of tricyclics may be a marker for less effective mental health care (Gibbons et al., 2005). Lethal access has major implications for suicide prevention, a topic discussed later in this chapter.

Suicide and Psychiatric Illness

Suicide is clearly associated with psychiatric illness; the WHO data suggest that worldwide, 90% of those who commit suicide had a psychiatric diagnosis at the time of death (Bertolote & Fleischmann, 2002). Psychiatric conditions that have high incidence of suicide include depression (both Unipolar and Bipolar), Schizophrenia, alcoholism, drug abuse, Panic Disorder, personality disorders, and Obsessive-Compulsive Disorder (Bertolote & Fleischmann, 2002; Lester, 1992). While it seems likely that clients with each of these disorders have increased suicidal risk, it is far more difficult to assess what percentage of persons who commit suicide have a diagnosable psychiatric disorder. An early Swedish study (Hagnell & Rorsman, 1979) found that 93% of

Table 16-1 Assessment of Suicide Potential

Name ______________________ Age ________ Sex ________ Date ________

Rater ______________ Evaluation ______________________ 1 2 Low 3 4 5 6 Medium 7 8 9 High

Suicide potential

Age and sex	________	Resources	________	Total	________
Symptoms	________	Prior suicidal behavior	________		
Stress	________	Medical status	________	Number of categories related	________
Acute vs. chronic	________	Communication aspects	________		
Suicidal plan	________	Reaction of significant other	________	Average	________

Rating for category

1. Age and sex (1–9) ☐
   - Male
     - 50 plus (7–9) ☐
     - 35–49 (4–6) ☐
     - 15–34 (1–3) ☐
   - Female
     - 50 plus (5–7) ☐
     - 35–49 (3–5) ☐
     - 15–34 (1–3) ☐
2. Symptoms (1–9) ☐
   - Severe depression: sleep disorder, anorexia, weight loss, withdrawal, despondency, loss of interest, apathy (7–9) ☐
   - Feelings of hopelessness, helplessness, exhaustion (7–9) ☐
   - Delusions, hallucination, loss of contact, disorientation (6–8) ☐
   - Compulsive gambler (6–8) ☐
   - Disorganization, confusion, chaos (5–7) ☐
   - Alcoholism, drug addiction, homosexuality (4–7) ☐
   - Agitation, tension, anxiety (4–6) ☐
   - Guilt, shame, embarrassment (4–6) ☐
   - Feelings of rage, anger, hostility, revenge (4–6) ☐
   - Poor impulse control, poor judgment (4–6) ☐
   - Frustrated dependency (4–6) ☐
   - Other (describe): ☐
3. Stress (1–9) ☐
   - Loss of loved person by death, divorce, separation (5–9) ☐
   - Loss of job, money, prestige, status (4–8) ☐
   - Sickness, serious illness, surgery, accident, loss of limb (3–7) ☐
   - Threat of prosecution, criminal involvement, exposure (4–6) ☐
   - Change(s) in life, environment, setting (4–6) ☐
   - Success, promotion, increased responsibilities (2–5) ☐
   - No significant stress (1–3) ☐
   - Other (describe): ☐
4. Acute versus chronic (1–9) ☐
   - Sharp, noticeable, and sudden onset of specific symptoms (1–9) ☐
   - Recurrent outbreak of similar symptoms (4–9) ☐
   - Recent increase in long-standing traits (4–7) ☐
   - No specific recent change (1–4) ☐
   - Other (describe): ☐
5. Suicidal plan (1–9) ☐
   - Lethality of proposed method—gun, jump, hanging, drowning, knife, poison, pills, aspirin (1–9) ☐
   - Availability of means in proposed method (1–9) ☐
   - Specific detail and clarity in organization of plan (1–9) ☐
   - Specificity in time planned (1–9) ☐
   - Bizarre plans (4–6) ☐
   - Rating of previous suicide attempt(s) (1–9) ☐
   - No plans (1–3) ☐
   - Other (describe): ☐

Rating for category

6. Resources (1–9) ☐
   - No sources of support (family, friends, agencies, employment) (7–9) ☐
   - Family and friends available, unwilling to help (4–7) ☐
   - Financial problem (4–7) ☐
   - Available professional help, agency, or therapist (2–4) ☐
   - Family and/or friends willing to help (1–3) ☐
   - Stable life history (1–3) ☐
   - Physician or clergy available (1–3) ☐
   - Employed (1–3) ☐
   - Finances no problem (1–3) ☐
   - Other (describe): ☐
7. Prior suicidal behavior (1–7) ☐
   - One or more prior attempts of high lethality (6–7) ☐
   - One or more prior attempts of low lethality (4–5) ☐
   - History of repeated threats and depression (3–5) ☐
   - No prior suicidal or depressed history (1–3) ☐
   - Other (describe):
8. Medical status (1–7) ☐
   - Chronic debilitating illness (5–7) ☐
   - Pattern of failure in previous therapy (4–6) ☐
   - Many repeated unsuccessful experiences with physicians (4–6) ☐
   - Psychosomatic illness (asthma, ulcer, etc.) (2–4) ☐
   - Chronic minor illness complaints, hypochondria (1–3) ☐
   - No medical problems (1–2) ☐
   - Other (describe): ☐
9. Communication aspects (1–7) ☐
   - Communication broken with rejection of efforts to reestablish by both patient and others (5–7) ☐
   - Communications have internalized goal (e.g., declaration of guilt, feelings of worthlessness, blame, shame) (4–7) ☐
   - Communications have interpersonalized goal (to cause guilt in others, to force behavior, etc.) (2–4) ☐
   - Communications directed toward world and people in general (3–5) ☐
   - Communications directed toward one or more specific persons (1–3) ☐
   - Other (describe): ☐
10. Reaction of significant other (1–7) ☐
    - Defensive, paranoid, rejected, punishing attitude (5–7) ☐
    - Denial of own or patient's need for help (5–7) ☐
    - No feelings of concern about the patient; does not understand the patient (4–6) ☐
    - Indecisiveness, feelings of helplessness (3–5) ☐
    - Alternation between feelings of anger and rejection and feelings of responsibility and desire to help (2–4) ☐
    - Sympathy and concern plus admission of need for help (1–3) ☐
    - Other (describe): ☐

Reprinted with permission from Los Angeles Suicide Prevention Center.

persons who completed suicide had previously received some kind of psychiatric diagnosis. Not surprisingly, most studies suggest that depression is commonly associated with both completed suicides (Barraclough, 1970) and suicide attempts (Chabrol & Moron, 1988). The Lundby study found that in a small, well-studied Swedish community, the diagnosis of either Unipolar or Bipolar Major Depressive Disorder increased suicide risk by 78 times compared to persons in the population with no psychiatric diagnosis (Hagnell, Lanke, & Rorsman, 1981). In general, suicide risk is increased in the presence of psychosis, major depression, poor impulse control, and a philosophical conviction that it is ethically acceptable to end an unsatisfactory life (Kishi & Kathol, 2002). The current WHO data suggest that mood disorders, schizophrenia, and substance-use disorders are the most prevalent diagnoses associated with completed suicide (Bertolote & Fleischman, 2002). Politically and religiously motivated murder-suicide has become more prevalent in recent years, leading to over 1,700 deaths in Afghanistan alone in 2007, and in some cases perpetrated by "orphans or mentally unstable teenagers recruited from asylums, orphanages, and ... refugee camps" (Rashid, 2008). Although an exceptionally important topic, this chapter will not address the complex issues (Townsend, 2007) raised by this tragic turn of events.

Bipolar Disorder

Although data are conflicting on whether suicide risk for bipolar depression is greater than for unipolar depression, clients with Bipolar Disorder have been known to have a much higher lifetime suicide risk than does the general population (Guze & Robin, 1970). Early work had suggested manic-depressive illness to be present in 46% of all persons who completed suicide (Robins, Murphy, Wilkinson, Glassner, & Kayes, 1959). More recent studies suggest that between 25% and 50% of clients with manic-depressive illness attempt suicide during their lives, the rates being higher for women than for men (Jamison, 2000). A current report indicates that 1 in 100 persons with Bipolar Disorder will make a suicide attempt and 3 in 1,000 people with Bipolar disorder will die through suicide annually, making their rate at least ten times higher than that of the general population (Dutta et al., 2007). Several studies suggest that persons with Bipolar II Disorder (Major Depressive Disorder combined with Hypomania, see Chapter 17) are at higher risk for suicide attempt than are persons with Bipolar I Disorder (Rihmer & Pestality, 1999).

Schizophrenia

Persons with schizophrenia are another group with a very high rate of suicide attempts (Funahashi, Ibuki, Damon, Nishimura, Domon, Nishimura, et al., 2000). Two studies have documented an 8% lifetime rate of successful suicide, with an attempt rate over four times higher (Allebeck & Wistedt, 1981; Roy, 1986). Suicide tends to be more common in younger males within the first 10 years of the onset of schizophrenia than in older individuals. In comparison to persons who do not have the diagnosis of schizophrenia, schizophrenic individuals are less likely to tell others of their intentions, and, perhaps not surprisingly, they are also depressed, socially isolated, more often college educated, and in significant fear of mental disintegration than are others. It is important for nurses to be aware that the suicide risk in schizophrenia is greatest during the post-inpatient hospitalization period (Carroll-Ghosh, Victor, & Bourgeois, 2003), and that, while a number of schizophrenic suicides occur during hospitalization, these are more often not in the hospital itself, but during escapes from involuntary confinement or while out on pass. A recent study in the United Kingdom found that approximately 10% of schizophrenic individuals committed suicide, and comorbid substance abuse was a related factor that complicated the social and medical conditions related to both treatment and prevention (Hunt, Kapur, Windfuhr, Robinson, Bickley, Flynn, et al., 2006).

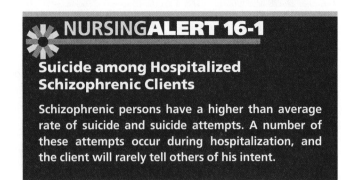

> **NURSING ALERT 16-1**
>
> **Suicide among Hospitalized Schizophrenic Clients**
>
> Schizophrenic persons have a higher than average rate of suicide and suicide attempts. A number of these attempts occur during hospitalization, and the client will rarely tell others of his intent.

Alcohol and Substance Abuse

It should not be a surprise that alcohol and substance abuse are strongly related to suicide, but the relationships are difficult to study and to describe. Alcohol probably plays a role in some suicidal decisions. Studies have shown that 30% to 40% of suicide victims have significant blood alcohol levels at postmortem examination (Varadaraz & Mendonca, 1987; Welte, Abel, & Wieczorek, 1988). Alcohol may be importantly involved in suicides that are impulsive and violent. One study in the 1980s found that 40% of persons attempting suicide acted within five minutes of considering self-harm (Williams, Davidson, & Montgomery, 1980). Such rapid decision making may be highly influenced by alcohol and other substances. Chronic alcohol dependency and abuse are clearly major risk factors for suicide. Alcoholics have been known to be four times more likely to commit suicide than are nonalcoholics and have a lifetime suicide risk that is much higher than that of the general population (Gipps, 1978; Ohara, Suzuki, Sugita, Kobayashi, Tamefusa, Hattori, et al., 1989). When viewed from a population perspective, alcohol abuse or dependency contribute to about 25% of suicides that occur in the United States (Carroll-Ghosh et al., 2003). In a sample of drug users with a criminal justice history, 63% of women and 47% of men reported suicidal thoughts or behaviors (Cottler, Campbell, Krishna, Cunningham-Williams, & Abdallah, 2005). Alcohol use was a predictor of suicide in this population. There is strong expert belief that alcohol abuse is associated with suicide among both the elderly and the very young. The findings of an association between depression, suicide, and alcoholism seem to hold across cultures as well.

Nonalcohol drug dependency and abuse is also related to suicide, especially in adolescents and young adults, as a significant percentage of adolescents who commit suicide have a history of substance abuse. Suicide attempts occur three times more often in adolescent substance abusers than in the general population, and there has been some evidence that suicidal ideation comes on only after drug use begins (Berman & Schwartz, 1990). While this latter finding does not establish that drug use leads to suicide, it does suggest that drug experiences may worsen depressive and other self-destructive feelings. Stimulant drugs may be particularly likely to provoke "post-high depression" that may lead to suicide for some individuals. Chemically dependent persons who commit suicide share some general characteristics: they tend to be young males who have a history of overdoses, who have cormorbid psychiatric disorders such as depression, and who have a recent history of an interpersonal loss (Carroll-Ghosh et al., 2003).

Conduct Disorder

Although depression and substance abuse figure strongly in the phenomenon of adolescent suicide, another DSM-IV diagnosis—Conduct Disorder—may play an even greater role. Conduct Disorder is a repetitive and persistent pattern of behavior in which the basic rights of others or major age-appropriate societal norms or rules are violated. Although Conduct Disorder may be one of the most common psychological findings among adolescent suicide victims, the not-unusual combination of Conduct Disorder, depression, and substance abuse is significantly associated with both the frequency and severity of suicide attempts (Carroll-Ghosh et al., 2003; Frances & Blumenthal, 1989). Completed suicide in this group was also found to be associated with access to firearms (Shah, Hoffman, Wake, & Marine, 2000).

Mixed Diagnoses

Although classifications such as the *Diagnostic and Statistical Manual of Mental Disorders, Fourth Edition-Text Revision* (DSM-IV-TR) and textbooks such as this one require that psychiatric diagnoses be neatly separated into discrete categories, clinicians caring for real-life clients much more commonly find mixtures and combinations of diagnoses present in the same person. Many separate conditions that predispose one to suicide can be found in individual clients. For example, it is not at all uncommon for persons with bipolar disease to abuse alcohol or other substances. This combination of morbidities significantly raises suicide risk (Carroll-Ghosh et al., 2003; Berglund, 1984). Rapid cycling Bipolar Disorder in an individual who also experiences panic attacks was found to be yet another combination posing significant suicide risk (Gao et al, 2009). Schizoaffective Disorder (see Chapter 17), a psychotic condition combining elements of major depression and schizophrenia, is a highly significant risk factor for suicide, especially in men. Finally, referring particularly to the elderly, Osgood described the combination of alcoholism, depression, and suicide as "the Deadly Triangle," implying that the combination of depression and alcohol abuse is particularly lethal among older individuals (Osgood, 1992). In general, although depression is certainly present in the vast majority of persons who complete suicide, other comorbidities are almost invariably present as well. A recent text reports that suicide completers under 30 years of age are likely to have substance abuse disorder as well as antisocial personality disorder, and that completers over the age of 30 years are more likely to have mood disorders (Andreasen & Black, 2006).

Medical Conditions and Suicide

Suicidal ideation and risk for suicide is perhaps higher among persons with chronic medical conditions, especially those that result in pain, serious risk to life, or severe physical limitations (Druss & Pincus, 2000). The best evidence supports a link between suicide and the following conditions: epilepsy, cerebrovascular disease, dementia, visual defect, multiple sclerosis, head injury, and brain tumor. With the exception of visual defect, these are all conditions in which brain centers affecting impulse, judgment, or affect might be involved. Two other conditions that appear to have increased suicide rates, lupus and Huntington's disease, may likewise affect both mood and overall cerebral functioning.

The suicide rate among clients with cancer is probably elevated, particularly in the first year after diagnosis (Allebeck, Bolund, & Ringback, 1989). Suicidal ideation and history of prior suicidal attempts are correlated with cancer diagnoses as well as other medical conditions, including asthma and bronchitis (Druss & Pincus, 2000).

THEORIES OF SUICIDE

In general, theories about why people commit suicide fall into three categories: sociological, psychological, and biochemical. Each of these is discussed separately.

Sociological Theory

In 1897, the French sociologist Emile Durkheim wrote a highly influential book entitled *Suicide* (Durkheim, 1951/1897). In this book, he argued that only social factors could explain suicide, and chief among these was *anomie*, which might be described as the combination of social disconnection and loss of societal control over individuals' impulsive behavior. In Durkheim's view, suicide often occurs because society fails to either control individual impulses or allow individuals a sense of social connectedness and hope.

Psychological Theory

There are numerous psychological models of suicide based on psychological theories as diverse as psychoanalysis and

RESEARCH Highlight 16–1

Caring for Patients with Suicidal Behavior: An Exploratory Study

STUDY PROBLEM/PURPOSE

To describe the challenges and experiences of frontline nurses in emergency departments who are called upon to care for patients presenting with suicidal attempts.

METHODS

Forty-two emergency department nurses completed a questionnaire asking them about their experiences with psychosocial care and their thoughts and feelings when caring for the suicidal patient.

FINDINGS

A majority of nurses reported having daily experiences with suicidal patients. The nurses identified that risk assessment is one of the important nursing goals when caring for such patients. Nurses identified that recognizing potential risk, providing a safe environment, and referral to psychiatric services is part of their work. The nurses did not identify meeting the clients' psychosocial needs as part of their care.

Nurses' feelings about suicidal patients varied and depended on the individual circumstances, however, nurses reported "uneasiness" in dealing with suicidal patients and frustration with patients who present multiple times with suicide attempts. Nurses tended to make judgments about the "genuineness" of the patients' attempts and distress. Further, nurses reported a lack of communication skills in dealing with uncooperative patients.

IMPLICATIONS

Nurses may be ill-equipped to deal with the complexities of patients presenting with suicidal attempts. Specialist education and preparation of emergency department staff is essential in meeting the needs of this vulnerable patient group.

Source: "Caring for Patients with Suicidal Behaviour: An exploratory study," by L. Doyle, B. Keogh, and J. Morrissey. 2007. *British Journal of Nursing*, *16*(29), 1218–1222.

RESEARCH Highlight 16–2

Emergency Department Visits for Suicidality

STUDY PROBLEM/PURPOSE

The researchers documented the characteristics of patients being treated for suicidality in hospital emergency departments, and recorded the treatments offered and disposition of the cases.

METHODS

A retrospective chart review of 163 cases who came to emergency departments and were seen by either ER staff or mental health professionals.

FINDINGS

Of the cases seen in the emergency departments, 1.1% were for suicidal injuries or behaviors, with men and women being seen in almost equal numbers. Fifty-one percent of those with suicidal ideation had a lethal plan. The most commonly used method of self-harm was drug/medication overdose.

Over one-third of patients seen were either admitted directly to a psychiatric unit for further evaluation (34.4%) or transferred to another facility for further evaluation (36.8%). Nineteen percent were discharged to home.

Emergency room staff tended to be more conservative in managing suicide cases than mental health professionals.

IMPLICATIONS

There is a role for liaison and collaborative consultations between psychiatric nurses and emergency department staff.

Source: Drew, B., Jones, S., Meldon, S. W., & Varley, J. D. (2006). Emergency Department Visits for Suicidality in Three Hospitals. *Archives of Psychiatric Nursing*, *20*(3), 117–125.

behavioral theories (described in Chapters 3 and 28). One integrative approach to modeling suicide was proposed by Schneidman (1987). His model suggests that three factors affect suicidal ideation: pain, perturbation, and press. In this model, pain is viewed as a psychological phenomenon but is unlikely to exclude physical pain. Perturbation is the degree of emotional distress reflected in the presence or absence of impulse control. Press is a concept describing the various stresses or pressures on an individual; these "presses" can come from inside the individual, from others, or from society as a whole. In Schneidman's view, suicide occurs when psychological pain results from blocked psychological needs in the context of high levels of perturbation (distress) and press (sense of overwhelming internal or external pressures).

Simpler psychological theories have been proposed that focus on depression alone. One major theory posits that depression is a major factor in suicide and that depression results from the belief, typically based on experience, that an individual is helpless to affect the outcome of his or her life events. In addition, it is theorized that depressed individuals tend to take psychological responsibility for their perceived failures. According to this "depression paradox theory" of suicide, the depressed person may be caught between strong

RESEARCH Highlight 16–3

The Relationship of Body Weight to Suicide Risk in Men and Women: Results of the U.S. National Health Interview Survey Linked Mortality File

PURPOSE

To examine the effects of body mass index on suicide risk for men and women.

METHODS

Data for the study are from combining the national health interview survey findings with the multiple cause of death file through the National Death Index.

FINDINGS

Relative body weight was associated with major depression, suicide attempts, and suicidal ideation. Among men, underweight was associated with elevated suicide risk, whereas both overweight and obese body mass indices were associated with reduced suicide risk. Among women, obesity was associated with reduced suicide risk.

CONCLUSIONS

There is need for further study to assess linkages between physical characteristics and suicide and depression. Nurses should use these findings to complete further assessments of clients who may be at risk.

Source: "The Relationship of Body Weight to Suicide Risk in Men and Women: Results of the U.S. National Health Interview Survey Linked Mortality File," by M. S. Kaplan, B. H. MacFarland, & N. Huguet, (2007), *Journal of Nervous and Mental Disease*, *195*(11), 948–951.

feelings of helplessness and equally strong feelings of responsibility. The bind generated by this conflict between feeling both responsible and helpless may lead people to feel that only suicide gives them a way out of their troubles (Lester, 1992).

Biological Explanations

Not content with sociological and psychological theories alone, many investigators have sought more strictly biological explanations of suicide. Since suicide is closely related to depression, both theoretically and empirically, and since depression has in many cases shown a strong relation to neurotransmitter imbalances, it is not surprising that much work has focused on serotonin metabolites in suicide. The literature is complex and unsettled, but the findings do show some striking consistencies. Serotonin is an important monoamine brain neurotransmitter, and it is readily metabolized to 5-hydroxyindoleacetic acid (5-HIAA), which circulates in blood and cerebrospinal fluid. In general, 5-HIAA levels in assayable body fluids are thought to reflect levels of brain serotonin (which cannot be directly measured). Multiple studies suggest that a subset of suicide attempters and completers, perhaps particularly those who use violent means of self-destruction, have very low 5-HIAA levels in the cerebrospinal fluid (Asberg, 1989). Increasingly sophisticated genetic studies have shown that clients with more than one suicide attempt have a higher-than-expected frequency of the "SS" form of a serotonin transporter gene that is active within the brain. While this gene type was also correlated with impulsive behavior, the authors concluded after a multivariate analysis that *both* impulsivity and the SS genotype were associated with repeated suicide attempts (Courtet, Picot, Bellivier, Torris, Jollant, Michelon, et al., 2004). Subsequent studies continue to implicate the serotonin transporter gene and the serotonin receptor in the genetics of suicidality, along with a variety of other biological pathways (Wasserman, Geijer, Sokolowski, Rozanov, & Wasserman, 2007).

A comprehensive biological theory of suicide has yet to emerge, though data suggesting that suicide risk may have a biological component are complemented by multiple studies showing an increased risk of suicide in families in which relatives have attempted suicide (Baldessarini & Hennen, 2004). Risk is even greater when suicide is completed. While environment likely plays some role in this familial association, these authors describe studies of twins and adoptive versus biological children that point to significant genetic influences. Since many of the psychiatric disorders associated with suicide (depression, Bipolar Disorder, schizophrenia) themselves have a genetic component, it has been very difficult to know what contribution genetics makes to suicide risk itself. Although a full-scale biological theory of suicide has yet to emerge from these neurotransmitter observations, scientists continue to be greatly interested in this area of research, and new results should be expected in the future.

Nursing Theory

Of all nursing theories, the work of Peplau speaks directly to the work of nurses in working with the suicidal and potentially suicidal client. Developing her theory of nursing in the 1950s, Peplau (1988) believed that nursing is therapeutic because it is a healing art, because nursing engages two or more people in an interaction with a common goal, and because both nurse and client learn and grow as a result of the nurse-client interaction. Peplau considers nursing to be a significant, interpersonal process; the tools of nursing are communication and interviewing skills, that is, tools of self.

There is strong evidence that one thing the nurse can do for the suicidal client is to form a significant, interpersonal relationship. Early studies of persons who were hospitalized because of failed suicide attempts indicated that those clients felt isolated and ignored during their hospital stays (Dunleavey, 1992) and that their major needs were to be loved, to maintain a high level of self-esteem, to begin to have control over their lives, and to be supported (Carrigan, 1994). Other

RESEARCH Highlight 16-4

Comparing Blogs of Depressed Men and Women

PURPOSE

To investigate and compare how men and women who self-identify as depressed describe their experiences on Internet blogs.

METHODS

The researchers used a qualitative content analysis method to determine themes and similarities/differences in the blogs written by men and women. They identified a sample of 45 blogs for each gender, based on finding reports that adequately described the "voice" and the experiences of the writers.

FINDINGS

A similar proportion of women and men (45% of women and 47.5% of men) discussed pharmaceuticals, while the genders differed in discussion of psychotherapy (48% of women and 15% of men) and violence and self-harm (7% of women and 37.5% of men).

CONCLUSIONS

The researchers noted that for men, suicide was a frequent topic of discussion. Comparison of women and men suggest that men are more likely than women to describe their experiences in terms of self-harm and violence against self, they are also more likely than women to attribute depression to situations outside their relationships and immediate experiences (the sad state of the world, for example). Research using Internet blogs and social networking Web sites is a very new approach, so it is still difficult to interpret findings. However, nurses should recognize that thoughts of suicide may occur in over one-third of men who self-identify as depressed.

Source: J. Clarke and G. van Anerom. A Comparison of Blogs by Depressed Men and Women. *Issues in Mental Health Nursing*, 2008, *29*(3), 243–264.

evaluations indicate that nurses consistently found that persons who exhibited self-harm behaviors and persons who did not readily form therapeutic alliances with their nurses were difficult to treat (Doyle, Keogh, & Morrissey, 2007; Gallop, Lancee, & Shuger, 1993). Researchers conclude that the nurse must take time with suicidal clients and engage them in interactions. Further, researchers recommend that there is a need for nurses to have a better understanding of clients who have attempted suicide. Authors who completed a current review of all literature on care of the suicidal patient conclude that "caring for suicidal people must be an interpersonal endeavor; and one personified by talking and listening" (Outcliffe & Stevenson, 2008, p. 942).

Peplau's theory provides direction on how to intervene. First, the nurse and client meet as strangers. The nurse provides time, support, and interactions aimed at assisting the client to identify problems and concerns and what resources can be used to meet the client's needs. The nurse and client clarify each other's perceptions and expectations. The nurse will make clear to the client that she will both protect him from self-harm and continue to provide opportunity for interaction and unconditional support. The nurse will assist the client to take advantage of all available services: hospitalization, if indicated; family supports; group therapy; medications; and community services. The client may learn a new independence and develop self-care skills. When the client has resolved his initial suicidal crisis, and the underlying depression and distress have been addressed, the nurse can then terminate the relationship, ensuring that the client has a support system and knows where he can call for help and receive help should the need arise again.

The art of nursing, in this case, is the art of being in a relationship with another who is in need. While other nursing theories—most notably Watson's, Parse's, and Erickson's—are grounded in the concepts of caring, presence, and nurturing, respectively, the basic work of Peplau provides a foundation and framework for all nursing care of the suicidal client.

SPECIAL POPULATIONS

There are three populations that merit attention because of their elevated risk for suicide or the fact that many overlook their calls for help. These are adolescents/young adults, the elderly, and the incarcerated and military combatants.

Adolescents and Young Adults

I knew just how to go about it.

The minute the car tires crunched off down the drive and the sound of the motor faded, I jumped out of bed and hurried into my white blouse and green figured skirt and black raincoat. The raincoat felt damp still, from the day before, but that would soon cease to matter.

I went downstairs and picked up a pale blue envelope from the dining room table and scrawled on the back, in large painstaking letters: I am going for a long walk.

I propped the message where my mother would see it the minute she came in.

Then I laughed.

I had forgotten the most important thing.

I ran upstairs and dragged a chair into my mother's closet. Then I climbed up and reached for the small green strongbox on the top shelf. I could have torn the metal cover off with my bare hands, the lock was so feeble, but I wanted to do things in a calm, orderly way.

Wheatfield with Crows by Vincent Van Gogh

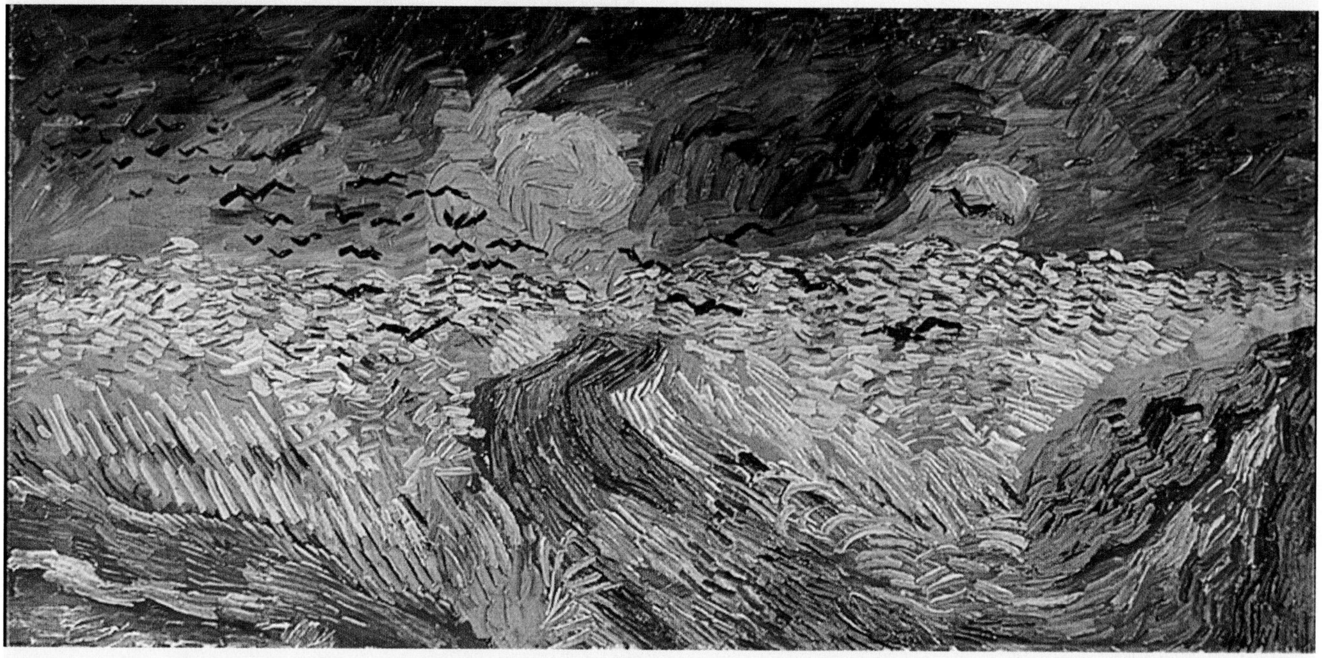

Courtesy: Art Resource, NY. Van Gogh Museum, Amsterdam, The Netherlands.

The last of Van Gogh's paintings, this was painted only a few days before his suicide. It is hard not to see death in this painting. The sky is ominously bearing down on the dry and yellowed wheat; a green road seems to go nowhere; the crows disappear into the sky at the upper right of a picture that has no focus or center. Even the brushstrokes seem undirected and despairing.

I pulled out my mother's upper right-hand bureau drawer and slipped the blue jewelry box from its hiding place under the scented Irish linen handkerchiefs. I unpinned the little key from the dark velvet. Then I unlocked the strongbox and took out the bottle of new pills. There were more than I had hoped.

There were at least fifty.

If I had waited until my mother doled them out to me, night by night, it would have taken me fifty nights to save up enough. And in fifty nights, college would have opened, and my brother would have come back from Germany, and it would be too late.

I pinned the key back in the jewelry box among the clutter of inexpensive chains and rings, put the jewelry box back in the drawer under the handkerchiefs, returned the strongbox to the closet shelf and set the chair on the rug in the exact spot I had dragged it from.

Then I went downstairs and into the kitchen. I turned on the tap and poured myself a tall glass of water. Then I took the glass of water and the bottle of pills and went down into the cellar.

A dim, undersea light filtered through the slits of the cellar windows. Behind the oil burner, a dark gap showed in the wall at about shoulder height and ran back under the breezeway, out of sight. The breezeway had been added to the house after the cellar was dug, and built out over this secret earth bottomed crevice.

A few old, rotting fireplace logs blocked the hole mouth. I shoved them back a bit. Then I set the glass of water and the bottle of pills side by side on the flat surface of one of the logs and started to heave myself up.

It took me a good while to heft my body into the gap, but at last, after many tries, I managed it, and crouched at the mouth of the darkness, like a troll.

The earth seemed friendly under my bare feet, but cold. I wondered how long it had been since this particular square of soil had seen the sun.

Then, one after the other, I lugged the heavy, dust-covered logs across the hole mouth. The dark felt thick as velvet. I reached for the glass and bottle, and carefully, on my knees, with bent head, crawled to the farthest wall.

Cobwebs touched my face with the softness of moths. Wrapping my black coat round me like my own sweet shadow, I unscrewed the bottle of pills and started taking them swiftly, between gulps of water, one by one by one.

Sylvia

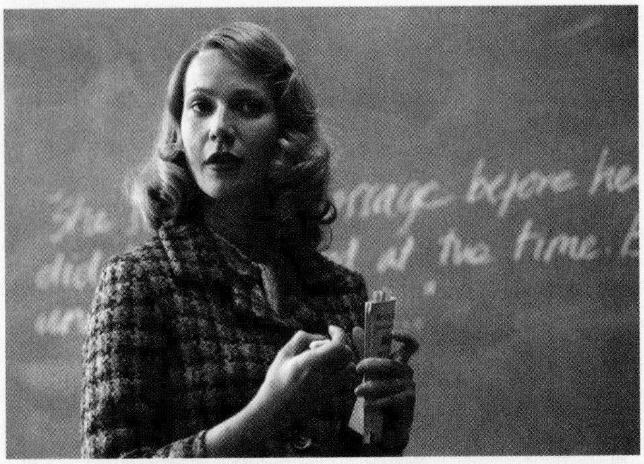

Courtesy: Focus Features/The Kobal Collection/The Picture Desk

One of the twentieth century's most famous victims of suicide, poet Sylvia Plath struggled with depression for years. Here, as portrayed by Gwyneth Paltrow in *Sylvia*, the life-long feelings of despair that haunted Plath seem palpably visible.

At first nothing happened, but as I approached the bottom of the bottle, red and blue lights began to flash before my eyes. The bottle slid from my fingers and I lay down.

*The silence drew off, baring the pebbles and shells and all the tatty wreckage of my life. Then, at the rim of vision, it gathered itself, and in one sweeping tide, rushed me to sleep.**

(Plath, 1971, 189–190)

In this passage, from her fictional work "The Bell Jar", Sylvia Plath has captured some of the essential elements of adolescent suicide. Drug ingestions are common in suicide attempts among the young, particularly young women, and the home is the most common suicide site. The attempt described here seems particularly serious; adolescent ingestions more typically occur in the presence of others and are of relatively low lethality. Studies suggest that 8% to 9% of high school students have made one or more suicide attempts (Harkavy-Friedman, Asnis, Boeck, & DiFiore, 1987), and other studies report that 1 out of every 15 youths in the United States responds on interview that they do not expect to live much past 30 years. Forty-three percent of those who were "fatalists" forecast suicide as a likely death (Jameison & Romer, 2008). While most youth suicide attempts do not result in death, the triad of homicide, accident, and suicide is by far the leading cause of death in adolescents and young adults. Indeed, there is persuasive sociological theory that homicide and suicide are closely related phenomena. This theory is based on observations that suicide rates are often inversely related to homicide rates; that is, geographic regions with low suicide rates tend to have high homicide rates (Unnithan, Huff-Corzine, Corzine, & Whitt, 1994). Furthermore, data show that when follow-up is extended over four decades, suicide attempt by ingestion of drugs is associated with a significant lifetime risk of completed suicide (Suominen, Isometsa, Suikas, Haukka, Achte, & Longqvist, 2004).

*From *The Bell Jar* by Sylvia Plath. Copyright © 1971 by Harper & Row, Publishers, Inc. Reprinted with permission from HarperCollins Publishers, Inc.

NURSING**ALERT** 16-2

Adolescent Suicide

Most adolescent suicide completers have never received mental health treatment, although the majority of these adolescents had exhibited psychiatric symptoms prior to their deaths.

The Elderly

A SUMMER TRAGEDY

Old Jeff Patton, the black share farmer, fumbled with his bow tie. His fingers trembled and the high stiff collar pinched his throat. A fellow loses his hand for such vanities after thirty or forty years of simple life. Once a year, or maybe twice if there's a wedding among his kinfolks, he may spruce up; but generally fancy clothes do nothing but adorn the wall of the big room and feed the moths. That had been Jeff Patton's experience. He had not worn his stiff-bosomed shirt more than a dozen times in all his married life....

"Jennie," he called.

"What's that, Jeff?" His wife's shrunken voice came out of the adjoining room like an echo. It was hardly bigger than a whisper.

"I reckon you'll have to he'p me wid this heah bow tie, baby," he said meekly. "Dog if I can hitch it up."

Her answer was not strong enough to reach him, but presently the old woman came to the door, feeling her way with a stick. She had a wasted, dead-leaf appearance. Her body, as scrawny and gnarled as a string bean, seemed less than nothing in the ocean of frayed and faded petticoats that surrounded her. These hung an inch or two above the tops of her heavy unlaced shoes and showed little grotesque piles where the stockings had fallen down from her negligible legs.

Jennie sat on the side of the bed and old Jeff Patton got down on one knee while she tied the bow knot. It was a slow and painful ordeal for each of them in this position.

Jeff's bones cracked, his knee ached, and it was only after a half dozen attempts that Jennie worked a semblance of a bow into the tie....

Jeff opened the door and helped his wife into the car. A quick shudder passed over him. Jesus! ...

"How come you shaking so?" Jennie whispered.

"I don't know," he said.

"You mus' be scairt, Jeff."

"No, baby, I ain't scairt.... "

"You mustn't cry, baby," he said to his wife. "We gotta be strong. We can't break down.... "

Jeff thought of the handicaps, the near impossibility, of making another crop with his leg bothering him more and more each week. Then there was always the chance that he would have another stroke, like the one that had made him lame. Another one might kill him. The least it could do would be to leave him helpless. Jeff gasped—Lord, Jesus! He could not bear to think of being helpless, like a baby, on Jennie's hands. Frail, blind Jennie....

Below, the water of the stream boomed, a soft thunder in the deep channel. Jeff ran the car onto the clay slope, pointed it directly toward the stream and put his foot heavily on the accelerator. The little car leaped furiously down the steep incline toward the water. The movement was nearly as swift and direct as a fall. The two old black folks, sitting quietly side by side, showed no excitement. In another instant the car hit the water and dropped immediately out of sight.

*A little later it lodged in the mud of a shallow place. One wheel of the crushed and upturned little Ford became visible above the rushing water.**

(Bontemps, 1961, pp. 253–262)

Writing over 40 years ago, Arna Bontemps raised the issue of suicide among the elderly, a problem that has only recently received significant attention. As Frank and Lester observed 17 years after this story was written, suicide in older individuals does tend to be a summer tragedy, peaking somewhat in May (Lester, 1992). Suicide among the elderly is a much greater problem in the isolated Western states (Arizona, Wyoming, Montana, and Alaska) than it is in the South, which, at least in urban areas, has long had a lower suicide rate than other areas in the country (Osgood, 1992). Couple suicide, as in Bontemps's story, is actually a very rare event. Between 1980 and 1987, Wickett (1989) was able to document only 97 U.S. cases, and the method almost always involved firearms. Rare as they may be, couple suicides typically involve all of the elements of tragedy found in Jeff and Jennie's story: unemployment, physical loss, financial troubles, recent emotional loss, and an event occurring in the morning (Fishbain & Aldrich, 1985). In real-life double suicides, alcohol is commonly involved, but as in Jeff and Jennie's story, depression and guilt are not typically prominent.

Elderly suicide more commonly affects individuals living alone and is an especially serious problem for men over age 75. Individual suicides among the elderly are related to depression as well as to alcohol. The problem of suicide among the elderly is arguably much greater than reflected in statistics if one includes deaths from self-starvation and medication refusal, common self-willed forms of death among older adults. Since the geriatric population is growing steadily, it is likely that the problem of suicide among the elderly will increase in visibility even though current trends show a downward rate in elderly suicides.

*From "The Old South" by A. Bontemps, in *Death in Literature* (pp. 253–262). Anthologized by R. Weir, 1961, New York: Columbia University Press.

RESEARCH Highlight 16–5

Suicidal Ideation among Elderly Homecare Patients

STUDY PURPOSE

Researchers sought to determine the prevalence, correlates, and naturalistic course of suicidal ideation in a sample of elderly adults receiving care from homecare services.

METHODS

Researchers interviewed 539 newly admitted patients to a home care service, using standard interviews to categorize the patients as either having suicidal ideation (in the previous month) or not. For those with suicidal ideation, patients were classified as having passive ideation or active ideation. Active ideation was further categorized as with or without poor impulse control, and as having or not having a suicide plan.

FINDINGS

Of the sample interviewed, 10.6% were assessed as having passive suicidal ideation, and 1.2% as having active suicidal ideation. Factors that were associated with suicidal ideation included: lower subjective social support, greater medical comorbidity, and higher depression severity than found in the general sample. At one year, suicidal ideation persisted for 36.7% of those at first interview, and the overall suicidal ideation rate at one year was 5.6%.

IMPLICATIONS

The elderly homecare population has increased risk of suicidal ideation and this ideation persists over time. Nurses must make appropriate assessments and provide supports and referrals when caring for this group.

Source: "Suicidal Ideation among Elderly Homecare Patients" by P. J. Raye, B.S. Meyers, J. Rowe, M. Heo, & M. L. Bruce, 2007. *International Journal of Geriatric Psychiatry, (22)*, 32–37.

Conventional preventive efforts seem not to effectively reach the elderly. For example, only 2% of all calls to crisis hotlines are said to be made by persons over the age of 60 years (Osgood, 1992), although self-rated depression is the strongest predictor of suicide in the elderly population (Garand, Mitchell, Dietrick, Hiijjawi, & Pan, 2006). There is a developing nursing role in activities that serve as preventive efforts for the elderly. These include increasing participation in adult day care and other socialization activities, increasing pet ownership and pet visitation programs, and actively seeking and treating depression in the elderly. Perhaps not surprisingly, physical illness, financial stress, unemployment (for persons over 50 but younger than retirement age), and family stress have been found more frequently in case control studies comparing the families of suicide victims with others (Duberstein, Conwell, Conner, Eberly, & Caine, 2004). While such studies have a serious risk of bias (because family members of recent suicides may believe that stresses lead to suicide and may be more likely to report these than families in which no suicide has occurred), they also point to risk factors amenable to intervention. The presence of a gun in the house, as for younger individuals, poses a significant threat for suicide in the elderly as well. In one sample of elders, 19.7% reported having a handgun in the house, and an additional 8% had another kind of firearm (Oslin, Zubritsky, Brown, Mullaby, Puliafico, & Ten Have, 2004). Guns were just as likely to be found in homes where elders reported depression, suicide ideation, or other psychological distress. These data emphasize the importance of screening for both suicidal ideation and firearm presence among elderly clients.

The Incarcerated and Military Combatants

BEHIND BARS

In a West Coast community, after smoking "crack," a 34-year-old man developed a toxic psychosis that caused hallucinations and paranoid delusions. He heard the voice of his daughter calling. He phoned her but he was so confused he could not recognize her voice. He entered his mother's room at 3:00 A.M., holding a knife in one hand and a razor in the other, and threatened to cut his wrists. His mother was able to calm him down and get him to drop his weapons. His sister called the police and stated that her brother and the family wanted him to be admitted to a psychiatric hospital. Sheriff's deputies arrived and obtained his history. When they ran a police check they discovered that he had an outstanding traffic warrant and decided to take him to jail instead of a psychiatric hospital.

The booking officer noted the history and added that he thought the man was a homosexual. He requested a mental health evaluation because he felt that the man was mentally ill and suicidal. A call was made to summon a nurse to evaluate him, but apparently she did not feel that there was any urgency to this request; she made other rounds first and these delayed her for a long time. During this time the man claimed that he was being gassed through the vents in his cell and complained of loud noise when in fact he was in a completely quiet area....

*Two hours later when the nurse appeared, she saw the man lying on his cot and because she assumed he was asleep, she did not awaken him or schedule a watch so she could be notified when he awoke. Forty-five minutes later he was found hanging in his cell.**

(Lester & Danto, 1993, pp. 9–10)

The suicide rate for incarcerated persons is much higher than for the population as a whole, but, as in the case presented here, suicide events are much more common in local jails and holding facilities than they are in prisons. Although there are exceptions—rates may be particularly high in units for psychiatrically disturbed inmates and on "death row"—suicide rates in federal and state prisons are generally not much different than those in the general population. One group of researchers provided a list of six characteristics that, in combination, serve as a predictor of prisoner suicide: 40+ years of age, homelessness, history of psychiatric care, history of drug abuse, prior incarceration, and violent offense (Blaauw, Kerkhof, & Hayes, 2005). In addition, there have been very high reported suicide rates among youthful offenders placed in facilities for adults (Lester & Danto, 1993), a practice that is not as frequent currently as in the past. A national survey in Great Britain confirmed the importance of prisoner suicide in that country as well (Shaw, Baker, Hunt, Moloney, & Appleby, 2004). As in the preceding "Behind Bars" example, hanging or self-strangulation was the cause of death in 92% of fatalities.

Nurses are often major care providers in local jails and so may be the first to recognize the potential for suicide. Failure to recognize risk may result in not only potentially avoidable loss of life, as in this case, but also in serious legal liability. A recent study of suicides in the California prison system estimated that 60% of the prisoner suicides were foreseeable and preventable (Patterson & Hughes, 2008).

While military combatants are often volunteers, the conditions of military service can be harsh, and—as is the case for incarcerated persons—freedoms that civilians take for granted are often severely limited by military command. Suicide risk among soldiers during peacetime is generally somewhat lower than that in the age and sex-matched general population. Pre-Iraq war suicide rates for U.S. Army soldiers have averaged between 10.5 and 11

*From *Suicide Behind Bars* by D. Lester and B. Danto, 1993, Philadelphia: Charles Press, Publishers. Reprinted with permission.

per 100,000 compared with civilian population rates of about 17.5 per 100,000 (Nelson, 2004). During the Iraq war in 2003, rates increased to at least 13.5 per 100,000 troops, with some unclassified deaths still under investigation. Many of the same risk factors important in civilian life apply to military suicides: depression, personal losses, financial and legal concerns, and firearm availability. Unlike prisoners, military combatants do not represent a notably high-risk group for suicide, but military caregivers must be alert to suicidal risk among service personnel. Recently, the popular media has drawn increased attention to the needs of servicemen and women in relation to mental health care needs generally and suicide prevention specifically. While military medical personnel are responding to these needs currently, it will be several years before data on the experiences of these individuals will be known. Recently, one research team reported on the experiences of past veterans who were studied over a 12-year period (Kaplan, Huguet, McFarland, & Newson, 2007). The researchers found that veterans in the United States had a higher risk of suicide than did nonveterans, and that veterans were twice as likely to die from suicide than nonveterans. The factors that contributed to the highest risk were being a white male, having less than 12 years of education, and having activity limitation (presumably the result of service-related injury).

SUICIDE SURVIVORS

In recent years, more attention has been given to the needs of **suicide survivors**, the friends and family of an individual who dies from suicide. The normal process of bereavement has been discussed elsewhere in this text (Chapter 14), and evidence from a number of studies has suggested that the process of grief after suicidal loss is not fundamentally different from that after any other death (Van der Wal, 1990). Nonetheless, the suddenness and, on occasion, the violence of suicide may constitute particular stresses in the grieving process. Over the past two or three decades, many self-help groups have been formed to allow survivors to share experiences with others and to channel anger and sadness into socially helpful activities. It is thought that suicide bereavement is different than natural loss, particularly because those close to the suicide victim experience social stigma and respond with a variety of coping mechanisms (Cvinar, 2005). Some survivors have written of their experiences in an effort to assist others with the grieving process.

It is important to remember that while both suicide attempts and successful suicide are extremely stressful events for family members and friends, they also are exceptionally stressful for caregivers of these individuals (Lafayette & Stern, 2004). Consider the following case report (Dell & O'Brien, 2003):

> *CASE: A 26-year-old primigravida at 12 weeks' gestation presented for emergency psychiatric evaluation after discontinuing psychotropic medications when starting prenatal care. She developed worsening depression and was suicidal. She was admitted to an inpatient psychiatric unit, medication was reinitiated, and she appeared to stabilize well enough to be followed as an outpatient. Two days after discharge, she shot herself in the left chest, resulting in her death and that of her fetus.*

It is hard to believe that anyone working on the inpatient unit would not have been devastated by the experience described in this case.

NURSINGTIP 16-1

How to Help Survivors of Suicide

- Give survivors the opportunity to talk. Allow them to determine how much or how little they wish to share.
- Do not intimidate or seek to find blame. Try to see the situation through the survivor's eyes.
- Allow the individual the opportunity to express the anger that often accompanies the grieving process. Reassure the survivor that these are normal feelings and emotions.
- Offer information and provide practical help. Educate the survivor on literature, community resources, and available support groups.
- Provide the survivor with time to heal. Do not suggest, "You should be over this by now." Offer unconditional support as they move through the period of bereavement.
- Do not abandon the survivor. Send cards, call, or visit. Offer oneself, but allow the survivor to refuse invitations. Keep offering oneself over time.

From "Exploring Widows' Experiences After the Suicide of Their Spouse," by B. J. Smith, A. M. Mitchell, A. A. Bruno, and R. E. Constantino, 1995, *Journal of Psychological Nursing and Mental Health Services*, 33, 10. Reprinted with permission.

REFLECTIVE THINKING 16-1

A Discussion of Euthanasia

Suicide has long been regarded as a crime, both in Christian doctrine and in English Common Law, and many contemporary authors argue equally eloquently against the moral acceptance of suicide. However, there seems little doubt that academic and public views of suicide have become more liberal during recent past decades—as evidence of this liberalization, psychologists have suggested "rational choice" theories of suicide (Lester, 1988), and, perhaps more importantly, there has been a growing acceptance of the legality and even desirability of **euthanasia**, or the act of killing or permitting a death for reasons of mercy. Since most cases of euthanasia involve the elderly and the terminally ill, many have expressed concerns that euthanasia enthusiasts may have social ends (reducing the number of expensive and dependent individuals) more in view than altruistic ones (reducing individuals' pain and suffering). Nonetheless, even in relatively conservative medical circles there is conditional acceptance of the principles of assisted dying (Lancet editors, 1995b). This willingness to admit "euthanasia openly (and more honestly) into all . . . future discussions of end-of-life decisions affecting competent adults" (Lancet editors, 1995b, p. 259) has already found expression in a number of states. In 1995, Oregon voters narrowly approved a ballot measure authorizing physician-assisted suicide for the terminally ill. In a 2000 study of oncologists in the United States, researchers reported that 22.5% supported the use of physician-assisted suicide for terminally ill patients experiencing unremitting pain and 6.5% supported euthanasia (Emanuel, Fairclough, Clarridge, Blum, Bruera, Penley, et al., 2000). The Netherlands was among the first countries to liberalize laws and practices relating to assisted suicide, but the actual number of clients and physicians involved seems to have remained relatively small. Euthanasia is clearly an issue that deeply divides practitioners of medicine and nursing. The ethical, moral, and religious problems it raises are unlikely to recede.

Data from the Netherlands (where assisted suicide is legal) show that only 37% of requests for physician assistance are actually granted (Haverkate, Onwuteaka-Philipsen, van Der Heide, Kostense, van Der Wal, & van Der Maas, et al., 2000). Persons with recognized depression or other mental health diagnoses are said to be among those whose requests are most commonly refused by physicians. These individuals are also judged less likely to be truly terminally ill. A report from Oregon based on surveys of hospice nurses and social workers documented that out of 82 patients whose assisted suicide was recalled, 63 decisions had been formally discussed at a multidisciplinary conference. Nearly all cases had been informally discussed by hospice staff prior to provision of lethal medication, and nurses reported that these clients—rather than being depressed—were primarily concerned about retaining control over end of life (Ganzini, Harvath, Jackson, Goy, Miller, & Delorit, 2002). Assisted suicide remains highly controversial both in the Netherlands (van Kolfschooten, 2003) and in the United States (Steinbrook, 2002). In 2001, the attorney general reversed a previous Justice Department ruling and asserted that the use of controlled substances for assisting suicide was a violation of controlled substances regulations. Subsequent legal actions have kept the Oregon "Death with Dignity" act in an uncertain legal position (Walsh & Hendrickson, 2003).

Each nurse must examine her own views, feelings, and moral convictions in relation to euthanasia.

Refer to the ethical principles described in Chapter 9 to assist you in determining the actions you believe are appropriate for you as a nurse and as a citizen.

REFLECTIVE THINKING 16-2

Antidepressants and Suicide

A major controversy concerns whether some antidepressant medications increase risk for suicide when used in children and adolescents. The British government has concluded that paroxetine (6/2003), venlafaxine (10/2003), ertraline (12/2003), and citalopram (12/2003) are all associated with increased risk and should not be used in the young (Abbott, 2003). The U.S. Food and Drug Administration (FDA) has not taken such a strong stand, but it has required warnings to be placed on these medications. There are conflicting data available showing that SSRI medications such as those listed here *decrease* suicidal ideation in some persons but are associated with an *increased* risk of suicidal acts (Healy & Whitaker, 2003). Fluoxetine seems not to be associated with increased suicidal risk and continues to be prescribed to young persons. These data emphasize the importance of continuing surveillance for suicidal ideation and other risk factors in all clients treated for depression.

Given conflicting data and knowledge that some persons may be helped by use of these antidepressants, what is your view about when such medications should or should not be used? What factors do you consider most important in our efforts to help others and to do no harm?

RESEARCH Highlight 16–6

Nurses' Experiences of Suicide and Suicide Attempts in an Acute Unit

STUDY PROBLEM/PURPOSE

The researchers conducted a qualitative study to understand the feelings nurses had when confronted with patient suicide or suicide attempts and to document the nurses' perceptions of level of support received when such events occurred.

METHODS

Researchers used a descriptive qualitative methodology and interviewed a volunteer, purposive sample of nine nurses who had worked in psychiatric care for at least three years and who had experienced a patient suicide or attempted suicide during that time period.

FINDINGS

Nurses described feelings of shock, anger, frustration and helplessness when confronting cases of patient suicide or suicide attempts. The anger nurses felt was often related to a strong sense of frustration. Nurses reflected that peer support was vital to their personal well-being. Peer support was often given in casual rather than formal ways. Nurses suggested that formal supports, having a break from the unit for a two- to three-day period, and team-building/supporting activities would be helpful.

IMPLICATIONS

Psychiatric nurses expressed the need to use services and request that services be provided in a formal way. The need for peer support and understanding is unquestioned.

Source: "Nurses' Experiences of Suicide and Suicide Attempts in an Acute Unit," F. Bohan & L. Doyle, 2008, *Mental Health Practice*, *11*(5), 12–16.

APPLICATION OF THE NURSING PROCESS 16-1

ASSESSMENT

Knowing the prevalence of suicide and the conditions under which it is likely to occur provides the nurse with only beginning information on nursing's unique role and contribution to client care. Because, by definition, nursing is "care of the human response to actual or potential health problems," the nurse must look at suicidal behaviors within the context of the individual's human response to the conditions in which he finds himself.

The nurse must begin her work with the client by making a clear assessment of not just the suicidal risk but also the individual's unique responses in his spiritual domain. Box 16-1 provides a series of factors to consider when conducting such as assessment and will help the nurse and client evaluate the individual's human response to his present life situations.

NURSING DIAGNOSIS

A common theme in all descriptions of the circumstances of suicide, and in both the sociological and psychological theories, is that the person attempting suicide feels helpless. Nursing literature has addressed these feelings from several perspectives, and a review of the relevant NANDA-I diagnoses provides insight. In 1994, introduction of a new diagnosis called *spiritual well-being* provoked an analysis of the then existing diagnoses of *spiritual distress*, *hopelessness*, and *powerlessness*. Examination of these diagnoses led nurses to identify the linkages among them. *Spiritual distress* is defined as an "Impaired ability to experience and

(*Continues*)

APPLICATION OF THE NURSING PROCESS 16-1 (Continued)

BOX 16-1
FACTORS FOR THE NURSE TO CONSIDER WHEN ASSESSING THE CLIENT'S SPIRITUAL DOMAIN

- Meaning and purpose in life
- Sense of the future
- Belief in ability to make changes or control one's situation
- Ability to feel joy and peace
- Ability to love self
- Connectedness with others
- Connectedness with a Higher Power
- Connectedness with nature
- Ability to forgive others and self

integrate meaning and purpose in life through connectedness with self, others, art, music, literature, nature, and/or a power greater than oneself" (Herdman, 2009, p. 301). *Hopelessness* is defined as "a subjective state in which an individual sees limited or no alternatives or personal choices available and is unable to mobilize energy on own behalf" (Herdman 2009, pg. 184). Lastly, *powerlessness* is defined as the "perception that one's own actions will not significantly affect an outcome; a perceived lack of control over a current situation or immediate happening" (Herdman, 2009). The common theme underlying these diagnoses is meaning and purpose in life. Without meaning and purpose, a person may become alienated from others and lose his sense of connectedness—the human response of *powerlessness*. Without meaning and purpose, a person may lose any positive sense of future and give up any belief that the world and those around him will meet his needs—the human response of *hopelessness*. Lastly, without meaning and purpose in life, a person may feel lack of inner strength and lack of his own sense of sacredness or mystery—the human response of *spiritual distress*. Thus, there seems a trio of responses that may even represent a continuum—alienation, despair, and distress of the human spirit. These are the human conditions present in circumstances where a person turns to suicide.

Although these three diagnoses have been approved for use for years, nurses have identified that these diagnoses are frequently missed in clients. Case studies compiled by Lunney over the years (2001) identify instances in which a client's hopelessness and calls for help were missed by nurses providing care that lacked sensitivity to these issues. For example, situations where a hospitalized client in critical care presents with progressive disinterest in her care, sleeping during her daughter's visits, making statements such as "I want to be done with this" and other negative comments, and withdrawing from nursing and medical staff. In such cases, nurses easily become too involved with other aspects of the client's care and do not consider a diagnosis of *hopelessness*. In other cases, nurses miss cues from clients such as comments like: "What's the use of living? I'm so old" and "I wish this were the end." Many nurses hear such comments and understand that the client needs care, but do not take full measures to assess potential for suicide. These examples underscore the need for nurses to develop sensitivity and to complete assessments when they have ideas that hopelessness may be present. It is imperative that nurses develop an awareness of suicide and risk for suicide in all clients in all clinical settings.

OUTCOME IDENTIFICATION

The immediate outcome for clients at risk for suicide includes preventing harm and ensuring client safety. Establishing a safe or reduced-risk environment is one means of increasing the chances of meeting this goal. An eventual decrease or elimination of the client's desire to commit suicide is an outcome that should also be identified as a goal to work toward.

PLANNING/INTERVENTION

While the majority of suicidal or potentially suicidal clients will in all likelihood need to be referred for evaluation, the nurse should nonetheless have a basic understanding of the principles of crisis management as they pertain to suicidal risk.

(*Continues*)

APPLICATION OF THE NURSING PROCESS 16-1 (Continued)

TERTIARY PREVENTION

One of the best reasons for studying the relationship of suicide to various physical, psychological, and social factors is to seek ways to prevent suicidal behavior. While improved treatment of suicide victims might not seem to really qualify as prevention, the term *tertiary prevention* is often given to such therapy. Over the past decades, there have indeed been advances both in trauma care and in the management of common ingestions. It is certainly likely that some persons who have attempted suicide survive today whereas they would have died in the past. Although no one would argue that tertiary prevention is sufficient, no doubt medical advances in the care of the acutely ill and injured will continue to be made.

BOX 16-2
CLUES TO SUICIDE

SYNDROMATIC CLUES

DEPRESSION

- Change in sleep patterns
- Loss of appetite and weight loss
- Complaints about illnesses, real or imaginary, or complaints about body aches and minor or major physical problems, real or imaginary
- Mood changes (sadness, lethargy)
- Loss of interest in usual activities
- Loss of energy and fatigue

ALCOHOLISM

- Increased drinking
- Physical dependence on alcohol
- Loss of control over drinking
- Lying and denial
- Hiding liquor
- Sneaking drinks
- Drinking in spite of medical admonitions against it
- Blackouts
- Hangovers
- Cuts, scratches, bruises, cigarette burns

VERBAL CLUES

- "I am going to kill myself."
- "I am going to commit suicide."
- "I want to end it all."
- "I've had it."
- "I've lived long enough. No more."
- "I'm tired of life."
- "I'm tired of living."
- "My family would be better off without me."
- "Nobody cares about me."
- "Who cares if I'm dead anyway?"
- "I won't be around much longer."
- "Pretty soon you won't have to worry about me anyway."

BEHAVIORAL CLUES

- Previous suicide attempts
- Buying a gun
- Stockpiling pills
- Giving away money or possessions
- Loss of interest in favorite activities, church, or family
- Making or changing a will
- Making funeral plans
- Suspicious behavior

SITUATIONAL CLUES

- Death of spouse, child, or close friend
- Death of a pet
- Major move
- Diagnosis of a terminal illness
- Retirement
- Flare-up with a friend or relative

(*Continues*)

APPLICATION OF THE NURSING PROCESS 16-1 (Continued)

SECONDARY PREVENTION

Secondary prevention focuses on persons who display recognizable risk factors or who have already survived suicide attempts. Some of these latter individuals go on to complete suicide, and they represent a particularly high-risk group for secondary preventive intervention. Other potential risk factors clearly include various psychiatric conditions associated with unusually high rates of suicide, or being in a defined high-risk situation by nature of age or geography. For example, elderly men living in rural areas of the American West have very high suicide risk (Osgood, 1992); these men may therefore be another target for secondary prevention.

For secondary prevention to be effective, mental health workers must have clear data that establish risk factors in the identified population and then develop programs aimed at reducing specific risk factors. Evaluation must be able to show that programs have reduced the suicide risk. Clearly, the more accurately risk can be predicted, the more focused preventive activities can be. Unfortunately, predicting suicide in specific individuals has proven a daunting or even impossible task. While previous suicide attempt(s) put an individual at very significantly increased risk for subsequent completed suicide, to date, no criteria have proven effective in identifying suicidal individuals, even among those hospitalized for severe depression. Consequently, if individuals at highest risk can rarely be identified, secondary prevention must target all patients with known risk factors, particularly Major Depressive Disorder. There is some evidence that the use of lithium (Althaus & Hegerl, 2003) or atypical antipsychotics (Barak, Mirecki, Knobler, Natan, & Aizenberg, 2004), when these are clinically indicated, can reduce suicidal risk. Programs targeted to depressed elderly individuals seem to have some effectiveness when the rate of suicidal ideation is used as an outcome measure (Bruce, Ten Have, Reynolds, Katz, Schulberg, Mulsant, et al., 2004).

Many mental health workers believe that improved detection and effective ongoing treatment of depression offer a real possibility to reduce suicide rates. Well-publicized national guidelines for depression treatment offer some hope of reducing suicide in treated clients. Based on this model of secondary prevention, Osgood offers the "Ten Common Characteristics of Persons Attempting Suicide," which may help guide efforts to detect persons at risk (see Box 16-3).

PRIMARY PREVENTION

Primary prevention describes preventive activities applied to the whole population, regardless of any demonstrable risk factors. Although primary prevention might seem futile, given that suicide is a relatively

BOX 16-3
TEN COMMON CHARACTERISTICS OF PERSONS ATTEMPTING SUICIDE

1. Unbearable psychological pain is the common stimulus.
2. Frustrated psychological need is the common stressor.
3. The common purpose is to seek a solution.
4. Cessation of consciousness is the common goal.
5. The common emotion is hopelessness-helplessness.
6. Ambivalence is the common internal attitude.
7. The common cognitive state is constriction.
8. Communication of intention is the common interpersonal act.
9. The common action is escape.
10. The common consistency is difficulty with lifelong coping patterns.

From *Suicide in Later Life* by N. Osgood. Copyright © 1992, by Jossey-Bass Inc., Publishers. Reprinted with permission from Jossey-Bass, Inc. First published by Lexington Books. All rights reserved.

(*Continues*)

APPLICATION OF THE NURSING PROCESS 16-1 (Continued)

rare occurrence in the general population, a number of primary prevention programs have actually been found effective in reducing suicides. The CDC (CDC, 2007) published guidelines for suicidal prevention among youth in 1994 and developed a national strategy for suicide prevention in 2001. There are three major areas of focus for primary prevention efforts: access control, media responsibility in reporting, and crisis intervention. Nurses can be involved as advocates for all three.

ACCESS CONTROL: Access control focuses on making it harder for people to gain access to lethal means. For example, over the past 30 years, many countries have greatly reduced carbon monoxide content in cooking gas for the purpose of preventing suicide. As a result, suicides due to oven-related asphyxiation decreased (Lester, 1990; Clarke & Mayhew, 1988; Yamasawa, Nishimukai, Ohbora, & Inoue, 1980). The comparable reduction of carbon monoxide in automobile exhaust (this reduction was done for environmental reasons rather than directly for suicide prevention) has also affected use of this suicide method (Mott, Wolfe, & Alverson, 2002; Lester, 1989). Several "waves" of suicide in specific locations have been stopped by blocking access to well-publicized sites for jumping or self-hanging (Beautrais, 2001; Berman, 1990). Unfortunately, when access is restored through deinstallation of safety barriers suicide rates have increased. (Beautrais, Gibb, Fergusson, Horwood, & Larkin, 2009).

Finally, while the data are challenged by some, much evidence supports the concept that reducing access to guns would significantly decrease the prevalence of suicide (Bridges & Kunselman, 2004; Ludwig & Cook, 2000; Lester, 1984). Guns are commonly available, highly lethal, and frequently used for suicidal purposes. Many have commented that restrictions of gun availability would likely constitute the strongest primary prevention possible (Cantor, 1990). Some critics of this form of primary prevention maintain that decreased lethal access such as might come about through tight gun control would have no overall effect on suicide because alternative methods would be chosen (Lester, 1992). Although this is likely true for some highly premeditated suicides, there is mounting evidence that reducing access to lethal means does reduce overall suicide rates, not just those due to the restricted method (Mann, J. J., Apter, A., Bertolote, J., Beautrais, A., Currier, D. Haas, A., et al., 2005); Lester & Murrell, 1980). In the United States, gun control has become a highly politicized issue, and it currently seems unlikely that there will be major federal or local efforts to reduce the availability of firearms. This is particularly unfortunate from a public health point of view since data also suggest gun control would reduce homicide rates as well.

MEDIA RESPONSIBILITY IN REPORTING: The issues of public knowledge and public reaction to suicide have drawn the attention of suicidologists. There is concern that suicide events can be reported to the public in ways that sensationalize suicide and, in fact, encourage vulnerable individuals to consider suicide as a way out of difficult life circumstances. There is some research evidence that this is true (Pirkis, Blood, Beautrais, Burgess, & Skehans, 2007). In addition, another study reported that media blackouts on reporting suicide did in fact lead to a decrease in suicide rates (Motto, 1970). The World Health Organization (WHO) recommends a human ecological approach to suicide prevention and includes responsible media reporting as one measure to impact overall suicide rates. (Bertolote & Fleischmann, 2002). The American Foundation for Suicide Prevention and the Annenberg Public Policy Center have produced reporting guidelines, but there have been no evaluations of their effects.

CRISIS INTERVENTION: Many communities have set up crisis intervention centers and telephone hotline services in an effort to provide resources for individuals in crisis who might otherwise have no nonsuicidal outlet for crises. Not surprisingly perhaps, given the relative rarity of suicide, only 6% to 11% of calls or visits to such centers in the past have been suicide related (Franklin, Comstock, Simmons, & Mason, 1989). The evidence that intervention centers and hotline services actually reduce suicide rates is at best equivocal. Data from one study support a significant reduction of suicide among young women (Miller, Coombs, Leeper, & Barton, 1984), but other evaluations have not found any effect on community suicide rates (Dew, Bromet,

(Continues)

APPLICATION OF THE NURSING PROCESS 16-1 (Continued)

Brent, & Greenhouse, 1987). Currently, such telephone call-in centers have been augmented with online Web-based counseling and online information sources (Martin, 2007). These online services reach literally thousands of people, largely youth, each month. While these programs have been evaluated to the extent possible and provide supports otherwise unavailable to the public, it remains impossible to establish direct links to suicide rates (Martin, 2007).

LISTENING TO THE CLIENT

Although data supporting the effectiveness of crisis intervention and hotlines in suicide prevention may be limited, there is little doubt that many suicides could be prevented if victims' warnings were heeded by friends, relatives, health care providers, and work colleagues. Although these reports are typically retrospective and subject to bias, friends and relatives consistently report that individuals committing suicide expressed thoughts of hopelessness, helplessness, suicide, and death. The elderly may be more likely to verbalize suicidal feelings than are the young, but all too often, even the most direct warnings are ignored.

ENCOURAGING HOSPITALIZATION

Most truly suicidal individuals should be hospitalized for their own protection. Hospitalization affords a safe environment in which subsequent risk can be assessed and ongoing intervention can be planned. Only when risk is judged to be minimal by highly experienced professional personnel should the option of hospitalization not be pursued. Many individuals will recognize that their own interests are best served by protective hospitalization, but for others, short-term involuntary commitment will be necessary.

RESTRICTING LETHAL ACCESS

Suicidal individuals should return to environments that have been made as safe as possible. In most cases, firearms should be removed from the access of the suicidal individual. Medication stockpiles should be

REFLECTIVE THINKING 16-3

Gun Control as Primary Prevention of Suicide

In 1992, the CDC established a Division of Violence Prevention as part of a national effort to view violence as a major U.S. public health problem. The division continues to support firearms research and has funded research that brought in the following findings: Guns kept in the home nearly triple the risk of homicide; guns in the home increase the risk of death from assault and the risk of suicide nearly fivefold. It was reported in 1995 (*Lancet* editors, 1995a) that the CDC's support of firearms research "has the gun lobby up in arms" (p. 563). The National Rifle Association (NRA) and a 500-member physician group called Doctors for Integrity in Research and Public Policy (DIRPP) has been campaigning against politicalization of the injury prevention program. The CDC staff state that it is not possible or creditable to address the problem of violence-related injuries without addressing the role firearms play in such injuries, and the World Health Organization now agrees. The only study to report a comparison of state firearms laws and the impact on suicide rates has shown that for both men and women, the suicide rates were higher in locations with the least firearms restrictions and that there was no evidence that firearms restrictions led to alternative suicide methods (Conner & Zhong, 2003)

As a nurse and as a citizen, what is your view regarding the role of public policy with regard to primary prevention of suicide by limiting access to firearms?

(*Continues*)

APPLICATION OF THE NURSING PROCESS 16-1 (Continued)

assessed and placed under others' supervision. Family and household members will likely need education to ensure their willingness to act in a potential victim's interests. Although nurses and mental health care workers do everything possible to protect the client and prevent suicidal death, the reader is cautioned that there are times when a person intent on killing himself will do so no matter what is done by professionals and family and friends.

ESTABLISHING A "SUICIDE CONTRACT" OR AGREEMENT

Most therapists agree that when clients readily agree to not harm themselves during a prescribed period, risk is decreased. Often such contracts are written and signed, and the client is assured he has someone to call if he cannot bear to be alone. However, Drew (2001) studied the use of no-suicide contracts in psychiatric inpatients units and found that clients with no-suicide contracts and with higher levels of ward restrictions on the unit had a higher likelihood of self-harm behaviors. This research indicates that in the inpatient settings, negotiation of a contract is probably a reflection of staff assessment that the client risk of self-harm was high.

DECREASING SOCIAL ISOLATION

Even if not hospitalized, suicidal individuals need to have a social network established. Persons in proximity to potentially suicidal clients must be aware of the need to not leave the individual alone. When such supportive networks of family and friends cannot be readily established, hospitalization must be considered.

DECREASING PSYCHOLOGICAL SYMPTOMS

Medication and psychotherapy should be used to reduce anxiety and stress. Depressive symptoms generally do not respond rapidly to medication, so monitoring is particularly important pending medication effects. Psychotherapy is often indicated and initially may focus on personal and social conditions that bring about and/or perpetuate suicidal thoughts. Cognitive-behavioral therapy may be particularly useful, as may techniques to deal with frustration and anger. Substance use and abuse are often involved and may require separate outpatient or inpatient interventions.

EVALUATION

The most obvious measure of success of interventions for suicidal clients is the prevention of suicide attempts or completions. The nurse should also carefully monitor the client's view of self and life situation to assess if the factors contributing to the client's suicidal ideations have changed in any way. The client should also be evaluated for restoration of some sense of hope and life meaning. Plans for ongoing care and evaluation, as well as involvement of family members and significant others, should be implemented for clients at continuing suicide risk.

NURSINGTIP 16-2

Suicide Precautions

- When a suicidal client is hospitalized, the nurse has a duty to protect the client from self-harm.
- The goal of suicide precautions is to create a safe environment.

Precautions usually include:

1. Removing sharp objects, such as knives, scissors, and mirrors from the client's possession and access
2. Removing toxic substances, such as drugs and alcohol, and ensuring that unit medications are locked
3. Removing clothing that could be used for self-destruction, such as neckties, belts, stockings, and the like
4. Placing the client under close supervision, including one-to-one supervision with a staff member

CARE PLANNING GUIDE 16-1 Suicidal Client

CLINICAL PICTURE

The clinical picture of a client with suicidal ideation is:

- Expresses feelings of depression and hopelessness
- Has lost a sense of purpose in life, lost a sense of future
- Has considered ending own life, may have a plan for carrying out suicide

COMMON NURSING DIAGNOSES

Nursing diagnoses most commonly employed for the suicidal client are:*

1. *Risk for suicide*
2. *Chronic, low self-esteem*

The following Care Planning Guide depict suggested interventions, rationales, outcomes, and discharge planning activities for such clients.

NURSING DIAGNOSIS 1: *RISK FOR SUICIDE*, RELATED TO SUICIDAL IDEATION

OUTCOMES

1. The client will verbalize suicidal intent with health care workers.
2. The client will contract for safety and will notify health care workers or significant others if ideation to harm self increases.
3. The client will begin to make plans to deal with the underlying depression.

NOC: *RISK CONTROL*

INTERVENTIONS (NIC: *SUICIDE PREVENTION*)	RATIONALE
• Monitor for presence of suicidal ideation	• Ongoing assessment allows for identification of changes from the baseline and provides current state data.
• If suicidal ideation is present, ask follow-up questions to appraise for the presence of a plan and a viable means to carry out a suicide.	• A thorough plan and a means to carry it out increase the danger of success.
• Appraise the status of social supports.	• Social supports are an essential component of assisting a very depressed person through the worst part of an illness.
• Discuss a safety contract.	• Alliance with the health care team is built into the contract if the client can agree to it.
• Use empathetic listening and communication techniques.	• These actions convey genuine caring and concern when the client cannot care for self.
• Hospitalize if there is real danger of self-harm.	• Hospitalization is necessary to prevent self-harm.
• Remove any article that could be used in self-injury and assign a staff person to sit with the client.	• These actions convey a sense of caring for the client's safety.
• Reassure that feelings of hopelessness and despair remit with antidepressant medication.	• A sense of hope is provided based on realistic treatment outcomes.
• Convey a sense of unconditional acceptance and being fully present for the client and his or her needs.	• Therapeutic presence is a nursing intervention conveying connection of one human being to another.
• Monitor suicidal potential on an ongoing basis until approximately 14 to 21 days after medication has been initiated, and on an as-needed basis	• Clients are most at risk when energy level rises as the client begins to respond to antidepressant medication, yet the mood has not altered.

*Diagnoses common for the depressed client (see Chapter 14) should also be considered.

(*Continues*)

CARE PLANNING GUIDE 16-1 Continued

NURSING DIAGNOSIS 2: *CHRONIC LOW SELF-ESTEEM*, RELATED TO EXAGGERATED AND OFTEN UNFOUNDED FEELINGS OF SHAME/GUILT

OUTCOMES

1. Client will decrease the number of self-negating comments.
2. Client will identify own strengths.

NOC: *SELF-ESTEEM*

INTERVENTIONS (NIC: *SELF-ESTEEM ENHANCEMENT*)	RATIONALE
• Assess thought patterns for reality.	• Depressed and suicidal clients tend to ruminate on negative thoughts.
• Assist to set realistic expectations of self.	• Realistic expectations of self assist in reality-testing the negative thoughts.
• Encourage to attend groups or activities to break the pattern of self-criticism.	• Attention directed outside self will result in diminished intrusive thoughts.
• Evaluate the frequency of occurrence of negative thoughts as treatment progresses.	• Such evaluations allow for assessment of the success of milieu and medical treatment.

LONG-TERM CONSIDERATIONS FOR THE SUICIDAL CLIENT

1. Inpatient hospitalization as required for safety.
2. Individual therapy to provide support and follow symptoms.
3. Treatment for underlying depression.
4. Refer to community-based support groups.
5. Ensure that the client has a suicidal "hotline" or "helpline" that is available 24/7.

Note: The care planning guides have been adapted from *Plans of Care for Specialty Practice: Psychiatric Mental Health Nursing* by M. Coler, and K. G. Vincent, 1995, Clifton Park, NY: Delmar, Cengage Learning.

NURSING CARE PLAN: NURSING PROCESS FORMAT 16-1

Penny is a 17-year-old woman who was brought to the emergency department by her mother. Penny had ingested an unknown quantity of medications from the family's medicine cabinet and was found unresponsive by her mother when the mother returned home from work. Penny was treated medically and has been referred to the mental health unit for hospitalization.

ASSESSMENT

Jane is a psychiatric nurse who will be Penny's primary nurse. Jane observes that Penny is withdrawn. Penny's physical appearance is disheveled; her eyes are reddened as if she has been crying recently. Penny avoids eye contact and does not speak much. Penny tells Jane that she is tired, that she has not slept. Penny does not answer the question "Do you feel you could or would harm yourself again tonight?"

(*Continues*)

NURSING CARE PLAN: NURSING PROCESS FORMAT 16-1 (Continued)

NURSING DIAGNOSIS 1 *Risk for self-directed violence*, related to psychological dysfunction (suicide attempt).

OUTCOMES	NIC	NURSING ACTIONS	EVALUATION
• Penny will not harm herself further while in the hospital. • Penny will make a verbal contract to not harm herself for the next 4 days.	• Suicide prevention	• Initiate suicide precautions to ensure Penny's safety. For example, institute one-to-one monitoring, removing all potentially harmful items from the environment. • Begin to establish trust with Penny by approaching her in a nonjudgmental manner. • Penny will sign a written contract to not hurt herself at any time in the next 4 months. • Establish in each 24-hour period Penny's verbal contract to not harm herself. • Offer positive encouragement to Penny for remaining free of injury and/or for taking a positive interest in herself.	Penny did not harm herself during the hospital stay. Penny did make a verbal contract with the nurse by the second hospital day that she would not harm herself while in the hospital. Penny did sign a written contract to call a hotline number rather than make another attempt.

NURSING DIAGNOSIS 2 *Ineffective coping*, related to situational crisis (suicide attempt), as evidenced by destructive behavior and inability to ask for help.

OUTCOMES	NIC	NURSING ACTIONS	EVALUATION
• Penny will verbalize one positive statement about herself. • Penny will begin to examine her coping skills and consider alternatives.	• Coping enhancement • Support system enhancement	• Permit Penny to be herself. • Promote Penny's control by giving her choices of daily activities and of conversation topics. • Develop a positive relationship with Penny by remaining caring and truthful in interactions, by actively listening when Penny wants to talk, and by remaining attentive when Penny wishes to be silent.	Penny did respond to the nurse and entered into a relationship with the nurse. Penny began to describe her interests, her feelings. Penny accepted individual therapy and agreed to weekly sessions.

(*Continues*)

NURSING CARE PLAN: NURSING PROCESS FORMAT 16-1 (Continued)

OUTCOMES	NIC	NURSING ACTIONS	EVALUATION
		• Encourage Penny to view others as a source of support and assistance. • Encourage Penny to enter therapy on an ongoing basis.	

REFLECTIVE QUESTIONS

1. **ASSESSMENT**
   Would you also assess Penny's family situation for possible clues into her present psychological state? What other contacts (friends, school, boyfriend) would you pursue?
2. **NURSING DIAGNOSIS**
   What family-oriented diagnoses might be uncovered in Penny's case?
3. **OUTCOMES**
   What outcomes would you identify for a longer-term period (perhaps two weeks and beyond)? Are there family-oriented outcomes that you would include?
4. **NURSING ACTIONS**
   Identify family interventions that might help in Penny's situation.
5. **EVALUATION**
   How would you plan follow-up care and evaluation for Penny and her family once she is discharged?

NURSING CARE PLAN: CONCEPT MAP FORMAT 16-1

Suicidal Client

BACKGROUND INFORMATION

Gloria is admitted to the psychiatric unit, having been stabilized in the medical floor for having taken an overdose of aspirin and vodka—a serious suicidal attempt. Gloria came in for help after the ingestion, only because before the drugs took their full effect, Gloria called her friend May and told her what she had done. May intervened and her actions saved Gloria's life. Gloria is a 30-year-old, single professional who has had a history of mood swings and depression in the past. She has not been on any medication and had not been in treatment for a mental health or psychiatric problem. She has a few close female friends, she does not date, nor does she have a boyfriend. She remains distant from her parents, who live in a city about 500 miles away.

Coming to the psychiatric unit, Gloria appears tired and fatigued. She tells Margaret, her nurse, that she just wants to sleep. She states that she is not hungry, has no interest in any activities this evening, and wishes to remain alone. She refuses dinner, and goes to bed at 8 P.M. Gloria was not interactive with Margaret or anyone else on the unit, but she did comment that she did a "stupid thing" and that was what brought her to the hospital.

(Continues)

NURSING CARE PLAN: CONCEPT MAP FORMAT 16-1 (Continued)

INITIAL ASSESSMENT AND REFLECTION

Margaret understands that Gloria has carried out a serious suicidal attempt. Margaret and the psychiatrist have discussed the matter of Gloria's safety and have decided that Gloria should be on a suicidal watch. Margaret will assign a technician to sit with Gloria during the night. Also, as it is the unit's policy for all clients, there are no sharp objects permitted on the unit, and the staff have access to all rooms because there are no locks that could keep the staff away.

Margaret understands Gloria's lack of energy and withdrawal, because these are common symptoms of someone who is depressed. Margaret knows that it will take some time for her to develop a therapeutic relationship with Gloria, because Gloria has closed out the rest of the world.

INITIAL REVIEW OF NURSING DIAGNOSES

The nursing diagnoses and issues that are prominent are:

- Risk for self-directed violence related to suicidal ideation
- Risk for situational low self-esteem related to expression of shame, doing something stupid

PRIORITIES OF CARE

The concept map indicates that the focal issues point to the low self-esteem. However, Margaret knows that the risk for self-directed violence is real and that her care must provide safety for Gloria while supporting her self-esteem.

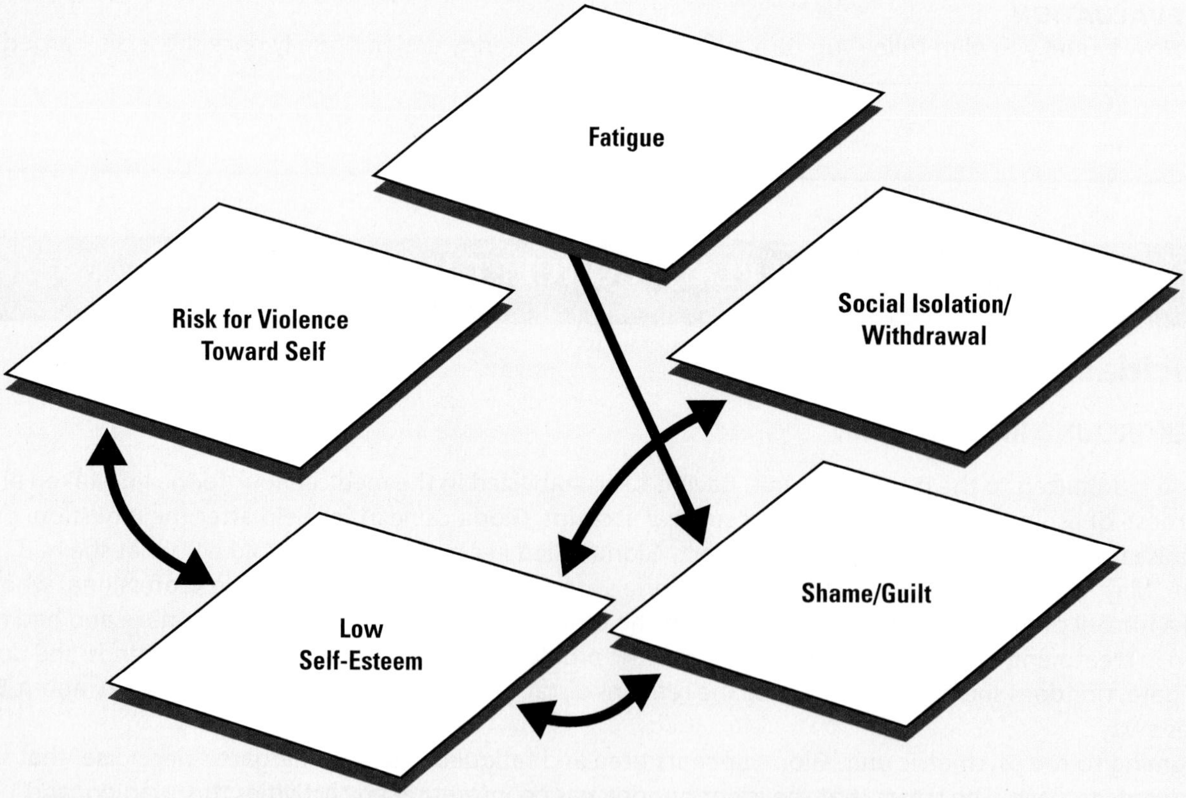

CONCEPT MAP OF ISSUES AND PROBLEMS. (DELMAR CENGAGE LEARNING.)

(Continues)

NURSING CARE PLAN: CONCEPT MAP FORMAT 16-1 (Continued)

NURSING INTERVENTIONS

Margaret tells Gloria that she will provide for a technician to "sit" with her and stay at her doorway through the night. Gloria responds, "That isn't necessary. You all have other things to do." Margaret responds in a kind and caring manner that the staff will stay with her to provide for her own safety and support and to "be there" for her at all times. Further, Margaret states, "We are here for you, and we care about your well-being and your recovery."

Margaret plans to maintain presence for Gloria now and to assure her that medications will help her in the way she feels. Margaret will not dwell on the hopelessness and depression, but will try to direct Gloria toward activities. At the same time, Margaret knows that the risk for suicide is greatest at the time when a client begins to feel more energy, thus a continual assessment and monitoring is definitely needed.

OUTCOMES/EVALUATION

Gloria progresses over the next three days. She is taking antidepressant medications and has begun daily group therapy sessions on the unit. She appears somewhat more sociable, in that she will acknowledge others on the unit. She remains on suicide precautions, and Margaret believes that this is still appropriate. She considers a no-suicide contract, but decides against bringing it up. Margaret will wait until Gloria expresses insight as to her suicide attempt and a desire to call for help. At day three in the hospital, that has not yet happened. Margaret decides to spend at least one-half hour of focused time with Gloria each day to develop a trusting relationship with her, to redirect Gloria's energies toward social and group activities, and to set the stage for Gloria to begin to talk about her feelings and expectations. Margaret, appropriately, takes her directions from the client and is not attempting to move the process along faster than her client can handle.

KEY CONCEPTS

- Suicide is an event rooted in fear, anger, despair, and loss of human touch and solace.
- The nurse must understand her own feelings about death, despair, and the human spirit to enter into a therapeutic relationship with a suicidal client.
- Suicide accounts for 13 deaths per 100,000 in the United States, with the rates for adolescents and the elderly (particularly elderly men) higher than the national average.
- Suicide attempts are much more common than completed suicides, with estimates ranging from 2.9% to as high as 10% of populations studied.
- Suicide is clearly associated with other psychiatric illnesses, including depression, bipolar disorders, schizophrenia, and substance abuse.
- Some persons with chronic illnesses have an increased risk for suicide; these include persons with epilepsy, cerebrovascular disease, dementia, multiple sclerosis, head injury, and brain tumor.
- Theories of suicide include sociological, psychological, and biological perspectives.
- The nursing diagnoses of *powerlessness, hopelessness,* and *spiritual distress* represent the human conditions of alienation, despair, and spiritual distress, which are linked to suicide.
- Preventive services include all levels of prevention: tertiary, secondary, and primary.
- Nursing management of clients at risk for suicide centers on protecting from harm and beginning to decrease isolation and psychological symptoms.
- Nursing theories that focus on the nurse-client relationship and the need to develop trust are helpful to guide interventions.
- Special populations requiring nursing care include adolescents, the elderly, the incarcerated, and family members and friends of those who attempt or complete suicide.

REVIEW QUESTIONS

1. The nurse conducts a complete physical and mental health assessment on a client admitted to the psychiatric unit with suicidal ideations. The primary purpose for conducting a complete physical assessment is to determine which of the following?
   1. It is a requirement of the hospital
   2. To establish a baseline for future treatments
   3. To determine if there are other medical conditions present
   4. To determine if the client has signs of previous attempts of self-harm
2. A depressed client tells the nurse that nothing will help and he still plans to kill himself. Which of the following statements by the client indicates that he is still suicidal?
   1. The client states that he is unable to enjoy eating anymore.
   2. The client states that he is unable to get a good night's sleep.
   3. The client states that no one cares about him.
   4. The client states he will purchase a gun once he is discharged.
3. A client is admitted to the unit after a failed suicide attempt. The nurse in developing the care plan would include which of the following as a priority short-term goal?
   1. Client will lead at least one group activity
   2. Client will be discharged within two days of admission
   3. Client will discuss suicidal thoughts with the nurse
   4. Client will express guilt over attempting suicide and disappointing family members
4. A client is admitted after a suicide attempt. The nurse would allow the client to keep which of the following items in his room?
   1. Shaving cream and razor
   2. Mediations he brought to the hospital
   3. Cigarettes and lighter
   4. Magazines and books
5. A new client is admitted to the psychiatric unit after attempting suicide. Which of the following clients would be an appropriate roommate?
   1. A client who is in an acute manic state
   2. Another client who has attempted suicide
   3. A client treated for PTSD and is awaiting discharge
   4. A schizophrenic client who is actively hallucinating
6. On the day of discharge a female client begins giving her belongings away to other patients. The client states, "I won't need these things anymore." The priority nursing intervention would be to do which of the following?
   1. Tell the client not to give her things away because she may need them.
   2. Thank the client for the nice watch she gave the nurse.
   3. Ask the client why she wants to give away her possessions.
   4. Reassess the client for possible suicidal ideations.
7. The priority nursing diagnosis for a client admitted after a suicide attempt would be which of the following?
   1. Risk for self-harm
   2. Alteration in body image
   3. Ineffective family coping
   4. Disturbed interpersonal relationships

LEARNING ACTIVITIES

1. What is your attitude toward suicide? What do you need to do before you approach a suicidal client?
2. Describe the conditions under which suicide is most likely to occur.
3. What groups in the United States have the highest prevalence of suicide? Suicide attempts?
4. Describe the way a worker on a telephone hotline would assess the suicidal risk in a caller.
5. Use theory to provide an explanation for why a person would choose suicide.
6. Identify the means of validating the presence of the nursing diagnoses of *hopelessness, powerlessness,* and *spiritual distress.*
7. Evaluate how nursing theory helps you in your work to establish a therapeutic relationship with a client.
8. What can be done (and what is being done) to prevent suicide in your community?
9. What are your personal attitudes and beliefs regarding assisted suicide?

*Study*WARE™ CONNECTION

Using your *Study*WARE™ CD-ROM

1. Complete the Crossword activity for this chapter.
2. Complete the Quiz for this chapter in Test Mode.
3. Explore the other games and activities that support this chapter.

VIDEO LINK

Read and contemplate the following questions about Evelyn, the client experiencing suicide ideation. Then watch the video "Major Depressive Disorder/Suicide" on your *Study*-WARE™ CD-ROM to observe Evelyn discussing her experience. Consider these questions prior to listening to the psychiatrist's analysis:

1. How did Evelyn describe her suicidal ideation?
2. How did she describe her feelings as she suffers from a Major Depressive Disorder?
3. What is the prevalence of suicide risk for individuals suffering from this disorder?
4. Assess Evelyn's status by means of a suicide risk assessment tool.
5. If you were answering a telephone hotline, describe how you would assess the suicide risk in a caller.
6. Do you know the means of providing a safe environment for someone in your community?
7. Evelyn chose to be admitted to a psychiatric institute; what restrictions do you think were put into place in order to keep her safe?
8. At what point in her depression was Evelyn at greatest risk of suicide?
9. How would you evaluate the meaning and purpose in Evelyn's life? Develop a plan of care to engage in a therapeutic relationship with Evelyn. Assess your own feelings of death, despair, and the human spirit as you become part of this therapeutic process.
10. Would group therapy have been beneficial for Evelyn when she was first admitted to hospital?
11. What are the typical initial inventions for a client who is profoundly depressed?
12. Develop a plan of care for Evelyn during her hospital stay and in preparation for discharge.
13. What did she identify as being particularly therapeutic during her hospital stay?
14. What resources are available in your community to assist a family when a mother is suffering from a Major Depressive Disorder and is at risk for suicide?
15. On her discharge, Evelyn focused on prevention; she addressed the stigma involved in mental illness. Preventative services include all levels of prevention: primary, tertiary, and secondary levels. What does your community provide in this regard?

REFERENCES

Abbott, A. (2203). British panel bans use of antidepressants to treat children. *Nature, 423*(6942), 792.

Allebeck, P., Bolund, C., & Ringback, G. (1989). Increased suicide rate in cancer patients. *Journal of Clinical Epidemiology, 42,* 611–616.

Allebeck, P., & Wistedt, B. (1981). Mortality in schizophrenia. *Archives of General Psychiatry, 43,* 650–653.

Althaus, D., & Hegerl, U. (2003). The evaluation of suicide prevention activities: State of the art. *World Journal of Biological Psychiatry,* 4(4), 156–165.

Andreason, N. C., & Black, D. W. (2006). *Introductory textbook of psychiatry* (4th ed.). Washington, DC: American Psychiatric Publishing, Inc.

Asberg, M. (1989). Neurotransmitter monoamine metabolites in the cerebrospinal fluid as risk factors for suicidal behavior. In *Alcohol, Drug Abuse and Mental Health Administration, Report of the Secretary's Task Force on Youth Suicide. Vol. 2: Risk factors for youth suicide* (DHHA Publication No. ADM 89–1623, pp. 193–212). Washington, DC: U.S. Government Printing Office.

Bagley, C. (1985). Psychosocial correlates of suicide behaviors in an urban population. *Crisis, 6,* 63–67.

Baldessarini, R. J., & Hennen, J. (2004). Genetics of suicide: An overview. *Harvard Review of Psychiatry, 12*(1), 1–13.

Barak, Y., Mireck, I., Knobler, H. Y., Natan, Z., & Aizenberg, D. (2004). Suicidality and second generation antipsychotics in schizophrenic patients: A case-controlled retrospective study during a 5-year period. *Psychopharmacology,* E-pub ahead of print.

Barraclough, B. (1970). The diagnostic classification and psychiatric treatment of 100 suicides. In R. Fox (Ed.), *Proceedings of the fifth international conference for suicide prevention* (pp. 129–132). Vienna: IASP.

Beautrais, A.L. (2001) Effectiveness of barriers at suicide jumping sites: a case study. *Australian and New Zealand Journal of Psychiatry, 35,* 557–562.

Beautrais, A. L., Gibb, S. J., Fergusson, D. M., Horwood, L. J., Larkin, G. L. (2009). Removing bridge barriers stimulates suicides: An unfortunate natural experiment. *Australian and New Zealand Journal of Psychiatry. 43*, 495–497.

Berglund, M. (1984). Suicide in alcoholism: A prospective study of 88 suicides: The multidimensional diagnosis at first admission. *Archives of General Psychiatry, 41*, 888–891.

Berman, A. (Ed). (1990). *Suicide prevention: Case consultation*. New York: Springer.

Berman, A., & Jobes, D. A. (1991). *Adolescent suicide*. Washington, DC: American Psychiatric Press.

Berman, A. N., & Schwartz, R. (1990). Suicide attempts among adolescent drug users. *American Journal of Diseases of Children, 144*, 310–314.

Bertolote, J. M., & Fleischman, A. (2002). Suicide and psychiatric diagnosis: A worldwide perspective. *World Psychiatry, 1*(3), 181–185.

Blaauw, E., Kerkhof, A. J., & Hayes, L. M., (2005). Demographic, clinical and psychiatric factors related to inmate suicide. *Suicide and Life Threatening Behavior, 35*(1), 63–75.

Brezo, J., Paris, J., Tremblay, R., Vitaro, E., Hebert, M., & Turecki, G. (2008). Predicting suicide attempts in young adults with histories of childhood abuse. *British Journal of Psychiatry, 193*(2), 134–139.

Bridges, F. S., & Kunselman, J. C. (2004). Gun availability and use of guns for suicide, homicide and murder in Canada. *Perceptual and Motor Skills, 98*, 594–498.

Bruce, M. L., Ten Have, T. R., Reynolds, C. F., III, Katz, H., Schulberg, H. C., Mulsant, B. H., et al. (2004). Reducing suicidal ideation and depressive symptoms in depressed older primary care patients: A randomized controlled trial. *Journal of the American Medical Association, 291*(9), 1081–1091.

Cantor, P. C. (1990). Intervention strategies: Environmental risk reduction for youth suicide. In *Alcohol, Drug Abuse and Mental Health Administration, Report of the Secretary's Task Force on Youth Suicide. Vol. 3: Prevention and intervention in youth suicide* (DHHA Publication No. ADM 89–1623, pp. 285–293). Washington, DC: U.S. Government Printing Office.

Carpenter, K. M., Hasin, D. S., Allison, D. B., & Faith, M. S. (2000). Relationships between obesity and DSM-IV major depressive disorder, suicide ideation, and suicide attempts: Results from a general population study. *American Journal of Public Health, 90*(2), 251–257.

Carrigan, J.T. (1994). The psychosocial need of patients who have attempted suicide by overdose. *Journal of Advanced Nursing, 20*, 635–742.

Carroll-Ghosh, T., Victor, B. S., & Bourgeois, J. A. (2003). Suicide. In R. E. Hales and S. C. Yudofsky, *Textbook of Clinical Psychiatry* (4th ed.). Washington, DC: American Psychiatric Publishing, Inc.

Centers for Disease Control and Prevention (2007). Suicide facts at a glance. Available from URL: http://www.cdc.gov/ncipc/dvp/Suicide/SuicideDataSheet.pdf. Accessed June 30, 2008.

Chabrol, H., & Moron, P. (1988). Depressive disorders in 100 adolescents who attempted suicide. *American Journal of Psychiatry, 145*, 379.

Chesley, K., & Loring-McNulty, N. E. (2003). Process and suicide: Perspective of the suicide attempter. *Journal of the American Psychiatric Nurses' Association, 9*(2), 41–45.

Clarke, R. N., & Mayhew, P. (1988). The British gas suicide stay and its criminological implications. *Crime and Justice, 10*, 79–116.

Conner, K. R., & Zhong, Y. (2003). State firearm laws and suicides in men and women. *American Journal of Preventive Medicine, 25*(4), 320–324.

Cottler, L. B., Campbell, W., Krishna, V. A. S., Cunningham-Williams, R. M., & Abdallah, A. B. (2005). Predictors of high rates of suicidal ideation among drug users. *Journal of Nervous and Mental Disorders, 193*(7), 431–437.

Courtet, P., Picot, M. D., Bellivier, F., Torris, S., Jollant, F., Michelon, C., et al. (2004). Serotonin transporter gene may be involved in short-term risk of subsequent suicide attempts. *Biological Psychiatry, 55*(1), 46–51.

Cvinar, J. G. (2005). Do suicide survivors suffer social stigma: A review of the literature. *Perspectives in Psychiatric Care, 41*(1), 14–21.

Dell, D. L., & O'Brien, B. W. (2003). Suicide in pregnancy. *Obstetrics and Gynecology, 102*(6), 306–309.

Dew, M. A., Bromet, E. J., Brent, D., & Greenhouse, J. B. (1987). A qualitative literature review of the effectiveness of suicide prevention centers. *Journal of Consulting and Clinical Psychiatry, 55*, 239–244.

Doyle L., Keogh, B., &. Morrissey, J. (2007). Caring for patients with suicidal behavior: An exploratory study. *British Journal of Nursing, 16*(29), 1218–1222.

Drew, B. L. (2001). Self-harm behavior and no-suicide contracting in psychiatric inpatient settings. *Archives of Psychiatric Nursing, 15*(3), 99–106.

Druss, B., & Pincus, H. (2000). Suicidal ideation and suicide attempts in general medical illnesses. *Archives of Internal Medicine, 160*(10), 1522–1526.

Duberstein, P. R., Conwell, Y., Conner, K. R., Eberly, S., & Caine, E. D. (2004). Suicide at 50 years of age and older: Perceived physical illness, family discord, and financial status. *Psychological Medicine, 34*(1), 37–46.

Duberstein, P. R., Conwell, Y., Seidlitz, L., Denning, D. G., Dox, C., & Caine, E. D. (2000). Personality traits and suicidal behavior and ideation in depressed inpatients 50 years of age and older. *Journal of Gerontology, Series B, Psychological Sciences and Social Sciences, 55B*(1), 18–26.

Dunleavey, R. (1992). An adequate response to a cry for help? Parasuicide patients' perception of their nursing care. *Professional Nurse, 7*, 213–215.

Durkheim, E. (1951). *Suicide, a study in sociology* (J. S. Spaulding & G. Simpson, Trans.; G. Simpson, Ed.). New York: Free Press.

Dutta, R., Boydell, J., Kennedy, N., Van Os, J., Fearon, P., & Murray, R.M. (2007). Suicide and other causes of mortality in bipolar disorder: A longitudinal study. *Psychological Medicine, 37*, 839–847.

Emanuel, E., Fairclough, D., Clarridge, B., Blum, D., Bruera, F., Penley, W., Schnipper, I., & Mayer, R., (2000). Attitudes and practices of U.S. oncologists regarding euthanasia and physician-assisted suicide. *Annals of Internal Medicine, 133*(7), 527–532.

Fishbain, D. A., & Aldrich, T. E. (1985). Suicide pack. *Journal of Clinical Psychiatry, 46*, 11–15.

Frances, A., & Blumenthal, S. J. (1989). Personality as a predictor of youth suicide. In *Alcohol, Drug Abuse, and Mental Health Administration, Report of the Secretary's Task Force on Youth Suicide. Vol. 2: Risk factors for youth suicide* (DHHS Publication No. ADM 89-1622, pp. 160–171). Washington, DC: U.S. Government Printing Office.

Franklin, J. L., Comstock, B. S., Simmons, J. T., & Mason, M. (1989). Characteristics of suicide preventions, intervention programs: Analysis of a survey. In *Alcohol, Drug Abuse, and Mental Health Administration, Report of the Secretary's Task Force on Youth Suicide* (Vol. 3, pp. 93–102). Washington, DC: U.S. Government Printing Office.

Funahashi, T., Ibuki, Y., Damon, Y., Nishimura, T. Y., Domon, Y., Nishimura, T., et al. (2000). A clinical study on suicide among schizophrenics. *Psychiatry and Clinical Neurosciences, 54*(2), 173–179.

Gallop, R., Lancee, W., & Shuger, G. (1993). Residents' and nurses' perceptions of difficult-to-treat short-stay patients. *Hospital and Community Psychiatry, 44*, 352–357.

Ganzini, L., Harvath, T. A., Jackson, A., Goy, E. R., Miller, L. L., & Delorit, M. A. (2002). Experiences of Oregon nurses and social workers with hospice patients who requested assistance with suicide. *New England Journal of Medicine, 347*(8), 582–588.

Gao, K., Tolliver, B. K., Kemp, D. E., Ganocy, S. J., Bilali, S., Brady, K. L., Findling, R. L., & Calabrese, J. R. (2009) Correlates of historical suicide attempt in rapid-cycling bipolar disorder: A cross-sectional assessment. *Journal of Clinical Psychiatry. 70,* 1032–1040.

Garand, L., Mitchell, A. M., Dietrick, A., Hiijjawi, S. P., & Pan, D. (2006). Suicide in older adults: Nursing assessment of suicide risk. *Issues in Mental Health Nursing, 27,* 355–370.

Gibbons, R. D., Brown, C. H., Hur, K., Marcus, S. M., Bhaumik, D. K., Erkens, J. A., et al. (2007). Early evidence on the effects of regulators' suicidality warnings on SSRI prescriptions and suicide in children and adolescents. *American Journal of Psychiatry, 164*(9), 1356–1363.

Gibbons, R. D., Hur, K., Bhaumik, D. K., & Mann, J. J. (2005). The relationship between antidepressant medication use and rate of suicide. *Archives of General Psychiatry, 62*(2), 165–172.

Gipps, C. H. (1978). Alcohol, diseases of alcoholics, and alcoholic liver disease. *Netherlands Journal of Medicine, 21,* 83–90.

Guze, S. B., & Robin, E. (1970). Suicide and primary affective disorders. *British Journal of Psychiatry, 117,* 437–438.

Hagnell, O., Lanke, J., & Rorsman, B. (1981). Suicide rates in the Lundby study: Mental illness as a risk factor for suicide. *Neuropsychobiology, 7,* 248–253.

Hagnell, O., & Rorsman, B. (1979). Suicide in the Lundby study. *Neuropsychobiology, 5,* 61–73.

Harkavy-Friedman, J., Asnis, G., Boeck, M., & DiFiore, J. (1987). Prevalence of specific suicidal behaviors in a high school sample. *American Journal of Psychiatry, 144,* 1203–1206.

Haverkate, I., Onwuteaka-Philipsen, B. D., van Der Heide, A., Kostense, P. J., van Der Wal, G., & van Der Maas, P. J. (2000). Refused and granted requests for euthanasia and assisted suicide in the Netherlands: Interview study with structured questionnaire. *British Medical Journal, 321*(7265), 865–866.

Hawton, K., & Vislisel, L. (1999) Suicide in nurses. *Suicide and Life-Threatening Behavior, 29,* 86–95.

Healy, D., & Whitaker, C. (2003). Antidepressants and suicide: Risk-benefit conundrums. *Journal of Psychiatry and Neurology, 28*(5), 331–337.

Herdman, H. (Ed). (2009). *Nursing diagnoses: Definitions and classifications: 2009–2011.* Oxford: Wiley Blackwell.

Hunt, I. M., Kapur, N., Windfuhr, K., Robinson, J., Bickley, H., Flynn, S., et al. (2006). National confidential inquiry into suicide and homicide by people with mental illness. *Journal of Psychiatric Practice, 2*(3), 139–147.

Jameison, P. E., & Romer, D. (2008). Unrealistic fatalism in U.S. youth ages 12–22: Prevalence and characteristics. *Journal of Adolescent Health, 42*(2), 154–160.

Jamison, K. R. (2000). Suicide and bipolar disorder. *Journal of Clinical Psychiatry, 61*(Suppl. 9), 47–51.

Joyce, B., & Wallbridge, H. (2003). Effects of suicidal behavior on a psychiatric unit nursing team. *Journal of Psychosocial Nursing and Mental Health Services, 41*(3), 14–23, 42–43.

Kaplan, M. S., Hugeut, N., McFarland, B. H., & Newson, J. T. (2007) Suicide among veterans: A prospective population-based study. *Journal of Epidemiology and Community Health, 61*(7), 619–624.

Kishi, Y., & Kathol, R. G. (2002). Assessment of patients who attempt suicide. *Primary Care Companion of the Journal of Clinical Psychiatry,* 4(4), 132–136.

Kposawa, A. J. (2000). Marital status and suicide in the National Longitudinal Mortality Study. *Journal of Epidemiology and Community Health, 54*(4), 254–261.

Lafayette, J. M., & Stern, T. A. (2004). The impact of a patient's suicide on psychiatric trainees: A case study and review of the literature. *Harvard Review of Psychiatry, 12*(1), 49–55.

Lancet editors. (1995a). U.S. gun lobby takes aim at CDC injury centre. *The Lancet, 346,* 563–564.

Lancet editors. (1995b). The final autonomy. *The Lancet, 346,* 259.

Larkin, G. L., Smith, R. P., & Beautrais, A. L. (2008). Trends in U.S. emergency department visits for suicide attempts: 1992–2001. *Crisis, 29*(2), 73–80.

Lester, D. (1984). *Gun control.* Springfield: Charles C. Thomas.

Lester, D. (1988). Rational choice theory and suicide. *Activitas Nervosa Superior, 30,* 309–312.

Lester, D. (1989). Suicide by car exhaust. *Perceptual and Motor Skills, 68,* 442.

Lester, D. (1990). The effects of detoxification of domestic gas on suicide in the United States. *American Journal of Public Health, 80,* 80–81.

Lester, D. (1992). *Why people kill themselves* (3rd ed.). Springfield, IL: Charles C. Thomas.

Lester, D., & Danto, D. L. (1993). *Suicide behind bars.* Philadelphia: Charles Press.

Lester, D., & Murrell, M. E. (1980). The influence of gun control laws on suicidal behaviors. *American Journal of Psychiatry, 137,* 121–122.

Levav, I., Magnes, J., Aisenberg, E., & Rosenblum, I. (1988). Sociodemographic correlates of suicidal ideation and reported attempts. *Israel Journal of Psychiatry, 25,* 38–45.

Lewis, G., & Sloggett, A. (1998). Suicide, deprivation, and unemployment: Record of linage study. *British Medical Journal, 317*(7168), 1283–1286.

Ludwig, J., & Cook, P. J. (2000). Homicide and suicide rates associated with implementation of the Brady Violence Prevention Act. *JAMA, 284,* 585–591.

Lunney, M. (2001). *Critical thinking and nursing diagnosis: Case studies and analysis.* Philadelphia: Nursecom, Inc.

Luoma, J. B., & Pearson, J. L. (2002). Suicide and marital status in the United States, 1991–1996: Is widowhood a risk factor? *American Journal of Public Health, 92*(9), 1518–1522.

Mann, J. J., Apter, A., Bertolote, J., Beautrais, A., Currier, D. Haas, A. et al. (2005). Suicide prevention strategies: A systematic review. *JAMA, 294*(16), 2063–2074.

Martin, G. (2007). Success! The Australian National Youth Suicide Prevention Strategy (1995–2000) worked. But what exactly made the difference? *Australian e-Journal for the Advancement of Mental Health, 6*(3), 1–5.

McKeown, R. E., Cuffe, S. P., & Schulz, R. M. (2006). U.S. suicide rates by age group, 1970–2002: An examination of recent trends. *American Journal of Public Health, 96*(10), 1744–1751.

Miller, H. L., Coombs, S. W., Leeper, J. D., & Barton, S. N. (1984). An analysis of the effect of suicide prevention facilities on suicide rates in the U.S. *American Journal of Public Health, 74,* 340–343.

Moscicki, E. K., O'Carrol, P., Rae, D. S., Locke, B. Z., Roy, A., & Regier, D. A. (1988). Suicide attempts in the Epidemiological Catchment Area Study. *Yale Journal of Biology and Medicine, 61,* 259–268.

Mott, J. A., Wolfe, M. I., & Alverson, C. J. (2002). National vehicle emissions policies and practices and U.S. carbon monoxide-related mortality. *JAMA, 288,* 988–995.

Motto, J. A. (1970). Newspaper influences on suicide: A controlled study. *Archives of General Psychiatry, 23,*(2), 143–148.

National Institutes of Mental Health. (2008). Suicide in the U.S.: Statistics and Prevention. URL: http://www.nimh.gov/health/publications/suicide-in-the-us-statistics-and-prevention.shtml.

Nelson, R. (2004). Suicide rates rise among soldiers in Iraq. *The Lancet, 363,* 300.

Ohara, K., Suzuki, Y., Sugita, T., Kobayashi, K., Tamefusa, K., Hattori, S., et al. (1989). Mortality among alcoholics discharged from a Japanese hospital. *British Journal of Psychiatry, 84*, 287–291.

Osgood, N. (1992). *Suicide in later life.* Lexington: Lexington Books.

Oslin, D. W., Zubritsky, C., Brown, G., Mullaby, M., Puliafico, A., & Ten Have, T. (2004). Managing suicide risk in late life: Access to firearms as a public health risk. *American Journal of Geriatric Psychiatry, 12*(1), 30–36.

Outcliffe, J. R., & Stevenson, C. (2008). Feeling our way in the dark: The psychiatric nursing care of suicidal people – a literature review. *International Journal of Nursing Studies, 45*(6), 942–953.

Patterson, R. F., & Hughes, K. (2008). Review of completed suicides in the California Department of Corrections and Rehabilitation, 1999 to 2004. *Psychiatric Services, 59*(6), 676–682.

Peplau, H. (1988). The art and science of nursing: Similarities, differences and relations. *Nursing Science Quarterly, 1*, 8–15.

Phillips, D. P., & Ruth, T. E. (1993). Adequacy of official statistics for scientific research and public policy. *Suicide and Life-Threatening Behavior, 23*(4), 307–319.

Pirkis, J., Blood, R. W., Beautrais, A., Burgess, P., & Skehans, J. (2007) Media guidelines on the reporting of suicide. *Crisis, 27*(2), 82–87.

Rashid, A. (2008). Jihadi suicide bombers: The new wave. *New York Review of Books, LV*(10), 17–22.

Rihmer, Z., & Pestality, P. (1999). Bipolar disorder and suicidal behavior. *Psychiatric Clinics of North America, 22*(3), 667–673.

Robins, E., Murphy, G. E., Wilkinson, R. N., Glassner, S., & Kayes, J. (1959). Some clinical considerations in prevention of suicide based on a study of 134 successful suicides. *American Journal of Public Health, 49*, 888–899.

Robins, L. N., & Regier, D. A. (Eds.). (1991). *Psychiatric disorders in America.* New York: Free Press.

Roy, A. (1986). Depression, attempted suicide and suicide in chronic schizophrenia. *Psychiatric Clinics of North America, 9*, 193–206.

Safer, D. J. (1997). Self-reported suicide attempts by adolescents. *Annals of Clinical Psychiatry, 9*(4), 263–269.

Saluatore, T. (2000). Elder suicide. *Home Healthcare Nurse, 18*(3), 180–188.

Schneider, K. L., & Shenassa, E. (2008). Correlates of suicide ideation in a population-based sample of cancer patients. *Journal of Psychosocial Oncology, 26*(2), 49–62.

Schneidman, E. S. (1987). A psychological approach to suicide. In G. R. Vardenbos & B. K. Bryant (Eds.), *Cataclysms, crises, and catastrophes: Psychology in action.* Washington, DC: American Psychological Association.

Schwartz, A. J. (2006). Four eras of study of college student suicide in the United States, 1920–2004). *Journal of American College Health, 54*, 353–356.

Schwenk, T. L., Coyne, J., & Fechner-Bates, S. (1996). Differences between detected and undetected patients in primary care and depressed psychiatric patients. *General Hospital Psychiatry, 18*(6), 407–415..

Shah, S., Hoffman, R. E., Wake, L. & Marine, W. M. (2000). Adolescent suicide and household access to firearms in Colorado: Results of a case-control study. *Journal of Adolescent Health, 26*(3), 157–163.

Shaw, J., Baker, D., Hunt, I. M., Moloney, A., & Appleby, L. (2004). Suicide by prisoners: National clinical survey. *British Journal of Psychiatry, 184*, 263–267.

Smith, B. J., Mitchell, A., Bruno, A., & Constantino, R. (1995). Exploring widows' experiences after the suicide of their spouse. *Journal of Psychosocial Nursing and Mental Health Services, 33*, 10–15.

Steinbrook, R. (2002). Physician-assisted suicide in Oregon—an uncertain future. *New England Journal of Medicine, 346*(6), 460–464.

Suominen, K., Isometsa, E., Suikas, J., Haukka, J., Achte, K., & Longqvist, J. (2004). Completed suicide after a suicide attempt: A 37-year follow-up study. *American Journal of Psychiatry, 151*(3), 562–563.

Townsend, E. (2007). Suicide terrorists: Are they suicidal? *Suicide and Life Threatening Behavior, 37*(1), 35–49.

U.S. Centers for Disease Control and Prevention. (1994). Programs for the prevention of suicide among young adults. *Morbidity and Mortality Weekly Review, 43*(RR-6), 1–7.

Unnithan, P. M., Huff-Corzine, L., Corzine, J., & Whitt, H. P. (1994). *The currents of lethal violence.* Albany, NY: SUNY.

Valuck, R. J., Libby, A. M., Orton, H. D., Morrato, E. H., Allen, R., & Baldessarini, R. J. (2007). Spillover effects on treatment of adult depression in primary care after FDA advisory on risk of pediatric suicidality with SSRIs. *American Journal of Psychiatry, 164*(8), 1198–1205.

Van der Wal, J. (1990). The aftermath of suicide: A review of empirical evidence. *Omega, 20*, 149–171.

van Kolfschooten, F. (2003). Dutch television report stirs up euthanasia controversy. *The Lancet, 361*(9366), 1352–1353.

Varadaraz, R., & Mendonca, J. (1987). A survey of blood alcohol levels in self-poisoning cases. *Advances in Alcohol and Substance Abuse, 7*(1), 63–69.

Walsh, E., & Hendrickson, S. (2003). Oregon update. *British Medical Journal, 327*(7425), E256.

Wasserman, D., Geijer, T., Sokolowski, M., Rozanov, V., & Wasserman, J. (2007). Nature and nurture in suicidal behavior, the role of genetics: Some novel findings concerning personality traits and neural conduction. *Physiology and Behavior, 92*(1-2), 245–249.

Welte, J., Abel, E., & Wieczorek, W. (1988). The role of alcohol in suicides in Erie county, NY, 1972–1984. *Public Health Reports, 103*, 648–652.

Wickett, A. (1989). *Double exit.* Eugene, OR: Hemlock Society.

Williams, C., Davidson, J., & Montgomery, I. (1980). Impulsive suicidal behavior. *Journal of Clinical Psychology, 36*, 90–104.

Yamasawa, K., Nishimukai, J., Ohbora, Y., & Inoue, K. (1980). A statistical study of suicide through intoxication. *Acta Medicinae Legalis et Socalis, 30*, 187–192.

LITERARY REFERENCES

Anonymous. (1970). Death in the first person. *American Journal of Nursing, 70*, 336.

Bontemps, A. (1961). The old south. Anthologized in R. Weir, *Death in Literature* (pp. 253–262). New York: Columbia University Press.

Lester, D., & Danto, B. (1993). *Suicide behind bars.* Philadelphia: Charles Press.

Plath, S. (1971). *The bell jar.* New York: Harper & Row.

SUGGESTED READINGS

Joiner, T., (2005). *Why people die by suicide.* Cambridge: Harvard University Press.

Lieberman., L. (2005). *Leaving you: The cultural meaning of suicide.* Chicago: Ivan Dee.

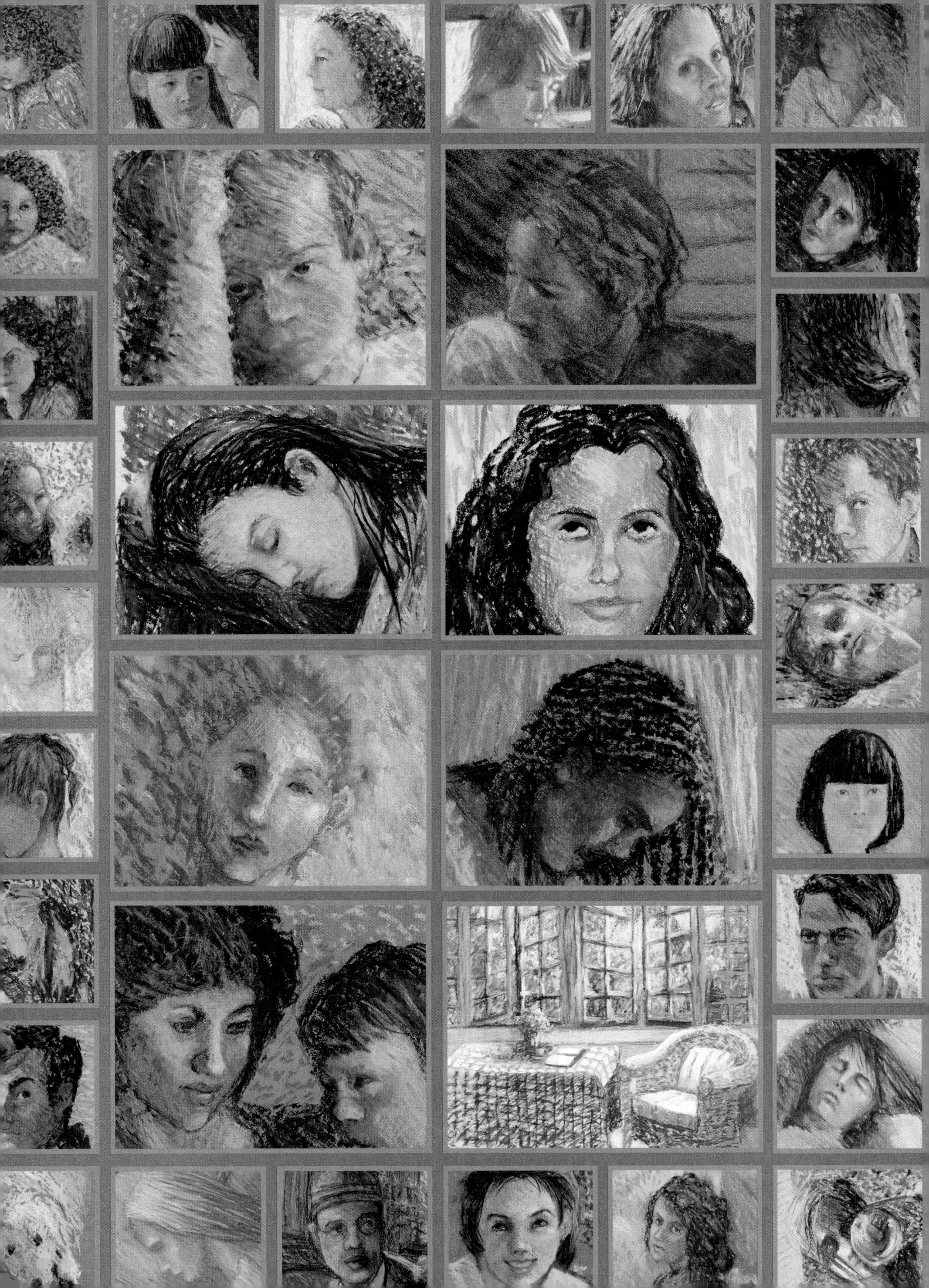

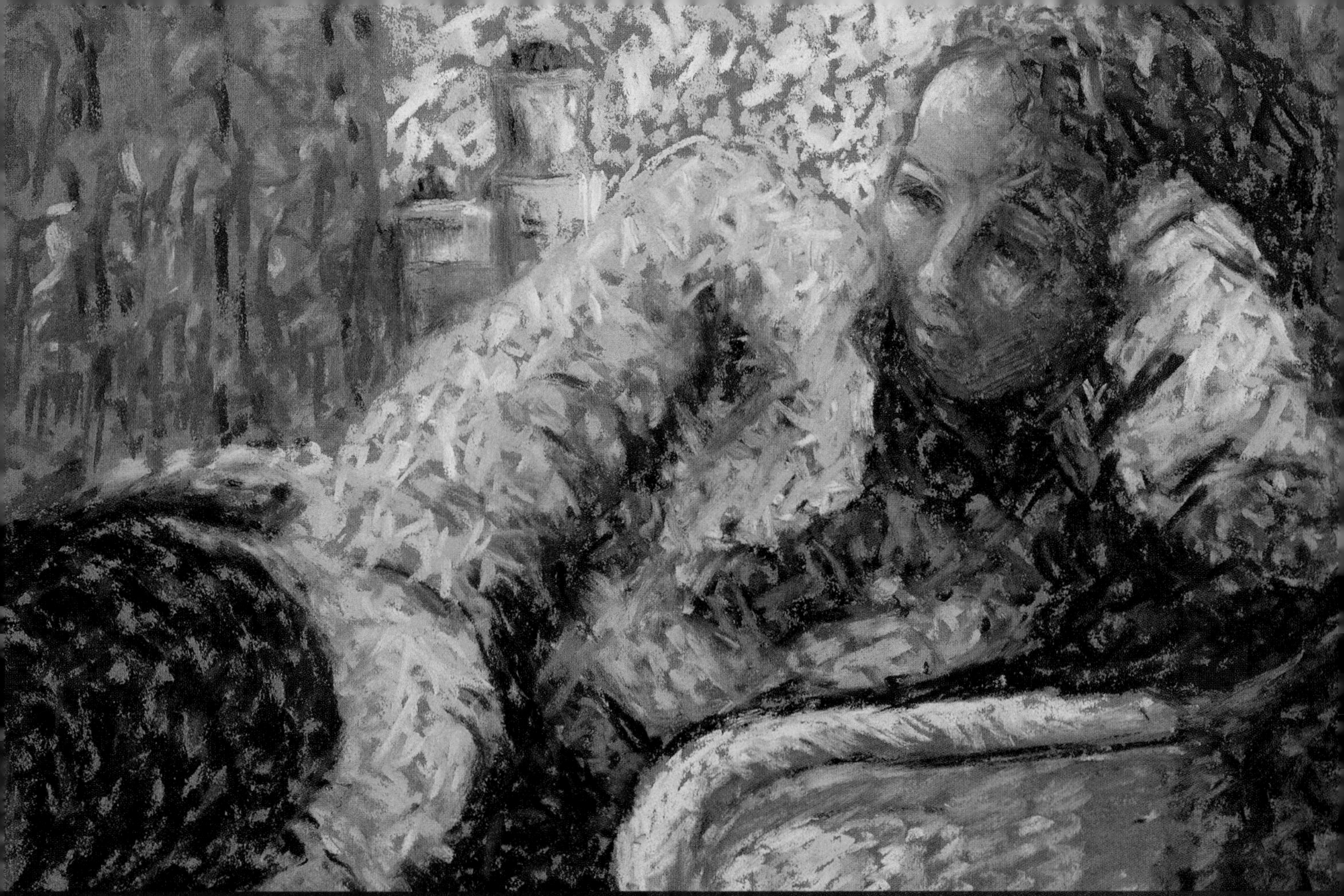

I Did Nothing

Chemical Substances in Your Life

If you are reading this textbook while drinking a cup of coffee or tea, or (we hope not!) smoking a cigarette, sipping a glass of wine, or drinking a can of beer, you are using the most commonly abused substances in the United States. Chemical substances are a part of our lives. While this chapter is primarily about substances of abuse, it is surely a fact that medications, both over-the-counter and prescription drugs, are a part of our social environment.

Before reading this chapter:

- ***Look in your refrigerator and food cabinets and identify any food or drink that is known to contain habituating substances such as alcohol or caffeine.***
- ***Look in your medicine cabinet and identify the number and kind of prescription and over-the-counter drugs.***
- ***Take note over the next week of how often you:***
    - ***–Use a drug or chemical substance***
    - ***–Are offered a drug or chemical substance by another person***
    - ***–See an advertisement for a drug or chemical substance***
- ***Document for yourself the number and kind of chemical substances in your personal environment.***

CHAPTER 17

The Client Who Abuses Chemical Substances

Noreen Cavan Frisch
Lawrence E. Frisch

CHAPTER OUTLINE

COMPETENCIES

Upon completion of this chapter, the reader should be able to:

1. Describe the widespread nature of substance abuse in historical and modern cultures.
2. List the types of substances subject to misuse and abuse.
3. Define and differentiate between the terms *tolerance*, *withdrawal*, *dependence*, *craving*, and *addiction*.
4. Identify the effects, withdrawal symptoms, patterns of abuse, and means of treatment for nicotine, alcohol, cocaine, and opiate abuse.
5. Explain the philosophy and treatment approach of Alcoholics Anonymous and 12-step programs.
6. Explain the relationship between chemical abuse and family dysfunction.
7. Explain the dynamics of codependency.
8. Employ nursing theory and diagnoses to plan care for the individual and family unit affected by chemical abuse.

KEY TERMS

Addiction
Alcoholism
Codependence
Craving
Drug Dependence
Drug Use
Substance Abuse
Tolerance
Withdrawal

While all psychiatric disorders reflect a complex interplay of interpersonal, genetic, and sociocultural factors, perhaps nowhere is this complexity so evident as in the disorders of substance use and dependence. As an introduction to the substance-related disorders, this chapter focuses on some of the most important issues. Five substances are considered in detail: nicotine, alcohol, cocaine, methamphetamines, and opiates. This discussion outlines the most common and dangerous substances abused in modern society and provides a broad understanding of the social, psychiatric, and nursing challenges posed by substance use.

The chapter begins with a general discussion of four basic topics: the widespread (if not universal) nature of substance use in human cultures, the very large number of substances subject to misuse and abuse, the varied range of drug effects and dependency symptoms, and the challenges of changing substance-using and substance-abusing behavior.

Following this overview, discussion is devoted to each of five specific substances and to the topic of multiple-drug abuse. Consideration is then given to issues of preventing substance abuse and dependency and the role of families or significant others in substance abuse. Independent and collaborative nursing roles of caring for clients and families are examined in the context of nursing theory and diagnosis in planning and evaluating care for individuals and for families.

DEFINITIONS RELATED TO SUBSTANCE ABUSE

One of the difficult problems in coming to an understanding of substance-related disorders is agreeing on definitions of various terms used to describe excessive drug use—these include *use, abuse, tolerance, withdrawal, dependence, craving,* and *addiction.*

Drug use refers to any taking of a drug. **Substance abuse** is quite different from use alone and may be defined in a number of ways. The following definition has been presented in the *Diagnostic and Statistical Manual, Fourth Edition-Text Revision* (DSM-IV-TR): "A maladaptive pattern of substance use leading to a clinically significant impairment or distress, manifested by one (or more) of the following ... (1) recurrent substance use resulting in a failure to fulfill major role obligations at work, school, or home ... (2) recurrent substance use in situations in which it is physically hazardous ... (3) recurrent substance-related legal problems ... (4) continued substance use despite having persistent or recurrent social or interpersonal problems caused or exacerbated by the effects of the substance" (American Psychiatric Association, 2000, p. 199).

In this definition, diagnosing abuse requires that use continue despite real or potential harm. The *Tenth Revision of the International Classification of Diseases* (ICD-10) explicitly incorporates this idea of harm by making reference to "harmful use" of drugs. In ICD-10, *harmful use* is defined as use causing actual physical or mental damage to the using individual. The ICD-10 definition is somewhat more restrictive than the DSM view of abuse. Under the DSM definition, abusers need not actually harm themselves; they only have to use a drug in potentially hazardous ways. For purposes of this text, abuse will be defined in accord with the DSM criteria, so that abuse refers to situations where a drug or substance is used in situations of real or potential harm.

BOX 17-1
BEHAVIORS ASSOCIATED WITH DRUG DEPENDENCE

- Develop tolerance to drug effects
- Manifest withdrawal from a drug
- Use more drug than intended
- Try persistently or unsuccessfully to cut down on use
- Spend significant amount of time using or trying to obtain the drug
- Give up important activities because of the drug
- Continue to use a drug despite knowing it is causing physical or psychological problem(s)

Tolerance is an acquired resistance to the effects of a drug and is defined in DSM-IV-TR as either needing to increase drug dosage to achieve a given effect or finding decreasing effect from a continuing fixed dosage (American Psychiatric Association, 2000). **Withdrawal** is a maladaptive behavioral change, with physiological and cognitive concomitants, that occurs when the blood or tissue concentrations of the substance decline in an individual who had maintained prolonged heavy use of the substance (American Psychiatric Association, 2000, p. 194). The symptoms of withdrawal are relieved by additional doses of the drug. **Drug dependence** occurs when individuals exhibit a set of behaviors associated with inability to control use of the drug. These behaviors are listed in Box 17-1. The DSM-IV-TR definition of dependence requires that three or more of these characteristics occur within one year and be related to one drug.

Craving is a term often used to describe some of the behavior of individuals who abuse or are dependent on drugs (Richardson, Baillie, Reid, Morley, Teesson, Sannibale, et al., 2008). Although a totally satisfactory definition of craving has never been offered, it is often taken to describe "the strong, almost overpowering urge for opiates experienced by opiate-dependent clients during acute withdrawal. It has subsequently found favor as a description of the desire to use any abused substance at any time" (Bauer, 1992). Probably because of difficulties with definition, the word *craving* has not found its way into the definition of dependence.

Addiction is an even more difficult term to define. Some have suggested that addiction may be diagnosed when both tolerance and withdrawal are present (Grinspoon & Bakalar, 1992). Others have diagnosed addiction only when an individual demonstrates inability to abstain from drug use in addition to displaying evidence of both tolerance and withdrawal (Jellinek, 1960). Still others define addiction as the combination of drug craving, compulsive use, and relapse after withdrawal (Rinaldi, Steindler, Wilford, & Goodwin, 1988). Partly because it has proven difficult to define reproducibly, *addiction* is not a term used in DSM-IV-TR. Instead, DSM-IV-TR defines "physiological dependence," in which either tolerance or withdrawal (or both) are included among the three or more criteria used to establish an individual's diagnosis of dependence. In contrast, if neither tolerance nor withdrawal has occurred but criteria for dependence are otherwise met, the condition is described as "without physiological dependence." While widely accepted, the DSM-IV-TR concept of dependence assumes that the same definition can apply to all substances—a concept that has been challenged by some researchers (Etter, 2008; Budney, 2006; Hughes, 2006).

SUBSTANCE USE AND ABUSE IN SOCIETY

Since the 1980s, there has been such emphasis on controlling drug use in America that it is easy to think drugs are something new and unique. There certainly were importantly unique aspects to drug use in the late twentieth century, and these will certainly continue well into the twenty-first century. As with other consumer goods, drugs are currently available in unprecedented variety, potency, and abundance. In nineteenth-century America, drug users likely had fewer drugs from which to choose, but access was probably easier. In nineteenth-century America, neither alcohol, nor cocaine, nor opiates were restricted in any effective way, and both adults and children had relatively free access to these substances. Morphine, one of the products of nineteenth-century chemical technology, was widely used during the Civil War to relieve the pain of battlefield injuries. By the end of the century, 500,000 pounds of opium were imported yearly into the United States and distributed uncontrolled as opium, morphine, or codeine (Musto, 1992). Pure preparations of cocaine became readily available only after the 1880s. Coca-Cola (whose manufacturers voluntarily removed cocaine from the formula in 1903) was only one of many cocaine-containing "tonics" advertised and marketed as stimulants.

The use of drugs seems to have been part of the human condition since earliest human prehistory. The *Old Testament* vividly describes drunkenness and attributes to Noah the discovery of grapes and wine. Indeed, by the time the *Old Testament* was written, the consumption of alcohol had long been a source of both consolation and misery. Beer and wine were produced and consumed by the ancient Egyptians many centuries before the story of Noah was set in writing. Early humans made fermented liquors from algae, tree saps, rice, and numerous fruits, and, in fact, there probably has never been a time since the Bronze Age when humans have not had access to alcohol.

It is harder to trace the past history of other drugs, but archeological evidence suggests coca use in what is now Peru (coca is the leaf from which cocaine is made) for at least the past 5,000 years. However improbable it might seem that early humans would fail to recognize the psychoactive properties of the common hemp plant, Sufi legend claims that marijuana consumption began only 1,000 years ago. Much firmer evidence suggests that tobacco use had its origins at least 7,000 years earlier. Opium use is mentioned in *The Odyssey*, and opium was an important item of commerce throughout the Mediterranean region over 3,500 years ago. The cultivation of opium poppies in Europe can be traced back even further, to Paleolithic and Neolithic times; it is highly likely that Stone Age people had discovered narcotics long before their twentieth-century descendants declared war on the drugs (Siegel, 1989).

While use of drugs has been clearly established in the earliest epochs of human history, it is much harder to document drug dependency and abuse. It is difficult to imagine that earlier cultures were more successful in avoiding at least some of the complications of drug use seen today.

ABUSED SUBSTANCES

Psychoactive substances used and abused by humans have their origins either as plant products or as modern laboratory chemicals. Most substances can be classified primarily as stimulant drugs, hallucinogens, or central nervous system (CNS) depressants. Stimulants act on brain neurotransmitter receptors to produce excitation, increased alertness, aggressiveness, and decreased food intake. Hallucinogens produce perceptual and sensory alterations that may involve any sensory modality (vision, hearing, smell, touch, or taste) and frequently result in hallucinations. Depressants act to decrease CNS functioning, and as with alcohol, their initial effect may be stimulation if inhibitory brain centers are depressed first. Many drugs have several effects, particularly in higher doses. For example, amphetamines are stimulants that may cause psychosis and hallucinations in high doses; marijuana is both a hallucinogen and a depressant; and nicotine has both stimulant and depressant characteristics. Table 17-1 lists a representative sampling of frequently abused substances.

Table 17-1 Some Frequently Abused Substances

Depressants	Alcohol, opium, morphine, heroin, barbiturates, benzodiazepines, volatile inhalants
Stimulants	Amphetamines, cocaine, crack, phencyclidine (PCP), nicotine, caffeine
Hallucinogens	LSD, mescaline, psilocybin MDMA (Ecstasy)

Despite concerns over increased use of cocaine and hallucinogens in the United States, the most commonly utilized psychoactive substances are most certainly caffeine, nicotine, alcohol, marijuana, and volatile inhalants. Although much evidence suggests that caffeine is habituating and there is a caffeine withdrawal syndrome, psychiatric practice and DSM-IV do not recognize caffeine dependency as a psychiatric condition. Nicotine and alcohol dependence and abuse, however, are clearly defined as disorders and continue to constitute major health problems. Although experts dispute whether marijuana causes withdrawal symptoms, DSM-IV-TR does define both cannabis (marijuana) dependence and cannabis abuse. Volatile inhalants (paint, glue) are other frequently abused substances whose use may lead not only to intoxication but also occasionally to death.

Individuals become dependent on and abuse substances because these substances act on the brain, most often by producing pleasant sensations or experiences. Not only do wild animals indulge in drug-seeking behavior (birds, for example, will eat some berries only after they ferment), but laboratory animals can easily be induced to self-administer drugs in ways that mimic human dependence and abuse. In such laboratory experiments, drugs can be administered directly into specific sites in an animal's brain. Such experiments clearly show that only when a drug is administered into specific brain areas can dependence and abuse be elicited. These experiments suggest that very specific brain centers are involved in dependence. Many psychologists now believe that the brain has built-in "reward centers" that when stimulated electrically or chemically, result in inherently pleasurable stimuli (Delgado, 2007). The best theory of substance dependence is that a variety of abused drugs can stimulate brain reward systems, in the process producing a desired "high" (Boutrel, 2008). Under this hypothesis, pleasurable sensations are actually produced by the brain itself; the drug is only a means to stimulate the necessary brain centers. While most data supporting this hypothesis are based on animal studies, there are also human experiments showing that electrical brain stimulation of discrete "pleasure centers" can produce sensations of intense pleasure (Heath, 1964). In both humans and animals, these centers are widely distributed in the brainstem, midbrain, and forebrain. Scattered and separated from one another as they are, these pleasure centers appear to share neural connections of the so-called dopaminergic brain pathways (Schultz, 2001). This dopaminergic connection means that most of these centers seem to be influenced by the neurotransmitter dopamine.

It was long ago suggested that humans who abuse drugs may have defective abilities to stimulate their pleasure centers through ordinary daily activities and as a result require the more intense stimulation of drug administration (Weiss, Mirin, Michael, & Sollogrub, 1986). Although this idea is far from universally accepted, it offers one attractive explanation for how brain function and psychological behavior might be linked, especially as newer genetic studies show that drug abuse susceptibility may not be substance-specific (Uhl, 2004).

EFFORTS TO CONTROL SUBSTANCE ABUSE

Many societies and cultures have made strong efforts to control substance use and abuse. Because of the power that substance dependence can exert over human behavior, it is perhaps not surprising that historical efforts to reduce drug use and abuse have met with, at best, limited success. Some of these efforts are described in the following section.

Control of Tobacco Use

While efforts to ban smoking in public places seemed relatively successful in the 1990s, prior similar rulings failed from the very earliest days of tobacco use. In 1639, the director-general of New Amsterdam (later to become New York City) banned smoking. The city's smokers—most of its male inhabitants—protested by camping outside his office to overturn the edict (Siegel, 1989). By the middle of the seventeenth century, the addictive nature of tobacco was recognized in Europe, and official edicts banning smoking existed in Bavaria, Saxony, Zurich, and other states. Punishments against smokers were introduced in Russia and Turkey, yet tobacco use continued (Siegel, 1989).

It is probable that no other drug has ever become so widely abused so quickly as did tobacco. Neither King James's condemnation of 1604 nor his heavy taxation stopped the widespread adoption of tobacco use in England. Papal encyclicals in 1642 and 1650 were similarly unsuccessful in changing patterns of increasing use in Catholic countries (Woods, 1993). Recent trends of increasing cigarette use among young persons despite unprecedented educational efforts testify to the immense difficulties of reducing tobacco consumption.

Control of Alcohol Use

Prohibitions have been notably unsuccessful in controlling use of alcohol. Although most Americans identify prohibition with the Eighteenth Amendment of 1920, there was actually a strong prohibition movement in the mid-nineteenth century that led to antiliquor laws in a majority of states. It is likely that prohibition gained popularity because of serious and widespread alcohol abuse—in the early nineteenth century, Americans were consuming an astonishing yearly average of seven gallons of 200-proof alcohol (Zimring & Hawkins, 1992). Consumption did significantly decrease over the following century, but only to about two gallons per capita on the eve of Prohibition in 1920. Historians dispute the degree to which state and local antiliquor laws were responsible for this decline in use.

The evidence suggests that national Prohibition did result in a further, though temporary, decrease in American per-capita consumption of alcohol (Lender & Martin, 1987). After Prohibition began in 1920, deaths from cirrhosis declined, as did hospital admissions for alcoholic psychosis and arrests for disorderly conduct (Zimring & Hawkins, 1992). Religious use of alcohol was allowed and, interestingly, accounted for almost a million gallons of wine during Prohibition's early years. Ultimately, the voting public found diminishing enthusiasm for restrictions on alcohol use, and the Eighteenth Amendment was repealed in 1933. As one historian has observed, Prohibition proved to Americans that "as bad as a drug might be, there could be laws that were worse" (Zimring & Hawkins, 1992, p. 69).

Control of Cocaine and Opiate Use

The Harrison Act of 1914 prohibited the sale of narcotics and cocaine without prescription. Prior to this legislation, both cocaine and opiates could be easily purchased in pharmacies and were widely and legally used by Americans of all social classes. It is thought by some that heroin addiction became less common after the Harrison Act was passed, but many experts believe that formal prohibition of narcotics has had no significant effect on abuse frequency. The cocaine story is similar. The 1914 prohibition of cocaine dramatically increased street prices, and by the 1930s, usage seems to have declined significantly. There was little or no decline in total drug use—many users switched to less expensive heroin, whereas those whose doctors would supply stimulant needs by prescription began to use amphetamines (synthetic drugs providing much of the high of cocaine, but lasting far longer). Widespread marketing and prescription of amphetamines began in the 1920s, and by 1932 these drugs were made available by inhaler for rapid absorption and psychoactive effect. Amphetamine use declined in the 1960s as these drugs became subject to more stringent control. At the same time, cocaine use increased, at first steadily, then at a rapidly accelerating pace, to the very high levels seen in the 1980s and early 1990s. Cocaine use was increasing dramatically when President Nixon first announced and then declared victory in his "War Against Drugs," and increased even more dramatically during First Lady Nancy Reagan's "Just Say No" campaign. If Americans were saying "No" to anything during the 1980s, it was not cocaine (Woods, 1993). Despite major governmental efforts, it seems highly unlikely that prohibition has had a significant effect on the long-term use of either heroin or cocaine in the United States.

SPECIFIC ABUSED SUBSTANCES

In this section, five of the most commonly abused drugs are discussed. The purpose is to provide the reader with background and understanding of the unique properties and difficulties encountered during withdrawal and treatment for nicotine, alcohol, cocaine, methamphetamines and opiates.

NICOTINE

ON QUITTING SMOKING

At that time I didn't know whether I liked or hated the taste of cigarettes and the condition produced by nicotine. When I discovered that I really hated it all, it was much worse. That was when I was about twenty. For several weeks I suffered from a violent sore throat accompanied by fever. The doctor ordered me to stay in bed and to give up smoking entirely. I remember being struck by the word entirely, which the fever made more vivid. I saw a great void and no means of resisting the fearful oppression which emptiness always produces.

*... I was in a state of fearful agitation. I thought: "As it's so bad for me I won't smoke any more, but I must first have just one last smoke." I lit a cigarette and at once all my excitement died down, though the fever seemed to get worse.... I smoked my cigarette solemnly to the end as if I were fulfilling a vow. And though it caused me agony I smoked many more during that illness ... [which] was the direct cause of my second trouble: the trouble I took trying to rid myself of the first. My days became filled with cigarettes and resolutions to give up smoking, and to make a clean sweep of it, that is more or less what they are still. The dance of the last cigarette which began when I was twenty has not reached its last figure yet.... I may as well say that for some time past I have been smoking a great many cigarettes and have given up calling them the last.**

(Svevo, 1958, pp. 5–26)

Writing of a life lived (or imagined) many years ago, Italo Svevo captures with irony and in remarkably modern terms the smoker's experience: the ambivalence, the multiple broken resolutions to have "just one more," the endless "quit dates." In a similarly ironic vein, Svevo's English contemporary Oscar Wilde wrote that cigarettes are the perfect pleasure: "They are exquisite and they leave one completely unsatisfied." (Wilde, 1993) Few drugs have the addictive potential of nicotine. Whereas only a small percentage of persons who have used cocaine or alcohol become addicted, by far the majority of tobacco users are physiologically dependent on this substance (Jarvik & Schneider, 1992). While nicotine may not be the direct cause of tobacco-related deaths, tobacco kills 70 times more people every year than do heroin and cocaine combined. The economic and social costs of tobacco dependence are immense.

Even addiction experts have been slow to recognize that nicotine is a powerfully addictive substance capable of producing both tolerance and withdrawal symptoms. Perhaps the widespread social acceptance of smoking has, until recently, made it difficult to acknowledge that nicotine is no less an abused substance than heroin or cocaine. There is little doubt that potent advertising techniques lent a social status to tobacco that continues to make it seem different from street drugs. Such ads proclaim one brand better than another in "taste" or image; the accompanying photographs or, more recently, cartoons are given the nonverbal task of advertising the smoker's high.

Effects

When tolerance limits unpleasant side effects, the "full effect" of nicotine may be surprisingly similar to that of other abused substances. Research indicates that human subjects not only like intravenously administered nicotine as well as morphine or cocaine (Jesinski, Johnson, & Henningfield, 1984), but also sometimes have difficulty in distinguishing which drug they have actually been given because the highs of all three are perceived as similar (Rosencrans & Chance, 1977).

The net result of nicotine intoxication is a peculiar combination of subjective relaxation and excitement. While nicotine users often claim that smoking relieves anxiety, in most cases the perceived anxiety is actually the effect of periodic nicotine withdrawal, an anxiety directly relievable only via nicotine. Users also claim that nicotine alerts them and helps performance, and psychological studies do suggest that nicotine improves performance in some motor tasks (Edwards, Wesnes, Warburton, & Gale, 1985) but not in tasks that are cognitively related. Nicotine does decrease appetite, perhaps more in females than males (Grunberg, 1990).

*From *Confessions of Zeno*, by I. Svevo. Translated by Beryl deZoete. Copyright © 1930, renewed 1958. Reprinted with permission from Alfred A. Knopf, a division of Random House, Inc.

Dependence and Withdrawal

Nicotine withdrawal was clinically described as early as 1942 (Johnston, 1985). However, for the next 35 years, symptoms of withdrawal were attributed, both by scientists and by the public, purely to psychological distress. More recent investigations have established a wide range of withdrawal symptoms: mood change, exhibited by irritability, frustration, anger, anxiety, or depression; physiological symptoms such as drowsiness, fatigue, restlessness, difficulty concentrating, or hunger; and measurable physiological changes such as weight gain, decrease in pulse, EEG alterations, performance deficit, and increased sweating (Jarvik & Schneider, 1992). DSM-IV-TR establishes the following criteria for the diagnosis of Nicotine Withdrawal (American Psychiatric Association, 2000):

- Daily use of nicotine for at least several weeks
- Abrupt cessation or reduction of use followed within 24 hours by four or more of the following symptoms: dysphoria or depression, insomnia, irritability, anxiety, difficulty concentrating, restlessness, decreased heart rate, increased appetite, or weight gain

Since nicotine is too physically and psychologically addicting to be abused without resulting in dependence, there is little distinction between nicotine abuse and dependence. Dependence is defined similarly to that for all other substances and may include tolerance, withdrawal, the use of larger quantities than desired (Svevo's perpetual "last cigarette"), continuing unsuccessful efforts to quit, chain smoking, and continuing use despite widespread knowledge of medical harm. Nicotine tolerance is defined by the absence of common side effects despite high dosage: nausea, dizziness, and rapid heart rate. Withdrawal commonly occurs even with brief abstinence, as in nonsmoking workplaces or airplane rides. In contrast to alcohol, methamphetamines, and many other abused substances, nicotine itself does not appear to cause significant physical harm, though there remains some controversy about whether smoking during pregnancy has lasting effects on child development (Winzer-Serhan, 2008). Nicotine's greatest harm comes from its tobacco-associated delivery system, though greater experience with long-term pharmacological nicotine replacement may uncover underappreciated risks.

Treatment of Dependence

It is estimated that between 80% and 90% of regular smokers have Nicotine Dependence (American Psychiatric Association, 2000, p. 268). The occurrence of withdrawal contributes to the great difficulties many individuals have in discontinuing nicotine use. Failure rates for organized quitting (efforts to bring a cohort of people through cessation efforts together) are very high, frequently 70% to 80%. The use of telephone "quit lines" and even the Internet have been shown to significantly increase rates of abstinence (Stead, Perera, & Lancaster, 2006; Brendryen & Kraft, 2008). Specialized modalities such as acupuncture and hypnosis have yet to be shown generally more effective than other techniques (Green & Lynn, 2000; White, Rampes, & Campbell, 2006). Most successful ex-smokers have simply stopped on their own. For many others, the use of nicotine replacement (gum, patches, or sprays) is an attractive option to help control nicotine withdrawal in the early weeks of quitting. Short-term quit rates are approximately doubled with the use of nicotine replacement. Long-term benefits are less-well established, but at least one recent multinational study suggests that replacement may have benefit beyond the acute stage (West & Zhou, 2007). A variety of antidepressant medications have been shown to be of modest value in smoking cessation, with bupropion having the strongest evidence favoring its use. Varenicline, a drug that stimulates and blocks nicotine-binding receptors, appears to be the most effective currently available pharmacological treatment (Nides, 2008). For smokers willing to quit, relapse remains the greatest problem. Withdrawal is not the only factor in relapse; many people relapse because they find themselves in situations that they habitually associate with smoking—for example, drinking alcohol or having a morning cup of coffee (Bottoroff, Johnson, Irwin, & Ratner, 2000). Behavioral programs have been designed to reduce relapse by recognizing and training for these occurrences, and such programs may prove to have a lasting effect by teaching skills for avoiding relapse in specific high-risk situations (Prochazka, 2000). Both evidence and expert opinion strongly support combining behavioral interventions (including telephone-based "quit lines") with any pharmacological intervention such as nicotine replacement, bupropion, or varenicline.

Nurse's Role in Nicotine Abuse

Probably the most significant role of nurses in nicotine use and abuse is that of client education and prevention of nicotine use (Percival, 2003). While virtually all of the American population has heard of the negative health effects caused by smoking, cigarettes and cigars are still quite popular. Nurses are involved in each level of prevention:

- Primary prevention: community-wide education efforts to prevent individuals (particularly children) from becoming smokers
- Secondary prevention: encouraging smokers to quit smoking through involvement in cessation programs, for example, during pregnancy (Johnson, Ratner, Bottoroff, & Dahinten, 2000; Crawford, Tolosa, & Goldenberg, 2008)
- Tertiary prevention: unbiased treatment for those who have smoking-related disease (i.e., providing quality care to those with emphysema, lung cancer, and heart disease)

Focusing on primary prevention is the activity likely to have the greatest effect on the greatest number of individuals. Antismoking efforts in schools and advocacy for no-smoking legislation in public buildings are examples of wide-reaching primary prevention efforts.

Nurses and Smoking

In as much as nurses must be engaged in smoking cessation, it is unfortunate to note that 15% of RNs and 28% of LPNs are themselves smokers (http://www.nursingworld.org, retrieved July 2008). These rates are the highest among health professionals. Concern about worker health and safety, exposure to second-hand smoke, and the need for nurses to be involved in supporting others to quit smoking provided the impetus for the American Nurses Association (ANA) and the American Nurses Foundation to found the Tobacco Free Nurses Project (TFN), a resource center for nurses. The Tobacco Free Nurses' mission is to ensure that the nursing profession is prepared to actively promote health by reducing nurses' barriers to involvement in tobacco control, including lack of education, smoking among professionals, and lack of nursing leadership. A major goal of TFN is supporting and assisting smoking cessation efforts of nurses and nursing students. The ANA is joined by other nursing organizations in this effort, including the American Association of Colleges of Nursing. Further information can be found at the following Web site: http://www.nursingworld.org.

ALCOHOL

UNDER THE INFLUENCE

My father drank. He drank as a gut-punched boxer gasps for breath, as a starving dog gobbles food—compulsively, secretly, in pain and trembling. I use the past tense not because he ever quit drinking but because he quit living. That is how the story ends for my father, age sixty-four, heart bursting, body cooling and forsaken on the linoleum of my brother's trailer. The story continues for my brother, my sister, my mother, and me, and will continue so long as memory holds.

In the perennial present of memory, I slip into the garage or barn to see my father tipping back the flat green bottles of wine, the brown cylinders of whiskey, the cans of beer disguised in paper bags. His Adam's apple bobs, the liquid gurgles, he wipes the sandy-haired back of a hand over his lips, and then, his bloodshot gaze bumping into me, he stashes the bottle or can inside his jacket, under the workbench, between two bales of hay, and we both pretend the moment has not occurred.

"What's up, buddy?" he says, thick-tongued and edgy.

"Sky's up," I answer, playing along.

"And don't forget prices," he grumbles. "Prices are always up. And taxes." ...

I still shy away from nightclubs, from bars, from parties where the solvent is alcohol. My friends puzzle over this, but it is no more peculiar than for a man to shy away from the lions' den after seeing his father torn apart. I took my own first drink at the age of twenty-one, half a glass of burgundy. I knew the odds of my becoming an alcoholic were four times higher than for the sons of nonalcoholic fathers. So I sipped warily.

Lost Weekend

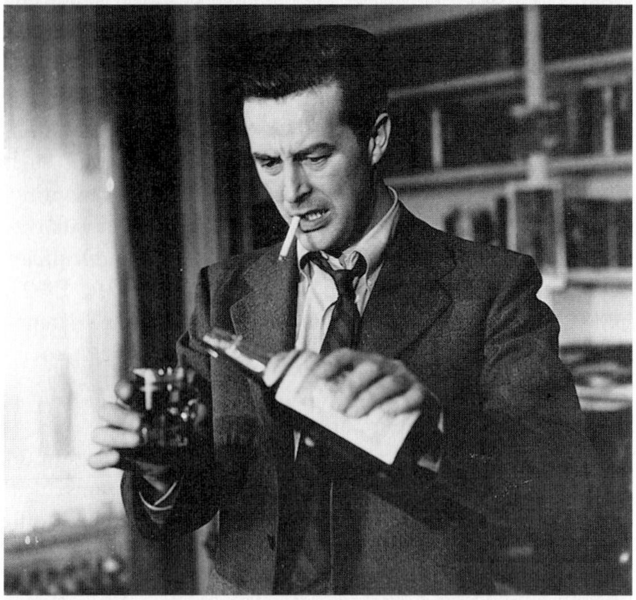

Source: Paramount (Courtesy: The Kobal Collection)

Alcoholism is featured in many movies. The real trauma of the disease and its effects on individuals and families, however, is frequently underplayed by the media.

*I still do—once a week, perhaps, a glass of wine, a can of beer, nothing stronger, nothing more. I listen for the turning of a key in my brain.**

(Sanders, 1989, pp. 68–75)

Alcohol is such a widely abused substance that there are almost as many "Under the Influence" stories as there are families. Father could have been (and often is) mother, brother, sister, uncle, or grandfather.

Effects

Alcohol is so widely used in American society that virtually all persons are familiar with common effects of acute alcohol intoxication. In most people, alcohol produces varying degrees of talkativeness, disinhibited behavior, uncoordination, irritability and combativeness, slurred speech, and drowsiness, depending on dose and individual susceptibility. Even in fairly small doses, alcohol significantly impedes motor and cognitive function. There is good correlation between measured blood alcohol levels and symptoms, but only in nondependent drinkers. Tolerance to alcohol develops with continued use, and tolerant individuals can perform surprisingly well at blood levels that would produce stupor, if not death, in nontolerant persons (Victor, 1992).

*From "Under the Influence," by S. R. Sanders. Copyright © 1989 by *Harper's Magazine*. All rights reserved. Reprinted from the November issue with special permission.

NURSINGALERT 17-1

Alcohol-Induced Hypoglycemia

A blood sugar determination should always be done on persons brought to medical attention for alcohol-related symptoms because alcohol can significantly lower blood sugar, and symptoms of such hypoglycemia can easily be mistaken for intoxication.

One of the remarkable pharmacological facts about alcohol is its biochemical simplicity: a pair of carbon atoms, a single oxygen atom, and a few hydrogens. Many simple substances have effects on the CNS by dissolving in the lipid layers of brain cells. Indeed, in high doses, ethanol clearly *does* act by dissolving in the lipid membranes that separate cells (Goldstein, Chin, & Lyon, 1982). However, at relatively low doses, other mechanisms are required to explain alcohol's effects. These mechanisms are incompletely understood, but do involve a variety of brain neurotransmitter systems. Chief among these is the glutamate system, especially through the methyl aspartate (NMDA) receptor (Krystal, Pertrakis, Krupitsky, Schutz, Trevisan, & D'Sousa, 2003). Alcohol strongly inhibits this major system that is closely linked to memory and a variety of other brain functions (Vengeliene, Bilbao, Molander, & Spanagel, 2008). Functional MRI studies of humans given alcohol show that alcohol stimulates reward systems in the striatum and reduces limbic system fear responses to stimuli that otherwise would provoke anxiety (Gilman, Ramchandani, Davis, Bjork, & Hommer, 2008).

The chronic effects of alcohol are also highly complicated. Chronic alcohol abuse may produce serious damage to the bone marrow, heart, liver, pancreas, stomach, intestines, reproductive tract, and developing embryo. Even in the absence of nutritional/vitamin deficiency, alcohol abuse frequently leads to brain damage and cognitive impairment (Harper 2007); there is some suggestion that women are at higher risk for neurotoxicity than are men (Hommer, 2003). Other neurological complications of alcoholism are often due to associated nutritional deficiencies and may affect many different parts of the nervous system. Two of these complications are summarized in Box 17-2.

Long-term excessive alcohol consumption is associated with an increase in the rates of certain cancers, particularly esophageal, mouth, laryngeal (Bagnardi, Blangiardo, La Vecchia, & Corrao, 2001) and colonic (Mizoue, Inoue, Wakai, Nagata, Shimazu, Tsuji, et al., 2008). The social and psychological effects of chronic alcohol abuse are widespread and profound. They include job loss, family disintegration, homelessness, depression, ill health, violence, accidents, and multiple concomitant psychiatric disorders. Chronic alcohol use does not cause all of these consequences, but it is strongly associated with a wide range of social dysfunction and pathology.

BOX 17-2
NEUROLOGICAL COMPLICATIONS OF CHRONIC ALCOHOLISM

Korsakoff's Syndrome—Dementia with profound loss of recent memory.

- Symptoms: amnesia, dementia, psychosis
- Cause: alcoholism, nutritional deficiency
- Treatment: supportive care
- Prognosis: poor for cognitive recovery

Wernicke's Encephalopathy—Delirium with cranial nerve dysfunction.

- Symptoms: mental status changes, paralysis of extraocular eye movements leading to disconjugate gaze
- Cause: thiamine deficiency due to poor diet
- Treatment: thiamine. Giving glucose without thiamine leads to permanent neurological damage
- Prognosis: excellent with early thiamine administration, but may also have Korsakoff's Syndrome

Dependence and Withdrawal

Alcohol withdrawal is often called delirium tremens (DTs). Because withdrawal from alcohol is so often similar to withdrawal from other substances, terms like DTs are best avoided in favor of the more generic term of withdrawal. Alcohol withdrawal symptoms typically include sweating, rapid pulse, tremor, sleep disorder, nausea or vomiting, and agitation. The rarest and most dramatic symptoms of alcohol withdrawal include seizures and hallucinations involving animals, frequently spiders or other insects. In Mark Twain's classic novel *Adventures of Huckleberry Finn*, Huck describes his father's dramatic and frightening alcoholic hallucinations:

YELLING ABOUT SNAKES

*I don't know how long I was asleep, but all of a sudden there was an awful scream and I was up. There was pap looking wild, and skipping around every which way and yelling about snakes. He said they was crawling up his legs; and then he would give a jump and scream, and say one had bit him on the cheek—but I couldn't see no snakes. He started and run round and round the cabin, hollering "Take him off! take him off! he's biting me on the neck!" I never see a man look so wild in the eyes.**

(Twain, 1987, p. 36)

*From *The Adventures of Huckleberry Finn*, by M. Twain. Translated/Edited by Walter Hunter Blair, Copyright © 1987 by the Mark Twain Foundation and Regents of the University of California Press. Reprinted with permission.

This sort of delirium occurs in only a small proportion of those withdrawing from alcohol, and its occurrence is often a sign of coexisting serious, though often alcohol-related, medical illness. Common underlying conditions predisposing to delirium include liver disease, pneumonia, gastrointestinal (GI) bleeding, hypoglycemia, and electrolyte imbalance. Clients presenting with withdrawal-associated delirium should be carefully monitored for medical problems and treated vigorously. Treatment typically includes medications to suppress agitation (chlordiazepoxide is most commonly used), fluids, and nutritional support including thiamine and other vitamins. Abnormal mental status must not be assumed to be due solely to alcohol withdrawal—conditions such as head injury, subdural hematoma, and meningitis should be excluded via appropriate testing.

DSM-IV-TR criteria for alcohol abuse and dependence are similar to those for other substances. Abuse is typically diagnosed when alcohol use leads to work problems, hazardous practices (such as driving under the influence), legal difficulties, or continuing use in the face of physical or social problems due to alcohol. Alcohol Dependence is diagnosed on the basis of three or more symptoms from a list that includes withdrawal, tolerance, greater-than-intended use, unsuccessful attempts to control use, and giving up of other activities in favor of alcohol use. Goodwin (1992) offers a simpler definition of **alcoholism**: "a compulsion to drink alcohol, causing harm to self or others" (p. 144).

NURSINGTIP 17-1

The Client in Alcohol Withdrawal

GOALS OF CARE

- Decrease the physical need for alcohol
- Monitor withdrawal
- Prevent alcohol withdrawal delirium
- Control symptoms and prevent injury

COMMON SEQUENCE OF WITHDRAWAL (UNTREATED)

1. Tremulousness (the shakes)
    - Onset: 3 to 36 hours after last dose (drink)
    - Symptoms: tremors, anorexia, insomnia, tachycardia, agitation, increased blood pressure, anxiety, nausea and vomiting
2. Acute hallucinations
    - Onset: any time after tremors have begun
    - Symptoms: psychomotor agitation; auditory hallucinations
3. Alcohol withdrawal delirium (delirium tremens)
    - Onset: 24 to 72 hours after last drink
    - Symptoms: disorientation, delusions, hallucinations (most often visual, but can be tactile), delirium, severe agitation, fever, perspiration, tachycardia, seizures (either petit mal or grand mal)

Dependency on alcohol is more common among men than women and affects up to 14% of the U.S. population at some time in their lives (American Psychiatric Association, 2000). It has been suggested that alcoholism can be classified into two varieties: Type I alcoholism involves men and women equally, is associated with environmental stresses such as poverty, and tends to be relatively mild. Type II alcoholism is well described in the excerpt from Scott Russell Sanders: It affects primarily men, begins in the twenties or earlier, and is associated with binge drinking. Type II alcoholism tends to run in families, and there is evolving evidence for genetic factors in many cases (Mayfield, Harris, & Schuckit, 2008).

Some experts feel that the inclusion of most women alcohol abusers in the Type I classification may underestimate the seriousness of alcohol dependence in women. Women seem to metabolize alcohol differently than do men and attain higher blood levels with lower intake (Frezza, DiPadova, Pozzato, Terpin, Bargona, 1990). Although women are proportionately more likely than men to be steady rather than binge drinkers, liver disease and other complications seem to occur at lower drinking intensities in women. While women alcohol abusers do drink less, they are

REFLECTIVE THINKING 17-1

Acetaldehyde

Alcohol is metabolized in the body to the substance *acetaldehyde*, which in turn is further metabolized and excreted. Acetaldehyde is a toxic substance that in large doses causes flushing, nausea, and sleepiness. Acetaldehyde is a strongly psychoactive substance. Some scientists speculate that it is acetaldehyde formed from alcohol that leads to alcohol dependence, not the alcohol itself. However, alcohol consumption is not the only source of acetaldehyde—smoking produces significant blood levels of acetaldehyde. Studies in animals suggest that the combination of acetaldehyde and nicotine may have unusually high addictive potential (Belluzzi, Wang, & Leslie, 2005).

As a result of these studies, it has been suggested that acetaldehyde may be a major link between the two most common American addictions: tobacco and alcohol. This link may operate through the inhibition of the monoamine oxidase enzyme (MAO) system by metabolites of acetaldehyde (Van Amsterdam, Talhout, Vleeming, & Opperhuizen, 2006). MAO inhibition appears to increase the risk of nicotine addiction (Talhout, Opperhuizen, & van Amsterdam, 2007) and—while not clearly related to acetaldehyde among Type II alcoholics—MAO inhibition is also a characteristic finding among persons with this diagnosis (Demir, Ucar, Ulug, Ulusoy, Sevinc, & Batur, 2002) and may be linked to the addictive nature of drinking in this group.

Consider what implications this information has for drug prevention and drug treatment.

Absinthe Drinker by Degas

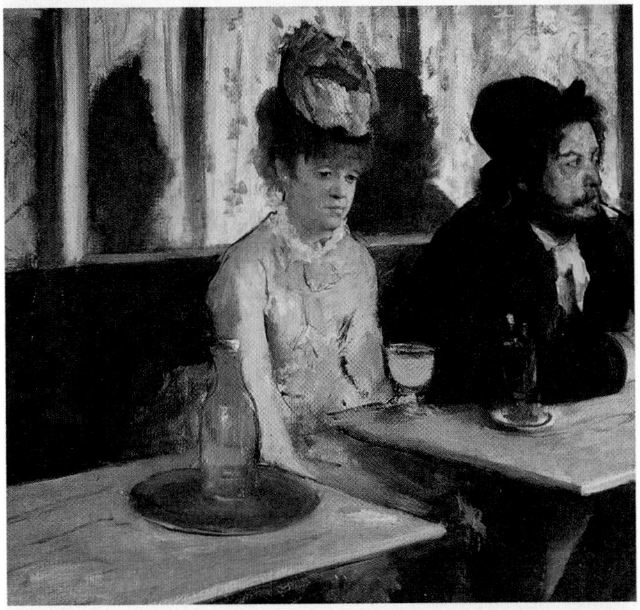

Courtesy: Réunion des Musées Nationaux/Art Resource, NY

Absinthe (wormwood) was widely used as an intoxicant in nineteenth-century Europe. This painting hints at withdrawal and social isolation in a young woman who seems well dressed but lost in her (drugged?) thoughts. Absinthe frequently produced permanent brain

also more likely to start at a later age, to drink privately, and to be socially isolated (Lex, 1992). Some data suggest that these observations apply primarily to older women and that, in recent years, not only has alcohol abuse become more common among women, but also women are beginning to drink at a younger age and drink more heavily than in the past. Any such change in drinking patterns may have a serious long-term impact on the health of alcohol-abusing women, especially as these women advance into middle and old age (Blum, Nielson, & Riggs, 2000; Epstein, Fischer-Elber, & Al-Otaiba, 2007).

Clients rarely present for health or mental health care complaining of alcohol abuse or dependence. Even clients who present to emergency facilities intoxicated or with high blood alcohol levels often deny that their alcohol use is compulsive or represents a problem. Yet, because of associated medical problems, alcohol abusers commonly seek health care—90% of alcoholics have significant medical problems in addition to their alcohol dependency (Schuckit, 1992). The four-item CAGE questionnaire (Ewing, 1984) in Box 17-3 is often used to screen medical clients for alcohol abuse.

"Yes" answers to two or more items on the CAGE constitute a positive response, and in some populations, a positive response is over 90% sensitive in detecting individuals with alcohol problems (Chang & Kosten, 1992). A longer

BOX 17-3
CAGE QUESTIONNAIRE

- **C** Have you ever felt you should **c**ut down on your drinking?
- **A** Have people **a**nnoyed you by criticizing your drinking?
- **G** Have you ever felt bad or **g**uilty about drinking?
- **E** Have you ever taken a drink the first thing in the morning to steady your nerves or get rid of a hangover (**e**ye opener)?

From "Detecting Alcoholism: The CAGE Questionnaire," by J. A. Ewing, 1984, *Journal of the American Medical Association*, *252*, 1905–1907. Copyright © 1984, American Medical Association. Reprinted with permission.

questionnaire, the Michigan Alcohol Screening Test (MAST), is more sensitive but takes more time to administer (Schuckit & Irwin, 1988). Screening tools such as the CAGE or MAST can be used to identify persons at potential risk for alcohol dependence; however, the actual diagnosis should be made by a trained interviewer using accepted criteria such as those in DSM-IV-TR. Although screening can be effective in identifying persons at risk for alcohol abuse, it is frequently not performed in actual clinical practice, especially for women clients (Svikis & Reid-Quinones, 2003). Effective screening can also be performed with biological tests such as the Carbohydrate Deficient Transferrin and the Early Detection of Alcohol Consumption tests. These tests are approved by the FDA but are not frequently used in clinical practice because of cost and lack of provider awareness (Montalto & Bean, 2003).

Treatment of Dependence

As is demonstrated in the story of Scott Sanders's father, alcohol dependency, or alcoholism, is a condition that persists and develops over many years. There may be a wide array of crises in the life of an alcoholic, but as with many chronic illnesses, the pattern of the disease is to vary in severity over a lifetime. Schuckit (1992) has provided a summary of the typical pattern of Type II alcoholism in men (see Table 17-2). In addition, Table 17-3 presents phases of alcoholism, taken from the experiences of many, which document a common evolution in drinking behaviors from moderate drinking to chronic alcoholism.

Any consideration of treatment must take some account of where in the alcoholic "natural history" an individual is, his personal goals for behavioral change, and the likelihood of spontaneous remission. Although studies on remission are difficult to interpret unless criteria for definition are strictly adhered to, a number of studies have shown that 10% to 30% of alcoholics will experience long-term abstention with no formal treatment (Vaillant, 1982). Sanders's father was "dry" for 15 years and only relapsed and died after retirement allowed him to move back to the community in which his drinking had begun five decades before.

Therapy for alcohol abuse and dependency most commonly begins with a four- to five-day drug detoxification wherein

TABLE 17-2 Natural History of Primary Alcoholism in Men

1. Age of first drink	12–14 years
2. Age first intoxicated	14–18 years
3. Age of first minor alcohol problem (missed school or work due to drinking behavior)	18–25 years
4. Usual age of first major problem (lost job because of drinking behavior)	28–30 years
5. Usual age entering treatment	40 years
6. Usual age of death (leading causes: years heart disease, cancer, accidents, suicide)	55–60 years
7. Year abstinence alternates with active drinking	Any
8. "Spontaneous remission" rate or response to nonspecific intervention	10%–30%

From "Treatment of Alcoholism in Office and Outpatient Settings," by M.A. Schuckit, in *Medical Diagnosis and Treatment of Alcoholism* (p. 369). Edited by J. H. Mendelson and N. K. Mello, Copyright © 1972. Reprinted with permission from the McGraw-Hill Companies.

alcohol is replaced by a benzodiazepine in rapidly decreasing dosages. Detoxification may sometimes take place outside the hospital, but many individuals require brief hospitalization for either safety or success. Detoxification is followed by a treatment program involving some mixture of counseling, group support, and medication. Schuckit (1992) has summarized six issues that may be useful in forming the basis of alcohol counseling:

- Using free time constructively now that alcohol is no longer available
- Remaining sober while interacting with heavy-drinking friends
- Reestablishing ties with significant others, including the spouse, children, and parents, recognizing that the absence of alcohol will uncover many problems that have built up for years
- Learning how to say no to drinking at a party
- Handling stress
- Coping with general life problems, including the possible need to change jobs (vocational counseling), money management, and learning to deal with the sexual difficulties that often develop in the context of heavy drinking

ALCOHOLICS ANONYMOUS Alcoholics Anonymous (A.A.) is a self-help organization of persons who come together to assist one another in dealing with their drinking problems. Alcoholics Anonymous is nonprofessional, self-supporting,

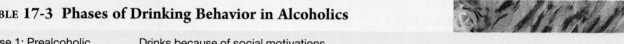

TABLE 17-3 Phases of Drinking Behavior in Alcoholics

Phase 1: Prealcoholic	Drinks because of social motivations Finds that alcohol relieves stress Over time, needs to increase the amount of alcohol needed for relief May be told by others that his drinking is too heavy or too frequent Can be described as the "nonaddicted heavy drinker"
Phase 2: Early alcoholic	Begins to drink alone Becomes preoccupied with the supply of drinks Hides bottles of alcohol at work, home, or car Wakes up in the morning and needs a drink to control tremors (the eye-opener) May experience blackouts (memory loss for immediate past events) Uses denial as a defense mechanism and does not admit to being dependent on alcohol
Phase 3: True alcoholic	Completely loses control over ability to choose whether or not to drink Goes out on binge-drinking episodes; stops drinking only when too sick to take another drink Experiences the following: isolation from others, aggression, loss of interest in any activity that once brought pleasure, impotence/frigidity, nutritional impairment In this phase, most who were gainfully employed have lost their jobs, many have lost their families, and all have lost their self-esteem
Phase 4: Chronic alcoholic	Over time, the individual's continuous use of alcohol leads to extensive emotional disorganization May exhibit impairment of reality testing; regression; or loss of a sense of ethics Physically the individual exhibits disorders of the CNS (bilateral, progressive neuritis of the lower extremities; temporary nerve palsies) and liver and vascular disease

From Rutgers University Center of Alcohol Studies, Piscataway, NJ 08854. In *Quarterly Journal of Studies on Alcohol* (currently *Journal of Studies on Alcohol*), *13*, 673–684, by E. M. Jellinek. Copyright © 1952 by *Journal of Studies on Alcohol*. Reprinted with permission.

nondenominational, apolitical, and multicultural. The A.A. program is based on 12 steps that offer the individual a way of living without alcohol (Box 17-4). Each person considering joining A.A. is encouraged to seek a sponsor, another A.A. member willing to offer support to the new member in following the A.A. treatment program. Alcoholics Anonymous sponsors meetings in nearly every community in the United States. Meetings may include speakers who tell their personal stories of recovery and may include discussions among several members. The objective is to assist each person by providing a close bond among people. Through A.A., the individual accepts that, while he did not choose to become an alcoholic, he has complete responsibility for his own recovery.

Group support for alcoholics, recommended for all persons dealing with alcoholism, almost always includes A.A. Available data suggest that alcoholics who become A.A. members have a 40% to 50% chance of long-term abstention (Emrick, 1987), but the evidence supporting effectiveness of A.A. or other 12-step programs is weak by contemporary standards (Ferri, Amato, & Davoli, 2006). Some alcohol-dependent individuals, particularly younger men, have difficulty accepting the strongly religious flavor of A.A. (Boscarino, 1980). However, for those who join, A.A. offers a strong support program with daily meetings, a remarkably widespread and accepting network, and no-cost treatment.

Medication Along with formal counseling and A.A., medication may usefully play a role in the management of alcohol dependence. After acute detoxification, there is generally no role for benzodiazepine medications or sleeping pills. Insomnia (not an uncommon problem) in this setting may require treatment to prevent relapse (Arnedt, Conroy, & Brower, 2007). Buspirone may be of value when anxiety is a major psychological symptom (Kranzler, Burleson, Del Boca, Babor, Korner, Brown, et al., 1994), and while antidepressant medications are used for persons who clearly have Major Depressive Disorder (Muhonen, Lonnqvist, Juva, & Alho, 2008), they are not otherwise indicated for the treatment of alcohol abuse or dependence (Kranzler et al., 1994). Disulfiram (Antabuse) is still occasionally prescribed for the prevention of relapse in alcohol abuse. The drug inhibits a major enzyme in the pathway that metabolizes alcohol; as a result, toxic metabolites of alcohol accumulate in the body, and a person who drinks while taking disulfiram becomes physically ill, typically with flushing, nausea, and vomiting lasting for up to an hour. The effects of disulfiram persist at least 72 hours after the most recent dose, so disulfiram cannot be conveniently stopped to facilitate an unplanned binge. At one time, the use of disulfiram was common, but its popularity has fallen in recent years for at least three reasons. First, studies have failed to show much benefit in the majority of individuals who receive disulfiram (Fuller, Branchley, & Brightwell, 1986). Second, the side effects of disulfiram toxicity may be serious and may involve rare complications including serious neurological dysfunction and fatal liver disease. Finally, persons who relapse on alcohol, particularly those with significant underlying medical disorders, may become dangerously ill from the combination of disulfiram and alcohol.

Numerous medications are currently being explored as adjunctive treatment for alcohol abuse (Miller, 2008). Among these are naltrexone (especially in a long-acting injection form), gabapentin, topiramate, and namentin. The combination of naltrexone (an opioid antagonist) and psychological/behavioral therapy has been shown to be particularly effective in at least one large study (Anton et al., 2006). Targeting pharmacotherapy to specific symptoms (i.e., cravings) may be particularly useful; new anticonvulsants such as topiramate may play a role in such targeted therapy (Johnson, Rosenthal, Capece, Wiegand, Mao, Beyers, et al., 2008).

Naltrexone is the most widely used of several new drugs that may help prevent relapse in alcohol abusers. Naltrexone

BOX 17-4
THE TWELVE STEPS OF ALCOHOLICS ANONYMOUS

1. We admitted we were powerless over alcohol—that our lives had become unmanageable.
2. Came to believe that a power greater than ourselves could restore us to sanity.
3. Made a decision to turn our will and our lives over to the care of God as we understood Him.
4. Made a searching and fearless moral inventory of ourselves.
5. Admitted to God, to ourselves, and to another human being the exact nature of our wrongs.
6. Were entirely ready to have God remove all these defects of character.
7. Humbly asked Him to remove our shortcomings.
8. Made a list of all persons we had harmed, and became willing to make amends to them all.
9. Made direct amends to such people wherever possible, except when to do so would injure them or others.
10. Continued to take personal inventory and when we were wrong promptly admitted it.
11. Sought through prayer and meditation to improve our conscious contact with God *as we understood Him,* praying only for knowledge of His will for us and the power to carry that out.
12. Having had a spiritual awakening as the result of these steps, we tried to carry this message to alcoholics and to practice these principles in all our affairs.

The Twelve Steps are reprinted with permission of Alcoholics Anonymous World Services, Inc. (A.A.W.S) Permission to reprint the Twelve Steps does not mean that A.A.W.S. has reviewed or approved the contents of this publication, nor that A.A.W.S. agrees with the views expressed herein. A.A. is a program of recovery from alcoholism *only*—use of the Twelve Steps in connection with programs and activities that are patterned after A.A. but which address other problems, or in any other non-A.A. context, does not imply otherwise.

is a long-acting, orally administered antagonist of opiate effects that has found a role in preventing relapse among opiate abusers. While the reasons for effectiveness are not yet clear, naltrexone also has some benefit in preventing alcohol craving and relapse (Medical Letter, 1995). Naltrexone seems to work best when combined with supportive psychotherapy (O'Malley, Jaffe, Chang, Schottenfeld, Meyer, & Rounsaville, 1992). Naltrexone is expensive and carries a risk of producing unanticipated opiate withdrawal in clients who, unknown to their physicians, also abuse these drugs. Acamprosate, clinically available in Europe and currently under investigation in the United States, works to reduce craving for alcohol through its effects on NMDA receptors. Acamprosate has more promise than other pharmacological treatments for alcohol dependence, but it is effective in less than 50% of individuals to whom it is administered. Long-term benefits remain uncertain but may be enhanced by counseling and 12-step enrollment (Fiellin, Reid, & O'Connor, 2000).

Given that no universally effective treatment for alcoholism has been developed, it has been standard practice to try to match clients to a treatment program based on perceptions of how well that program might fit their personal characteristics. The 1998 MATCH study randomly assigned alcohol-dependent individuals to one of three treatment programs: cognitive behavioral therapy, 12-step, and motivational enhancement (Anonymous, 2000). Treatments were provided for both outpatients and inpatients, and follow-up continued for up to three years. At one and three years, there were no significant differences in effectiveness among any of the three treatments. None of the factors evaluated at entry (including gender, cognitive impairment, spirituality, motivation, social network support, level of anger, interpersonal dependency, prior A.A. involvement, social functioning, personality disorder or other psychiatric disorder, readiness to change) strongly predicted differential; success in any of the three treatments. The authors concluded that matching clients to programs had very little benefit.

Special Treatment Issues for Women Most studies on alcohol treatment effectiveness have included few women (Vanicelli & Nash, 1984). Programs targeted to the special problems of alcohol abuse in women can be effective in reducing drinking in this group, even when limited to gathering information about antipartum drinking habits (Chang, Wilkins-Haug, Berman, & Goetz, 1999). Women who abuse alcohol seem to have a very high incidence of past history of physical and sexual abuse. Successful treatment of alcohol dependence in women may require sensitivity to these issues of emotional and physical trauma (Bower, 1994). These issues are addressed more fully in Chapter 26 of this text. Further, use of alcohol during pregnancy has a significant effect on the developing fetus and may lead to Fetal Alcohol Spectrum Disorders. Fetal Alcohol Syndrome, the most severe of these disorders, can result in mental retardation, behavioral consequences, and other developmental disorders that may lead to life-long functional impairment (Spohr, Willms, & Steinhausen, 2007).

Nurse's Role in Alcohol Abuse

Nurses are involved in giving care at every phase of alcohol dependence (Littlejohn & Holloway, 2008), three of which are discussed here. Two are distinct phases in which the nurse provides in-hospital care: the acute phase, when the client is under care during the period of withdrawal; and the recovery phase, when the client and providers are establishing a treatment plan for immediate follow-up to hospital care. The third phase takes place in the community, when the nurse may follow a client to encourage compliance with a treatment plan and also engage in community-wide alcohol abuse prevention activities. Each of these phases is discussed following.

In the acute phase, the nurse's role is collaborative, monitoring the client's withdrawal from alcohol and taking steps to provide interventions to prevent DTs. Nursing care is provided usually through established protocols, as a physician's order is needed to carry out appropriate treatments. The goals of nursing care are to:

- Prevent alcohol withdrawal delirium through administration of drugs that duplicate the depressant action of alcohol on the CNS.
- Correct fluid and electrolyte imbalances. Because alcoholics are often overhydrated, electrolytes must be determined by blood chemistries and corrective action must be taken.
- Perform diagnostic measures such as evaluating the client for medical conditions associated with alcoholism, such as liver damage, pancreatitis, and altered blood glucose levels; evaluating the client for nervous system disorders associated with chronic alcohol use, such as peripheral polyneuritis and temporary nerve palsies; and evaluating nutritional status, particularly vitamin deficiency (B complex).

Further, the nurse must establish rapport with the client and initiate the follow-up plan for recovery from alcoholism. The nurse must recognize that the client will cope according to established patterns. The most frequent defense mechanism used by the alcoholic is denial, and the nurse should expect to encounter it. The client will very likely deny that the alcoholism is a significant problem—he may state that he can handle his condition himself, or may flatly deny that there is a condition needing follow-up care. The nursing approach should be firm and based in reality, but should also indicate to the client that the nurse cares about his recovery. The alcoholic has lost much or all of his self-esteem; the nurse must provide a balance of reality and caring so the client has the opportunity to choose recovery.

In the recovery phase, the nurse must work with an interdisciplinary team to develop a discharge plan. Almost always, the client is invited to attend A.A. or a similar self-help group. The nurse must be aware of the fact that the risk for the alcoholic in the initial stage of recovery is returning to social and work settings in which others are drinking. A.A. attempts to break the cycle by providing the client with an alternative social environment where

NURSINGTIP 17-2

Denial: Living with Alcoholism

It is important to remember that many alcohol abusers strongly deny their alcohol-related problems. Consider the following:

*Again his hands shook too much for him to run a saw, to make his precious miniature furniture, to drive straight down back roads. Again he wound up in the ditch, in the hospital, in jail, in treatment centers. Again he shouted and wept. Again he lied. "I never touched a drop," he swore. "Your mother's making it up."**

(Sanders, 1989, p. 74)

nondrinking behavior is reinforced. Initial meetings of A.A. and treatment with a therapist or counselor should be scheduled while the client is in hospital. The nurse ensures that the client has a plan for where to obtain help before leaving a hospital setting.

In the community setting, the nurse may work to support the client's individual recovery and may also work to support the client's family's needs in dealing with alcohol addiction. An outpatient treatment center may provide a space for A.A. meetings, individual therapy and counseling, and referral to community services. A nurse working in such a setting will be part of a treatment team and will collaborate with others in the approach used. Issues specifically related to family needs are discussed later in this chapter. Primary prevention programs, those related to community-wide prevention of alcohol abuse, are also important. Projects such as enforcement of drinking laws to prevent underage drinking and programs such as educational activities geared to teach responsible drinking behavior to college students are examples of such preventative activities.

Nursing and "Brief Intervention"

In recent years, it has been recognized that so-called brief intervention can be highly effective in changing client behavior (Kaner, Beyer, Dickinson, Pienar, Campbell, Schlesinger, et al., 2007). Brief intervention is typically limited to four or fewer sessions lasting only a few minutes each. Nurses can effectively apply this technique in clinical practice, often best at times of perceived client vulnerability, such as following an alcohol-related injury (Dyehouse & Sommers, 1998). Brief intervention is often based on the FRAMES model:

Feedback—to emphasize to the client that her drinking puts her at risk of serious consequences.

Responsibility—to stress that only the client can change behavior: "It is your decision—no one else can make you change."

Advice to change—to offer ways that clients can reduce risk such as adapting "low risk" drinking patterns. For alcohol-dependent clients, abstinence may be the only "low risk" pattern.

Menu of ways to reduce drinking. These may include keeping a diary of drinking patterns, setting a limit on alcohol intake, identifying and avoiding situations most likely to lead to drinking, and pacing drinking behaviors by practices such as diluting drinks, and sipping rather than drinking.

Empathic counseling—focusing on warmth and understanding rather than confrontation and blame.

Self-efficacy—giving a message of empowerment, emphasizing client strengths, and eliciting client "buy in" by helping clients to express sentiments such as "I know my drinking is unhealthy and I need to change" or "I plan to do the following to reduce my drinking."

This model works particularly well when clients express readiness to change their behavior, but it can also help move clients from a precontemplative state to a willingness to consider behavior change. Brief intervention has been extensively used with alcohol problems, but may apply equally well to other forms of substance abuse, including smoking (Dyehouse & Sommers, 1998).

COCAINE

"MY PRECIOUS MARTY"—SIGMUND FREUD WRITES TO HIS FIANCÉE

*I first took 0.05 gram of cocainum muriaticum in a 1% water solution when I was slightly out of sorts due to fatigue. The solution is rather viscous, slightly opalescent, and with an unusual aromatic smell. At first the taste is bitter but this then changes to a series of very nice aromatic flavors.... A few minutes after taking the cocaine one suddenly feels light and exhilarated. The lips and palate feel first furry and then warm, and if one drinks cold water it feels warm to the lips but cold to the throat. But on some occasions the main feeling is a rather pleasant coolness in mouth and throat.**

(Clark, 1980, p. 59)

April 21, 1884—I am also toying with a project and a hope which I will tell you about; perhaps nothing will

*From *Freud: The Man and the Cause*, by R. W. Clark, 1980, New York: Random House.

*come of this, either. It is a therapeutic experiment. I have been reading about cocaine, the effective ingredient of coca leaves, which some Indian tribes chew in order to make themselves resistant to privation and fatigue. A German has tested this stuff on soldiers and reported that it has really rendered them strong and capable of endurance. I have now ordered some of it and for obvious reasons am going to try it out on cases of heart disease, then on nervous exhaustion, particularly in the awful condition following withdrawal of morphine.... There may be any number of other people experimenting on it already ... but ... as you know an experimenter's temperament requires two basic qualities: optimism in attempt, criticism in work.**

(Freud, 1960, pp. 107–108)

June 2, 1884—Woe to you, my Princess, when I come. I will kiss you quite red and feed you till you are plump. And if you are forward, you shall see who is the stronger, a gentle little girl who doesn't eat enough or a big wild man who has cocaine in his body. In my last severe depression I took coca again and a small dose lifted me to the heights in a wonderful fashion. I am just now busy collecting the literature for a song of praise to this magical substance.†

(Clark, 1980, p. 59)

*June 29, 1884—If you really insist on meeting me at the station, I cannot stop you.... I won't be tired because I shall be traveling under the influence of coca, in order to curb my terrible impatience.**

(Freud, 1960, p. 115)

*May 17, 1885—Yesterday I received from Berlin a very flattering letter.... When the letter came I was suffering from migraine.... I took some cocaine, watched the migraine vanish at once ... but I was so wound up that I had to go on working and writing and couldn't get to sleep before four in the morning.**

(Freud, 1960, p. 145)

*February 2, 1886—The bit of cocaine I have just taken is making me talkative, my little woman. I will go on writing and comment on your criticism of my wretched self. Do you realize how strangely a human being is constructed, that his virtues are often the seed of his downfall and his faults the source of his happiness?**

(Freud, 1960, pp. 200–207)

*From *Letters of Sigmund Freud*, by S. Freud, 1975/1960, New York: Basic Books.
†From *Freud: The Man and the Cause*, by R. W. Clark, 1980, New York: Random House.

In 1881, Sigmund Freud received his medical degree and almost immediately fell in love with Martha Bernays. Marriage was impossible without a solid career and income, and so Freud sought a subject for scientific study that would potentially bring him both fame and fortune. Whereas the development of psychoanalysis would much later be the real source of Freud's fame, the study of cocaine was his first prominent—and controversial—accomplishment. He published several scientific papers on cocaine and was among the first to recognize cocaine's potential role as a local anesthetic agent for eye surgery. He also self-administered cocaine in an effort to cure migraine and depression. By 1887, he had come to recognize that the use of cocaine was not without serious risks (Brain & Coward, 1989).

As he himself suggested in his April 21 letter to Martha, Freud was not unique in his pioneering enthusiasm for cocaine. Only a few years later, John Pemberton offered prohibition-minded Americans a new alcohol-free "temperance drink" compounded from caffeine and cocaine. Each 8-ounce glass of Coca-Cola contained 60 mg of cocaine, about the dose Freud recommended for depression (Gold, 1992). Freud could have met his own 200 mg cocaine needs with just under four Coca-Cola bottles a day. For 25 years, until cocaine was removed from the formula, many Americans found Coca-Cola to be very much "the real thing."

Over the next 90 years, the side effects and addictive nature of cocaine seem to have been largely forgotten. The 1980 edition of the *Comprehensive Textbook of Psychiatry* claimed that "used no more than two or three times a week cocaine creates no serious problems. In daily and fairly large amounts, it can produce minor psychological disturbances. Chronic cocaine abuse usually does not appear as a medical problem" (Gold, 1992, p. 206). Only 14 years later, DSM-IV turned these "minor psychological disturbances" into 10 diagnoses: Cocaine Intoxication, Cocaine Withdrawal, Cocaine Intoxication Delirium, Cocaine-Induced Psychotic Disorder (with and without delusions and hallucinations), Cocaine-Induced Mood Disorder, Cocaine-Induced Anxiety Disorder, Cocaine-Induced Sexual Dysfunction, Cocaine-Induced Sleep Disorder, and Cocaine-Related Disorder Not Otherwise Specified. (American Psychiatric Association, 1994). For associated medical problems, DSM-IV-TR now details sinusitis, nasal irritation and bleeding, perforated nasal septum, pneumonia, bronchitis, weight loss, chest pain, pneumothorax, myocardial infarction, sudden death, stroke, seizures, cardiac arrhythmias, premature labor and delivery, and acquired immunodeficiency syndrome (AIDS; American Psychiatric Association, 2000). This is a lengthy list for a drug that only a few years before had been authoritatively declared free of adverse medical side effects.

Effects

Cocaine acts in the brain's reward centers to block the reuptake of neurotransmitters, especially norepinephrine and dopamine (see Figure 17-1). This results in excess stimulation of these reward centers by these two excitatory neurotransmitters. In consequence, the brain mediates a release of stress

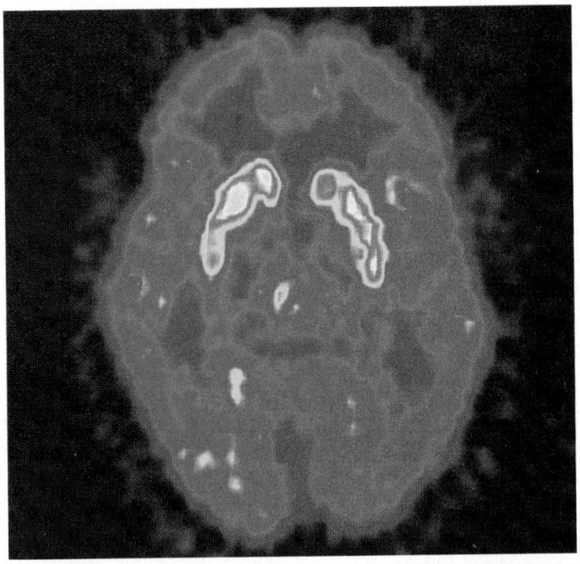

FIGURE 17-1 **Positron Emission Scan showing cocaine binding at dopamine-rich sites. This positron emission tomography (PET) shows that cocaine binds to specific brain locations, primarily at dopamine-rich sites in the basal ganglia (white, orange, and yellow areas on the scan). Green areas show lower density binding, and no binding occurs in the ventricles and other blue areas. The maximum binding is in the basal ganglia nuclei, which appear white.** (FROM "ADDICTION BRAIN MECHANISMS AND THEIR RELATED IMPLICATIONS," BY D.J. NUTT. ELSEVIER (*LANCET, 347*, 33–35, 1996). REPRINTED WITH PERMISSION.)

hormones including epinephrine. There is some evidence that cocaine has effects on brain serotonin pathways as well (Muller, Carey, & Huston, 2003). Psychological effects of cocaine are listed in Box 17-5.

BOX 17-5
PSYCHOLOGICAL EFFECTS OF COCAINE: LOW TO AVERAGE DOSES (25–150 MG)

Generally enjoyable effects with great increase in self-image. Rapid onset of a high with the following components:

- Euphoria, seldom dysphoria
- Increased sense of energy
- Enhanced mental acuity
- Increased sensory awareness (sexual, auditory, tactile, visual)
- Decreased appetite (anorexia)
- Increased anxiety and suspiciousness
- Decreased need for sleep
- Postponement of fatigue
- Increased self-confidence, egocentricity
- Delusions—dependence
- Physical symptoms of generalized sympathetic discharge

From *Substance Abuse: A Comprehensive Textbook* (2nd ed.), by J. H. Lowinson, 1992, Baltimore: Williams and Wilkins. Reprinted with permission.

Especially in higher dosages, the effects of cocaine on bodily drives are very strong. One authority reports that "so powerful is the direct stimulation provided by cocaine that sleep, safety, money, morality, loved ones, responsibility, even survival become largely irrelevant to the cocaine user" (Gold, 1992, p. 208). In animal studies, given a choice between cocaine and food or sex, rats choose cocaine until they die from overdose or starvation (Siegel, 1989).

Why has medical opinion shifted so strongly between 1980 and 1994 from nonchalance to a view that cocaine is a serious and dangerous drug of abuse? The answer is, in part, crack. Crack is a crystallized form of cocaine that can be smoked, gives a brief (5- to 10-minute) but almost instantaneous high, and provides cocaine blood levels as high or higher than those that result from intravenous administration. Noncrack cocaine is most commonly inhaled—"snorted"—into the nose, as a (usually impure) powder. Oral administration, as in the original Coca-Cola, has a relatively lower potential for producing dependence than does snorting, in which larger amounts of the drug are carried quickly to the brain. Smoked cocaine—most commonly, crack—has a much higher addictive potential than does any other means of administration

Another reason for the shift in medical opinion has been the recognition that cocaine can be physically dangerous—even occasionally when used for medically appropriate indications such as anesthesia of the nose during ENT surgery. Cocaine has been associated with chest pain due to myocardial infarction, other coronary syndromes, and aortic dissection (Frishman, Del Vecchio, Sanal, & Ismail, 2003). Cocaine is also responsible for ischemic and hemorrhagic strokes among users. Use of crack cocaine may increase the risk of these adverse events, but they also have been reported with intranasal use of cocaine powder (Vasica & Tennant, 2002).

Dependence and Withdrawal

Perhaps because some heavy cocaine users do not seem to have withdrawal symptoms, it was once thought that physiological dependence on cocaine was rare. When withdrawal symptoms occur, they include fatigue, vivid or unpleasant dreams, sleep disturbance, increased appetite, and psychomotor changes, either agitation or retardation. Symptoms typically occur a few hours to several days after the prior dose, but with large or repetitive doses may occur almost immediately after a cocaine high. Craving for cocaine is very common but is not included by DSM-IV-TR among symptoms meeting criteria for withdrawal. Two withdrawal symptoms following reduction of cocaine dose are required to make a diagnosis of withdrawal.

The DSM-IV-TR criteria for cocaine dependence and abuse are similar to those for other substances. DSM-IV-TR describes inability to resist cocaine when it is available as an early sign of dependence (American Psychiatric Association, 2000). Tolerance is common, leading to escalating dosage, and larger amounts of money are often required to support a growing cocaine dependence. While the initial experience or experiences with high-dose cocaine may produce highly pleasurable euphoria, subsequent drug use rarely leads to an equally powerful high. Increasing doses or repetitive binging may come closer to replicating initial feelings, and this desire for recapturing vivid memories of intoxication may be a strong impetus for compulsive use (Gold, 1992).

Treatment of Dependence

Withdrawal from cocaine is rarely physically dangerous; cocaine deaths occur from the drug itself, not its absence. The major challenge in treatment is to prevent relapse. Most clients with crack dependency need inpatient care because of both the intensity of drug cravings that crack provokes and the severity of the postintoxication psychological "crash" that occurs during withdrawal. Day hospitalization is another alternative that offers many of the advantages of inpatient treatment at lower costs (Alterman, O'Brien, McLellan, August, Snider, Droba, et al., 1994). Voucher-based programs reward users for abstinence while in outpatient treatment. This "community reinforcement therapy" significantly reduces cocaine use while payments continue, but has not been associated with sustained effectiveness (Higgins, Heil, Dantona, Donham, Matthews, & Badger, 2007). Counseling focuses on recognizing and avoiding situations that might lead to renewed use. This often requires changing friends, living situations, and jobs. Depression is often a problem and may benefit from psychological or medical treatment. Cocaine Anonymous programs, self-help groups patterned after A.A., are helpful for many in preventing relapse.

Cocaine abuse differs from many other forms of substance abuse in that women are as commonly represented among abusers as are men. Programs specifically designed to address women's needs and concerns may be more attractive to and effective for female abusers (Hughes, Coletti, Neri, Urmann, Stahl, Aialian, et al., 1995; Stecker, Han, Curran, & Booth, 2007). Overall, retention is a major problem for all cocaine treatment programs. Effectiveness of treatment is strongly related to motivation and to the level of functioning that the dependent individual had prior to becoming involved with cocaine. With increasing motivation and higher precocaine levels of functioning, treatment outcomes improve.

There is currently no proven pharmacotherapy for cocaine dependence, but a variety of treatments have been proposed and are under study (Karila, Gorelick, Weinstein, Noble, Benyamina, Coscas, et al., 2008). Topiramate, an anticonvulsant with many psychiatric uses, appears to have some benefit in reducing craving and promoting abstinence (Reis, Castro, Faria, & Laranjeira, 2008). Research is underway to find other medications effective in reducing cocaine craving, and there is considerable interest in a vaccine that could reduce the psychological effects of cocaine. At least one such vaccine has been developed and is currently being tested on humans (Bunce, Loudon, Akers, Dobson, & Wood, 2003).

Nurse's Role in Cocaine Abuse

The nurse working in a chemical dependency unit will provide direct care to clients experiencing intense cravings for the drug and a sometimes overwhelming sense of depression related to the crash of not having another dose. The client may wish to stop his own use of the drug, but such recovery involves changing the client's lifestyle completely. The nurse must work with a treatment team, helping the client to choose recovery and then place himself in settings where recovery is possible. Changing jobs, living situations, and friends is not an easy task. Group support such as that of Cocaine Anonymous is helpful. The nurse is always in a collaborative role, working with other professionals, including addictions counselors, to help the client choose recovery. The nurse also has a role in assessing for depression, as cocaine users frequently experience depression during recovery.

METHAMPHETAMINE

HOWARD

Howard has thirteen aliases, all backed up by Washington State driver's licenses. Howard A. Schultz is his current favorite identity. He paid one of his runners two grams for the date of birth, address, and Social Security number of the Starbucks coffee mogul.

He sometimes worries that he has stuck with this moniker too long. He enjoys being well known—he craves the underground fame, is proud of his place in tweeker lore—but he also recognizes the hazards of being the top cook in ... the county that leads the western United States in methamphetamine production, Methlehem County.

*... To the outside eye Howard looks depleted and decrepit, wheezing like a man dying from the plague, but inside he feels dynamic and destined for greatness, ruling the world like a man holding the hammer of the gods. As dopamine surges through his brain cells he is proud that he is zooming on his own homemade fuel, euphoric that he is wildly free, confident that he can outsmart the cops every time.... "I am, I am Superman, and I can do anything"**

(Lindquist, 2007, pp. 10–11, 18–19)

"Tweeker" is a slang term for heavy methamphetamine users. *The King of Methlehem*, written by Mark Lindquist, a prosecuting attorney in Washington State, vividly describes Howard's efforts to stay out of jail and to live life as both a tweeker and "top cook" despite having the pot-smoking lawyer-turned-detective Wyatt James (perhaps an amalgam of "good guy" Wyatt Earp and "bad guy" Jesse James?) hot on his heels. Written by the head of a major drug prosecution unit who moonlights as a novelist of Pacific Northwest

*From Book is *The King of Methlehem* by M. Lindquist, 2007, New York: Simon and Schuster.

low-life, it seems likely that the vivid descriptions of methamphetamine cooking and tweeker low life are true to life. Or perhaps more accurately, true to death.

Amphetamines, including methamphetamine, have in recent years become much more widespread drugs of abuse. While chemically distinct from cocaine, methamphetamine acts similarly on a variety of brain receptors, producing much the same effect as does cocaine. Like freebase ("crack") cocaine, methamphetamine can be snorted, smoked, or injected. Unlike cocaine, which has its origins in South America, methamphetamine can be synthesized from chemical precursors in decentralized relatively low-technology "labs" that can be readily hidden from law enforcement agencies. Methamphetamine precursors have, until recently, been readily available in common cold remedies. Restrictions on the sale of these medications (as well as other precursors such as ephedrine) have temporarily reduced methamphetamine use in some (Cunningham & Liu, 2008) but not all (Brandenburg, Brown, Arneson, & Arneson, 2007) studies. To date, each reduction has been associated with a "rebound" as new sources of precursors find their way into the drug market.

Following initial chemical synthesis in the late nineteenth century, it was recognized that methamphetamine could be used as a stimulant. There was widespread military use of amphetamines during World War II. After the war, large stockpiles in Japan came onto the civilian market and were responsible for local abuse. While methamphetamine spread to the United States in the 1950s, it long remained largely restricted to California, especially among motorcycle gang members. During the "Desert Storm" campaign there was significant use of amphetamines by U.S. combat personnel to prevent fatigue during extended operations (Emonson & Vanderbeek, 1995), but it is not clear to what extent, if any, military experiences contributed to more widespread domestic usage. In the past three decades, there has been a spread of methamphetamine availability and consumption over much of the United States, as well as in Canada, Asia, and Europe.

Effects

While the subjective effects of methamphetamine are similar to those of cocaine, they last much longer. The half-life of methamphetamine is between 10 and 20 hours, compared to 60–90 minutes for cocaine. As a result, the behavioral and health consequences of methamphetamine may be more severe than are those attributable to cocaine. The most striking health consequence is loss of teeth due to a combination of chronic dry mouth and poor oral hygiene ("meth mouth"). Methamphetamine usage is associated with compulsive sexual behavior that may lead to serious consequences such as infection with HIV. Of most importance, methamphetamine appears to be associated with long-term or even permanent brain changes that may have important behavioral consequences. These changes are seen in a variety of animal models as well as in humans, and may or may not be reversible with prolonged abstinence (Scott, Woods, Matt, Meyer, Heaton, Atkinson, et al., 2007).

Dependence and Withdrawal

Chronic use of methamphetamine leads to downregulation of brain dopamine receptors. This means that users experience diminished pleasure responses to normal activities and can achieve pleasure primarily through repeated use of methamphetamine. The effects of this downregulation are often coupled with changes in the frontal lobes that may interfere with drug-related decision-making and, when present, may increase the likelihood of relapse (Paulus, Tapert, & Schuckit, 2005). Perhaps not surprisingly given these effects on brain functioning, methamphetamine use is associated with changes in memory and decision-making that may persist despite subsequent abstinence (McCann, Kuwabara, Kumar, Palermo, Abbey, Brasic, et al., 2008). Because of its long half-life, methamphetamine withdrawal takes place over a much longer period than for many other drugs—the first phase lasting for 7–10 days, followed by a second, less-intense phase of several weeks duration (McGregor, Srisurapanont, Jittiwutikarn, Laobhripatr, Wongtan, & White, 2005). Major withdrawal effects include fatigue, increased appetite, and a variety of symptoms of depression. There is evidence from electroencephalogram studies that withdrawal is associated with a clinical encephalopathy that affects thinking, memory, and decision-making (Newton, Cook, Kalechstein, Duran, Monroy, Ling, et al., 2003). Medications like mirtazapine and modafinil have been used to increase alertness during withdrawal, but their effectiveness for improving cognitive functioning remains to be proven. Providing effective drug-related counseling can be very difficult in the face of the cognitive impairment induced by methamphetamine and its withdrawal state.

Acute Methamphetamine Toxicity

Since the effects of methamphetamine are long-lasting, it is not a surprise that nurses working in psychiatric emergency services are not infrequently required to treat persons who are acutely intoxicated with this substance. Methamphetamine intoxication can present with agitation, psychosis, and/or a variety of nonpsychiatric conditions such as seizures, stroke, or coronary artery spasm. Emergency personnel will attend to these physical risks initially, providing airway support, blood pressure monitoring, cardiac assessment, and seizure control as needed. Droperidol (most commonly used as an antinausea medication) or haloperidol (a first generation antipsychotic) inhibit brain dopamine, and are most commonly used to sedate patients whose agitation is due to methamphetamine. Benzodiazepines may be combined with these drugs, and are nearly always added to the treatment regimen when seizures occur. Psychosis is significantly more common among methamphetamine users than the general population (McKetin, Kelly, & McLaren, 2006) and may accompany acute methamphetamine toxicity.

Treatment of Dependence

Not all methamphetamine users necessarily meet DSM criteria for dependence, however use of crystalline methamphetamine and administration by means other than oral ingestion are risk factors for dependence (McKetin et al., 2006). The management of methamphetamine dependence is similar to that outlined for cocaine in the preceding section. Methamphetamine users are probably more likely than cocaine users to have significant cognitive impairment (Homer, Solomon, Moeller, Mascia, DeRaleau, & Halkitis, 2008), and this impairment may influence the choice of treatment. Cognitively based treatments (such as cognitive behavioral therapy) may be less effective in individuals whose ability to sequence and reason is impaired. Despite such concerns, current evidence supports the effectiveness of cognitive therapies in the management of methamphetamine dependence and addiction (Lee & Rawson, 2008).

Nurse's Role in Methamphetamine Abuse

Nurses in many settings will encounter patients using methamphetamine and will be in a supportive role regarding the treatments cited previously. Community nurses need to be mindful of the presenting symptoms of agitation, aggressive behavior, rapid mood swings, hypertension, and tachycardia (Getting, Grady, & Nowosadzka, 2006), and can make referrals for individuals using meth. When the user is a child/youth, school and parental authorities need to become part of the treatment plan. Nurses in emergency departments will be involved in caring for such individuals who can present with a variety of health problems and may become combative. Setting boundaries, placing meth users in private rooms, and avoiding stimuli may be useful, however restraints are sometimes necessary to provide for staff and patient safety. Nurses can advocate for prevention through participation in community educational programs, particularly those directed toward youth, and public health programs geared at restricting access to meth and its component parts.

Opiates

I DID ABSOLUTELY NOTHING

*I lived in one room in the Native Quarter of Tangier. I had not taken a bath in a year nor changed my clothes or removed them except to stick a needle every hour into the fibrous grey wooden flesh of terminal addiction. I never cleaned or dusted the room. Empty ampule boxes and garbage piled to the ceiling. Light and water long since turned off for non payment. I did absolutely nothing. I could look at the end of my shoe for eight hours. I was only roused to action when the hourglass of junk ran out. If a friend came to visit and they rarely did since who or what was left to visit I sat there not caring that he had entered my field of vision a grey screen always blanker and fainter and not caring when he walked out of it. If he had died on the spot I would have sat there looking at my shoe waiting to go through his pockets. Wouldn't you? Because I never had enough junk—no one ever does. Thirty grains of morphine a day and it still was not enough. And long waits in front of the drugstore. Delay is a rule in the junk business. The Man is never on time. This is no accident. There are no accidents in the junk world. The addict is taught again and again exactly what will happen if he does not score for his junk ration. Get up that money or else. And suddenly my habit began to jump and jump. Forty, sixty grains a day. And it still was not enough. And I could not pay.**

(Burroughs, 1960, p. 18)

William Burroughs's testimony is particularly extraordinary because despite living under degrading circumstances in New York and North Africa, he still managed to be a major novelist, writer, and cult figure of the "beat" generation. As an author, Burroughs consciously cultivated the image of an outlaw, a man of evil and degradation. But however much he struck the literary pose of one who has purposefully chosen ugliness and self-destruction, drug dependency governed his life. He had left the protected world of Harvard for a life of filth and poverty, where his only certainty was withdrawal:

*I was an addict for fifteen years. When I say addict I mean an addict to junk (generic term for opium and/or derivatives including all synthetics from demerol to palfium). I have used junk in many forms: morphine, heroin, dilaudid, eukodal, pantapon, diocodid, diosane, opium, demerol, dolophine, palfium. I have smoked junk, eaten it, sniffed it, injected it in vein-skin-muscle, inserted it in rectal suppositories. The needle is not important ... the result is the same: addiction.**

(Burroughs, 1960, p. 18)

Effects

There are many opiates, all chemical derivatives of opium. Opium, in turn, is derived from a milky secretion produced by the poppy flower's seed pods as they ripen. Small amounts of opium are found in poppy seeds and in other poppies, but the opium poppy—native to what is now Turkey—has by far the highest concentration. By some extraordinary biological coincidence, opium and its derivatives are a perfect fit for chemical receptor molecules in the nervous system of animals. Animals have a complex neurotransmitter system that regulates pain and activity and is known as the endorphin system. Opiates fit into the endorphin receptors as a key fits into a lock, and fitting into that lock, they have profound effects on the brain. Stimulation of endorphin (usually called opiate) receptors produces a wide variety of changes in the nervous system—perception of pain is diminished, a sense of comfort or pleasure is established, bodily functions slow down, and the brain vomiting center is stimulated. Opiates have important medical use in relieving pain and apprehension. They are also widely abused because of their euphoric properties—they make some users feel contented and free of worry and, depending on the dose and rapidity of administration, may give users a "rush" of intense pleasure. This rush seems to come primarily after intravenous administration and explains the continuing popularity of this exceedingly dangerous means of administering drugs.

Dependence and Withdrawal

As Burroughs implies, withdrawal is a phenomenon well known both to opiate abusers and care providers. Symptoms of withdrawal include depression, restlessness, nausea or vomiting, muscle aches, tearing or nasal discharge, dilated pupils, "gooseflesh," sweating, diarrhea, yawning, fever, and insomnia. Perhaps Burroughs was exaggerating when he claimed to need hourly injections; withdrawal usually occurs 6 to 24 hours after a previous dose and is unlikely to occur at hourly intervals. Still, most addicts make every effort to avoid withdrawal and whenever possible provide themselves with opiates on a schedule that prevents the profoundly uncomfortable symptoms of withdrawal.

Tolerance is highly characteristic of opiate use. Burroughs describes his escalating dose of morphine. Addicts may come to require exceedingly high (and expensive) doses after a relatively brief time. In experimental studies, volunteers can be made tolerant to huge morphine doses (up to 500 mg/day) in only a little more than a week (Jaffe, 1990).

Technically, dependence can be demonstrated even after only one dose of morphine (see Figure 17-2). If a narcotic antagonist (a drug that blocks the effects of opiates) is given soon after a single dose of morphine, mild withdrawal symptoms can be produced. This rapid development of dependence is of no clinical significance, but chronic or dependent users may have very protracted withdrawal that occurs in two phases. The first phase includes the acute symptoms discussed in the previous section and is over in a few days; the second phase may last for six months. Symptoms of the second phase include vague malaise, depression, changes in appetite, and measurable differences in temperature and respiration (Jaffe, 1990).

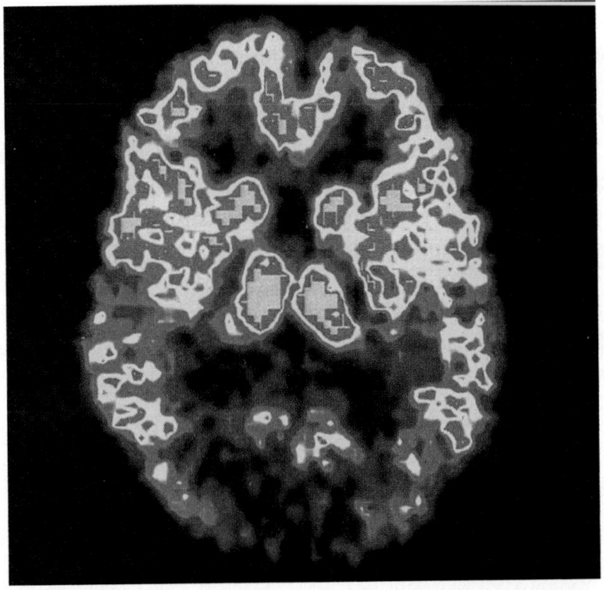

FIGURE 17-2 **This PET scan shows the wide distribution of opioid binding sites. The highest opioid binding is represented by pink, yellow, and red/orange. Blue and green areas bind the least amount of opioid** (FROM "ADDICTION BRAIN MECHANISMS AND THEIR RELATED IMPLICATIONS," BY D. J. NUTT. ELSEVIER (*LANCET*, 347, 33–35, 1996). REPRINTED WITH PERMISSION.)

It seems that only some persons become dependent on opiates despite experimentation. There was widespread opiate use among U.S. servicemen in Vietnam, but only about half of those who used heroin became dependent. Persons who used heroin multiple times were more likely to become dependent while in Vietnam, but many spontaneously stopped use when they returned to the United States (Robins, 1979). DSM-IV-TR defines opiate abuse as occurring in persons who use opiates rarely but find themselves in social or legal difficulties because of that use. The presence of withdrawal or tolerance is far more likely to suggest dependence rather than merely abuse.

Treatment of Dependence

In the second passage from William Burroughs quoted previously, Burroughs claims that "The needle is not important." According to this view, the addict seeks only the chemical reaction of opiates with his or her endorphin receptors. Burroughs reports that addiction follows whatever the form of the substance used. However, while these pharmacological actions of opiates are undoubtedly of very great importance in leading to dependence, opiate addiction is a complex physical, psychological, and social phenomenon in which the *setting*—often including drug injection paraphernalia—is very important. Opiate users constitute a subculture with defined interactions, rituals, and hierarchies. Successful treatment must recognize that opiate abuse is a way of life that for the addict to say, "I did absolutely nothing," really means, "I lived for opiates and nothing else." Treatment must not only separate the abuser from his or her junk, but it must also help supply human and spiritual content to a life that would otherwise be spent "looking at the end of a shoe for eight hours."

When opiate-dependent individuals seek treatment, the primary therapeutic decision is whether the goal should be detoxification or substitution of oral methadone for injected opiates. The principles of detoxification are not fundamentally different for opiates than they are for alcohol, tobacco, or cocaine—drug usage is stopped, and any withdrawal symptoms are managed by medical intervention. Because opiate withdrawal symptoms are common and may be severe, specialized therapeutic and pharmacological approaches have been developed to facilitate detoxification (Vining, Kosten, & Kleber, 1988).

Methadone maintenance is an entirely different concept that bypasses detoxification but substitutes a "more acceptable" substance—medically prescribed methadone—for street opiates. Methadone is a long-acting orally administered opiate that can indefinitely suppress both the symptoms of withdrawal and the craving for intravenous fast-acting opiates such as heroin. At least in dependent individuals, oral methadone seems not to produce euphoria or sedation. It does, however, block opiate receptors so that while on methadone, further doses of intravenous heroin have little psychological or physical effect. In this way, not only does methadone reduce or eliminate opiate craving, but it also makes further administration of the opiate drug less attractive. The experience of 30 years suggests that in most cases methadone is safe and does not impair normal client functioning (Lowinson, Marion, Joseph, & Dole, 1992).

One of the strongest arguments in favor of methadone maintenance is that to the extent it is effective, it reduces injection drug use and hence decreases the risk of human immunodeficiency virus (HIV) transmission. Methadone maintenance has been a controversial therapy because it involves the legalized supply of prescription narcotics to clients whose only disease is opiate dependence. There is also little doubt that some of the methadone prescribed in maintenance programs is diverted onto the street, where it becomes part of the fabric of illegal abuse. If the goal is to keep opiate-dependent persons free of injection drugs, functional, and employable, then methadone maintenance has a useful role. The administration of methadone programs is complicated by the realities of current substance abuse. Abuse involving multiple drugs—often mixtures of heroin and cocaine—is very common. Methadone maintenance is, by its nature, focused on opiates alone, but opiate users are also frequently and simultaneously abusing cocaine, amphetamines, marijuana, and alcohol. As is discussed in the following section, many methadone programs have adapted to the special needs of multidrug abuse (Joseph & Appel, 1985).

While methadone maintenance is strongly advocated by some, many experts equally strongly endorse the alternative goal of detoxification followed by abstinence. The principles of this latter approach are very similar to those employed in alcohol and cocaine treatment. As with these substances, successful treatment seems to require a combination of psychotherapy; attention to social, vocational, and spiritual well-being; and involvement in a 12-step group. The drug buprenorphine is an alternative to methadone that may be more acceptable to clinicians for whom abstinence is an important goal. Buprenorphine is a substance that taken orally binds to opiate receptors in the brain, but—unlike methadone—does not produce any significant "high." Under the brand name Suboxone, it is combined with an opiate antagonist so that even if injected it has no euphoric effects. For these reasons, it is preferred by many clinicians who begin treatment with detoxification (usually on an inpatient basis) and then prescribe daily buprenorphine administration with periodic urine testing to assure that no other drugs are being consumed. The approach is very similar to that used for methadone, except that clients are often given several weeks of medication to take home and are followed at longer intervals than is customary in methadone treatment. Since buprenorphine is not regulated as stringently as is methadone, it can be administered by any physician who has taken a prescribed instructional course on its usage. While each physician who receives training can treat only a limited number of clients, the ability of generalist physicians such as family doctors and internists to offer treatment potentially expands access to effective treatment. Current evidence suggests that methadone may be more effective than is buprenorphine (Connock, Juarez-Garcia, Jowett, Frew, Liu, Taylor, et al., 2007), but the potential for easier (or perhaps less stigmatized) access to treatment may make buprenorphine the rehabilitation treatment of choice for some. Increasing numbers of drug-related deaths associated with methadone (Graham, Merlo, Goldberger, & Gold, 2008; Shields, Hunsaker Iii, Corey, Ward, & Stewart, 2007) have raised concerns about the safety of current methadone provision models—especially when these result in diversion onto the street. While fatalities do occur with buprenorphine abuse (perhaps especially when not compounded with naloxone), a study in France—where buprenorphine is widely used by general practitioners (Fatseas & Auriacombe, 2007)—found the buprenorphine-associated fatality rate to be about one-third that of methadone (Auriacombe, Franques, & Tignol 2001).

Candy

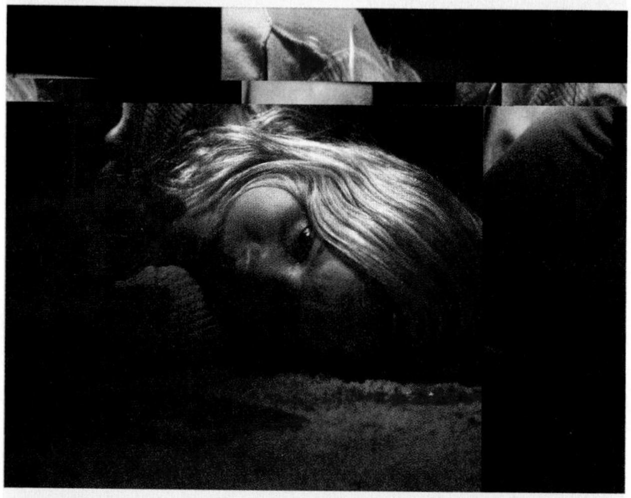

Courtesy: Renaissance Films/Paradigm Hyde Films/The Kobal Collection

Candy, a film about heroin addiction, stars Abbie Cornish as a young middle class woman who marries an addict (played by Heath Ledger) and follows him into a self-destructive life. In the still from this highly realistic movie, we see Cornish strung out on heroin.

Nurse's Role in Opiate Abuse

The nurse has a similar role in treating the opiate addict as in treating the alcoholic. The nurse may be involved with caring for the client in acute withdrawal, initial recovery, and long-term maintenance. In acute recovery, the nurse must monitor the withdrawal and ensure client safety. If methadone is used, the nurse will monitor the dose and effect. The nurse is almost always in a collaborative role, working with addictions counselors and other professionals to assist the client to choose recovery and then find a living situation where recovery is possible.

Prescription drug abuse, particularly the abuse of opiates prescribed for chronic pain, has been a growing concern. While some persons may successfully order illicit substances from international sources on the Internet (Larson, 2002), the majority are prescribed by community physician offices—many of which likely employ nurses (Miller & Greenfeld, 2004). Nurses who work in settings where chronic pain is treated have to be aware of the important need to balance a duty to relieve suffering with a responsibility to not dispense controlled substances to persons likely to abuse them. No completely effective screening tool exists to separate those persons susceptible to dependency/abuse from those with pain who appear not to be susceptible, but nurses can work together with prescribing physicians to optimize the responsible prescribing of opiate medications for persons in pain (Nicholson, 2003).

Other Commonly Abused Substances

Hallucinogens

Hallucinogens are substances such as lysergic acid diethylamide (LSD), mescaline, peyote, psilocybin, and MDMA (Ecstasy) that, when ingested, cause disturbances of perception or frank hallucinations. Hallucinogens were widely used in the 1960s, and reports suggest that they are once again relatively popularly abused substances. Although tolerance to hallucinogen use develops quite quickly, dependence is rarely seen. Hallucinogen use is most commonly intermittent, often punctuated by long periods of abstinence. Injury from these drugs typically results from dangerous behaviors that occur when under the immediate influence, for example driving or diving off a building or other high place under the delusion that the individual can fly. Such abuse may result in serious injury or death. In contrast, violent behavior, though reported occasionally, is not frequent.

Inhalants

Inhalants are volatile chemical substances found most often as solvents in common household and industrial products: paints (especially aerosol spray paints), glue, and gasoline. Inhalants produce significant behavioral and psychological changes that may be variable or even seemingly opposite, depending both on the individual and the substance. Among these behavioral changes are aggressiveness, apathy, and poor judgment. Inhalants also produce neurological signs and symptoms, including dizziness, incoordination, slurred speech, unsteady gait, tremor, weakness, and stupor or coma. Hallucinations often result from inhalant use, and injury may occur because of impaired judgment. Death may occasionally occur from lung or heart complications. Long-term use of inhalants can lead to permanent neurological damage including brain atrophy and dysfunction. Inhalants are most often used by adolescents, frequently as part of group activities. Inhalant use is widespread and potentially dangerous, but only a relatively small proportion of users become dependent. Inhalants are frequently used in settings in which other drugs are not readily available. The ready availability of organic solvents makes controlling legal access to these drugs very difficult.

Cannabis (Marijuana)

Cannabis, also called hemp or "pot" or "weed," is a plant whose leaves, stems, and resin contain a variety of psychoactive substances that may be smoked or eaten. The effects of cannabis use include euphoria and impairments in memory, judgment, sensory perceptions, and motor skills. Hallucinations may occur, but symptoms of anxiety and dysphoria are more common psychiatric consequences. Cannabis is not regarded as a hallucinogen. While physiological dependence on cannabis probably does not occur, psychological dependence is not uncommon and may have a significant negative effect on personal and social functioning.

In recent years, it has become apparent that the effects of cannabis on the brain are mediated by receptors that bind to this drug. In turn, these receptors exist because the brain utilizes a variety of endogenous cannabinoids as part of its internal signaling processes. It remains incompletely understood precisely what the function of cannabinoid signaling is in the brain, but some research connects these substances to internal "reward" systems that influence behavioral choices (Solinas, Goldberg, & Piomelli, 2008). Endocannabinoids seem to have inhibitory effects on brain neurons, modulating the effects of other neurotransmitters in a unique way known as retrograde signaling (Nicoll & Alger, 2004). Endocannabinoids seem to be involved in suppressing prior memories of unpleasant events, and so may be involved in the development of Post-Traumatic Stress Disorder. They also appear to play a role in the regulation of eating, though their relationship to obesity and eating disorders remains incompletely worked out. There is emerging evidence that marijuana usage is linked to the development of psychosis in some susceptible individuals (Semple, McIntosh, & Lawrie, 2005), suggesting that regulation of endogenous cannabinoids may play a role in the genesis of mania and schizophrenia (Leweke & Koethe, 2008).

MULTIPLE DRUGS, MULTIPLE DIAGNOSES

Out of the dozens of substances that humans commonly abuse, this chapter has focused on the four most commonly used and widely abused: nicotine, alcohol, cocaine, and opiates. Nutt and colleagues have constructed a multicategory matrix comparing dependency (on the Y axis) with physical harm (on the X axis; Nutt, King, Saulsbury, & Blakemore, 2007). This matrix provides an expert assessment of the relative risks of single drug usage, but it doesn't address the complexities of multidrug usage. In line with the consumer society of the twenty-first century, in which few people limit their consumption to one product, it is not at all unusual for any combination of these and other substances to be abused simultaneously. One important study that addressed multiple drug use was the Treatment Outcome Prospective Study (TOPS), which reported its findings in 1989 (Hubbard, Marsden, Rachal, Harwood, Cavannaugh, & Ginzburg). TOPS enrolled 10,000 participants in methadone programs and ambulatory and inpatient treatment centers. Thirty percent were women and 25% were under 21 years of age; the majority were male and over 21 years old. A large proportion of all enrolled participants were members of U.S. ethnic minorities. Thirty-one percent had been referred to their programs by the courts. In an analysis of multidrug use, methadone clinic enrollees differed somewhat from those in other treatment programs. Not surprisingly, the participants in methadone clinics were primarily heroin users; but even in methadone programs, 20% of individuals were heavy users of multiple drugs, and 50% used alcohol, cocaine, or marijuana in addition to heroin. Participants in nonmethadone programs were even more likely to be multiple-drug users.

While multidrug abuse is a real and growing problem, it is also important to realize that many drug-dependent clients have other psychiatric problems in addition to drug dependence. The Epidemiologic Catchment Area Study found that more than 50% of substance-abusing individuals also had other psychiatric diagnoses. This study and others have reported a strong link between anxiety disorders, depression, mania, schizophrenia, and substance use (Beeder & Millman, 1992). Personality disorders are very common, with borderline and antisocial personalities strongly represented, the latter especially in opiate abusers (Nace, Davis, & Gaspari, 1991). Not surprisingly, it may be difficult for even experienced psychiatric diagnosticians to decide whether depression or anxiety is caused by drug dependence or was a problem before the dependence began. Some clients use substances to self-medicate their symptoms of depression or to suppress hallucinations. In such an individual, effective treatment of the primary underlying psychiatric diagnosis may occasionally eliminate the major motivation to use drugs. In the majority of dually diagnosed individuals, the combination of abuse and other psychiatric disorders merely complicates both diagnosis and treatment. Potentially successful programs, such as 12-step programs or methadone treatment, may be resisted by paranoid or antisocial clients. Dually diagnosed persons take immense amount of staff time in programs that are increasingly underfunded and understaffed. An equally important concern is that substance abuse may be significantly underrecognized in clients with other psychiatric disorders. The failure to recognize a comorbid substance abuse diagnosis may greatly interfere with treatment effectiveness for the presenting psychiatric problem (Beeder & Millman, 1992).

SUBSTANCE ABUSE AS A SOCIAL PROBLEM

Substance abuse is a serious and perplexing social problem that is by no means solely (or perhaps even primarily) psychiatric in its nature. The issues surrounding substance abuse raise important questions about law, individual rights and freedom, and the social role of productive work versus the pursuit of pleasure. Substance abuse challenges society to address issues of homelessness, poverty, alienation, and the spread of infectious diseases, including hepatitis B, AIDS, and tuberculosis including its multidrug-resistant forms. There is no easy answer to the nearly universal and timeless problem of substance abuse. Strict controls have yet to work, perhaps because, as some have argued, they have not yet been strict enough or perhaps because, as others claim, criminal elements have achieved too great an influence over politicians and police. Some have argued for moving beyond limited methadone maintenance to a legalization of virtually all abused substances as long as access is restricted to adult use only. Comparable arguments were first made more than 150 years ago by the English political philosopher John Stuart Mill, and they continue to prove attractive to liberal and libertarian Americans alike.

Economists approach drug social policy through the concept of "elasticity of demand." Put most simply, this is the degree to which a rise in price will affect the quantity of a product demanded by consumers. Fuel prices, as it turns out, have a relatively low demand elasticity: there are no cheaper substitutes for gasoline; buying a new high-mileage car is expensive; the bus is often inconvenient; and we have to get to work somehow. So we may drive a little less, but overall as fuel prices go up our demand for gas stays fairly stable: the elasticity of our purchasing is low. The same is not true for the price of tobacco products—especially for young people. A planned rise in prices due to increased tobacco taxes significantly reduces the number of cigarette packages that young people will buy. They may switch to cheaper "complementary" products (bidis, roll-your-own, try to find smuggled products, or perhaps still-expensive generic cigarettes), but on the balance smoking among the young has a relatively high elasticity: prices go up and quantity demanded goes down.

Economists determine elasticity by actually measuring prices and consumption, which is not easy to do for the purchase of street drugs. It appears, however, that the demand elasticity of most drugs is very much like that of tobacco—when prices go up demand drops and/or people switch to less expensive complementary alternatives (Grossman, Chaloupka, & Shim, 2002). For example, demand for cocaine may be influenced by the price of methamphetamine, and vice versa. Demand elasticity works in the opposite direction as well—when prices drop, demand rises.

Economists argue further that legalization with prices set purely on acquisition/production costs will significantly drop consumer costs—hence raising the quantity of drugs demanded, but shifting demand from the streets into legal channels (Mamber, 2006). Most people would find this an unsatisfactory policy—its outcome potentially being quite similar to the early nineteenth-century U.S. experience with alcohol noted earlier in this chapter: low prices, no excise taxes, no age limits on drinking, and per capita 200-proof consumption of seven gallons yearly. Mirroring current public policy for both tobacco and alcohol and combining legalization with hefty taxation could keep prices high as long as

Blow

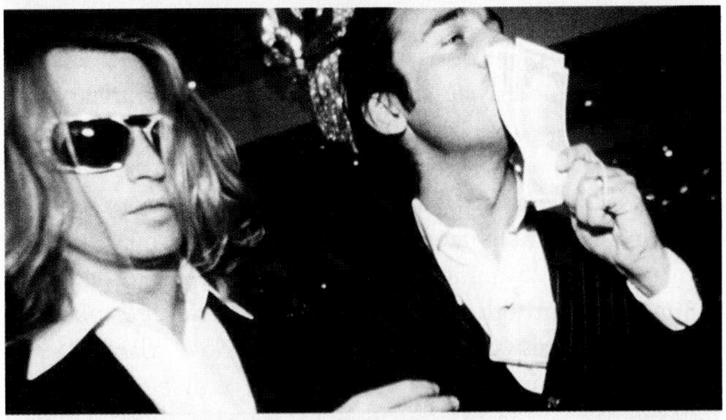

Courtesy: New Line/Avery Pix/The Kobal Collection

In *Blow*, Johnny Depp plays a drug trafficker in love with money (and, of course, women). *Blow* is a reminder of the violent hold that drug distribution has on all who come in contact with cocaine and other illegal substances of abuse

some of the taxation revenues were used to make street sales risky enough (prosecution and fines) that prices on the street stayed high. The reader will have to make up his or her mind about the desirability of legalization, because there are no comprehensive models anywhere in the world demonstrating that it is a workable policy. Currently, neither political nor public opinion supports legalization, and while relaxation of marijuana enforcement may continue, it seems highly unlikely that any country will adopt wholesale drug legalization in the near future.

Siegel (1989) has proposed a quite different solution to addressing the seemingly irrepressible human need for intoxication. In his view, legalization is flawed, at least in part because drugs are not safe, because of demand elasticity their use would likely increase under legalization, and the process of legalization puts "the government seal of approval on such appealing yet imperfect substances" (p. 299). Instead of legalizing current substances, Siegel proposes that society devote some of its scientific skill to developing safer and better ones. Even assuming that the "perfect drug" could be found—a drug highly appealing and safe for short- and long-term use—it is unclear that society is likely to endorse its legal use. Still, at this time there are no "good" drugs. Each has its health risks, its tolerance, its withdrawal symptoms, and its dependent users. This reality is unlikely to change as far into the twenty-first century as it is now possible to see.

SUBSTANCE ABUSE AS A PUBLIC HEALTH PROBLEM

An alternative view to substance abuse is emerging that bypasses the contentious question of legalization and focuses on the public health concept of "harm reduction" (Ball, 2007). Harm reduction focuses on injection drug use and seeks to stop the spread of HIV through needle sharing and other risky practices. The World Health Organization has been a leader in the definition of harm reduction and, according to Ball, has defined six key elements in this public health model:

- Reducing HIV transmission through a series of public health activities including needle and syringe access, safe sharps disposal, drug treatment programs including (for opiates) methadone and/or buprenorphine, and condom availability;
- Effective clinical management of HIV/AIDS, end-of-life care, chronic pain, other substance use (including alcohol), and other mental health disorders such as depression;
- Creating health care service models that incorporate the preceding two elements along with assured availability of necessary drugs including methadone and buprenorphine into a system that includes peer outreach, HIV treatment, addiction management, and a clear definition of the minimum level of service available to all;
- Assuring the availability of human resources—surely including mental health-educated nurses—to carry out harm-reduction services;
- "Supportive policy, legal and social environment, including policies that ensure equitable access to HIV services for drug users; laws that do not compromise access to HIV services for drug users through criminalization and marginalization; and campaigns to reduce stigma and discrimination, related particularly to health services and workers";
- Assuring the availability and staffing of appropriate systems for disease surveillance and the assessment of service effectiveness.

Many would describe this vision of harm reduction as highly idealistic, but it has evolved in the face of devastating world-wide spread of HIV among injection drug users. Iran, China, and Vietnam, three countries with very high rates of injection drug-related HIV spread and very strong reliance on criminalization of drug use, have adopted national harm-reduction policies (Hammett, Wu, Duc, Stephens, Sullivan, Liu, et al., 2008; Committee on the Prevention of HIV Infection, 2006). Many other countries, especially in Europe, have endorsed harm reduction as key elements of their policy toward illicit drugs (Ball, 2007 as evidence mounts for the effectiveness of these programs (Committee on the Prevention of HIV Infection, 2006; Ritter & Cameron, 2006). Hilton and colleagues and Pauly and Gladstone have usefully reviewed strategies and theories of harm reduction from a nursing perspective (Hilton, Thompson, Moore-Dempsey, & Janzen, 2001; Pauly, 2008; Pauly & Gladstone, 2008). Much of the success of harm reduction in several Asian countries has been due to the extremely hard work of dedicated community health nurses (Limbu, 2008). Other successful "grass roots" efforts involving peer counselors and family members have been described (Ngo, Schmich, Higgs, & Fischer, 2008). While Pauly correctly cautions that we have a need to better understand the role nurses can play in harm reduction, this strategy offers hope worldwide in our collective efforts to overcome two of humanity's most serious current challenges: the spread of HIV and the personal and social destructiveness of drug dependencies.

IMPACT OF DRUG USE/ABUSE ON FAMILIES

The impact of substance abuse goes beyond the individual abuser. Each person is a member of a family unit, a social group, and society, such that the result of addiction and chemical dependency extend to those in the person's immediate and sometimes not-so-immediate environment.

FAMILY DYSFUNCTION

FATHER

He weaves past into the house, where he slumps into his overstuffed chair and falls asleep.... All evening, until our bedtimes, we tiptoe past him, as past a snoring dragon. Then we curl in our fearful sheets, listening. Eventually he wakes with a grunt, Mother slings accusations at him, he snarls back, she yells, he growls, their voices clashing. Before long, she retreats to their bedroom, sobbing—not from the blows of fists, for he never strikes her, but from the force of words.... Whatever my brother and sister and mother may be thinking on their own rumpled pillows, I lie there hating him, loving him, fearing him, knowing I have failed him. I tell myself he drinks to ease an ache that gnaws at his belly, an ache I must have caused by disappointing him somehow, a murderous ache I should be able to relieve by doing all my chores, earning A's in school, winning baseball games, fixing the broken washer and the burst pipes, bringing in money to fill his empty wallet....

*When the drink made him weepy, Father would pack a bag and kiss each of us children on the head, and announce from the front door that he was moving out. "Where to?" we demanded, fearful each time that he would leave for good as Mr. Sampson had roared away for good in his diesel truck. "Someplace where I won't get hounded every minute," Father would answer, his jaw quivering.... We bawled and bawled, wondering if he would ever come back. He always did come back, a day or a week later, but each time there was a sliver less of him.**

(Sanders, 1989, p. 73)

The effects of alcoholism on families has been well documented. Family disruption related to alcoholism is a serious, complex, and pervasive social problem. Alcoholism is linked to violence, disrupted family roles, impaired family communication, and some physical and psychological illnesses such as depression, GI disturbances, and asthma/emphysema (Lindeman, Hawks, & Bartek, 1994). Similarly, consequences of alcoholism all too often result in chaotic, disorganized, and dysfunctional family units. Children reared in homes where one parent is an alcoholic exhibit stress and express a lack of ability to get along with others, as well as a lack of feelings of attachment toward their parents. Adolescents from alcoholic families are reported to exhibit low levels of warmth, awareness, understanding, trust, respect, and kindness toward others when compared to adolescents from families without alcohol abuse (Scavnicky-Mylant, 1990). Characteristics inherent in the diagnosis of *dysfunctional family processes related to alcoholism* (Herdman, 2009) are presented in Box 17-6. Major defining characteristics of this nursing diagnosis are also presented. Review of these family characteristics indicates that the family milieu is such that the needs of family members cannot be met without dealing first with the alcohol abuse and the family characteristics that support the abuse. While less research exists on family dysfunction when drugs other than alcohol are involved, the dysfunctional family unit is the same in any situation where the need to obtain drugs/chemicals takes precedence over the need to nurture and support the development of each family member.

BOX 17-6
CONCEPTS INHERENT IN THE DEFINITION OF THE NURSING DIAGNOSIS DYSFUNCTIONAL FAMILY PROCESSES RELATED TO ALCOHOLISM

- Affects psychosocial function of family
- Dysfunction
- Denial of problem
- Chronicity
- Pervades all family functions
- Conflict
- Disorganization of family unit
- Ineffective problem-solving style
- Family experiences series of crises
- Difficulty in escaping dysfunctional system
- Insidious process
- Affects spiritual functioning of family
- Creates lifetime self-perpetuating pattern
- Lack of protective, stable family unit
- Ineffective support systems
- Affects physiological functioning of family members

From "The Alcoholic Family: A Nursing Diagnosis Validation Study," by M. Lindeman, J. H. Hawks, and J. K. Bartek, 1994, *Nursing Diagnosis*, 5, 65–73. Reprinted with permission.

*From "Under the Influence," by S. R. Sanders. Copyright © 1989 by *Harper's Magazine*. All rights reserved. Reprinted from the November issue with special permission.

Codependence

Codependence is a term used to describe the cluster of behaviors exhibited by family members/significant others (most often a spouse) of one who is chemically addicted that serve to enable the alcoholic or addict to continue using the substance. Codependent behaviors serve to satisfy the needs of the family member to feel loved, important, and needed. The codependent behaviors of a spouse of an alcoholic typically are those enabling behaviors that permit the alcoholic to avoid the logical consequences of drinking. For example, if a husband is unable to go to work due to a hangover and his wife calls his office while he sleeps to tell his coworkers that he has the flu and cannot come to work today, the wife has enabled the alcoholic to be irresponsible. Further, examination of the dynamics of her motivations will almost always demonstrate that she has a need to do good things for others and defines her own self-worth only in terms of caring for and caring about others *at the exclusion of her own needs for self-development and fulfillment.* Codependence should not be confused with altruistic, prosocial behaviors that are performed on the basis of a genuine desire to serve the greater good by acts of kindness and compassion. The difference is that the codependent person performs the acts to meet her own needs and loses her sense of self by defining her self-worth in relation to what others think. The codependent person lacks ability to form intimate relationships with others, as she develops only one part of her personality to the exclusion of others.

Family members who assist an alcoholic or drug addict in maintaining addictive behaviors only aid their loved one in the general downward spiral of chemical dependence. These family members must be taught how to let the addict suffer the logical consequences of addictive behaviors and to remove themselves personally from the disease, the behaviors, and the shame that the addict experiences. Family members need help to realize that there is hope for recovery only if and when the addict himself is willing to stop the addiction. Enabling behaviors serve only to keep the addict from having to confront his behaviors and further keep the enabler from coming to terms with her own unmet needs for acknowledgment, love, intimacy, and personal growth.

A nurse working with any family where alcohol or drugs are used must become familiar with the dynamics of codependence and the means to assist family members even when the addicted individual refuses help. National self-help groups such as Al-Anon and Alateen (which help family members, friends, and teens who have an alcoholic relative or friend), Cocaine Anonymous, Narcotics Anonymous, and Co-dependents Anonymous are some of the many groups to which referrals can be made.

BOX 17-7
EXAMPLES OF THE DEFINING CHARACTERISTICS OF THE NURSING DIAGNOSIS DYSFUNCTIONAL FAMILY PROCESSES: RELATED TO ABUSE OF ALCOHOL

- Deterioration in family relationships
- Disturbed family dynamics
- Marital problems
- Ineffective spousal communication
- Inconsistent parenting
- Family denial
- Intimacy dysfunction
- Closed communication system
- Loss of control of drinking
- Rationalization
- Broken promises
- Inability to meet emotional needs of members
- Manipulation
- Inappropriate expression of anger
- Dependency
- Enabling behaviors
- Decreased self-esteem
- Frustration
- Powerlessness
- Tension
- Insecurity

From "The Alcoholic Family: A Nursing Diagnosis Validation Study," by M. Lindeman, J. H. Hawks, and J. K. Bartek, 1994, *Nursing Diagnosis*, 5, 65–73. Reprinted with permission.

Nursing Theory and Psychological Theory

Nurses may use any nursing theory in understanding the addicted client and in planning interventions. In some cases, a psychological theory may also be used to guide practice. Theory helps the nurse put the complex problems faced by clients and families in perspective. In addition, theory helps the nurse understand the addiction and accompanying behaviors, as well as helps to frame interventions in light of that understanding. An example follows:

> *If the nurse seeks to understand the drinking behavior of an alcoholic, she can frame the behavior in terms of behavioral theory: heavy-drinking behaviors related to a positive reinforcement history for drinking behaviors. Here, the nurse will look at the societal reinforcements for drinking—drinking heavily at parties, being taken out for drinks after work, and so on—as factors that contributed to alcoholism. Interventions would be aimed at changing environmental factors that reinforced drinking. In contrast, the same nurse can frame the heavy-drinking behaviors in terms of psychoanalytic theory and view the heavy-drinking*

behaviors as related to unmet needs for oral gratification. Here, the heavy-drinking behaviors are seen as symptoms of an underlying problem, and interventions would be aimed at meeting the developmental needs from the psychoanalytic perspective.

Interpersonal nursing theory guides the nurse to see the addict as an individual, a human being who has succumbed to the effects of a chemical and lost much of his humanity in the process—as William Burroughs asked when describing his addicted life, "Who or what was left to visit?" It is difficult to establish a relationship with one who is chemically dependent; however, the individual's recovery is almost certainly dependent on his ability to bond with others and to find a life worth living outside the drug world. Interpersonal theory suggests that the nurse approach the client as a caring human being, placing the full responsibility for the client's recovery in his own hands. The nurse can then provide caring, support, and, above all, honesty in all matters relating to recovery. One theme that seems to recur in work with addicted persons is that they do not see themselves as worthy of other persons' caring and attention. Years of abuse lead the person to lose self-esteem; many describe themselves as merely a shell. It is the goal of nursing interventions, then, to assist the client to regain himself, to find the humanness that was once there and literally build a new life.

APPLICATION OF THE NURSING PROCESS 17-1

A nurse in any setting in virtually every field of nursing will encounter chemical dependency in the course of routine work. Clearly, one recognizes that a nurse working in a chemical dependency unit will encounter addictions. However, few stop to recognize that every nurse in an emergency department, on a medical floor, in home care, or in the schools will be faced with alcohol or drug dependency.

To be adequately prepared to meet the needs of the client and family, the nurse must first make herself ready and willing to view chemical dependency as a disease and know that the client who wishes to recover has options that only he can take. The nurse can play a major role in directing the client to recovery programs and directing the family members to deal with their own dysfunction whether or not the client chooses to deal with his addiction.

ASSESSMENT

Assessment begins with a client history. The nurse should always inquire about use of alcohol and other substances. The nurse should begin with questions such as "Do you drink alcohol?" If the answer is "yes," follow-up questions such as "How much do you drink each week?" "Do you drink every day?" "Have you ever had trouble at work related to your drinking?" and "Have you missed work or school over the last month because of drinking?" should be asked to obtain a clearer picture of the degree to which alcohol plays a role in the client's life. Further questions such as "Do you take medications regularly?" "Do you use street drugs?" and "Have you used street drugs in the past?" help the nurse to obtain information regarding other addictive drugs. Lastly, questions about smoking and caffeine use are also indicated.

If the client has been using addictive substances regularly or if the client is admitted to a chemical dependency treatment unit, the nurse must assess closely for specific symptoms of withdrawal, described earlier in this chapter.

NURSING DIAGNOSIS

There are several nursing diagnoses that are common in situations of addictions. These relate to both client and family. A list is presented in Box 17-8.

OUTCOME IDENTIFICATION

The expected outcome of treatment for any chemical dependence is that the client chooses recovery and establishes a lifestyle that does not require use of addictive substances. There are, however, several outcomes of care viewing the recovery as a life-long process with several steps leading to complete recovery. A first expected outcome is the safe withdrawal from the addictive substance. A second outcome is that the client will choose recovery and begin to plan changes in his life based on finding needed supports to avoid

(*Continues*)

APPLICATION OF THE NURSING PROCESS 17-1 (Continued)

BOX 17-8
COMMONLY USED NURSING DIAGNOSES FOR CLIENTS ADDICTED TO CHEMICAL SUBSTANCES

PSYCHOSOCIAL DIAGNOSES

- *Ineffective coping*
- *Ineffective denial*
- *Dysfunctional family processes*
- *Chronic low self-esteem*
- *Social isolation*
- *Powerlessness*
- *Hopelessness*
- *Spiritual distress*

PHYSIOLOGICAL DIAGNOSES

- *Imbalanced nutrition, less than body requirements*
- *Risk for infection*

using the substance. A third expected outcome is that the client will remain free of the substance, first for one day, then for every other day of his life.

Caring for families, the nurse may identify an expected outcome that the family members will not take on the addict's illness; rather, the family will provide support for recovery and seek healthy family functioning whether the addict chooses recovery or not.

PLANNING/INTERVENTIONS

Interventions will be based on the setting in which the nurse finds herself and the availability of drug treatment programs. In many situations, the nurse will function in a collaborative role rather than as the primary care provider.

Nursing interventions include establishing a relationship with the client that is based on trust, grounded in reality, and characterized by firm kindness. Remembering that denial is the most commonly used defense mechanism by one who is addicted, the nurse must approach the client in a manner to challenge such denial.

Nursing interventions, then, must encourage a successful treatment plan: helping the client to make significant changes in lifestyle, friends, job, and so on are needed. Referrals to groups such as A.A. along with encouragement to enter into a long-term program (such as a 12-step program) are important nursing activities.

EVALUATION

Evaluation is based on expected outcomes. Many persons addicted to alcohol or drugs or both, choose recovery, but many do so only after several tries. The nurse must always be ready to help a client toward recovery at the level that the client wants.

CARE PLANNING GUIDE 17-1 Client Abusing Substances: Alcohol Abuse

CLINICAL PICTURE

The presenting pattern of a client who abuses alcohol is:

- A history of heavy drinking, such that the drinking impairs functioning (missed work, missed school)
- Evidence of alcohol intoxication or withdrawal, or both
- Denial of impact the drinking has on own life
- Family dysfunctions related to the alcohol abuse
- May have history of violent behavior associated with intoxication

COMMON NURSING DIAGNOSES

The nursing diagnoses most commonly employed for the client abusing alcohol are:

1. *Ineffective denial*
2. *Dysfunctional family processes*

The following Care Planning Guides depict suggested interventions, rationales, outcomes, and discharge planning for such clients.

NURSING DIAGNOSIS 1: *INEFFECTIVE DENIAL*, RELATED TO THREAT OF LOSS OF ALCOHOL FOR STRESS RELIEF PURPOSES

OUTCOMES

1. The client will verbalize facts of alcohol use.
2. The client will verbalize dependence on alcohol and accept the need for treatment.

NOC: *ACCEPTANCE: HEALTH STATUS*

INTERVENTIONS (NIC: *SUBSTANCE USE TREATMENT; TEACHING: DISEASE PROCESS*)	RATIONALE
• Assist the client to identify the use of denial as a substitute for confronting the problem and monitor the level or degree of denial.	• Denial is symptomatic of the disease; it can be mild/moderate/intense and tends to become more extreme as the alcoholism progresses.
• Determine the details about alcohol use; do not accept rationalizing statements about why the client is using alcohol; use confrontation as a communication technique.	• Denial can be reinforced by a nurse's avoidance of open and honest communication about alcohol or other drug use.
• Present specific facts about alcoholism and the disease.	• Education and knowledge of the disease is critical for the client's recovery.
• Involve family members in education about the disease.	• Family members may also be in denial and may impede treatment.
• Work with other members of the health care team to plan appropriate treatments and referrals.	• A multidisciplinary approach works best in planning treatment and in confronting denial, because continued denial is hard to maintain when there is strong concurrence among health care providers.

NURSING DIAGNOSIS 2: *DYSFUNCTIONAL FAMILY PROCESSSES:* RELATED TO FAMILY PATTERNS THAT SUSTAIN ALCOHOLISM

OUTCOMES

1. Family members will communicate openly about the alcoholism.
2. Family members will identify factors that affect care.
3. Family members will adopt behaviors that support recovery.

(*Continues*)

CARE PLANNING GUIDE 17-1 Continued

NOC: *FAMILY NORMALIZATION*

INTERVENTIONS (NIC: *FAMILY PROCESS MAINTENANCE; FAMILY INTEGRITY PROMOTION*)	RATIONALE
• Monitor family dynamics (roles, degree of impairment, degree of denial, degree of enabling behaviors).	• Family dynamics will determine the type, immediacy, and urgency of treatment needed.
• Appraise for physical violence, risk of violence, and degree of safety among family members.	• Immediate removal of dependent children and spouse may be recommended to ensure physical safety.
• Teach the family about the disease and the dynamics that sustain it.	• Knowledge is vital for the family members to support recovery, rather than to enable the alcoholic behaviors.
• Use therapeutic messages to convey that family members did not cause and are not responsible for the member's illness (alcoholism) or recovery.	• Family members often feel responsible and accountable; the alcoholic member often tells them it is their fault.
• Refer to community supports such as Al-Anon and Alateen where the family can interact with others dealing with the same issues.	• These groups represent ongoing support systems for a lifelong recovery process.

Note: The care planning guides have been adapted from *Plans for Care for Speciality Practice: Psychiatric Mental Health Nursing*, by M. Coler and K. Vincent, 1995, Clifton Park, NY: Delmar, Cengage Learning.

CARE PLANNING GUIDE 17-2 Client Abusing Substances: Cocaine Abuse

CLINICAL PICTURE

The presenting pattern of a client who abuses cocaine is:

- At the time of intoxication: affective/cognitive symptoms—euphoria, anxiety, psychomotor agitation; physical symptoms—may have pupillary dilatation, perspiration, chills, muscular weakness, respiratory depression, cardiac arrhythmia
- Impaired social functioning as the client relinquishes needs for safety and security for behaviors required to satisfy drug craving

COMMON NURSING DIAGONOSES

Nursing diagnoses most commonly used for the client abusing cocaine are:

1. *Risk for injury*
2. *Ineffective denial*

The Care Planning Guide that follows presents suggestions for interventions with rationales.

(*Continues*)

CARE PLANNING GUIDE 17-2 Continued

NURSING DIAGNOSIS: *RISK FOR INJURY,* RELATED TO EXTREME EFFORTS TO OBTAIN THE DRUG AND THE EXTREME EFFECTS AND SIDE EFFECTS OF THE DRUG

NOC: *RISK CONTROL: DRUG USE*

INTERVENTIONS (NIC: *SUBSTANCE ABUSE TREATMENT*)	RATIONALE
• Appraise the level of dependence—use, frequency, route, craving pattern.	• To make appropriate treatment referral, the level of dependence must be known.
• Refer to community supports, psychoeducation groups, and specific drug abuse groups; ensure that the client receives accurate information about cocaine use.	• Such groups provide accurate information about use of cocaine and the risks, as well as the hope for recovery.
• Provide for one-to-one counseling; encourage the client to engage in self-protecting behaviors.	• Over time, a one-to-one relationship with a counselor will increase chance of recovery.
• Refer to programs such as Cocaine Anonymous.	• The client will benefit from support of another who has maintained long-term sobriety.

See the Care Planning Guide for *ineffective denial* on page 434

Note: The care planning guides have been adapted from *Plans for Care for Speciality Practice: Psychiatric Mental Health Nursing*, by M. Coler and K. Vincent, 1995, Clifton Park, NY: Delmar, Cengage Learning.

CARE PLANNING GUIDE 17-3 Client Abusing Substances: Opioid Abuse

CLINICAL PICTURE

The behavior pattern that the client who is currently abusing opioids is:

- Confusion, slowed speech, delusions, hallucinations, memory deficit, and inaccurate interpretation of the environment.

COMMON NURSING DIAGNOSES

The commonly used nursing diagnoses for such clients are:

1. *Disturbed thought processes*
2. *Dysfunctional family processes*
3. *Ineffective denial*

The nursing interventions for *dysfunctional family processes* and *ineffective denial* can be derived from the Care Planning Guides on pages 434–435. Suggestions for care planning for the *disturbed thought processes* are presented in the Care Planning Guide that follows.

NURSING DIAGNOSIS: *DISTURBED THOUGHT PROCESSES,* RELATED TO CHEMICAL INTOXICATION

OUTCOMES

- The client will remain in a sheltered, safe environment.
- The client will have no or mild indicators of substance withdrawal.

(*Continues*)

CARE PLANNING GUIDE 17-3 Continued

NOC: *SUBSTANCE WITHDRAWAL SEVERITY*

INTERVENTIONS (NIC: *SUBSTANCE ABUSE TREATMENT: DRUG WITHDRAWAL*)	RATIONALE
• Monitor changes in thought processes in relation to the degree of intoxication or state of withdrawal.	• Allows for early identification of changes from baseline and contributes to individualized treatment plans.
• Treat the client for his physical needs, keep external stimuli to a minimum, and do not engage in confrontation or lengthy discussion with the client at this time.	• The client has altered thought processes due to an intoxication. The nursing care should deal with the intoxication and plan for the longer term treatment once the immediate intoxication has been treated. The client will not know that his thoughts are altered from reality and may react unexpectedly to interactions with others.
• Administer medications as per protocols for detoxification.	• Medications are used to avoid or eliminate severe withdrawal symptoms that could be life-threatening.
• Protect the client from harm to self and to others.	• Inaccurate perception of reality may cause the client to react defensively or violently.
• Work with an interdisciplinary team and community resources to recommend ongoing treatment.	• Opioid dependency requires the care of those who specialize in such treatment. The client will need long-term treatment and continued support for recovery.

LONG-TERM CONSIDERATIONS FOR THE CLIENT WHO ABUSES SUBSTANCES

Recognizing that chemical dependency is a lifelong disease, and that, ultimately, clients must make their own choices about recovery and are accountable for their own choices, the nurse should:

1. Initiate and maintain interdisciplinary collaboration for the client's treatment.
2. Arrange support for ongoing treatment.
3. Refer clients to ongoing community support groups, such as A.A.
4. Support the client to make choices helpful to his or her own recovery.
5. Support the family to make choices for their own health.

Note: The care planning guides have been adapted from *Plans for Care for Speciality Practice: Psychiatric Mental Health Nursing*, by M. Coler and K. Vincent, 1995, Clifton Park, NY: Delmar, Cengage Learning.

NURSING CARE PLAN: NURSING PROCESS FORMAT 17-1

In the excerpts presented in the discussion of alcoholism and its effects on families, Sanders and his father represent a family who could be encountered by a nurse. In his younger years, the father is presented as a man consumed by alcoholism—a husband/father who slips into the garage or barn to drink, who sleeps in a drunken stupor on the living room couch, who fights with his wife, who packs his bags to leave the family home, who then returns to his dysfunctional home. This father, however, stayed dry for 15 years, following the death of his own brother from alcohol abuse. The father's retirement signaled a return to his previous

(*Continues*)

NURSING CARE PLAN: NURSING PROCESS FORMAT 17-1 (Continued)

home (Mississippi) and a return to drinking. We are told, "He gave up his identity along with his job." Sanders visits his father only to discover, quite unexpectedly, that his father has resumed drinking and that his mother has been too distraught (or codependent) to tell her son that the father's illness has reemerged.

Based on the son's interpretation, the nurse would want to validate that the drinking behavior resumed because of a loss of direction or self-esteem, or both.

Further, the nurse would assess the personal significance to the father of his move back to Mississippi: What are the factors (social, environmental, familial) in Mississippi that contribute to drinking behaviors of this man? His personal history is important. Further, the wife's behavior is important to assess. Her son writes that she is "distraught." Assessment of her level of stress, her support, and verbal/physical abuse needs to be performed.

Imagine nurses are giving care to the Kerwin family, a family with an alcoholic father. The father, a retired mechanic, has moved the family to a smaller town. His increased drinking has disrupted family functioning. This family is going through similar experiences as those described by Sanders. The son has called a community health nurse to assist the family.

ASSESSMENT

The Kerwin family is undergoing confusion. The father of the family has alcoholism, and his drinking has disrupted family functioning. The father drinks in secrecy, but he is overtly impaired. The mother and wife alternates between anger, tears, and frustration. The father is drinking heavily, apparently as a result of his retirement from work.

NURSING DIAGNOSIS 1 Father: *Ineffective coping,* related to situational crisis (loss of social role and loss of support system), as evidenced by inability to meet role expectations (of father and retiree).

OUTCOMES	NIC	NURSING ACTIONS	EVALUATION
• Client will willingly participate in a treatment program within the next 3 weeks. • Client will choose recovery. • Within 2 weeks, client entered a program and began attending A.A. • Client will identify: (1) one negative effect of excessive alcohol consumption, and (2) two positive personal strengths. • Client will identify one behavior other than drinking to deal with life stressors.	• Coping enhancement • Substance use (alcohol) treatment	• Approach the client nonjudgmentally and establish a professional relationship. • Discuss alcoholism as a disease that is treatable. • Encourage the client to self-admit to a treatment program. • Offer referral to the program. • Encourage client to talk about himself and his life. • Point out personal strengths and positive traits, such as the fact that client stopped drinking for 15 years, he has his physical health at this time, and he has a good understanding of his disease.	The client began to think about his drinking as an illness; he admitted that the drinking was out of his control. He stated he could choose whether or not to take a drink, but if he did take but one drink, he could not choose when to stop drinking. Provide firm grounding in reality when the client uses denial by pointing out his behaviors and their effects.

(*Continues*)

NURSING CARE PLAN: NURSING PROCESS FORMAT 17-1 (Continued)

OUTCOMES	NIC	NURSING ACTIONS	EVALUATION
		• Introduce client to A.A., encourage him to talk with his A.A. sponsor; help him to see that A.A. is a support group where individuals help one another to stop drinking.	

NURSING DIAGNOSIS 2 Mother: *Fear*, related to living in unknown/unpredictable situations due to spouse's drinking behavior, as evidenced by her behavior described by son as "distraught" and past history of spousal fights during active drinking.

OUTCOMES	NIC	NURSING ACTIONS	EVALUATION
• Within 1 week, client will verbalize her fears. • Within 2 weeks, client will identify codependent behaviors and begin to take steps to meet her own needs for safety and security.	• Counseling • Substance use treatment	• Provide positive encouragement for client to talk with nurse; remain nonjudgmental, establish trust, and use interpersonal communication to affirm positive regard. • Help Mrs. Kerwin to recognize that alcoholism is a family disease that affects family function, and appraise the client's desire to participate in a support program; and encourage her to accept Al-Anon groups by explaining that many others in her situation have found support there. • Reaffirm client's personal integrity by letting her make her own choices. Give the control of decisions and treatment to her. Let her know you are there to assist.	Client almost immediately opened up to the nurse. She disclosed personal information regarding herself and her family. She is unhappy and is willing to consider a change but is afraid. She accepted information about Al-Anon. She asked the nurse to introduce her to one person from Al-Anon.

NURSING DIAGNOSIS 3 Family: *Dysfunctional family process:* related to abuse of alcohol, as evidenced by deterioration in family relationships, ineffective spousal communication, denial of problems, and enabling behaviors.

(*Continues*)

NURSING CARE PLAN: NURSING PROCESS FORMAT 17-1 (Continued)

OUTCOMES	NIC	NURSING ACTIONS	EVALUATION
• The family members will acknowledge to one another that they have a member with alcoholism and that this fact has affected their functioning for years.	• Mutual goal setting • Substance use treatment • Family process maintenance	• Visit with each family member individually and ask the family members if they would like to meet with the nurse as a group. • Provide information on the behaviors common in families experiencing alcoholism: enabling behaviors, use of denial, inability to communicate with one another, and fear of family violence. • Discuss strategies for normalization of family life.	Within 3 weeks time, the nurse had established a nurse-client relationship with each family member. The family members listened to and received written information on the behaviors of families dealing with alcoholism, but were not willing to talk with the nurse or any other counselor as group.

REFLECTIVE QUESTIONS

1. **ASSESSMENT**
   What other factors (e.g., input from the father's former coworkers) would help give a complete assessment picture of the father's apparent substance abuse?
2. **NURSING DIAGNOSIS**
   How can a nurse be truly holistic with this family?
3. **OUTCOMES**
   There were several clients in this situation. How often do we consider spouses, partners, children, and friends in treatment plans? How often should we?
4. **NURSING ACTIONS**
   How do nurses deal with "solutionless" problems?
5. **EVALUATION**
   How do you help a family or individual begin a lifelong process of recovery? Is the nurse's work ever done?

NURSING CARE PLAN: CONCEPT MAP FORMAT 17-1

Family with an Alcoholic Member

BACKGROUND INFORMATION

Don is a professional man who has a drinking problem. In fact, he has been a heavy drinker for years and has managed to cover up his problem with an engaging personality and superb insights on how to get people to work with him in teams, and cover for him when he is unable to complete his work. He is married, with two school-aged children. His wife has expressed deep concern over his drinking behaviors, because he

(Continues)

NURSING CARE PLAN: CONCEPT MAP FORMAT 17-1 (Continued)

drinks two to five drinks per night at home and sometimes goes to a bar and drinks more. On weekends, he drinks more heavily, and his wife, Betty, has to drive him home because she believes (correctly) that it is not safe for him to drive. Betty has confronted him about his drinking, and he becomes angry and loud, stating he just likes a drink or two and tells Betty she should stay out of his business.

A crisis has just presented itself for Don's family—Don was stopped for driving while intoxicated and has received both a fine (which he can pay) and a suspension of his driver's license for six months. Don is in denial that his drinking patterns are severe or even problematic. Betty sees the problem and doesn't really know where to turn. Betty is further concerned that Don will drive without a license, compounding the problems he currently faces. Both are worried that others (neighbors, community members, or relatives) might learn of Don's troubles, and both have the feeling that alcoholism is an embarrassing condition.

Don was required by the Department of Motor Vehicles to go to a class, and there he was provided information about A.A. and other community treatment options for alcoholism. Don informs Betty of the information and tells her that he will not attend because A.A. is not for people like him. There is a community clinic that treats chemical addictions that both Don and Betty know about and this clinic was on the list of referrals that Don received.

Betty decides to go and talk with a nurse at the community clinic, knowing that Don wouldn't go. Betty is gainfully employed and sees herself as an independent, modern woman. The nurse, Bruce, welcomes her and begins by getting some basic information.

Betty has been in the role of enabling Don to continue drinking and maintaining the semblance of success by doing the following: calling into work and telling the boss he is sick when he has a hangover; paying bills for his car and insurance and, one time, covering up for a minor accident he had by not claiming the accident on the car insurance; explaining to the children that their father needs a lot of rest and time off and making excuses for Don's failure to attend the children's school events. Betty has never felt physically vulnerable. Don has never hit her, but she does relate that she "backs off" every time there is a confrontation because she has seen it as her role to "keep the peace."

INITIAL ASSESSMENT AND REFLECTION

Bruce sees the patterns of a dysfunctional family, where Betty's behaviors are sustaining Don's illness and his denial. Betty is willing to admit there is a problem, but she is concerned about the family's reputation in the community. She doesn't want to hurt the children, and she has accepted the role of keeping the peace in the family. Betty is also concerned that she would be responsible if she behaved in a way such that Don lost his job.

INITIAL REVIEW OF NURSING DIAGNOSES

The nursing diagnoses and issues that Bruce considered are:

1. *Dysfunctional family processes*
2. *Ineffective denial* (Don)
3. *Deficient knowledge regarding* the disease and its management (Don and Betty)

PRIORITIES OF CARE

The concept map points to two focal areas: dysfunctional family processes and deficient knowledge regarding the disease of alcoholism. Bruce decides he must focus on the deficient knowledge at this time, because Betty needs to understand the nature of the disease, the role that good-intentioned family members play in enabling denial of the illness, and Don's lack of control over his drinking behaviors.

(*Continues*)

NURSING CARE PLAN: CONCEPT MAP FORMAT 17-1 (Continued)

NURSING INTERVENTIONS

Bruce begins by opening up the idea that alcoholism is a family problem, and that the behaviors of all members of the family are critical in the long-term recovery of the individual with the disease. He also opens up the idea that denial plays a very strong role in the dynamic of alcoholism and that the denial is the single most difficult issue in the beginning of treatment. Lastly, he points out that some of Betty's behaviors (calling in sick for Don when she knows he is not sick) work to enable Don to maintain a state of denial. Bruce was beginning a teaching/educational session by trying to uncover what level of knowledge Betty had and what level of information she was ready to accept. Bruce noted that Betty listened, took it all in, and seemed to understand, but did not say much. Bruce stated, "I know this is a crisis for you and your family right now. Further, I know I've given you a lot of information. The bottom line is that, from what you tell me, your husband has a disease and only he can bring this disease under control. Your behaviors can either assist him to stay in denial or push him toward understanding the logical consequences of this illness."

Bruce provided Betty with information about Al-Anon, a support group for family members of alcoholics, and offered himself as a resource to Betty in the future. Bruce gave Betty his business card and also asked if he could call her in a week's time for follow-up. Betty agreed to the follow-up phone call.

OUTCOME EVALUATION

This case illustrates a one time intervention with a family experiencing alcoholism. Bruce acted appropriately to provide information and accept Betty for who she was and where she was with her knowledge about the disease. Bruce understood the need for time to take in a new interpretation of one's own family. He provided referrals to community supports, and he established the follow-up phone call as a means to reach out to a client who may have great difficulty reaching out again. The fact that Betty agreed to a follow-up call from Bruce is positive. It opens the door to what might be a long recovery and healing process for Betty and her husband as well.

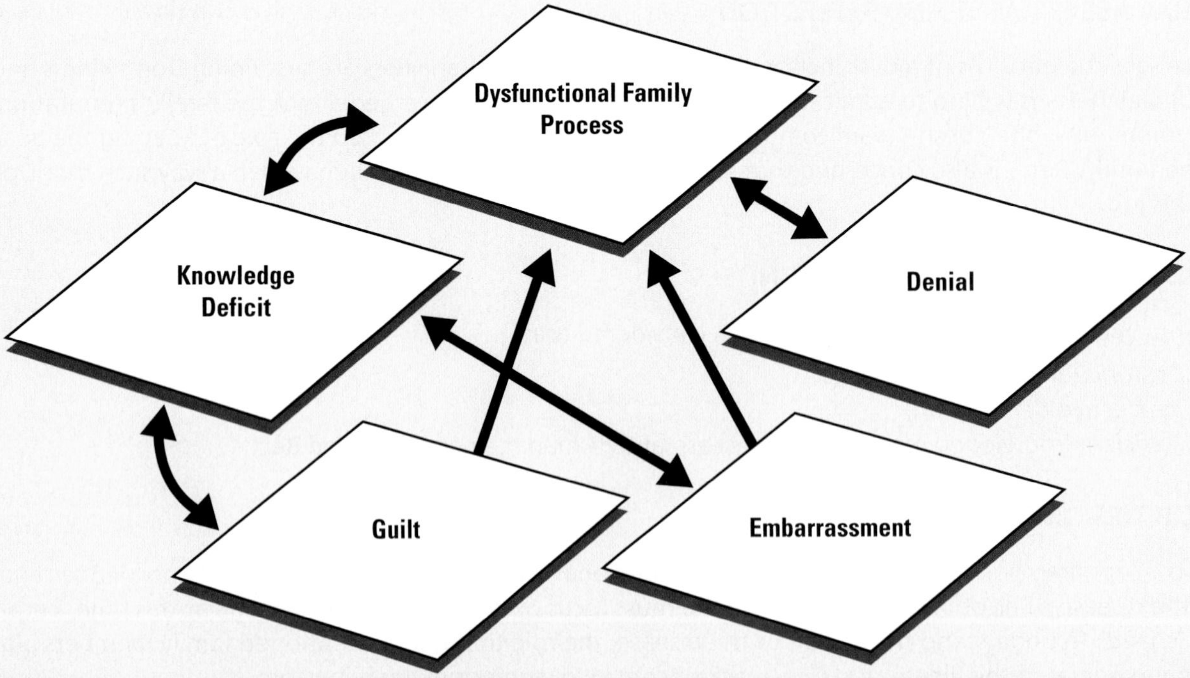

CONCEPT MAP OF ISSUES AND PROBLEMS (DELMAR/CENGAGE LEARNING.)

KEY CONCEPTS

- Substance abuse has been a part of human society since early human history.
- Most abused substances can be classified as stimulants, hallucinogens, or CNS depressants.
- Drug use refers to the taking of the drug; abuse refers to a maladaptive pattern of continued use despite real or potential harm.
- Tolerance is an acquired resistance to a drug's effects; withdrawal is a condition that occurs when stopping a drug results in a drug-specific set of symptoms that would be relieved by taking additional doses of the drug.
- Nicotine is the most commonly abused substance in the United States, with clear addictive properties.
- Alcohol abuse is typically diagnosed when alcohol use leads to work problems, hazardous practices, legal difficulties, or continuing use in the face of physical or social problems.
- Ninety percent of alcoholics have significant medical problems in addition to their alcohol dependence; thus, nurses come into contact with alcoholics in virtually every nursing specialty.
- Screening questionnaires like CAGE provide a means of identifying those who require referral.
- Treatment for alcohol dependence begins with a drug detoxification and is followed by counseling, group support, and medication.
- Alcoholics Anonymous (A.A.), based on 12 steps, provides individuals with group support and a method of learning to live without drinking.
- Cocaine, which affects the brain's reward centers, produces a high that includes a feeling of improved self-image and increased euphoria. In the form of crack, cocaine has exceedingly high addictive potential.
- Tolerance to cocaine is common, with persons reporting that their initial experiences of pleasure and euphoria are almost never replicated with continuing use.
- Opiates, which have important medical uses in relieving pain and apprehension, are widely abused because of their euphoric properties.
- The opiate addict has a need for increasingly higher doses and experiences distressing symptoms that occur anytime between 6 and 24 hours after the previous dose.
- Opiate addiction is a complex physical, psychological, and social phenomenon; treatment involves detoxification and helping the person to find human and spiritual content in a life that has been devoid of everything but the opiate subculture.
- Multidrug use is a growing problem in the United States.
- Many individuals who abuse substances have other psychiatric diagnoses as well.
- *Codependence* is a term used to describe the behaviors of family members who enable the addicted person to maintain the addiction while serving to satisfy the family members' needs to feel loved, important, and needed.
- Drug abuse affects families and is linked to violence, disrupted family roles, and impaired family communications.
- Both nursing theory and psychological theory guide the nurse in understanding the client and family and in planning interventions.

REVIEW QUESTIONS

1. When reviewing a client's chart, the nurse notes that the client had previously been prescribed Antabuse. The nurse knows that this medication is most often prescribed for which of the following disorders?
   1. Anxiety
   2. Alcoholism
   3. Depression
   4. Schizophrenia

2. A client who has a history of cocaine abuse is being discharged from a treatment facility. The discharge teaching by the nurse would include encouraging the client to do which of the following?
   1. Participate in an exercise program
   2. Divorce his wife who is still abusing cocaine
   3. Reduce the amount of drug consumption to prevent relapse
   4. Contact his primary care provider if he experiences flu symptoms

3. A client is admitted to the emergency department after a car accident. The nursing assessment reveals that the client has sustained a head injury and has several lacerations on his face and upper extremities. Laboratory results confirm that the client has heroin in his system. A priority nursing intervention would include which of the following?
   1. Refer the client to the mental health unit
   2. Clean and dress wounds to prevent infection
   3. Check vital signs and neurological signs
   4. Assure that the client is made comfortable

4. A client has been referred to a chemical rehabilitation facility by a judge after her involvement in a vehicle accident that killed two people. While in the facility the client is withdrawn and depressed. In a conversation with the nurse, the client states, "I'm no good. I am a drunk like my father. The world would be better without me." How should the nurse respond to the client's statement?
1. "Research shows that alcoholism runs in many families."
2. "The accident wasn't your fault so don't be sad."
3. "Are you having thoughts about hurting yourself?"
4. "My father was also an alcoholic. That's why I don't drink."

5. Which of the following is a priority in the discharge instructions for a client who has been prescribed Antabuse?
1. Follow a high calorie and high protein diet
2. Avoid food, drinks, and other products containing alcohol
3. Contact the primary care provider if the client experiences the desire to drink
4. Avoid driving or working with machinery

6. While caring for a client who was admitted to the hospital for chemical abuse, a therapeutic intervention for addressing the client's use of denial as an ego defense mechanism is which of the following?
1. Serve as the client's rescuer
2. Confront the client's behavior
3. Provide sympathy for the client
4. Tell the client he is a liar

7. A client is admitted for opioid intoxication. The nursing assessment would reveal which of the following?
1. Hypotension, nausea, confusion, and flight of ideas
2. Muscle stiffness, blurred vision, slowed speech, and confusion
3. Confusion, slowed speech, delusions, hallucinations, and memory deficit
4. Nausea, vomiting, confusion, and inaccurate interpretation of the environment

8. A nurse is developing a care plan for a client for opioid abuse. A priority nursing diagnosis would be which of the following?
1. Ineffective denial
2. Altered thought process
3. Dysfunctional family processes
4. Alteration in body image

9. A couple comes to the clinic for counseling. The wife begins to cry and states to the nurse, "My husband has a problem. He uses drugs. Lately he has been using more and more. He has emptied our savings account and begun taking items from our home to sell them so he can get more drugs." The nurse assesses that the husband has developed which of the following?
1. Addiction to drugs
2. Tolerance to the drug
3. Aversion to the drug
4. Love for the drug

LEARNING ACTIVITIES

1. Describe the nature of substance abuse in your home town, in your local high school, and on your college campus.

2. List the commonly abused substances in your region.

3. Identify factors that contribute to use and continued abuse of drugs in your community.

4. Identify community efforts to prevent as well as to treat drug abuse.

5. Identify the effects, withdrawal, and patterns of abuse for nicotine, alcohol, cocaine, and opiates.

6. Explain the major treatment approaches for drug dependence.

7. Examine the effects of alcohol or drug abuse on families and children in your community. What is being done to support families/children? What could the nurse do as a client advocate?

8. Use nursing theory to develop a care plan/treatment approach for a client you have seen with drug dependency.

*Study*WARE™ CONNECTION

Using your *Study*WARE™ CD-ROM

1. Complete the Concentration activity for this chapter.
2. Complete the Quiz for this chapter in Test Mode.
3. Explore the other games and activities that support this chapter.

VIDEO LINK

Read and contemplate the following questions about Tim, the client experiencing Alcohol Dependency. Then watch the video "Substance Related Disorders: Substance Dependence" on your *Study*WARE™ CD-ROM to observe Tim's interview with a psychiatrist. Consider these questions prior to listening to the psychiatrist's analysis.

1. Most substances are classified, how would we classify alcohol?
2. How is the diagnosis of alcoholism made?
3. What would the CAGE questionnaire reveal about Tim's drinking?
4. Is Tim fitting into the stages of the Natural History of Alcoholism in men?
5. Is he fitting into the profile of the Phases of Drinking Behavior in Alcoholics?
6. Tim describes himself as feeling forlorn: Can a diagnosis of depression be made if he is drinking?
7. How does Tim describe his path to alcohol tolerance?
8. What social and psychological effects has Tim's chronic alcoholism caused?
9. What do you think is the most dangerous effect of Tim's drinking to date?
10. Has Tim experienced withdrawal? What are typical symptoms of withdrawal?
11. What brought Tim to seek assistance at this point?
12. How does he describe the difference between Alcoholics Anonymous and Treatment programs?
13. Do you feel that Tim is aware of the seriousness of his addiction? Does he intend to stop drinking?
14. Describe the usual medical routine for treating someone during alcohol withdrawal.
15. Describe the measures that nurses can take to help clients cope with alcohol withdrawal and the period immediately following alcohol withdrawal.

REFERENCES

Alterman, A. I., O'Brien, C. P., McLellan, A. T., August, D. S., Snider, E. C., Droba, M., et al. (1994). Effectiveness and costs of inpatient versus day hospital cocaine rehabilitation. *Journal of Nervous and Mental Disease, 182*, 157–163.

American Psychiatric Association. (1994). *Diagnostic and statistical manual of mental disorders* (4th ed.). Washington, DC: Author.

American Psychiatric Association. (2000). *Diagnostic and statistical manual of mental disorders* (4th ed.-Text Revision). Washington, DC: Author.

Anonymous. (2000). Research refines alcoholism treatment options. *Alcohol Research Health, 24*(1), 53–61.

Anton, R. F., O'Malley, S. S., Ciraulo, D. A., Cisler, R. A., Couper, D., Donovan, D. M., et al. (2006). Combined pharmacotherapies and behavioral interventions for alcohol dependence: The COMBINE study: randomized controlled trial. *JAMA, 295*(17), 2003–2017.

Arnedt, J. T., Conroy, D. A., & Brower, K. J. (2007). Treatment options for sleep disturbances during alcohol recovery. *Journal of Addictive Diseases, 26*(4), 41–54.

Auriacombe M., Franques P., & Tignol J. (2001) Deaths attributable to methadone vs buprenorphine in France. *JAMA*, 285,45.

Bagnardi, V., Blangiardo, M., La Vecchia, C., & Corrao, G. (2001). A meta-analysis of alcohol drinking and cancer risk. *British Journal of Cancer, 85*(11), 1700–1705.

Ball, A. L. (2007). HIV, injecting drug use and harm reduction: A public health response. *Addiction, 102*(5), 684–690.

Bauer, L. O. (1992). Psychobiology of craving. In J. Lowinson, P., Ruiz, R. Millman, & J. Langrod (Eds.), *Substance abuse: A comprehensive textbook* (2nd ed., pp. 51–55). Baltimore: Williams & Wilkins.

Beeder, A. B., & Millman, R. B. (1992). Treatment of patients with psychopathology and substance abuse. In J. Lowinson, P. Ruiz, R. Millman, & J. Langrod (Eds.), *Substance abuse: A comprehensive textbook* (2nd ed., pp. 675–689). Baltimore: Williams & Wilkins.

Belluzzi, J. D., Wang, R., & Leslie, F. M. (2005). Acetaldehyde enhances acquisition of nicotine self-administration in adolescent rats. *Neuropsychopharmacology, 30*(4), 705–712.

Blum, L. H., Nielson, N. H., Riggs, J. A. (2000). Alcoholism and alcohol abuse among women: Report of the Council on Scientific Affairs, American Medical Association. *Journal of Women's Health, 7*(7), 861–871.

Boscarino, J. (1980). Factors related to stable and unstable affiliation with Alcoholics Anonymous. *International Journal of Addiction, 15*, 839–848.

Bottoroff, J. L., Johnson, J. L., Irwin, L. G., & Ratner, P. A. (2000). Narratives of smoking relapse: The stories of postpartum women. *Research in Nursing and Health, 23*(2), 121–134.

Boutrel, B. (2008). A neuropeptide-centric view of psychostimulant addiction. *British Journal of Pharmacology, 154*(2), 343–357.

Bower, B. (1994). Assaults may amplify female alcoholism. *Science News, 146*, 5.

Brain, P. F., & Coward, G. A. (1989). A review of the history, actions, and legitimate uses of cocaine. *Journal of Substance Abuse, 1*, 431–451.

Brandenburg, M. A., Brown, S. J., Arneson, W. L., & Arneson, D. L. (2007). The association of pseudoephedrine sales restrictions on emergency department urine drug screen results in Oklahoma. *Journal of the Oklahoma State Medical Association, 100*(11), 436–439.

Brendryen, H., & Kraft, P. (2008). Happy ending: A. randomized controlled trial of a digital multi-media smoking cessation intervention. *Addiction, 103*(3), 478–84; discussion 485–486.

Budney, A. J. (2006). Are specific dependence criteria necessary for different substances: How can research on cannabis inform this issue? *Addiction, 101 Suppl. 1*, 125–133.

Bunce, C. J., Loudon, P. T., Akers, C., Dobson, J., & Wood, D. M. (2003). Development of vaccines to help treat drug dependence. *Current Opinions in Molecular Therapy, 5*(1), 58–63,

Chang, G., & Kosten, T. (1992). Emergency management of acute drug intoxication. In J. Lowinson, P. Ruiz. R. Millman, & J. Langrod (Eds.), *Substance abuse: A comprehensive textbook* (2nd ed., pp. 437–445). Baltimore: Williams & Wilkins.

Chang, G., Wilkins-Haug, L., Berman, S., & Goetz, M. A. (1999). Brief intervention for alcohol use in pregnancy: A randomized trial. *Addiction, 94*(10), 1499–1508.

Committee on the Prevention of HIV Infection among Injecting Drug Users in High-Risk Countries. (2006). *Prevention of HIV infection among injecting drug users in high-risk countries: Assessing the evidence.* Washington, DC: National Academy Press.

Connock, M., Juarez-Garcia, A., Jowett, S., Frew, E., Liu, Z., Taylor, R. J., et al. (2007). Methadone and buprenorphine for the management of opioid dependence: A. systematic review and economic evaluation. *Health Technology Assessment, 11*(9), 1–171, iii–iv.

Crawford, J. T., Tolosa, J. E., & Goldenberg, R. L. (2008). Smoking cessation in pregnancy: Why, how, and what next. *Clinical Obstetrics and Gynecology, 51*(2), 419–435.

Cunningham, J. K., & Liu, L. M. (2008). Impact of methamphetamine precursor chemical legislation, a suppression policy, on the demand for drug treatment. *Social Science and Medicine, 66*(7), 1463–1473.

Delgado, M. R. (2007). Reward-related responses in the human striatum. *Annals of the New York Academy of Sciences, 1104*, 70–88.

Demir, B., Ucar, G., Ulug, B., Ulusoy, S., Sevinc, I., & Batur, S. (2002). Platelet monoamine oxidase activity in alcoholism subtypes: Relationship to personality traits and executive functions. *Alcohol and Alcoholism, 37*(6), 597–602.

Dyehouse, J. M., & Sommers, M. S. (1998). Brief intervention after alcohol-related injuries. *Nursing Clinics of North America, 33*(1), 93–104.

Edwards, J. A., Wesnes, K., Warburton, D. M., & Gale, A. (1985). Evidence of more rapid stimulus evaluation following cigarette smoking. *Addictive Behaviors, 10*, 113–126.

Emonson, D. L., & Vanderbeek, R. D. (1995). The use of amphetamines in U.S. Air Force tactical operations during Desert Shield and Storm. *Aviation Space and Environmental Medicine, 66*(3), 260–263.

Emrick, C. D. (1987). Alcoholics Anonymous affiliation process and effectiveness as treatment. *Alcohol, Clinical and Experimental Research, 11*, 416–423.

Epstein, E. E., Fischer-Elber, K., & Al-Otaiba, Z. (2007). Women, aging, and alcohol use disorders. *Journal of Women and Aging, 19*(1–2), 31–48.

Etter, J. F. (2008). [Commentary] The importance of reaching a consensual definition of dependence and of communicating this knowledge to the public. *Addiction, 103*(7), 1224–1225.

Ewing, J. A. (1984). Detecting alcoholism: The CAGE questionnaire. *Journal of the American Medical Association, 252*, 1905–1907.

Fatseas, M., & Auriacombe, M. (2007). Why buprenorphine is so successful in treating opiate addiction in France. *Current Psychiatry Reports, 9*(5), 358–364.

Feillin, D. A., Reid, M. C., O'Connor, P. G. (2000). New therapies for alcohol problems: Application to primary care. *American Journal of Medicine, 108*(3), 227–237.

Ferri, M., Amato, L., & Davoli, M. (2006). Alcoholics Anonymous and other 12-step programmes for alcohol dependence. *Cochrane Database of Systematic Reviews, 3*.

Frezza, M., DiPadova, C., Pozzato, G., Terpin, M., Bargona, E., Lieber, C. S. (1990). High blood alcohol levels in women: The role of decreased gastric alcohol dehydrogenase activity and first-pass metabolism. *New England Journal of Medicine, 322*, 95–99.

Frishman, W. H., Del Vecchio, A., Sanal, S., & Ismail, A. (2003). Cardiovascular manifestations of substance abuse part 1: Cocaine. *Heart Disease, 5*(3), 187–201.

Fuller, R. K., Branchley, L., & Brightwell, D. R. (1986). Disulfiram treatment of alcoholism: A Veteran's Administration cooperative study. *Journal of the American Medical Association, 256*, 1449–1455.

Gettig, J. P., Grady, S. E., & Nowosadzka, N. (2006) Methamphetamines: Putting the brakes on speed. *Journal of School Nursing, 22*(2), 66–73.

Gilman, J. M., Ramchandani, V. A., Davis, M. B., Bjork, J. M., & Hommer, D. W. (2008). Why we like to drink: A functional magnetic resonance imaging study of the rewarding and anxiolytic effects of alcohol. *Journal of Neurosciences, 28*(18), 4583–4591.

Gold, M. S. (1992). Cocaine (and crack): Clinical aspects. In J. Lowinson, P. Ruiz, R. Millman, & J. Langrod (Eds.), *Substance abuse: A comprehensive textbook* (2nd ed., pp. 205–206). Baltimore: Williams & Wilkins.

Goldstein, D. B., Chin, J. H., & Lyon, R. C. (1982). Ethanol disordering of spin-labeled mouse brain membranes—correlation with genetically-determined ethanol sensitivity of mice. *Proceedings of the National Academy of Science USA, 79*, 4231–4233.

Goodwin, D. W. (1992). Alcohol: Clinical aspects. In J. Lowinson, P. Ruiz, R. Millman, & J. Langrod (Eds.), *Substance abuse: A comprehensive textbook* (2nd ed.). Baltimore: Williams & Wilkins.

Graham, N. A., Merlo, L. J., Goldberger, B. A., & Gold, M. S. (2008). Methadone- and heroin-related deaths in Florida. *American Journal of Drug and Alcohol Abuse, 34*(3), 347–353.

Green, J. P., & Lynn, S. J. (2000). Hypnosis and suggestion-based approaches to smoking cessation: An examination of the evidence. *International Journal of Clinical Hypnosis, 48*(2), 195–224.

Grinspoon, L., & Bakalar, J. B. (1992). Marijuana. In J. Lowinson, P. Ruiz, R. Millman, & J. Langrod (Eds.), *Substance abuse: A comprehensive textbook* (2nd ed., pp. 236–246). Baltimore: Williams & Wilkins.

Grossman, M., Chaloupka, F. J., & Shim, K. (2002). Illegal drug use and public policy. *Health Affairs (Millwood), 21*(2), 134–145.

Grunberg, N. E. (1990). The inverse relationship between tobacco use and body weight. In L. T. Koslowski, H. M. Annis, & H. D. Cappell (Eds.), *Research advances in alcohol and drug problems* (Vol. 10, pp. 273–315). New York: Plenum.

Hammett, T. M., Wu, Z., Duc, T. T., Stephens, D., Sullivan, S., Liu, W., et al. (2008). "Social evils" and harm reduction: The evolving policy environment for human immunodeficiency virus prevention among injection drug users in China and Vietnam. *Addiction, 103*(1), 137–145.

Harper C. (2007) The neurotoxicity of alcohol. *Human Experimental Toxicology*, 26, 251–7.

Heath, R. G. (1964). Pleasure response of human beings to direct stimulation of the brain. In R. G. Heath (Ed.), *The role of pleasure in behavior* (pp. 219–243). New York: Hoeber.

Herdman, H. (Ed). (2009). *Nursing diagnoses: Definitions and classifications.* Oxford: Wiley Blackwell.

Higgins, S. T., Heil, S. H., Dantona, R., Donham, R., Matthews, M., & Badger, G. J. (2007). Effects of varying the monetary value of voucher-based incentives on abstinence achieved during and following treatment among cocaine-dependent outpatients. *Addiction, 102*(2), 271–281.

Hilton, B. A., Thompson, R., Moore-Dempsey, L., & Janzen, R. G. (2001). Harm reduction theories and strategies for control of human immunodeficiency virus: A review of the literature. *Journal of Advanced Nursing, 33*(3), 357–370.

Homer, B. D., Solomon, T. M., Moeller, R. W., Mascia, A., DeRaleau, L., & Halkitis, P. N. (2008). Methamphetamine abuse and impairment of social functioning: A review of the underlying neurophysiological causes and behavioral implications. *Psychological Bulletin, 134*(2), 301–310.

Hommer, D. W. (2003). Male and female sensitivity to alcohol-induced brain damage. *Alcohol Research and Health, 27*(2), 181–185.

Hubbard, R. I., Marsden, M. E., Rachal, J. V., Harwood, H. J., Cavannaugh, E. R., & Ginzburg, H. M. (1989). *Drug abuse treatment: A national study of effectiveness.* University of North Carolina at Chapel Hill Press.

Hughes, J. R. (2006). Should criteria for drug dependence differ across drugs? *Addiction, 101 Suppl. 1,* 134–141.

Hughes, P. H., Coletti, S. D., Neri, R. L., Urmann, C. F., Stahl, S., Aialian, D. M., et al. (1995). Retaining cocaine abusing women in a therapeutic community: The effect of a child live-in program. *American Journal of Public Health, 85,* 1149–1152.

Jaffe, J. H. (1990). Drug addiction and drug abuse. In A. G. Gilman, T. W. Rall, A. S. Nies, & P. Taylor (Eds.), *Goodman and Gilman's the pharmacological basis of therapeutics* (8th ed., pp. 311–331). New York: Pergamon.

Jarvik, M. E., & Schneider, N. G. (1992). Nicotine. In J. Lowinson, P. Ruiz, R. Millman, & J. Langrod (Eds.), *Substance abuse: A comprehensive textbook* (2nd ed., pp. 334–356). Baltimore: Williams & Wilkins.

Jellinek, E. M. (1952). Phases of alcohol addition. *Quarterly Journal of Studies on Alcohol, 13,* 673–684.

Jellinek, E. M. (1960). *The disease concept of alcoholism.* New Brunswick, NJ: Jillhouse.

Jesinski, D. R., Johnson, R. E., & Henningfield, J. E. (1984). Abuse liability assessment in human subjects. *Trends in Pharmacological Science, 5,* 96–200.

Johnson, B. A., Rosenthal, N., Capece, J. A., Wiegand, F., Mao, L., Beyers, K., et al. (2008). Improvement of physical health and quality of life of alcohol-dependent individuals with topiramate treatment: U.S. multisite randomized controlled trial. *Archives of Internal Medicine, 168*(11), 1188–1199.

Johnson, J. L., Rattner, P. A., Bottoroff, J. L., & Dahinten, S. (2000). Preventing smoking relapse in postpartum women. *Nursing Research, 49*(1), 44–52.

Johnston, L. M. (1985). Tobacco smoking and nicotine. *Lancet, 2,* 742.

Joseph, H., & Appel, P. (1985). Alcoholism and methadone treatment: Consequences for the patient and the program. *American Journal of Drug and Alcohol Abuse, 11,* 37–53.

Kaner, E. F., Beyer, F., Dickinson, H. O., Pienar, E., Campbell, F., Schlesinger, C., et al. (2007). Effectiveness of brief alcohol interventions in primary care populations. *Cochrane Database of Systematic Reviews* (2).

Karila, L., Gorelick, D., Weinstein, A., Noble, F., Benyamina, A., Coscas, S., et al. (2008). New treatments for cocaine dependence: A.A. focused review. *International Journal of Neuropsychopharmacology, 11*(3), 425–438.

Kranzler, H. R., Burleson, J. A., Del Boca, F. K., Babor, T. F., Korner, P., Brown, J., et al. (1994). Buspirone treatment of anxious alcoholics. A placebo-controlled trial. *Archives of General Psychiatry, 51,* 720–731.

Krystal, J. H., Pertrakis, I. L., Krupitsky, E., Schutz, C., Trevisan, L., & D'Sousa, D. (2003). NMDA receptor antagonism and the ethanol intoxication signal: From alcoholism risk to pharmacology. *Annals of the New York Academy of Sciences, 1003,* 176–184.

Larson, B. S. (2002). Medications through the Internet: What clinicians and patients need to know. *Journal of Pain, Palliative Care and Pharmacotherapy, 16*(2), 49–57.

Lee, N. K., & Rawson, R. A. (2008). A systematic review of cognitive and behavioural therapies for methamphetamine dependence. *Drug and Alcohol Review, 27*(3), 309–317.

Lender, M. E., & Martin, J. K. (1987). *Drinking in America: A history.* New York: Free Press.

Leweke, F. M., & Koethe, D. (2008). Cannabis and psychiatric disorders: It is not only addiction. *Addiction Biology, 13*(2), 264–275.

Lex, B. W. (1992). Alcohol problems in special populations. In J. H. Mendelson & N. K. Mello (Eds.), *Medical diagnosis and treatment of alcoholism* (pp. 71–154). New York: McGraw-Hill.

Limbu, B. (2008). The role of community-based nurses in harm reduction for HIV prevention: A South East and South Asia case study. *International Journal of Drug Policy, 19,* 211–213.

Lindeman, M., Hawks, J. H., & Bartek, J. K. (1994). The alcoholic family: A nursing diagnosis validation study. *Nursing Diagnosis, 5,* 65–73.

Littlejohn, C., & Holloway, A. (2008). Nursing interventions for preventing alcohol-related harm. *British Journal of Nursing, 17*(1), 53–59.

Lowinson, J. H. (1992). *Substance abuse: A comprehensive textbook* (2nd ed.). Baltimore: Williams and Wilkins.

Lowinson, J. H., Marion, I. J., Joseph, H., & Dole, V. P. (1992). Methadone maintenance. In J. Lowinson, P. Ruiz, R. Millman, & J. Langrod (Eds.), *Substance abuse: A comprehensive textbook* (2nd ed., pp. 550–561). Baltimore: Williams & Wilkins.

Mamber, N. (2006). Coke and smack at the drugstore: Harm reductive drug legalization: An alternative to a criminalization society. *Cornell Journal of Law and Public Policy, 15*(3), 619–664.

Mayfield, R. D., Harris, R. A., & Schuckit, M. A. (2008). Genetic factors influencing alcohol dependence. *British Journal of Pharmacology, 154*(2), 275–287.

McCann, U. D., Kuwabara, H., Kumar, A., Palermo, M., Abbey, R., Brasic, J., et al. (2008). Persistent cognitive and dopamine transporter deficits in abstinent methamphetamine users. *Synapse, 62*(2), 91–100.

McGregor, C., Srisurapanont, M., Jittiwutikarn, J., Laobhripatr, S., Wongtan, T., & White, J. M. (2005). The nature, time course and severity of methamphetamine withdrawal. *Addiction, 100*(9), 1320–1329.

McKetin, R., Kelly, E., & McLaren, J. (2006). The relationship between crystalline methamphetamine use and methamphetamine dependence. *Drug and Alcohol Dependency, 85*(3), 198–204.

Medical Letter. (1995). Naltrexone for alcohol dependence. *Medical Letter on Drugs and Therapeutics, 37,* 64–66.

Meredith, C. W., Jaffe, C., Ang-Lee, K., & Saxon, A. J. (2005). Implications of chronic methamphetamine use: Literature review. *Harvard Review of Psychiatry, 13*(3), 141–154.

Miller, G. (2008). Psychopharmacology. Tackling alcoholism with drugs. *Science, 320*(5873), 168–170.

Miller, N. S., & Greenfeld, A. (2004). Patients' characteristics and risk factors for development of dependence on hydrocodone and oxycodone. *American Journal of Therapeutics, 11*(1), 26–32.

Mizoue, T., Inoue, M., Wakai, K., Nagata, C., Shimazu, T., Tsuji, I., et al. (2008). Alcohol drinking and colorectal cancer in Japanese: A pooled analysis of results from five cohort studies. *American Journal of Epidemiology, 167*(12), 1397–1406.

Montalto, N. J., & Bean, P. (2003). Use of contemporary biomarkers in the detection of chronic alcohol use. *Medical Science Monitor, 9*(12), 285–290.

Muhonen, L. H., Lonnqvist, J., Juva, K., & Alho, H. (2008). Double-blind, randomized comparison of memantine and escitalopram for the treatment of major depressive disorder comorbid with alcohol dependence. *Journal of Clinical Psychiatry, 69*(3), 392–399.

Muller, C. P., Carey, R. J., & Huston, J. P. (2003). Serotonin as an important mediator of cocaine's behavioral effects. *Drugs Today, 39*(7), 497–511.

Musto, D. F. (1992). Historical perspectives on alcohol and drug abuse. In J. Lowinson, P. Ruiz. R. Millman, & J. Langrod (Eds.), *Substance abuse: A comprehensive textbook* (2nd ed.). Baltimore: Williams & Wilkins.

Nace, E. P., Davis, C. W., & Gaspari, J. P. (1991). Axis II comorbidity in substance abusers. *American Journal of Psychiatry, 148,* 118–120.

Newton, T. F., Cook, I. A., Kalechstein, A. D., Duran, S., Monroy, F., Ling, W., et al. (2003). Quantitative EEG abnormalities in recently abstinent methamphetamine dependent individuals. *Clinical Neurophysiology, 114*(3), 410–415.

Ngo, A. D., Schmich, L., Higgs, P., & Fischer, A. (2008). Qualitative evaluation of a peer-based needle syringe programme in Vietnam. *International Journal of Drug Policy, 20,* 179–182.

Nichols, M. R. (1999). The use of bupropion hydrochloride for smoking cessation therapy. *Clinical Excellence for Nurse Practitioners,* 3(6), 317–322.

Nicholson, B. (2003). Responsible prescribing of opioids for the management of chronic pain. *Drugs, 63*(1), 17–32.

Nicoll, R. A., & Alger, B. E. (2004). The brain's own marijuana. *Scientific American, 291*(6), 68–75.

Nides, M. (2008). Update on pharmacologic options for smoking cessation treatment. *American Journal of Medicine, 121*(4 Supplement 1), S20–31.

Nutt, D. J. (1996). Addiction brain mechanism and their related implications. *Lancet, 347,* 33–35.

Nutt, D., King, L. A., Saulsbury, W., & Blakemore, C. (2007). Development of a rational scale to assess the harm of drugs of potential misuse. *Lancet, 369*(9566), 1047–1053.

O'Malley, S. S., Jaffe, A. J., Chang, G., Schottenfeld, R. S., Meyer, R. E., & Rounsaville, B. (1992). Naltrexone and coping skills therapy for alcohol dependence: A controlled study. *Archives of General Psychiatry, 49,* 881–887.

Paulus, M. P., Tapert, S. F., & Schuckit, M. A. (2005). Neural activation patterns of methamphetamine-dependent subjects during decision making predict relapse. *Archives of General Psychiatry, 62*(7), 761–768.

Pauly, B. B. (2008). Shifting moral values to enhance access to health care: Harm reduction as a context for ethical nursing practice. *International Journal of Drug Policy, 19*(3), 195–204.

Pauly, B. B., & Goldstone, I. (2008). Harm reduction in nursing practice: Current status and future directions. *International Journal of Drug Policy, 19*(3), 179–182.

Percival, J. (2003). The place of pharmacotherapy product in smoking cessation. *Professional Nurse, 19*(2), 113–117.

Prochazka, A. V. (2000). New developments in smoking cessation. *Chest, 117*(Suppl. 1), 1695–1755.

Raloff, J. (1994). Cigarettes: Are they doubly addictive? *Science News, 145,* 294.

Reis, A. D., Castro, L. A., Faria, R., & Laranjeira, R. (2008). Craving decrease with topiramate in outpatient treatment for cocaine dependence: An open label trial. *Revista Brasileira de Psiquiatria, 30*(2), 132–135.

Richardson, K., Baillie, A., Reid, S., Morley, K., Teesson, M., Sannibale, C., et al. (2008). Do acamprosate or naltrexone have an effect on daily drinking by reducing craving for alcohol? *Addiction, 103*(6), 953–959.

Rinaldi, R. C., Steindler, E. M., Wilford, B. B., & Goodwin, D. (1988). Clarification and standardization of substance abuse terminology. *Journal of the American Medical Association, 259,* 555–567.

Ritter, A, Cameron, J. (2006) A review of the efficacy and effectiveness of harm reduction strategies for alcohol, tobacco and illicit drugs. *Drug and Alcohol Reviews,* 25(6), 611–624.

Robins, L. N. (1979). Addict careers. In R. I. Dupont, A. Goldstein, & J. O'Donnell (Eds.), *Handbook on drug abuse* (pp. 325–336). Washington, DC: U.S. Government Printing Office.

Rosencrans, J. A., & Chance, W. T. (1977). Cholinergic and noncholinergic aspects of the discriminative stimulus properties of nicotine. In H. Lai (Ed.), *Discriminative stimulus properties of drugs* (pp. 155–186). New York: Plenum.

Scavnicky-Mylant, M. (1990). The process of coping among young adult children of alcoholics. *Journal of Studies on Alcohol, 43,* 119–128.

Schuckit, M. A. (1992). Treatment of alcoholism in office and outpatient settings. In J. H. Mendelson & N. K. Mello (Eds.), *Medical diagnosis and treatment of alcoholism* (pp. 363–392). New York: McGraw-Hill.

Schuckit, M. A., & Irwin, M. (1988). Diagnosis of alcoholism. *Medical Clinics of North America, 72,* 1133–1153.

Schultz, W. (2001). Reward signaling by dopamine neurons. *Neuroscientist,* 7(4), 293–302.

Scott, J. C., Woods, S. P., Matt, G. E., Meyer, R. A., Heaton, R. K., Atkinson, J. H., et al. (2007). Neurocognitive effects of methamphetamine: A critical review and meta-analysis. *Neuropsychology Review, 17*(3), 275–297.

Semple, D. M., McIntosh, A. M., & Lawrie, S. M. (2005). Cannabis as a risk factor for psychosis: Systematic review. *Journal of Psychopharmacology, 19*(2), 187–194.

Shields, L. B., Hunsaker Iii, J. C., Corey, T. S., Ward, M. K., & Stewart, D. (2007). Methadone toxicity fatalities: A review of medical examiner cases in a large metropolitan area. *Journal of Forensic Sciences, 52*(6), 1389–1395.

Siegel, R. K. (1989). *Intoxication.* New York: E. P. Dutton.

Solinas, M., Goldberg, S. R., & Piomelli, D. (2008). The endocannabinoid system in brain reward processes. *British Journal of Pharmacology, 154*(2), 369–383.

Spohr, H. L., Willms, J., & Steinhausen, H. C. (2007). Fetal alcohol spectrum disorders in young adulthood. *Journal of Pediatrics, 150*(2), 175–179.

Stead, L. F., Perera, R., & Lancaster, T. (2006). Telephone counselling for smoking cessation. *Cochrane Database of Systematic Reviews,* (3).

Stecker, T., Han, X., Curran, G. M., & Booth, B. M. (2007). Characteristics of women seeking intensive outpatient substance use treatment in the VA. *Journal of Women's Health (Larchmont), 16*(10), 1478–1484.

Svikis, D. S., & Reid-Quinones, K. (2003). Screening and prevention of alcohol and drug use disorders in women. *Obstetrics and Gynecological Clinics of North America, 30*(3), 447–468.

Talhout, R., Opperhuizen, A., & van Amsterdam, J. G. (2007). Role of acetaldehyde in tobacco smoke addiction. *European Neuropsychopharmacology, 17*(10), 627–636.

Uhl, G. R. (2004). Molecular genetics of substance abuse vulnerability: Remarkable recent convergence of genome scan results. *Annals of the New York Academy of Sciences, 1025,* 1–13.

Vaillant, G. E. (1982). Natural history of male alcoholism. *Archives of General Psychiatry, 39,* 127–133.

van Amsterdam, J., Talhout, R., Vleeming, W., & Opperhuizen, A. (2006). Contribution of monoamine oxidase (MAO) inhibition to tobacco and alcohol addiction. *Life Sciences, 79*(21), 1969–1973.

Vanicelli, M., & Nash, L. (1984). Effect of sex bias on women's studies on alcoholism. *Alcoholism, Clinical and Experimental Research, 8,* 334–336.

Vasica, G., & Tennant, C. C. (2002). Cocaine use and cardiovascular complications. *Medical Journal of Australia, 177*(5), 260–262.

Vengeliene, V., Bilbao, A., Molander, A., & Spanagel, R. (2008). Neuropharmacology of alcohol addiction. *British Journal of Pharmacology, 154*(2), 299–315.

Victor, M. (1992). The effects of alcohol on the nervous system. In J. H. Mendelson & N. K. Mello (Eds.), *Medical diagnosis and treatment of alcoholism* (pp. 201–262). New York: McGraw-Hill.
Vining, E., Kosten, T. R., & Kleber, H. G. (1988). Clinical utility of rapid clonidine-naltrexone detoxification for opioid abusers. *British Journal of Addiction, 83,* 567–575.
Weiss, R. D., Mirin, S. M., Michael, J. I., & Sollogrub, A. C. (1986). Psychopathology in chronic cocaine abusers. *American Journal of Drug and Alcohol Abuse, 12,* 17–29.
West, R., & Zhou, X. (2007). Is nicotine replacement therapy for smoking cessation effective in the "real world"? Findings from a prospective multinational cohort study. *Thorax, 62*(11), 998–1002.
White, A. R., Rampes, H., & Campbell, J. L. (2006). Acupuncture and related interventions for smoking cessation. *Cochrane Database of Systematic Reviews* (1).
Winzer-Serhan, U. H. (2008). Long-term consequences of maternal smoking and developmental chronic nicotine exposure. *Frontiers in Bioscience, 13,* 636–649.
Woods, G. (1993). *Drug abuse in society.* Santa Barbara, CA: ABC-CLIO.
Zimring, F. E., & Hawkins, G. (1992). *The search for rational drug control.* Cambridge: Cambridge University Press.

LITERARY REFERENCES

Burroughs, W. (1960). Deposition: Testimony concerning a sickness. *Evergreen Review, 4,* 18.
Clark, R. W. (1980). *Freud: The man and the cause.* New York: Random House.
Freud, S. (1975/1960). *Letters of Sigmund Freud.* (J. Stern, Trans.). New York: Basic Books.
Sanders, S. R. (1989, November). Under the influence. *Harper's Magazine,* 68–75.
Svevo, I. (1958). *Confessions of Zeno.* New York: Vintage.
Twain, M. (1987). *The adventures of Huckleberry Finn.* Berkeley: University of California Press.
Wilde, O (1993). *The picture of Dorian Gray.* New York: Dover, p. 78.

SUGGESTED READINGS

Committee on the Prevention of HIV Infection among Injecting Drug Users in High-Risk Countries. (2006). *Prevention of HIV infection among injecting drug users in high-risk countries: Assessing the evidence.* Washington: National Academy Press. Available online at URL: http://www.nap.edu/catalog.php?record_id=11731#toc, as accessed 7/7/2008.
Mate, G. (2008). *In the realm of hungry ghosts: Close encounters with addiction.* Toronto: Knopf Canada.
Weaver, A. (2007). *Gone to the crazies: A memoir.* New York: Harper Collins.

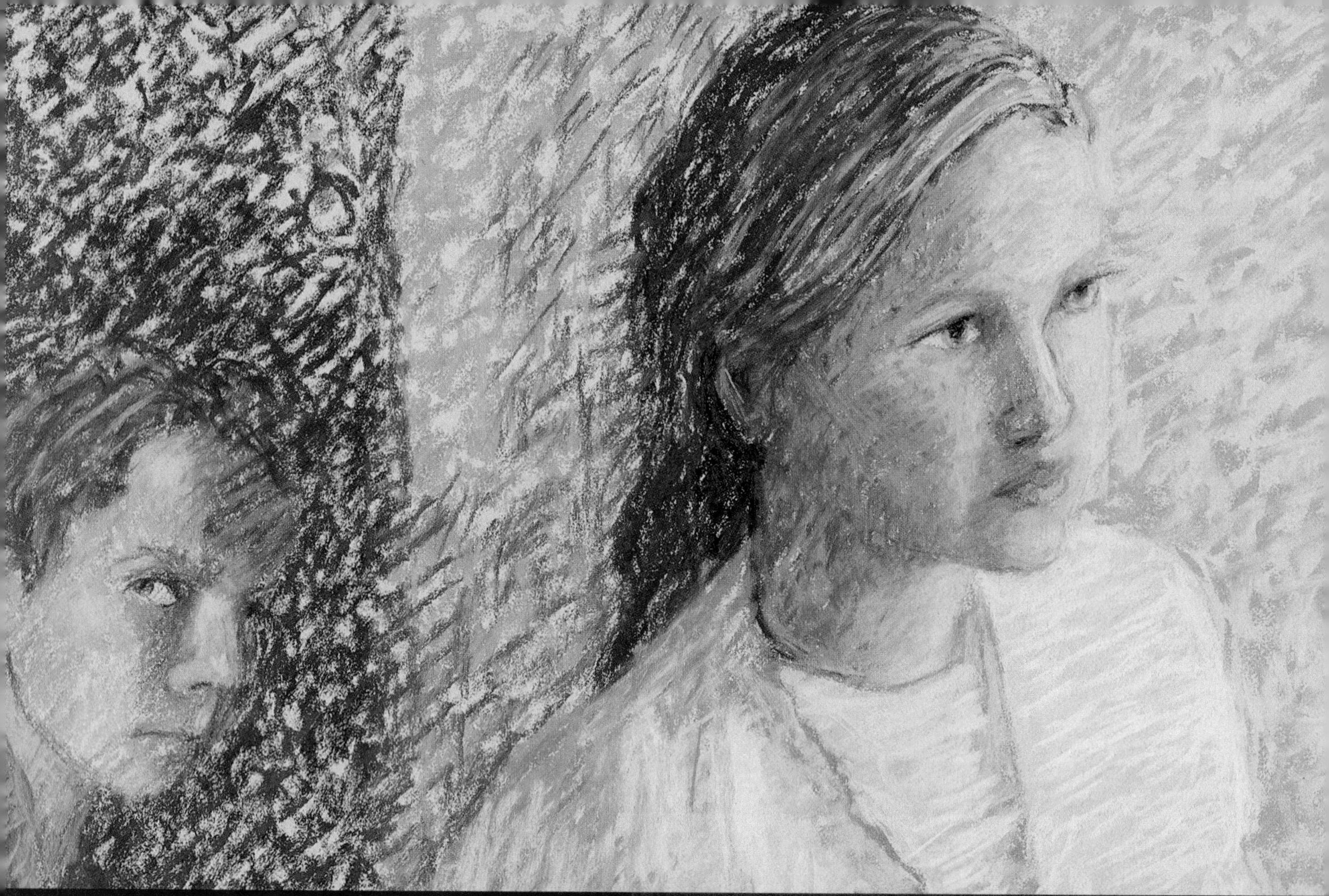

Personality and You

Boundaries

Consider the following:

- ***What qualities do you present to others?***
- ***How would your best friend describe you?***
- ***How would your teachers/boss describe you?***

Can you identify any experiences that you believe shaped your personality?

Is your personality like that of one of your parents? Your siblings?

Recognize that each person has a number of characteristics that make up who he is and how he presents himself to the world. In this chapter, we explore personality characteristics that are dysfunctional and learn how to identify normal variations from disorders.

CHAPTER 18

The Client with a Personality Disorder

LAWRENCE E. FRISCH

CHAPTER OUTLINE

COMPETENCIES

Upon completion of this chapter, the reader should be able to:

1. Define *personality*, *personality trait*, and *personality disorder*.
2. Differentiate between a person with eccentric personality traits and a person with a personality disorder.
3. Identify characteristics of specific personality disorders.
4. Describe how early childhood influences can affect personality development.
5. Use nursing theory to understand a client with a personality disorder and to plan appropriate nursing interventions.

KEY TERMS

Antisocial Personality Disorder
Avoidant Personality Disorder
Borderline Personality Disorder
Dependent Personality Disorder
Histrionic Personality Disorder
Narcissistic Personality Disorder
Obsessive-Compulsive Personality Disorder
Paranoid Personality Disorder
Passive-Aggressive Personality Disorder
Personality
Personality Disorder
Personality Traits
Schizoid Personality Disorder
Schizotypal Personality Disorder

A dictionary definition of **personality** reads: "habitual patterns and qualities of behavior of any individual as expressed by physical and mental activities and attitudes; distinctive individual qualities of a person" (Guralnik, 1982, p. 1062). Every person has his own personality, and by this we mean that each individual has characteristic **personality traits** or qualities that make him unique. Living in a society as diverse as the modern United States, one can observe a wide variation in personality traits. Some persons are shy and retiring, others loud and boisterous; some persons are full of humor, others rather morose; some are spontaneous in action, others thoughtful and considered. All of these traits could be used to describe a person's personality, and each individual has a number of characteristics contributing to his personality as a whole. Personality traits tend to be stable patterns over time and influence how a person looks, behaves, and reacts to life's events.

Clusters of personality traits are sometimes used to describe a person's personality style. An individual might be described as flexible, resourceful, and compassionate if he has a style that exhibits these rather healthy characteristics. In contrast, some individuals have developed personality styles that demonstrate unhealthy characteristics—styles that limit the ability to function in society. Such an individual is said to have a personality disorder.

A **personality disorder** is defined by the *Diagnostic and Statistical Manual, Fourth Edition-Text Revision* (DSM-IV-TR) as "an enduring pattern of inner experience and behavior that deviates markedly from the expectations of the individual's culture, is pervasive and inflexible, has an onset in adolescence or early adulthood, is stable over time, and leads to distress or impairment" (American Psychiatric Association, 2000, p. 686). As detailed in Chapter 5 of this text, personality disorders are identified on Axis II of DSM. In general, personality disorders seem to derive from interactions among an individual's temperament, family upbringing, and life experiences. In turn, they strongly color an affected individual's reaction to stress, illness, and other psychiatric disorders. The multiaxial approach has been adopted by DSM to emphasize that Axis I disorders (primary psychiatric diagnoses such as Depression, Mania, Schizophrenia, Panic Disorder) are constant across all personality types, but their impact on the individual and their management are strongly influenced by underlying personality factors.

There are several personality disorders identified in DSM that present rather commonly to the nurse in both psychiatric and general nursing practice. These personality disorders are categorized into three clusters, each with somewhat similar characteristics. The clusters are based on behaviors observed and are (1) dramatic and emotional, (2) odd and eccentric, and (3) anxiety and fear based. Table 18-1 offers a summary of personality disorders grouped by cluster. The

NURSINGTIP 18-1

As Axis II disorders, personality disorders are NOT illnesses or conditions that a person acquires at some point in his/her life—personality disorders are descriptions of the characteristics that an individual has and expresses that make up the whole of who the individual is. These characteristics impact virtually every other aspect of the person's psychosocial functioning.

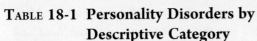

Table 18-1 Personality Disorders by Descriptive Category

DESCRIPTION	PERSONALITY DISORDER
Dramatic and emotional	Borderline Personality Disorder Narcissistic Personality Disorder Histrionic Personality Disorder Antisocial Personality Disorder
Odd and eccentric	Schizoid Personality Disorder Schizotypal Personality Disorder Paranoid Personality Disorder
Anxiety and fear based	Obsessive-Compulsive Personality Disorder Avoidant Personality Disorder Dependent Personality Disorder Passive-Aggressive or Negativistic Personality Disorder*

*Passive-Aggressive Personality Disorder was removed from the list of personality disorders in DSM-IV and is included in DSM-IV-TR as a category requiring further study.

important factor for the nurse to understand is that a personality disorder is identified only if the cluster of personality traits observed clearly leads to distress or impairment. Many, even most, persons have some elements of a disordered personality in their own makeups. Although these personality elements may cause occasional personal or social difficulties, unless they constitute "inflexible and pervasive" patterns *and* lead to "clinically significant distress or impairment," they do not constitute a personality disorder.

This chapter identifies and describes 11 personality disorders in detail. The clinical descriptions of personality disorders are often dry and remote, and nurses may approach the understanding of personality disorders as purely an exercise in memorizing lengthy names and unusual characteristics and behaviors. These conditions are too interesting, vivid, and important to be studied in this abstract way, however. In an effort to bring the reader some "flavor" of these disorders, this discussion provides the name of the personality disorder followed by a literary excerpt that presents behaviors consistent with the personality disorder described. A textbook description of the disorder then follows.

DRAMATIC AND EMOTIONAL PERSONALITY CLUSTER

The common theme of these personality disorders is the inability to establish and maintain close interpersonal relationships. The individual with one of these personality disorders exhibits labile mood swings, for example, going from laughter to tears in seconds. Behavior often appears calculated or cunning to accomplish a goal, such as maintaining the attention of others or gaining power or domination over others.

Borderline Personality Disorder

ANNIE

She was laughing. At first he thought she might be crying, but she was laughing....

She laughed and kicked her legs and gave off an air, an odor, of intense fleshy heat. I won't survive this one, she giggled....

At Christmas, somehow, they lost contact with each other. Days passed. Twelve days. Fifteen. His widowed mother came to visit them in the big red-brick colonial in Lathrup Park, and his wife's sister and her husband and two young children, and his oldest boy, a freshman at Swarthmore, brought his Japanese roommate home with him; life grew dense, robustly complicated. He telephoned her at the apartment but no one answered....

A girl in a raw unfinished painting. Like the crude canvases on exhibit at the gallery, that day he had drifted by: something vulgar and exciting about the mere droop of a shoulder, the indifference of a strand of hair blown into her eyes. And the dirt-edged fingernails. And the shoes with the run-over heels. She was raw, unfinished, lazy, slangy, vulgar, crude, mouthing in her cheerful insouciant voice certain words and phrases [he] would never have said aloud in the presence of a member of the opposite sex; but at the same time it excited him to know that she was highly intelligent, and really well-educated, with a master's degree in art history and a studied, if rather flippant, familiarity with the monstrousness of contemporary art. He could not determine whether she was as impoverished as she appeared or whether it was a pose, an act....

It excited him to imagine her haphazard, promiscuous life; he knew she was entirely without guilt or shame or self-consciousness, as if, born of a different generation, she were of a different species as well....

In early March he saw her again, but only for lunch. She insisted he return to the gallery to see their current show—ugly, frantic, oversized hunks of sheet metal and aluminum, seemingly thrown at will onto the floor....

He led her to his car. They were both smiling.

Where are we going? she asked....

He watched her face as he drove along Washburn Lane, which was graveled and tranquil and hilly. Is this—? Do you live—? she asked. He brought her to the big red-brick colonial he had bought nearly fifteen years ago; it seemed to him that the house had never looked more handsome, and the surrounding trees and blossoming shrubs had never looked more beautiful....

But—Where is—Aren't you afraid—?

There's no one home, he said.

He led her through the foyer, into the living room with its thick wine-colored rug, its gleaming furniture, its many windows. He led her through the formal dining room and into the walnut-paneled recreation room where his wife had hung lithographs and had arranged innumerable plants, some of them hanging from the ceiling in clay pots, spidery-leafed, lovely. He saw the girl's eyes dart from place to place....

She asked him why he had brought her here and he said he didn't know....

Then she kicked about, and laughed, and chattered. He was sleepy, pleasantly sleepy. He did not mind her chatter, her high spirits. While she spoke of one thing or another ... he watched through half-closed eyes the play of shadows on the ceiling....

His snoring disturbed him. For an instant he woke, then sank again into a warm grayish ether ... then his snoring woke him again and he sat up.

Annie?

Her things were still lying on the floor. The red blouse lay draped across a chintz-covered easy chair whose bright red and orange flowers, glazed, dramatic, seemed to be throbbing with energy. Annie? Are you in the bathroom?

The bathroom door was ajar, the light was not on. He got up. He saw that it was after two. A mild sensation of panic rose in his chest, for no reason. He was safe. They were safe here. No one would be home for hours.... The house was silent. It was empty.

He thought: What if she steals something?

But that was ridiculous and cruel. Annie would never do anything like that.

No one was in this bathroom, which was his wife's. He went to a closet and got a robe and put it on, and went out into the hallway, calling Annie?—Honey?—and knew, before he turned the knob to his own bathroom, that she was in there and that she would not respond. Annie? What's wrong?

The light switch to the bathroom operated a fan; the fan was on; he pressed his ear against the door and listened. Had she taken a shower? He didn't think so. Had not heard any noises. Annie, he said, rattling the knob, are you in there, is anything wrong? He waited. He heard the fan whirring. Annie? His voice was edged with impatience. Annie, will you unlock the door? Is anything wrong?

She said something—the words were sharp and unintelligible.

Annie? What? What did you say? ...

Again her high, sharp voice. It sounded like an animal's shriek. But the words were unintelligible....

He heard the lock being turned, suddenly.

He opened the door.

She must have taken the razor blade out of his razor, which she had found in the medicine cabinet. Must have leaned over the sink and made one quick, deft, hard slash with it—cutting the fingers of her right hand also. The razor blade slipped from her then and fell into the sink. There was blood on the powder-blue porcelain of the sink and the toilet, and on the fluffy black rug, and on the mirror, and on the blue-and-white tiled walls. When he opened the door and saw her, she screamed, made a move as if to strike him with her bleeding arm, and for an instant he could not think: could not think: what had happened, what was happening, what had this girl done to him? Her face was wet and distorted. Ugly. She was sobbing, whimpering. There was blood, bright blood, smeared on her breasts and belly and thighs: he had never seen anything so repulsive in his life....

He was paralyzed. Yet, in the next instant, a part of him came to life. He grabbed a towel and wrapped it around her arm, struggling with her. Stop! Stand still! For God's sake! ...

Why did you do it? Why? Why? You're crazy! You're sick! This is a—this is a terrible, terrible—a terrible thing, a crazy thing—

Her teeth were chattering. She had begun to shiver convulsively ... I hate you—I don't want to live—

She pushed past him, she staggered into the bedroom. The towel came loose. He ran after her and grabbed her and held the towel against the wound again, wrapping it tight, so tight she flinched. His brain reeled. He saw blood, splotches of blood, starlike splashes on the carpet, on the yellow satin bedspread that had been pulled onto the floor....

After some time the bleeding was under control. He got another towel, from his wife's bathroom, and wrapped it around her arm again. It stained, but not so quickly. The bleeding was under control; She was not going to die.

*He had forced her to sit down. He crouched over her, breathing hard, holding her in place. What if she sprang up, what if she ran away?—through the house? He held her still. She was spiritless, weak. Her eyes were closed. In a softer voice he said, as if speaking to a child: Poor Annie, poor sweet girl, why did you do it, why, why did you want to hurt yourself, why did you do something so ugly? ... It was an ugly, ugly thing to do.**

(Oates, 1981, pp. 509–518)

*From "The Tryst," in *Sentimental Education*, by Joyce Carol Oates, 1981.

This excerpt from "The Tryst" is profoundly shocking. The reader certainly agrees with John that Annie's cutting herself is as ugly as it is totally unexpected. Why, indeed, did Annie want to hurt herself? One very plausible explanation is that Annie has the psychological condition known as **Borderline Personality Disorder** (BPD). The essential features of BPD are patterns of unstable interpersonal relationships and self-image, efforts to avoid being abandoned, and impulsive actions. Annie's impulsive swings of emotion from childish laughter to abject despondency are highly characteristic of BPD. Recurrent self-mutilating behavior, especially cutting, is another important BPD characteristic. It seems likely that Annie chose to cut herself out of fear of rejection. Finding herself suddenly in the physical setting of a traditional middle-class marriage—expensive suburban house, custom-decorated bedroom, manicured lawns, grown children, and an aging lover—she surely recognized a relationship with little future.

Borderline individuals develop a life-long pattern of "unstable and intense interpersonal relationships" accompanied by "frantic efforts to avoid real or imagined abandonment." They frequently have "marked reactivity of moods (e.g., intense episodic dysphoria, irritability, or anxiety usually lasting a few hours and only rarely more than a few days)" (American Psychiatric Association, 2000, p. 707). Like Annie, many borderline individuals enter (often repeatedly) into imprudent sexual liaisons, and they also commonly display other impulsive behavior: substance use, reckless spending, unsafe driving, and binge eating. Borderline persons are frequently angry, most often with those closest to them or trying to help them. Depression, a sense of emptiness, and an "unstable self-image or sense of self" are other frequent accompaniments of BPD. Annie's appearance and behavior—"raw, unfinished, lazy, slangy, vulgar, crude"—might suggest an "unstable self-image" or might merely reflect what could be considered her Bohemian "artsy" lifestyle. Unlike Annie, who apparently has finished her master's degree, persons with BPD may often have a history of giving up or quitting projects prior to achieving success (e.g., quitting school right before graduation).

Head-On

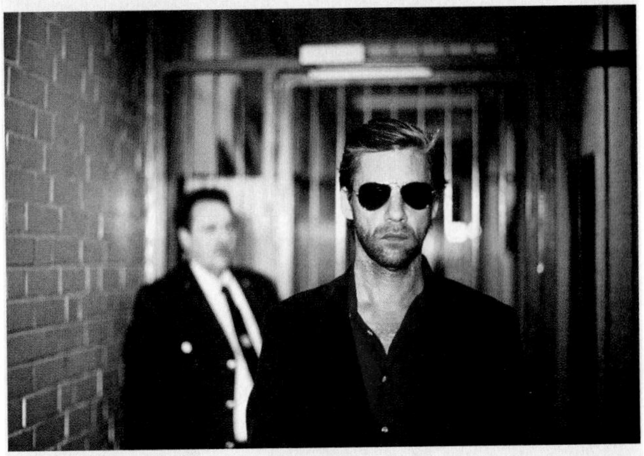

Courtesy: NDR/PanFilm/The Kobal Collection

In *Head On* (*Gegen die Wand*), a German film about Turkish immigrants, the two main characters have sociopathic tendencies (he) and borderline personality disorder (she). Relationships here are inevitably complicated by personality disorders and the special difficulties of living as an immigrant in a Germany highly ambivalent toward its many Turkish "guest workers."

Etiology

Although the precise cause of BPD remains unknown, it is generally assumed that BPD is an acquired condition deriving from the experience of growing up in a chaotic and often violent family (Zanarini, 2000). Functional MRI studies complement PET scan research (Lis, Greenfield, Hanry, Guile, & Dougherty, 2007) and show that under laboratory conditions leading to "negative emotions" persons with BPD show significantly less activity in the frontal lobe areas that inhibit emotional responses than do normals (Silbersweig, Clarkin, Goldstein, Kernberg, Tuescher, Levy, et al., 2007). Such findings may, of course, result from learned patterns due to past experience, or they may have some genetic component (Silbersweig et al., 2007). First-degree relatives (parents, siblings, or children) of individuals with BPD are about five times more likely to have this diagnosis than are less closely related individuals. This tendency for the disorder to cluster in families could be due to either environmental or genetic factors, but most experts currently stress the importance of environmental determinants. Such determinants include chaos in the family, which may manifest as fighting, infidelity, suicide or suicide attempts, and problems with the law, including imprisonment. It is perhaps not surprising that individuals with BPD are much more likely to suffer from mood disorders (depression), substance abuse disorders, or other associated personality disorders, particularly Antisocial Personality Disorder, than are individuals without BPD. One author describes the family history of the borderline personality as a "disaster a day" and likens the resultant family life to the plot of a television soap opera (Benjamin, 1993). Issues of abandonment are common, and most adults with BPD have some history of feeling abandoned, fearful, and unprotected as children. A childhood history of physical and/or sexual abuse is also common (Horstfall, 1999). The early life of individuals with BPD may also be deficient in experiences that enhance normal personality development (Helgeland & Torgersen, 2004). These include school success and talents in art or other areas of accomplishment. While environmental factors almost certainly play a decisive role in the expression of this disorder, genetic factors may be involved as well. Several studies suggest that genetic changes in the serotonin transporter protein (see earlier discussions on suicide in Chapter 16) may be associated with BPD (Ni, Chan, Bulgin,

BOX 18-1
ESSENTIAL FEATURES OF BORDERLINE PERSONALITY DISORDER

- Frantic efforts to avoid real or imagined abandonment
- Pattern of unstable interpersonal relationships
- Unstable self-image or sense of self
- Impulsivity in at least two areas that are potentially self-damaging (spending, sex, substance abuse, reckless driving, binge eating)
- Recurrent suicidal behaviors, gestures, or threats or self-mutilating behavior
- Chronic feelings of emptiness
- Inappropriate anger or difficulty controlling anger
- Transient, stress-related paranoid ideation

Sicard, Bismil, McMain et al., 2006). These findings remain preliminary and have not yet been adequately confirmed (Pascual, Soler, Barrachina, Campins, Alvarez, Perez, et al., 2008).

The concept "borderline" derives from observations made during psychoanalysis—under the stress of psychoanalytic treatment, these individuals often develop characteristics of psychosis, such as losing touch with reality, hallucinations, or delusions. This potential for developing dissociative symptoms under stress remains one of the DSM-IV-TR defining criteria. To early psychiatrists, these individuals seemed to be "borderline" between persons with "neurosis" (a term now rarely used) and psychosis. It is estimated that about 2% of the general population will meet criteria for a diagnosis of BPD; the majority of persons diagnosed are women (American Psychiatric Association, 2000).

As clients, borderline individuals are often very difficult, demanding, and emotional. They are frequently annoyed *with* and angry *at* their nurses and physicians, and in response, they may provoke angry and rejecting responses from their caretakers. Because individuals with BPD have difficulty maintaining healthy relationships with anyone, including health care providers, they often receive fragmented (and expensive) care in multiple facilities. One authority states:

> *The medical setting provides fertile soil for borderline people to experience regressive emotional states. They are unclear as to the source of the physical and emotional discomfort of illness, tending to blame their pain on others; and they may react to painful interventions as specifically motivated hostile acts. Borderline patients are intolerant of groups in general and become confused in the hospital where their care is divided among a variety of doctors, nurses, consultants, and other medical personnel. They respond by simplifying this collection of persons into allies and enemies and proceed with desperate attempts to enlist the former to save them from the latter.**
>
> (Nardo, 1986, pp. 59–60)

The major physical risk for individuals with BPD is suicide. Although attempts are much more common than completed suicides, there is a real risk of suicide success, either intentional or unintentional. Because of extreme emotional liability and the frequent association with substance abuse, suicide may be very difficult to predict or prevent in BPD, as was seen in Annie's case. Although the overall pattern of behavior in BPD is quite stable over time, the intensity of borderline behavior often decreases with age. Borderline individuals tend to become relatively more functional and to have less risk of attempted and completed suicide as they reach their thirties, forties, and beyond (American Psychiatric Association, 2000).

Persons with BPD are often seen by care providers as being unusually difficult clients. Similarly, persons with BPD find the health care delivery system discriminatory, blaming, and inaccessible. Their perceptions may significantly affect the quantity of health care and support received (Nehls, 1999). BPD is the Axis II disorder that more commonly requires specific treatment, partly because of the frequency of suicide and self-mutilating behaviors. Treatment includes psychotherapy (which generally must be consistent and focused on increasing self-esteem and motivation) and medication. A structured form of group therapy combining elements of cognitive behavioral training with life skills has been shown to be effective in producing adaptive change over a period of at least a year (Blum, St John, Pfohl, Stuart, McCormick, Allen, et al., 2008). This therapy is called *dialectical behavior therapy*, first described and developed by Linehan, Armstrong, and Suarez (1991) and usually consists of once-weekly individual therapy sessions and twice-weekly group sessions, along with crisis interventions as needed and other supports (Phillips, Yen & Gunderson, 2003). Cognitive behavioral therapy alone has also been shown to be effective in improving outcomes over time (Davidson, Norrie, Tyrer, Gumley, Tata, Murray, et al., 2006).

A variety of medications in nearly all categories (antidepressants, atypical neuroleptics, anxidytics, and mood stabilizers) have shown some effectiveness with selected groups of clients with BPD. Medication is often selected based on Axis I comorbid diagnoses (Soloff, 2000; Zanarini, Frankenburg, Hennen, & Silk, 2004), but several studies have suggested

*From "The Personality in the Medical Setting," by J. M. Nardo. In H. K. Brodie & J. L. Houpt (Eds.), *Consultation-Liaison Psychiatry and Behavioral Medicine*, 1986, New York: Basic Books.

RESEARCH Highlight 18–1

To Tame a Volcano: Patients with Borderline Personality Disorder and Their Perceptions of Suffering

STUDY PROBLEM/PURPOSE

The researchers sought to investigate life situations, suffering, and perceptions of encounter with psychiatric care held by patients with Borderline Personality Disorder (BPD). Specifically, the researchers wanted to know how suffering is experienced by these patients, how they experience their life situation and their encounters with psychiatric care.

METHODS

Researchers conducted interviews with 10 women who had been in treatment for 12 months or longer and who met DSM IV criteria for BPD. The study method was a phenomenological hermeneutic interpretation of the narrative interview data.

FINDINGS

The data indicated there are three main themes that describe the experiences of these women: "life on the edge," "struggle for health and dignity," and "the good and the bad act of psychiatric care in the drama of suffering." The narratives, or the voices of these patients reveal intense suffering and emotional pain. An array of emotions was described, including anxiety, emptiness, hopelessness, meaninglessness, anger, and powerlessness. In the face of these emotions, the patients experienced a struggle to be normal. The women reported mood changes and ambivalence—from despair/suffering to a struggle for a life worth living. The women provided insights into their perceptions of role of psychiatric professionals who sometimes come across as non-caring and disrespectful and acting in ways that did not permit the patient to make her own decisions.

IMPLICATIONS

The researchers discuss the findings encouraging us to fully understand the pain and suffering patients with BPD may be experiencing, and to recognize that these patients are dealing with universal life struggles: longing for life, yet fearing death and fearing life.

Given that nurses and other health professionals find BPD patients difficult to care for, it is important for nurses to attempt to understand the client's behaviors and feelings, for an understanding of the client's experiences will assist nurses to provide care that is both appropriate and compassionate.

Source: Perseius, K., & Asberg, E. (2005). To Tame a Volcano: Patients with Borderline Personality Disorder and Their Perceptions of Suffering. *Archives of Psychiatric Nursing*, 19(4), 160–168.

that the atypical neuroleptic olanzepine can benefit a wide range of symptoms (Bogenschutz & George Nurnberg, 2004). Persons with this disorder commonly receive long-term counseling along with treatment with multiple medications—not infrequently four or more (Zanarini et al., 2004). The antiseizure medication lamotrigine is undergoing evaluation for its effectiveness in this condition (Green, 2003). Lamotrigine is effective in reducing aggression and impulsivity (Leiberich, Nickel, Tritt, & Gil, 2008) and may be an attractive treatment since it is not associated with weight gain. Current evidence-based drug treatment preferences are for atypical neuroleptics and anticonvulsants (Abraham & Calabrese, 2008).

Narcissistic Personality Disorder

In Greek mythology, Narcissus is a young man of great beauty who, long before the invention of proper mirrors, happens to see his own image reflected in a pool of water. He is so enchanted with what he sees that he dies of a broken heart — madly in love with the image of himself that he is unable to reach in the depths of the pool. Not surprisingly, many young women had similarly fallen in love with Narcissus earlier in his short life. Perhaps the most tragic of these, Echo, declares her love for him and is spurned. Being a wood nymph, she disappears into the woods to waste away in mourning. Thus, the story of Narcissus provides the diagnostic title of a personality disorder for individuals demonstrating similar characteristics and having similar impact on the lives of others. Consider the following excerpt.

"TELL ME, IS DORIAN GRAY VERY FOND OF YOU?"

The painter [Basil Hallward] considered for a few moments ... I know he likes me. Of course I flatter him dreadfully ... As a rule, he is charming to me, and we sit in the studio and talk of a thousand things. Now and then, however, he is horribly thoughtless, and seems to take a real delight in giving me pain. Then I feel, Harry, that I have given away my whole soul to some one who treats it as if it were a flower to put in his coat, a bit of decoration to charm his vanity, an ornament for a summer's day." ...

As they entered they saw Dorian Gray. He was seated at the piano, with his back to them, turning over the pages of a volume of Schumann's "Forest Scenes." ... Hallward looked for a long time at Dorian Gray, and then for a long time at the picture [of Dorian which he had been painting], biting the end of one of his huge brushes and frowning. "It is quite finished," he cried at last, and stooping down he wrote his name in long vermilion letters on the left-hand corner of the canvas.

Lord Harry came over and examined the picture... "My dear fellow, I congratulate you most warmly," he said. "It is the finest portrait of modern times. Mr. Gray, come over and look at yourself."...

Dorian ... passed listlessly in front of his picture and turned towards it. When he saw it he drew back, and his cheeks flushed for a moment with pleasure. A look of joy came into his eyes, as if he had recognized himself for the first time. He stood there motionless and in wonder, dimly conscious that Hallward was speaking to him, but not catching the meaning of his words. The sense of his own beauty came on him like a revelation ... as he stood gazing at the shadow of his own loveliness...

*"Don't you like it?" cried Hallward at last, stung a little by the lad's silence, not understanding what it meant ... "How sad it is!" murmured Dorian Gray with his eyes still fixed upon his own portrait. "How sad it is! I shall grow old, and horrible, and dreadful. But this picture will remain always young. It will never be older than this particular day of June.... If it were only the other way! If it were I who was to be always young, and the picture that was to grow old! For that—for that—I would give everything! Yes, there is nothing in the whole world I would not give! I would give my soul for that!"**

(Wilde, 1890)

Very likely, Dorian Grey has **Narcissistic Personality Disorder**, the essential features of which are self-centeredness and inflated self-esteem, both beginning by early adulthood. Individuals with Narcissistic Personality Disorder typically overestimate their abilities, feel superior to others, and demand admiration. They invariably expect special treatment and have a lack of empathy toward others (American Psychiatric Association, 2000). These individuals are often highly sensitive to the criticism of others and frequently have difficulty in establishing close relationships. Dorian's relationships are all one sided, exploitative, and highly destructive to those around him.

While DSM-IV-TR requires that only five of eight criteria be present to make the diagnosis of Narcissistic Personality Disorder, Dorian may well meet all of these. In addition to lack of empathy, he has a grandiose sense of self-importance, he believes he is special and unique and should associate with important people, and he requires excessive admiration. In addition, his interpersonal relationships are highly exploitative and his behavior is arrogant. Dorian is certainly preoccupied with fantasies of unlimited and lasting beauty and, as the story of Dorain Gray continues, he loses his soul in search of lasting beauty and youth.

*From: *The Picture of Dorian Gray, by Oscar Wilde,* (1890), Chapter 1, retrieved from Authorama. Classic literature free of copyright, (http://www.authorama.com/the-picture-of-dorian-gray-1.html)

BOX 18-2
ESSENTIAL FEATURES OF NARCISSISTIC PERSONALITY DISORDER

- Has a grandiose sense of self-importance
- Is preoccupied with fantasies of unlimited success, power, brilliance, beauty, or ideal love
- Believes he or she is unique and special and should only associate with others who are special or high-status people
- Requires admiration of others
- Has a sense of entitlement
- Is interpersonally exploitive
- Lacks empathy
- Shows arrogance

From the *Diagnostic and Statistical Manual of Mental Disorders-TR* (4th ed.). Copyright © 2000. Reprinted with permission from the American Psychiatric Association.

Etiology

The developmental history of persons with Narcissistic Personality Disorder typically shows a pattern of selfless love and adoration from a significant adult, such that the child escapes reality-based experiences. At the same time, the child experiences an ever-present threat of criticism for not being perfect. Benjamin (1993) states that the "rich and famous are particularly vulnerable to developing Narcissistic Personality Disorder in adulthood" (p. 146) because of the attention, devotion, and nurturance given celebrities by the American public.

To others, narcissistic individuals appear arrogant, conceited, insensitive, and ruthless. Unlike individuals with BPD, who are relatively susceptible to psychotic episodes, narcissistic persons have developed a stable personality structure, but the rigidity of that personality hides extreme vulnerability to any experience that threatens their sense of self-perfection. Narcissistic individuals often use fantasy and daydreams to cope with such stressful experience; the content of these daydreams and fantasies frequently incorporates themes of self-admiration, power, revenge, and personal entitlement (Raskin & Novacek, 1991). Under stress, narcissistic individuals may demonstrate varying degrees of anxiety or depression. Physical illness is often a severe challenge for narcissistic individuals who typically have as much trouble with medical and nursing practitioners as they do with their own illness. Indeed, persons with narcissistic personality disorder are vulnerable to intense reactions when in situations where their self-image is compromised (Phillips et al., 2003). Narcissistic persons are often highly critical and competitive, and caregivers can readily come into conflict with them if the providers allow their own feelings of authority or importance to come to the surface. Along with illness, aging is a major stress for those with Narcissistic Personality Disorder.

These individuals are often extraordinarily reluctant to accept or accommodate to the declining capabilities brought on by aging. To deal with a client who has a Narcissistic Personality Disorder, the nurse must understand the personality dynamics behind the person's anger and criticism. The nurse should take an unemotional but supportive approach.

In comparison to other personality disorders, Narcissistic Personality Disorder is relatively rare. The prevalence of Narcissistic Personality Disorder in the general population is estimated to be less than 1%, with a majority of those diagnosed being male (American Psychiatric Association, 2000). However, since many individuals with this disorder have significant difficulties adjusting to life stresses, Narcissistic Personality Disorder will be seen with more frequency in mental health practice than expected given the 1% figure.

Narcissus

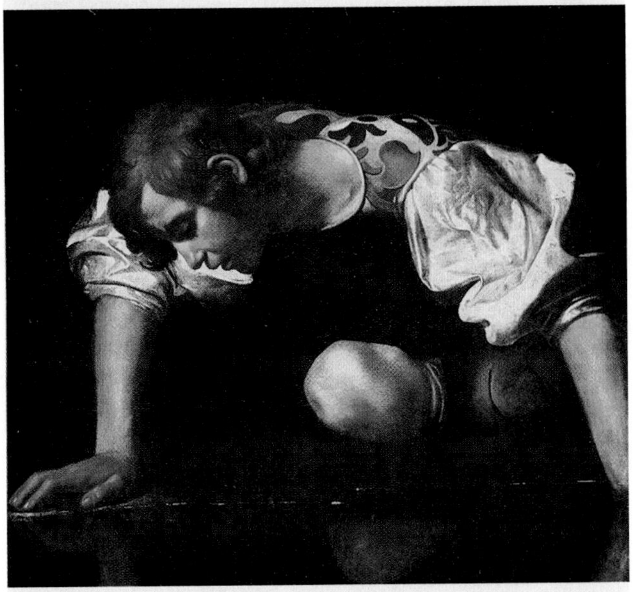

Caravaggio, Michaelangelo Merisida (1573-1610) *Narcissus*. Galleria Nazionale d'Arte Antica, Rome, Italy. Courtesy Scala/Art Resource, NY.

Narcissus is the youth who believes he is so beautiful that he spends his days admiring his own image. In this painting, Narcissus is depicted as a handsome young man of the era. Today, we would be more likely to see narcissistic behavior at the health club, where both young and old strive for physical perfection, and some become so engrossed in their own beauty and attractiveness that they find little time for developing interpersonal relationships.

Histrionic Personality Disorder

WHO IS SHE?

"And who is she? What does she do?"

"She's an English girl, an actress: sings at the Lady Windermere—hot stuff, believe me!"

"That doesn't sound much like an English girl, I must say."

"Eventually she's got a bit of French in her. Her mother was French."

A few minutes later, Sally herself arrived.

"Am I terribly late, Fritz darling?"

"Only half of an hour, I suppose," Fritz drawled, beaming with proprietary pleasure. "May I introduce Mr. Isherwood—Miss Bowles? Mr. Isherwood is commonly known as Chris."

"I'm not," I said. "Fritz is about the only person who's ever called me Chris in my life."

Sally laughed. She was dressed in black silk, with a small cape over her shoulders and a little cap like a page-boy's stuck jauntily on one side of her head:

"Do you mind if I use your telephone, sweet?"

"Sure. Go right ahead." Fritz caught my eye. "Come into the other room, Chris. I want to show you something." He was evidently longing to hear my first impressions of Sally, his new acquisition.

"For heaven's sake, don't leave me alone with this man!" she exclaimed. "Or he'll seduce me down the telephone. He's most terribly passionate."

As she dialed the number, I noticed that her finger-nails were painted emerald green, a colour unfortunately chosen, for it called attention to her hands, which were much stained by cigarette-smoking and as dirty as a little girl's. She was dark enough to be Fritz's sister. Her face was long and thin, powdered dead white. She had very large brown eyes which should have been darker, to match her hair and the pencil she used for her eyebrows.

"Hiloo," she cooed, pursing her brilliant cherry lips as though she was going to kiss the mouthpiece: "Ist dass Du, mein Liebling?" Her mouth opened in a fatuously sweet smile. Fritz and I sat watching her, like a performance at the theatre. "Was wollen wir machen, Morgen Abend? Oh, Wie wunderbar ... Nein, nein, ich werde bleiben Heute Abend zu Hause. Ja, ja, ich werde wirklich bleiben zu Hause ... Auf Wiedersehen, mein Liebling...."

She hung up the receiver and turned to us triumphantly.

"That's the man I slept with last night," she announced. "He makes love marvelously. He's an absolute genius at business and he's terribly rich—" She came and sat down on the sofa beside Fritz, sinking back into the cushions

BOX 18-3
ESSENTIAL FEATURES OF HISTRIONIC PERSONALITY DISORDER

- Is uncomfortable in situations in which he or she is not the center of attention
- Displays inappropriate sexually seductive or provocative behavior
- Has rapid shifts of emotion
- Uses physical appearance to draw attention to self
- Shows dramatization or exaggerated expression of emotion
- Is suggestible
- Considers relationships to be more intimate than they really are

*with a sigh: "Give me some coffee, will you, darling? I'm simply dying of thirst."**

(Isherwood, 1989, pp. 22–23)

Sally's personality is characterized by dramatic extremes of expression; being around her seems to Fritz and Christopher "like [watching] a performance at the theater." This sense of performance strongly suggests that Sally has **Histrionic Personality Disorder**. Both Sally's behavior and appearance are quite typical of this disorder: dramatic dress, striking makeup, theatrical entrance, seductive boasting about sexual promiscuity. Individuals with Histrionic Personality Disorder constantly seek attention through excesses of emotional expression. They crave being the center of attention and, like Sally, often gain attention by talking or behaving seductively and dressing in ways that call attention to themselves. Speech in Histrionic Personality Disorder is dramatic, exaggerated, but shallow—for Sally, everyone is "darling" or "sweet," or (since this episode was set in pre-World War II Berlin) "*liebling*." Sally is not just thirsty, but "simply dying of thirst." Individuals with this disorder are often highly suggestible. Later in the story, Christopher says to Sally, "What I really like about you is that you're so awfully easy to take in. People who never get taken in are so dreary" (Isherwood, 1989, p. 69). Histrionic persons may frequently cause embarrassment to others by dramatic public displays of affection directed toward individuals they know only distantly.

There is clearly some similarity between Histrionic Personality Disorder and Borderline Personality Disorder: Both are characterized by rapid emotional swings, seductive behavior, and inability to form close interpersonal relationships. The distinguishing borderline characteristic is marked shifts in feelings about others, usually based on some perception of rejection. Histrionic individuals also shift emotions rapidly (e.g., moving almost instantaneously from loud laughter to tears), but their primary aim is to keep themselves the focus of attention. It is not uncommon for persons to have characteristics of both Borderline and Histrionic Personality Disorders, and certain DSM-IV Axis I disorders (particularly Somatization Disorder, Conversion Disorder, and Major Depressive Disorder) are relatively common among histrionic individuals (Benjamin, 1993).

Gypsy

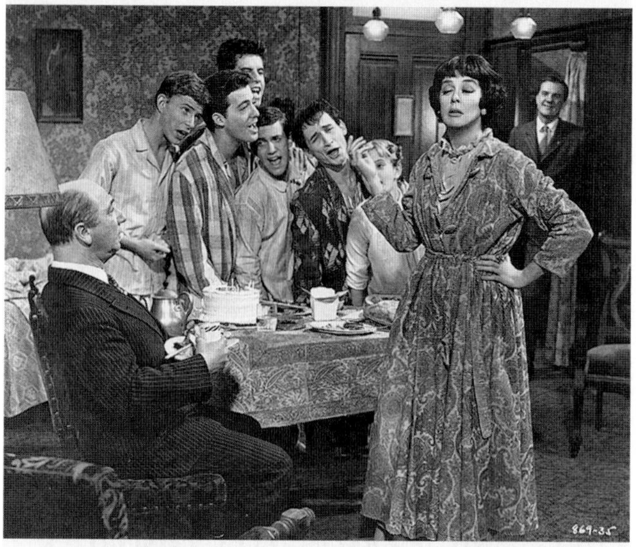

Source: Warner Brothers (Courtesy: The Kobal Collection).

A histrionic personality, Mama Rose, finds herself to be the center of attention.

Etiology

The adult with Histrionic Personality Disorder has probably been brought up with the sense that his or her value is based on good looks and ability to entertain others. Histrionic personality is sometimes an asset in a theatrical career, but for most individuals, Histrionic Personality Disorder seriously interferes with life goals and intimate relationships. For both the German, Fritz, and the Englishman, Christopher, Sally's behavior was intriguingly exotic: "She's got a bit of French in her," Fritz offers in trying to explain Sally's histrionic performances. Cultures certainly differ in the degree of flamboyance and emotional expressiveness that is considered normal. These cultural differences always need to be considered before making any personality disorder diagnosis, but it is likely that Sally's extremes of expression would fall outside the norms in any modern culture. All personality disorder

*From *The Berlin Stories*, by Christopher Isherwood, Copyright © 1935. Reprinted with permission from New Directions Publishing Corporation.

REFLECTIVE THINKING 18-1

Histrionic Personality Disorder

In health care settings, a person with Histrionic Personality Disorder will become frustrated easily when she is not able to maintain attention on herself. You must both understand the client's need for attention and provide realistic care, such as setting limits regarding your availability and taking time to let the client know what is possible and not possible. How could you ensure that your nursing care remains objective and appropriate when caring for a client with a histrionic personality who seems to be in need of constant attention?

diagnoses require that the condition lead to "significant distress or impairment in social, occupational, or other important areas of functioning" (American Psychiatric Association, 2000, p. 686). Isherwood's (1989) account of Sally Bowles paints her as generally successful and happy, though at one point she observes: "Sometimes I feel I'm no damn use at anything.... Why, I can't even keep a man faithful to me for the inside of a month" (p. 41). Despite Isherwood's sympathetic portrayal, it seems inevitable that Sally's histrionic personality will eventually cause her significant distress or functional impairment. The features of histrionic personality disorder reflect the person's "insecurity about their value as being anything other than a fetching companion" (Phillips et al., 2003, p. 819).

Data from the general population estimate the prevalence of Histrionic Personality Disorder to be 2% to 3%, with some studies reporting equal prevalence among males and females and other studies of clinical populations reporting a higher prevalence among women (American Psychiatric Association, 2000). Histrionic personality in men differs somewhat from that in women. The male histrionic typically focuses on "macho" behavior and talk, often involving physical or athletic prowess. In men, Histrionic Personality Disorder may seem to overlap with Narcissistic Personality Disorder. The histrionic male seeks continually to be the center of attention, whereas the narcissistic male primarily seeks power and domination over others. As with other personality disorders, the stress of illness or surgery can lead to behaviors that threaten good outcomes and challenge the patience and therapeutic ingenuity of nursing care providers (Smith, Chakraburatty, Nelson, & Paradis, 2000).

Antisocial Personality Disorder

CONFESSIONS OF A "CON MAN"

I am only able to live in conditions that leave my spirit and imagination completely free; and so it is that the memory of my years in prison is actually less hateful to me than the recollection of the slavery and fear to which my sensitive boyish soul was subjected through the ostensibly honourable discipline in the small square white schoolhouse down there in the town. And ... it is not surprising that I soon hit on the idea of escaping from school more often than on Sundays and holidays.

In carrying out this idea I was helped a good deal by a playful diversion I had long indulged in—the imitation of my father's handwriting. A father is the natural and nearest model for the growing boy who is striving to adapt himself to the adult world. Similarity of physique and the mystery of their relationship incline the boy to admire in his parent's conduct all that he himself is still incapable of and to strive to imitate it—or rather it is, perhaps, his very admiration that unconsciously leads him to develop along the lines heredity has laid down. Even when I was still making great hens' tracks on my lined slate, I already dreamed of guiding a steel pen with my father's swiftness and sureness; and many were the pages I covered later with efforts to copy his hand from memory, my fingers grasping the pen in the same delicate fashion as his. His writing was not, in fact, hard to imitate, for my poor father wrote a childish, copybook and, quite undeveloped hand, its only peculiarity being that the letters were very tiny and separated by long hairlines to an extent I have never seen anywhere else. This mannerism I quickly mastered to perfection. As for the signature "E. Krull," in contrast to the angular Gothic letters of the text it had a Latin cast. It was surrounded by a perfect cloud of flourishes, which at first sight looked difficult to copy, but were in reality so simple in conception that with them I succeeded best of all. The lower half of the E made a wide sweep to the right, in whose ample lap, so to speak, the short syllable of the last name was neatly cradled.... The whole signature was higher than it was long, it was naive and baroque; thus it lent itself so well to my purpose that in the end its inventor would have certified my product as his own. But what was more obvious, once I had acquired this skill for my own entertainment, than to put it to work in the interests of my intellectual freedom? "On the 7th instant," I wrote, "my son Felix was afflicted by severe stomach cramps which compelled him to stay away from school, to the regret of yours—E. Krull." And again: "An infected gumboil, together with a sprained right arm, compelled Felix to keep his room from the 10th to the 14th of this month. Therefore, much to our regret, he was unable to attend school. Respectfully yours—E. Krull." When this succeeded, nothing prevented me from spending the school hours of one

BOX 18-4
ESSENTIAL FEATURES OF ANTISOCIAL PERSONALITY DISORDER

- A pervasive pattern of disregard for and violation of the rights of others
- Repeated acts that are grounds for arrest
- Repeated lying, use of aliases, or conning others
- Impulsivity or failure to plan ahead
- Repeated physical fights or assaults
- Reckless disregard for safety of self or others
- Failure to sustain consistent work behavior or honor financial obligations
- Lack of remorse [at] having hurt, mistreated, or stolen from another

From the *Diagnostic and Statistical Manual of Mental Disorder – TR* (4th ed.). Copyright © 2000. Reprinted with permission from the American Psychiatric Association.

*day or even of several wandering freely outside the town or lying stretched out in a green field, in the whispering shade of the leaves, dreaming the dreams of youth.**

(Mann, 1970, pp. 31–33)

Used as an adjective, the word *confidence* in this excerpt means to swindle or cheat. Today, the slang term conman is more frequently used. It certainly is natural, as Felix states, for a young boy to seek to imitate his father; however, this is hardly an excuse for forgery. As he grows up, Felix constantly manipulates, lies, steals, and seduces—all without remorse, even when (as he casually indicates in the excerpt) he ends up in prison as a result. Unlike many persons with **Antisocial Personality Disorder**, Felix seems never to have been violent. Felix manipulates his way out of military draft to avoid the inconvenience of service; others with Antisocial Personality Disorder thrive on the opportunities for violent behavior that military service provides. Much fiction and many films focus on the violence associated with this disorder. *Pulp Fiction*, *Reservoir Dogs*, and *The Godfather* are three films that depict remorseless violence. Chapter 33 in this text lists a number of other films, some requiring quite a strong stomach to watch. Felix Krull reminds us that violence, although common, is not necessary for a diagnosis of Antisocial Personality Disorder to be made—persistent disregard for the rights and well-being of others can manifest itself through charm and manipulation as well as through violence.

Along with a pattern of "pervasive ... disregard for and violation of the rights of others," at least three of the characteristics in Box 18-4 must be present to diagnose Antisocial Personality Disorder.

In addition, the person's antisocial behavior must have begun before age 15 and at that time have met the criteria for Adolescent Conduct Disorder (see Chapter 24).

Etiology

Family history of adults with Antisocial Personality Disorder shows a pattern of violence, neglect, and, frequently, alcoholism. The child may have been a victim of physical abuse or have watched violent parents in their interactions with each other. Adolescent Conduct Disorder—a prerequisite to the adult diagnosis—includes such behaviors as bullying, cruelty to people and animals, stealing or otherwise damaging property, truancy, and running away from home. It has been suggested that adults with Antisocial Personality Disorder often have had inordinate control over their families when they were children and adolescents, often because of parental negligence or absence (Benjamin, 1993). In this way, patterns of coercion may begin at a very early age. Environment clearly plays an important role in the development of Adolescent Conduct Disorder and Antisocial Personality Disorder. Adoption studies indicate that both genetic and environmental factors contribute to risk for this disorder, which clearly has a tendency to occur repeatedly in families (American Psychiatric Association, 2000).

Fox Butterfield has written about a single remarkably violent family in which the disorder can be traced back as far as 1820. Summing up the current evidence for how antisocial behavior is transmitted from generation to generation, he comments:

*Everything criminologists have learned in recent research is that most adolescents who become delinquents, and the overwhelming majority of adults who commit violent crimes, started very young. They were the impulsive, aggressive, irritable children who would not obey their parents, bullied their neighbors and acted out when they got to school. Because they were accustomed to getting their way by physical force, they see no reason to change. They actually like the way they act, and this makes it increasingly difficult to reverse their antisocial proclivities.... Many factors go into producing personality: temperament, the genetic component you are born with; the neighborhood in which you grow up; and perhaps most important, the style of your parents.**

(Butterfield, 1994, p. 327)

Antisocial Personality Disorder is one of the conditions specifically studied in the Epidemiologic Catchment Area

*From *Confessions of Felix Krull, Confidence Man*, by Thomas Mann and H. T Lowe-Porter, Copyright © 1955, renewed 1983. Reprinted with permission from Alfred A. Knopf, a division of Random House, Inc.

*From *All God's Children: The Bosker Family and the American Tradition of Violence*, by F. Butterfield (p. 327), 1994, New York: Knopf.

(ECA) Study of psychiatric disorders in the community (see Chapter 8). One of the major findings of the ECA study was that less than half of persons with Antisocial Personality Disorder have significant criminal records. The most common symptoms are "job troubles (94%), violence (85%), multiple moving traffic offenses (72%), and severe marital difficulties (desertion, multiple separations or divorces, multiple infidelities, found in 67%)" (Robins, Tipp, & Przybeck, 1991, p. 260). The ECA study also clearly showed that this disorder tends to improve with age: The average duration of symptoms was 19 years, but almost no individuals displayed significant antisocial behavior after their mid-thirties (Robins et al., 1991). Men have a significantly higher prevalence of Antisocial Personality Disorder than do women, but the ECA study data suggest that the prevalence may be rising among women. The overall prevalence of the disorder may also be increasing (Robins et al., 1991, p. 271). The prevalence is currently estimated to be about 3% in males and 1% in females (American Psychiatric Association, 2000).

Not surprisingly, when psychiatric diagnoses are sought among persons serving sentences in prison, Antisocial Personality Disorder is significantly overrepresented. In a summary of reported surveys involving 23,000 of an estimated 9 million worldwide prison population, 47% of prisoners were thought to have Antisocial Personality Disorder. There was a fairly wide discrepancy in diagnosis frequency among surveys from the 12 countries sampled, implying that somewhat different diagnostic criteria might have been used by different surveys (Fazel & Danesh, 2002). Intriguingly, there may even be structural brain differences between persons with antisocial personality disorder who are "caught in the act" and those who are not (Yang, Raine, Lencz, Bihrle, LaCasse, & Collettil, 2005). Duff (2003) has provided a model for using an interdisciplinary team to interact effectively with the range of personality disorders seen within a prison system. Some of these issues have also been addressed in the British context by Woods and Richards (2003), who also suggest an interdisciplinary approach rather than one based exclusively on nursing interventions.

Since substance abuse is very much a part of this disorder, nurses working in settings in which substance-abusing clients are treated, including emergency rooms, are particularly likely to encounter persons with Antisocial Personality Disorder. The client will view the nurse like anyone else, as a means of achieving his own goals. The client will look for alliances to obtain outcomes, such as admission to the hospital, a prescription for drugs, and relief from symptoms of illness. Violence and conning are very much a part of the lives of these individuals, and if the client does not get his way, nurses may on occasion be at physical risk from clients with this disorder. The nurse must recognize when she is dealing with a client with Antisocial Personality Disorder (Vaylor, 1999). Setting limits may require more than the nurse stating that something is so; the nurse may need to work with a team, including hospital security, when telling a client with antisocial personality that she cannot provide what he wants (Davon, 1994). (See also Chapter 32 for discussion on dealing with a violent client.)

NURSING TIP 18-2

Clients with Dramatic and Emotional Personality Disorders

The nurse caring for a client with any of the disorders from this cluster often becomes frustrated and angry because the client demands an excessive amount of time and attention. It often seems that, compared to other clients on a unit, the client with any of the personality disorders in this cluster has a minor problem and the nurse wants to give care to the other (seemingly more deserving) clients. Nurses should remember that clients with personality disorders have diagnosable problems; they cannot change who they are. These clients cannot graciously wait until the nurse attends to others; it is not part of their makeup to do so. The nurse will need to set limits, state clearly what she can and cannot do, and keep to her schedule. When the client complains about or criticizes the nurse, the nurse must understand that this, too, is part of the personality dynamics. Nurses must work as a team in caring for such individuals; each must avoid talking with other caregivers in a manner that criticizes the client for being who he is.

Treatment for clients with antisocial personality disorder remains difficult. In fact, there is little evidence that the disorder can be treated successfully. However, some reports suggest that when individuals with the condition are in confined settings (prisons or the military, for example) depressive and introspective concerns may emerge. When this occurs, confrontation by peers may bring about changes in behavior (Phillips et al., 2003).

ODD AND ECCENTRIC PERSONALITY CLUSTER

Individuals in this cluster have the characteristic of seeming unusual. They are often described by others as "different" or "somewhat odd." They tend to remain isolated from others, unconcerned about how others perceive them, and develop living patterns that appear disconnected and independent. Those with Paranoid Personality Disorder have a suspiciousness of others as well as an inability to trust.

SCHIZOID PERSONALITY DISORDER

PAUL'S CASE

It was Paul's afternoon to appear before the faculty of the Pittsburgh High School to account for his various misdemeanors. He had been suspended a week ago, and his father had called at the Principal's office and confessed his perplexity about his son. Paul entered the faculty-room suave and smiling. His clothes were a trifle outgrown, and the tan velvet on the collar of his open overcoat was frayed and worn, but for all that there was something of the dandy about him, and he wore an opal pin in his neatly knotted black four-in-hand, and a red carnation in his buttonhole. This latter adornment the faculty somehow felt was not properly significant of the contrite spirit befitting a boy under the ban of suspension....

When questioned by the Principal as to why he was there, Paul stated, politely enough, that he wanted to come back to school. This was a lie, but Paul was accustomed to lying; found it indeed, indispensable for overcoming friction. His teachers were asked to state their respective charges against him, which they did with such a rancor and aggrievedness as evinced that this was not a usual case. Disorder and impertinence were among the offenses named, yet each of his instructors felt that it was scarcely possible to put into words the real cause of the trouble, which lay in a sort of hysterically defiant manner of the boy's, in the contempt which they all knew he felt for them, and which he seemingly made not the least effort to conceal. Once, when he had been making a synopsis of a paragraph at the blackboard, his English teacher had stepped to his side and attempted to guide his hand. Paul had started back with a shudder and thrust his hands violently behind him.... In one way and another he had made all his teachers, men and women alike, conscious of the same feeling of physical aversion. In one class he habitually sat with his hand shading his eyes; in another he always looked out of the window during the recitation; in another he made a running commentary on the lecture, with humorous intent.

His teachers felt this afternoon that his whole attitude was symbolized by his shrug and his flippantly red carnation flower, and they fell upon him without mercy, his English teacher leading the pack. He stood through it smiling, his pale lips parted over his white teeth. (His lips were continually twitching, and he had a habit of raising his eyebrows that was contemptuous and irritating to the last degree.) Older boys than Paul had broken down and shed tears under that ordeal, but his set smile did not once desert him.... Paul was always smiling, always glancing about him seeming to feel that people might be watching him and trying to detect something. This conscious expression, since it was so far as possible from boyish mirthfulness, was usually attributed to insolence or "smartness." ...

*His teachers were in despair, and his drawing master voiced the feeling of them all when he declared there was something about the boy which none of them understood. He added: "I don't really believe that smile of his comes altogether from insolence; there's something sort of haunted about it. The boy is not strong, for one thing. There is something wrong about the fellow."**

(Cather, 1948, pp. 183–185)

Persons with **Schizoid Personality Disorder** are characterized by marked detachment from persons and events around them. They show little emotion, develop few close friendships, and most commonly spend time by themselves. In Willa Cather's description of "Paul's Case," Paul's teachers were offended by how little impact their criticism seemed to make on him. This lack of concern about either criticism or praise is one of the major characteristics of the schizoid personality. Schizoid individuals "usually display a 'bland' exterior without visible emotional reactivity and rarely reciprocate gestures or facial expressions such as smiles or nods.... They often display a constricted affect and appear cold and aloof" (American Psychiatric Association, 2000, p. 695). Paul exhibits a clear presence of aloofness and shows he does not care about the opinions of others, even his teachers. He responds neither to social cues of how to behave in class nor to social cues of how to behave in his current disciplinary hearing.

Paul's teachers are remarkably angry at him, but they have begun to recognize that his behavior does not merely derive from insolence or disrespect, such as one might see with Antisocial Personality Disorder, a much more common disorder. Paul's art teacher would seem to have gotten it nearly right: "I don't really believe that smile of his comes altogether from insolence;.... There is something wrong about the fellow."

Persons with Schizoid Personality Disorder might often inspire the comment, "There is something wrong about [him or her]." They do not seem to obtain satisfaction from being members of a family or social group. They are described as loners and therefore choose occupations and activities that call for a solitary lifestyle. Persons with Schizoid Personality Disorder seem oblivious to the subtleties of social interaction. They do not respond appropriately to social cues, coming across as inept or self-absorbed. Children and adolescents with Schizoid Personality Disorder stand out from their peers as loners and underachievers in school.

Etiology

Benjamin (1993) suggests that the child with Schizoid Personality Disorder would likely have grown up in a home that was orderly and formal, without much warmth, play, or spontaneous social interaction. The person with Schizoid Personality Disorder remains unattached to self or to others and probably learned behaviors from a parent who was withdrawn. The person with Schizoid Personality Disorder learns

*From "Paul's Case," in *Youth and the Bright Medusa* by Willa Cather (pp. 183–185), 1948, New York: Random House. Reprinted with permission.

to "expect nothing and give nothing" (Benjamin, 1993, p. 345). Further, clinicians note that persons with this disorder have little or no interest in developing relationships with others (Phillips et al., 2003).

In comparison to disorders in the dramatic and emotional cluster, Schizoid Personality Disorder is quite uncommon. As the name implies, persons with this disorder may sometimes closely resemble individuals with early schizophrenia. Most persons who develop schizophrenia gradually take on "negative" symptoms resembling, but ultimately more severe than, those of schizoid personality. As illustrated in Chapter 13, the contrast between preschizophrenic and postschizophrenic personality can be remarkable. In contrast, the personality of schizoid individuals remains constant from early adolescence or childhood. Thus, schizophrenia and Schizoid Personality Disorder can often be differentiated by their age of onset and the presence or absence of a premorbid normal state. Still, it is frequently not initially possible to distinguish early schizophrenia from a Schizoid Personality Disorder, and only time allows the distinction to be made: Schizophrenia is almost invariably relentlessly progressive, in contrast to the stable personality disorder. In reality, however, the two conditions are not completely separate; some individuals who develop schizophrenia seem to have had a long-standing schizoid personality. The relatively frequent occurrence of Schizoid Personality Disorder in relatives of individuals with Schizophrenia further suggests a significant etiologic association between the two. Like many other personality disorders, Schizoid Personality Disorder is diagnosed more frequently in males than females.

Nursing care for a client with Schizoid Personality Disorder is always marked by the inability to establish a nurse-client relationship. The client may describe a sense of being isolated, yet be unable to share emotions or experiences with others. The best nursing approach is to offer time and support to the client unconditionally; the client will be unable to respond in the way others do. Again, the nurse must be aware of the fact that the client is unable to change his basic personality. He may learn to change some behavioral characteristics, for example, the client may learn basic social skills. However, care should be directed to changing behavior that is causing the most disruption to the client's life, without attempting to change the client's personality.

BOX 18-5
ESSENTIAL FEATURES OF SCHIZOID PERSONALITY DISORDER

- Demonstrates pervasive pattern of detachment from social relationships
- Exhibits restricted range of emotions
- Must have four or more of the following:
  - Neither desires nor enjoys close relationships, including being part of a family
  - Chooses solitary activities
  - Has little (if any) interest in sexual experiences
  - Takes pleasure in few (if any) activities
  - Lacks close friends
  - Appears indifferent to praise or criticism
  - Shows emotional coldness

Schizotypal Personality Disorder

EGAEUS

My baptismal name is Egaeus; that of my family I will not mention. Yet there are no towers in the land more time-honored than my gloomy, gray, hereditary halls. Our line has been called a race of visionaries; and in many striking particulars—in the character of the family mansion—in the ... gallery of antique paintings ... and, lastly, in the very peculiar nature of the library's contents, there is more than sufficient evidence to warrant that belief.

The recollections of my earliest years are connected with that chamber, and with its volumes—of which latter I will say no more. Here died my mother. Herein I was born. But it is mere idleness to say that I had not lived before—that the soul has no previous existence. You deny it?—let us not argue the matter. Convinced myself, I seek not to convince. There is, however, a remembrance of aerial forms—of spiritual and meaning which will not be excluded; a memory like a shadow, vague, variable, indefinite, unsteady; and like a shadow, too, in the impossibility of my getting rid of it while the sunlight of my reason shall exist....

It is singular that as years rolled away, and the noon of manhood found me still in the mansion of my fathers ... the realities of the world affected me as visions ... while the wild ideas of the land of dreams became ... my everyday existence....

To muse for long unwearied hours with my attention riveted to some frivolous device on the margin, or in the typography of a book; to become absorbed for the better part of a summer's day, in a quaint shadow falling upon the tapestry, or upon the door; to lose myself for an entire night in watching the steady flame of a lamp; ... to repeat monotonously some common word, until the sound, by dint of frequent repetition, ceased to convey any idea whatever of the mind; ... such were a few of the most common and least pernicious vagaries induced by a condition of the *mental faculties ... certainly bidding defiance to anything like analysis or explanation.... In the strange anomaly of my existence, feelings with me, had never been of the heart, and my passions always were of the mind.**

(*Poe, 1983, pp. 208–213*)

Edgar Allan Poe's character Egaeus illustrates many of the features of **Schizotypal Personality Disorder**. Egaeus lacks the ability to form close relationships. His passions are only "of the mind"; he becomes engaged to his cousin Berenice when "in an evil moment, I spoke to her of marriage." His thoughts and language are distinctly odd; his speech is vague, difficult to follow, and overelaborate, probably even for Poe's time. He describes himself and his family as "visionaries," very likely meaning that they held unusual or superstitious beliefs, perhaps of magic or sorcery or communicating with the dead. Not only does Egaeus believe strongly in reincarnation, he speaks of hearing and seeing "aerial forms" (ghosts) too vivid to ignore "while the sunlight of my reason shall exist." He may not be obviously paranoid or suspicious, but he seems so confident that his beliefs in reincarnation will be challenged that he directly accuses the reader of not working hard enough to believe him: "It is mere idleness to say that I had not lived before.... You deny it? [reincarnation and spiritualism]—let us not argue the matter. Convinced myself, I seek not to convince." Egaeus is certainly far from friendly.

In addition to social and interpersonal deficits in close relationships, the DSM-IV-TR diagnosis of Schizotypal Personality Disorder requires a pattern of cognitive and perceptual distortions and eccentricities. These characteristics need to be traceable, as they are in Egaeus, to early adulthood and include at least five of nine diagnostic features. Such features include ideas of reference, odd or magical thinking, unusual perceptual experiences, odd speech, suspiciousness or paranoia, inappropriate affect, odd or eccentric behavior, lack of close friends, and excessive social anxiety. The individual with Schizotypal Personality Disorder shares with the person with Schizoid Personality Disorder a distinctly odd personality and a lack of close personal relationships. The schizotypal individual tends to have stranger and more overt thought processes along with magical thinking, paranoia, odd speech, and distorted (but not psychotic) beliefs. The schizoid individual withdraws into a cold, silent self, whereas the schizotypal individual enters a world that strikes us as bizarre and disordered.

Etiology

The cause of Schizotypal Personality Disorder is not known. There is, as in Egaeus's case, some tendency for the personality type to be found in more than one family member, but whether this represents a genetic clustering or the results of common upbringing is unknown. Schizophrenia (see Chapter 13) is also seen more commonly among the relatives of schizotypal individuals. While most persons with Schizotypal Personality Disorder maintain their personalities throughout adult life without developing schizophrenia, their deficits in social interactions are similar to those found in individuals with schizophrenia (Waldeck & Miller, 2000). Brain MRI and CT scanning also show important similarities between schizophrenia and Schizotypal Personality Disorder, though differences can be defined as well (Dickey, McCarley, & Shenton, 2002). Persons with both conditions share structural abnormalities in certain brain areas such as the superior temporal gyrus, parahippocampus, areas of the lateral ventricles, corpus callosum, thalamus, and septum pellucidum. Medical temporal lobe abnormalities are present in schizophrenia but lacking in those with Schizotypal Personality Disorder. The authors conclude from the reported studies that there are important similarities between the two disorders, and that Schizotypal Personality Disorder "probably represents a milder form ... along the schizophrenia continuum." Others report that "phenomenological, biological, genetic and treatment response" data support a link between Schizotypal disorder and schizophrenia (Phillips et al., 2003, p. 813). Schizotypal disorder is slightly more common in men than in women. Studies suggest that up to 3% of the population may suffer from Schizotypal Personality Disorder, making it perhaps the most common of the "odd" personalities. Not only is Schizotypal Personality Disorder common, it is also associated with extensive use of psychiatric services (Bender, Dolan, Skodal, Sanislow, Dyck, McGlashan, et al., 2001).

The nursing approach for a client with schizotypal personality is similar to the approach for a client with schizoid

BOX 18-6
ESSENTIAL FEATURES OF SCHIZOTYPAL PERSONALITY DISORDER

- Demonstrates pervasive pattern of acute discomfort with social and interpersonal relationships
- Exhibits cognitive or perceptual distortions and eccentricities of behavior
- Must exhibit five of the following:
  - Ideas of reference
  - Odd beliefs or magical thinking
  - Unusual perceptual experiences
  - Odd thinking and speech
  - Suspiciousness or paranoid ideation
  - Behavior or appearance that is odd, eccentric, or peculiar
  - Lack of close friends
  - Excessive social anxiety

From the *Diagnostic and Statistical Manual of Mental Disorders- TR* (4th ed.). Copyright © 2000. Reprinted with permission from the American Psychiatric Association.

*From "Berenice," by Edgar Allen Poe. In Viking Portable Library, by P. V. D. Stern (Ed.), 1945/1983, New York: Viking.

personality. The nurse should provide unconditional acceptance to the client for the person he is and not attempt to change the underlying personality. Characteristics and behaviors that cause the client difficulty can be addressed, and the client can be helped to focus on these specific behaviors. For example, if the client has difficulty communicating with others at work, a socialization group focusing on social communication skills might be helpful. If the client uses strange language that makes it difficult for others to understand him, the nurse may provide realistic feedback as to why others do not understand the client. The nurse's focus is on the behavior, not the personality.

Paranoid Personality Disorder

IVAN

His coat collar turned up, Ivan Gromov was splashing his way through the mud of alleys and back lanes one autumn morning to collect a fine from some tradesman or other. He was in a black mood as he always was in the mornings. In a certain alley he came across two convicts wearing foot-irons and escorted by four guards with rifles. Gromov had met convicts often enough before—they had always made him feel sympathetic and uncomfortable—but now this latest encounter had a peculiarly weird effect on him. Somehow it suddenly dawned on him that he himself might be clapped in irons and similarly hauled off to prison through the mud. He was passing the post office on his way home after paying this call when he met a police inspector of his acquaintance who gave him good day and walked a few steps down the street with him. This somehow struck Gromov as suspicious.... Was it so difficult to commit a crime accidentally and against one's will? Can false accusations—can judicial miscarriages, for that matter—really be ruled out? And hasn't immemorial folk wisdom taught that going to jail is like being poor; there isn't much you can do to escape from either? ...

He began seeking seclusion and avoiding people.... He was afraid of trickery: of having a bribe slipped surreptitiously into his pocket and then being caught, of making a chance error tantamount to forgery with official papers, or of losing someone else's money....

*In the early morning before sunrise, some stove-makers called on his landlady. They had come to rebuild the kitchen stove, as Gromov was well aware, but his fears told him that they were policemen in stove-makers' clothing. Stealing out of the flat, he dashed panic-stricken down the street without hat or coat. Barking dogs chased him, a man shouted somewhere behind him, the wind whistled in his ears, and Gromov thought that all the violence on earth had coiled itself together behind his back and was pursuing him.**

(*Chekhov, 1971, pp. 125–127*)

The Russian writer Chekhov, trained as a physician, was a keen observer of personality and personality types. In this excerpt from a short story, Ivan is convincingly portrayed as a man overcome by paranoia. Ivan begins to suspect that he might have done, or be accused of having done, something wrong. His fears of wrongful accusation increase steadily until his paranoia becomes so overwhelming that he finds himself committed to "Ward 6"—a primitive psychiatric hospital. Fearing imprisonment, Ivan ends up under psychiatric confinement.

Individuals with **Paranoid Personality Disorder** share Ivan's fears of others and their motives. From an early age, they tend to suspect that they are being exploited, or doubt the trustworthiness of friends. Essential characteristics of Paranoid Personality Disorder are listed in Box 18-8.

Chekhov implies that Ivan's symptoms are of fairly recent origin: "[Ivan] Gromov had met convicts often enough before—they had always made him feel sympathetic and uncomfortable—but now this latest encounter had a peculiarly weird effect on him. Somehow it suddenly dawned on him that he himself might be clapped in irons and similarly hauled off to prison through the mud." Today, the sudden development of paranoid ideas would strongly suggest chronic substance use, most commonly cocaine. Other medical conditions involving the central nervous system, particularly in the elderly, may also evoke paranoia. Chekhov provides little certainty about Ivan's actual diagnosis. He might have had a primary psychiatric disorder, or he might have been suffering from neurosyphilis, a common cause of paranoid delusions in the nineteenth century and still occasionally seen today. Individuals with Paranoid Personality Disorder have many of Ivan's traits but most commonly in a milder and more persistent form. Like Ivan, individuals with Paranoid Personality Disorder not infrequently develop brief psychoses under stress. Consider the following example:

A 60-year-old woman was brought to the psychiatric emergency room with a clinical picture suggesting paranoid schizophrenia. There was no previous history prior to several days before the visit when she became intensely delusional and agitated, fearing for her life. In the exploration of her persecutory thoughts, she reported that her persecutors had begun their assault by throwing her to the ground, taking her breath, and "wrenching" her chest. An electrocardiogram revealed a recent anterior wall myocardial infarction. When her medical illness was explained and she was transferred to the cardiac care unit, her

*From "Ward 6," in *The Oxford Chekhov* (Vol. VI, pp. 125–127), by Anton Chekhov, Copyright © 1971. Translated by R. Hingley, London: Oxford University Press. Reprinted with permission.

BOX 18-7
SIMILAR WORDS, DIFFERENT MEANINGS

1. What is the difference between the DSM diagnoses, *Schizophrenia* and two personality disorders with very similar names: *Schizoid* and *Schizotypal*?
   - *Schizophrenia* is a serious mental disorder that most commonly develops fairly suddenly in individuals who were previously quite normal. It tends to progress with time and to become dominated by "negative" symptoms that produce social withdrawal and significant impairment in cognitive and personal functioning.
   - *Schizoid Personality Disorder* is a long-standing stable disorder characterized by aloofness and reluctance to enter into social relationships. Persons with Schizoid Personality Disorder are loners who lack the ability for emotional involvement with others. While school failure is common, overall cognitive skills are generally unimpaired; occupational functioning may be surprisingly normal if an affected individual finds a job that allows him to function independently of others.
   - Persons with *Schizotypal Personality Disorder* share many of the features of Schizoid Personality Disorder. While also aloof and detached, schizotypal persons seem stranger than do those with schizoid personalities. Schizotypal individuals often have bizarre or mystical beliefs, odd speech and thinking patterns, and unusual behavior or dress. They often have some features that suggest schizophrenia—ideas of reference (beliefs that natural or historical phenomena have direct personal meaning) often occur, as do paranoia and suspiciousness. When present, both the ideas of reference and the paranoia are less intense than found in persons with Schizophrenia. When observed over time, symptoms of Schizotypal Personality Disorder are highly stable, in contrast to the steady worsening of individuals with Schizophrenia.
2. How are these disorders similar?
   - All three conditions—Schizophrenia, Schizoid Personality Disorder, and Schizotypal Personality Disorder—share marked detachment, oddness of behavior, and social dysfunction. Schizotypal Personality Disorder has even more similarities with Schizophrenia, which may include paranoia and ideas of reference.
3. How are these disorders different?
   - Schizophrenia differs from the two personality disorders by being a dynamic, evolving illness. Most persons with schizophrenia have normal personalities before they become ill; during the first months or years of their illness, they commonly experience serious loss of social and cognitive abilities. While persons with the two personality disorders may also be very socially handicapped, their conditions can often be traced to earliest childhood and are highly stable.
4. Can these three disorders coexist?
   - Yes. The odd ideas, beliefs, speech, and behavior of individuals with Schizotypal Personality Disorder may at times make it difficult to distinguish them from persons with Schizophrenia. Also, some individuals with either Schizoid or (especially) Schizotypal Personality Disorder may go on to develop Schizophrenia. Most schizotypal individuals could also meet criteria for Schizoid Personality Disorder, but in addition, they have the marked eccentricities of thought or behavior (or both) that characterize Schizotypal Personality Disorder.

*agitation and delusions disappeared, revealing her chronic but stable paranoid personality [disorder].**

(Nardo, 1986, p. 62)

In this fascinating case, a woman with a long-standing but unrecognized Paranoid Personality Disorder became psychotic under the stress of physical illness. Entering into her world, her caretakers were able to recognize the source of her decompensation: an acute myocardial infarction that had indeed thrown her to the ground and "wrenched" her chest several days before. Her delusional and psychotic response to this illness delayed treatment, but thoughtful and empathic interviewing allowed appropriate care to be given and full recovery to be made. In a setting lacking such able psychiatric assessment, this woman's delusions and evident psychosis would almost certainly have resulted in inappropriate care. Such, very possibly, was the fictional Ivan's fate in "Ward 6."

Etiology

Psychoanalysts believe that the childhood history of an adult with Paranoid Personality Disorder not infrequently includes a controlling parent who was abusive, cruel, or sadistic. From these experiences, the child learns to be fearful and mistrusting. In a very harsh upbringing, the child also learns not to ask for help, not to cry, and to remain independent (Benjamin, 1993). Paranoid Personality Disorder occurs in up to

*From "The Personality in the Medical Setting," by J. M. Nardo. In H. K. Brodie & J. L. Houpt (Eds.), *Consultation-Liaison Psychiatry and Behavioral Medicine*, 1986, New York: Basic Books.

BOX 18-8
ESSENTIAL FEATURES OF PARANOID PERSONALITY DISORDER

- Suspect, without sufficient basis, that others are exploiting, harming, or deceiving them
- Be preoccupied with unjustified doubts about the loyalty or trustworthiness of friends or associates
- Be reluctant to confide in others because of unwarranted fears that the information will be used maliciously against them
- Read hidden or demeaning or threatening meanings into benign remarks or events
- Persistently bear grudges
- Perceive attacks on their character or reputation that are not apparent to others
- Have recurrent suspicions, without justification, regarding fidelity of spouse or sexual partner

From the *Diagnostic and Statistical Manual of Mental Disorders,- TR,* (4th ed.). Copyright © 2000. Reprinted with permission from the American Psychiatric Association.

2.5% of the general population and much more frequently in both outpatient and inpatient psychiatric settings (American Psychiatric Association, 2000).

To care for a client with Paranoid Personality Disorder is challenging for the nurse. The nurse must understand that the client is suspicious, that he has long-standing patterns of interaction that will make him unable to respond to the nurse's offer of communication. The nurse should provide care and information to the client in a nonemotional and matter-of-fact manner. If the client is in for care because his behavior patterns are making life too difficult, the nurse should focus on the behaviors. For example, the client frequently does not know how he comes across to others. The nurse can provide clear and honest feedback. As with clients who have paranoid delusions (see Chapter 13), the nurse should not try to talk the client out of unfounded fears. Such discussions will only lead to the client becoming defensive.

The Assassination of Richard Nixon

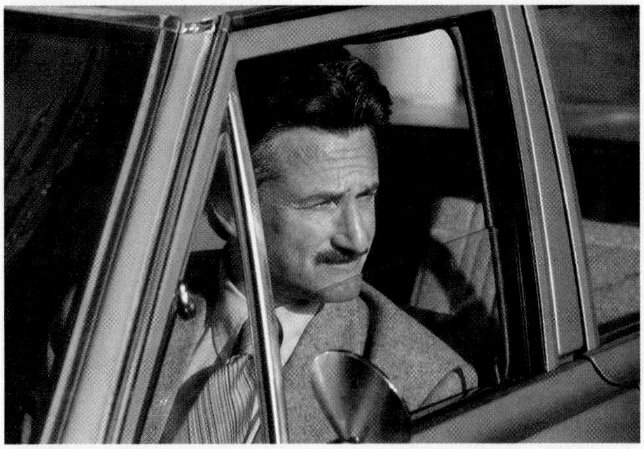

Source: Anhelo Productions. (Courtesy: The Kobal Collection.)

In *The Assassination of Richard Nixon*, Sean Penn plays a delusional Samuel Bicke whose paranoid personality disorder becomes increasingly delusional and leads to a plot to kill President Nixon. The movie is based on a true story and masterfully acted by Penn.

NURSINGTIP 18-3

Because patients with paranoid personality disorders will mistrust others, the best nursing approach will be straightforward, respectful, and unobtrusive.

ANXIETY- AND FEAR-BASED PERSONALITY CLUSTER

Persons with this cluster of personality disorders appear anxious or express fears that inhibit setting or attaining goals. This fear is not the suspiciousness of Paranoid Personality Disorder; rather, it is the fear that inhibits setting or attaining goals, or the fear of criticism or rejection.

Obsessive-Compulsive Personality Disorder

AKAKY AKAKYEVITCH

It would be hard to find a man who lived in his work as did Akaky Akakyevitch. To say that he was zealous in his work is not enough; no, he loved his work. In it, in that copying, he found a varied and agreeable world of his own. There was a look of enjoyment on his face; certain letters were favorites with him, and when he came to them he was delighted; he chuckled to himself and winked and moved his lips, so that it seemed as though every letter his pen was forming could be read in his face. If rewards had been given according to the measure of zeal in the service, he might to his amazement have even found himself a civil councillor; but all he gained in the service, as the wits, his fellow-clerks expressed it, was a buckle in his button-hole and a pain in his back. It cannot be said, however, that no notice had ever been taken of him. One director, being a good-natured man and anxious to reward him for his long service, sent him something a little more important than his ordinary copying; This cost him such an effort that it

NURSING TIP 18-4

Clients with Odd and Eccentric Personality Disorders

The nurse must approach clients with these personality disorders with the realization that the client will not respond to the nurse's efforts to build a relationship with the client. These clients are socially isolated, their behaviors lead others to avoid them, and they may have difficulties at work or school. They may seek mental health care because they are in distress for another reason, as, for example, the woman who experienced acute heart disease and became psychotic; or they may suffer from an Axis I disorder, depression being one of the most common. Clients with odd and eccentric personality disorders are frequently referred for mental health evaluation when they come up against a rigid system (e.g., schools, as in Paul's case in the excerpt under Schizoid Personality at the beginning of this section) where others notice the unusual aspects of the person's behavior and believe something is seriously wrong. The nurse should focus on the behaviors that are most disturbing or causing the most difficulty for the client and assess for other coexisting psychiatric and medical disorders.

threw him into a regular perspiration: he mopped his brow and said at last. "No, better let me copy something."

It seemed as though nothing in the world existed for him outside his copying.... On reaching home, he would sit down at once to the table, hurriedly sup his soup and eat a piece of beef with an onion. When he felt that his stomach was beginning to be full, he would rise up from the table, get out a bottle of ink and set to copying the papers he had brought home with him. When he had none to do, he would make a copy expressly for his own pleasure.

Akaky Akakyevitch had for some time been feeling that his back and shoulders were particularly nipped by the cold.... He wondered at last whether there were any defects in his overcoat. After examining it thoroughly in the privacy of his home, he discovered that in two or three places, to wit on the back and the shoulders, it had become a regular sieve; the cloth was so worn that you could see through it....

Then Akaky Akakyevitch saw that there was no escape from a new overcoat and he was utterly depressed. How indeed, for what, with what money could he get it? ... Akaky Akakyevitch had the habit every time he spent a ruble of putting aside two kopecks in a little locked-up box with a slit in the lid for slipping the money in. At the end of every half-year he would inspect the pile of coppers there and change them for small silver.

*... Another two or three months of partial fasting and Akaky Akakyevitch had actually saved up nearly eighty rubles.**

(Gogol, 1957, pp. 237–250)

This story, by the famous nineteenth-century Russian author Nicolai Gogol, is a reminder of how tedious it was to carry out business activities before the invention of typewriters, photocopiers, and word processing. Akaky is clearly preoccupied with his work, the proper performance of which demands compulsive attention. But, as his supervisors and fellow clerks observe, Akaky's compulsiveness goes beyond the requirements of his job. He has excluded leisure and friendships from his life, and he invariably takes his work home with him. Unlike a modern "workaholic," he is not trying to impress his supervisors or to distinguish himself by the quantity or quality of his work. As Gogol portrays him, Akaky is driven by a physical and psychological need to copy documents. The content is irrelevant to him; he has interest only in the physical form of the numbers and letters he writes, and perhaps in the identity of the persons to whom the documents are addressed. His compulsiveness extends to his personal finances. He carefully taxes himself 2% of all that he spends, but he has no long-term plans for how to use the money he saves. Individuals with **Obsessive-Compulsive Personality Disorder** (OCPD) tend, like Akaky, to hoard their money, and, also like him, they frequently find it difficult to discard old and worn-out possessions.

Such preoccupation with order, cleanliness, control, and perfectionism are characteristic of persons with Obsessive-Compulsive Personality Disorder. Persons with Obsessive-Compulsive Personality Disorder attempt to maintain control by attention to trivia, rules, detail, and procedures to the point where the reason for the activity is lost in the attention to form. Like Akaky, persons with Obsessive-Compulsive Personality Disorder are loyal to their work and may avoid leisure or pleasurable pursuits. Persons with this disorder often seem highly inflexible. As a result, they may initially have difficulty accepting the experience of physical illness. Hospitalization, medical visits, and other necessities of illness (and of aging) potentially threaten long-established routines and may be experienced as highly disruptive. With careful counseling, however, persons with Obsessive-Compulsive Personality Disorder can make extraordinarily compliant clients, especially when disorders like diabetes require careful self-management.

It is important to recognize that, despite a very similar name, Obsessive-Compulsive Personality Disorder is

*From "The Overcoat," in *The Overcoat and Other Tales of Good and Evil*, by Nicolai Gogol.

BOX 18-9
SIMILAR WORDS, DIFFERENT MEANINGS

1. What is the difference between the DSM diagnoses *Paranoid Schizophrenia* and *Paranoid Personality Disorder*?
   - *Paranoid Schizophrenia* is a term that applies to individuals with Schizophrenia whose delusions have paranoid content. These persons typically believe that others are intent on causing them harm, and because the paranoia is part of a psychotic disorder, it is expressed in bizarre thoughts and hallucinations. Persons afflicted with the paranoid type of Schizophrenia often experience their paranoid fears as voices threatening persecution or harm. These persons can become strongly aroused by their fear and as a result are often dangerous to others. As with other forms of Schizophrenia, the paranoid variety generally develops in an individual whose previous functioning was relatively normal.
   - Individuals with *Paranoid Personality Disorder* display a long-standing aloofness and unwillingness to trust others. They are suspicious, hypersensitive, and often hostile. This hostility frequently manifests itself as intense jealousy, particularly in marital relationships. Although individuals with this disorder may occasionally act out their paranoia either through individual violence or as members of a potentially violent "cult," persons with Paranoid Personality Disorder are generally more likely to express their disorder verbally. Although stress may bring on brief periods of psychosis, paranoid beliefs tend to be more unpleasant than irrational or bizarre; hallucinations and unpredictable behavior are generally absent.
2. How are these disorders similar?
   - Paranoia—the expression of distrust and suspiciousness—is common to both Paranoid Schizophrenia and Paranoid Personality Disorder. Individuals with either disorder can be very difficult to work with, either as a professional or as a family member.
3. How are these disorders different?
   - Paranoid Schizophrenia generally develops in an individual who was relatively normal before the onset of her illness. Paranoid Personality Disorder is a pervasive form of behavior that can often be traced to adolescence or even childhood and remains largely stable through a lifetime.
4. Can an individual have both Paranoid Schizophrenia and Paranoid Personality Disorder?
   - Yes. Some people who develop Paranoid Schizophrenia have had a history of Paranoid Personality Disorder.

distinct from Obsessive-Compulsive Disorder. In DSM-IV-TR, Obsessive-Compulsive Disorder is an Axis I anxiety diagnosis, whereas Obsessive-Compulsive Personality Disorder is an Axis II description of personality traits.

Etiology

Developmental history of an adult with Obsessive-Compulsive Personality Disorder often reveals a family in which it was expected that the child be perfect and adhere closely to rules. Adults report little warmth in their childhood homes and describe frequent punishment for failure to be perfect. Under such circumstances, praise is rarely received, and the child is strongly motivated to strive for carefully correct performance merely to avoid criticism (Benjamin, 1993). As noted previously, under some circumstances such as adjustment to the requirements of physical illness, the presence of obsessive-compulsive traits may be an asset. Despite the value of careful attention to detail, the constant striving for perfection that is characteristic of a personality disorder causes significant impairment in functioning. Whereas many persons have some obsessive-compulsive traits, the prevalence of frank Obsessive-Compulsive Personality Disorder in adults is only about 1%; the diagnosis is made twice as often for males as for females (American Psychiatric Association, 2000).

Clients with Obsessive-Compulsive Personality Disorder expect attention to detail. The nurse should recognize that order and rules are important to the client. The client is often prepared to do what is right for his health, but he expects clear and unconfused directions. When obsessive-compulsive behaviors cause personal difficulties, for example at work, school, or in hospital settings wherein the client is not in control, the nurse may assist the client to adapt by allowing the client to arrange aspects of the environment. The nurse also has a role in helping family members, teachers, and significant others in understanding why order is so important to the client.

Avoidant Personality Disorder

LAURA

Laura is seated in the delicate ivory chair at the small claw-foot table. She wears a dress of soft violet material for a kimono—her hair is tied back from her forehead with a ribbon. She is washing and polishing her collection of glass.

BOX 18-10
ESSENTIAL FEATURES OF OBSESSIVE-COMPULSIVE PERSONALITY DISORDER

- Is preoccupied with details, lists, rules, organization, or schedules
- Aspires to perfectionism that interferes with task completion
- Is excessively devoted to work and productivity
- Is overconscientious, scrupulous, and inflexible about matters of morality, ethics, or values
- Is unable to discard worn-out and worthless objects
- Is reluctant to delegate tasks
- Adopts a miserly spending style
- Is rigid and stubborn

From the *Diagnostic and Statistical Manual of Mental Disorders- TR* (4th ed.). Copyright 2000. Reprinted with permission from the American Psychiatric Association.

Amanda [her mother] appears on the fire escape steps. At the sound of her ascent, Laura catches her breath, thrusts the bowl of ornaments away, and seats herself stiffly before the diagram of the typewriter keyboard as though it held her spellbound....

LAURA: Hello, Mother, I was—[She makes a nervous gesture toward the chart on the wall. Amanda leans against the shut door and stares at Laura with a martyred look.]

AMANDA: Deception? Deception? [She slowly removes her hat and gloves, continuing the sweet suffering stare. She lets the hat and gloves fall on the floor—a bit of acting.]

LAURA: [shakily]: How was the D.A.R. meeting? [Amanda slowly opens her purse and removes a dainty white handkerchief which she shakes out delicately and delicately touches to her lips and nostrils.]
Didn't you go to the D.A.R. meeting, Mother?

AMANDA: [faintly, almost inaudibly];—No.—No. [then more forcibly:] I did not have the strength—to go to the D.A.R. In fact, I did not have the courage! I wanted to find a hole in the ground and hide myself in it forever! [She crosses slowly to the wall and removes the diagram of the typewriter keyboard. She holds it in front of her for a second, staring at it sweetly and sorrowfully—then bites her lips and tears it in two pieces.]

LAURA: [faintly] Why did you do that, Mother? [Amanda repeats the same procedure with the chart of the Gregg Alphabet.]
Why are you—

AMANDA: Why? Why? How old are you, Laura?

LAURA: Mother, you know my age.

AMANDA: I thought that you were an adult; it seems that I was mistaken. [She crosses slowly to the sofa and sinks down and stares at Laura.]

LAURA: Please don't stare at me, Mother. [Amanda closes her eyes and lowers her head. There is a ten second pause.]

AMANDA: What are we going to do, what is going to become of us, what is the future? [There is another pause.]

LAURA: Has something happened, Mother? [Amanda draws a long breath, takes out the handkerchief again, goes through the dabbing process.]

AMANDA: I'll be all right in a minute, I'm just bewildered—[she hesitates.]—by life ...

LAURA: Mother, I wish that you would tell me what's happened!

AMANDA: I went to the typing instructor and introduced myself as your mother. She didn't know who you were. "Wingfield," she said, "We don't have any such student enrolled at the school!"
I assured her she did, that you had been going to classes since early in January.

Heavy

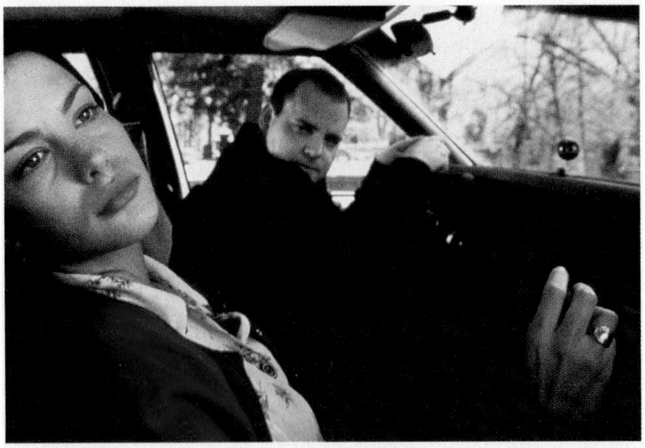

Source: Available Light (Courtesy: The Kobal Collection)

Victor and Callie, the two main characters in *Heavy* are made for each other only in Victor's fantasies. Overweight, bulimic, and despite his name, a loser, Victor also has Avoidant Personality Disorder. Unlikely to win the girl who haunts his sleeping and waking dreams, he is played here brilliantly by Pruitt Taylor Vince.

BOX 18-11
SIMILAR WORDS, DIFFERENT MEANINGS

1. What is the difference between the DSM diagnoses *Obsessive-Compulsive Disorder* and *Obsessive-Compulsive Personality Disorder*?
   - *Obsessive-Compulsive Disorder* (OCD) is one of the anxiety disorders. Although OCD may develop at any time in life, it tends to begin relatively acutely and may often improve either spontaneously or with therapy. The symptoms of OCD occur under quite specific stimuli (e.g., with fears of self-contamination), and the affected individual tries to relieve these symptoms by certain repeated actions (such as hand washing). The person who suffers from OCD generally recognizes that his fears are out of proportion to any real threat, but without therapy is often powerless to control those fears.
   - *Obsessive-Compulsive Personality Disorder* (OCPD) is an Axis II disorder in DSM-IV-TR. This means that it has developmental origins that can generally be traced back to young adulthood or even to childhood. Persons with OCPD tend to be rigid, perfectionistic, and distinctly uncomfortable if others fail to follow the patterns of activity or behavior that they demand. Individuals with OCPD often do not work well with others because they have great difficulty sharing or delegating. Individuals with OCPD typically lack interpersonal flexibility or the ability to negotiate.
2. How are these disorders similar?
   - OCD and OCPD may share patterns of rigidity; individuals with either disorder may hoard personal effects, clothing, or other items.
3. How are these disorders different?
   - In general, OCD and OCPD are quite distinct. The individual with OCD is usually psychologically normal except in situations that evoke their obsessions or compulsions. Consequently, many affected persons manage to successfully hide their symptoms from friends and family. A person with OCD symptoms that involve fear of contamination may be very uncomfortable if, for example, food is placed back on the table after having fallen on the floor. She may not care in the least if the candles are knocked off the table or the chairs are arranged in any arbitrary order. In contrast, an individual with OCPD may be exceedingly uncomfortable if papers, books, or furniture are moved in any way. She may insist on a rigid order of activities, for example, soup must never be eaten before salad, or the television must never be turned on before the windows are opened and the laundry folded. The rigidity of OCPD is generally extreme, unrelated to the specific anxieties or fears that characterize OCD, and applies to virtually all aspects of life and behavior.
4. Can a person have both OCD and OCPD?
   - Yes. Howard Hughes, described in the chapter on Obsessive-Compulsive Disorder, almost certainly also had characteristics of OCPD.

"I wonder," she said, "If you could be talking about that terribly shy little girl who dropped out of school after only a few days' attendance?"

"No," I said, "Laura, my daughter, has been going to school every day for the past six weeks!"

NURSINGTIP 18-5

Individuals with Obsessive-Compulsive Personality Disorder (OCPD) tend to be overly concerned with control—control of their own lives, their emotions, and other people. The nurse should give as much control to the client as is safe and reasonable, and avoid getting into power struggles with OCPD clients.

"Excuse me," she said. She took the attendance book out and there was your name, unmistakably printed, and all the dates you were absent until they decided that you had dropped out of school.

"I still said, No, there must have been some mistake! There must have been some mix-up in the records!"

And she said, "No—I remember her perfectly now. Her hands shook so that she couldn't hit the right keys! The first time we gave a speed test, she broke down completely—was sick at the stomach and almost had to be carried into the wash room! After that morning she never showed up any more. We phoned the house but never got any answer." ...

Laura, where have you been going when you've gone out pretending that you were going to business college?

*LAURA: I've just been going out walking.**

(*Williams, 1971, pp. 151–153*)

The major features of **Avoidant Personality Disorder** are social inhibition and feelings of inadequacy. Persons with this disorder avoid interpersonal situations at work or school that could lead to criticism or rejection. Affected individuals are shy, inhibited, and sometimes described as "invisible." They may turn down offers of advancement to avoid the risk of criticism or defeat. The affected individual perceives herself to be unappealing or inferior to others and is typically unwilling to take normal risks involved with employment or interpersonal relationships. This description fits Laura exceedingly well: She is shy, fearful, and, as becomes evident later in the play, unable to form relationships outside of the childlike imaginary world in which she lives. As her brother Tom observes:

*Laura is different from other girls.... She's terribly shy and lives in a world of her own and those things make her seem a little peculiar to people outside the house.... She lives in a world of her own—a world of little glass ornaments.... She plays old phonograph records and—that's about all.**

(*Williams, 1971, p. 153*)

Etiology

A person with Avoidant Personality Disorder often has a childhood history of being in a family where the opinions of others were held in high importance and the opinion of the child not highly regarded or noticed. As a result, the child is socialized to believe that public exposure can result in humiliation. The individual has a desire to be sociable but also a fear that being close to others may bring rejection or humiliation, or both. The family is the sole source of support for the person with Avoidant Personality Disorder, even if the family is critical and rejecting. The person with Avoidant Personality Disorder fears that those outside the family will reject him even more than does his own family (Benjamin, 1993).

Individuals with Avoidant Personality Disorder often perceive criticism when it is not intended by others. As with Laura, shyness is a major feature that often begins in early childhood and may increase significantly in adolescence. In contrast, normal childhood shyness decreases through adolescence and young adulthood. Shyness is a far more common trait than full-blown Avoidant Personality Disorder, a condition with a prevalence in the general population of something under 1%. Shyness and discomfort in socially demanding situations is also a major characteristic of social phobia (see Chapter 13). Although clients with the Axis II diagnosis of Avoidant Personality Disorder may also have elements of social phobia (Axis I) and may benefit from treatment for the condition, Avoidant Personality Disorder is lifelong and affects all settings, not only those involving performance and observations of others. Unlike many other personality disorders, this diagnosis is equally common among males as among females.

A client with Avoidant Personality Disorder will come across as shy and unwilling to try new things. The client's only source of support will be, as in Laura's case, her immediate family or very close friends. The nurse must engage the client's significant others in efforts to provide care. It is sometimes helpful to assist family members to understand the avoidant behaviors and help them to encourage the client to try out new things, as in Laura's case, going to school. The client may be receptive to establishing a relationship with the nurse, but the client will not give up her family supports or seek independence.

BOX 18-12
ESSENTIAL FEATURES OF AVOIDANT PERSONALITY DISORDER

- Is unwilling to get involved with people unless certain of being liked
- Shows restraint in intimate relationships for fear of being shamed or ridiculed
- Is inhibited in interpersonal relationships because of feelings of inadequacy
- Views self as socially inept and inferior to others
- Is unusually reluctant to take personal risks

From the *Diagnostic and Statistical Manual of Mental Disorder – TR* (4th ed.). Copyright © 2000. Reprinted with permission from the American Psychiatric Association.

Dependent Personality Disorder

EVELINE

She was about to explore another life with Frank. Frank was very kind, manly, open-hearted. She was to go away with him by the night-boat to be his wife and to live with him in Buenos Ayres where he had a home waiting for her.... Of course, her father had found out the affair and had forbidden her to have anything to say to him.... After that she had to meet her lover secretly.

The evening deepened in the avenue. The white of two letters in her lap grew indistinct. One was to [her brother]; the other was to her father.... As she mused the pitiful

*From *The Glass Menagerie* by Tennessee Williams. Copyright © 1945 by The University of the South and Edwin D. Williams. Reprinted by permission of New Directions Publishing Corporation.

> *vision of her mother's life laid its spell on the very quick of her being—that life of commonplace sacrifices closing in final craziness....*
>
> *She stood up in a sudden impulse of terror. Escape! She must escape! Frank would save her....*
>
> *She stood among the swaying crowd in the station at the North Wall. He held her hand and she knew that he was speaking to her, saying something about the passage over and over again.... She answered nothing. She felt her cheek pale and cold and, out of a maze of distress, she prayed to God to direct her, to show her what was her duty. The boat blew a long mournful whistle into the mist. If she went, to-morrow she would be on the sea with Frank, steaming towards Buenos Ayres.... A bell clanged upon her heart. She felt him seize her hand:—Come!*
>
> *No! No! No! It was impossible. Her hands clutched the iron in frenzy. Amid the seas she sent a cry of anguish!*
>
> *—Eveline! Evy!*
>
> *He rushed beyond the barrier and called to her to follow. He was shouted at to go on but he still called to her. She set her white face to him, passive, like a helpless animal. Her eyes gave him no sign of love or farewell or recognition.**
>
> *(Joyce, 1967, pp. 38–41)*

In this excerpt from Joyce's famous story in *The Dubliners,* Eveline is unable to decide or to act. She is in love with Frank, who has promised her a new life in Argentina, far from dreary, oppressive Ireland, but she cannot decide to go with him. She knows that women have been betrayed by men who promise marriage and then desert them far from their homes and family. Her own home offers little future other than the uncertain possibility of a dreary marriage to an unromantic, perhaps physically abusive husband. In the novel, Eveline stays with her father in Dublin, not because she chooses that life, but because she cannot choose. She lets her father dictate her life, and despite almost escaping, in the end she cannot make the separation from her past. The story leaves her both uncomfortable and helpless, but unable to respond with either "farewell or recognition."

A person with **Dependent Personality Disorder** has a need to be taken care of by others. The individual is clinging and submissive and fears separation from the known. Such persons have trouble making decisions and difficulty expressing disagreements with others. They feel unable to function alone and are not independent. They are willing to do what others want, particularly if such actions lead to others caring for them. As with other personality disorders, these characteristics must be present in sufficient degree that they significantly interfere with personal or social functioning.

*From "Eveline," in *The Dubliners,* by James Joyce. Copyright © 1916 by B. W. Heubsch. Definitive text Copyright © 1967 by the Estate of James Joyce. Reprinted with permission from Viking Penguin, a division of Penguin Books, USA Inc.

BOX 18-13
ESSENTIAL FEATURES OF DEPENDENT PERSONALITY DISORDER

- Has difficulty making everyday decisions
- Needs others to assume responsibility for major areas of his or her life
- Has difficulty expressing disagreement
- Has difficulty initiating projects
- Goes to excessive lengths to obtain nurturance from others
- Feels uncomfortable or helpless when alone
- Urgently seeks relationships as a source of care or support
- Is unrealistically preoccupied with fears of being left to take care of self

From the *Diagnostic and Statistical Manual of Mental Disorders- TR* (4th ed.). Copyright © 2000. Reprinted with permission from the American Psychiatric Association.

Etiology

One theory of Dependent Personality Disorder is that, in early childhood, parents did not stop nurturing the child when it was developmentally appropriate to do so. Instead of letting the toddler do things on his own, the caregivers offer too much protectiveness. The child becomes incompetent and begins to believe that he cannot do anything. There is overwhelming parental control and the only option for the developing child is submission. Cultural and social factors may certainly play a role. Some have argued that in our culture, women are encouraged to be dependent (Gilligan, 1982), thus it has been suggested that dependent personality disorder may represent an exaggerated or maladaptive variant of "normal" dependency (Phillips, et al., 2003). Not surprisingly, then, in clinical settings, the diagnosis is made more often for females than for males. Dependent Personality Disorder is one of the most frequently reported personality disorders encountered in mental health clinics (American Psychiatric Association, 2000). Individuals with highly dependent personalities frequently use illness to gain support and attention. There is potentially a strong tendency for individuals with Dependent Personality Disorder to develop Axis I somatoform disorders, especially when somatization brings them attention and support.

Nurses who encounter persons with Dependent Personality Disorder often become frustrated because the client does not demonstrate age-appropriate independence. Nurses must recognize that the client may, indeed, live a life of having others take charge. The client may come into nursing care only when he is physically ill or needs nurses to provide care because no one else in his world will do so at a given point in time. The nurse must set limits regarding what the nurse will do for the client and what the client is expected to do for himself.

Passive-Aggressive or Negativistic Personality Disorder

I AM A SPITEFUL MAN

I am a spiteful man ... I have been living like that for a long time now—twenty years. I am forty now. I used to be in the civil service, but no longer am. I was a spiteful official. I was rude and took pleasure in being so....

When petitioners would come to my desk for information I used to grind my teeth at them, and feel intense enjoyment when I succeeded in distressing someone. I was almost always successful. For the most part they were all timid people—of course, they were petitioners. But among the fops there was one officer in particular I could not endure. He simply would not be humble, and clanged his sword in a disgusting way. I carried on a war with him for eighteen months over that sword. At last I got the better of him. He left off clanking it....

*I was lying when I said just now that I was a spiteful official. I was lying out of spite. I was simply indulging myself with the petitioners and with the officer, but I could never really become spiteful.... Not only could I not become spiteful, I could not become anything: neither spiteful nor kind, neither a rascal nor an honest man, neither a hero nor an insect.... I am forty years old now, and forty years, after all is a whole lifetime; ... Who does live beyond forty? Answer that, sincerely and honestly. I will tell you who do: fools and worthless people do.... I have a right to say so, for I shall go on living to sixty myself. I'll live till seventy! till eighty!**

(Dostoevsky, 1960, pp. 3–5)

In *Notes from Underground,* Dostoevsky has created a character who is remarkable for his perversity and negative outlook on life. Few if any literary characters prior to *Notes* have been portrayed to be as unlikable and pathetic as is the narrator of this excerpt. One of the reasons it is so hard to respond positively to "the Underground Man" is the passive-aggressive way in which his self-hatred expresses itself. Passive-aggressive behavior creates anger in the persons to whom it is directed, and even the reader ultimately reacts with annoyance and anger. The DSM-IV-TR description of **Passive-Aggressive Personality Disorder** reflects Dostoevsky's character with remarkable accuracy: "These individuals ... may be sullen, irritable, impatient, argumentative, cynical, skeptical, and contrary ... [They may] feel cheated, unappreciated, and misunderstood and chronically complain to others" (American Psychiatric Association, 2000, p. 790). In DSM-IV-TR, Passive-Aggressive Personality Disorder was removed from the list of personality disorders and placed on the list of disorders requiring further research and investigation. Although a diagnosis of Passive-Aggressive Personality Disorder cannot be made (the correct diagnosis at this time is Personality Disorder, Not Otherwise Specified), the authors have included Passive-Aggressive Personality Disorder in this chapter because passive-aggressive behavior is seen relatively frequently in health care settings. The official diagnosis requires study to ensure consistency in definition and diagnosis, but the concept of the passive-aggressive individual is useful for the nurse to understand.

The individual with Passive-Aggressive Personality Disorder typically displays a combination of pervasive negativity with passive resistance to social and/or occupational demands. Such resistance to demands is often characterized by procrastination, stubbornness, and intentional inefficiency, particularly in response to demands made by authority figures. Passive-Aggressive Personality Disorder is sometimes also called negativistic personality disorder.

Etiology

The developmental history of persons with Passive-Aggressive Personality Disorder may include the abrupt loss of infantile and child nurturance followed by the imposition of unfair or excessive developmental demands. This developmental scenario may most frequently occur when a first-born child is displaced by the birth of a younger sibling. His resultant anger at being frustrated by his life events may be expressed passively. The child ultimately learns indirect ways of dealing with parents/authorities by taking a long time to complete tasks or doing them with obvious flaws (Benjamin, 1993).

To provide care to one with a passive-aggressive personality, the nurse must first evaluate her own feelings in reaction to the passive-aggressiveness. Typically, nurses find themselves angry at the client, and the client seems uncaring, devious, and even cruel. The nurse must have the ability to step back and recognize the passive-aggressive behavior and understand that the client's behavior is likely motivated by a negative view of self and the world. The individual with Passive-Aggressive Personality Disorder is unhappy with himself and with others in his life and will demonstrate his unhappiness through chronic complaints.

*From *Notes from Underground and the Grand Inquisitor*, by Fyodor Dostoevsky. Translated by Ralph E. Matlaw, Copyright © 1960, 1988 by E. P. Dutton. Reprinted with permission from Dutton Signet, a division of Penguin Books, USA Inc.

NURSING TIP 18-6

Clients with Anxiety- and Fear-Based Personality Disorders

Nurses must approach clients with this cluster of personality disorders from a perspective of caring and understanding. The client's anxieties, obsessions, and fears of failure are very real. The nurse may be able to help the client cope with his environment by giving the client control wherever possible and encouraging the client to manage his environment in his own way. Persons with an avoidant personality will need great patience and encouragement to take on even small responsibilities.

RESEARCH Highlight 18–2

The Validity of the DSV-IV Passive Aggressive (Negativistic) Personality Disorder

PURPOSE

Researchers conducted a study to evaluate the reliability and validity of the diagnosis, Passive-Aggressive (Negativistic) Personality Disorder.

METHODS

A large sample (over 1,000) of study subjects, who were solicited from a psychiatric outpatient facility in the North East, were interviewed and evaluated with the DSM criteria.

FINDINGS

The number of subjects that could be diagnosed with the disorder was 3.02% of the diagnostic criteria listed, two items were most strongly correlated to the diagnosis: "complaints of being misunderstood/unappreciated" and "sullen and argumentative." The diagnosis did show overlap with other personality disorders, notably BPD, Paranoid, and Avoidant.

IMPLICATIONS

There is need to further evaluate the usefulness of this diagnosis, however, the study provided some support for its use. Evaluation indicated more prominence of the "negativity" criteria than the "passively resists" criteria.

Source: O. H. Rotenstein, W. McDermut, A. Bergman, D. Young, M. Zimmerman, & I. Chelminski. (2007). The Validity of the DSM-IV Passive-Aggressive (Negativistic) Personality Disorder. *Journal of Personality Disorders*, *21*(1), 28–41.

Individuals with Passive-Aggressive Personality Disorder almost always provoke anger in others, including their nurses.

NURSING CARE

As emphasized in several of the previous individual discussions, nurses will likely encounter persons with personality disorders in virtually every area of practice. More often than not, the personality disorder is not the reason for the client's coming to medical or nursing attention; rather, the client presents for care of some other concurrent condition. The client with a personality disorder may present in a clinic with vague complaints or may present at a counseling center with depression. One author suggests that "early indicators that a personality disorder may be present include difficulty establishing a nurse-client relationship, disagreements among team members, a reluctance by the nurse to provide client care, or difficulty accomplishing treatment objectives" (Godfrey, 1991, p. 590). The goals of nursing care are first to recognize that the client has a personality disorder and second to provide care to minimize the negative impact of the client's behaviors.

Knowing that interpersonal difficulties are central problems for people who have personality disorders, it is not surprising that nurses report that it is both difficult and unsatisfying to work with such a population. One study documented that 84% of psychiatric nurses felt that dealing with this group of clients was more difficult than other client groups (Clearly, Siegfried, & Walter, 2002), and another report stated nurses see working with clients with personality disorders to be undesirable (Murphy & McVey, 2003). To assist nurses to undertake the task of working with these clients, Duff (2003) listed "self-awareness" (knowing one's own vulnerabilities and prejudices) and "systems awareness" (knowing how to work as a team and support other team members to function as a group) as essential. Further, Duff states that teams working with these clients need to be absolutely consistent and supportive of one another. There is a risk that individual nurses can feel stressed and isolated from coworkers, and nursing/mental health staff must guard against this. One group of authors reported that establishing a "personality disorder service," staffed with individuals who understood the dynamics of the disorders and worked together in meeting clients needs, was a successful model of care delivery that worked well in meeting client needs (Hitchcock, Isbell, & Loseby, 2007).

NURSING THEORY

The Modeling and Role-Modeling theory (Erickson, Tomlin, & Swain, 1983), with its emphasis on psychosocial development, will assist the nurse to explore the client's early experiences and to understand how such experiences impact on personality development and behavior patterns. For example, the character Eveline in the excerpt that illustrates dependent personality would be a case where knowledge of early years and adolescent development could form the basis for treatment choices. Presumably, Eveline (a young adult) has never been given choices over matters that affect her life. As a child, Eveline had no control over her lack of choices, but as an adult, Eveline could take some control over her own life. However, Eveline would have to be in enough discomfort (mental or physical) that she would be motivated to try something new, and she would have to trust someone enough to believe that that person would provide support to her during her process of changing. Counseling based on modeling her world would direct the nurse to see the events from Eveline's perspective and would ensure that the nurse interacting with Eveline understood that Eveline's condition is based on fear of independence and lack of self-esteem.

Martha Rogers's theory of unitary human beings has been used to assist psychiatric nurses to understand and intervene with clients with Borderline Personality Disorder (Thompson, 1990). The borderline client's behaviors, which include "rapid, radical shifts in mood, perception and behavior" (Thompson, 1990, p. 7), were interpreted from within the framework of human and environmental energy fields. The client with a borderline personality was viewed as having an energy field whose wave patterns change at an unusually rapid rate, which in turn affects the environmental energy field. This may explain why nursing staff often find the borderline client difficult to care for. It was proposed, however, that the nurse could maintain a sense of her own patterning and approach the client with a sense of calm. The interaction of the two energy fields could help produce calm in the client. Further, psychiatric nurses could attend to the environmental energy field, providing a borderline client with a space/room that the client could decorate and use as his own "personal space." Such an intervention would provide the client with both the security of having his own space and the safety of having an environment he can control. Use of Rogers's theory guides the nurse to a different understanding of clients with personality disorders and has great relevance in selection of interventions.

REFLECTIVE THINKING 18-2

Personality Disorders and You

Almost all students in the health fields begin to think about whether or not they have the condition, disease, or disorder that is the topic of their class discussions. For example, students studying cardiovascular disorders often begin to wonder if they have abnormal palpitations. Similarly, almost all students studying personality disorders start to place their own personality traits into one or another of the categories of disease. Please remember that the personality disorders described in this chapter refer to persistent personality traits and behaviors that lead to significant distress or impairment in the individual's functioning.

RESEARCH Highlight 18–3

Motivation for Treatment in Patients with Personality Disorders

STUDY PROBLEM/PURPOSE

A study was conducted to investigate associations between motivation for treatment and diagnosis of a personality disorder.

METHODS

A sample of over 1,000 patients was recruited from consecutive admissions to psychiatric clinics. Patients were assessed as having a personality disorder through interviews consistent with DSM-IV diagnostic criteria. The researchers assessed "symptom distress" through a standardized tool and developed a "motivation for treatment" questionnaire that was also administered. The motivation for treatment questionnaire included items on two factors: need for help and readiness for change.

FINDINGS

In the overall sample, only 28.1% of the patients did not have a diagnosable personality disorder. While many patients had more than one personality disorder, the authors devised mutually exclusive categories that provided the following data: 7.4% of the sample had PD in Cluster A; 20.5% in Cluster B and not A; 30.1% in cluster C but not A and B; and 14% had personality disorders that were not specified in the other groupings.

Patients with personality disorders scored higher than those without on the measures of motivation for change, including need for help and readiness for change. This higher degree of motivation is also associated with a higher degree of symptom distress perceived by the personality disorder patients.

IMPLICATIONS

Nurses and clinicians should recognize that motivation for treatment may not be a steady state, and thus, the motivation for treatment among personality disorder patients on admission may represent a critical time for engaging the client in reflection and behavioral change.

Source: "Motivation for Treatment in Patients with Personality Disorders," by N. van Beek & R. Verheul, 2008, *Journal of Personality Disorders, 22*(1), 89–100.

APPLICATION OF THE NURSING PROCESS 18-1

ASSESSMENT

Assessment of a client's behaviors through observation and history taking may suggest the presence of a personality disorder. A diagnosis of a personality disorder may be tentatively made by the nurse and confirmed through psychiatric evaluation. In some instances, psychological tests further add to data and to diagnostic certainty (Wiggins & Pincus, 1994). Personality disorders, by definition, develop in young adulthood or earlier in life. Personal history is therefore quite important to obtain, and often the client history can be augmented with information gathered through interview of family members, teachers, or others significant to the individual's life.

NURSING DIAGNOSIS

Whether or not a personality disorder is formally diagnosed, the nursing process typically results in the formulation of one or more nursing diagnoses. Table 18-2 lists common nursing diagnoses for clients with the DSM diagnoses of various personality disorders.

TABLE 18-2 Selected Personality Disorders with Expected Nursing Diagnoses

DISORDER	COMMON NURSING DIAGNOSES
Borderline Personality Disorder	*Risk for self-directed violence* *Risk for other-directed violence* *Ineffective coping* *Chronic low self-esteem* *Self-mutilation* *Impaired social interactions* *Hopelessness*
Narcissistic Personality Disorder	*Impaired social interaction* *Ineffective coping* *Ineffective denial*
Histrionic Personality Disorder	*Impaired social interaction* *Ineffective coping*
Antisocial Personality Disorder	*Risk for other-directed violence* *Ineffective denial* *Impaired social interaction*
Schizoid Personality Disorder	*Impaired social interaction* *Risk for loneliness* *Ineffective coping*
Paranoid Personality Disorder	*Fear* *Anxiety*
Obsessive-Compulsive Personality Disorder	*Anxiety* *Fear* *Chronic low self-esteem*

(Continues)

APPLICATION OF THE NURSING PROCESS 18-1 (Continued)

TABLE 18-2 (Continued)

DISORDER	COMMON NURSING DIAGNOSES
Avoidant Personality Disorder	*Fear* *Risk for loneliness* *Ineffective coping*
Dependent Personality Disorder	*Chronic low self-esteem* *Fear*
Passive-Aggressive or Negativistic Personality Disorder	*Ineffective coping* *Chronic low self-esteem* *Anxiety*

OUTCOME IDENTIFICATION

The goal of nursing care is to minimize the negative and self-defeating behaviors clients present. A positive outcome of care is that the client will experience a reduction in extreme behaviors and will increase effective coping strategies. The nurse must accept the client as he is and understand that the client will be unable to change his basic personality.

PLANNING/INTERVENTIONS

Some basic principles apply to all clients with personality disorders. The nurse must make clear what the nurse can and cannot do and approach the client in a professional, supportive, and nonjudgmental manner. Nurses must work with one another and the health care team to avoid being caught up in the client's manipulative behaviors, which could pit one staff member against another. The best nursing approach is one characterized by clear communication and expectations, setting limits when needed, and providing both structure and support. The nurse should recognize that clients with personality disorders are among the most "difficult" clients seen in clinical practice. The nurse will need a high degree of patience to provide comprehensive and accepted care in the presence of significant traits of personality disorders.

In some cases, the nurse may recommend and/or initiate treatment for one of these Axis II disorders. Psychotherapy is felt to be the treatment of choice for persons with schizoid, borderline, histrionic, narcissistic, dependent, passive-aggressive, and avoidant personality disorders (Andrews, 1993; Higgitt & Fonagy, 1992). However, research evidence for the effectiveness of psychotherapy in these conditions is based largely on case reports and is not strong. Other reports indicate that cognitive-behavioral therapy is successful in treating borderline (Linehan, 1987) and avoidant (Alden, 1989) personality disorders. (For a discussion of psychotherapy and cognitive-behavioral therapy, see Chapter 30 on individual therapy.) One author proposes "skills training" for selected clients since many with personality disorders have a long history of deficits in social functioning (Stanley, Bundy, & Beberman, 2001). Thus, one can consider interventions such as conversational skills training, social skills training, and anger management as potentially appropriate. Table 18-3 summarizes nursing interventions for working with clients with personality disorders.

(*Continues*)

APPLICATION OF THE NURSING PROCESS 18-1 (Continued)

NURSING TIP 18-7

Guidelines for Communicating with Clients Who Have a Personality Disorder

Guideline	Example (Do say this)	Example (Don't say this)
Communicate clearly; avoid ambiguity; give simple directions and messages.	"Today you are scheduled to attend the group therapy session at 10 A.M. I'll remind you 15 minutes early so you will get there on time."	"Maybe, if you're not too tired, you'd want to go to the group session at 10 A.M. I think it is a good idea for you to participate. Do you want me to tell you when it is time to go?"
Prevent or reduce manipulative behaviors (flattery, seductiveness, guilt instilling).	"You are telling me that I am the best nurse here, but really, we both know that the other nurses here are very, very good nurses."	"Why, thank you for the compliment! It's nice to know you think I'm the best."
Provide clear and consistent boundaries.	"No, it is not appropriate for me to give you my cell phone number. When I am not here, there are others with whom you can talk about your issues."	"You can call me whenever you just feel there is no one else to talk to."
Avoid arguments and power struggles with the client.	"I understand you may not agree, but that is the recommendation of the treatment team."	"No, I'm right on this and you are wrong. Can't you see your statements are illogical?"
Set an image of self-confidence and self-assurance.	"I've been a nurse long enough to know how to treat the clients in this clinic."	"Well, I've only been a nurse for one year... I'm just getting to learn what to do."

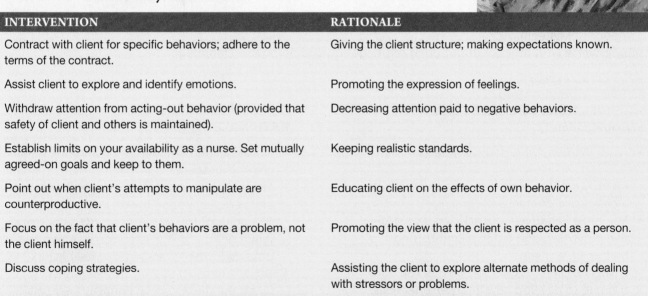

TABLE 18-3 Suggested Nursing Interventions for Clients with Personality Disorders

INTERVENTION	RATIONALE
Contract with client for specific behaviors; adhere to the terms of the contract.	Giving the client structure; making expectations known.
Assist client to explore and identify emotions.	Promoting the expression of feelings.
Withdraw attention from acting-out behavior (provided that safety of client and others is maintained).	Decreasing attention paid to negative behaviors.
Establish limits on your availability as a nurse. Set mutually agreed-on goals and keep to them.	Keeping realistic standards.
Point out when client's attempts to manipulate are counterproductive.	Educating client on the effects of own behavior.
Focus on the fact that client's behaviors are a problem, not the client himself.	Promoting the view that the client is respected as a person.
Discuss coping strategies.	Assisting the client to explore alternate methods of dealing with stressors or problems.

EVALUATION

As in all nursing care, evaluation is based on identified outcomes. The nurse should evaluate care realistically and recognize that if the client has been exposed to significant stress, care will be required over a time period of several weeks.

CARE PLANNING GUIDE 18-1 Client With A Personality Disorder: Antisocial Personality Disorder

CLINICAL PICTURE

The clinical picture of a client with Antisocial Personality Disorder includes:

- Inability to form lasting relationships with others
- Inability to sustain job performance
- Failure (repeatedly) to meet financial obligations
- Impulsiveness
- Lying and conning others for personal gain
- Lack of guilt/remorse

COMMON NURSING DIAGNOSES

Nursing diagnoses most frequently employed for Antisocial Personality Disorder are:

1. *Chronic low self-esteem*
2. *Risk for other directed violence*
3. *Ineffective copying*

The following Care Planning Guides suggest interventions, rationales, outcomes, and discharge planning for such clients.

Note: The care plans that follow are adapted from *Plans of Care for Specialty Practice: Psychiatric Mental Health Nursing*, by M. Coler and K. G. Vincent, 1995, Clifton Park, NY: Delmar, Cengage Learning.

NURSING DIAGNOSIS 1: *CHRONIC LOW SELF-ESTEEM*

OUTCOMES

1. The client will recognize that use of derogatory comments about others is a reflection of his or her own poor self-esteem.
2. Converse with others without using self-negating and derogatory language.

NOC: *SELF-ESTEEM*

INTERVENTIONS (NIC: *SELF-ESTEEM ENHANCEMENT*)	RATIONALE
• Assist in identifying positive aspects of self.	• Self-reflection and mastery over self-esteem are encouraged.
• Identify manipulative behavior and establish a behavioral contact.	• This assists in reality testing when behaviors and verbal dialogue are counterproductive.
• Minimize negative feedback, focus on positive behaviors, and enforce limit-setting in a matter-of-fact way.	• The goals of the therapeutic interaction are maintained and the attention is drawn to positive (rather than negative) behaviors.
• Assist the client to gain social skills; use skills training to develop new interpersonal skills.	• Social and copying skills training assist when the client's social behaviors are self-destructive and unproductive.
• Teach the difference between assertiveness and aggressiveness.	• Use of cognitive techniques assists in improving relationships with others and self-esteem.

Note: The care planning guides have been adapted from *Plans of Care for Speciality Practice: Psychiatric Mental Health Nursing*, by M. Coler, and K. G. Vincent, 1995, Clifton Park, NY: Delmar, Cengage Learning.

(*Continues*)

CARE PLANNING GUIDE 18-1 Continued

NURSING DIAGNOSIS 2: *RISK FOR OTHER DIRECTED VIOLENCE*

OUTCOMES

1. The client will identify situations that could precipitate into violence.
2. The client will acknowledge responsibility to maintain control over his or her own behavior.
3. The client will learn to verbalize his or her own needs with nonaggressive behaviors.

NOC: *AGGRESSION SELF CONTROL*

INTERVENTIONS (NIC: *ANGER CONTROL ASSISTANCE*)	RATIONALE
• Determine and document past history of violent behavior.	• The team needs to be aware of patterns of acting-out behaviors and the events that precipitate violence.
• Observe the client's behavior frequently; be aware of signs of escalating anger (clenched fists, pacing, loud verbalizations).	• The team can intervene if needed before violence takes place.
• Convey a trusting and consistent attitude by speaking in a calm manner; resist responding to provocative behavior or verbalizations of anger.	• The trusting attitude promotes self-worth and provides the basis for a therapeutic relationship. This provides opportunity for behavior change to form constructive relationships.
• Assist the client to identify the true object of his or her hostility.	• Displacement of anger can be an inappropriate use of defense mechanisms.
• Encourage appropriate verbalization of feelings.	• Talking about feelings increase self-awareness and the relationship of feelings and behaviors.
• Help to find alternate ways to express anger (exercise, assertiveness training, anger management programs).	• Alternate coping skills are essential to break the pattern of responding to stress and unmet needs with anger/violence.

NURSING DIAGNOSIS 3: *INEFFECTIVE COPING*

OUTCOMES

1. The client will identify past methods of coping and their outcome.
2. The client will verbalize need to develop new coping strategies.
3. The client will demonstrate different coping skills in therapeutic milieu and groups.

NOC: *COPING*

INTERVENTIONS (NIC: *COPING ENHANCEMENT*)	RATIONALE
• Review past acting-out, antisocial behaviors and their effects on relationships.	• This establishes a baseline assessment of coping behaviors.
• Explore alternate methods of coping that might have been used and the possible change in outcomes.	• This assists in identifying new ways of dealing with life stresses.

(*Continues*)

CARE PLANNING GUIDE 18-1 Continued

INTERVENTIONS (NIC: *COPING ENHANCEMENT*)	RATIONALE
• Encourage the client to keep a notebook of his or her own feelings and angry/hostile thoughts and the situation (context) that provoked these thoughts.	• This assists in reflecting what triggers aggressive/hostile thoughts and actions. A journal can provide the client with a beginning sense of control over finding alternative methods of dealing with these situations.
• Provide groups as a forum for emotional expression and reality testing.	• A therapeutic group is a safe place to try out new coping strategies.
• Recognize appropriate coping skills with positive feedback.	• Positive feedback reinforces the positive coping skills and enhances self-esteem.

LONG-TERM CONSIDERATIONS FOR CLIENTS WITH ANTISOCIAL PERSONALITY DISORDER

1. Clients should be referred to community resources for long-term follow-up and sustained growth in learning new coping skills and new patterns of relating to others.
2. Many clients will also need support from Alcoholics Anonymous, Narcotics Anonymous, or other drug treatment programs (see also Chapter 17).

CARE PLANNING GUIDE 18-2 Client with a Personality Disorder: Obsessive-Compulsive Personality Disorder (OCPD)

CLINICAL PICTURE

The clinical presentation of the client with OCPD includes:

- Preoccupations with lists, rules, details that result in a loss of the major point of the activities
- Vivid imagination
- Rigid perfectionism—often will fail to complete projects because of the inability to achieve high performance
- Heightened sense of responsibility

COMMON NURSING DIAGNOSES

Nursing diagnoses that are commonly used for OCPD include:

1. *Ineffective coping**
2. *Impaired social interaction*
3. *Chronic low self-esteem**
4. *Anxiety*
5. *Fear*

The following Care Planning Guides address two nursing diagnosis: impaired *social interaction* and *anxiety*.

NURSING DIAGNOSIS 1: *IMPAIRED SOCIAL INTERACTIONS*

OUTCOMES

1. The client will identify behaviors that interfere with social relationships.

*See care planning guides, Antisocial Personality Disorder.

(Continues)

CARE PLANNING GUIDE 18-2 Continued

2. The client will substitute constructive behaviors for those that interfere with socializations.
3. The client will enlist significant others in promotion of effective socializations.

NOC: *SOCIAL INVOLVEMENT*

INTERVENTIONS (NIC: *SOCIALIZATION ENHANCEMENT*)	RATIONALE
• Explore the quality of relationships at home, work, or school.	• Identify the environment where impaired social interactions occur.
• Assist the client to identify the character of present relationships and goals for future relationships.	• This employs the problem-solving technique of identifying difficulties and stating goals for the future.
• Get involved in a social skills building group that includes education on social skills, role playing, and peer support.	• The group can provide a supportive environment to learn socialization skills and to try them out in a safe, supportive environment.

NURSING DIAGNOSIS 2: *ANXIETY*

OUTCOMES

1. The client will use coping mechanisms that allow interactions with others and the environment with minimal anxiety.
2. The client will experience an increase in psychological/physiological comfort.

NOC: *ANXIETY SELF-CONTROL*

INTERVENTIONS (NIC: *ANXIETY REDUCTION*)	RATIONALE
• Monitor the level of anxiety and situations in which anxiety is increased/decreased.	• Allows for identification of changes from baseline and knowledge of the client's patterns.
• Stay with the client when he or she is anxious and present a calm presence.	• Provides reassurance and models calm behavior where anxiety does not escalate.
• Provide for a time-out activity when anxious—encourage slow deep breaths, and offer simple, repetitive tasks.	• Decreases sensory stimulation and discomfort may be eased.
• Assist in identifying stressors that cause anxiety, behaviors that result, and methods for diminishing the effect of stressors.	• Uses cognitive skills to understand behaviors and plan methods to cope with these stressors in new ways.

LONG-TERM CONSIDERATIONS FOR THE CLIENT WITH OCPD

1. Refer to ongoing therapy using a cognitive-behavioral approach.
2. Arrange for group therapy to encourage social support.
3. Encourage family therapy, when appropriate, with a goal that the family learn to provide support.

Note: The care planning guides have been adapted from *Plans of Care for Speciality Practice: Psychiatric Mental Health Nursing*, by M. Coler and K. G. Vincent, 1995, Clifton Park, NY: Delmar, Cengage Learning.

NURSING CARE PLAN: NURSING PROCESS FORMAT 18-1

For the case study, we will consider a character similar to "Annie" from the excerpt depicting Borderline Personality Disorder. June is a 24-year-old woman being seen after a suicide attempt. After the episode of her suicidal attempt/gesture, June is brought to a facility for physical treatment and psychiatric evaluation.

ASSESSMENT

June is a highly intelligent young woman. Her interests are eclectic and changeable: contemporary art and music, old classic cars, married men. She is careless about her personal appearance, but is able to attract a wide variety of gentlemen who are enticed by her reckless spirit and her energy. Her most recent social meeting is with Bill, a married stockbroker. Bill is horrified to find that June has attempted suicide. He finds her in his office, bleeding profusely from self-inflicted razor blade wounds to the wrists. June is making shrieking sounds, is shivering, and does not respond to Bill. Bill dials 911 to get June help. Her wrists are carefully stitched in the emergency room, and she is admitted to the psychiatric unit of the general hospital. She is minimally communicative.

NURSING DIAGNOSIS 1 *Risk for self-directed violence*, related to a history of self-destructive behavior.

OUTCOMES	NIC	NURSING ACTIONS	EVALUATION
• June will remain safely hospitalized for the next 3 days. • June will not mutilate herself further and will leave her current wounds alone during the next 5 days.	• Behavior management; self-harm • Environmental management: safety • Impulse control training	• Discuss with June the need to remain safe during her hospitalization. • Assist June in orienting herself to her room; explain the need for hospital care in relation to her need for safety. • Supervise June closely. • Clarify with June appropriate and expected behaviors specific to self-mutilation. • Discuss healing with June. • Gently set limits with June that she should leave her wounds alone and not further harm herself.	June remained safe in hospital and did not further harm herself. June did not disturb her wounds for 3 days.

NURSING DIAGNOSIS 2 *Impaired social interaction,* related to disturbed thought processes, as evidenced by inability to form supportive personal relationships with others.

OUTCOMES	NIC	NURSING ACTIONS	EVALUATION
• June will begin to communicate with her primary nurse within 24 hours.	• Presence • Socialization enhancement	• Offer self as truly interested in June. • Express unconditional acceptance in interactions with June. • Discuss potential breakdowns in communication	June was very slow to trust anyone. She refused to communicate for 3 days. She gradually opened up on day 4 to the nurse who sat quietly with June 30 minutes twice a day.

(Continues)

NURSING CARE PLAN: NURSING PROCESS FORMAT 18-1 (Continued)

OUTCOMES	NIC	NURSING ACTIONS	EVALUATION
		that June may find frustrating; explore how the nurse can foster communication.	The nurse praised June for her communication efforts.

NURSING DIAGNOSIS 3 *Ineffective coping,* related to chronic low self-esteem as evidenced by past behaviors of inflicting harm to self in stress-producing situations.

OUTCOMES	NIC	NURSING ACTIONS	EVALUATION
• Within 5 days, June will identify one cue that led her to her most recent self-mutilating behavior; June will identify two alternative behaviors other than directing violence toward self.	• Behavior management: self-harm • Support system enhancement	• Discuss with June the factors/situations and feelings that led up to her harming self. • Encourage June to express her feelings and anxieties. • Discuss behaviors to use when feeling out of control—phone call to primary nurse; identify a support system. • Identify with June resources she can immediately access including psych and crisis "hotlines."	The nurse continued to explore with June what precipitated the injury and what cues were present. June could not identify a specific cue, but did state she felt great anxiety at the time. June could not identify two alternative behaviors, but did agree that she could and would call the nurse or the psych hotline at the hospital if she felt "desperate."

REFLECTIVE QUESTIONS

1. **ASSESSMENT**
   What additional assessment information would be pertinent in planning care for June?
2. **NURSING DIAGNOSIS**
   In determining appropriate diagnoses, how does the nurse balance actual with potential problems? In the absence of client input, can a nurse determine the diagnosis of *spiritual distress?*
3. **OUTCOMES**
   Beyond safety, how do outcomes get prioritized? Do you agree with the priority order of outcomes as listed for June?
4. **NURSING ACTIONS**
   In addition to being self-destructive, June also had a variety of unattractive characteristics. How can a nurse be truly therapeutic when faced with such characteristics? What should the nurse do when a client acts in an embarrassing and inappropriate manner? How can a nurse best communicate with a noncommunicative client? Is nonverbal communication really noncommunicative?
5. **EVALUATION**
   What is June's long-term outcome likely to be?

NURSING CARE PLAN: CONCEPT MAP FORMAT 18-1

BACKGROUND INFORMATION

Mike is a single, adult male having some characteristics of dependency. Mike is coming for treatment in the outpatient clinic, because he has been unable to "set himself up" independently in the community. Bob is 30 years old, lives with his mother, and seems to seek a life of stability. He takes care of his mother's gardens when not at work, likes to spend time in computer "chat rooms," and works as a filing clerk in a major medical center hospital. He seems to have the capacity to go to college, but has not ever attended a full semester of coursework. He seeks therapy, but has no stated reason or outcome goals for therapy. He has health insurance through his employment that permits him to have 20 therapy sessions per year, so he is coming in for an insurance-permitted visit.

Mike learns that Mr. Bodin, RN, a certified psychiatric nurse, is scheduled to meet with him today and comes to meet the new nurse. Mike tells Mr. Bodin of the needs he has to make changes in his life, but relates that he needs to stay at home with his parents—he has promised his mother he will take care of her gardens and he will "be there" over time. His mother is now nearly 63 years old and has been widowed for five years. Mike is considering moving into an apartment of his own. There is a place in which he could live about one block from his mother's house, but he has been unable to decide whether or not this is a good idea. Mike has been considering this move for one year and has not drawn a conclusion. He asked Mr. Bodin to discuss this issue with him.

Mr. Bodin listens and provides encouragement for Mike to list the pro/cons of such a move. Mike does so but does not make a decision during the session. He tells Mr. Bodin that he will be back because he believes he needs more time. Even though Mr. Bodin makes an appointment to see Mike in two weeks, Mike calls Mr. Bodin's office daily to tell him about various aspects of his life—for example, Mike called to relate that he was able to visit the vacant apartment last night. Then he called the next day to say he determined that he could manage the costs of the rent on his current earnings, and that his mother thought it would be fine for him to move out, but maybe he would need to go to his mother's house for meals because he is not a good cook. Then two days later, Mike called to tell Mr. Bodin that the apartment has been rented by another person and that he had lost it, but maybe a different apartment would become available by the end of the month.

INITIAL ASSESSMENT AND REFLECTION

Mr. Bodin now has an appointment to see Mike next week. Mr. Bodin has identified the following behavior patterns in Mike: indecision and inability to make decisions about his own life. Strong affiliation needs are evidenced by the need to contact the nurse frequently and often wishing to engage in lengthy conversations with the nurse. He has asked for the nurse's home phone number and requests frequent appointments. In addition, Mr. Bodin noted the lack of age-appropriate independence from the family (particularly the mother) in a situation where the mother is able to care for herself and Mike has the financial means to live separately.

INITIAL REVIEW OF NURSING DIAGNOSES

Nursing diagnoses that Mr. Bodin identified for Mike are:

- *Chronic low self-esteem*
- *Decisional conflict*
- *Ineffective coping*

PRIORITIES OF CARE–NURSING INTERVENTIONS

The concept map indicates two focal areas for Mike. The first is the issue of low self-esteem and lack of self-confidence, which are prominent in all of his interactions and his inability to make decisions in his own best interest. The second focal area is the very strong need for positive affiliation. Mike calls the nurse often to

(*Continues*)

NURSING CARE PLAN: CONCEPT MAP FORMAT 18-1 (Continued)

gain acceptance, to validate that he is okay, and to use encounters with others as an external source of positive regard. Mr. Bodin has a goal to help Mike make these reassurances more internal and self-controlled.

NURSING INTERVENTIONS

Mr. Bodin will design individualized care by meeting Mike's affiliation needs through a supportive/friendly socialization group and setting limits on his (Mr. Bodin's) own ability to attend to all of Mike's needs. Secondly, he will design interventions to promote Mike to make decisions and stick with them. These will focus on issues of self-esteem and utilize interventions such as identifying positive aspects of self and assisting and reinforcing social participation.

Mr. Bodin recommends that Mike attend weekly socialization group meetings and reduces his individual appointments with Mike to one per month.

OUTCOME/EVALUATION

Mr. Bodin recognizes that the Dependent Personality Disorder traits are part of Mike's personality and that major changes in personality characteristics are unrealistic. His treatment goals are that Mike attend the groups sessions and begin to use other members of the group to meet his affiliation needs, and that Mike will begin to identify aspects of self.

Mr. Bodin does not set outcomes on the basis of Mike's behaviors (such as moving out of his mother's house and living in an apartment) as outcome criteria, because the underlying issue is self-esteem, not place of housing. Mr. Bodin will evaluate group sessions and his therapeutic interventions over time and expects that Mike will remain in treatment for six months or longer.

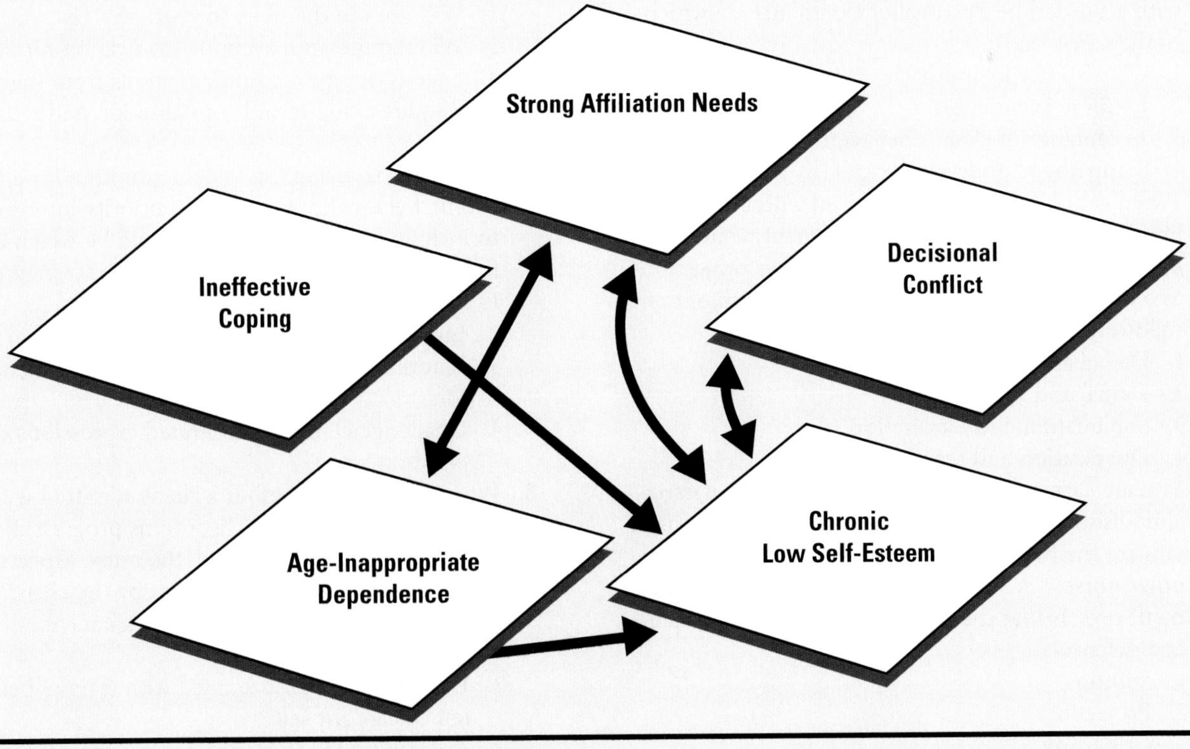

CONCEPT MAP OF ISSUES AND PROBLEMS (DELMAR/CENGAGE LEARNING.)

KEY CONCEPTS

- The term *personality* includes patterns of individual behavior expressed by physical and mental activities and attitudes.
- Personality style describes a cluster of personality traits exhibited by an individual.
- A personality disorder is described when a person has a personality style that deviates from the individual's culture and leads to distress or impairment.
- Personality disorders are divided into three clusters: odd and eccentric, dramatic and emotional, and anxiety and fear based.
- Nurses must recognize personality disorders in their clients and know that difficulty in establishing a nurse-client relationship, disagreement among team members regarding the client, personal reluctance to care for the client, or difficulty in reaching treatment goals may be warning signs that a personality disorder may be present.
- Psychotherapy and cognitive-behavioral therapy are thought to be the treatments of choice for personality disorders.
- Nursing theory directs the nurse to evaluate childhood development and its influence on personality development; further nursing theory directs the nurse to evaluate the client's current environment and its effect on behaviors.

REVIEW QUESTIONS

1. A 27-year-old male is admitted to the psychiatric unit with a diagnosis of Antisocial Personality. The nurse would plan to include which of the following on the nursing care?
1. Place client in seclusion
2. Establish clear and enforceable limits
3. Allow client to set his own daily schedule
4. Provide high protein and high calorie diet

2. A priority in the nursing care of a client diagnosed with a Borderline Personality would include which of the following?
1. Consistency in approach
2. Extreme friendliness
3. Acceptance of client's behaviors
4. Sympathetic understanding

3. When caring for a client diagnosed with a Borderline Personality, the nursing assessment would most likely reveal that the client not only uses projection as a defense mechanism but also uses which of the following?
1. Denial and dissociation
2. Denial and idealization
3. Sublimation and idealization
4. Dissociation and reaction formation

4. You are caring for a client diagnosed with a personality disorder. The client states, "I like you because you are the best nurse and much nicer than the other nurses." Your assessment of the client's statement reveals that the client is implementing which ego defense?"
1. Splitting
2. Projecting
3. Criticizing
4. Displacing

5. A client with Schizotypal Personality Disorder is admitted to the psychiatric unit. The nursing assessment would most likely reveal which of the following?
1. Labile affect
2. Self-centeredness
3. Need for immediate gratification
4. Social detachment

6. An important factor for the nurse to understand when planning care for a client diagnosed with a personality disorder is that the client:
1. Will not see the need to change
2. Will require antipsychotic medication for life
3. Eagerly accept recommendations from the nurse
4. Requires long-term hospitalization and rehabilitation

7. The nurse is caring for a client admitted for a Histrionic Personality Disorder. A priority intervention to include in the plan of care would be which of the following?
1. Respond to client's needs quickly
2. Limit setting on attention-seeking behaviors
3. Ignore inappropriate sexually seductive behaviors
4. Challenge client's exaggerated expressions of emotion

8. When evaluating whether a client admitted with a Dependent Personality Disorder is progressing toward accomplishing the goal, the nurse expects which of the following responses by the client?
1. Urgently seeks relationships as a source of care or support
2. Unrealistically preoccupied with fears of being left to care for self
3. Asks questions to clarify information that is not understood
4. Never disagrees with others even if own view is correct

9. When assessing a client with Antisocial Personality Disorder, the nurse would expect to find which of the following?
   1. Consistent work behavior
   2. Meticulous regarding plans for future
   3. Honest in relationships with others
   4. Disregard for and violation of the rights of others

10. A common nursing diagnosis for an individual with Dependent Personality Disorder would be which of the following?
    1. Low self-image
    2. Knowledge deficit
    3. Alteration in nutrition
    4. Isolation

LEARNING ACTIVITIES

1. Describe how the behaviors of unstable interpersonal relationships and self-image, efforts to avoid being abandoned, and impulsive acting out might be displayed by a woman with Borderline Personality Disorder who is brought to a hospital emergency room for treatment and evaluation of fainting and weakness.
2. Mr. R., a middle-aged man with a diagnosis of gastric ulcer, is in hospital care for evaluation of his ulcer. The nurse notes he has an air of self-importance, demands the nurse's time and attention, and expects particularly favorable treatment. Given that he has a narcissistic personality, what should the nurse expect related to Mr. R.'s being told he must accommodate his lifestyle and eating to his physical condition?
3. What would be a good approach for you as a nurse to use in establishing a therapeutic relationship with a client who has Histrionic Personality Disorder?
4. Identify at least one person you know who has characteristics of Antisocial Personality Disorder. Which characteristics? Explain.
5. Differentiate between Obsessive-Compulsive Personality Disorder and Obsessive-Compulsive Disorder.
6. Examine the DSM-IV-TR structure. Explain how Axis II disorders affect treatment and outcome for clients with both Axis I and Axis II disease.

*Study*WARE™ CONNECTION

Using your *Study*WARE™ CD-ROM

1. Complete the Concentration activity for this chapter.
2. Complete the Quiz for this chapter in Test Mode.
3. Explore the other games and activities that support this chapter.

VIDEO LINK

Read and contemplate the following questions about George, the client experiencing Antisocial Personality Disorder. Then watch the video "Antisocial Personality Disorder" on your *Study*WARE™ CD-ROM to observe George's interview with a psychiatrist. Consider these questions prior to listening to the psychiatrist's analysis:

1. Identify the chief characteristics of an Antisocial Personality Disorder.
2. Which of these characteristics does George exhibit?
3. How does George describe his feeling just prior to being admitted to the hospital?
4. What age is critical in the diagnosis of Antisocial Personality Disorder?
5. Adolescent Conduct Disorder is a prerequisite to the diagnosis of Antisocial Personality Disorder; what characteristics of this disorder are revealed through George's history?
6. Which two factors contribute to the risk for these disorders?
7. What is the prevalence of this disorder in males?
8. Which is the overwhelming emotion that George states he feels most of the time?
9. What is the main way that George has made his living?
10. What is the association between drugs and this disorder?
11. Describe George's demeanor throughout the interview. How does this influence your thoughts about him?
12. Do you think that George poses a threat to the nurses that are working with him?
13. He describes the nurses at this hospital in a positive way. What does he say about them?
14. Identify the therapeutic nursing interventions that are required for clients with this disorder.

REFERENCES

Abraham, P. F., & Calabrese, J. R. (2008). Evidenced-based pharmacologic treatment of borderline personality disorder: A shift from SSRIs to anticonvulsants and atypical antipsychotics? *Journal of Affective Disorders, 111,*(1) 21–30.

Alden, L. (1989). Short-term structured treatment for avoidant personality disorder. *Journal of Consulting and Clinical Psychology, 57,* 756–764.

American Psychiatric Association. (2000). *Diagnostic and statistical manual of mental disorders* (4th ed.-Text Revision). Washington, DC: Author.

Andrews, G. (1993). The benefits of psychotherapy. In N. Sartorius, G. Girolamo, G. Andrews, G. A. German, & L. Eisenberg (Eds.), *Treatment of mental disorders: A review of effectiveness* (pp. 235–247). Washington, DC: American Psychiatric Press.

Bender, D. S., Dolan, R. T., Skodal, A. E., Sanislow, C. A., Dyck, I. R., McGlashan, T., et al. (2001). Treatment utilization by patients with personality disorders. *America Journal of Psychiatry, 58*(2), 293–302.

Benjamin, L. S. (1993). *Interpersonal diagnosis and treatment of personality disorders.* New York: Guilford.

Blum, N., St John, D., Pfohl, B., Stuart, S., McCormick, B., Allen, J., et al. (2008). Systems Training for Emotional Predictability and Problem Solving (STEPPS) for outpatients with borderline personality disorder: A randomized controlled trial and 1-year follow-up. *American Journal of Psychiatry, 165*(4), 468–478.

Bogenschutz, M. P., & George Nurnberg, H. (2004). Olanzapine versus placebo in the treatment of borderline personality disorder. *Journal of Clinical Psychiatry, 65*(1), 104–109.

Clearly, M. Siegfried, N., & Walter, G. (2002). Experience, knowledge and attitudes of mental health staff regarding clients with borderline personality disorder. *International Journal of Mental Health Nursing, 11*(3), 186–191.

Coler, M., & Vincent, K. G. (1995). *Plans of care for speciality practice: Psychiatric mental health nursing.* Clifton Park, NY: Thomson Delmar Learning.

Davidson, K., Norrie, J., Tyrer, P., Gumley, A., Tata, P., Murray, H., et al. (2006). The effectiveness of cognitive behavior therapy for borderline personality disorder: Results from the borderline personality disorder study of cognitive therapy (BOSCOT) trial. *Journal of Personality Disord, 20*(5), 450–465.

Davon, A. L. (1994). The disruptive antisocial patients: Management strategies. *Nurse Manager, 25*(8), 46–51.

Dickey, C. C., McCarley, R. W., & Shenton, M. E. (2002). The brain in schizotypal personality disorder: A review of structural MRI and CT findings. *Harvard Review of Psychiatry, 19*(1), 1–15.

Duff, A. (2003). Managing personality disorders: Making positive connections. *Nursing Management, 10*(6), 27–31.

Erickson, H., Tomlin, E., & Swain, M. A. (1983). *The modeling and role-modeling theory: A paradigm for nursing.* Lexington, SC: Pine.

Fazel, S., & Danesh, J. (2002). Serious mental disorder in 23,000 prisoners: A systematic review of 62 surveys. *The Lancet, 359*(9322), 572–573.

Fraser, K., & Gallop, R. (1993). Nurses' confirming/discomfirming responses to patients diagnosed with borderline personality disorder. *Archives of Psychiatric Nursing, 7,* 336–341.

Gabbard, G. O., Coyne, L., Allen, J. G., Spohn, H., Colson, D. B., & Vary, M. (2000). Evaluation of intensive inpatient treatment of patients with severe personality disorders. *Psychiatric Services, 51*(7), 898–898.

Gallop, R., Lancee, W., & Shugar, G. (1993). Residents' and nurses' perceptions of difficult to treat short-stay patients. *Hospital and Community Psychiatry, 44,* 352–357.

Gilligan, C. (1982). *In a different voice: Psychological theory and women's development.* Cambridge, MA.: Harvard University Press.

Godfrey, M. (1991). Clients with personality disorders. In G. McFarland & M. D. Thomas (Eds.), *Psychiatric mental health nursing, application of the nursing process* (pp. 589–594). Philadelphia: Lippincott.

Green, B. (2003). Lamotrigine in mood disorders. *Current Medical Research Opinion, 19*(4), 272–277.

Guralnik, D. B. (Ed.). (1982). *Webster's new world dictionary of the American language.* New York: Simon & Schuster.

Helgeland, J. I., & Torgersen, S. (2004). Development antecedents of borderline personality disorder. *Comprehensive Psychiatry, 45*(2), 138–147.

Higgitt, A., & Fonagy, P. (1992). Psychotherapy in borderline and narcissistic personality disorder. *British Journal of Psychiatry, 161,* 23–43.

Hitchcock. R., Isbell, J., Loseby, J. (2007). Everybody's business: Developing a personality disorder service. *Mental Health Practice, 11*(2), 12–14.

Horstfall, J. (1999). Towards understanding some complex borderline behaviors. *Journal of Psychiatric Mental Health Nursing, 6*(6), 425–432.

Isherwood. C. (1989). *Berlin Stories.* New York: New Directions.

Leiberich, P. K., Nickel, M. K., Tritt, K., & Gil, F. P. (2008). Lamotrigine treatment of aggression in female borderline patients, Part II: An 18-month follow-up. *Journal of Psychopharmacology, 22*(7), 805–808.

Linehan, M. M. (1987). Dialectical behavioral therapy: A cognitive behavioral approach to parasuicide. *Journal of Personality Disorders, 1,* 228–333.

Linehan, M. M., Armstrong, H. E., Suarez, A., et al. (1991). Cognitive behavioral treatment of chronically parasuicidal borderline patients. *Archives of General Psychiatry, 48,* 1060–1064.

Lis, E., Greenfield, B., Hanry, M., Guile, J. M., & Dougherty, G. (2007). Neuroimaging and genetics of borderline personality disorder: a review. *Psychiatry & Neuroscience, 32*(3), 162–173.

Murphy, N., & McVey, D. (2003). The challenge of nursing personality-disordered patients. *British Journal of Forensic Practice, 5*(3), 21–27

Nehls, N. (1999). Borderline personality disorder: The voice of the patient. *Research in Nursing and Health, 22*(4), 285–293.

Ni, X., Chan, K., Bulgin, N., Sicard, T., Bismil, R., McMain, S., et al. (2006). Association between serotonin transporter gene and borderline personality disorder. *Journal of Psychiatric Research, 40*(5), 448–453.

Pascual, J. C., Soler, J., Barrachina, J., Campins, M. J., Alvarez, E., Perez, V., et al. (2008). Failure to detect an association between the serotonin transporter gene and borderline personality disorder. *Journal of Psychiatric Research, 42*(1), 87–88.

Phillips, K., Yen, S., & Gunderson, J.G. (2003). Personality disorders. In R. Hales and Yudofsky, S.C. (Eds.) *Textbook of clinical psychiatriy* (4th ed., pp. 803–832). Washington, DC: American Psychiatric Publishing, Inc.

Raskin, R., & Novacek, J. (1991). Narcissism and the use of fantasy. *Journal of Clinical Psychiatry, 47,* 490–499.

Robins, L. N., Tipp, J., & Przybeck, T. (1991). Antisocial personality. In L. N. Robins & D. A. Regier (Eds.), *Psychiatric disorders in America*. New York: Free Press.

Silbersweig, D., Clarkin, J. F., Goldstein, M., Kernberg, O. F., Tuescher, O., Levy, K. N., et al. (2007). Failure of frontolimbic inhibitory function in the context of negative emotion in borderline personality disorder. *American Journal of Psychiatry, 164*(12), 1832–1841.

Smith, C., Chakraburatty, A., Nelson, D., Paradis, I. (2000). Interventions for a heart transplant recipient with histrionic personality disorder. *Journal of Transplant Coordination, 9*(2), 109–113.

Soloff, P. H. (2000). Psychopharmacology of borderline personality disorder. *Psychiatric Clinics of North America, 23*(1), 169–192.

Stanley, B., Bundy, E., & Beberman, P. (2001). Skills training as an adjunctive treatment for personality disorders. *Journal of Psychiatric Practice, 7*(5), 324–335.

Thompson, J. E. (1990). Finding the borderline's border: Can Martha Rogers help? *Perspectives in Psychiatric Care, 26*, 7–10.

Vaylor, L. (1999). Antisocial personality disorder: Diagnostic, ethical, and treatment issues. *Issues in Mental Health Nursing, 20*(3), 247–258.

Waldeck, T. L., & Miller, C. S. (2000). Social skills deficits in schizotypal personality disorders. *Psychiatric Research, 93*(3), 237–246.

Wiggins, J. S., & Pincus, A. L. (1994). Personality structure and the structure of personality disorders. In P. Costa, Jr. & T. A. Widiger (Eds.), *Personality disorders and the five factor model of personality* (pp. 73–94). Washington, DC: American Psychological Association.

Woods, P., & Richards, D. (2003). Effectiveness of nursing interventions in people with personality disorders. *Journal of Advanced Nursing, 44*(2), 154–172.

Yang, Y., Raine, A., Lencz, T., Bihrle, S., LaCasse, L., & Colletti, P. (2005). Volume reduction in prefrontal gray matter in unsuccessful criminal psychopaths. *Biological Psychiatry, 57*(10), 1103–1108.

Zanarini, M. C. (2000). Childhood experiences associated with the development of borderline personality disorder. *Psychiatric Clinics of North America, 23*(1), 89–101.

Zanarini, M. C. (2004). Update on pharmacology of borderline personality disorder. *Current Psychiatry Reports, 6*(1), 66–70.

Zanarini, M. C., Frankenburg, F. R., Hennen, J., & Silk, K. R. (2004). Mental health service utilization by borderline personality disorder patients and Axis II comparison subjects followed prospectively for 6 years. *Journal of Clinical Psychiatry, 65*(1), 28–36.

LITERARY REFERENCES

Butterfield, F. (1994). *All God's children: The Bosket family and the American tradition of violence* (p. 327.). New York: Alfred A. Knopf.

Cather, W. (1948). Paul's case. In *Youth and the bright medusa* (pp. 183–185). New York: Random House.

Chekhov, A. (1971). Ward 6. In *The Oxford Chekhov* (Vol. 6, pp. 125–127). (Richard Hingley, Trans.). London: Oxford University Press.

Dostoevsky, F. (1960). Notes from underground. In *Notes from underground and the Grand Inquisitor* (pp. 3–5; R. E. Matlaw, Trans.). New York: Dutton Signet.

Gogol, N. (1957). The overcoat. In *The overcoat and other tales of good and evil* (pp. 237–250). New York: Bantam Doubleday Dell.

Isherwood, C. (1989). Sally Bowles. In *Berlin stories* (pp. 22–23; 89). New York: New Directions.

Joyce, J. (1967). Eveline. In *The Dubliners* (pp. 38–41). New York: Penguin Books.

Mann, T. (1970). *Confessions of Felix Krull, confidence man* (D. Lindley, Trans.). New York: Knopf.

Nardo, J. M. (1986). The personality in the medical setting: A psychodynamic understanding. In H. K. Brodie & J. L. Houpt (Eds.), *Consultation-liaison psychiatry and behavioral medicine*. New York: Basic Books.

Oates, J. C. (1981). The tryst. In *Sentimental education* (pp. 509–518). New York: Dutton Signet.

Poe, E. A. (1945/1983). Berenice. In P. V. D. Stern (Ed.), *Viking portable library* (pp. 208–213). New York: Viking.

Wilde, Oscar. (1890). *The picture of Dorian Gray*. Chapter 1, retrieved from Authorama. Classic literature free of copyright, http://www.authorama.com/the-picture-of-dorian-gray-1.html.

Williams, T. (1971). The glass menagerie. In *The theater of Tennessee Williams* (pp. 151–153). New York: New Directions.

SUGGESTED READINGS

Butterfield, F. (2008). *All God's children: The Bosket family and the American tradition of violence*. New York: Vintage.

Millon, T. et al. (2004). *Personality disorders in modern life*. Hoboken: Wiley.

Robinson, D.R. (2005). *Disordered personalities*. Port Huron, MI: Rapid Psychler.

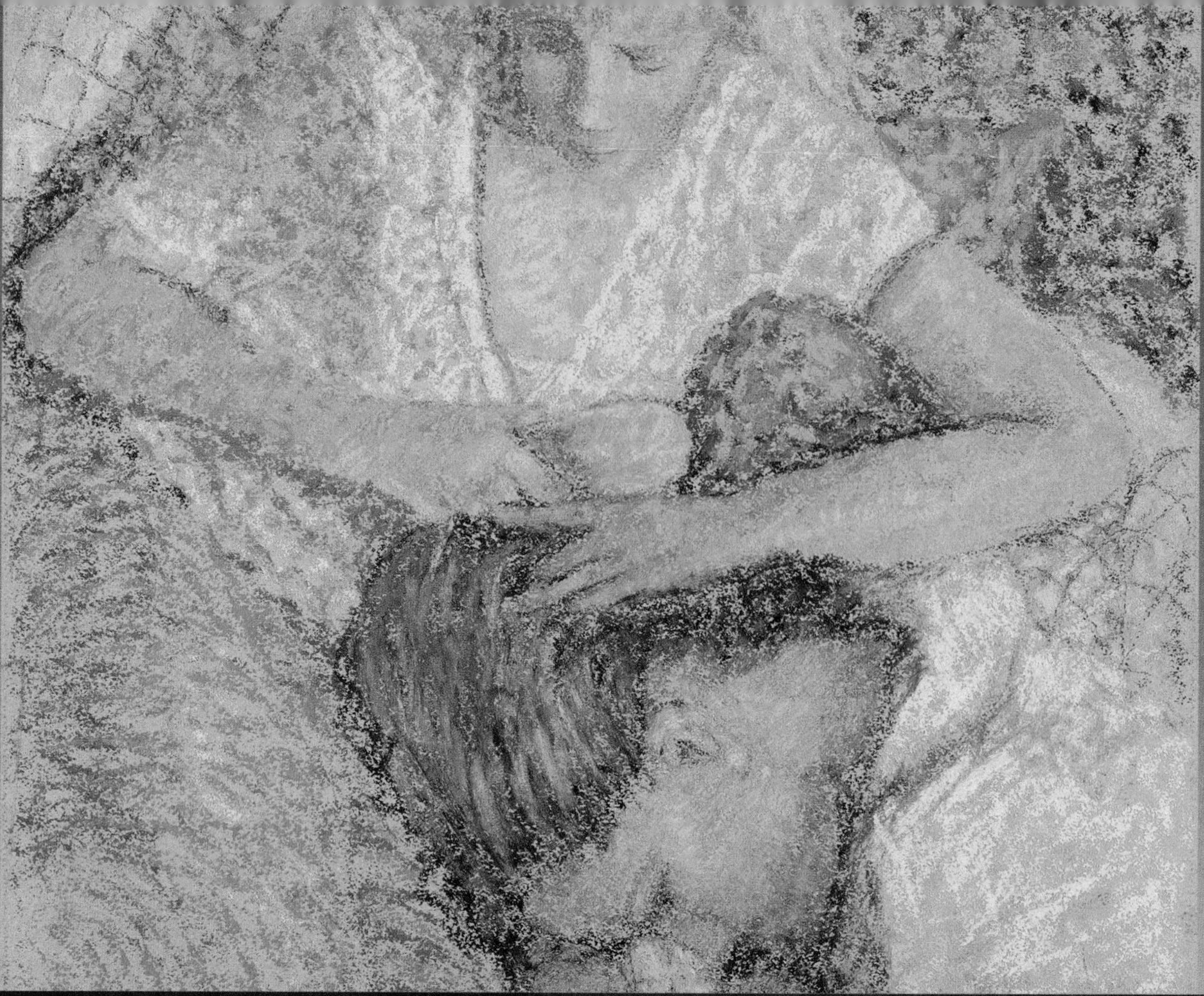

In Your Mind's Eye

It's All in His Head

During an evening change-of-shift report, the day shift nurse on a general medical-surgical unit makes the following observations:

In room 123 is Mr. S., a 37-year-old man admitted two days ago with severe back pain. He has been on bed rest and is being worked up for diagnosis. He complains of severe pain and inability to move that are not relieved by pain medication and muscle relaxants. He has also been complaining of intermittent paresthesias of the lower extremities. His neurological examinations and MRI are normal. The day-shift nurse says, "There is nothing wrong with him, we should discharge him. It's all in his head."

- *What is your reaction to this report?*
- *What are your feelings about this client?*
- *Do you have any explanations for what is going on with Mr. S.?*
- *How do you think a nurse should react to this report and to Mr. S.?*

In this chapter, you will learn of the psychological underpinnings of physical symptoms and specific psychiatric disorders that present as physical symptoms.

CHAPTER 19

The Client Experiencing a Somatoform, Factitious, or Dissociative Disorder

NOREEN CAVAN FRISCH
LAWRENCE E. FRISCH

CHAPTER OUTLINE

COMPETENCIES

Upon completion of this chapter, the reader should be able to:

1. Define *somatoform disorders* and distinguish among Somatization Disorder, Hypochondriasis, and Conversion Disorder.
2. Define *Factitious Disorder* (Munchausen's Syndrome) and *Munchausen's Syndrome by Proxy*.
3. Describe the presenting characteristics of an individual with Somatization Disorder who comes to an acute-care clinic for diagnosis and treatment.
4. Distinguish between Hypochondriasis and Anxiety Disorder.
5. Cite the major theoretical explanations for Hypochondriasis (psychoanalytic, behavioral, and biological).
6. Describe principles for the effective treatment of Hypochondriasis.
7. Provide an explanation for treatment of Conversion Disorder through direct explanation of the underlying conflict.
8. Differentiate between Factitious Disorder and malingering.
9. Utilize the nursing process and nursing theory to plan care for clients experiencing a somatoform disorder.
10. Use techniques of introspection and self-reflection to examine your own feelings with regard to clients whose physical complaints are results of psychiatric illness.

KEY TERMS

Amnesia
Conversion Disorder
Depersonalization
Dissociative Disorders
Dissociative Identity Disorder (DID)
Factitious Disorder
Fugue
Hypochondriasis
Malingering
Munchausen's Syndrome
Munchausen's Syndrome by Proxy
Somatization Disorder
Somatoform Disorders

This chapter considers a group of psychiatric disorders that have in common an emphasis on *physical* rather than *psychological* symptoms. Persons with these disorders typically present to one or more primary care providers and are usually managed without ever being seen by mental health practitioners. Clients with **somatoform disorders**, as this group of disorders is called, present with a variety of symptoms—symptoms not infrequently puzzling to their caretakers, highly disruptive to the lives of their sufferers, and often very difficult to distinguish from those of serious or life-threatening illness. Collectively, clients with the somatoform disorders are among the most difficult seen in general clinical practice. They are often dissatisfied with their care providers, and they are frequently certain that they have some serious condition that remains undiagnosed and untreated. Clients with somatoform disorders often move from provider to provider seeking new diagnoses and treatments. These clients truly believe they are seriously ill, and they make every effort to convince family members, nurses, and doctors of their need for care. Their efforts may result in hospitalizations, diagnostic procedures, and heroic treatments; rarely do they result in cure.

The somatoform disorders are a group of conditions in which symptoms suggest the presence of a general medical condition, but careful evaluation fails to find any evidence of a physical disorder sufficient to explain the complaints. Most experts feel that psychological factors account for the symptoms of somatoform disorders. This chapter considers three such disorders: Somatization Disorder, Hypochondriasis, and Conversion Disorder.

While disorders of another group, factitious disorders, are not classified as somatoform in the *Diagnostic and Statistical Manual, Fourth Edition-Text Revision* (DSM-IV-TR; American Psychiatric Association, 2000), they are also discussed in this chapter because they share certain similarities with the somatoform disorders. Persons with somatoform disorders truly believe themselves to be physically sick; they do not attempt to deceive their caretakers. In contrast, persons with factitious disorders typically fabricate their complaints and may even create physical findings, sometimes injuring themselves

REFLECTIVE THINKING 19-1

Feigning Illness

Some individuals purposefully try to deceive their health care providers and injure themselves to produce physical symptoms.

- **Why do you think someone would want to be ill?**
- **Can you provide a reason why someone would take a drug or toxin to produce symptoms?**

Try to understand the behaviors from the client's perspective. Talk to others in your class about such behaviors. Remember that in order to give care, a nurse must be willing to understand the client's subjective experiences.

by secretly self-administering drugs or toxins. In contrast to individuals with somatoform disorders, who honestly believe themselves to be physically ill, persons with factitious disorders purposefully try to deceive their caretakers into diagnosing and treating one or more medical conditions.

HISTORY OF SOMATOFORM DISORDERS

The terminology in this chapter derives from DSM-IV-TR, but medical practitioners have recognized somatoform disorders for hundreds, if not thousands, of years. The term *hysteria* was commonly applied to these conditions, particularly when they occurred in women. The ancient Greeks and Romans commonly used the diagnosis of hysteria, probably in turn having borrowed the concept from the more ancient Egyptians. The term itself is Greek, deriving from the word *hystera*, meaning "uterus." In these ancient cultures, hysteria was thought to occur when, under certain conditions, the uterus migrated from its usual place and attached itself to other bodily organs (Veith, 1965).

While for many centuries hysteria remained incompletely defined, its presumed origin in the uterus seems to have remained unchallenged until the late seventeenth century when Thomas Willis (best known for his description of the brain's blood supply—still today called the Circle of Willis) suggested that many cases of hysteria had their origin in the brain. Willis's equally famous contemporary Thomas Sydenham emphasized the importance of hysteria: "Of all the chronic diseases hysteria ... is the commonest" (Veith, 1965, p. 137). He developed a highly sophisticated "modern" view of this illness—that some persons experienced symptoms of "hysterical origin," that is, their pain and other symptoms had origins in the mind, not the body.

Over the next 200 years, ideas that the condition of hysteria was caused by the brain became accepted among many influential European and American physicians. The spectrum of hysterical symptoms was more accurately defined, and advances in medicine and neurology helped to more accurately distinguish organic from hysterical symptoms. The study of hysteria reached its clinical apex in Paris under the tutelage of Jean-Martin Charcot. Between 1862 and 1882, Charcot worked at the Salpêtrière Hospital, a huge asylum for neurologically and psychiatrically ill women. Faced with large numbers of ill persons, some with organic and others with hysterical symptoms, Charcot was able to define clinical characteristics of hysteria and increasingly to separate them from their organic "look-alikes." As a professor at the University of Paris, Charcot's personal fame attracted attention to the study of neurological disorders in general and of hysteria in particular (Veith, 1965).

But as medical practice became more sophisticated, it proved difficult to have no uniformly accepted theory of *how* mental processes could so strongly affect the physical body. The most influential of these theories was developed by the Viennese neurologist Sigmund Freud. Freud's brief study with Charcot was influential in directing his interest and attention to the causes of hysteria. On his return to Vienna, Freud began to search for psychological causes of hysteria in repressed memories of childhood events. He and his colleagues sought these repressed memories in dreams and through hypnosis. When such memories were explained to hysterical patients, their symptoms often seemed to improve or disappear. This clinical improvement was taken as evidence of the correctness of Freud's theories regarding the importance of unconscious, often sexually related memories in causing hysteria. While these "psychoanalytic" theories are no longer the only modern views of hysteria, through Freud's work it has become widely accepted that early childhood events may have lasting effects on mental and physical health.

Despite, or perhaps because of, this long history of interest in the relationship between the mind and somatic symptoms, the concept of somatoform diagnoses remains controversial. Starting about 2005, there has been considerable discussion in the literature about whether the next edition of DSM should include somatoform disorders on Axis 1 as primary diagnostic categories (Janca, 2005; Noyes, Stuart, & Watson, 2008). What impact this discussion will have on psychiatric classification and thinking remains unclear. The discussions in this chapter follow the more traditional viewpoint of DSM IV-R, but readers should be aware that changes in our understanding of these disorders (including whether some of them really "are" disorders) may be underway (Rief & Isaac, 2007).

SOMATIZATION DISORDER

Current psychiatric thinking has separated the diagnosis of Somatization Disorder from the general concept of hysteria (Stone, Hewett, Carson, Warlow, & Sharpe, 2008). **Somatization Disorder** is a somatoform disorder in which there are multiple physical complaints without an apparent physiological cause. Although most of the manifestations of hysteria are included in the diagnosis of Somatization Disorder, specific symptoms and behaviors are required for this diagnosis to be made. DSM-IV-TR requires that four basic criteria be met in order to diagnose Somatization Disorder; these are listed in Box 19-1.

BOX 19-1 DIAGNOSTIC CRITERIA FOR SOMATIZATION DISORDERS

1. A history of many physical complaints beginning before age 30 years that occur over a period of several years and result in treatment being sought or significant impairment in social, occupational, or other important areas of functioning.
2. A series of symptoms to include:
   - *Four pain symptoms:* A history of pain related to at least four different sites or functions (e.g., head, abdomen, back, joints, extremities, chest, rectum; during menstruation, during sexual intercourse, or during urination).
   - *Two gastrointestinal symptoms:* A history of at least two gastrointestinal symptoms other than pain (e.g., nausea, bloating, vomiting other than during pregnancy, diarrhea, or intolerance of several different foods).
   - *One sexual symptom:* Examples are sexual indifference, erectile or ejaculatory dysfunction, irregular menses, excessive menstrual bleeding, and vomiting throughout pregnancy.
   - *One pseudoneurological symptom:* A history of at least one symptom or deficit suggesting a neurological condition not limited to pain (conversion symptoms such as impaired coordination or balance, paralysis or localized weakness, difficulty swallowing or lump in throat, aphonia, urinary retention, hallucinations, loss of touch or pain sensation, double vision, blindness, deafness, or seizures; dissociative symptoms such as amnesia; or loss of consciousness other than fainting).
3. The symptoms cannot be explained fully by physical conditions, including drugs of abuse or medications.
4. The symptoms are not intentionally produced or feigned.

From the *Diagnostic and Statistical Manual of Mental Disorders* (4th ed.-TR). Copyright © 2000. Reprinted with permission from the American Psychiatric Association.

The complex diagnostic criteria reflect the great variety of symptoms that persons with Somatization Disorder manifest. Although the Countess in the following description does not describe enough symptoms to qualify for the diagnosis of Somatization Disorder by these criteria, the author, a physician who studied with Charcot in the 1880s, colorfully captures much of the flavor of this disorder:

WHAT IS THE MATTER WITH ME?

One of my last cases of appendicitis was, I think, the Countess who came to consult me, on the recommendation of Charcot, as she said. He used to send me patients now and then and I was of course most anxious to do my very best for her.... At first she did not know if she had appendicitis, nor did [I], but soon she was sure that she had it, and I that she had not. When I told her so with unwise abruptness she became very agitated. Professor Charcot had told her I was sure to find out what was the matter with her and that I would help her, and instead of that ... she burst into tears....

"What is the matter with me?" she sobbed, stretching out her two empty hands towards me with a gesture of despair....

She ceased to cry instantly. Wiping the last tears from her big eyes she said bravely:

"I can stand anything. I have already stood so much, don't be afraid, I am not going to cry any more. What is the matter with me?"

"Colitis."

Her eyes grew even larger than before, though I would have thought that to be impossible.

*"Colitis! That is exactly what I always thought! I am sure you are right! Tell me what is colitis?" I took good care to avoid that question, for I did not know it myself, nor did anybody else in those days. But I told her it lasted long and was difficult to cure, and I was right there. The Countess smiled amiably at me. And her husband who said it was nothing but nerves!**

(Munthe, 1975, pp. 43–46)

The Countess is less than 30 years old and has at least one gastrointestinal symptom (colitis) as well as pain. These symptoms are part of the spectrum of Somatization Disorder, and one suspects that further questioning of this woman could generate additional symptoms. In another example of Somatization Disorder, Alice James (the Countess's American contemporary) spent virtually her whole life as an invalid, the victim of pain, unexplained paralysis, menstrual disorder, and seemingly endless "doctor shopping." Alice's

*From *The Story of San Michele*, by A. Munthe, 1975, London:John Murray (Publishers, Ltd). Reprinted with permission.

illness is vividly revealed in letters to family members, including her brother, the famous Harvard psychologist William James. A selection of these letters follow:

TO HAVE A TORNADO GOING ON WITHIN ONE

December 23, 1884

Dear William

... My doctor came last week and examined me for an hour with a conscientiousness that my diaphragm has not hitherto been used to. When he came to the end he was as inscrutable as they always are and the little he told me I was too tired to understand. He is coming next week when as there won't be as much percussing and stethoscoping to be done I can get more out of him. I shall not tell you till then what he told me. I think he takes the gout as a foregone conclusion simply and is deciding what other complications there are. Meanwhile he has left me a pill of which he thinks all the world and I am to have my spine sponged with salt-water. I was much disappointed by his lack of remedial suggestions....

Always affectionately

Alice

January 31, 1885

My dear Aunt Kate.

... My doctor turned out as usual a fiasco an unprincipled one too. I could get nothing out of him and he slipped thro' my cramped and clinging grasp as skillfully as if his physical conformation had been that of an eel instead of a Dutch cheese—The gout he looks upon as a small part of my trouble, "it being complicated with an excessive nervous sensibility," but I could get no suggestions of any sort as to climate, baths, or diet from him. The truth was he was entirely puzzled about me and had not the manliness to say so. I got from him however a very thorough examination. He said I had no organic trouble, that my organs were simply disturbed in their functions. My legs are produced by a functional disturbance of the lower half of the spine. "Is this produced by gout?" "Oh! dear me yes I have seen people with their legs powerless for years from this cause!" He assured me that it did not lead to paralysis, a grim spectre which has been staring me in the face for a long time. My legs have been entirely useless for anything more than hobbling about the room for three months and a half and most of the time excessively painful. I asked the doctor whether it was not unusual for a person to be so ill and have no organic trouble and he said, "yes, very unusual indeed." ...

Yrs. as always

A.

November 21st, 23rd and 24th, 1885

My dearest Aunt,

Whether I am much better or not, I don't know, I am gradually getting stronger and am able to do a great deal more, but as always happens as my physical strength increases my nervous distress and susceptibility grows with it, so that from an inside view it is somewhat of an exchange of evils. To have a tornado going on within one, whilst one is chained to a sofa, is no joke, I can assure you....

Always very affectionately yr

A.

January 3rd, 4th, 1886

Dear William,

... Until lately every joint in my body was constantly pierced with rheumatic pains flying from my head to my feet, from my stomach to my hands, how I should have lived without salicene I don't know. The same betterment has taken place since I came to London that was so wonderfully marked when I was here four yrs. ago....

Always

Yr. loving sister

A.

September 10th, 1886

My dear William

... I thought it wrong, being so ill as I was last autumn, not to see a physician and find out whether my legs were getting to be a habit or not, so I called in Townsend who gave just the same diagnosis as Drs. Torrey and Garrod, a gouty diathesis complicated by an abnormally sensitive nervous organisation, the legs neurosis brought about by anxiety and strain. He assured me that they could not, the legs, be hurried that time would do it, assisted by his medicines, but I found that they were very strong tonics and that it was going to be only the old Neftel system, drugs instead of battery so I gave him up. I was very glad that I went to him however, as he gave me much good advice and relieved my mind about the genuiness of my legs. He said what I have been told often before that I should be much better at any rate, when I reached middle life, this seems highly probable as I have had sixteen periods the last year....

Yr loving sister

Alice—

June 16, 1887

Dear William and Alice,

... I have been running down very much the last six weeks, and had a bad little illness last week; but Katharine is come to the rescue.... Before K. arrived I fell so low as

to send for an M.D. who had been variously and highly recommended. After examining my heart, which he seemed to consider an unnecessarily vivacious organ, he looked at me and asked, "Does the protuberance of your eyeballs increase rapidly?" I am only sorry, not to be able to gratify William, by saying that my reply was "Yes"; but truth forbids. He also remarked, "You won't die, but you will live, suffering to the end." ...

Yours as ever
Alice.

November 15, 1887

Dear Aunt Kate.

... I have constant "attacks" of all descriptions, more frequent than ever, but not so bad at the time and I get up from them quicker and feel stronger in the intervals. They are extremely inconvenient and I much prefer the rarer kind. My new doctor ... gave a very remarkable diagnosis of my case and nature after seeing me once for 20 minutes during which time I lay with my eyes shut in explosions of laughter owing to the comicality of his manner. I shall give him a good trial....

Always your loving niece
*A**

(Yeazell, 1981, pp. 100–109)

While it is risky to attempt diagnosis more than 100 years after the fact, it seems unlikely that "gout" would today be considered a reasonable diagnosis for Alice. It also seems very improbable that multiple distinguished American and English physicians of this very sophisticated age would have overlooked an organic cause for her difficulty walking. While, for example, a disease such as rheumatoid arthritis might have explained many of Alice's extremity pains, photographs still available today show no evidence of deformity and make such illnesses unlikely. One doctor even asked about "protuberance of your eyeballs," very likely entertaining a diagnosis of hyperthyroidism as a cause of her leg weakness and "abnormally sensitive nervous organisation." DSM-IV-TR stresses the need to exclude complex medical problems such as hyperthyroidism, which may masquerade as Somatization Disorder (American Psychiatric Association, 2000). Today, it is highly likely that Alice's lengthy illness, with its "'attacks' of all descriptions ... every joint in my body ... constantly pierced with rheumatic pains flying from my head to my feet, from my stomach to my hands ... sixteen periods in one year" and unexplained paralysis, would be diagnosed as Somatization Disorder.

Clients with Somatization Disorder frequently describe their illness dramatically, sometimes with inappropriate laughter (as Alice describes in her November 15, 1887, letter). Both the Countess and Alice emphasize multiple contacts with physicians, and Alice details a seemingly endless parade of diagnostic and therapeutic efforts. In modern times, these women likely would have received an extensive battery of diagnostic testing, including X-rays, hospitalizations, and even surgery. Alice tried numerous pills, electrical treatments, and physical therapies. Today, she would have had far more treatments from which to choose, but her chances of receiving benefits from modern treatments are probably no higher now than a century ago.

Epidemiology and Cause

Somatization Disorder occurs far more frequently among women than men. The Epidemiologic Catchment Area Study found a gender ratio of 10 to 1, but overall found Somatization Disorder to be rare, occurring in only 0.13% of individuals (Robins & Regier, 1991). Other studies have found Somatization Disorder in up to 2% of women (American Psychiatric Association, 2000). Studies of primary care medical populations have found that a strict diagnosis of Somatization Disorder applies to only a minority of clients who present with medically unexplained symptoms (Jackson & Kroenke, 2008). These patients were often judged "difficult" by their physicians, tended to have symptoms that persisted over time despite reassurance, and often had coexisting mental illness, particularly depression or anxiety (Henningson, Jakobsen, Schiltenwolf, & Weiss, 2005).

The exact cause of Somatization Disorder is not known, but it clearly tends to occur in families (Yutzy, 2003). In early studies the disorder was shown to occur frequently in families in which Antisocial Personality Disorder could be diagnosed in both female and male relatives (Guze, Cloninger, Martin, & Clayton, 1985). Others report that subsequent studies have documented that children of patients with Somatization Disorder have a higher chance of developing the disorder than their counterparts growing up in families without the disorder (Lantz, 2008; Oyama, Paltoo, & Greengold, 2007). Such clustering in families does not establish whether Somatization Disorder is caused by genetics, environment, or some combination of both. Studies have often been used to try to separate the genetic and environmental causes of complex psychological disorders, and these studies often involve twins who were separated early in life and reared in different families. Such twin studies on Somatization Disorder have concluded that both heredity and environment contribute to the development of the disorder (Bohman, Cloninger, von Knorring, & Siquardsson, 1984).

Neuropsychological testing has shown patterns of cerebral dysfunction that seem to be typical of Somatization Disorder. In comparison to controls, individuals with Somatization Disorder have subtle but unique abnormalities on tests of nondominant-hemisphere function (Flor-Henry, Fromm-Auch, Tapper, & Schopflocher, 1981). While such findings are of interest, they do not allow much understanding of the causation of Somatization Disorder. However, unless some more specific testing of this sort is incorporated into the diagnostic process, many will continue to argue that Somatization Disorder ought best to be

*From *The Death and Letters of Alice James*, by R. B. Yeazell, 1981, Berkeley:University of California Press. Reprinted with permission.

termed "medically unexplained symptoms" and removed from the category of psychiatric diagnoses (Hatcher & Arroll, 2008).

Some authors have suggested that individuals with this disorder learn at an early age to express emotional distress through somatization. Such complaints may bring them support and comfort that they may not otherwise receive (Quill, 1985). While most care providers associate relatively young age with a diagnosis of Somatization Disorder, somatoform conditions are not uncommon at all ages, including the geriatric population (Wijeratne, Brodaty, & Hickie, 2003).

TREATMENT

As implied earlier, effective treatment for Somatization Disorder is difficult. There are a series of challenges to be overcome in managing individuals with Somatization Disorder. First is establishing the diagnosis. Screening instruments can be useful in suggesting the diagnosis of Somatization Disorder. However, even when the diagnosis is made with reasonable certainty, clinicians must always be alert to the continuing possibility of undiagnosed physical illness. In actuality, though, undiagnosed psychiatric illness (especially depression) is more likely—especially among clients managed by generalist providers (Hatcher & Arroll, 2008). Somatization Disorder frequently remains a tentative diagnosis subject to modification if new symptoms or signs emerge. A diagnosis of Somatization Disorder does not protect individuals from other independent conditions. After years of suffering without any medical explanation, Alice James was found to have breast cancer, from which she eventually died; her last years were spent in severe pain, but she was seemingly happy that she had finally developed a medically diagnosable illness.

Keeping an appropriate level of vigilance in the face of seemingly endless subjective complaints is yet another challenge in caring for these clients. Most authorities recommend that persons with Somatization Disorder be encouraged to make regular scheduled clinical visits at which their problems and symptoms are reviewed. Such regular visits offer support without requiring clients to have new or more severe symptoms in order to receive medical or nursing attention.

Finally, caretaker fatigue is a major challenge in managing the needs of these clients. Clients with Somatization Disorder can be exceedingly demanding, manipulative, and occasionally seductive. It is probable that care for this problem is best given by a team of professionals, perhaps including one or more nurses, physicians, and mental health workers. Effective communication between client and provider and among varied providers is a major challenge in providing quality care. Maynard (2003) has offered a nurse practitioner's perspective on the assessment and management of somatization. She emphasizes that the care provider must have a management plan that emphasizes client needs, an empathic relationship with the client, and the ability to set goals and establish boundaries/limits while providing care.

The Barretts of Wimpole Street

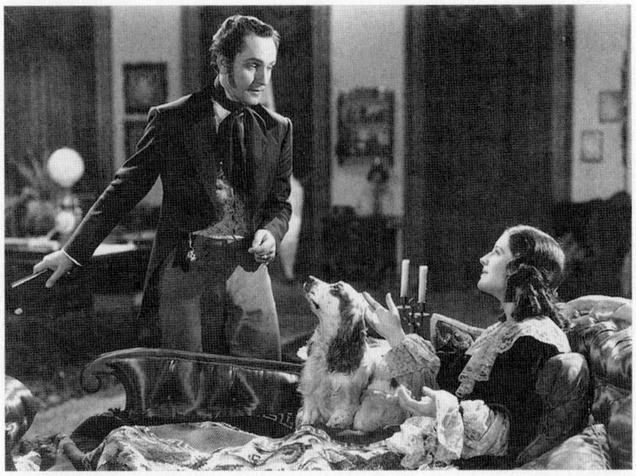

Source: MGM (Courtesy: The Kobal Collection).

Elizabeth Barrett spent much of her youth in bed with undiagnosed somatic symptoms until she fell in love with Robert Browning. She improved greatly after their marriage, and both went on to become major nineteenth-century English poets.

Psychotherapy

While there have been many claims for specific treatment methods, none has been shown to be uniquely effective (Kellner, 1989). Three therapeutic goals seem to be of value for any approach to treatment (Martin & Yutzy, 1994):

1. Establishing a firm therapeutic alliance with the client
2. Educating the client regarding the manifestations of Somatization Disorder
3. Providing consistent reassurance to the client

One of the major problems with psychotherapy for this disorder is that many clients do not believe they are psychologically ill. Their symptoms feel physical, and they are often highly reluctant to accept either psychiatric diagnosis or treatment. Both individual and group therapy have been tried, but there is little other than anecdotal data to suggest benefit from either approach. At least one study suggests that primary health care providers can effectively care for clients with Somatization Disorder, utilizing where necessary the consultative services of a psychiatrist (Smith, Monson, & Ray, 1986). This study randomly divided clients into a "usual care" group and a group followed by primary care providers with explicit therapeutic goals set by a psychiatric consultant. The consultant psychiatrist specifically suggested that clients be seen regularly by appointment (so as not to require the presence of symptoms in order to be given medical care), be examined carefully on each visit, and not be subjected to extensive investigations or to hospitalization unless medically essential. While outcomes were largely measured in terms of cost of care, clients treated with such a medically oriented approach seemed to do well and incurred significantly fewer medical expenses.

In Somatization Disorder, cognitive-behavioral therapy has been evaluated in numerous controlled trials and generally shown to be effective in reducing symptoms and disability (Sumathipala, 2007). A major problem with such studies is that participants in studies have agreed to accept cognitive-behavioral therapy. Like Alice James, many clients are too convinced of the physical nature of their complaints to agree to psychological treatment (Kroenke & Swindle, 2000). Studies in actual primary care practice are starting to emerge, however, showing the value of cognitive behavioral therapy in the community (Martin, Rauh, Fichter, & Rief, 2007).

HYPOCHONDRIASIS

Hypochondriasis is, like hysteria, a condition that has been diagnosed for hundreds, if not thousands, of years. As with hysteria, the medical meaning of Hypochondriasis has changed significantly over the centuries. Only since the early 1820s has this diagnosis come to resemble the current definition (Veith, 1965). Presently, Hypochondriasis is regarded as "the preoccupation with the fear of having, or the idea that one has, a serious disease based on the person's misinterpretation of bodily symptoms or bodily functions" (American Psychiatric Association, 2000, p. 504). Persons with Anxiety Disorder also have fears, including sometimes fears that they may become ill or die; however, Hypochondriasis differs from Anxiety Disorder in that persons with Hypochondriasis have anxieties limited to fear of illness, *and* their fear arises from actual bodily symptoms rather than from more general concerns about contamination. The DSM-IV-TR criteria for Hypochondriasis are presented in Box 19-2.

BOX 19-2 DIAGNOSTIC CRITERIA FOR HYPOCHONDRIASIS

- Preoccupation with fears of having, or the idea that one has, a serious disease based on the person's misinterpretation of bodily symptoms.
- The preoccupation persists despite appropriate medical evaluation and reassurance.
- The belief in the first criterion is not of delusional intensity.
- The preoccupation causes clinically significant distress or impairment in social, occupational, or other important areas of functioning.
- The duration of the disturbance is at least six months.
- The preoccupation is not better accounted for by another psychological disorder.

It is also important that comprehensive medical evaluation reveal no medical condition to account for the symptoms. Although Hypochondriasis may still exist in persons who have definable general medical conditions, concerns about health in persons with such conditions are most often *not* Hypochondriasis, but, rather, represent either appropriate worries about sickness or a form of affective disorder. As noted in Box 19-2, the belief in or about illness must not be delusional. This means that individuals with Hypochondriasis typically recognize that their worries are out of proportion to the probability that they truly have the feared illness or condition. Delusional individuals cannot be dissuaded from the conviction that they are ill, no matter how improbable the illness given their symptoms and signs.

Persons with Hypochondriasis differ somewhat in the content of their fears and worries. Some focus their concerns on a single disease (cancer or heart disease) and seek confirmation of their fears in minimal symptoms or alterations of normal bodily function. Others focus on a variety of symptoms—a cough, a skipped heart beat, skin blemishes or moles, or fatigue. In either case, clinical reassurance (from examination or often from multiple noninvasive and invasive tests) is temporary at best. The worries about health recur and tend to become a major focus of the individual's life and daily routine. It often becomes difficult for persons with Hypochondriasis to function normally in their social and occupational roles, and this disorder can lead to invalidism. While DSM-IV-TR criteria usually allow a clear distinction between Hypochondriasis and Somatization Disorder, both of the cases of Somatization Disorder discussed earlier in this chapter might be equally well taken as examples of Hypochondriasis: the Countess with her focus on "appendicitis" and "colitis" and Alice James with her multiple somatic complaints leading to a life as an invalid. Hypochondriasis and invalidism seemed to have occurred with some frequency in the latter years of the nineteenth century, seemingly often among the very famous. For example, Charles Darwin had numerous anxieties about his health, which lasted from his youth into very old age:

DARWIN

*I was also troubled with palpitations and pain about the heart, and like many a young ignorant man, especially one with a smattering of medical knowledge, was convinced that I had heart disease. I did not consult any doctor, as I fully expected to hear the verdict that I was not fit for the voyage, and I was resolved to go at all hazards.**

(Colp, 1977, p. 9)

Here is an excerpt from one of several recent biographies focusing on the famous biologist's enigmatic lifelong "illnesses":

Charles Darwin suffered chronic ill-health from the age of thirty until he was sixty. During the last decade of his

*From *To Be an Invalid*, by R. Colp, Copyright 1977. Reprinted with permission from the University of Chicago Press.

life, however, he was much better, and he lived to be seventy-three. In the Darwin archives there are plentiful papers giving detailed information about his condition, often monthly and for some periods even day by day.

The symptoms on which attention has tended to be concentrated and with which in later years Darwin himself was constantly preoccupied are the gastric ones, which afflicted him especially at night. They included flatulence, gastric pain and a symptom variously referred to as sickness and vomiting.

By far the most complete description of the symptoms is given in a long account Darwin wrote on 20 May 1865. Representative extracts from the first half, with his numerous insertions placed here in brackets, run as follows: "For 25 years extreme spasmodic daily and nightly flatulence; occasional vomiting, on two occasions prolonged during months. Vomiting preceded by shivering (hysterical crying) dying sensations (or half-faint) ... ringing in ears, treading on air and vision (focus and black dots) ... (nervousness when E. leaves me)—What I vomit intensely acid, slimy (sometimes bitter) consider teeth. Doctors (puzzled) say suppressed gout—No organic mischief...."

*During the course of his life Darwin consulted most of the leading physicians and surgeons of his day, but none of them ever found anything organically wrong. Although a number of physical illnesses that could not have been diagnosed last century have since been proposed—for example chronic cholecystitis, hiatus hernia, arsenic poisoning ... nearly every medically qualified man who has written on the subject is inclined to the view, with a variable degree of conviction, that Darwin's symptoms were mainly, if not entirely, psychogenic.**

(Bowlby, 1991, pp. 6–8)

Epidemiology and Cause

Very little is known about the epidemiology of Hypochondriasis. The Epidemiologic Catchment Area Study did not ask about this condition, but the prevalence of Hypochondriasis in general medical practice is said to range from 4% to 9% (American Psychiatric Association, 2000). It is likely that Hypochondriasis is similarly much more prevalent than is Somatization Disorder.

Almost all current theories suggest that Hypochondriasis is a condition resulting from psychological causes. Psychoanalysts have a number of causative theories that include the concept that repressed anger and hostility are displaced into physical symptoms so that they can be safely, if indirectly, communicated to others (Brown & Vaillant, 1981). Freud's emphasis was on the displacement of sexual drive into "narcissistic libido," a more complex theory that also suggested that Hypochondriasis reflects the repression and redirection of feelings toward others (Nemiah, 1985). Other psychological theories suggest that the hypochondriacal individual has low self-esteem and finds it easier to believe there is something wrong with his body than with his fundamental personality makeup (McCranie, 1979).

More recent theories suggest that hypochondriacal behavior is learned through the repetition of rewards—either the attention of parents and caretakers or rewards from internal stimuli resulting from anxiety: "Hypochondriasis can then be characterized by a vicious cycle of anxiety and somatic sensations leading to more anxiety, and with more frequent repetitions of this cycle, an overlearned pattern of behavior occurs in a rapid and predictable sequence" (Iezzi & Adams, 1993, p. 177). Both from such personal experience and from watching others who gain attention via their physical symptoms, an individual may come to develop Hypochondriasis.

An influential alternative view of Hypochondriasis has been that these individuals learn to be excessively sensitive to normal bodily sensations, and this sensitivity may be further enhanced by fear resulting from the incorrect perception of the significance of such sensations (Barsky & Klerman, 1983). Some psychologists believe that such hypersensitivity may have a neurophysiological basis in reduced central nervous system (CNS) inhibition of sensations that originate in somatic or visceral neural pathways (Ludwig, 1972). Hypochondriasis has much in common with anxiety disorder including phobias, and future research could possibly change the way that hypochondriasis is classified (Fineberg, Saxena, Zohar, & Craig, 2007).

Treatment

Some data indicate that persons who enter therapy early in the course of Hypochondriasis have a better prognosis and

BOX 19-3
PRINCIPLES OF EFFECTIVE TREATMENT FOR HYPOCHONDRIASIS

- Treatment begins with a physical examination and diagnostic tests for physical disease.
- Concurrent psychiatric disorders (particularly anxiety and depression) should be treated as indicated.
- The client should become knowledgeable about the condition of Hypochondriasis as the client needs to understand how his or her perception of bodily sensations leads to overemphasis on illness and disease.
- Symptoms should be acknowledged as real not imaginary, prolonged, troublesome, but not serious or dangerous.

*From *Charles Darwin: A New Life*, by John Bowlby, Copyright © 1990 by R. P. L. Bowlby, R. J. M. Bowlby, and A. Gatling. Reprinted with permission from W. W. Norton & Company, Inc.

outcome than do those who continue to receive only somatic evaluations and treatments. The principles of effective treatment are summarized in Box 19-3.

Success in treatment requires that the individual abandon any belief that she has a dangerous undiagnosed condition. This is often the greatest therapeutic challenge, usually accomplished only after establishment of client trust in the health care providers, reassurance regarding physical health, and the individual's understanding of how her own perception of her body leads to overemphasis on symptoms and illness. A review of treatment effectiveness more generally in somatoform disorders suggests that cognitive behavioral therapy has the strongest evidence supporting it with some studies also suggesting value for antidepressant medication treatment (Kroenke, 2007). This same stronger evidence for cognitive behavioral therapy appears to be true for Somatization Disorder as well (Thomson & Page, 2007).

If, as suggested previously, Hypochondriasis shares characteristics with anxiety disorders, one might expect treatments such as SSRI medication to be effective for Hypochondriasis, and limited data does support such effectiveness (Greeven, van Balkom, Visser, Merkelbach, van Rood, van Dyck, et al. 2007; Fallon, Schneier, Marshall, Campeas, Vermes, Goetz, et al., 1996). However, some data also suggest that psychotherapy improves Somatization Disorder (Ben-Tovim & Esterman, 1998). Perhaps another consideration to treatment is the fact that, when asked, a majority of clients state that they preferred cognitive-behavioral therapy to drug treatment (Walker, Vincent, Furer, Cox & Kjornisted, 1999).

CONVERSION DISORDER

The DSM-IV-TR concept of **Conversion Disorder** includes most of the dramatic manifestations of the old diagnosis of *hysteria*. Conversion Disorder is a condition in which patients exhibit symptoms that cannot be explained by any medical or neurological condition. These symptoms often include seizures (convulsions) but may include "impaired coordination or balance, paralysis or localized weakness, aphonia, difficulty swallowing or a sensation of a lump in the throat, and urinary retention. Sensory symptoms of deficits include loss of touch or pain sensation, double vision, blindness, deafness, and hallucinations" (American Psychiatric Association, 2000, p. 493). The specific diagnostic criteria are presented in Box 19-4.

While there are many possible conversion symptoms, the most common are loss of vision, loss of hearing, limb paralysis, and glove and stocking anesthesia, that is, numbness of hands and feet. Two specific features are central to the concept of Conversion Disorder:

1. No medical condition explains the observed symptoms, and
2. Symptoms occur as the result of psychological factors

The concept of conversion derives from psychoanalytic ideas that an individual with these symptoms is caught between conflicting desires or needs, some or all of which may be unrecognized or unconscious. The emergence of physical symptoms is thought to keep the unconscious conflict from surfacing into consciousness, where the resultant anxiety might be too strong for the individual to manage. The following excerpt from a play illustrates these concepts. In this play written soon after World War II, the American soldier Coney has become paralyzed after a South Seas battle with Japanese forces in which his fellow soldier, Finch, is killed. Coney could have helped Finch get medical help, but chose instead to run to safety, taking with him maps that could not be allowed to fall into enemy hands. The doctor soon recognizes that Coney's paralysis resulted from repressed memories of his flight and Finch's death. Coney is dimly aware of the psychological conflicts that led to his paralysis, but can describe them only vaguely as a "bad feeling." By helping Coney remember the details of Finch's death, the doctor is eventually able to bring the "bad feeling" out into the open and to cure Coney of his Conversion Disorder:

BOX 19-4 DIAGNOSTIC CRITERIA FOR CONVERSION DISORDER

- One or more symptoms or deficits affecting voluntary motor or sensory function that suggest a neurological or other general medical condition.
- Psychological factors are judged to be associated with the symptom or deficit because the initiation or exacerbation of the symptom or deficit is preceded by conflicts or other stressors.
- The symptom or deficit is not intentionally produced or feigned.
- The symptom or deficit cannot, after appropriate investigation, be fully explained by a general medical condition, the direct effects of a substance, or a culturally sanctioned behavior or experience.
- The symptom or deficit causes clinically significant distress or impairment or warrants medical evaluation.
- The symptom or deficit is not limited to pain or sexual dysfunction, does not occur exclusively during the course of Somatization Disorder, and is not better accounted for by another mental disorder.

From the *Diagnostic and Statistical Manual of Mental Disorders* (4th ed.-TR). Copyright © 2000. Reprinted with permission from the American Psychiatric Association.

WHY CAN'T YOU WALK, CONEY?

CONEY [turning] I should have stayed with him.

DOCTOR If you'd stayed with him the maps would be lost. The maps were your job and the job comes first....

CONEY He's dead....

DOCTOR Finch knew he had to get those maps. He told you to take them and go, didn't he? Didn't he, Coney? ...

CONEY I shouldn't've left him....

DOCTOR Coney, do you remember how you got off that island? ...

CONEY I remember being taken off the plane.

DOCTOR You weren't shot, were you?

CONEY No.

DOCTOR Then why can't you walk, Coney?

CONEY I don't know. I don't know....

DOCTOR Do you remember waking up in the hospital? Do you remember waking up with that bad feeling?

CONEY Yes.

[Slight pause. The Doctor walks next to the bed.]

DOCTOR Coney, when did you first get that bad feeling?

CONEY It was—I don't know.

DOCTOR Coney—[He sits down] did you first get it right after Finch was shot?

CONEY No.

DOCTOR What did you think of when Finch was shot?

CONEY I don't know.

DOCTOR You said you remember everything that happened. And you do. You remember that too. You remember how you felt when Finch was shot, don't you, Coney? Don't you?

CONEY [sitting bolt upright] Yes. [A long pause. His hands twist his robe and then lay still. With dead, flat tones] When we were looking for the map case, he said—he started to say: You lousy yellow Jew bastard. He only said you lousy yellow jerk, but he started to say you lousy yellow Jew bastard. So I knew. I knew.

DOCTOR You knew what?

CONEY I knew he'd lied when—when he said he didn't care. When he said people were people to him. I knew he lied. I knew he hated me because I was a Jew so—I was glad when he was shot.

[The Doctor straightens up.]

DOCTOR Did you leave him there because you were glad?

CONEY Oh, no!

DOCTOR You got over it.

CONEY I was—I was sorry I felt glad. I was ashamed.

DOCTOR Did you leave him because you were ashamed?

CONEY No.

DOCTOR Because you were afraid?

CONEY No.

DOCTOR No. You left him because that was what you had to do. Because you were a good soldier. [Pause] You left him and you ran through the jungle, didn't you? ...

CONEY Yes.

DOCTOR So your legs were all right.

CONEY Yes....

DOCTOR And you remember now, you remember that nothing happened to your legs at all, did it?

CONEY No, sir.

DOCTOR But you had to be carried here.

CONEY Yes, sir.

DOCTOR Why?

CONEY Because I can't walk.

DOCTOR Why can't you walk?

CONEY I don't know.

*DOCTOR I do. It's because you didn't want to, isn't it Coney? Because you knew if you couldn't walk, then you couldn't leave Finch. That's it, isn't it?**

(Laurents, 1946, pp. 56–63)

Epidemiology and Cause

The epidemiology of Conversion Disorder is incompletely understood, partly because of the difficulties of defining the condition and hence establishing accurate diagnosis. Few patients can afford the intensive evaluation and treatment of psychoanalysis, and hence it is likely that milder forms of conversion go unrecognized and untreated. One early study found that 25% of hospitalized women (many of whom were in the hospital only for normal childbirth) had previously suffered from one or more conversion symptoms (Cloninger, 1985). Another report indicated that conversion symptoms are not at all unusual among hospitalized patients (Folks, Ford, & Regan, 1984). Community studies have provided much lower but highly variable estimates of the prevalence of Conversion Disorder, ranging from 11 to 300 per 100,000 persons (Martin & Yutzy, 1994). Some of this variability seems to be explained by social class and status. While Freud thought Conversion Disorder to be rare among the poor, available data from research indicates that clients with Conversion Disorder are much more likely to be poor, uneducated, and often from rural backgrounds (Iezzi & Adams, 1993). There is much debate about whether or not Conversion Disorder is found more frequently in women, but at least some evidence suggests a relatively equal sex distribution (Iezzi & Adams, 1993), while others report women are diagnosed more often than men (Yutzy, 2003). Experts report that about 5%–24% of psychiatric outpatients, 5%–14% of general hospital patients, and 1%–3% of outpatient psychiatric referrals have a history of conversion symptoms (Yutzy, 2003).

*From *Home of the Brave*, by Arthur Laurents, Copyright 1946. Foreword by Robert Garland. Reprinted with permission from Random House, Inc.

The classical psychoanalytic theories of Conversion Disorder stress trauma due to childhood sexual experiences, real or imagined. Repression of the feelings associated with such sexual trauma leads to the bizarre symptoms often seen in conversion. Psychoanalytic theory assumes that through repression, childhood memories become unconscious but still need to be expressed in some overt way. Since bringing these memories into consciousness would cause great anxiety and fear, they manifest themselves as conversion symptoms. More recent psychoanalysts have suggested that strong nonsexual feelings of aggression or dependency (such as Coney's conflict and anger in the previous excerpt) can also result in conversion symptoms. Not all psychologists have accepted psychoanalytic explanations for Conversion Disorder. Some psychologists have viewed conversion symptoms as primarily manipulative, as a means to get attention or care, while others see these symptoms as learned responses to behavior that is reinforced by others.

Some neuropsychologists have focused on one of the characteristic features of Conversion Disorder—a surprising indifference that many clients show toward their symptoms. This indifference is often termed *la belle indifference* and is particularly striking when encountered. For example, persons who find themselves unable to move or see seem remarkably unconcerned about the disability. Such indifference, while highly characteristic of Conversion Disorder, can also be seen in medically ill clients whose symptoms give rise to strong denial. Some studies have suggested that in individuals with Conversion Disorder, such indifference is not solely psychological in origin but results from CNS inhibition of sensory inputs. In this theory, clients with Conversion Disorder have localized brain dysfunction that affects sensory perception and reduces their likelihood of recognizing the seriousness of their symptoms (Iezzi & Adams, 1993). Multiple studies suggesting that conversion symptoms are far more likely to occur on the left side of the body than is explainable by chance may add weight to such a neurophysiological theory of Conversion Disorder (Bishop, Mobley, & Far, 1978). Recent developments in neuroimaging techniques have generated increased interest in the conversion disorders (Aybeck, Kanaan, & David, 2008) and led to the recognition that these states are associated with distinct abnormalities in brain function. For example, paralysis like Coney's is associated with different patterns of brain activation than is seen during normal attempts to move affected muscles (Stone, Zeman, Simonotto, Meyer, Azuma, Flett, & Sharpe, 2007). Persons who have conversion-related loss of sensation do not activate their sensory cortex when the involved limb is stimulated—presumably due to some kind of inhibitory signals acting in pre-cortical brain areas (Ghaffar, Staines, & Feinstein, 2006).

Diagnosis

In many cases the diagnosis of conversion disorder is not easy. Leary (2003) raises related issues based on a child with conversion symptoms who received an extensive battery of noncontributory tests before the diagnosis was definitively made. Accurate diagnosis requires experience and close observation. Most conversion symptoms are similar to, but do not exactly mimic, those of the true physical disorders. Subtle findings (eye movements in pseudoseizures, the absence of certain abnormal neurological findings in multiple sclerosis presentations) can help make the diagnosis. If obtained within 15–20 minutes after the acute episode, blood determination of prolactin can help distinguish pseudoseizures from true epileptic convulsions (Chen, So, & Fisher, 2005), but equally effective tools are rarely available for other conversion symptoms.

Conversion reactions may present in unanticipated ways such as with an apparent club foot seemingly needing surgery (Michelson, 2000). It is important to recognize the difference between conversion and factitious disorders (see next section). Individuals with factitious disorders consciously feign having a condition such as a club foot so that they will receive treatment such as surgery. Most psychiatrists believe that conversion disorders are not feigned but derive from inherent psychological conflicts that manifest themselves physically. If there had been a real Coney, he would presumably have experienced his paralysis no differently whether due to a conversion reaction or a more "physical" neurological disorder. Sometimes only a period of prolonged observation (as in *Why Can't You Walk, Coney?*) will allow a diagnosis of conversion to be made. Heruti and colleagues (2002) from Israel describe a group of 34 individuals admitted to rehabilitation facilities with severe impairments of mobility. These persons presented with neurological symptoms that after extensive inpatient evaluation were felt to be due to conversion reaction (Heruti, Reznik, Adunski, Levy, Weingarden, & Ohry, 2002). Unlike Coney, half of these individuals had no functional improvement during their rehabilitation admission, though the authors concluded that these 30 clients comprised less than 1% of the entire population of rehabilitation clients seen during this period. The relative rarity of this disorder heightens the importance of clinical vigilance in suspecting and making the diagnosis.

Treatment

The recognition that an individual's physical symptoms and signs are due to conversion often makes caretakers angry. Nurses need to identify this anger and approach the client without confrontation. For some individuals, symptoms resolve without any treatment (Folks et al., 1984), but while strong evidence of effectiveness is lacking, expert opinion supports the use of psychotherapy, and where symptoms are severe, first-generation antipsychotics (Allin, Streeruwitz, & Curtis, 2005). If symptoms do persist for long periods of time, chronicity and poor outcome may develop. Acute conversion often responds, as did Coney's in the previous excerpt, to direct explanation of the underlying psychological conflicts. More chronic conversion symptoms are more difficult to treat with such explanation and may require prolonged therapy. "Faith healing" and exorcism have been traditional approaches to conversion symptoms, and these emotionally charged catharses are often effective in relieving symptoms.

FACTITIOUS DISORDER

As noted earlier in this chapter, **Factitious Disorder** involves physical or psychological symptoms that are intentionally produced in order to gain attention from potential caregivers. The *intention* to fabricate symptoms distinguishes factitious disorders from the somatoform disorders. **Malingering** also involves the fabrication of symptoms, but here the purpose is to achieve some objective goal such as financial compensation or avoiding work. Individuals with Factitious Disorder may present with a complex mixture of real and feigned symptoms, for example, fabricated seizures in a person with prior epilepsy and an abnormal electroencephalogram (Chabolla, Krahn, So, & Rummans, 1996). This complex interweaving of truth and falsehood is often accompanied by dramatic embellishment of details and by outright lies. Whereas DSM-IV-TR uses the term Factitious Disorder, many clinicians prefer to call this disorder **Munchausen's Syndrome**, a name suggested in 1951 when Asher first clearly described persons with this dramatic condition:

> *The patient showing the syndrome is admitted to hospital with apparent acute illness supported by a plausible and dramatic history. Usually his story is largely made up of falsehoods; he is found to have attended, and deceived, an astounding number of other hospitals.... It is almost impossible to be certain of the diagnosis at first, and it requires a bold casualty officer to refuse admission.... It must be recognized that these patients are often quite ill, although their illness is shrouded by duplicity and distortion.... Often a real organic lesion from the past has left some genuine physical signs which the patient uses.... Most cases resemble organic emergencies. Well-known varieties are: 1. The acute abdominal type. ... 2. The haemorrhagic type, who specialise in bleeding from lungs or stomach. ... 3. The neurological type, presenting with paroxysmal headache, loss of consciousness or peculiar fits. The most remarkable feature of the syndrome is the apparent senselessness of it. Unlike the malingerer, who may gain a definite end, these patients often seem to gain nothing except the discomfiture of unnecessary investigations or operations. Their initial tolerance to the more brutish hospital measures is remarkable, yet they commonly discharge themselves after a few days with operation wounds scarcely healed, or intravenous drips still running.**
>
> (Asher, 1951, p. 340)

Munchausen's Syndrome is named after an eighteenth-century personage, Baron Munchausen, whose devious exploits, fabrications, and trickeries—real and imagined—were widely popularized in Europe and have remained of sufficient interest to serve as the subject of director Terry Gilliam's 1989 film *The Adventures of Baron Munchausen*. Factitious Disorder seems to be relatively rare, but most nurses eventually encounter one or more clients with this condition.

While Munchausen's Syndrome is probably more common, there has been increasing interest in another Factitious Disorder known as **Munchausen's Syndrome by Proxy**. This is a form of child abuse in which a parent, usually the mother, falsely reports a story of childhood illness that may result in unnecessary medical investigations or treatments. As in Munchausen's Syndrome, the reports of illness may contain elaborate falsifications, and clinical personnel may fail to recognize the deception for many months or years. Frequently, harm may come to a child from either unnecessary interventions or the parent's efforts to induce the appearance of symptoms through various toxins, drugs, or physical manipulations.

*From "Munchausen Syndrome," by R. Asher, Copyright © 1951. Reprinted with permission from Elsevier (*Lancet, 1*, p. 340).

REFLECTIVE THINKING 19-2

Munchausen's Syndrome by Proxy

Consider the discussion of Munchausen's Syndrome by Proxy. How would you react to a parent who has intentionally induced symptoms in his child, so the child appears ill?

EPIDEMIOLOGY AND CAUSE

The actual prevalence of Factitious Disorder is not known, due to both the fact that the diagnosis may not be made and the fact that the chronic forms of the disorder may be over reported when a client who is diagnosed by one provider moves on to obtain care somewhere else and is reported again. The disorder, however, is more common among men than among women (American Psychiatric Association, 2000).

The factors leading to Factitious Disorder are unclear, but possible predisposing factors listed in DSM-IV-TR include the presence of other mental disorders and/or general medical conditions during childhood or adolescence that led to extensive treatments and hospitalizations; a grudge against the medical profession; employment in medically related work; the presence of a severe personality disorder; and an important relationship with a physician in the past.

TREATMENT

The nature of the disorder makes it almost impossible to treat, and treatment is almost always unsatisfactory with very little evidence to define effective treatment practices (Eastwood & Bisson, 2008). Clients, particularly those who develop a chronic form of the disorder, develop lifelong patterns of hospitalization, willingness to submit to invasive diagnostic and surgical procedures, and an unending list of

NURSINGALERT 19-1

Munchausen's Syndrome by Proxy

Munchausen's Syndrome by Proxy is, like any other form of child abuse, reportable to Children's Protective Services.

symptoms. When the factitious nature of the symptoms is discovered, the clients will most often discharge themselves against medical advice and move to other clinics and other locations to receive care where they are not known.

DISSOCIATIVE DISORDERS

Dissociative Disorders are a group of uncommonly recognized conditions that are fascinating, highly controversial, and frequently discussed in the popular media. The dissociative disorders also form the subject matter for a number of books and films, some of the latter of which are reviewed in this text. Certainly, students who see the films *Sybil* or *Three Faces of Eve* will want to know more about the Dissociative Disorder they depict. The book by Oxnam referenced under "Suggested Readings" describes in lucid detail the author's multiple personalities—characteristic of the psychiatrically controversial dissociative identity disorder discussed next.

DSM-IV TR includes four specific diagnoses under the category Dissociative Disorders. These include Dissociative Amnesia, Dissociative Fugue, Depersonalization Disorder, and Dissociative Identity Disorder. There is also a fifth category for Dissociative Disorder that does not meet criteria for any of these other four.

Amnesia is the loss of memory, sometimes concerning events that are particularly traumatic or frightening. **Fugue** is sudden unexplained travel away from home or normal environment; fugue is usually associated with confusion about past identity or, more rarely, with the assumption of a completely new personal identity. **Depersonalization** refers to either persistent or recurrent feelings of being separated from one's normal mental functions, or feeling as if one is outside one's body.

Each of these symptoms—amnesia, fugue, and depersonalization—can be part of other psychological conditions, most commonly, anxiety or somatoform disorders. Historically, these conditions have often been considered to be part of the spectrum of "hysteria," but this diagnosis, so important in the development of psychoanalysis, is no longer part of the DSM-IV-TR diagnostic vocabulary. Symptoms that were once considered "hysterical" are now commonly ascribed to a range of disorders, including Dissociative Disorders.

Amnesia, fugue, and depersonalization all refer to quite specific and circumscribed symptoms for which there are no alternative physical or psychological explanations.

AMNESIA

Dissociative Amnesia is a form of memory loss that is not associated with discernible neurologic disease—in particular head trauma—and is assumed to have a psychological basis (Brandt & Van Gorp, 2006). When amnesia follows a blow to the head or a stroke, it is considered a neurological rather than a psychological condition. Such amnesia due to physical trauma is almost invariably "retrograde": memories that were created before the physical injury are lost for a period of time. Dissociative Amnesia associated with psychological trauma is generally "anterograde": memory is lost for a period after the traumatic event. Clients with dissociative amnesia usually retain the ability to learn new information, a skill that is often impaired in those with non-dissociative amnesia. A careful assessment will occasionally determine that both physical trauma and Dissociative Amnesia (triggered by the psychological trauma of an accident or assault) have occurred together. Memory deficits are also seen in persons with a variety of other neurological and psychiatric conditions. For example, persons with dementia often have memory loss, but this is generally quite global and not restricted to a specific period of time. Alcoholics and other substance abusers will frequently have periods of amnesia related to heavy substance use. These amnesic episodes are not regarded as dissociative. Neuropsychologists can generally distinguish among the various forms of memory loss to determine which have organic basis and which are likely to be dissociative (Serra, Fadda, Buccione, Caltagirone, & Carlesimo, 2007).

FUGUE

As with amnesia, fugue behavior is not solely a dissociative phenomenon but may also occur in other conditions. For example, elements of fugue—undirected wandering—may be seen during some forms of complex partial seizures (temporal lobe epilepsy). Psychiatrists and neurologists can usually separate relatively brief neurologically mediated fugue states from the more prolonged wanderings of a person in dissociative fugue. In many situations the challenge is to identify that an individual is actually in a fugue state since these persons may function remarkably normally until detailed questioning reveals that they don't know who they are or why they are in that place. Remarkably, other than identity confusion, their orientation and global mental functioning may be entirely intact—a marked contrast to the wandering seen among individuals with Alzheimer's or other forms of dementia who typically have quite global cognitive impairments.

DEPERSONALIZATION

Persons experiencing depersonalization feel as if they are living in a dream or even a film. They may feel as if they are watching themselves from a vantage point outside their own bodies. In particular, they describe a dulling of all emotional experiences—quite different from the anhedonia reported by persons with depression. While full understanding of this disorder remains elusive, depersonalization is associated with measurable changes in memory formation and attention (Guralnik, Giesbrecht, Knutelska, Sirroff, & Simeon, 2007). Functional magnetic resonance imaging also confirms the subjective dulling of emotion that persons with depersonalization report. Compared to controls, these individuals process verbal material with emotional content quite differently and without activation of areas of the brain normally involved in emotional processing (Medford, Brierley, Bramer, Bullmore, David & Phillips, 2006). Depersonalization does, of course, occur in normal individuals, with or without use of psychoactive substances, and it may be a component of "flashback" experiences that occur months or years after prior hallucinogen use. Many individuals also describe panic attacks that describe depersonalization as part of these. Depersonalization becomes a disorder when it occurs frequently or interferes significantly with an individual's life.

Dissociative phenomena including fugue, amnesia, and depersonalization can be seen as part of trance-like states that occur normally in some individuals and are commonly seen in a variety of religious and cultural observances. Dissociation is only regarded as abnormal if it is prolonged, leads to distress or social dysfunction, and has not occurred as part of culturally normative ceremonies or practices.

DISSOCIATIVE IDENTITY DISORDER

Dissociative Identity Disorder (DID) is by far the most complex and controversial of the dissociative disorders. Formerly termed Multiple Personality Disorder, DID refers to individuals who possess two or more distinct identities, at least two of which periodically take control of the individual's behavior—typically not at the same time. Periods of amnesia are found in DID and may be quite extensive. The expression of multiple identities (personalities) may be exceedingly dramatic and even colorful. Each identity may have a separate name, gender, voice, or set of psychological symptoms. While not part of the diagnostic criteria for DID, there is often a reported history of severe psychological, physical, or sexual trauma or abuse in early childhood. These memories may be highly repressed, "known" only to some of the individual's identities, and highly difficult to corroborate through independent witnesses. Such memories may emerge only after long periods of intense psychotherapy.

There has been immense controversy about such repressed memories. Experts differ in their opinions as to whether the remembered abuse actually happened, or whether such "memories" are actually created during the process of psychotherapy. There are few areas of mental health practice in which expert opinion has been so strongly divided and forcefully expressed. Whether or not repressed memory can and does occur is of great legal and ethical importance (McAllister, 2000)

Those who believe in the ability of psychotherapy to identify true repressed memories defend their viewpoint on the high frequency of *known* child abuse and sexual molestation. For every case that is detected there must surely be some that are unreported and unprosecuted. There is no doubt that perpetrators of childhood abuse go to great lengths to deny their involvement, and abuse frequently is revealed (and admitted by the perpetrator), but victims find their experiences too terrible to remember. They bury these memories deep in the unconscious—only to have them emerge later as elements of dissociative behavior.

The opponents of repressed memories feel that most memories of prior abuse are subtly suggested to highly suggestible individuals by generally well-meaning therapists. Sometimes these memories are recognized during therapy involving hypnosis, when suggestibility is perhaps at its highest. Additionally, persons who can be readily hypnotized may often be more suggestible than the average person. Close corroborative investigation makes it seem likely that some persons—especially those with DID—have not really experienced the abuse that they describe vividly to their psychological interviewers.

Unfortunately, since many repressed memories recall criminal acts (physical or especially, sexual assault), courts frequently need to judge the truth of allegations based solely on memories recalled during the course of psychotherapy for dissociative symptoms. Many believe that in at least some cases, innocent persons have been punished for crimes that were incorrectly "recalled" from amnestic memory during psychotherapy for dissociative disorders.

Does Dissociative Identity Disorder Really Exist?

There is little doubt that a phenomenon related to Dissociative Identity or multiple personality does exist. There is an immensely long history, in nearly all cultures, of reports of "possession" and exorcism; these, and spiritual mediumship/shamanism are likely related to but not identical with dissociative phenomena (Moreira-Almeida, Neto, & Cardeña, 2008). There is reason to believe that at least one of the most prominent cases of DID, the multiple personalities of a woman given the name of "Sybil" and made the subject of a best-selling book and widely viewed movie, were at least in part an artifact of her psychotherapy. In an interview, the psychiatrist, Herbert Spiegel, recalls his own work with the real Sybil and raises significant questions about the accuracy of the written descriptions of Sybil's illness and course of psychotherapy for Multiple Personality Disorder—now DID. While Dr. Spiegel's recollections don't fully discredit the diagnosis of DID, others have been more assertive in their challenge and have argued that DID and the concept of repressed sexual abuse are both unscientific myths. There have been both sensational legal settlements and thoughtful essays detailing unquestioned errors in the recovery of repressed memory.

There is, however, considerable evidence for what some have termed *False Memory Syndrome* in which memories, particularly of repressed physical or sexual abuse, come to play a major role in a person's self-image and daily life, but appear not to be objectively true. In few areas of psychiatry are opinions so strongly divided between those who question the existence, perhaps not primarily of DID, but of its origins in childhood abuse and those who feel that such abuse is extraordinarily common and devastating in its effects. Despite skepticism and controversy over repressed memories and DID, many persons and their therapists believe that their symptoms have, in fact, been caused by profound repressed psychological trauma during childhood. Readers who like to peruse the Internet will find intriguing sites created by persons who view themselves as having multiple personalities.

Psychiatrists disagree about whether there is sufficient evidence to justify the inclusion of DID within DSM. Coons (1998) has been a strong advocate and argues that not only does this disorder exist, but between 5% and 10% of persons with psychiatric disorders have some form of Dissociative Disorder. Others have concurred with this estimate (Elmore, 2000). In contrast, a survey of nearly 400 U.S. psychiatrists found that only a quarter felt that DID and Dissociative Amnesia were "supported by strong evidence of scientific validity" (Pope, Oliva, Hudson, Bodkin, & Gruber, 1999). While dissociative disorders have captured public and legal attention, it seems unlikely that this degree of uncertainly among psychiatrists will be resolved in the near future.

TREATMENT

There is no good evidence that supports the use of medication in treating DID. Psychotherapy has been the major form of treatment used and remains the treatment of choice for most therapists. The role of hypnosis remains controversial partly because of concerns that hypnosis may increase the risk of creating false memories.

> **BOX 19-5**
> **HOW DOES DISSOCIATIVE IDENTITY DISORDER OR MULTIPLE PERSONALITY DISORDER DIFFER FROM SCHIZOPHRENIA?**
>
> In Chapter 13, we emphasize the difference between DID ("disorders of multiple personalities") and schizophrenia. Schizophrenia does not mean split personality as in Dr. Jekyll and Mr. Hyde (Robert Lewis Stevenson's classic short novel describing a fictional character with DID). Instead, schizophrenia is a term chosen to emphasize the serious effects of this disorder on language and thought. Persons with DID retain full control of their thought processes, though they may be amnestic for major periods of their lives. DSM-IV adapted the term *Dissociative Identity Disorder* at least in part because in psychological terms an individual has only one personality but may have a number of independent identities. The older term (Multiple Personality Disorder) was apparently felt to misrepresent the unity of personality.

NURSING CARE AND SOMATOFORM DISORDERS

One of the great challenges in nursing is to care for and care about a difficult client—a client who does not respond in the manner expected or one who does not have the same values and goals that nurses generally hold. Although all nursing theories and stated philosophies of nursing include care of each individual as a unique and whole person, nurses frequently find themselves to be judgmental, particularly when it comes to caring for a client with a somatoform disorder. The client with such a disorder tests the patience of nurses and the ethic that nursing must provide unconditional *care*. It is important to explore nurses' experiences with such clients and to understand the nurses' feelings and attitudes. Further, it is equally important to revisit basic nursing philosophies that underlie modern theories of care.

Nurses and other health care providers have limited resources (time, energy, emotions, and finances) with which

> **REFLECTIVE THINKING 19-3**
> **Somatoform Disorder**
>
> Take a moment to stop and reflect on the information you have read in the chapter so far, and ask yourself the following questions:
>
> - What emotions have you experienced? List them for yourself and reflect on the source of each.
> - Do the descriptions of somatoform disorders make you angry? If yes, what is the source of your anger?
> - Do you find that the clients described are believable?
> - Can you begin to understand the world experience of someone who is suffering from any one of these disorders?
> - How much do you value health, rather than illness, in yourself? In others?
> - How much do you value independence in yourself? In others?
>
> Consider your answers and recognize that there are no right or wrong answers to these questions. Know that if you know yourself and understand your reactions to clients with these disorders, you will be in a much better position to provide professional and therapeutic care.

to provide care to clients. Studies have indicated that there are persons who "over utilize" health care services. For example, data such as early findings that 13% of adults in an HMO made 31% of the office visits and accounted for 35% of hospital admissions and 30% of the surgeries (McFarland, Freeborn, Mullody, & Pope, 1985) lead many to conclude that such clients are indeed taking or demanding, or both, more than their "fair share." More recently, health policy reports continue to document, for example, that most medical emergency departments provide services to a relatively small number of frequent users who account for a disproportionately large number of visits (Shumway, Boccelar, O'Brien, & Okin, 2008). Health care providers, particularly primary care providers, find themselves frustrated with such clients. These clients seem to demand something of them that they are unable or unwilling to give. Nursing authors commented: "If you often feel frustrated by somatizing patients, you're hardly alone" (Ford, Katon, & Lipkin, 1993, p. 31). Each nurse must explore the personal meaning of this frustration, recognizing that clients with somatoform disorders are psychiatrically ill and greatly in need of care. For many, the frustration comes from not knowing what to do and from being uncomfortable with the psychiatric nature of the physical problem. The following discussion of nursing theory and approaches may help to empower nurses to provide quality, professional care.

NURSING THEORY

Nursing as caring is an important concept when dealing with clients with somatoform disorders. Caring means that the nurse will try to understand the client as she is, accept her personality, her complaints, and her need for care. Often, clients with somatization have low self-esteem, repressed hostility, and guilt derived from a dysfunctional family background (Roberts, 1994). A nurse must see through the presenting symptoms in order to begin caring for the person behind the presenting illness.

Caring means that the nurse will bring a presence, an acceptance, and a sense of compassion and concern. Watson's Theory of Human Care draws attention to the need for care, not cure. However, another important component of Watson's theory is that "caring can be effectively demonstrated and practiced only interpersonally" (Talento, 1995). Clients with somatoform disorders will not enter into relationships readily or readily express emotions. The challenge, then, is to give care and to present a healing presence without making demands on the client that he be someone or something he is unable to be.

In addition to the concept of nursing as caring, some of the ideas basic to the Modeling and Role-Modeling theory (Erickson, Tomlin, & Swain, 1983) are also helpful. Modeling the client's world means understanding the world from the client's perspective. A nurse must attempt to know the client's subjective experience of her illness, her disability, her needs for care and services. More than likely, much of the nurse's frustration with the somatizing client is the nurse's inability to comprehend how and why the client reacts to her life situations in the manner she does. The best advice coming from the Modeling and Role-Modeling theory is to *listen* to the client and begin to build a nurse-client relationship based on trust. Nurses need to understand that by building such a relationship they are, indeed, providing nursing care. Further, from the perspective of this theory, when a client is in impoverishment, that is, in a state where she is unable to mobilize any of her own resources to deal with life's stressors (see Chapter 3), the nurse is guided to provide direct physical care. It becomes clear that a client presenting with Somatization Disorder is quite often in impoverishment. At that time, direct nursing care would be offered by a nurse using this theory.

NURSING TIP 19-1

Caring for Someone with Somatoform Disorder

The following are ways to provide a healing presence without demanding the client be someone he is not:

- Know yourself
- Read the descriptions of the somatoform disorders
- Reread them
- Tell yourself and your colleagues that these clients are psychiatrically ill
- Try to empathize with the client by feeling and understanding the client's pain
- Consider the client's day-to-day life
- Compare the client's life to your own
- Tell yourself to remember you became a nurse to care about people and to provide compassion

REFLECTIVE THINKING 19-4

Factitious Disorder

How can nurses manage their personal feelings in order to provide sensitive nursing care to clients presenting with Factitious Disorder?

- **How would you react to the client?**
- **Does your institution have counseling or support services that nurses might use if faced with a situation such as that described in the Research Highlight?**

RESEARCH Highlight 19-1

Efficacy of Treatment for Somataform Disorders

STUDY PROBLEM/PURPOSE

The researcher conducted a review of 34 randomized controlled clinical trials (RCTs published over a 10-year period and accounting for nearly 4,000 patients) to evaluate the effectiveness of treatments provided.

METHOD

RCTs were identified through a literature search using MEDLINE and the diagnostic labels of somataform disorders.

FINDINGS

In a vast majority of the studies evaluating the efficacy of cognitive behavioral therapy (11 of 13), the therapy was found to be effective. Drug therapy (antidepressants) was also found to be useful, but in a smaller number of RCTs. The author concludes that cognitive behavioral therapy is the best established treatment for somataform disorders. Preliminary, though nonconclusive evidence suggests antidepressants may be effective.

IMPLICATIONS

Increasingly, nurses need to be aware of the evidence presented in randomized controlled trials, and summary data from such trials should provide a basis on which to suggest and monitor treatment plans.

Source: "Efficacy of Treatment for Somataform Disorders: A Review of Randomized Controlled Trials," by K. Kroeke, 2007, *Psychosomatic Medicine*, *69*, 881–888.

The Special Case of Factitious Disorder

Many of the nursing approaches and nursing theories discussed previously for somatoform disorders also apply to clients with Factitious Disorder. However, there seems an even greater reluctance on the part of nurses to truly *care* for clients who feign illnesses. A 1994 report from a group of critical care nurses describes the nurses' reactions to a client with significant psychiatric disease. The nurses were angry (in their words, "furious") and in a state of "shock and disbelief" that they had been fooled by this client (Miller & Cabeza-Stradi, 1994). These nurses recommended that all who provided care to a client with Factitious Disorder participate in discussion sessions to explore their own feelings and reactions and share their perceptions of the situation. Clearly, there is an important aspect of caring for the caregiver here, in that nurses need support from one another in dealing with such a difficult and hard-to-comprehend client. These nurses tended to blame themselves for having been taken in by a client who was lying; they felt betrayed. It would perhaps be helpful if these nurses remembered that clients with factitious disorders are excellent actors. These clients do "take people in"; the acting and lying are part of the illness. Questions these critical care nurses could ask themselves are:

- Does this client need a nurse?
- Do I believe that this client is ill?
- Can a mental disorder ever take precedence over physical problems?
- How do I feel when the client does not want to get well?

There is a very important need for nurses outside of psychiatry to have compassion for and understanding of a client whose disorder is not physical in nature.

APPLICATION OF THE NURSING PROCESS 19-1

ASSESSMENT

Nursing care must begin with an assessment of the client, both his physical condition and the psychosocial aspects of his functioning. While the nurse will be working in a collaborative role with physicians and other professionals in any case as complicated as a Somatoform or Factitious Disorder, specific nursing assessment includes questioning about the family history and family interaction patterns, sociocultural history and its influence on values and beliefs, current life stressors and past methods of coping, and the significance of the current illness/symptoms to the client. Assessment questions are presented in Box 19-6.

(*Continues*)

APPLICATION OF THE NURSING PROCESS 19-1 (Continued)

BOX 19-6
ASSESSMENT QUESTIONS FOR SOMATIZING CLIENTS

FAMILY HISTORY

Please tell me about your family:

- Who do you consider to be your family?
- Do you live with family members? Friends? By yourself?
- Do other members of your family have medical illnesses?
- Does anyone in your family have the same symptoms as you?
- Where do members of your family go to receive care?
- Who have you told that you are ill?
- How often do you interact with family members/significant others?
- Has the interaction changed since you have become ill?

SOCIOCULTURAL HISTORY

- How do you interpret your illness/symptoms?
- Have you known others who have similar problems?
- How is your illness/symptom interpreted within your family? By your friends?
- How does your illness/symptom affect how others treat you?
- Do members of your family share the same values? Or are they different in their thinking?

CURRENT STRESSORS

- What are the current stresses in your life?
- What would you do if you needed medical attention in the middle of the night?
- What would you say is your method of dealing with stress?
- Do you have health insurance?
- Are you able to obtain the care you think you need?
- What do you expect from care in this hospital (clinic)?

SIGNIFICANCE OF THE SOMATIZATION

- How do you interpret your symptoms?
- What is the significance of this hospitalization for you?
- Have you experienced these or similar symptoms in the past?

NURSING DIAGNOSIS

In addition to the nursing diagnoses related to the specific physical condition/symptoms displayed by the client, the psychosocial nursing diagnoses that need to be considered include the following:

- *Disturbed body image*
- *Chronic low self-esteem*
- *Ineffective coping*
- *Hopelessness*
- *Powerlessness*
- *Spiritual distress*
- *Social isolation*

(Continues)

APPLICATION OF THE NURSING PROCESS 19-1 (Continued)

Nursing diagnoses specifically for the family may also include *interrupted family processes* and *caregiver role strain*. Each of these diagnoses, when validated, could lead to specific interventions based on the client's readiness to acknowledge feelings and accept a path toward greater health. For example, the client that relates she feels socially isolated and wishes to engage in more frequent interactions with others can be assisted to identify means to accomplish this within the parameters of her lifestyle and symptoms. The client who relates she has a poor image of her own body may be encouraged to see the positive qualities and strengths she does have. Consideration of the nursing diagnoses listed helps the nurse consider the range of problems his client may face and then helps in determining what appropriate nursing actions to take.

OUTCOME IDENTIFICATION

Outcome for clients with somatoform or factitious disorders will not realistically be perfect physical and psychological health. Short-term treatment goals make more sense, for example, stating as an outcome that a client who has Somatization Disorder "will maintain independent functioning in between weekly visits to the clinic" may be a realistic goal. The nurse should discuss outcomes with the client and set out mutually agreed-on goals. Goals should focus on care, not cure.

PLANNING/INTERVENTIONS

In all cases, the nurse should begin by establishing a caring and trusting nurse-client relationship, understanding full well that many of these clients will not reciprocate. In many cases, listening to the client and attempting to understand the client's experience is the best nursing intervention one has to offer. In cases where specific diagnoses (such as social isolation) and goals are identified, nursing interventions will be to work with the client to solve the identified problem (for example, wanting increased interaction with others).

Financial resources almost inevitably become a source of concern for clients who cannot work and must pay bills for numerous health care problems. Nurses must be aware of community services and will need to make referrals to social workers and others who can assist the client to obtain health care and services to meet other basic needs.

EVALUATION

Evaluate care for somatizing clients based on short-term, identifiable goals. Ask the client what he thinks can be expected and continue to offer compassionate care, recognizing that these are chronic diseases that require management over time.

CARE PLANNING GUIDE 19-1 Client with a Somatoform Disorder: Hypochondriasis

CLINICAL PICTURE

The clinical picture of a client with Hypochondriasis includes:

- Preoccupation with the fear that one has a serious disease
- Lack of diagnostic findings on clinical and laboratory tests
- Failure to develop the feared disease
- Duration for at least six months

(Continues)

CARE PLANNING GUIDE 19-1 Continued

NURSING DIAGNOSES

The nursing diagnoses most commonly employed for such client are:

1. *Anxiety*
2. *Fear*

Note: The care plans that follow have been adapted from *Plans of Care for Specialty Practice: Psychiatric Mental Health Nursing*, by M. Coler and K. G. Vincent, 1995, Clifton Park, NY: Delmar, Cengage Learning.

NURSING DIAGNOSIS 1: *ANXIETY*

OUTCOMES

1. The client will verbally and behaviorally demonstrate a decrease in anxiety.
2. The client will use adaptive coping strategies (such as relaxation, biofeedback, reality testing, problem solving, and leisure activities).

NOC: *ANXIETY SELF-CONTROL*

INTERVENTIONS (NIC: *ANXIETY REDUCTION*)	RATIONALE
• Conduct (or refer the client to a practitioner to conduct) a thorough physical examination.	• Assessment is needed to rule out physiological conditions.
• Plan psychotherapeutic interventions.	• Psychotherapy will help to identify underlying depression and causes of anxiety.
• Consider medication as treatment for anxiety or depression, or both.	• Medication may be helpful in controlling symptoms.
• Teach self-control strategies (relaxation, biofeedback, cognitive reframing).	• These strategies may help to decrease symptoms.
• Teach problem-solving strategies.	• This provides adaptive ways of solving conflicts.
• Teach strategies for developing an unencumbering daily routine.	• Thinking in a state of anxiety is diffuse and can be focused by routines to avoid confusion.

NURSING DIAGNOSIS 2: *FEAR RELATED TO PRECEIVED THREAT OF ILLNESS*

OUTCOMES

1. The client will identify the object of fear.
2. The client will assume control over the fear.
3. The client identify the significance of fear to life's goals.

NOC: *FEAR SELF-CONTROL*

INTERVENTIONS (NIC: *COGNITIVE RESTRUCTURING*)	RATIONALE
• Monitor the background of fear and its intensity.	• Ongoing assessment determines if the fear is based on misconception, lack of knowledge, or classical conditioning.
• Determine the extent of victimization by fear production techniques of external sources.	• Fear-producing techniques are used by individuals to control others' behaviors.

(*Continues*)

CARE PLANNING GUIDE 19-1 Continued

INTERVENTIONS (NIC: *COGNITIVE RESTRUCTURING*)	RATIONALE
• Refer for short-term psychotherapy.	• Psychotherapy will help the client to identify the object of the fear.
• Examine the significance of the object of the fear.	• Frequently, the greater the significance, the greater the distortion and the greater the fear.
• Teach the physiological responses to fear.	• Knowledge of the physiological responses helps one to get control over them.
• Relate cultural concepts to conditions under which fear arises.	• The origin of fear may be different from one culture to another.

LONG-TERM CONSIDERATIONS FOR THE CLIENT WITH HYPOCHONDRIASIS

1. Evaluate periodically for evidence of depression and anxiety.
2. Provide for long-term follow-up for medications and psychotherapy, because this is a chronic disease.

NURSING CARE PLAN: NURSING PROCESS FORMAT 19-1

Similar to the descriptions of health/illness in the letters of Alice James, we will consider Betty as a modern-day woman who is coming to a clinic for a work-up for the following symptoms: functional disturbance of lower extremities, including weakness, intermittent partial paralysis and numbness of lower extremities, and pain with movement; multiple vague discomforts, including head and foot pain; stomach pain; and episodes of nausea and vomiting, "heart trouble," and palpitations.

ASSESSMENT

Betty has had multiple medical work-ups and evaluations. She has seen several subspecialists, and there is no known physiological cause for all of her symptoms; however, she does carry a diagnosis of gout. Betty readily talks about her symptoms and seems pleased that her nurse wants to hear of her situation. However, Betty does not wish to talk about any feelings or her family background. Betty has been suffering with various physical complaints for 20 years and believes her symptoms have worsened with time. Betty expresses a sense that she will never get better but does not express feelings of despair or sadness when describing this. Betty denies stress in her life, although she does admit to having few friends and no support system. Further, there are few activities Betty enjoys. She rarely leaves her house and receives no visitors. When the nurse asked Betty, "If you were sick in the middle of the night and needed help, do you have a friend you could call who would come to help you?" Betty responded, "No, there is no one to call."

NURSING DIAGNOSIS 1 *Social isolation*, related to inability to engage in satisfying personal relationships, as evidenced by absence of supportive significant others.

(Continues)

NURSING CARE PLAN: NURSING PROCESS FORMAT 19-1 (Continued)

OUTCOMES	NIC	NURSING ACTIONS	EVALUATION
• Betty will reciprocate in establishing a nurse-client relationship. • Betty will interact with one individual who is not a member of the health care team during the week in between regular visits to the clinic.	• Socialization enhancement • Social support enhancement	• Establish a positive nurse-client relationship by offering time to meet with Betty each week, expressing positive regard, and listening to her experiences. • Help Betty to identify someone she could consider a friend—a neighbor, a relative—someone with whom she could interact. Explore the ways Betty could reach out to this person—by telephone, letter writing. • Given Betty's physical health, explore with her the option of interacting with persons over the World Wide Web through e-mail, discussion groups, and chat rooms.	Betty seemed quite willing to talk with the nurse, although her interactions seemed guarded and she did not disclose more about herself and family. When Betty arrived at the clinic, she did ask to see the nurse. Betty was unwilling or unable to identify a person with whom she could interact other than the nurse and health care workers at the clinic; however, she did become interested in computer-based communications. She had a computer and began to interact via a discussion group related to literature. Betty related that she enjoyed this activity.

NURSING DIAGNOSIS 2 *Powerlessness*, related to lifestyle of helplessness, as evidenced, by passivity.

OUTCOMES	NIC	NURSING ACTIONS	EVALUATION
• Betty will feel in control of some aspects of her life within 2 months. • Betty will identify two of her day-to-day activities over which she has choices.	• Cognitive structuring	• Provide caring interactions and support. • Engage Betty in conversation and reflection regarding what she does and how she can make some decisions.	Betty stated she has choices over what she reads and what she eats. She has only begun to see that even given her physical symptoms, she does have some choices. The condition of *powerlessness* still exists; continued interventions are needed.

REFLECTIVE QUESTIONS

1. **ASSESSMENT**
   What other factors in Betty's environment should be considered when planning her care? Should the nurse pursue questions about Betty's family?

(*Continues*)

NURSING CARE PLAN: NURSING PROCESS FORMAT 19-1 (Continued)

2. **NURSING DIAGNOSIS**
   Are there other diagnoses that would apply to Betty?
3. **OUTCOMES**
   Do you believe a nurse can enter into a relationship with Betty? What are the obstacles? Do you think Betty is trustworthy?
4. **NURSING ACTIONS**
   What can you really do to empower another person?
   Do you think helping someone make choices in day-to-day life has anything to do with powerlessness?
5. **EVALUATION**
   Does it seem like a good idea to bring social interaction to someone over the Internet?

NURSING CARE PLAN: CONCEPT MAP FORMAT 19-1

Somatization Disorder

BACKGROUND INFORMATION

Linda is a 40-year-old married woman with a long history of medical complaints. She has experienced abdominal pain on and off for as long as she can remember. She had an appendectomy in her late twenties of an apparently normal appendix. She has received medical evaluations for severe headaches, joint pain, and pain during menstruation, that have not resulted in clear physical diagnoses. She has food intolerance that seems to shift between milk products, meat, and nuts. Her complaints regarding these foods range from nausea and vomiting to bloating. She believes she is allergic to many substances, including wool, grasses, perfumes and household cleaning products, as well as being allergic to cats and dogs. Currently she is experiencing numbness and tingling in her right hand, of five days duration. Linda relates that she is unable to use the hand and expresses great difficulty because she cannot drive due to her inability to use her hand.

She has been unable work as an adult because of her long history of physical complaints. She has no children herself, but does have a niece who lives nearby who comes to visit her regularly to assist her with household tasks. Her spouse works at a professional job and is supportive of her need for medical care, often taking her to the doctor and assisting her to make appointments to be seen. Further family history reveals that Linda's mother also suffers from multiple ailments, and her mother had never been diagnosed with a clear physical condition. Linda's mother had been living in an assisted living apartment, but has just been transferred to a home where more extended care can be provided.

Linda is being evaluated neurologically for her complaints of numbness and tingling at a specialty clinic. Her nurse, Wendy, is supporting her through this process. Wendy notes that Linda's medical history includes a diagnosis, made five years earlier, of Somatization Disorder. Wendy learns from Linda that Linda sees herself to be chronically ill and severely impaired. Further, Linda states she lives in fear of being exposed to an allergen that could result in respiratory distress. Lastly, Linda states she has seen many physicians and nurses in her time and has never found one health care professional that understands her problems, thus she constantly looks for someone who can help her.

INITIAL ASSESSMENT AND REFLECTION

Wendy reflects on the presenting symptoms and obvious need for comprehensive evaluation. Further, Wendy notes the issues with a long history of somatization, impairment, and chronicity. Other issues stand

(Continues)

NURSING CARE PLAN: CONCEPT MAP FORMAT 19-1 (Continued)

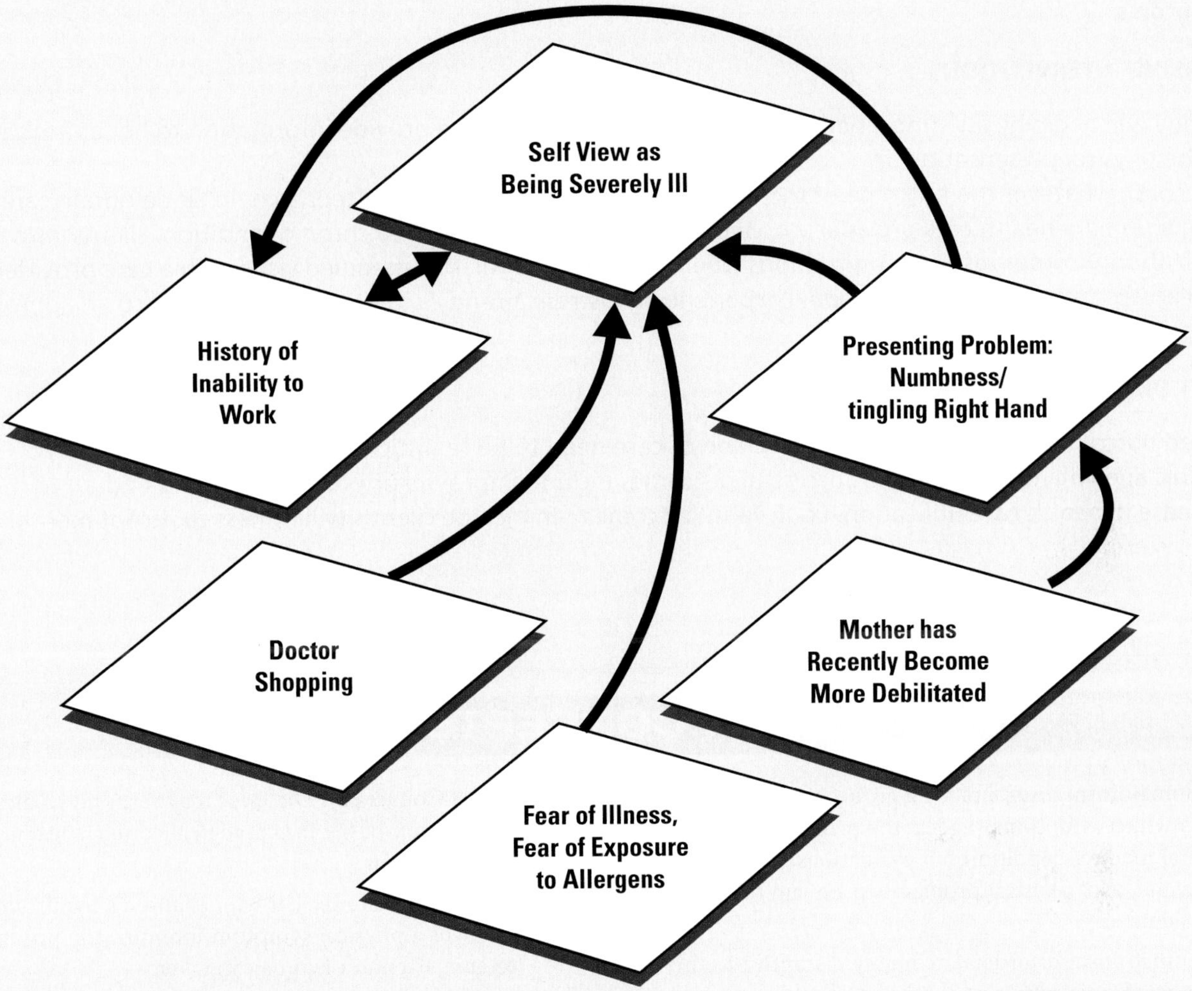

Concept Map of Issues and Problems (DELMAR/CENGAGE LEARNING.)

out in Wendy's assessment: Linda's view of herself as being chronically ill and a current situation of family stress that may be related to Linda's mother needing a different level of care.

INITIAL REVIEW OF NURSING DIAGNOSES

The concept map indicates that Linda's view of self as severely ill may be the central issue regarding her need for care. Wendy considers the following nursing diagnoses:

1. *Powerlessness* related to view of self as severely, chronically ill and being unable to recover.
2. *Disturbed Sensory Perception (tactile: numbness and tingling in right hand)* related to unknown origin.
3. *Risk for injury, (right hand)* related to lack of sensations.

PRIORITIES OF CARE

Wendy recognizes that there are two important issues in Linda's care. First, Linda does not experience sensations in her right hand and is at risk for injury and in need of thorough evaluation. Second, Linda truly sees herself as a severely ill person, needing care, attention, and support. Wendy understands that

(Continues)

NURSING CARE PLAN: CONCEPT MAP FORMAT 19-1 (Continued)

even if the presenting problem turns out to be a result of a psychiatric condition, caring for the physical condition is required in the same manner one would use for any other client with similar presenting symptoms.

NURSING INTERVENTIONS

Wendy will begin by assisting Linda to schedule diagnostic tests and provide information to her as indicated by the physical presentation.

Second, whatever the outcome of the diagnostic tests, Wendy will take steps to help Linda obtain care from a primary health care provider who will manage Linda's illness. As a chronic condition, clients with Somatization Disorder respond to situations where they have regularly scheduled visits with a care provider who accepts the client as an individual experiencing distress. Wendy's role would be referral to an appropriate primary care provider or clinic.

OUTCOMES/EVALUATION

Stated outcomes of treatment and evaluation of care need to be realistic. Somatization Disorder is chronic and will not be "cured." Successful outcomes include improved physical functioning and a decrease in health care utilization. Long-term outcomes can include client's willingness to accept mental health care.

KEY CONCEPTS

- Somatoform disorders are a group of conditions in which symptoms suggest the presence of a general medical condition but evaluations fail to find evidence of physical problems to explain the complaint.
- Somatoform disorders are highly disruptive to the lives of their sufferers, puzzling to health care providers, and difficult to distinguish from major physical illnesses.
- Somatization Disorder exists when there is a history of physical complaints beginning before age 30, with a series of specific symptoms that cannot be explained and are not intentionally produced.
- Somatization Disorder is usually treated in general medical clinics, not mental health clinics; regularly scheduled appointments are recommended.
- Conversion Disorder has two specific features: no medical condition explains the symptoms and the symptoms occur as a result of psychological factors.
- *La belle indifference* is a characteristic of at least some clients with Conversion Disorder, describing the fact that they show surprising indifference toward their symptoms.
- Acute Conversion Disorder may respond to direct explanation of the psychological conflicts leading to the symptoms.
- Factitious Disorder (or Munchausen's Syndrome) involves a physical symptom intentionally produced to gain attention from a caretaker.
- Munchausen's Syndrome by Proxy is a form of child abuse whereby an individual (usually a parent) intentionally produces symptoms of illness in a child under his or her care.
- Nurses must examine their own feelings in relation to being asked to provide care to clients with somatoform and factitious disorders.
- The goal of nurse-client interactions dealing with clients who have somatoform and factitious disorders should be *care* and not *cure*.
- Dissociative disorders include conditions of amnesia, fugue states, and depersonalization that are specific and circumscribed symptoms.
- Dissociative Identity Disorder is a condition where an individual possess two or more distinct personalities.

REVIEW QUESTIONS

1. A client is admitted to the unit for treatment of a Conversion Disorder characterized by numbness of hands and feet, known as stocking and glove anesthesia. Which of the following diagnosis would be most appropriate for this client?
   1. Risk for self-directed harm
   2. Confusion and disorientation
   3. Ineffective individual coping
   4. Dysfunctional skeletal system

2. The nurse is caring for a client who is experiencing hysterical blindness after witnessing a tragic car accident. The nursing assessment would most likely reveal which of the following?
   1. Altered body image
   2. Increased serum electrolytes
   3. Sensory loss of the optical nerves
   4. No significant physical or laboratory findings

3. During a physical examination, the nurse notes that the client is unable to move her left leg. When asked to walk across the room, the client drags the leg. A diagnosis of Conversion Disorder is made. When asked about walking, the client states she has no difficulty. The nurse recognizes that the client's response is an example of which of the following?
   1. Denial
   2. Confabulation
   3. *La belle indifference*
   4. *Folie a deux*

4. A nursing student caring for a client with Somatization Disorder asks her instructor how this disorder differs from a Factitious Disorder. The best response by the instructor would be which of the following?
   1. Both disorders are identical and the terms are used interchangeably.
   2. Clients with Somatization Disorder genuinely believe they have an illness, while a client with a Factitious Disorder involves physical or psychological symptoms that are intentionally produced in order to gain attention from potential caregivers.
   3. Clients with a Factitious Disorder genuinely believe they have an illness, while a Somatization Disorder involves physical or psychological symptoms that are intentionally produced in order to gain attention from potential caregivers.
   4. A Factitious Disorder is a psychological disorder caused by a physical illness, while a Somatic Disorder is a disorder that only presents itself sometimes in the patient.

5. An outcome objective appropriate for a client treated for a Somatization Disorder would be which of the following?
   1. Client will experience less fear and anxiety
   2. Client will attend individual and group therapy sessions
   3. Client will discuss the side effects of medications
   4. Client will verbally and behaviorally demonstrate a decrease in anxiety

6. A young college student visits the campus health center nurse. The student is very upset and reports to the nurse that she was driving to school this morning because she was scheduled to take her final exam but she found herself on the other side of the city. She began crying and stated, "I don't remember driving in that direction. I have missed my exam and my teacher won't believe what happened." The nurse assesses that the client has experienced which of the following?
   1. A dissociative experience
   2. A conversion experience
   3. An hysterical experience
   4. A psychotic episode

LEARNING ACTIVITIES

1. Describe the differences between Somatization Disorder, Conversion Disorder, Hypochondriasis, and Factitious Disorder.

2. Explain the principles of treatment for managing clients with Somatization Disorder in a general medical clinic.

3. Do you believe a nurse practitioner is in the best position to care for somatizing clients?

4. What would you tell the critical care nurses quoted in this chapter regarding care of a client with Factitious Disorder?

5. Which nursing theories do you believe are most beneficial when working with a client with Somatoform Disorder?

StudyWARE™ CONNECTION

Using your StudyWARE™ CD-ROM

1. Complete the Flashcard activity for this chapter.
2. Complete the Quiz for this chapter in Test Mode.
3. Explore the other games and activities that support this chapter.

REFERENCES

Allen, L. S., Escobar, J. I., Lehrer, P. M., Gara, M. A. & Woolfolk, R. L. (2002). Psychosocial treatments for multiple unexplained physical symptoms: A review of the literature. *Psychosomatic Medicine, 64*(6), 939–950.

Allin, M., Streeruwitz, A., & Curtis, V. (2005). Progress in understanding conversion disorder. *Neuropsychiatric Disease Treatment, 1*(3), 205–209.

American Psychiatric Association. (2000). *Diagnostic and statistical manual of mental disorders* (Fourth Edition-Text Revision). Washington, DC: Author.

Aybek, S., Kanaan, R. A., David, A. S. (2008) The neuropsychiatry of conversion disorder. *Current Opinions in Psychiatry, 21*(3), 275–280.

Barsky, A. J., & Klerman, G. L. (1983). Overview: Hypochondriasis, bodily complaints and somatic styles. *American Journal of Psychiatry, 140,* 273–283.

Ben-Tovim, D. I., & Esterman, A. (1998). Zero progress with hypochrondriasis. *Lancet, 352*(0143), 1798–1799.

Bishop, E. R., Jr., Mobley, M. C., & Far, W. F., Jr. (1978). Lateralization of conversion symptoms. *Comprehensive Psychiatry, 19,* 393–396.

Bohman, M., Cloninger, C. R., von Knorring, A. L., & Siquardsson, S. (1984). An adoption study of somatoform disorders, III: Cross-fostering analysis and genetic relationship to alcoholism and criminality. *Archives of General Psychiatry, 41,* 872–878.

Brandt, J., & Van Gorp, W. G. (2006) Functional "psychogenic" amnesia. *Seminars in Neurology, 26*(3), 331–340.

Brown, H. N., & Vaillant, G. E. (1981). Hypochondriasis. *Archives of Internal Medicine, 141,* 723–726.

Chabolla, D. R., Krahn, L. E., So, E. L., & Rummons, T. A. (1996). Psychogenic neuroleptic seizures. *Mayo Clinic Proceedings, 71*(5), 493–500.

Chen, D. K., So, Y. T., & Fisher, R. S. (2005). Use of serum prolactin in diagnosing epileptic seizures: Report of the Therapeutics and Technology Assessment Subcommittee of the American Academy of Neurology. *Neurology, 65*(5), 668–675.

Cloninger, C. R. (1985). Somatoform and dissociate disorders. In G. Winokur & P. J. Clayton (Eds.), *The medical basis of psychiatry* (pp. 123–151). Philadelphia: W. B. Saunders.

Coler, M., & Vincent, K. G. (1995). *Plans of care for specialty practice: Psychiatric mental health nursing.* Clifton Park, NY: Thomson Delmar Learning.

Coons, P. M. (1998). The dissociative disorders. Rarely considered and underdiagnosed. *Psychiatric Clinics of North America, 21*(3), 637–648.

Eastwood S., & Bisson J. I.(2008) Management of factitious disorders: A systematic review. *Psychotherapy and Psychosomatics, 77*(4), 209–218.

Elmore, J. L. (2000). Dissociative spectrum disorders in the primary care setting. *Primary Care Companion to the Journal of Clinical Psychiatry, 2*(2), 37–41.

Erickson, H., Tomlin, E., & Swain, M. (1983). *Modeling and role-modeling: A theory and paradigm for nursing.* Lexington, KY: Pine Press.

Fallon, B. A., Schneier, F. R., Marshall, R., Campeas, R., Vermes, D., Goetz, D., et al. (1996). The pharmacotherapy of hypochondriasis. *Psychopharmacology Bulletin, 132*(4), 607–611.

Fineberg, N. A., Saxena, S., Zoha, J., & Craig, K. J. (2007). Obsessive compulsive disorders: boundary issues. *CNS Spectrum, 12,* 367–375.

Flor-Henry, P., Fromm-Auch, D., Tapper, M., Schopflocher, D. (1981). A neuropsychological study of the stable syndrome of hysteria. *Biological Psychiatry, 16,* 601–626.

Folks, D. G., Ford, C. V., & Regan, W. M. (1984). Conversion symptoms in a general hospital. *Psychosomatics, 25,* 285–295.

Ford, C., Katon, W., & Lipkin, M., Jr. (1993). Managing somatization and hypochondriasis. *Patient Care, 27,* 31–34, 37, 40.

Ghaffar, O., Staines, W. R., & Feinstein, A. (2006) Unexplained neurologic symptoms: An fMRI study of sensory conversion disorder. *Neurology, 67*(11), 2036–2038.

Greeven, A., van Balkom, A. J., Visser, S., Merkelbach, J. W., van Rood, Y. R., van Dyck, R., et al. (2007). Cognitive behavior therapy and paroxetine in the treatment of hypochondriasis: A randomized controlled trial. *American Journal of Psychiatry, 164*(1), 91–99.

Guralnik, O., Giesbrecht, T., Knutelska, M., Sirroff, B., & Simeon, D. (2007) Cognitive functioning in depersonalization disorder. *Journal of Nervous and Mental Disease, 195*(12), 983–988.

Guze, S. B., Cloninger, C. R., Martin, R. L., & Clayton, P. J. (1985). A follow-up and family study of Briquet's syndrome. *British Journal of Psychiatry, 149,* 17–23.

Hatcher, S., & Arroll, B. (2008). Assessment and management of medically unexplained symptoms. *British Medical Journal, 336*(7653), 1124–1128.

Henningsen P., Jakobsen, T., Schiltenwolf, M., & Weiss, M. G. (2005). Somatization revisited: Diagnosis and perceived causes of common mental disorders. *Journal of Nervous and Mental Disorders, 193*(2), 85–92.

Heruti, R., Reznik, J., Adunski A., Levy, A., Weingarden, H., & Ohry, A. (2002). Conversion motor paralysis disorder: Analysis of 34 consecutive referrals. *Spinal Cord, 40*(7), 335–340.

Iezzi, A., & Adams, H. E. (1993). Somatoform and factitious disorders. In P. B. Surker & H. E. Adams (Eds.), *Comprehensive handbook of psychopathology* (2nd ed., p. 170). New York: Plenum.

Jackson, J. L., & Kroenke, K. (2008). Prevalence, impact, and prognosis of multisomatoform disorder in primary care: A 5-year follow-up study. *Psychosomatic Medicine, 70*(4), 430–434.

Janca, A. (2005). Rethinking somatoform disorders. *Current Opinion in Psychiatry, 18*(1) 65–71.

Kellner, R. (1989). Hypochondriasis and body dysmorphic disorders. In *Treatments of psychiatric disorders: A task force report of the American Psychiatric Associagtion* (Vol. 3). Washington, DC: American Psychiatric Association.

Kluft, R. P. (1999). An overview of the psychotherapy of dissociative identity disorder. *American Journal of Psychiatry, 3*(3), 289–319.

Kroenke, J., & Swindle, R. (2000). Cognitive-behavioral therapy for somatization and symptom syndromes: A critical review of controlled clinical trials. *Psychotherapy and Psychosomatics, 69*(14), 205–215.

Kroenke, K. (2007). Efficacy of treatment for somatoform disorders: A review of randomized controlled trials. *Psychosomatic Medicine, 69*(9), 881–888.

Lantz, M. (2008). Somatization disorder: Where the patient has multiple medical problems and ongoing somatic complaints. *Clinical Geriatrics, 16*(2), 21–23.

Leary, P. M. (2003). Conversion disorder in childhood—diagnosed too late, investigated too much? *Journal of the Royal Society of Medicine, 96*(9), 436–438.

Ludwig, A. M. (1972). Hysteria: A neurobiological theory. *Archives of General Psychiatry, 17*, 771–777.

Martin, A., Rauh, E., Fichter, M., & Rief, W. (2007). A one-session treatment for patients suffering from medically unexplained symptoms in primary care: A randomized clinical trial. *Psychosomatics, 48*(4), 294–303.

Martin, R. M., & Yutzy, S. H. (1994). Somatoform disorders. In R. E. Hales, S. C. Yudofsky, & J. A. Talbott (Eds.), *The American Psychiatric Press textbook of psychiatry* (2nd ed.). Washington, DC: American Psychiatric Association.

Maynard, C. K. (2003). Assess and manage somatization. *Nurse Practitioner, 28*(4), 20–29.

McAllister, M. M. (2000). Dissociative identity disorder: A literature review. *Journal of Psychiatric and Mental Health Nursing, 7*(1), 25–33.

McCranie, E. J. (1979). Hypochondriacal neurosis. *Psychosomatics, 20*, 11–15.

McFarland, B., Freeborn, D., Mulloly, J., & Pope, C. (1985). Utilization patterns among long term enrollees in a prepaid group practice health maintenance organization. *Medicare Care, 23*, 762–767.

Medford, N., Brierley, B., Brammer, M., Bullmore, E.T., David, A. S., & Phillips, M. L. (2006). Emotional memory in depersonalization disorder: a functional MRI study. *Psychiatry Research, 148*, 93–102.

Michelson, J. D. (2000). Psychogenic equinovarus: The importance of recognition and non-operative management. *Foot and Ankle International, 21*(1), 31–37.

Miller, M., & Cabeza-Stradi, S. (1994). Addiction to surgery: A nursing dilemma. *Critical Care Nurse, 14*, 44–47.

Moreira-Almeida, A., Neto, F. L., & Cardeña, E. (2008). Comparison of Brazilian spiritist mediumship and dissociative identity disorder. *Journal of Nervous and Mental Diseases, 196*(5), 420–424.

Nemiah, J. C. (1985). Somatoform disorders. In H. I. Kaplan & B. J. Saddock (Eds.), *Comprehensive textbook of psychiatry* (4th ed., pp. 924–942). Baltimore: Williams & Wilkins.

Noyes, R. (1999). The relationship of hypochondriasis to anxiety disorders. *General Hospital Psychiatry, 21*(1), 8–17.

Noyes, R., Jr, Stuart, S. P., & Watson, D. B. (2008). A reconceptualization of the somatoform disorders. *Psychosomatics, 49*(1), 14–22.

Oyama, O., Paltoo, C., & Greengold, J. (2007). Somataform disorders. *American Family Physician, 76*(9), 1333–1339.

Pope, H. G., Jr., Oliva, P. S., Hudson J. I., Bodkin, J. A., & Gruber, A. J. (1999). Attitudes toward DSB-IV dissociative disorders diagnoses among board-certified American psychiatrists. *American Journal of Psychiatry, 256*(2), 312–323.

Quill, T. E. (1985). Somatization disorder. One of medicine's blind spots. *Journal of the American Medical Association, 254*, 3075–3079.

Rief, W., & Isaac, M. (2007). Are somatoform disorders "mental disorders"? A contribution to the current debate. *Current Opinion in Psychiatry, 20*(2), 143–146.

Roberts, S. (1994). Somatization in primary care: The common presentation of psychosocial problems through physical complaints. *Nurse Practitioner, 19*, 47–55.

Robins, L. N., & Regier, D. A. (1991). *Psychiatric disorders in America.* New York: Free Press.

Serra, L., Fadda, L., Buccione, I., Caltagirone, C., & Carlesimo, G. A. (2007). Psychogenic and organic amnesia: A multidimensional assessment of clinical, neuroradiological, neuropsychological and psychopathological features. *Behavioural Neurology, 18*(1), 53–64.

Shumway, M., Boccellar, A., O'Brien, K., & Okin, R. (2008). Cost-effectiveness of clinical case management for Emergency Department frequent users: Results of a randomized trial. *American Journal of Emergency Medicine, 26*(2), 155–164.

Smith, G. R., Monson, R. A., & Ray, D. C. (1986). Psychiatric consultation in somatization disorder. *New England Journal of Medicine, 314*, 1407–1413.

Smith R. C., Gardiner, A. C., Armatti, S., Johnson, M., Lyles, J. S., Given, C. W., et al. (2001). Screening for high utilizing somatizing patients using a prediction rule derived from the management information system of an HMO: A preliminary study. *Medical Care, 39*(9), 968–978.

Stone, J., Hewett, R., Carson, A., Warlow, C., & Sharpe, M. (2008). The "disappearance" of hysteria: Historical mystery or illusion? *Journal of the Royal Society of Medicine, 101*(1), 12–18.

Stone, J., Zeman, A., Simonotto, E., Meyer, M., Azuma, R., Flett, S., & Sharpe, M. (2007). FMRI in patients with motor conversion symptoms and controls with simulated weakness. *Psychosomatic Medicine, 69*(9), 961–969.

Sumathipala, A. (2007). What is the evidence for the efficacy of treatments for somatoform disorders? A critical review of previous intervention studies. *Psychosomatic Medicine, 69*(9), 889–900.

Talento, B. (1995). Jean Watson. In J. George (Ed.), *Nursing theories, the base for professional practice* (4th ed., pp. 317–333). Norwalk, CT: Appleton & Lange.

Thomson, A. B., & Page, L. A. (2007). Psychotherapies for hypochondriasis. *Cochrane Database of Systematic Reviews*(4).

Veith, I. (1965). *Hysteria: The history of a disease.* Chicago: University of Chicago Press.

Walker, J., Vincent, N., Furer, P., Cox, B., & Kjornisted, K. (1999). Treatment preferences in hypochondriasis. *Journal of Behavioral Therapy and Experimental Psychiatry, 30*(4), 251–258.

Wijeratne, C., Brodaty, H., & Hickie, I. (2003). The neglect of somatoform disorders by old age psychiatry: Some explanations and suggestions for future research. *International Journal of Geriatric Psychiatry, 18*(9), 812–819.

Yutzy, S. H. (2003). Somataform disorders. In R. E. Hales and S. C. Yudofsky (Eds.). *Textbook of clinical psychiatry* (4th ed., pp. 659–690). Washington, DC: American Psychiatric Publishing.

LITERARY REFERENCES

Asher, R. (1951). Munchausen syndrome. *Lancet, 1,* 339–341.

Bowlby, J. (1991). *Charles Darwin: A new life.* New York: W. W. Norton.

Colp, R. (1977). *To be an invalid.* Chicago: University of Chicago Press.

Laurents, A. (1946). *Home of the brave.* New York: Random House.

Munthe, A. (1975). *The story of San Michele.* London: John Murray.

Yeazell, R. B. (Ed.). (1981). *The death and letters of Alice James.* Berkeley: University of California Press.

SUGGESTED READINGS

Feldman, M. D., & Feldman, J. M. (1998). *Stranger than fiction: When our minds betray us.* Washington, D.C.: APA Press.

Oxnam, R. B. (2005). *A fractured mind: My life with multiple personality disorder.* New York: Hyperion.

Starcevic, V., et al. (2001). *Hypochondriasis: New perspectives on an ancient malady.* Oxford: Oxford University Press.

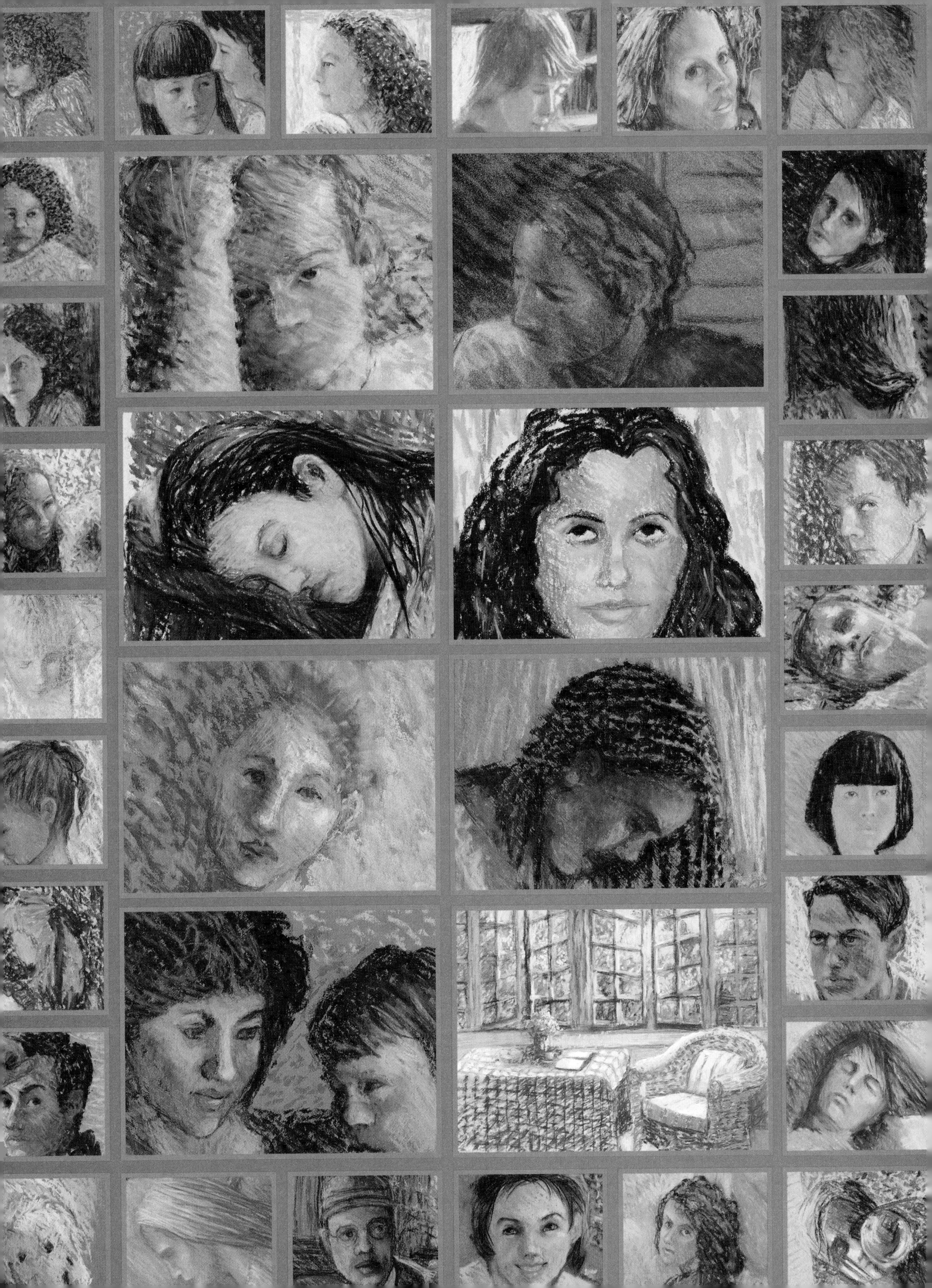

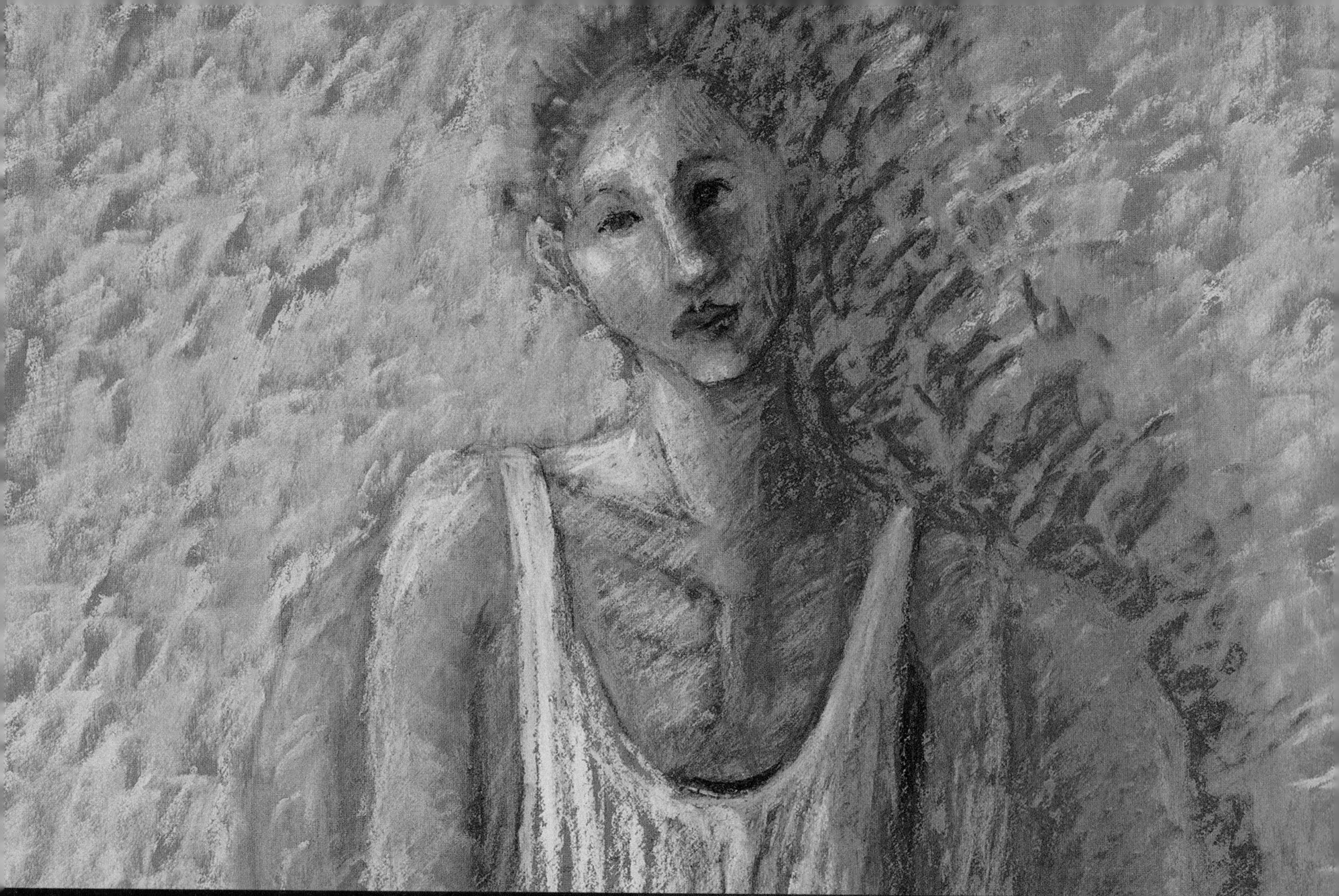

Just Five More Pounds

Finding Balance

Many people these days talk about finding balance in the hectic world of modern life. The idea of balance assumes that people are able to regulate their activities in a way that produces or promotes health. Consider your own life in terms of a balance between needs for sleep, exercise, and rest.

- *Do you meet your physiological needs in these areas? If not, what is stopping you from finding your own balance in this regard?*

Consider your own need for food and nutrition. Nutrients are essential for physical health; social aspects of food and eating contribute to mental health.

- *Do you meet your physical and social needs in relation to your food and eating habits?*
- *Are there aspects of your food habits that you would like to change? If yes, what do you need to do to make the change?*

Lastly, consider your own sexual identity and needs for intimacy.

- *Have you found a balance in your relationships that results in personal health?*

As you reflect on your own life and lifestyle, examine how much or how little you believe you can control your own behaviors in areas of sleep, eating, and sexuality. In this chapter, we examine common disorders, many quite debilitating, that can be grouped as disorders of regulation. Being honest about your own ability and success in these areas will assist you to learn about these disorders and provide empathy to clients.

CHAPTER 20

The Client with Disorders of Self-Regulation: Sleep Disorders, Eating Disorders, and Sexual Disorders

NOREEN CAVAN FRISCH
LAWRENCE E. FRISCH

CHAPTER OUTLINE

COMPETENCIES

Upon completion of this chapter, the reader should be able to:

1. Describe normal sleep cycles and changes in sleep cycles expected in aging.
2. Assess clients for the presence of Insomnia
3. Provide a sleep hygiene regimen for clients with disturbed sleep.
4. Define *Primary Hypersomnia*.
5. Identify parasomnias and provide appropriate nursing interventions and support.
6. Assess clients for the presence of Bulimia Nervosa and Anorexia Nervosa.
7. Plan nursing care for clients with eating disorders, including nutritional rehabilitation, psychotherapy, maintenance, and follow-up care.
8. Assess clients for *ineffective sexuality pattern*, *sexual dysfunction*, and sexual disorders.
9. Utilize nursing theory and the nursing process in planning and providing care for clients with disorders of regulation.

KEY TERMS

Anorexia Nervosa
Breathing-Related Sleep Disorders
Bulimia Nervosa
Cataplexy
Dyssomnias
Exhibitionism
Fetishism
Frotteurism
Gender Dysphoria
Gender Identity
Gender Identity Disorder
Gender Role
Hypoactive Sexual Desire Disorder
Insomnia
Narcolepsy
Nightmares
Normal Sexual Behavior
Paraphilias
Parasomnias
Pedophilia
Primary Hypersomnia
Primary Insomnia
Restless Legs Syndrome
Sexual Dysfunction
Sexual Masochism
Sexual Sadism
Sleep Hygiene
Sleep Latency
Sleep Paralysis
Sleep Terrors
Sleepwalking
Transvestic Fetishism
Voyeurism

Sleeping, eating, and sexual function are basic human drives that are closely related to good physical and mental health. Both psychological disorders and physical illnesses often manifest as disturbances in any or all of these functions. But, even in the absence of more general psychiatric or physiological diagnoses, independent disorders of sleeping, eating, and sexual function can occur. These disorders may present in psychiatric nursing practice or in the course of giving care to clients in other settings. The purpose of this chapter is to provide an introduction to some of the most common disorders of regulation.

SLEEP DISORDERS

SO INESTIMABLE A JEWEL

*Do but consider what an excellent thing sleep is: it is so inestimable a jewel that, if a tyrant would give his crown for an hour's slumber, it cannot be bought; of so beautiful a shape is it, that though a man lie with an Empress, his heart cannot beat quiet till he leaves her embracements to be at rest with the other: yea, so greatly indebted are we to this kinsman of death, that we owe ... half our life to him: and there is good cause why we should do so: for sleep is the golden chain that ties health and our bodies together. Who complains of want? of wounds? of cares? of great men's oppressions? of captivity? whilst he sleepeth? Beggars in their beds take as much pleasure as kings: can we therefore surfeit of this delicate ambrosia?**

(Dekker, 1982, p. 138)

Although sleep is not always the exquisite release from daily cares that Thomas Dekker describes writing four

*From "On Sleep," by T. Dekker. In *Night Walks: A Bedside Companion* (p. 138), by J. C. Oates (Ed.), 1982, Princeton, NJ: Ontario Review Press. Reprinted with permission.

centuries ago, he is certainly correct in describing high-quality sleep as "an excellent thing." As common as sleep is in everyone's life, it is remarkable how much is still unknown about its nature and functions. The physiological function of sleep remains a mystery, and there is remarkably little evidence that even prolonged sleep deprivation is physically harmful, at least in young and healthy individuals. Nonetheless, most people feel highly unwell when they are deprived of sleep.

In recent years, many hospitals and medical centers have developed sleep study programs to evaluate persons who complain of sleep-related disorders. Sleep has become a scientific and medical study of its own, and many nurses now work exclusively with individuals whose only problem is disturbed sleep. The discussion in this section on sleep disorders is divided into two parts: the first addressing **dyssomnias**, those conditions in which there is an abnormality in the amount, quality, or timing of sleep, and the second addressing **parasomnias**, those conditions in which the client exhibits abnormal behavioral or physiological events in association with sleep. First, however, normal sleep cycles are reviewed.

Normal Sleep Cycles

There are five sleep stages identified by changes in brain wave patterns that are measured by electroencephalographic (EEG) recordings. Stages 1 through 4 are characterized by increasingly slow brain wave patterns and coincide with deepened sleep. Stage 5 is rapid-eye-movement (REM) sleep and is characterized by vivid dreams and a comparably faster brain wave pattern that resembles awake states. Persons typically pass through each of the five stages in cycles of one to two hours. There is marked individual variation in the time spent in each sleep cycle; however, most persons will experience all of the sleep stages in the course of a night's sleep. Older adults experience sleep pattern changes with aging and will awaken several times during the night. Sleep is needed for body restoration and repair, and the subjective sense of being well rested is central to a person's perception of well-being. Temporary disruption of sleep patterns requires nursing support and attention; true sleep disorders require both accurate nursing assessment and care as well as referral for specialist evaluation and treatment.

REFLECTIVE THINKING 20-1

Sleepiness

Have you ever experienced a situation in which:

- You were driving home from a trip late at night feeling tired and unable to stay awake? You opened the car window to let cold air in, turned the radio up, yawned, and continued to drive?
- You could not stay awake in a class lecture, and even though you tried to listen to the topic or discussion, you found your head nodding and your eyes closing?
- You went to bed early the night before an important event knowing that a good night's sleep would help you during the event, only to find that you could not get to sleep until the early hours of the morning?

If you have experienced any of these situations (and almost all of us have), you have an understanding of the feelings of sleep deprivation, sleepiness at times when you need to be awake, and arousal at times when you need to be asleep. Consider these isolated incidents from your own life as compounded or exaggerated when you think of the day-to-day lives of persons with sleep disorders.

Dyssomnias

The conditions discussed in the following represent the most common abnormalities of amount, quality, and timing of sleep; they are insomnias and daytime sleepiness.

Insomnia is a sleep disorder characterized by difficulty in initiating or maintaining sleep. Insomnia is considered a psychological problem if it lasts sufficiently long (one month or more) and leads to impairment in functioning. The term **Primary Insomnia** is given to the condition in which there are no known external causes of the inability to sleep; for example, there are psychological disorders (Post-Traumatic Stress Disorder), physical disorders (those resulting in pain or discomfort), or medications or substances (caffeine) that affect sleep. Primary Insomnia refers only to those situations in which there is no other condition responsible for the sleep difficulties. The following passage describes the experience of insomnia, an experience probably familiar to most readers of this book at least on some nights.

INSOMNIA

It's three or four in the morning.
There's a bird squawking and beating
its wings in the chimney, louder
than the jealous noise of dreams:
a boy turning into a dog.
The changing profile of a man on the wall.
These have nothing to do
with my life here in bed, next to
this other dreamer: he lifts his head,
looks me in the eye, rows away.
He hears the bird but prefers to think
it's hallucination. I kick the sheets away,
spend the night eliminating
possibilities. I don't want to walk
around with this bird's bad dream.
Anyway, it's another day.

There's dew on the stack of logs.
There's the sound of wings
trying to fly. A strong smell of ash
lifts through the house.
*A lime-colored sun wheels through the sky.**

(Mishkin, 1982, pp. 251–252)

In her poem entitled "Insomnia," Julia Mishkin describes a sleepless night during which the softest of noises—the sound of a bird fluttering in the fireplace chimney—is enough to keep her awake and actively engaged in the process of "eliminating possibilities." Her sleeping partner apparently wakes up enough to listen, concludes the sounds are imaginary, and "rows away" back to sleep, leaving the poet alone in bed with her night thoughts. She might choose to get up, get a flashlight, and check the chimney, but she does not "want to walk around," she tells us, "with this bird's bad dream." In contrast, the famous nineteenth-century novelist Charles Dickens spent his sleepless nights far from his own chimney, walking around dark and dangerous London until he, too, found himself seemingly in the middle of someone else's nightmare:

NIGHT WALKS

Some years ago, a temporary inability to sleep, referable to a distressing impression, caused me to walk about the streets all night, for a series of several nights. The disorder might have taken a long time to conquer, if it had been faintly experimented on in bed; but, it was soon defeated by the brisk treatment of getting up directly after lying down, and going out, and coming home tired at sunrise.

... My principal object being to get through the night, the pursuit of it brought me into sympathetic relations with people who have no other object every night of the year.

The month was March, and the weather damp, cloudy, and cold. The sun not rising before half-past five, the night perspective looked sufficiently long at half-past twelve: which was about my time for confronting it.

The restlessness of a great city, and the way in which it tumbles and tosses before it can get to sleep, formed one of the first entertainments offered to the contemplation of us houseless people. It lasted about two hours....

When a church clock strikes, on houseless ears in the dead of night, it may at first be mistaken for company and hailed as such....

*Once—it was after leaving the Abbey and turning my face north—I came to the great steps of St. Martin's church as the clock was striking Three. Suddenly, a thing that in a moment more I should have trodden upon without seeing, rose up at my feet with a cry of loneliness and houselessness, struck out of it by the bell, the like of which I never heard. We then stood face to face looking at one another, frightened by one another. The creature was like a beetle-browed hair-lipped youth of twenty.**

(Dickens, 1982, pp. 3–12)

Both Mishkin and Dickens describe common experiences of sleeplessness: a desire to sleep, preoccupation with thoughts on retiring, an interest in getting up and walking about (repressed by the poet and indulged in by the novelist), and a sense of the waking night world as threatening and ultimately nightmarelike.

On occasion, almost everyone experiences difficulties getting to sleep or staying asleep. Even a few days of insomnia, as Dickens describes, while acutely unpleasant, are far from abnormal. Insomnia is considered a psychological problem if it lasts sufficiently long to impair functioning. Although impairment may result from complaints of daytime sleepiness, individuals with insomnia rarely have objectively detectable daytime sleepiness (American Psychiatric Association, 2000). In many individuals, insomnia does lead to anxiety, arousal, and preoccupation with the process of falling to sleep. As Dickens observed about his brief bout with insomnia, "The disorder might have taken a long time to conquer, if it had been faintly experimented on in bed." An astute psychologist, Dickens recognized that worrying about sleeplessness while in bed can prolong an episode of insomnia. Some individuals fall asleep easily and remain asleep through the night but do not feel in the morning as if they have had a restful or restorative night of sleep.

Primary Insomnia is usually diagnosed on the basis of an individual's subjective complaint, but quality and quantity of sleep are difficult to judge objectively outside the sleep laboratory. Many people overestimate the amount of sleep they need and underestimate the amount they actually get during a restless night. Requirements for sleep vary widely. Most adults need the traditional seven to nine hours of sleep a night, but some adults are "short sleepers" and function well on only three or four hours. Persons who function well despite little sleep are not diagnosed with Primary Insomnia.

Primary Insomnia is diagnosed only when no other psychological, medical, or substance-related condition is responsible for sleep difficulties. Substance use is often a cause of sleep disturbance. Alcohol and caffeine are both commonly associated with sleep disorders, and use of stimulant drugs such as diet pills, amphetamines, and cocaine may be falsely denied. While prescription sleep medications (most commonly benzodiazepines) may have a role in short-term treatment of insomnia, their side effects may include insomnia, especially when long-term use leads to habituation and withdrawal symptoms. Mood disorders, both depression and

*From "Insomnia," by J. Mishkin. In *Night Walks: A Bedside Companion* (pp. 251–252), by J. C. Oates (Ed.), 1982, Princeton, NJ: Ontario Review Press. Reprinted with permission.

*From "Night Walks," by C. Dickens. In *Night Walks: A Bedside Companion* (pp. 3–12), by J. C. Oates (Ed.), 1982, Princeton, NJ: Ontario Review Press. Reprinted with permission.

mania, may affect the need for and quality of sleep, and these must be carefully excluded in evaluating and treating sleep complaints.

Primary Insomnia in the Elderly: Special Considerations

The National Institutes of Health (NIH) convened an expert panel on sleep disturbance in older people (1990). This panel reached a number of conclusions. First, sleep problems are common but probably not inevitable among older individuals. As the panelists observed (NIH, 1990, p.2):

> *A large proportion of older people are at risk for disturbances of sleep that may be caused by many factors such as retirement and changes in social patterns, death of spouse and close friends, increased use of medications, concurrent diseases and changes in circadian rhythms. While changes in sleep patterns have been viewed as part of the normal aging process, new information indicates that many of these disturbances may be related to pathological processes that are associated with aging.*

Estimates are that disturbances of sleep, including but not limited to Primary Insomnia, afflict more than half of the people aged 65 years and older who live at home and about two-thirds of those who live in long-term care facilities. In addition to affecting the quality of life, troubled sleep has been associated with excess mortality among the elderly, though a causal relationship has not been proven. A single case report documents the resolution of suicidal ideation in an elderly man whose sleep disorder was successfully treated (Krahn, Miller, & Bergstrom, 2008). Multiple drug treatment of the elderly is extremely common, and sedative-hypnotics are among the most frequently prescribed medications for these individuals. There is currently little evidence that medications are useful in improving the sleep of the older individual, and they may be particularly harmful by increasing the risk of falls and by interacting with other prescription and nonprescription medications. Over-the-counter sleep preparations such as diphenhydramine may be troublesome in the elderly person since they have anticholinergic effects that may influence vision and excretory function. The effectiveness of such over-the-counter substances for inducing sleep in older persons remains unproven, and risks have been well documented—especially for hospitalized clients (Fosnight, Holder, Allen, & Hazelett, 2004).

Treatment for Insomnia

Insomnia is often treated with techniques of **sleep hygiene**—specific activities that assist many persons to achieve restful sleep. While there is no standard sleep hygiene regimen, the recommendations presented in Box 20-1 are often employed and are felt to be clinically useful. With the use of sleep hygiene techniques, most people should be able to overcome Primary Insomnia after a short period. These techniques have been used and evaluated positively by nurses working with elderly hospitalized patients (Lareau, Benson, Watcharotone, & Manguba, 2008) and in nursing home clients (Alessi, Martin, Webber, Cynthia Kim, Harker, & Josephson, 2005). In addition, nurse researchers report that the use of music at bedtime can positively impact sleep quality (Harmat, Takacs, & Bodzs, 2008). The use of nonprescription medications, including the unregulated drug melatonin, is of unproven benefit.

Prescription medications have been widely used for insomnia, but data supporting their long-term efficacy is sparse. Systematic review of the use of a variety of benzodiazepines (among the most commonly used drugs for insomnia) show a beneficial effect on the time required to fall asleep and total sleep time (Holbrook, Crowther, Lotter, Cheng, & King, 2000). In contrast, persons receiving benzodiazepines reported more daytime sleepiness and dizziness than those given placebo. Zolpidem and zaleplon may have somewhat fewer side effects, but despite frequent prescription by physicians, there is still little evidence supporting their long-term use in insomnia. The FDA has approved only eszopiclone (Lunesta) for long term use. This medication appears to have quite good efficacy for treating insomnia when evaluated over a six-month period (Krystal, Walsh, Lasha, Caron, Amato, Wessel, et al., 2003). While it is likely that most persons with insomnia are treated with medication, multiple studies show a small but significant benefit from cognitive behavioral therapy (Montgomery & Dennis, 2003). Cognitive behavioral therapy is likely to have fewer side effects and may have lower long-term costs. A "primary care" cognitive therapy has been described that appears to have good short-term efficacy for managing uncomplicated adult Primary Insomnia in outpatient practice (Edinger & Sampson, 2003). In recent years it has become apparent that long-term use of medications (including eszopiclone) may be associated with depression in some individuals (Kripke, 2007). In March 2007, the FDA issued a warning for all sleep medications that cited potential risks of allergies and of complex sleep-related behaviors including driving an automobile while asleep. While it might appear that for many persons the benefits of cognitive behavioral therapy could outweigh potential risks, because of the high prevalence of sleep disorders and the immediate effectiveness of drug treatment, prescription hypnotic drugs continue to be used extensively worldwide.

NURSING TIP 20-1

Melatonin

While not proven to be useful in treating insomnia, melatonin has been shown useful when jet travel, shift work (common in hospital employment), or other temporary factors disrupt the normal day-night sleepiness cycle.

BOX 20-1
TECHNIQUES OF SLEEP HYGIENE

- Restrict bed and bedroom to sleep and sexual activities. Do not read, watch television, or do other activities in bed. If sleepless, do not lie in bed for hours staring at the walls or clock. If you do not fall asleep after 15 or 20 minutes, it is best to get up and do something quiet until you become drowsy.
- Try to get up at the same time each day, regardless of when you went to bed. This will help establish a sleep-wake rhythm.
- Exercise each day, preferably in late afternoon or early evening.
- Make sure the bedroom is quiet, dark, and comfortable in temperature (around 65°F).
- A light snack may help, possibly with warm milk; a heavy meal will not. If gastroesophageal reflux (an occasional physical cause of insomnia) has been diagnosed, never eat within three hours of sleeping.
- Avoid daytime napping.
- Caffeine in the evening disturbs sleep, even if you do not think so! Alcohol causes fragmented sleep, especially if consumed immediately before sleep, but also earlier in the day.
- If your alarm clock's ticking keeps you awake at night, get a quieter one. Position the clock so that you cannot see it.
- It is sometimes possible to break the cycle of insomnia by deliberately staying awake for an entire night.

Daytime Sleepiness

Three conditions in which a person experiences excessive sleepiness during the day, often unrelated to the amount and quality of sleep at night are discussed following. These are Primary Hypersomnia, Narcolepsy, and Breathing-Related Sleep Disorder. To begin the discussion, consider the following:

HE'S GONE TO SLEEP AGAIN

"Damn that boy, he's gone to sleep again."

So the stout gentleman put on his spectacles, and Mr. Pickwick pulled out his glass, and everybody stood up in the carriage, and looked over somebody else's shoulder at the evolutions of the military.

"Joe, Joe!" said the stout gentleman, when the citadel was taken, and the besiegers and besieged sat down to dinner. "Damn that boy, he's gone to sleep again. Be good enough to pinch him, Sir—in the leg, if you please; nothing else wakes him—thank you. Undo the hamper, Joe."

The fat boy, who had been effectually roused by the compression of a portion of his leg, between the finger and thumb of Mr. Winkle, rolled off the box again, and proceeded to unpack the hamper, with more expedition than could have been expected from his previous inactivity....

"Now, Joe, knives and forks." The knives and forks were handed in, and the ladies and gentlemen inside, and Mr. Winkle on the box, were each furnished with those useful implements.

"Now, Joe, the fowls. Damn that boy; he's gone to sleep again. Joe!, Joe! ...

"Very extraordinary boy, that," said Mr. Pickwick, "does he always sleep in this way?"

"Sleep!" said the old gentleman, "he's always asleep. Goes on errands fast asleep, and snores as he waits at table." ...

*As the Pickwickians turned round to take a last glimpse of it, the setting sun. ... fell upon the form of the fat boy. His head was sunk upon his bosom; and he slumbered again.**

(Dickens, 1969, pp. 64–69)

Remaining awake when fatigued is among the hardest of human activities:

Captain Harold Doud, attached to the Japanese Army from 1934 to 1935, tells of his conversation with a Captain Teshima. During peacetime maneuvers the troops "twice went three days and two nights without sleep except what could be snatched during ten-minute halts and brief lulls in the situation. Sometimes the men slept while walking. Our junior lieutenant caused much amusement by marching squarely into a lumber pile on the side of the road while sound asleep." When camp was finally struck, still no one got a chance to sleep; they were all assigned to outpost and patrol duty. "'But why not let some of them sleep?" I asked. "Oh no!" he said. "That is not necessary. They already know how to sleep. They need training in how to stay awake.'"†

(Benedict, 1974, p. 181)

Joe, the "fat boy" in Charles Dickens's *The Pickwick Papers*, has profound daytime sleepiness, marked obesity, and loud snoring. He falls asleep in a moment and sleeps through every possible daytime disturbance, including military drills

*From *The Posthumous Papers of the Pickwick Club*, by Charles Dickens, 1969, New York: Oxford University Press.

†From *The Chrysanthemum and the Sword*, by Ruth Benedict. Copyright © 1946 by Ruth Benedict, received 1974 by Donald G. Freeman. Reprinted with permission from Houghton Mifflin Company. All rights reserved.

RESEARCH Highlight 20-1

Sleep Quality, Depression, Anxiety, and Fatigue among Nurses

STUDY PROBLEM/PURPOSE

The researchers sought to examine the shift-related differences in chronic fatigue and the contributions of sleep quality, anxiety, and depression in a sample of critical care nurses.

METHODS

Using a descriptive research design, the researchers obtained a random sample of 262 female critical care nurses who worked full-time, and administered standardized measures of fatigue, depression, sleep quality, and anxiety. Researchers also obtained demographic and work-related data from the population. Data were evaluated to determine the relationships between fatigue and the other variables, as well as make comparisons between day shift and night shift workers.

FINDINGS

A majority of nurses in the sample worked the night shift. Sixty-eight percent of the nurses met the criteria for poor sleepers; 23% met the criteria for mild, moderate, or severe depression; and 32% met the criteria for mild or moderate anxiety. Nurses who worked permanent night shifts had significantly poorer sleep quality and more depression than did day-shift workers. Chronic fatigue was found to be directly related to poor sleep, anxiety, and depression. Day-shift and night-shift workers had similar levels of chronic fatigue.

IMPLICATIONS

Sleep disturbances and depression may be common in critical care nurses and could be an occupational hazard for nurses in other settings as well. The associated feelings of chronic fatigue could certainly impede the nurses' ability to function optimally and to care for clients. Nurses should adopt a self-care regimen to nurture quality sleep and to assess self for fatigue, depression, and anxiety.

Source: "Correlates of Fatigue in Critical Care Nurses," by Jeanne S. Ruggiero, 2003, *Research in Nursing and Health*, *26*, pp. 434–444.

and the firing of cannons. Joe has been thought to have a Breathing-Related Sleep Disorder, "Pickwickian syndrome," a condition of alveolar hypoventilation secondary to massive obesity. Individuals with Pickwickian syndrome breathe very shallowly and are sleepy because of carbon dioxide (CO_2) narcosis: They breathe so little they are unable to blow off CO_2, which in the resulting high concentrations acts very much like a general anesthetic and produces sleepiness. This life-threatening medical syndrome was named after Dickens's vivid description in *The Pickwick Papers*. Whether or not he is truly Pickwickian, Joe snores loudly and may have obstructive sleep apnea, another cause of daytime sleepiness. Obstructive sleep apnea is a Breathing-Related Sleep Disorder caused by upper airway obstruction during sleep and is discussed in more detail following. In the novel, Joe receives from Charles Dickens a colorful nineteenth-century description of his sleep disorder; from a modern perspective, he also needs a careful medical evaluation and probably a sleep laboratory study to determine the cause of his recurrent sleep attacks.

Even after such a comprehensive evaluation, some individuals have no obvious explanation for daytime sleepiness. Their nighttime sleep is normal, so they are not suffering from insomnia. They do not have obstructive sleep apnea, are not Pickwickian, and have no psychological disorder such as depression that can account for their symptoms. They do not have a substance-related disorder such as occurs in users of depressant drugs or those on withdrawal from stimulants. They do not suffer from another sleep disorder, yet the condition exists and results in impairment of daily activities; these individuals have **Primary Hypersomnia**—daytime sleepiness for which there is no external or physiological explanation.

In Primary Hypersomnia, formal sleep studies are essentially normal except that **sleep latency** (the time it takes to fall asleep) is decreased, consistent with increased daytime sleepiness. No REM sleep occurs during daytime sleep episodes. Primary Hypersomnia is relatively rare, but does occur in about 10% of persons referred to sleep centers for evaluation (American Psychiatric Association, 2000). One of the most critical issues in management is to ensure that persons with excessive daytime sleepiness not engage in activities, particularly driving, since a sleep attack could put them or others at risk. Many states have laws requiring health care professionals to report individuals with potential for loss of consciousness during driving.

Treatment for daytime sleepiness is not well established; however, stimulant drugs may be useful. Careful medical and sleep evaluation can assist in excluding potentially treatable physiological conditions such as obstructive sleep apnea.

Narcolepsy is another primary sleep disorder in which individuals frequently have three different and quite striking sleep-related symptoms. First, like Joe, they have the frequent recurrence of irresistible need for brief episodes of sleep. They awaken from these feeling remarkably refreshed and rarely report daytime sleepiness except immediately prior to one of these episodes. Second, narcoleptic persons often have vivid dreamlike states as they are falling asleep or waking up. These states typically include hallucinatory experiences in which elements of the real world around them are mixed with dream images. **Sleep paralysis**—the sensation of being unable to move, speak, or breathe—may accompany these states and may provoke great fear. Third, individuals with Narcolepsy may have episodes of **cataplexy**, which is defined as the sudden loss of muscle power at times of sudden emotion, often laughter or fear. These persons may drop things or even fall to the ground, but unlike a simple faint, they never lose consciousness during a cataleptic episode.

RESEARCH Highlight 20–2

Fatigue and Sleep Quality in Nurses

STUDY PROBLEM/PURPOSE

Nurse researchers sought to evaluate the differences of nurses' perceptions of fatigue comparing day-shift and night-shift workers.

METHODS

A study sample of 90 night-shift nurses and 100 day-shift nurses were recruited for the study. These nurses responded to two questionnaires assessing perception of fatigue and sleep quality. Statistical comparisons were done to compare the two groups.

FINDINGS

Compared to day-shift nurses, night-shift nurses experience more fatigue and poorer sleep quality. In addition, night-shift nurses had poorer sleep duration and were more likely to use sleep medications. Also, night-shift nurses reported greater daytime dysfunction than their day-shift counterparts. There were two predictors of fatigue in night-shift nurses: use of sleeping medication and reports of daytime dysfunction.

Interestingly, nurses with more than 20 years of experience perceived greater fatigue and poorer sleep quality than nurses with less than 20 years of experience. Also, for nurses with less than nine years of experience, there were no differences in perception of fatigue or sleep quality.

CONCLUSIONS/IMPLICATIONS

The researchers concluded that studies are needed to determine appropriate interventions for nurses working shifts. While sleep disturbances may be an unavoidable occupational hazard for nurses, it is very important to address this issue in terms of both client safety and nurse self-care.

Source: "Fatigue and Sleep Quality in Nurses," by K. Kunert, M. L. King, and F. W. Kolkhorst, 2007, *Journal of Psychosocial Nursing & Mental Health Services*, *45*(8), 30–37.

Narcolepsy is rare, occurring in only about one per thousand individuals. Since there is strong evidence for a hereditary predisposition, Narcolepsy is relatively common among close relatives of affected individuals. The disorder is diagnosed on the basis of a history that includes sleep attacks, usually with cataplexy or hallucinations with or without sleep paralysis. Formal sleep studies confirm the diagnosis by measuring how long it takes the individual to fall asleep. The consequences of Narcolepsy can be severe. Individuals with this disorder should generally not drive or operate dangerous machinery, as they are at risk for falling asleep and injuring themselves or others. There is a significant association with other psychological disorders, including Major Depressive Disorder. Treatment has traditionally involved daytime use of stimulant drugs, typically amphetamines. However, to minimize unacceptable side effects, the development of tolerance, and potential dependency or drug diversion, current management generally substitutes either the non-amphetamine "wakefulness promoting agent" modafinil (a non-controlled substance) or gamma hydroxybutyrate (a controlled "Schedule 3" drug with significant abuse potential) when treating daytime sleepiness (Bhat & El Sohl, 2008). Gamma hydroxybutyrate or the addition of antidepressants may be needed to treat cataplexy. Pressure may increase to place controls on modafinil as it is increasingly being used as a "lifestyle drug" to alleviate daytime sleepiness having nonclinical origins (in many cases due to staying awake late and/or arising early; Lawton, 2006).

Breathing-Related Sleep Disorders primarily comprise the diagnosis of obstructive sleep apnea. In this condition the tissues of the upper airway relax so profoundly during deep sleep that they collapse and obstruct the flow of air into the lungs. When obstruction is only partial, snoring results, but when complete, the client often arouses from sleep. Such arousals may occur many times during the night and may significantly interfere with rest. Persons with obstructive sleep apnea are at increased risk for hypertension, some forms of heart disease, and daytime sleepiness (which may lead to injuries at work or on the highway). While not itself a psychiatric disorder, obstructive sleep apnea is potentially important to psychiatric nurses because of emerging evidence that it may increase the risk of depression in affected individuals (Kawahara, Akashiba, Akahoshi, & Horie, 2005; Krahn, Miller, & Bergstrom, 2008). Treatment for sleep apnea is indicated when formal sleep studies (usually performed during overnight sleep laboratory observations) document severe and frequent apneic episodes. Treatment usually consists of nightly use of positive airway pressure applied through a mask or nasal cannula. Surgery is occasionally recommended for very severe symptoms unresponsive to simpler treatments.

PARASOMNIAS

Individuals with parasomnias suffer from profoundly disturbed sleep, most commonly nightmares, sleep terrors, or sleepwalking. The increasingly recognized "restless legs syndrome" is sometimes classified among the parasomnias. Of these four conditions, nightmares would seem to be the most common, occasionally affecting up to half of all persons.

Nightmares are exceedingly vivid dreams from which the individual wakens in fear, often with signs of autonomic nervous system hyperactivity: sweating and tachycardia. The content of nightmares is often inherently frightening: a physical attack or pursuit by another person, animal, or frightening "monster." One of the important characteristics of nightmares is that, on awakening, the individual has good recall of the nightmare content. This recall is often accompanied by persistent anxiety that may inhibit return to sleep.

Persons with recurrent nightmares that interfere with sleep and social functioning may have Nightmare Disorder, a DSM-IV-TR diagnosis.

Sleep terrors are a related parasomnia in which there is *no recall* of the sleep-related event. Individuals experiencing sleep terrors rouse suddenly from sleep with a cry or scream. They typically sit up in bed in apparent terror: sweaty, pupils dilated, tachypneic, and tachycardic. Usually, the affected individual cannot be awakened during a terror but gradually calms and returns to sleep. If awakened at the time, he has only fragmentary recall of the episode without prominent dream imagery, and on arising in the morning, has virtually no memory of what may have happened. Some individuals with sleep terrors will have prominent physical activity including motions of physical fighting. In such cases, the distinction between sleep terrors and sleepwalking may become blurred. Sleep terrors are fairly commonly seen in children and typically resolve by adolescence. Adult-onset sleep terrors may also occur.

A SCREAM IN THE NIGHT

The car door opened. "Wssht" said Miss Finan, scuttling out again. "I've just remembered. Not last night, but two weeks ago. And once before that. A scream, you said?"

Mrs. Hazlitt stood up. Almost unable to speak, for the tears that suddenly wrenched her throat, she described it.

*"That's it, just what I told my niece on the phone next morning. Like nothing human, and yet it was. I'd taken my Seconal too early, so there I was wide awake again, lying there just thinking, when it came. 'Auntie,' she tried to tell me, 'it was just one of the sirens. Or hoodlums maybe.'" Miss Finan reached up very slowly and settled her hat.... "But I've laid awake on this street too many years, I said, not to know what I hear.... Like somebody in a fit, it was. We'd a sexton at church taken that way, with epilepsy once. And it stopped short like that, just as if somebody'd clapped a hand over its mouth, poor devil."**

(Calisher, 1982, p. 40)

Mrs. Hazlitt and her elderly neighbor are discussing a strange and curiously recurrent night noise that Mrs. Hazlitt fears might be the scream of a neighbor in danger. Miss Finan is struck by how short the sound was and speculates that it might have come from some neighbor experiencing an epileptic seizure. It seems likely that these women heard a neighbor suffering from sleep terrors, a condition in which the sleeper awakens screaming.

Whereas nightmares are difficult to confuse with other disorders, night terrors have a more extensive differential diagnosis. Central nervous system injury, infection, or tumor can occasionally produce night terrorlike episodes. Epileptic seizures not infrequently occur during sleep and, as the elderly Miss Finan suggests, can be difficult to distinguish from night terrors. Often only EEG studies at home or in the sleep laboratory can make this distinction. Medications, particularly in the elderly, can produce symptoms of either nightmares or night terrors that disappear or are greatly attenuated with drug withdrawal.

Sleepwalking involves a pattern of behavior usually including getting out of bed, walking around in the bedroom or on occasion outside of the bedroom, and then returning to bed. During these episodes, the individual is not fully conscious but on occasion may perform remarkably coherent activities such as eating or talking. Some persons may be able to carry on rudimentary conversations during a sleepwalking episode. Sometimes sleepwalking behaviors are bizarre and stereotyped, occasionally including behavior such as urinating in unusual places. Episodes of this sort require careful evaluation, often with ambulatory EEG monitoring, to distinguish them from temporal lobe epilepsy. Like persons with sleep terrors, sleepwalkers are difficult to arouse during an episode and if awakened are often confused and without any specific recall of the events that led to their behaviors. In the morning, they have little or no recall of what has happened to them. Sometimes, the affected individual may awaken spontaneously in the middle of a sleepwalking episode, occasionally completely out of her house and in a strange environment. Frequently, a sleepwalker awakens in the morning to find herself sleeping in an entirely different bed or room than where she fell asleep the previous night. Sleepwalking occurs in up to 7% of individuals and, like sleep terrors, is much more common in children than in adults (American Psychiatric Association, 2000). A recent FDA advisory has called attention to "sleepdriving"—a parasomnia variant of sleepwalking which may be linked to the use of some medications given for insomnia (Anonymous, 2007).

Restless Legs Syndrome (RLS) is a condition associated with poor sleep for both an individual and, often, anyone who shares his or her bed. People with RLS describe uncomfortable sensations in their legs when at rest that require them to move nearly constantly. This movement and the sensation that stimulates it typically interfere with both falling asleep and staying asleep. While the usual movements in RLS are voluntary, many affected individuals also experience frequent *involuntary* leg movements during sleep. RLS is common and may affect 10% of the population to some degree. Women may be somewhat more commonly affected than are men. The cause of RLS is unknown, though genetic factors are clearly involved, and specific chromosome sites conferring excess risks have been identified. Iron deficiency, kidney problems, diabetes, and certain medications may contribute to RLS, but in the majority of individuals no cause is determined.

Treatment for Parasomnias

Treatment is rarely indicated for sleep terrors. Nightmares often necessitate reassurance, especially in children. Occasionally nightmares reflect significant anxieties or unrecognized traumatic experiences. Sympathetic interviewing and counseling may be effective in evaluating and treating

*From "The Scream on Fifty-Seventh Street," by H. Calisher. In *Night Walks: A Bedside Companion* (p. 40), by J. C. Oates (Ed.), 1982, Princeton, NJ: Ontario Review Press. Reprinted with permission.

nightmares. Sleepwalking potentially poses some danger to the sleepwalker, and good management often requires special efforts to ensure protection from injury during an episode. Such protection is particularly important if the sleepwalker ventures out of the house or is at risk of falling down stairs. Treatment for adult parasomnias must be given in the relative absence of a strong evidence base. Prazosin has been used in nightmares due to Post-Traumatic Stress Disorder (Dierks, Jordan, & Sheehan, 2007), and benzodiazepines (Schenck and Mahowald, 1996) are frequently employed when parasomnias could be injurious to the sleeper (most commonly in sleepwalking) or to others. Some data supports the use of hypnosis in management of parasomnias (Hauri, Silber, & Boeve, 2007). For Restless Leg Syndrome a variety of drugs, including anti-parkinsonians, benzodiazepines, opiates, and anticonvulsants have been used. Much remains to be learned about this relatively common disorder (Trotti, Bhadriraju, & Rye, 2008).

APPLICATION OF THE NURSING PROCESS 20-1

All standardized nursing history tools include questions related to a client's sleep and rest patterns. *Disturbed sleep pattern* was accepted as a nursing diagnosis in the 1970s, indicating the nursing role in maintenance of sleep in support of the general health and well-being of clients. In the updated NANDA-I (Herdman, 2009) taxonomy, *Insomnia, Sleep deprivation* and *Readiness for enhanced sleep* are currently listed as diagnoses. Currently, NANDA-I defines *Sleep pattern disturbance* as "Time-limited interruptions of sleep amount and quality due to external factors" (p. 117). Whereas, *Insomnia* is defined as a "disruption in amount and quality of sleep that impairs functioning" (p. 115). Prolonged periods of time without sleep is addressed in the diagnosis Sleep deprivation. *Sleep* is listed as a diagnostic concept to address such nursing concerns (Herdman, 2009). The nurse has a clear role to assess the sleep patterns, quality of sleep, and duration of sleep in all clients. Care of one who is diagnosed with a sleep disorder will be collaborative, and the nurse will participate in an interdisciplinary team providing treatment.

ASSESSMENT

The nurse must always assess the client's sleeping patterns in completing any nursing history. Suggestions for obtaining information are presented in Box 20-2.

BOX 20-2
ASSESSMENT OF SLEEP PATTERNS

It is not enough to ask, "Did you sleep well last night?" A nurse must inquire if the client has/had difficulty falling asleep, experiences early awakening without the ability to return to sleep, and feels well rested in the morning. Further, the nurse should ask if the client feels fatigued and sleepy during the day. Questions for the nurse to ask are:

- How long does it take you to fall asleep at night?
- Do you awaken during the night? If yes, how many times in a typical night?
- If you do awaken at night, can you get back to sleep?
- Do you feel well rested in the morning?
- Do you have enough energy to perform your tasks during the day?
- Do you find yourself nodding off or sleeping during classes or meetings or while watching TV or movies?

Evaluate with the client whether there have been any environmental changes associated with the bedroom or household that could be influencing changes in sleep cycle. Questions for the nurse to ask are:

- Have you changed where you sleep?
- Have there been any changes in your household that could affect your sleeping?
- Have there been any changes in your environment (neighbors, traffic) that could affect your sleeping?

Determine whether there have been any emotional stressors that could be contributing to an inability to sleep. A question for the nurse to ask is:

- Do you find yourself awake at night worrying about a problem or an upcoming activity?

(*Continues*)

APPLICATION OF THE NURSING PROCESS 20-1 (Continued)

NURSING DIAGNOSIS

The nurse must first determine if the client has a sleep disturbance that can be addressed by nursing care or if the client requires referral to a sleep specialist. If the client experiences Sleep deprivation or Insomnia (the condition where he is unable to obtain restorative sleep) or is experiencing nightmares or sleep terrors, the nurse may make the nursing diagnoses and begin intervention. However, if the nurse suspects that the client has a Breathing-Related Sleep Disorder, Narcolepsy, episodes of sleepwalking, or Restless Leg Syndrome, the nurse should make a referral to a sleep specialist or other appropriate caregivers.

OUTCOME IDENTIFICATION

If the nurse is initiating treatment for a sleep deprivation, as may be the case in a DSM-IV-TR diagnosis such as Primary Insomnia, the expected outcome will be that within two weeks the client will experience restorative sleep and will describe falling asleep easily and waking up feeling rested. If the nurse is initiating treatment for a condition such as nightmares, the expected outcome is that the client will understand the disorder and establish means of coping with it within his family.

PLANNING/INTERVENTIONS

For Primary Insomnia, the best intervention is a standard sleep hygiene protocol, such as the one presented in Box 20-1. The nurse should educate the client and family about the condition and explain that a sleep hygiene protocol is a series of techniques that have been useful to many. The nurse should then help the client to individualize the protocol to fit his own environment and personality. Further, the nurse may suggest complementary modalities, such as guided relaxation, music therapy, or massage, that have been helpful for many who are unable to get to sleep (see Chapter 33 for complementary modalities).

For a client experiencing nightmares or sleep terrors, the nurse has two important interventions. First, support and reassurance for the anxiety that these conditions provoke are needed. The nurse should develop a supportive relationship with both the client and family and help the family to maintain a sense of calm regarding the disorder. Second, the nurse should provide education on the disorder to the client and family so that they have a better understanding of the condition. If the nurse suspects the nightmares or sleep terrors are a result of other trauma, anxieties, or delusions, the nurse must refer the client for further assessment and evaluation.

EVALUATION

Evaluation of nursing care will be done on the basis of achieving expected outcomes. The nurse should remember that the subjective experience of sleep, sleepiness, and rest is of utmost importance; that is, the outcomes may not be directly observed. The nurse must validate with the client that there has or has not been improvement.

CARE PLANNING GUIDE 20-1 Client with a Sleep Disorder

CLINICAL PICTURE

The clinical picture of a client with sleep disturbances includes:

- Sleep deprivation or Insomnia
- Fatigue

(Continues)

CARE PLANNING GUIDE 20-1 Continued

- Impaired social interaction
- Ineffective role performance

COMMON NURSING DIAGNOSES

Nursing diagnoses most frequently used are:

1. *Sleep deprivation*
2. *Anxiety*
3. *Ineffective individual coping*

The following Care Planning Guide suggests interventions, rationales, outcomes, and discharge planning for such clients, as related to the primary diagnosis of sleep pattern disturbances.

NURSING DIAGNOSIS 1: *SLEEP DEPRIVATION*

OUTCOMES

1. The client will develop a regular sleep schedule and will awake in the morning feeling rested.

NOC: *SLEEP*

INTERVENTION (NIC: *SLEEP ENHANCEMENT*)	RATIONALE
• Monitor the client's current sleep pattern and the duration.	• Helps the client identify problem areas; allows for identification of changes from baseline.
• Discuss previous methods used/tried to promote sleep.	• Encourages use of successful coping methods.
• Assist client to identify life stressors.	• Evaluates potential problem area that could be affecting sleep.
• Encourage a regular sleep pattern—going to bed and getting up at the same time each day.	• A regular sleep pattern develops regular, predictable patterns.
• Develop a bedtime schedule, such as taking a warm bath, eating a light snack, drinking a glass of milk, listening to music, or reading.	• A bedtime schedule provides consistent cues that the client will identify with sleep.
• Explain the effects of drugs and alcohol on sleeping patterns; encourage the client to avoid drugs/alcohol.	• Promotes the body's natural sleep cycle.
• Encourage the client to avoid daytime napping.	• Avoids further disruption in sleep patterns.
• Discuss the role of diet and exercise.	• Promotes a balance among exercise, sleep, and rest. Encourages good nutrition.

LONG-TERM CONSIDERATIONS FOR THE CLIENT WITH A SLEEP DISORDER

1. Clients will need time to repattern sleep. Establishing a routine will take cooperation of others in the family, such that information to family members may be needed.
2. Some clients will require additional support for nursing diagnoses of impaired coping, anxiety, or drug abuse/misuse (for example, caffeine) that contribute to the problem.

Note: The care planning guides have been adapted from *Plans of Care for Speciality Practice: Psychiatric Mental Health Nursing*, by M. Coler and K. G. Vincent, 1995, Clifton Park, NY: Delmar Cengage Learning.

NURSING CARE PLAN: NURSING PROCESS FORMAT 20-1

Fred is a 65-year-old, retired man who lives with his wife in a comfortable home they have owned for more than 40 years. He is an active member of his community, being involved in civic clubs and church activities. Fred is in good health, as is his wife. They have a stable retirement income. They have two grown children and three grandchildren who live in another city. Fred makes an appointment to talk with the nurse at the Senior Citizens' Center because he is unable to sleep at night and explains that the problem has been worsening over the last two weeks.

ASSESSMENT

Taking a detailed nursing history, the nurse learns that Fred has several concerns about his sleep; specifically, Fred explains that he just does not "sleep well anymore." He says, "I wake up several times during the night, sometimes I have dreams that I am with several other people—but I can't quite make out or remember what the dreams are about. Noise in the neighborhood bothers me—when I hear a bus go down the street I can't go back to sleep." Fred stays in bed about seven hours but believes he gets very little sleep; he gets up in the morning feeling tired and tries to nap in the afternoon to keep himself going.

On further questioning, the nurse learns that Fred often eats a snack before retiring; takes a daily walk, usually in the morning; sleeps with his wife in their bedroom, where they have a TV on which they often watch a late show before going to sleep. He retires at about 11:00 P.M.

NURSING DIAGNOSIS

Insomnia, related to inadequate sleep hygiene as evidenced by subjective reports of not sleeping well, waking up during the night, awakening during the night without ability to go back to sleep, and feeling tired in the morning and throughout the day.

OUTCOMES	NIC	NURSING ACTIONS	EVALUATION
By 2 weeks' time, Fred will experience restful sleep and feel rested on awakening.	• Sleep enhancement	• Establish a sleep hygiene protocol with Fred that includes: – Taking some form of physical exercise, such as Fred's daily walk, in the early evening. – Eating an evening meal around 7:00 P.M. and then having only a drink of warm milk before bedtime. – Keeping his bed reserved for sleep, therefore watching TV in the living room and retiring to bed when feeling sleepy. – Running a fan in the bedroom to provide good circulation of air and to provide a background "white" noise that could help eliminate disturbances of street noise. – Refraining from afternoon naps, at least until nighttime sleep is reestablished. • Educate Fred on what is known regarding sleep patterns in persons of his age group.	With establishment of the change in patterns, Fred reported he was able to sleep better at night. Within 2 weeks, Fred felt he had received restful sleep for the first time in months. Fred also reported feeling reassured that it was "normal" for him to be awakening frequently during the night. Fred did not know that most people develop different sleeping patterns in their 60s than they had in their 40s.

(Continues)

NURSING CARE PLAN: NURSING PROCESS FORMAT 20-1 (Continued)

REFLECTIVE QUESTIONS

1. **ASSESSMENT**
   Would you also question Fred's wife about his sleeping patterns? What questions should you ask about the physical environment of Fred's bedroom?
2. **NURSING DIAGNOSIS**
   Are there other diagnoses the nurse should look for in Fred? How do we know the nurse is not missing something important in Fred's emotional life?
3. **OUTCOMES**
   Is it too much to expect that the nurse and Fred together can change this pattern?
4. **NURSING ACTIONS**
   How should the nurse provide this sleep hygiene protocol to Fred? Should she write it out? Put it on a graph? Put it on a timetable? How would the nurse decide? Should Fred's wife be involved? In what way?
5. **EVALUATION**
   If the interventions used did not work, what else could the nurse do or suggest?

NURSING CARE PLAN: CONCEPT MAP FORMAT 20-1

Sleep Disorder

BACKGROUND INFORMATION

Vera is a Registered Nurse who is single with no children and who enjoys her nursing job. She graduated two years ago and feels comfortable with her work routine. She works at a large medical center and is assigned to a surgical floor with clients who have had abdominal and gastrointestinal surgeries. She works rotating shifts, often 12 hours or more per day. On occasion (at least once every two weeks) she works back-to-back double shifts, thereby being at work in excess of 16 hours in one day. She is talking with the employee health nurse at her hospital today, Ms. Frank, because she needs to check in for her annual TB testing and to schedule her CPR recertification. When asked about her basic health status, she reports to the nurse that over the past two months she has noticed that she is awakening from sleep with worry over her job performance—she finds herself awake at night wondering if she had given the correct medication, if she had completed all her charting, or if she had left something undone. She describes herself as a very busy person. She frequently "eats on the run" and recognizes that she does not always eat healthy foods. She drinks a lot of coffee when at work to "keep going" and drinks beer at home to "relax." Vera says she feels irritable at times and has been increasingly fatigued on her days off. Vera comments to Ms. Frank, "I should know better than to keep this lifestyle, but what am I to do?"

INITIAL ASSESSMENT AND REFLECTION

Ms. Frank recognizes the issues many nurses have in finding a balance between work and home life. She also is very much aware that the increased work hours may provide real benefits for Vera, such as increased experience, increased pay, and a focus in her life. Ms. Frank, however, is concerned that Vera is adopting a schedule that cannot be sustained over time, and sees that Vera herself has commented that her schedule is not good for her in the long run.

(Continues)

NURSING CARE PLAN: CONCEPT MAP FORMAT 20-1 (Continued)

INITIAL REVIEW OF NURSING DIAGNOSES

The initial nursing diagnoses to be considered are:

- *Sleep deprivation,* related to sustained circadian asynchrony secondary to work as evidenced by awakenings at night without being able to return to sleep
- *Imbalanced nutrition less than body requirements* related to perceived demands on time as evidenced intake of non-nutritious diet, increased caffeine intake
- *Fatigue* related to sleep deprivation as evidenced by reports of increasing fatigue on days off
- *Stress overload* related to competing demands as evidenced by reported worry over job performance

CONCEPT MAP OF ISSUES AND PROBLEMS

Ms. Frank draws a concept map to identify the focal issues and to set the priorities of care.

PRIORITIES OF CARE

The concept map points to the fact that sleep is the focal issue for Vera. Other areas that require attention to enhance health status (nutrition, anxiety) should be addressed once the need for sleep is addressed.

NURSING INTERVENTIONS

Ms. Frank uses the concept map as an illustration for Vera to reflect and review her own situation. Vera agrees that the relationships Ms. Frank suggested are true and stated, "I never really sat down to look at myself that way! I know I need to slow down and take care of myself."

With this, Ms. Frank suggested the steps for sleep hygiene discussed in Box 20-1.

OUTCOMES/EVALUATION

Vera left Ms. Frank's office with her concept map and her own sense that she could enhance her well-being.

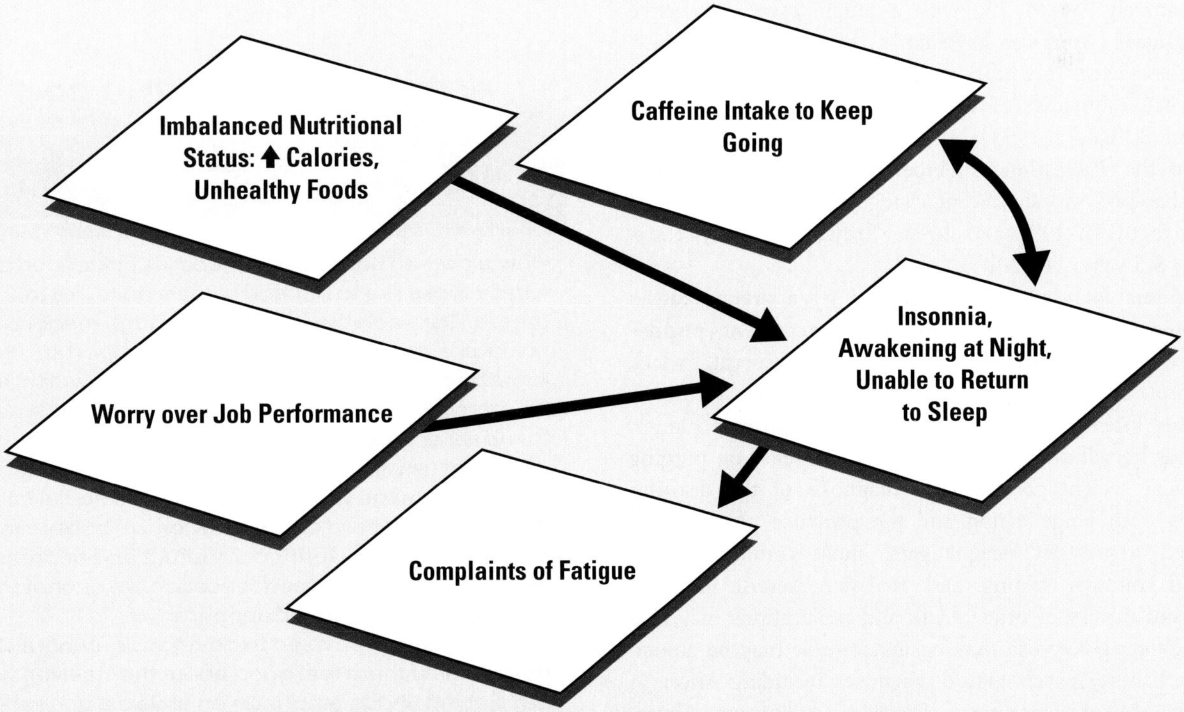

CONCEPT MAP OF ISSUES AND PROBLEMS (DELMAR/CENGAGE LEARNING.)

EATING DISORDERS

Two eating disorders are described in this chapter: Bulimia Nervosa and Anorexia Nervosa. Before reading about this ever-prevalent problem, read and consider the Reflective Thinking on body image and self-worth.

BULIMIA NERVOSA

FOOD FRENZY

As I opened the refrigerator door, my stomach growled with anticipation.... Suddenly, I realized I'd gone too far. In two minutes I had destroyed an all-day effort to avoid eating. Well, no need to get depressed. I might as well eat my fill of everything now. I'll just have to get rid of it later. I knew how. I'd done it dozens of times before.

Mindlessly, I began shoveling handfuls of food into my mouth. I devoured huge amounts of leftovers from Christmas dinner, breakfast, and even from days before.... *

(O'Neill, 1982, pp. xii–xiv)

In this episode, the author describes the experience of what the *Diagnostic and Statistical Manual of Mental Disorders, Fourth Edition-Text Revision* (DSM-IV-TR) now terms **Bulimia Nervosa**. Fasting, binging, and purging, three major aspects of Bulimia Nervosa, are illustrated. There is the ever-present risk of discovery by parents or other family members. DSM-IV-TR states that the prevalence of Bulimia Nervosa among adolescent and young adult females is approximately 1% to 3%, with a much lower prevalence among males (American Psychiatric Association, 2000). Several cross-sectional studies have offered somewhat lower prevalence estimates (Hoek, 1991; Warheit, Langer, Zimmerman, & Biafora, 1993), but recent reassessments seem to confirm the 1% estimates (Hoek & van Hoeken, 2003). There has been no significant change in U.S. prevalence of bulimia between 1990 and 2004 (Crowther, Armey, Luce, Dalton, & Leahey, T., 2004).

Bulimia Nervosa is characterized by a preoccupation with weight and bodily appearance and by recurrent episodes of binge eating dominated, as in the previous excerpt, by lack of control. The young woman, Cherry Boone, goes to the refrigerator intending only to sample the Christmas dinner. She finds herself unable to stop eating and relies on purging to achieve weight control. The diagnosis of the disorder requires both binge eating and the presence of behaviors intended to restrict weight gain, most commonly self-induced vomiting, fasting, and excessive exercise. Laxative abuse and misuse of other drugs and medications may also occur. Bulimia Nervosa may occur alone or may be associated with other psychological diagnoses including Anorexia Nervosa, Major Depressive Disorder, Substance Abuse, Obsessive-Compulsive Disorder, and Borderline Personality Disorder. While DSM-IV-TR requires that the full spectrum of binging and purging behaviors be present at least twice weekly for three months to make the diagnosis, many individuals report milder or less frequent manifestations of the eating disorder. Not surprisingly, these manifestations may

*From *Starving for Attention*, by S. B. O'Neill, 1982, New York: Continuum. Reprinted with permission.

The Meaning of Life

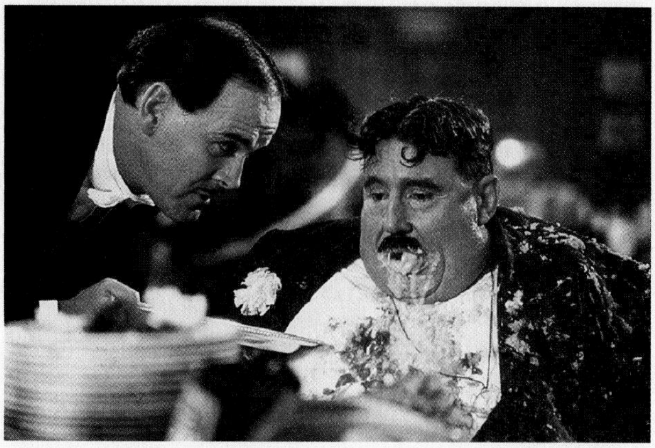

Courtesy: Universal/Celandine/Monty Python/The Kobal Collection

Binging and purging, common in many eating disorders, are generally hidden behaviors, rarely observed by the nurse.

REFLECTIVE THINKING 20-2

Body Image and Self-Worth

How a person perceives her body is influenced by what it looks like to her and what it looks like to others. Our society teaches us through media and social pressures that body image is important. Feeling attractive is an important part of self-worth, and for many, feeling attractive means matching a certain ideal appearance.

Most of us will never be able to look like this ideal, but the message we get is that we risk social failure if we do not try hard enough. When we believe this message, we may feel incompetent and depressed and have low self-esteem because we cannot meet impossible standards of appearance.

Women and men need to develop personal skills that will help them feel good about themselves without placing undue emphasis on physical appearance. No one should rely on dieting, exercising, and dressing to determine their self-worth.

be much more common than fully developed Bulimia Nervosa (Langer, Warheit, & Zimmerman, 1991).

The consequences of Bulimia Nervosa depend on its severity, duration, and associated psychological disorders. Recurrent vomiting leads to erosion of dental enamel and tooth decay, and may occasionally result in stone formation in the salivary glands. Salivary gland enlargement is common and, along with enamel erosion, may be a helpful diagnostic clue when physical examination is performed for some unrelated reason. Frequent vomiting and weight loss may lead to electrolyte disturbances that can result in heart arrhythmias (Roseborough & Felix, 1994), however, despite the difficulties of studying outcomes in this often secret disorder, the literature does not suggest increased mortality from bulimia (Berkman, Lohr, & Bulik, 2007).

Depression often complicates bulimia and may lead to suicide attempts or to completed suicide (Fedorowicz, Falissard, Foulon, Dardennes, Divac, Guelfi, et al., 2007). Bulimic individuals commonly use psychoactive substances that affect appetite and weight. Tobacco is probably the most common of such abused substances and is linked to increased suicide risk (Fedorowicz et al., 2007), but bulimia is also strikingly common among cocaine abusers (Walfish, Stenmark, Sarco, Shealy, & Krone, 1992). Nurses and other health professionals must be vigilant to detect bulimia in a variety of clinical settings and to recognize complications of bulimia as causes of otherwise-unexplained serious illness (Myer & O'Brien, 1993). While bulimic individuals may be very evasive in their actual binging and purging activities, direct clinical questioning seems to be remarkably effective in screening for bulimia. Freund and coworkers have suggested that two specific questions are particularly useful (Freund, Graham, Lesky, & Moskowitz, 1993). In these authors' study, a "no" response to the question "Are you satisfied with your eating patterns?" or a "yes" response to "Do you ever eat in secret?" had a sensitivity of 1.00 and a specificity of 0.90 for bulimia. In other words, 100% of bulimic individuals were either unsatisfied with their eating patterns or reported eating in secret (or both). Only 10% of nonbulimic persons answered similarly. Because Bulimia Nervosa is rare in most clinical settings, positive answers to such screening questions are commonly "false positives," detecting individuals who, on further questioning, do not have bulimia. Nonetheless, the authors strongly endorse the incorporation of these two screening questions into routine clinical interviews of women. Longer screening instruments such as "SCOFF" (see Nursing Tip 20-3) and the much longer Eating Disorder Examination Questinnaire (EDE-Q; Mond, Hay, Rodgers, Owen, & Beumont, 2004) have been developed for use in primary care (Mond, Myers, Crosby, Hay, Rodgers, Morgan, et al., 2008), but at least the shorter of these has not yet been shown to have significant advantages over the two-question version given in Nursing Tip 20-3.

NURSINGTIP 20-2

Body Image

Here are some hints that can help in developing a positive body image:

- Learn to like yourself as you are.
- Set realistic goals.
- Learn about good nutrition and exercise.
- If you are a woman, expect that you may experience normal monthly changes in weight and shape.
- Listen to your body. Eat when you are hungry, and only then.
- When life proves stressful, learn to ask for support from friends and family.

Remember the Three A's:

Attention: Listen to and respond to internal cues; know when your body is hungry and when it is tired.

Appreciation: Honor and appreciate the pleasures your body can provide.

Acceptance: Accept yourself for what you are. Do not long for the unattainable; having a wish "magically" come true does not lead to happiness, but leads to more unattainable wishes.

NURSINGTIP 20-3

Screening Questions for Persons with Bulimia

1. Are you satisfied with your eating patterns?
2. Do you ever eat in secret?

Note that 100% of persons with Bulimia Nervosa will answer "no" to question #1 and "yes," to question #2.

The SCOFF Questionnaire:

S – Do you make yourself **S**ick because you feel uncomfortably full?

C – Do you worry you have lost **C**ontrol over how much you eat?

O – Have you recently lost more than **O**ne *stone* (14 pounds) in a 3-month period?

F – Do you believe yourself to be **F**at when others say you are too thin?

F – Would you say that **F**ood dominates your life?

"Yes" answers to two or more of these is a positive response. A positive response is found in 72% of persons with bulimia. Seventy-three percent of persons without bulimia will have fewer than two "Yes" answers.

Mond, J. M., Hay, P. J., Rodgers, B., Owen, C., & Beumont, P. J. (2004). Validity of the Eating Disorder Examination Questionnaire (EDE-Q) in screening for eating disorders in community samples. *Behav Res Ther*, 42(5), 551–567.

Treatment

Both psychological and pharmacological treatments for Bulimia Nervosa have been used and studied. Numerous studies have shown that antidepressant medications, particularly selective serotonin reuptake inhibitors (SSRIs), are useful in the management of bulimia (Crow & Mitchell, 1994). While a variety of SSRI medications are commonly used to treat bulimia, only the use of fluoxetine (Prozac) is supported by strong evidence (Lilly, 2003). Various forms of psychotherapy have been used for bulimia, and in one study, structured cognitive-behavioral therapy was found to be more effective than antidepressants alone (Pyle, Mitchell, Eckert, Hatsukami, Pomeroy, & Zimmerman, 1990). Multiple studies, including a number of good experimental quality, have shown cognitive-behavioral therapy to have good short-term benefit in reducing the frequency and severity of bulimic symptoms (White, 1999). Comorbid depression is associated with less satisfactory treatment outcome in bulimia (Berkman, Bulik, Brownley, Lohr, Sedway, Rooks, et al., 2006).

Few long-term follow-up studies have been done, but the available evidence supports the idea that about half of male bulimic clients improve over a follow-up period of 10 or more years (Mehler, 2003), whereas the remainder continue to engage in at least some bulimic behaviors. Such failure to improve may be associated with comorbid substance abuse and a long-term duration of symptoms before initial diagnosis and treatment (Keel, Mitchell, Miller-Davis, & Crow, 1999). Failure to improve is also specifically associated with Borderline, Narcissistic, and Antisocial Personality Disorders, Impulsivity, and Depression (Mehler, 2003).

Anorexia Nervosa

There is a strong association between Bulimia Nervosa and Anorexia Nervosa, an association illustrated by another quote from *Starving for Attention*:

I'LL TELL YOU IF I NEED A DOCTOR!

*"There is nothing wrong with me! I'm just thin! I don't feel sick and I don't need to see the doctor! ... "It's my body!" I argued. "I know how I feel, and I'm not sick! I'm not hurting anyone else by being thin, so why should it bother you? I'll tell you if I need a doctor."**

(O'Neill, 1982, p. 55)

In the first excerpt from *Starving for Attention*, Cherry Boone describes the binging and purging of Bulimia Nervosa. In this second excerpt, she argues with her parents, who have discovered how emaciated she is. They begin a medical evaluation that results in the additional diagnosis of **Anorexia Nervosa**. Anorexia Nervosa, frequently termed anorexia, is a serious medical-psychological condition characterized by a profound disturbance in body image. Persons with Anorexia Nervosa view themselves as undesirably fat even when they, like Cherry, become clinically emaciated. These individuals do not lose their appetite for food (the strict meaning of the word "anorexia"), but, like Cherry, actively starve themselves in an effort to keep from gaining weight. Some anorexic individuals control their weight through dieting and exercising alone; others combine this restriction with episodes of binge eating and purging.

Anorexia results in profound bodily changes. The most apparent change is weight loss, which may reach levels of profound emaciation before being detected by friends, family members, or even health care providers. The diagnosis of Anorexia Nervosa requires that weight be 15% below that expected for age and height, but many anorexic individuals experience much greater weight loss. In women, malnutrition typically results in menstrual dysfunction; most women stop menstruating altogether. The skin becomes dry and frequently is covered with fine downy hair called lanugo. Because of fat loss and metabolic changes, anorexic individuals frequently complain of feeling cold. Recurrent syncope is not uncommon, and cardiac dysrhythmias may occur from electrolyte imbalance. Bradycardia is almost always present, partly due to the commonly associated rigorous exercise regimens adopted by many anorexics but probably also as a direct response to starvation (Kollai, Bonyhay, Jokkel, & Szonyi, 1994). Osteoporosis is common and may result in bone fractures (Salisbury & Mitchell, 1991). Writing in the European nursing literature, Vestergaard and colleagues (2003) counsel a high index of suspicion for anorexia and bulimia whenever young women present with fractures, especially those that occur after relatively minor trauma.

In addition to 15% weight loss and cessation of menstrual cycle (in women), requirements for diagnosis include documentation of an intense fear of gaining weight *and* either a disturbed experience of body weight or shape *or* denial of the seriousness of the individual's current low weight (American Psychiatric Association, 2000). Cherry's "There is nothing wrong with me! I'm just thin! I don't feel sick and I don't need to see the doctor!" is a highly typical response of anorexic individuals when challenged with the reality of their physical emaciation.

Differential Diagnosis

Weight loss alone does not permit a diagnosis of Anorexia Nervosa. Weight loss can occur from a wide variety of medical and psychiatric conditions, including intestinal malabsorption, brain tumors (Chipkevitch, 1994), cancer, chronic bacterial infections, human immunodeficiency virus (HIV)-associated conditions, and autoimmune disorders. Depressed, schizophrenic, and obsessive-compulsive individuals may sometimes experience significant weight loss as a manifestation of their psychological conditions. On occasion, distinguishing these psychological conditions from Anorexia Nervosa may be difficult. Usually, medical and psychiatric consultation can rapidly establish a diagnosis of Anorexia Nervosa by ruling out other potential causes of weight loss.

*From: *Starving for Attention*, by S. B. O'Neill, 1982, Reprinted with permission. New York: Continuum.

The Perceived Need for Weight Control

The precise cause of Anorexia Nervosa remains unknown. Psychoanalysts have stressed that weight control in Anorexia Nervosa derives from a desire to suppress adult sexual development and responsibility (Wilson, Hogan, & Mintz, 1985). Such desire for suppression in turn is thought to derive from early childhood sexual experiences, perhaps including seeing the mother's abdomen enlarge during pregnancy.

The psychoanalytic view is only one of a number of competing psychological explanations for Anorexia Nervosa. It has long been taught by some psychologists that Anorexia Nervosa is a developmental disorder deriving from disordered family structure and functioning. Family systems theorists have suggested that the condition arises in a family structure characterized by marital discord, strong emphasis on control, and overprotectiveness. More socially oriented theorists have stressed how pressures to achieve success, competence, and societally defined attractiveness can lead, especially in women, to compulsive efforts to control weight. This is especially true given strong social identification of thinness with attractiveness (Palmer, 1990).

Other theorists stress that anorexic individuals manifest very strong perfectionist tendencies and that failing to achieve complete control in other aspects of their lives leads them to attempt to gain full control of their eating and weight. Cherry had a particularly strong need for control and perfection. In other chapters of her book, she describes experiences of growing up in a Hollywood environment that strongly emphasized personal appearance. She and her sisters performed on television with their father, Pat Boone, a nationally famous singer and celebrity. While anecdotes do support the concept that a perfectionistic upbringing in high-achieving families may lead to eating disorders, more formal studies of families of anorexic individuals failed to show any distinct pattern of family interaction (Rastam & Gillberg, 1991).

In contrast to psychodynamic explanations, other psychologists have offered cognitive and behavioral models. Some of these emphasize the important role that film, photography, and, especially, advertising images of thinness play in leading to anorexia (Bruch, 1978). Bruch has further suggested that anorexic individuals have a combination of poor self-esteem, distorted self-image, and an inability to process *interoceptive stimuli* such as the sensations of being hungry and full (Bruch, 1973). Such discussions of self-image and misperceived stimuli raise the possibility that a definable neurological or endocrine abnormality underlies some cases of anorexia (Braun & Chouinard, 1992). This possibility of organic causation has been considered for many years with varying degrees of enthusiasm. For example, between 1920 and 1945, physicians commonly regarded anorexia as an endocrine disorder and experimented with numerous (unsuccessful) hormonal treatments (Vandereycken & Van Deth, 1994). More recent evaluations of individuals with anorexia reveal significant abnormalities in all major neuroendocrine pathways and in a variety of major neurotransmitter systems (Study Group on Anorexia Nervosa, 1995). Whether any or all of these abnormalities are a *cause* of anorexia or merely *result from* the disorder remains unknown. Aberrations in luteinizing hormone (LH), follicle-stimulating hormone (FSH), and gonadotrophin-releasing hormone (GnRH; all hormones involved in regulating sexual function) are common in anorexia, and, like the loss of periods in affected women, may occur *before* significant weight loss takes place (Pope & Hudson, 1989). Reported neurotransmitter abnormalities suggest that there may be a link between Anorexia Nervosa and Major Depressive Disorder, but it remains unclear whether these findings are primary abnormalities or are the result of starvation. There is some interest in the role that endocannabinoids (see Chapter 4) may play in anorexia and its potential treatment (Fride, Bregman, & Kirkham, 2005), but investigations in this area are still preliminary.

Genetic studies have often been used to help distinguish organic (hereditary) from environmental causes of psychological disorders. Such studies, while difficult to perform without bias, do suggest that some individuals may be genetically predisposed to develop anorexia (Strober, 1991). Twin studies, for example, show that when one sibling has anorexia, there are higher rates of anorexia in identical (monozygotic) than in fraternal (dizygotic) sibling twins. Such studies suggest a definite genetic contribution to the development of anorexia (Treasure & Holland, 1990).

Joughin and colleagues have emphasized that anorexia may sometimes present in individuals over the age of 30 years (Joughin, Crisp, Gowers, & Bhat, 1991). Anorexia in this older age group may be much harder to diagnose, partly because it is often an unsuspected diagnosis, and may have a significantly worse prognosis than when it occurs in adolescence and young adulthood.

History of Anorexia as a Disorder

Anorexia is not a "new" disorder. Modern understanding of anorexia began in 1868 when William Gull addressed the British Medical Association on the subject of mesenteric tuberculosis (Gull, 1868). In an era in which systemic tuberculosis frequently caused profound weight loss, he cautioned his fellow doctors against assuming that all anorexic patients suffered from tuberculosis. In his lecture, he briefly described "young women emaciated to the last degree through hysteric apepsia," a reference frequently taken to be the first scientific recognition of anorexia. Five years later, a French psychiatrist and contemporary of Charcot, Ernest Lasègue, wrote a paper describing eight individuals ages 18 to 32 years who today would be recognized as having Anorexia Nervosa. He even used the word *anorexia* in his description, though influenced by the terminology of his era, he called the condition "hysterical anorexia." But while Gull and Lasègue were the first to provide clinical descriptions of anorexia, the famous Romantic poet George Byron (1788–1824) almost certainly suffered from anorexia more than 60 years before his countryman Gull described the disorder:

> *Born with a club foot and being a "fat bashful boy," Byron suffered on account of his outward appearance. His notorious sexual escapades during his adolescence, however,*

*seem to indicate that women found him attractive.... He was obviously upset about his fatness and decided to drastically reduce weight. About this endeavour he made a bet with an acquaintance, which he won by a fanatic regime of strict dieting and violent exercise. Within a few months ... acquaintances found, according to his own saying, "great difficulty in acknowledging me to be the same person." The weight reduction did not satisfy. Like a "leguminous-eating ascetic," as he called himself, he persevered anxiously to remain so.... For the rest of his life he remained obsessed by fear of fatness and preoccupied with food.... Initially his diet consisted of biscuits and soda water, later of purely vegetarian meals or potatoes mashed in vinegar. To appease his hunger he chewed tobacco or smoked cigars, but occasionally gave himself up to an abundant meal (then "I gorge like an Arab or a Boa snake," he wrote). For this reason Byron took refuge in vomiting and purgative pills or consumed quantities of vinegar.... At the end of his life ... he was described as "unnaturally thin."**

(Vanderycken & Van Deth, 1994, pp. 227–228)

At times, Byron's food preoccupations seem to have made their way into his poetry. For example, his satirical poem "Don Juan" describes an episode of cannibalism among shipwrecked sailors who "perish'd, suffering madly,/ For having us'd their appetites so sadly" (from Lord Byron, "Don Juan," Canto 2, LXXX). In Byron's poem, as in his life, eating led to suffering, even "suffering madly."

Treatment

Numerous medications have been studied for treatment of anorexia: hormones, antidepressants, antipsychotics, and gastrointestinal motility enhancers. None has shown any consistent benefit (Crow & Mitchell, 1994). Where depression coexists, antidepressants are likely to be of significant benefit, but these may have only limited effect on the anorexic process itself. One group of researchers found strong evidence for the co-occurrence of Anorexia Nervosa and Obsessive-Compulsive Disorder (Thiel, Broocks, Ohlmeier, Jacoby, & Schussler, 1995). These authors also found that obsessive-compulsive symptoms were more likely in clients whose anorexia was most severe. Since Obsessive-Compulsive Disorder is typically drug responsive (Chapter 12), certain clients may benefit significantly from carefully chosen pharmacotherapy. For most individuals, however, psychotherapy is the mainstay of treatment. Profoundly emaciated individuals are almost invariably hospitalized and managed with a combination of behavioral therapy and, where necessary, forced feeding (Agras, 1987). Cognitive therapy, clearly effective in bulimia, is thought to be helpful in Anorexia, especially in combination with behavioral approaches (Powers & Powers, 1984). When the individual is severely emaciated, efforts to restore positive nutritional balance take precedence over psychological issues. The nurse's role is often to ensure that the individual receives and retains appropriate nourishment. Most of these individuals will receive care from a team, including experts in psychiatry or psychology, nursing, and nutrition. Overall, treatment for anorexia is less effective than treatment for bulimia (Berkman et al., 2006), and treatment failure in anorexia is relatively common (Kaye, Klump, Frank, & Strober, 2000).

*From *Fasting Saints to Anorexic Girls*, by W. Vanderycken and R. Van Deth, 1994. Reprinted with permission from the Continuum International Publishing Group.

Three Dancers

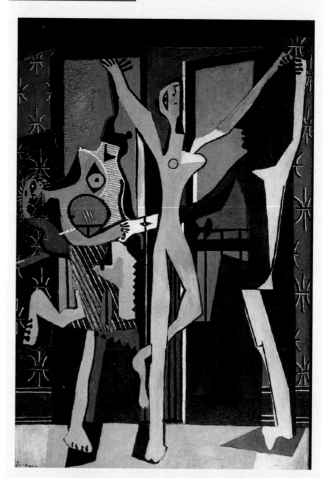

Only the still-large left breast suggests that this remarkably thin, hairless, central dancer does not have anorexia. Picasso's interests are primarily in the forms and colors of his canvas, but surely it was the anorexic appearance of this woman that caught his artistic fancy.

APPLICATION OF THE NURSING PROCESS 20-2

The majority of affected individuals may be treated as outpatients, and the nurse often has an important role in this setting. Frequently, as in the inpatient setting, a team of professionals works together to supervise the affected individual's recovery. Therapeutic goals will differ from program to program, but will certainly include the necessity of ensuring adequate caloric intake and documenting weight gain. Individuals with eating disorders are typically made exceedingly anxious by eating and will often try to deceive their caretakers by hiding food or falsifying their weight. The nurse will have to balance her important "policing" role with the likewise-important task of gaining the individual's trust and confidence (Chitty, 1991). Further important tasks in the management of these clients include addressing needs for exercise (usually at a level much less than the individual had previously engaged in), building self-esteem, and helping the individual to achieve a more normal sense of body image.

ASSESSMENT

The nurse will begin with an assessment and then identify nursing diagnoses that present for the individual client. The nurse will need to know the weight history, eating and purging experiences, and the degree of distress and/or anxiety the client is experiencing. Further, the nurse should identify the motivation for treatment, understanding that most individuals with eating disorders are highly ambivalent toward treatment. Authors have advised that motivation can be considered as inversely proportional to the level of ambivalence the client experiences (Love & Seaton, 1991). Listing the advantages and disadvantages of treatment can serve to explore background and readiness for change.

NURSING DIAGNOSIS

Common nursing diagnoses associated with eating disorders are presented in Box 20-3. The nurse can focus care on these human responses to the eating disorder and begin to plan interventions aimed at the client's priority of need.

BOX 20-3
COMMON NURSING DIAGNOSES FOR PERSONS WITH EATING DISORDERS

1. *Imbalanced nutrition: less than body requirements*
2. *Disturbed body image*
3. *Chronic low self-esteem*
4. *Social isolation*
5. *Ineffective health maintenance*

From Herdman, H., (Ed), 2009, *Nursing Diagnoses: Definitions and Classification, 2009–2011*,Oxford:Wiley-Blackwell.

OUTCOME IDENTIFICATION

The nurse must identify realistic outcomes of care, recognizing that eating disorders are complex, chronic diseases. It is best to focus on short-term outcomes, such as the client will take in 1,200 calories per day for the next week; the client will gain weight to return to a regular menstrual cycle; or the client will identify one positive aspect of her body unrelated to weight.

PLANNING/INTERVENTIONS

Nursing care can be viewed as taking place during four stages of treatment: nutritional rehabilitation, psychotherapy, maintenance, and follow-up care (Cahill, 1994). The first, nutritional rehabilitation, begins with diagnosis and sometimes with hospital admission. The priority here is to establish nutrition adequate to stop

(*Continues*)

APPLICATION OF THE NURSING PROCESS 20-2 (Continued)

starvation. During this phase, the nurse may need to take on the role of guardian and promote the client's physical well-being by monitoring food intake and weight gain (Irwin, 1993). Once an appropriate eating pattern is established, the client will enter a stage of treatment focusing on psychotherapy. Interventions that raise self-esteem and increase assertiveness are helpful, as are recreational therapies that provide a balance of exercise with rest and nutrition. Group and individual therapy would be initiated during this phase. Maintenance involves the client in learning to monitor and take control of her own eating patterns (Cahill, 1994). The client must develop internal strategies to meet her needs for nutrition and her desire to feel good about herself. The nurse should remember that personal stress and anxiety seem to increase the client's need to eat less and/or purge or vomit. Stress reduction techniques, then, may prove appropriate in helping the client find balances in her life. Further, it has been noted that persons with eating disorders frequently have little or no experiences with events or services that put one in touch with one's own body, for example with massage therapy, having a professional manicure, or having one's hair shampooed at a salon (Irwin, 1993). These activities may help the client to focus on her body in a positive way and can be encouraged. Above all, nurses interacting with clients with eating disorders can offer presence, role modeling of healthy eating/exercise behaviors, and emotional and psychological support. Further, nurses provide flexibility, empathy, and rational limit setting for one who is out of control but has a strong need to be in control (Love & Seaton, 1991). A recent investigation of nursing activities supportive of clients with eating disorders revealed that nurses provide empathy, surveillance, and constant, ever-present care (Ryan, Malson, Clarke, Anderson, & Kohn, 2006). Thus, a very important nursing role is to develop a positive therapeutic relationship with the client, based on nurses' knowledge and understanding of individuals as a result of their constant presence with the clients.

EVALUATION

Evaluation of the individual nursing care plans is done on the basis of stated outcomes. In evaluating treatment, however, the nurse must recognize the numerous challenges that still exist in dealing with this complex disorder.

CARE PLANNING GUIDE 20-2 Client with an Eating Disorder: Anorexia Nervosa

CLINICAL PICTURE

The clinical picture of a client with Anorexia Nervosa includes:

- Preoccupation with physical appearance
- Preoccupation with eating or food preparation, or both
- Secretive or solitary eating behaviors
- Verbalizations of fears of gaining weight
- Prolonged or excessive exercise programs
- Use of cigarettes or alcohol, or both, to diminish hunger

Note: The care plans that follow are adapted from *Plans of Care for Specialty Practice: Psychiatric Mental Health Nursing*, by M. Coler and K. G. Vincent, 1995, Clifton Park, NY: Thomson Delmar Learning.

(*Continues*)

CARE PLANNING GUIDE 20-2 Continued

COMMON NURSING DIAGNOSES

Nursing diagnoses most commonly used for such clients are:

1. *Imbalanced nutrition: less than body requirements*
2. *Disturbed body image*

The following Care Planning Guides suggest interventions, rationales, outcomes, and discharge planning for such clients.

NURSING DIAGNOSIS 1: *IMBALANCED NUTRITION, LESS THAN BODY REQUIREMENTS*

OUTCOMES

1. The client will increase intake of food.
2. The client will gain weight, as appropriate.
3. The client will identify eating patterns that contribute to under eating.
4. The client will decrease exercise/physical activity to a balance for exercise and nutrition.

NOC: *NUTRITION STATUS*

INTERVENTIONS (NIC: *NUTRITION MANAGEMENT*)	RATIONALE
• Encourage eating well—three small meals per day, with nutritious snacks of fruits/vegetables.	• Meal planning experience is often lacking.
• Offer nutritional counseling.	• Nutritional counseling educates the client regarding dietary needs for physiologic health.
• Plan daily exercise that will be appropriate.	• Conservation or utilization of calories must be in balance with caloric intake and body needs.
• Structure mealtimes with the client.	• Solitary eating encourages unhealthy patterns.

NURSING DIAGNOSIS 2: *DISTURBED BODY IMAGE*

OUTCOMES

1. The client will set realistic goals regarding body size.
2. The client will identify social/cultural issues that encourage thinness.
3. The client will accept positive features of own body.

NOC: BODY IMAGE

INTERVENTIONS (NIC: BODY IMAGE *ENHANCEMENT; SELF-AWARENESS ENHANCEMENT*)	RATIONALE
• Discuss factors that influence perceptions of desirable shape.	• Understanding conflicting messages helps to sort them out.
• Encourage emphasis on positive body attributes.	• Recognition of positive attributes encourages self-esteem.
• Work toward acceptance of body—determine if the client is responding to own or other's acceptance of our body.	• Acceptance of own body builds self-esteem. If the client is other-directed, assist the client to identify how others view her in realistic terms.

CARE PLANNING GUIDE 20-2 Continued

LONG-TERM CONSIDERATIONS FOR THE CLIENT WITH ANOREXIA NERVOSA

1. Encourage psychotherapy—long-term insight therapy.
2. Arrange for medical supervision of condition.

NURSING CARE PLAN: NURSING PROCESS FORMAT 20-2

Marcia is a 22-year-old university student who comes to the student health center for evaluation of upper respiratory symptoms. She has been coughing and has had "cold symptoms" for three days. She is uncomfortable and unable to sleep well at night because coughing keeps her awake. She expresses worry that she will not do well on her upcoming tests because she is not able to adequately prepare for them.

ASSESSMENT

Taking her history, the nurse, David, documents that Marcia is 5 feet 7 inches tall and weighs 95 pounds. Inquiring about recent weight gain or loss, the nurse learns that Marcia has just gained five pounds, and Marcia expresses some concern over that fact. The nurse begins to ask questions regarding nutrition and food intake, to which Marcia responds, "I've come here for my cold, I don't want to talk with you about my eating!"

NURSING DIAGNOSES

- *Ineffective protection*, related to inadequate nutrition, as evidenced by cough, cold symptoms.
- *Fear*, related to uncertainty over ability to perform on upcoming exams.
- *Imbalanced nutrition: less than body requirements*, related to inadequate food intake as evidenced by body weight under ideal (diagnosis needing validation).

OUTCOMES	NIC	NURSING ACTIONS	EVALUATION
• Cough and cold symptoms will subside. • Marcia will feel in control of her physical symptoms and attend to her studies. • Marcia will return to the clinic in a few days for further interaction with the nurse.	• Teaching: Disease process • Anxiety reduction • Nutrition management	• Instruct on measures to minimize cold symptoms and cough, such as increasing fluids. • Provide reassurance to Marcia that she will feel better soon and will be able to return to her normal pattern by providing information on what to expect from the physical illness. • Plan to discuss Marcia's eating habits when Marcia returns to the clinic.	Marcia's physical health problem improved and she returned to the clinic for follow-up. The nurse was unable to validate whether an eating disorder existed.

(*Continues*)

NURSING CARE PLAN: NURSING PROCESS FORMAT 20-2 (Continued)

REFLECTIVE QUESTIONS

1. **ASSESSMENT**
   What other factors (family, friends, daily habits, or sleep patterns) would you assess to get a more complete picture of Marcia's health?
2. **NURSING DIAGNOSIS**
   Why did the nurse focus only on the cold and cough? Do you think there is enough information to make a diagnosis of an eating disorder?
3. **OUTCOMES**
   Are these the outcomes you would have written? How do we really plan care for a chronic condition? Is it appropriate to merely suggest that the client return? Is the nurse trying to establish trust or do you think something else is going on?
4. **NURSING ACTIONS**
   How would you go about obtaining enough information to validate a diagnosis of altered nutrition?
5. **EVALUATION**
   What do you think would have happened if the nurse focused on Marcia's weight during this first encounter? How long do you think it will take to be able to diagnose and address Marcia's weight and eating patterns?

NURSING CARE PLAN: CONCEPT MAP FORMAT 20-2

Eating Disorder

BACKGROUND INFORMATION

Mary is a 15-year-old high school student who likes athletics (basketball, swimming, and track). She was "grounded" from playing this fall after she had surgery for a knee injury. She was unable to play any sport for the entire semester and was interviewed by the school nurse, who asked her how things were going, given that she was still recovering from the operation. Mary told the nurse that although she could attend classes at school, she went home afterward and had little to do that she felt was enjoyable. Mary told the nurse that she has lost her appetite, has stopped eating, and has lost weight (about 15 pounds). The nurse noticed that Mary had become increasingly more concerned about her appearance and that Mary was worried about her hair and clothes. The nurse asked Mary to talk about what else was going on in her life. Mary related that she wanted to be noticed and liked by the popular group of students in her school. Without being on a team, Mary found herself to be more isolated from the others. Mary said, "I feel like I am watching the other kids from outside—like I'm not really a part of the group anymore." Mary stated that she wants to look better so others will notice her, and she said she believes she needs to lose about five more pounds to look "okay." When the nurse asked Mary if she felt depressed, Mary said, "Not really."

INITIAL ASSESSMENT AND REFLECTIONS

The school nurse sees that Mary has lost a considerable amount of weight. In one semester Mary has gone from weighing 126 pounds to barely 105 pounds. Mary used to look athletic and fit and now she appears frail. The weight loss and lack of appetite are of concern, as is the lingering issue of Mary's being removed from others and possibly depressed.

(Continues)

NURSING CARE PLAN: CONCEPT MAP FORMAT 20-2 (Continued)

INITIAL REVIEW OF NURSING DIAGNOSES

The nurse identifies the following nursing diagnoses:

- *Imbalanced nutrition: less than body requirements*, related to perceived need to lose weight
- *Social isolation*, related to low self-esteem
- *Situational low self-esteem*, related to change in athletic role and accompanying concerns about being noticed by others, wanting to be popular

The nurse completes a concept map of the issues and problems noted.

PRIORITIES OF CARE

The concept map points to the weight loss as the focal issue. However, the factors and issues impacting the weight loss are self-esteem, social isolation, and feelings of powerlessness. The nurse uses this information to plan care that addresses the weight loss as a problem in the context of understanding that the root causes of the problem are the other issues going on in Mary's life. Thus, the concept map helps to illustrate that Mary's situation must be viewed holistically, and treatment should address each aspect of her life.

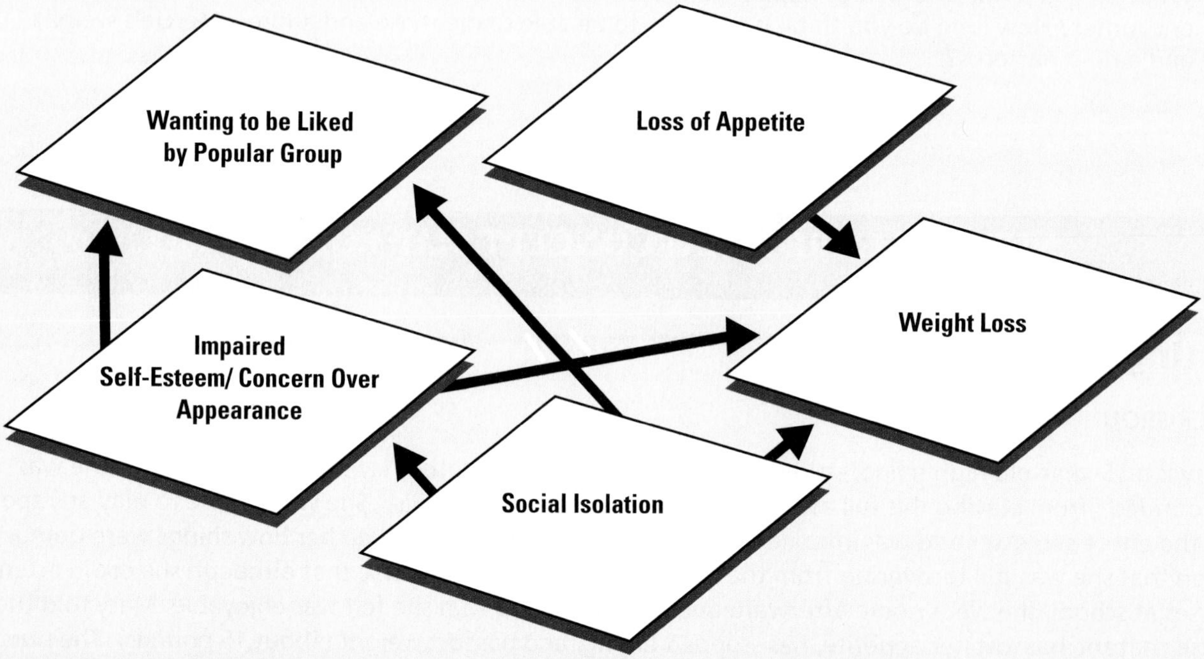

CONCEPT MAP OF ISSUES AND PROBLEMS (DELMAR/CENGAGE LEARNING.)

NURSING INTERVENTIONS

Although Mary can (and will) be referred to her family doctor for care and supervision, the nurse has developed a plan at school to address socialization, self-esteem, and nutrition. The nurse's plan is to encourage Mary to become involved in school and after-school activities with others that do not require the kind of physical ability needed to be on the sports teams. She will also provide Mary with information on basic nutrition and encourage healthy eating.

OUTCOMES/EVALUTION

Evaluation of Mary's care will be based on goals that Mary and her health care provider make regarding her need for adequate nutrition and weight gain. The school nurse will monitor Mary's activities at school and her social behaviors.

SEXUAL DISORDERS

Sexuality is part of any person's personality. It is an important dimension of a person, and influences how that person views herself and presents herself to others. It is quite impossible to define "normal" sexual behaviors and attitudes, as these are highly dependent on personal/family values, culture, and societal views. Sexual identity includes **gender identity** (internal sense that one is male or female) and **gender role** (learned expressions of maleness or femaleness). One author suggests that **normal sexual behavior** [for adults] is any sexual act that is consensual, lacks force, is mutually satisfying to both partners, and is conducted in private (Goldstein, 1976).

Sexual dysfunction occurs when a person experiences problems with any aspect of sexuality. According to NANDA International (Herdman, 2009), sexual dysfunction is the state in which an individual experiences a "change in sexual function during the sexual response phases of desire, excitation, and/or orgasm that is viewed as unsatisfying, unrewarding, inadequate" (p. 196). Some persons with sexual dysfunction will readily seek counseling; however, many will be reluctant to discuss sexual concerns with anyone. Nurses and health care providers must be willing to take a sexual history in their general assessments of individuals to determine if their clients are experiencing sexual dysfunction or some identified sexual disorder.

TAKING A SEXUAL HISTORY

The nurse must remember that sexuality is among the most personal and private areas of human life, and few individuals will volunteer information about sexual functioning or sexual thoughts unless explicitly asked. Many nurses and doctors are uncomfortable asking questions related to sexuality, and as a result, these questions frequently remain unaddressed during clinical encounters. Asking is important, however, and may even be life-saving when HIV infection is involved. Nurses should evaluate their own feelings regarding discussing sexuality and attempt to identify personal factors that may help or inhibit one's ability to provide care.

Many persons seek medical care with somatic complaints as an excuse to discuss issues of sexual functioning but are too embarrassed to raise their sexual concerns unless asked specifically about them. As a result, taking a sexual history is a highly important task in a clinical nursing evaluation. The sexual history may be quite brief or it may include a wide variety of questions; the length of the interview should be tailored to the client's interest, need, and presenting concerns.

Three important topics of the sexual history are sexual functioning; sexual thoughts, fantasies, and behaviors; and sexual preferences. Although many, if not most, individuals are sexually involved and sexually competent, have sexual thoughts and behaviors, and are comfortable with their sexual choices and gender assignment, a careful sexual history will occasionally discover problems in one or more of these areas of sexual being. Further, once the nurse asks questions that open the topic of sexuality as appropriate for discussion, clients may be able to express needs for education/information or the desire for sex counseling or support, or both.

SPECIFIC SEXUAL DISORDERS

Sexual disorders fall into two basic categories: (1) disorders of sexual functioning and (2) **paraphilias**, or disorders of sexual thought, fantasy, and behavior. The disorders of functioning include difficulties with sexual interest, arousal, and orgasm. Paraphilias include Exhibitionism, Fetishism, Pedophilia, Sadism, and Masochism. These terms are defined more explicitly later in this section. DSM-IV-TR also includes a third category, termed Gender Identity Disorder, which is considered briefly in this chapter.

Disorders of Sexual Functioning

The human sexual response typically occurs in four sequential stages: sexual interest or desire, sexual excitement, orgasm, and resolution. Sexual dysfunction may manifest itself as a disorder of interest or desire, a physical disorder of erection in men or vaginismus in women, a dysfunction in orgasmic response, or in men, premature ejaculation and in women, a painful response to intercourse. These dysfunctions correspond fairly closely to the stages of sexual response. Sexual dysfunctions may be entirely somatic—that is, have no discernible physical cause—or may clearly be the result of a physical disorder. Whatever their causation, as with most psychological conditions, a diagnosis of dysfunction or disorder is made only when the observed problem causes significant discomfort to the involved individual or couple. Many individuals report sexual "difficulties" that they integrate quite comfortably into their lives. In taking a sexual history, the nurse must be alert to the human responses of both accommodation and denial. Many individuals come to accept or accommodate aspects of their lives—including what might otherwise be termed sexual dysfunction—that would prove difficult for others to accept. For some, however, such accommodation really represents a form of denial: The problem actually is causing problems in personal life or relationships, but acknowledging this reality would prove too painful. Accommodation is usually a healthy response, whereas denial is generally dysfunctional. The nurse should not overlook the presence of denial, but she should be very careful to avoid challenging or threatening this psychological defense mechanism without a clear psychotherapeutic plan.

Disorders of Desire

There is a wide variation in normal human sexual interest, and this variation is in turn influenced by a huge variety of extrapersonal factors, including age, health, leisure, and availability of potential partners. On occasion, disorders of sexual desire reflect other sexual disorders: If intercourse is painful, nonorgasmic, or consistently embarrassing (as with premature ejaculation), there will be decreased motivation to seek sexual opportunities. The San Francisco newspaper columnist Arthur Hoppe not infrequently found variations in human sexual interest to be apt subjects for his satirical humor:

DR. PETTIBONE

Dr. Homer T. Pettibone is executive director of the United Anti-Sex Drive, a social-consciousness-raising organization. "Once again ... we are appealing to sectarians of all faiths ... to see sex for what it is. It is a monumental waste of time."

Dr. Pettibone said the most recent studies showed that Americans, who are not even French, devoted 3.2 hours per day—or 20 percent of their waking time—to thinking about, talking about, reading about, viewing depictions of, preparing for, attempting to avoid or indulging in (on fleeting occasions) sex.

"Any individual who renounces sex thereby immediately increases his or her overall efficiency 20 percent," he pointed out. "And that's seven days a week. Here at last is the secret to power, fame and fortune in one easy step."

*Members of Dr. Pettibone's organization are only too eager to testify to the benefits of celibacy: "I was a poor, friendless $100-a-week stock clerk until I gave up sex," says Bert L. of Flint, Mich. "With the time I saved I was able to complete a correspondence course in accounting. I am now a bookkeeper for a large pet firm. Last year alone, I was able to embezzle $43,578 and two parakeets."**

(Hoppe, 1979, p. 35)

While Dr. Pettibone, Bert L., and the easy adoption of celibacy are probably equally products of Hoppe's imagination, his essay emphasizes the important interplay of sexual thoughts, sexual fantasies, and sexual desire. Outside of religious orders, relatively few people choose, like Bert L. of Flint, Mich., to purposefully renounce sex drive, and for some individuals with a disorder of sexual desire, an endocrinological dysfunction may contribute to symptoms. For example, elevations of the hormone prolactin—sometimes due to a small pituitary tumor—may greatly reduce libido or sexual interest. In both men and women, testosterone levels seem to be directly linked to sexual drive, and any process that leads to a reduction in testosterone, such as prolactin excess or "normal" aging, may decrease sexual interest. There is currently an increasing interest in androgen supplementation (most commonly testosterone and dihydroepiandrosterone sulfate [DHEAS]) to counteract the effects of aging on sexual function. Currently, however, there is no good evidence that DHEASs improve libido (Huppert, Van Niekork, & Herbert, 2000). Whether, and under what circumstances, elderly men or women should receive testosterone supplementation remains uncertain (Sternbach, 1998; Redmond, 1999; Gruenewald & Matsumoto, 2003). Recent studies in men suggest little benefit (Emmelot-Vonk, Verhaar, Nakhai Pour, Aleman, Lock, Bosch, et al., 2008).

*From A. Hoppe, April 17, 1979, Copyright © *San Francisco Chronicle*, p. 35. Reprinted with permission.

REFLECTIVE THINKING 20-3

Erectile Dysfunction, Male Menopause, and the "Medicalization" of Sexual Dysfunction

Few readers of this text will be unaware of the existence of the drug sildenafil, better known by the brand name of Viagra, or of its competitors Cialis and Levitra. The over $1 billion yearly profit that Pfizer has made since Viagra's introduction indicates clients' and doctors' new perception that sexual dysfunction is a physical disorder and not primarily a psychiatric one. Although Pfizer has decided not to get Viagra licensed for use in women (Mayor, 2004), "off label" use in women as treatment of sexual dysfunction is probably not uncommon and is supported by at least some evidence (Berman, Berman, Toler, Gill, Haughie, & Sildenafil Study Group, 2003). Competitive alternatives to sildenafil are now on the market, and sildenafil has been frequently sold over the Internet without the need for a physician visit (Kahan, Seftil, and Resnick, 2000). Other medications with some evidence of benefit in treating hypoactive sexual disorder in women include bupropion (Segraves, Croft, Kavoussi, Ascher, Batey, Foster, et al., 2001) and a variety of androgen preparations (Segraves, 2003). Androgens, primarily testosterone, have also been prescribed for men to treat the decreased sexual desire that frequently accompanies aging. While androgen treatment can improve libido in some men, the long-term safety of this treatment remains unknown, with relatively few individuals carefully followed for 10 or more years (Morley & Perry, 2003). Despite uncertainties about safety, the concept of "andropause" has become established in both the popular and the medical press (Peate, 2003). Many physicians offer testosterone prescriptions to men with hypoactive sexual desire, and the popular media features descriptions of clinics specializing in andropause management. Some experts have expressed concerns about the wisdom of "medicalizing" human sexual experience through treating common disorders with potent (and expensive) drugs (Bancroft, 2002). Given the linked combination of high profit and high consumer demand, it seems very unlikely that the near future will see any reversal of this trend.

How do you think the use of Viagra has impacted the public's perception of sexuality?

What role do you believe medications should have in supporting sexual functions?

However, most persons with what DSM-IV-TR terms **Hypoactive Sexual Desire Disorder** are not elderly and many have no demonstrable hormonal abnormalities. The disorder is diagnosed when the affected individual reports significant distress or disturbance in interpersonal relationships and when the evaluating clinician assesses subjectively that sexual desire is truly less than would be normal for that individual. Because there is such a wide range of normal sexual interest, interpersonal difficulties often result when two sexual partners have significantly different levels of interest that are well within the normal range. For instance, one partner may have an "excessive" interest or need for sexual expression. While the other partner's sexual desire may be completely normal, interpersonal difficulties arise from unwillingness (or inability) to meet unusually frequent sexual demands. The evaluating clinician must also be careful to ask about physical conditions, affective disorders, and, especially, substance use; each of these may have a significant effect on sexual desire. Nonetheless, for carefully selected pre- and post-menopausal women with hypoactive sexual desire the use of testosterone can have a modest benefit without evident short-term risk (Davis, Papalia, Norman, O'Neill, Redelman, Williamson, et al., 2008).

Premature Ejaculation

Premature ejaculation is defined as male orgasm and ejaculation taking place with minimal physical stimulation and before it is expected or desired. Premature Ejaculation, one of the most common sexual dysfunctions, may cause significant psychological distress for both sexual partners. Because there are no standards for the duration of any of the four stages of sexual functioning, Premature Ejaculation has to be defined subjectively. Almost all men experience significant variability in the length of time between arousal and ejaculation; in general, that time is shortest in youth, with a new partner, under situations of poor privacy, and after relatively long sexual abstinence. It is not unusual for any of a variety of circumstances to lead to relatively brief and self-limited episodes of premature ejaculation. A disorder of Premature Ejaculation should be defined only when the complaint is persistent, psychologically troublesome, and not due to a chemical substance (some medications and opioid withdrawal can occasionally be causes).

For many men, the reassurance of a normal examination is sufficient to relieve an episode of premature ejaculation. As with other sexual disorders, there is often an element of ongoing anxiety about performance that can respond to brief counseling. Often, this counseling can involve the sexual partner, who may not have a complete understanding of the frequently self-limited nature of this disorder. The use of condoms may somewhat decrease physical sensation and moderately prolong the time between penetration and ejaculation. Topical anesthetic cream may have the same function, and newer preparations are in development (Morales, Barada, & Wyllie, 2007). In many circumstances, especially when symptoms have been prolonged and particularly troublesome, specialized evaluation and treatment are indicated. Often reflecting the work of the sexual therapists Masters and Johnson, sexual counselors have developed fairly standardized protocols for the management of common disorders of sexual functioning, including premature ejaculation. Confronted with a client whose symptoms do not readily respond to reassurance, the nurse might urge consultation with an experienced sex therapist.

Alternatives to sex therapy include daily use of SSRI antidepressants. Although perhaps for obvious reasons studies have proven difficult to evaluate rigorously, several of the SSRI medications (which have delayed ejaculation as a generally undesirable side effect) have been found clinically useful, with paroxetine the most effective (Waldinger, 2007). Studies are underway to identify on-demand SSRI regimens that are effective, but so far none is equivalent to daily administration. The opioid-like drug tramadol has shown some effectiveness if taken one to two hours before intercourse (Salem, Wilson, Bissada, Delk, Hellstrom, & Cleves, 2008).

Paraphilias

Sexuality is such a private part of human life that most persons know very little about unusual sexual behavior. Some paraphilias and their definitions are found in Box 20-4.

EXHIBITIONISM Many women have, at some time in their lives, been confronted by **Exhibitionism**, or a male exposing himself. When asked to describe the sexual excitement deriving from their behavior, some exhibitionists describe a desire to shock their victims, whereas others fantasize that their displays will result in sexual interest. Exhibitionism rarely results in any response other than fear or disgust, and most exhibitionists do not pursue their sexual overtures more aggressively. Rape, for example, almost never results from an exhibitionistic encounter. Unless arrested, few exhibitionists come to professional attention, and outside a forensic setting, few nurses will come into clinical contact with this paraphilia.

TRANSVESTIC FETISHISM In recent years, cross-dressing has been sympathetically portrayed in popular films. *The Crying Game* (1992) featured a homosexual transvestite who astonishes both the movie's hero and audience by revealing his male identity. While some homosexuals do dress as women, individuals with **Transvestic Fetishism** are more commonly heterosexual males. The movie *Ed Wood* (1994) offers a convincing view of Transvestic Fetishism. In this film, Ed Wood (a real-life 1950s novelist and director of low-budget films) is sympathetically portrayed as an otherwise normal heterosexual who is possessed by the desire to wear women's clothing. Rudolph Grey's biography of Ed Wood includes lengthy interviews with Wood's wife, Kathy, and with numerous Hollywood actors and friends:

NIGHTMARE OF ECSTASY

KATHY WOOD When he was a kid growing up in Poughkeepsie, he was always interested in the movies, especially the westerns.... Eddie told me that his mother did dress him as a girl when he was two, three or four, so maybe she's responsible.... He didn't embarrass me too much with it ... it was kind of a put-on half the time.... . And nobody took offense at it. Nobody at all.

BOX 20-4
PARAPHILIAS

- **Exhibitionism:** Exposing one's genitals to a stranger. This exposure may actually occur or it may be only a sexually exciting fantasy.
- **Fetishism:** Sexual arousal occurring from contact with a nonliving object, often an article of clothing. Individuals with fetishism often cannot achieve sexual excitement without the presence of such objects.
- **Frotteurism:** Recurrent sexual touching of a nonconsenting individual, usually a stranger and usually in a crowded public place.
- **Pedophilia:** Sexual interests directed primarily or exclusively toward children. As with other paraphilias, there may only be recurrent fantasies or urges but no abnormal behavior.
- **Sexual Masochism:** Sexual excitement resulting from being the recipient of physical suffering. Masochistic individuals may overtly seek out forms of physical abuse (commonly by asking to be beaten, bound, or otherwise physically humiliated) or they may only fantasize about such experiences.
- **Sexual Sadism:** Sexual excitement resulting from fantasizing about or participating in the infliction of suffering on others. In its extreme forms, Sexual Sadism may result in severe injury or even death.
- **Voyeurism:** Observing or fantasizing about observing others disrobing, naked, or involved in sexual activity.
- **Transvestic Fetishism:** Cross-dressing or fantasies about cross-dressing; usually a male dressing in women's clothes. Transvestic Fetishism varies from the wearing of a single inconspicuous item of clothing to complete cross-dressing.
- **Other paraphilias:** Urophilia (fascination with urine and urination), necrophilia (real or fantasized sexual interests in the dead), zoophilia (sexual involvement with animals), and telephonic scatologia (sexual excitement from obscene telephone calls).

JOE ROBERTSON We were both in the Marine Corps, he was in the invasion of Tarawa. 4000 Marines went in ... 400 came out. He was one of the 400. He was wearing pink panties and a pink bra underneath his battle fatigues. And he said to me, "Thank God Joe I got out, because I wanted to be killed. I didn't want to be wounded because I could never explain my pink panties and pink bra." ....

Ed knew Danny Kaye, who was also a transvestite .... And he'd [Wood] say he could write much better if he could wear my angora sweater. He would work for hours, sitting there, saying that it felt good...

*HARRY THOMAS .... Ed said, "Harry, come over and pick up the script." So he gave me the address, I went over there and knocked on the door. This beautifully dressed person comes to the door. Polished nails, hair all grown down. I said, "Oh, I beg your pardon, is your brother home?" "You mean Eddie?" "Yes, Eddie, is he home?" She says, "Oh, come in and have a cup of tea, he'll be here in a little while." I sat there, and she poured me a cup of tea, she was prancing around and changing garments, the ermine coat, all this, and I said, "I'm getting a little perturbed. I have a lot of appointments, do you think he'll be very much longer?" She says, "Oh, no, he'll be here soon." Suddenly, she comes out of a sliding door, and says, "I am Ed Wood."**

(Gray, 1992, pp. 16–42)

Other films with significant cross-dressing scenes include *Paris Is Burning* (1991), a documentary about New York City transvestite dances; *Philadelphia* (1993); and *Just One of the Girls* (1993). The last of these describes a high school student who cross-dresses to avoid a run-in with the neighborhood tough. In his female guise he meets, and eventually wins the heart of, the school's prettiest girl. *Just One of the Girls* effectively conveys one of the major characteristics of Transvestic Fetishism—the common onset of this disorder in adolescence. Cross-dressing often begins in private, and, as in Ed Wood and *Just One of the Girls*, the individual does not "come out" publically until late adolescence or young adulthood. For some cross-dressers, the involved articles of clothing are erotic fetishes—sources of sexual excitement. However, as both Ed Wood and *Nightmare of Ecstasy* convincingly show, the wearing of female clothing is frequently experienced as more a source of emotional comfort.

While, like Ed Wood, most persons with Transvestic Fetishism are fully comfortable as social and sexual males, occasionally cross-dressing individuals do develop a strong desire to live as a female. DSM-IV-TR categorizes these persons—some of whom may eventually seek sex-changing surgery—as having **gender dysphoria**. Whether or not they are comfortable with their genetic gender assignment, transvestic fetishists may find illness and hospitalization particularly distressing. Like Marine Corporal Ed Wood at age 18, cross-dressers may fear discovery if they are injured or become ill: "I didn't want to be wounded because I could never explain

*From *Nightmare of Ecstasy: The Life and Art of Edward D. Wood, Jr.*, by R. Gray, 1994, Portland, OR: Feral House Press. Reprinted with permission.

my pink panties and pink bra." Worse, they may fear the hospital as a place where cross-dressing, an important source of comfort, can be neither acknowledged nor practiced. A thorough history can help the nurse recognize a client's special needs for comforting objects or clothing.

PEDOPHILIA Of all the paraphilias, **pedophilia** is probably the diagnosis that is of most concern to the nonclinical public. Recent revelations of large-scale abuse of children by Catholic priests have brought this disorder to attention and emphasized how persistent pedophilic abuse may be over time in those afflicted with the disorder. Suggestions that a U.S. Congressman was involved in pedophilic behaviors offers a reminder that, while uncommon, this condition is widespread in the population. What this public awareness fails to recognize is that much sexual *assault* involving children is perpetrated by family members or other caretakers. Pedophilia is a particularly complex topic because its definition involves interest or preoccupation, but not necessarily behavior (DSM-IVR requires for diagnosis only that an individual with recurrent sexual urges or fantasies involving children suffer "marked distress" or interpersonal difficulty). Not all sexual crimes against children are committed by pedophiles (some sexual offenders will prey on anyone who is available to them), and many pedophiles never engage in behaviors harmful to children (though this latter conclusion is difficult to substantiate since the prevalence of pedophilia among noncriminal offenders is unknown [Seto, 2004]). Most pedophiles have one or more other paraphilias such as **Voyeurism** or **Frotteurism**, and consequently—except in the context of incest or involvement of older children—are more likely to engage in touching behaviors than penetrative sex.

If the prevalence of pedophilia is uncertain, the frequency of harm that it causes is somewhat better known. About 15% of all adults report being sexually touched by an older person during childhood with likelihood being greater among children growing up in poverty (Fagan, Wise, Schmidt, & Berlin, 2002). As discussed further in Chapter 26, sexual abuse in childhood may have significant adverse psychological outcomes in adult years.

Understanding of the cause of pedophilia remains elusive. Sixty percent of child molesters report that they themselves were victims of child sexual abuse, a much higher percentage than found among opiate abusers or normal controls. These studies suggest that while a history of child sexual abuse may increase risk of pedophilia, frequency of criminal offense is not increased by a personal history of molestation (Lamberg, 2005). Recent studies document functional differences in brains of pedophiles compared with normals (Cantor, Kabani, Christensen, Zipursky, Barbaree, Dickey, et al., 2008). When pedophiles are shown nonsexual photographs of children, functional magnetic resonance imaging demonstrates activation in the amygdala (see Chapter 4) significantly more than in nonoffenders (Sartorius, Ruf, Kief, Demirakca, Bailer, Ende, et al, 2008). These studies raise important ethical questions about guilt and responsibility, and they offer a somewhat chilling prospect of a potential pedophile "lie detector" test that might be used (or misused) for screening or prosecuting. Nonetheless, they also suggest that prior sexual experiences and/or other factors leave a measureable trace in our very basic emotional structuring. Since the amygdala is a core generator of emotions, these studies also help explain why pedophilia is highly recurrent in many individuals and often requires long-term treatment. Evidence for the effectiveness of psychological treatment of pedophilia remains scant (Kenworthy, Adams, Bilby, Brooks-Gordon, Fenton, 2004), although cognitive behavioral therapy and group therapy are often used in treatment (Studer & Alwyn, 2006). Since some studies show a strong correlation between pedophilia and substance abuse, treatment plans need to address dual diagnoses where needed (Hughes, 2007). Available data suggests that recidivism is a major problem for pedophilic offenders. In a six-year follow-up study, more than half of offenders sentenced to maximum security prisons had subsequent criminal convictions, and over a third had repeat sexual offenses (Hughes, 2007). Whether this degree of recidivism is seen among persons with less serious initial offenses is unclear, but clearly preventing repeat offense is a major goal of treatment. For this reason, many pedophile offenders are subject to hormonal therapy in an attempt to directly modify sexual behavior. There is some evidence that hormonal therapy with each of several agents (leuprolide, triptorelin, cyproterone—not available in the United States—or medroxyprogesterone) can be effective in reducing, but not eliminating, sexual recidivism (Hughes, 2007). Preliminary studies suggest a role for the anti-epileptic drug topiramate and perhaps for SSRI antidepressants (Hall & Hall, 2007). However, without willing cooperation, no treatment is likely to succeed over time. Even surgical castration, occasionally still used, has occasionally been ineffective in preventing repeat offense if the perpetrator obtains testosterone supplementation either through ill-advised medical treatment or illicitly (Hall & Hall, 2007). Until treatments can be better shown to prevent recurrent offenses, pedophiles who have committed crimes against children but who are not incarcerated should be kept away from unsupervised contact with children. Many pedophiles work or volunteer in settings that afford them opportunities for close interactions with children that may lead to criminal abuse. While screening questionnaires have been developed that can identify persons with pedophilic traits (Kolton, Boer, & Boer, 2001), it is unlikely that these will or should come into common usage in screening babysitters, scout masters, clergy, and others who can (and have) perpetrated pedophilic abuse. Many states have implemented "Megan's Laws," named after a young girl who was raped and murdered by a predatory neighbor who—unbeknownst to anyone in the neighborhood—had a past history of criminal sexual offenses. Megan's Laws typically require that neighbors be warned whenever a convicted sexual offender takes residence in a neighborhood. Whether these laws will have any effect on recurrent offenses remains to be seen. It is clear from recent lawsuits and public apologies that when Catholic bishops reassigned offending clergy to other distant parishes—often after "successful" treatment—but gave no warnings to at-risk families, recurrence of offense not infrequently followed. Pedophilia involving the Internet is an evolving and highly complex problem potentially involving child pornography and, even more troublesome, newly available ways for intent pedophiles to gain access to unsuspecting children (Malesky, 2007). Pedophilia resulting in criminal acts is a serious public health problem common enough that every nurse will almost certainly encounter both its victims and its perpetrators not infrequently during a career.

Sexual Sadism **Sexual Sadism** is defined as persistent fantasies or behaviors involving the infliction of suffering on others. **Sexual Masochism** is a reciprocal disorder in which fantasies and/or behaviors involve being the recipient of physical abuse or humiliation. The word *sadism* derives from the family name of Donatien-Alphonse-François de Sade, whose sexual exploits and writings led to his lengthy imprisonment in eighteenth-century France and, ever since, to his great notoriety as a writer and exemplar of evil. Sade's multiple imprisonments were for debt, attempted poisoning, and sodomy (until the present century, a serious crime throughout Europe). He was also been accused but not convicted of beating, cutting, and otherwise abusing prostitutes. Released from the Bastille during the French Revolution, he narrowly escaped a death sentence, was finally rejailed in 1801, and was committed to a mental institution two years later. Apparently quite sane, but regarded as a serious moral menace, he remained comfortably housed in this asylum until his death in 1814—"helping to stage plays which the hospital's director regarded as a form of therapy" (de Sade/D. Coward trans., 1992, p. xv). There is little in the historical record to prove that Sade's actual behavior was particularly vicious, and he claimed as much in a letter to his wife (whose family had aggressively sought his imprisonment):

> *Yes, I am a libertine, I admit it freely. I have dreamed of doing everything that it is possible to dream of in that line. But I most certainly have not done all the things I dreamt of and never shall.**
>
> (*de Sade/D. Coward. trans., 1992, p. xvii*)

Whatever his actual behavior, Sade's writings were, and remain, profoundly shocking in their imaginings of sexual violence. *The Misfortune of Virtue* was written while he was imprisoned in the Bastille and is far less "sadistic" than much of his later work. Part of the plot involves a young servant woman, Sophie, who is falsely accused of murdering the woman for whom she works. The victim's son, the real murderer, surprises Sophie in the woods, ties her to a tree, and assisted by friends proceeds to punish her for his mother's murder. Sade's writing combines murder, bondage, flagellation, and a fascination with the victim's suffering. These are the elements of sadism, and even if Sade had "most certainly ... not done all the things [he] dreamt of," others at that time and since have both fantasized and enacted scenes of sexual sadism.

Sadism and masochism are often combined in the same individual. One of the most striking sadomasochists of recent times was Percy Grainger, a famous pianist and composer who died in 1961:

> *Grainger was one of the eccentrics of music—a gangling figure with an aquiline face and a formidable mop of hair; a vegetarian; a health faddist; a man who likely as not would hike from concert to concert with a knapsack on his back, and a whale of a pianist.... Grainger was one of the most gifted pianists of the century ... who forged his own style and expressed it with amazing skill, personality and vigor.**
>
> (*Schonberg in T. P. Lewis, 1992, pp. 12–13*)

Unlike Sade, whose sadism probably expressed itself primarily with prostitutes and in his imagination, Grainger seems to have confined his sadomasochistic behavior to ongoing relationships, including his 33-year marriage. In his will, Grainger directed "that the flesh be removed from my bones and the flesh destroyed" (Bird, 1976, p. 248). This dying request (never granted) symbolized much of his behavior in life:

> *Grainger liked to flagellate himself or to be beaten by another.... These acts were obsessively documented in his letters to his lover, the pianist Karen Holten (with whom he seems also to have enjoyed normal sexual relations) ... in reality he practised such monstrosities on himself, branding his own nipple with a hot key and forcing needles through his breasts.*†
>
> (*B. Morton in T. P. Lewis, 1992, pp. 33–34*)

Grainger's sadomasochism appears to have been confined to relationships with consenting partners. There seems no evidence that either he or his several partners were ever seriously injured or that he imposed his sexual preferences on others without due warning. Long before their marriage, for example, his wife-to-be received a lengthy letter detailing his sexual appetites and fascinations:

> *"Despite many statements to the contrary, [she] did walk into wedlock fully aware of Grainger's lust for bizarre, even brutal sex acts"***
>
> (*Gillies & Pear, 1994, pp. 94–100*)

*From *The Misfortune of Virtue, and Other Early Tales*, by Marquis de Sade, 1992. Translated and edited by D. Coward, Oxford: Oxford University Press. Reprinted with permission.

*From "To Half Fight Nature: Percy Grainger," by B. Morton. In *A Guide to the Music of Percy Grainger*, edited by T. P. Lewis, 1992, White Plains, NY: ProAm Music Resources.

†From "Percy Grainger," by H. C. Shonberg. In *A Guide to the Music of Percy Grainger*, edited by T. P. Lewis, 1992, White Plains, NY: ProAm Music Resources.

**From *The All-Round Man: Selected Papers of Percy Grainger, 1914–1961*, by M. Gilles and D. Pear, 1994, London: Clarendon Press.

La Pianist (The Piano Teacher)

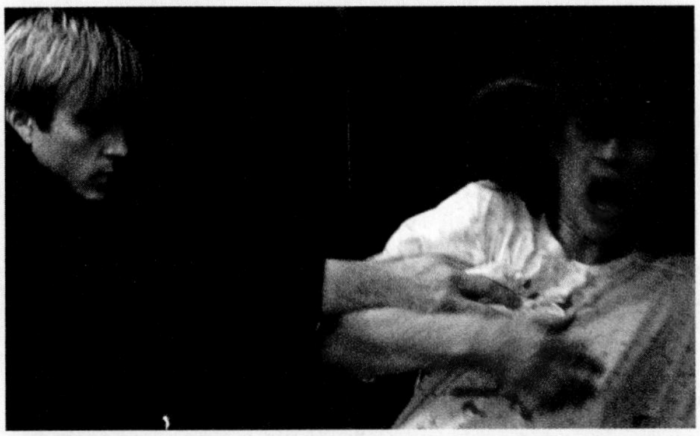

Source: Studio Canal + Centre National de la Cinematographie. (Courtesy: The Kobal Collection)

Viennese piano professor Erika Kohut (Isabelle Huppert) seeks domination over her students—and over her intrusively controlling mother. Beneath her tightly-controlled exterior is an unfeeling sado-masochistic core revealed when a young and narcissistic student finds himself attracted to her. Huppert's portrayal of obsessive sado-masochism is brilliant.

It is likely that some individuals express Sexual Sadism or Sexual Masochism only in fantasy. For others, pornography may be a vehicle for such sexual drives. Yet others may find themselves subject to sadistic or masochistic urges that they strive to repress; some of these individuals may seek therapy and in this manner come to clinical attention. Others may become the perpetrators of sexual crimes on nonconsenting victims. While the majority of sexual sadists are probably harmless—like Sade, expressing themselves more in fantasy than in reality—there is no doubt that some sadistic individuals represent very dangerous risks to society. Psychiatrists and psychiatric nurses may play a role in evaluating the societal risk posed by sadistic individuals who have committed sex crimes. This task is exceedingly difficult and risks wrongly imprisoning a person who may pose little risk of perpetrating serious harm. There is limited evidence that Sexual Sadism can be modified by treatment, and for some individuals, lengthy incarceration may be society's best protection against dangerous behavior. When such behavior results in harm to others, and when there is little motivation for change, incarceration may offer the only hope of preventing catastrophe.

The average nurse is relatively unlikely to be involved in ongoing treatment of these individuals, many of whom will be treated in specialist or forensic psychiatric units. It is important to recognize that paraphilic behavior often seems bizarre, repulsive, "perverted," and physically and morally offensive. It is not wrong for the nurse to be shocked or offended by the behavior of some individuals. Sadism, particularly when directed against nonconsenting victims, is revolting, as is child sexual abuse, sometimes an accompaniment of pedophilia. Occasionally, paraphilias seem quite harmless and even of some social value as stimuli to artistic creativity. For example, while the idea of Pedophilia is deeply disturbing to most adults, it is well to remember that one of this era's most popular books, *Alice in Wonderland*, was written by Charles Dodgson (pen name, Lewis Carroll), a shy bachelor whose passion was to befriend young girls and photograph them nude (Cohen, 1979).

We do not yet know what causes some individuals to act criminally, aggressively, or *evilly*, but as an editorialist for the *Lancet* observed, perhaps in the not-distant future "evil ... may even prove reversible" (Anonymous, 1996, p. 1). In pursuit of such a potentially optimistic vision, one of humankind's goals must be to identify and, where possible, to correct the genetic, social, and psychological antecedents of evil behavior. Our survival as a society requires no less.

As with many other psychological disorders manifesting primarily as unusual behavior, the cause of paraphilias remains unknown. Psychoanalytic theory traces Fetishism and cross-dressing to severe castration anxiety during the oedipal phase of early childhood, with the chosen object replacing the missing penis. Other explanations for paraphilias also focus on early childhood experiences and evoke pleasurable reactions to early cross-dressing or sexual encounters with other children as sources of subsequent transvestism or Pedophilia (Becker & Kavoussi, 1994). The reader may remember the excerpt from *Nightmare of Ecstasy* quoted earlier where Ed Wood's wife suggested a similar etiology for his cross-dressing: "His mother did dress him as a girl when he was two, three or four, so maybe she's responsible." These conditions are very deeply a part of the individual's self-image, probably indeed implying an origin in early childhood. While insight-oriented psychotherapy has occasionally proven effective with paraphilias, programs that combine behaviorally oriented counseling with appropriate pharmacological interventions may be the most effective (Marshall, Jones, Ward, Johnston, & Barbaree, 1991).

Other Disorders

DSM-IV-TR recognizes **Gender Identity Disorder**, a condition in which an individual feels himself or herself to be a member of the opposite sex and desires gender change, as a psychiatric disorder. Homosexuality is not defined as a disorder because it has become clear that a psychiatric disorder, by definition, requires that the individual experience some degree of personal, vocational, or social dysfunction. However, there are some individuals who have difficulty in accepting their sexual orientation, whether it be heterosexual or homosexual; these persons do qualify for a sexual disorder diagnosis, but only on the basis of their distress. Sexual and Gender Identity Disorders imply marked, persistent distress about sexual orientation.

APPLICATION OF THE NURSING PROCESS 20-3

No matter where the nurse works in clinical practice, she will encounter individuals in various states of sexual dysfunction or disorder. It is the nurse's role to support clients in their quest for physical and emotional health, and this most certainly includes sexual health. All aspects of human sexuality can be affected by illness or injury, and illness or injury may cause a change in perception of self or in participation in sexual activity (Lubkin, 1990).

ASSESSMENT

The nursing role is to identify in conjunction with the client whether a dysfunction or disorder exists and to refer to the most appropriate resource for the client's care. Should any of the diagnoses of sexual disorders discussed in this chapter be uncovered, the nurse will function in a collaborative role and will refer the client to a sex therapist or other specialist. In other cases, however, assessment will indicate that the client has neither a dysfunction nor a disorder but, rather, wishes to discuss a sexual concern. The nurse will be able to provide an empathic understanding of the issues raised and relay needed information.

NURSING DIAGNOSIS

The nursing diagnosis of *Ineffective sexuality patterns* has been defined as the state in which an individual expresses "concern regarding own sexuality" (Herdman, 2009, p. 229). It has been difficult for nurses to differentiate this diagnosis from the general diagnosis of *Sexual dysfunction*. One researcher suggested that one diagnosis, *Altered sexuality patterns*, be used by nurses to encompass both a change in sexual patterns and the concerns related to that change (LeMone, 1993). In the 1990s, LeMone & Weber (1995) conducted a gender-specific validation study of the meaning of the new, proposed nursing diagnosis of *Altered sexuality patterns*. These defining characteristics represent definitions of *sexuality patterns* and provide a basis for nurses to plan general nursing care, though the current descriptor of the diagnosis has been changed from *altered* to *ineffective*. The diagnoses of *Ineffective sexuality pattern* and *Sexual dysfunction* remain on the current list (Herdman, 2009).

OUTCOME IDENTIFICATION

The nurse planning independent nursing care for the client with *Ineffective sexuality pattern* will identify outcomes with the client. For example, if a client wishes to discuss a sexual concern, the outcome will be that the client was given the opportunity to discuss and reflect upon sexuality.

PLANNING/INTERVENTIONS

Nursing theories that provide for unconditional acceptance and support may prove most helpful in guiding nursing care, as issues of a sexual nature will rarely be discussed in situations other than those of complete trust. The most commonly used nursing intervention for the diagnosis of *Ineffective sexuality patterns* is active listening.

EVALUATION

Individuals who present with a psychiatric diagnosis of sexual disorder will require referral to a psychiatrist, psychologist, or sex therapist. Therefore, in addition to knowledge of sexual health and dysfunction, it is essential that the nurse have knowledge of the identified sexual disorders. Follow-up with other health care team members will help ensure continuity of care.

CARE PLANNING GUIDE 20-3 Sexual Dysfunction

CLINICAL PICTURE

The clinical picture of the client presenting with sexual dysfunction includes:
- Deficient or absent sexual desires
- Persistent aversion to genital sexual contact
- Recurrent or persistent failure to attain physiological response of sexual excitement
- Recurrent or persistent absence of, or delay in, achieving an orgasm
- Recurrent or persistent genital pain
- Premature ejaculation in males
- Involuntary, interfering vaginal spasms in females

COMMON NURSING DIAGNOSES

Nursing diagnoses most frequently employed for sexual dysfunction are:
1. *Sexual dysfunction*
2. *Ineffective sexuality pattern*

The following Care Planning Guides suggest interventions, rationales, outcomes, and discharge planning for such clients.

NURSING DIAGNOSIS 1: *SEXUAL DYSFUNCTION*

OUTCOMES

The client will be able to experience sexual pleasure.

NOC: *SEXUAL FUNCTIONING*

INTERVENTIONS (NIC: *SEXUAL COUNSELING*)	RATIONALE
• Discuss existing, intact sexual responses.	• The existing responses indicate at what level to begin therapeutic intervention.
• Monitor for organic, psychological, or social etiological factors.	• The type and extent of etiology will serve as an indicator of what is physically feasible to attain.
• Appraise the relationship between etiological factors and sexual dysfunction.	• These relationships will determine the focus of the psychotherapy.
• Discuss the client's and significant other's attitudes regarding the sexual dysfunction.	• Provides an opportunity to express attitudes; attitude is important in determining if and when psychotherapy is indicated.
• Identify for cultural and religious attitudes toward sexual function.	• Culture and religious beliefs have a profound influence on sexual behavior and must be considered in the therapeutic plan.
• Provide anticipatory guidance if the dysfunction is physiologically based.	• Knowledge of the repercussions of the effect of physiological changes will aid the client in planning an acceptable alternative lifestyle.
• Explain the influence of attitudes on behavior.	• Such knowledge will help the client adapt to personally and culturally acceptable behavior.
• Involve the client and partner in psychotherapy if dysfunction affects the relationship.	• Communication regarding dysfunction and plans for interventions are essential to building a healthy, mutually acceptable sexual relationship.

(*Continues*)

CARE PLANNING GUIDE 20-3 Continued

NURSING DIAGNOSIS 2: *INEFFECTIVE SEXUALITY PATTERNS*

OUTCOMES

The client will attain sexual pleasure.

NOC: *SEXUAL FUNCTION*

INTERVENTION (NIC: *TEACHING SEXUALITY*)	RATIONALE
• Explain the relationship over etiological factors and concern over the client's sexuality.	• The etiology is directly related to the intensity of the behavior.
• Discuss attitudes relative to cultural and religious dictates.	• Attitude is determined by cultural and religious factors that may directly influence change in sexuality patterns.
• Teach preventative measures.	• Seeking professional help for sexuality patterns provides opportunity to teach about illness prevention and contraception.
• Teach assertiveness as needed.	• Altered sexual patterns may be a signal by a passive partner of abuse or violence. In such a setting, assertiveness can become a survival mechanism.
• Refer for supportive individual or group therapy.	• Individual therapy and supportive group therapy provide opportunity for exploring sexual conflicts in a safe, controlled environment.

LONG-TERM CONSIDERATIONS FOR THE CLIENT WITH SEXUAL DYSFUNCTION

1. Continue therapy.
2. Refer the client to a sex therapist.
3. Refer the client for appropriate medical interventions.

Treatment of sexual dysfunction is beyond the scope of practice of nonspecialist nurses. The nurse's primary role is assessment, education, and referral.

Note: The care plans are adapted from *Plans of Care for Specialty Practice: Psychiatric Mental Health Nursing*, by M. Coler and K. G. Vincent, 1995, Clifton Park, NY: Delmar Cengage Learning.

NURSING CARE PLAN: NURSING PROCESS FORMAT 20-3

Ken is an 18-year-old man. He comes to see a nurse for an employment physical. In the process of taking a general nursing history, the nurse asks questions related to sexual health. Specifically, she asks Ken if he is sexually active and if he has any concerns over matters of sexual health. Ken responds that, indeed, he does have some concerns. He describes having ambivalence over his sexual preferences; he has had a personal

(*Continues*)

NURSING CARE PLAN: NURSING PROCESS FORMAT 20-3 (Continued)

history of both heterosexual and homosexual encounters. He is not sure which is more comfortable for him. He feels pressured to decide what his preferences are. He discloses that he has always been somewhat "preoccupied" with academic and work successes, so that he has had somewhat limited social interactions. He does not feel that he has a strong sexual drive and states he has never had anyone with whom he could discuss these issues. His family includes parents (married and living together), two brothers who are both heterosexual, and one young sister who is 11 years old. Ken believes that no one in his family would either understand or support his exploring his sexual concerns.

NURSING DIAGNOSIS *Ineffective sexuality pattern,* related to conflicts with sexual orientation, as evidenced by reported concerns over sexual behaviors and activities.

OUTCOMES	NIC	NURSING ACTIONS	EVALUATION
• Client will explore his own sexuality and will reflect on issues to gain insight regarding his un-comfortable feelings.	• Sexual counseling	• Let the client know that the nurse is willing to talk about these matters as a professional. Make sure he knows that all discussions are/will be confidential and that the nurse can assist him in exploring his concerns and his feelings. • Make an appointment for Ken to talk with the nurse the following week. • Provide a safe environment where Ken can describe his very personal, sexual concerns in the presence of a caring professional. • Encourage Ken to discuss his sexuality as well as his relationships with others in both a social and a sexual sense. • Help Ken understand where the "pressure to decide" on his personal sexual preferences is coming from.	Ken returned to talk with the nurse for three appointments. He talked freely only after the first meeting. He disclosed that he had felt pressure from peers and his parents to declare his sexual preference and that he believed that sexuality was not as important to him as it seemed to be to others. He stated he did not need to deal with these issues with the nurse again, although he was grateful for the oppor-tunity to explore them. He stated he felt much less anxious about his sexuality at this time.

REFLECTIVE QUESTIONS

1. **ASSESSMENT**
   Do you feel that Ken's current sexual status needs further exploration? Does it seem worthwhile to assess other aspects of his life as well?

2. **NURSING DIAGNOSIS**
   Is this the correct diagnosis? Could you make another diagnosis based on the information you have been given?

(*Continues*)

NURSING CARE PLAN: NURSING PROCESS FORMAT 20-3 (Continued)

3. **OUTCOMES**
Is it appropriate to have as an outcome that the client will explore something rather than that the client will do something? Why or why not?
4. **NURSING ACTIONS**
Should the nurse be thinking of something else?
5. **EVALUATION**
Is this client ready to terminate sessions with the nurse? Have the nurse and client achieved a good outcome?

NURSING CARE PLAN: CONCEPT MAP FORMAT 20-3

Sexual Dysfunction

BACKGROUND INFORMATION

Diane is a 40-year-old woman who describes herself as having lost interest in sexual expressions/activities. She is talking with a nurse at the clinic where she goes for primary care. The nurse, Helen, has been offering classes for women undergoing menopause to assist them in understanding the physiological changes of "change of life." Diane expresses some of her concerns and feelings to Helen because she has not had anyone to talk with about personal issues before. For the past 15 or so years, Diane says that her children had been the focus of her life, and now that they are growing up, they are needing her less. Diane feels fatigued and not happy about her life at this time. Diane believes that she has lost interest in previously enjoyable activities. She is married and has been for over 20 years. She and her husband get along reasonably well, but Diane is feeling somewhat unhappy in her marriage. Diane tells the nurse that she likes to think of herself as "pretty" but is uncomfortable with bodily changes common to middle-age. She doesn't want to engage in sexual activities but feels that she should want to. She is unable to talk to her husband about her feelings, and asks Helen if other women feel the same way as she does.

INITIAL ASSESSMENT AND REFLECTION

Nurse Helen understands that Diane is talking to her about issues that Diane has not talked about with others. Helen recognizes that Diane has the characteristics of ineffective sexual pattern, and is also concerned about issues of self-esteem, body image, and the effects these concerns can have on Diane's marriage.

INITIAL REVIEW OF NURSING DIAGNOSES

The nurse identifies the following nursing diagnoses:
- *Ineffective sexuality pattern*
- *Chronic low self-esteem*
- *Disturbed body image*

(Continues)

NURSING CARE PLAN: CONCEPT MAP FORMAT 20-3 (Continued)

The following concept map reveals the relationships that point to the priorities of care:

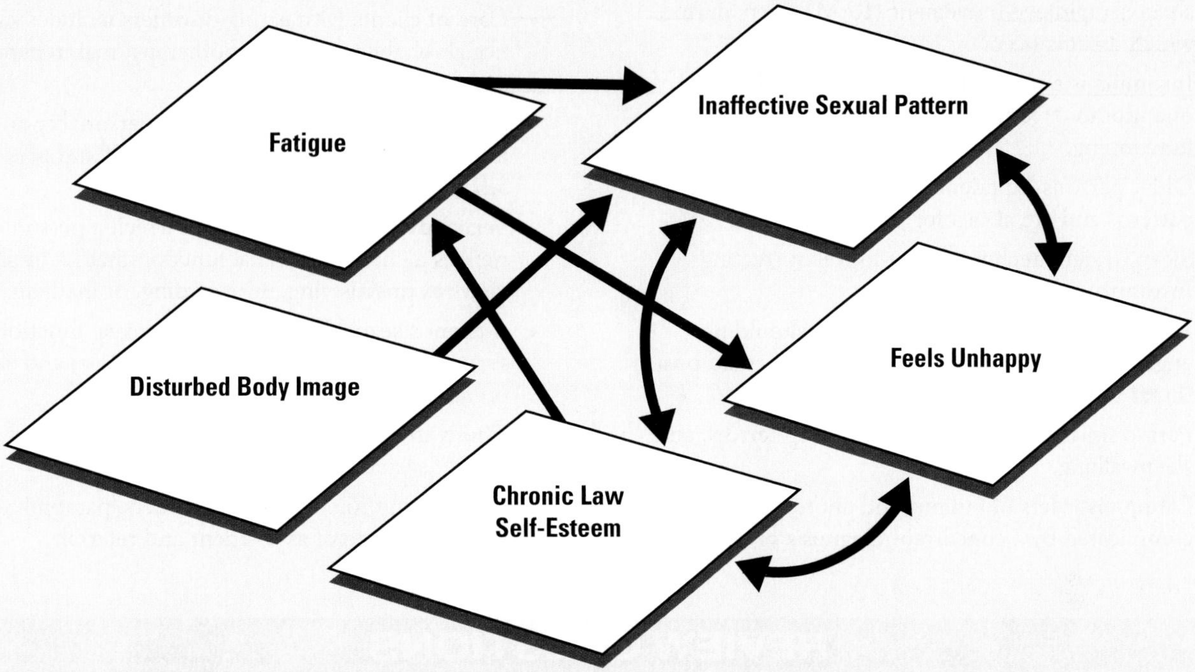

CONCEPT MAP OF ISSUES AND PROBLEMS (DELMAR/CENGAGE LEARNING.)

PRIORITIES OF CARE

The concept map points to the focal issues of impaired sexual patterns, and this focal issue is affirmed by Diane's discussion of her sexual issues with the nurse. However, the concept map also indicates that self-esteem, body image, and feelings of fatigue/unhappiness all contribute to the impaired sexual functions. Nurse Helen will choose nursing interventions based on the holistic assessment provided and deal with the focal issue and the other issues of body image and self-esteem at the same time.

NURSING INTERVENTIONS

Nursing interventions that Helen planned focus on the basic activities a nurse can provide related to sexual counseling: establishing a trusting nurse-client therapeutic relationship, permitting the client to ask and receive answers to any questions related to sexual functioning, being ready to explore the effects that changes in sexuality can have on significant others, helping the client to express the grief/anger that alterations in body appearance/functioning can have on sexuality, and referring the client to a sex therapist, as appropriate. Further, Helen planned interventions related to self-esteem and body image: identifying strengths, conveying Diane's ability to handle her own life situations, exploring reasons for self-criticism, and assisting Diane to discuss bodily changes affected by healthy aging.

OUTCOMES/EVALUTION

Helen began by providing a private place and time for Diane to explore her issues related to disinterest in sexuality. Diane asked many questions about the common issues related to sexuality in peri- and postmenopausal women (vaginal dryness, concerns about appearance, concerns about changes in relationships). When Helen answered Diane's questions, it seemed that Diane become increasingly relieved to know that what she was experiencing was not unusual for women in situations similar to her own. Helen provided sexual counseling for three sessions where Diane could explain her feelings, seek factual information, and reflect on her own marriage and relationships. Helen focused Diane to reflect on her areas of strength: health, fitness, and independence, and encouraged Diane to think of herself as moving into late middle-age as a healthy woman. At the end of this time, Diane expressed no need to further explore sexual issues and declined the offer for referral to a sexual therapist.

KEY CONCEPTS

- Sleep occurs in five stages, with marked individual variation in time spent in each sleep cycle. Stage 5 sleep is rapid-eye-movement (REM) sleep, during which dreams occur.
- Insomnia is a psychiatric problem when it lasts one month or longer and leads to impairment of functioning.
- Older persons experience changing of their sleep patterns and are at risk for Insomnia.
- Sleep hygiene techniques are useful in treating Insomnia.
- Persons with Primary Hypersomnia should not engage in activities where a sleep attack could pose a threat to self or others (such as driving).
- Parasomnias include nightmares, sleep terrors, and sleepwalking.
- Eating disorders of bulimia and anorexia are often complicated by a concurrent diagnosis of depression, low self-esteem, and the client's strong denial of the problem.
- Care of clients with eating disorders includes nutritional rehabilitation, psychotherapy, maintenance, and follow-up.
- Sexuality is part of each person's personality and influences how each person views self and presents self to others.
- Sexual dysfunction is a state in which a person experiences a change in sexual function that he or she views as unsatisfying, unrewarding, or inadequate.
- A client's sexual history includes sexual functioning; sexual thoughts, fantasies, and behaviors; and sexual preferences.
- There are two categories of sexual disorders: disorders of sexual functioning and paraphilias.
- The nursing role in sexual disorders/paraphilias is most often one of assessment and referral.

REVIEW QUESTIONS

1. A nurse is developing a care plan for a client being admitted for Anorexia Nervosa. Which of the following will be the most difficult nursing diagnosis to successfully resolve?
   1. Disturbed body image
   2. Alteration in nutrition
   3. Knowledge deficit
   4. Social isolation

2. The nurse conducts a complete physical and mental health assessment on a client diagnosed with Anorexia Nervosa who is admitted to the psychiatric unit. The primary purpose for conducting a complete physical assessment is which of the following?
   1. It is a requirement of the hospital
   2. To establish a baseline for future treatments
   3. To determine whether the client has been physically abused
   4. To determine if there are other medical conditions present

3. The advance practice nurse is meeting with a new client who is being seen for sexual dysfunction. The primary goal of therapy will be which of the following?
   1. Restoring the client's sexual function
   2. Assisting the client to resolve any sexual conflicts
   3. Promoting a more satisfactory life style
   4. Preventing further sexual dysfunction

4. A client arrives at the clinic and complains to the nurse that he has been having difficulty sleeping at night. He states, "My job is very intense. I have to leave for work at 6 A.M. and the day is nonstop. I work late many evenings and when I get home I have to make myself do my daily exercise. I watch the news and cook dinner. After dinner, I have a light dessert with a cup of coffee." The nurse's recommendation would be which of the following?
   1. "Maybe you should consider changing jobs."
   2. "You should probably have your doctor prescribe a sleeping pill for you."
   3. "As an adult you do not need more than three to four hours of sleep at night."
   4. "You should not drink coffee late at night because it is a stimulant."

5. A client is admitted for bulimia. After lunch, the nurse finds the client in the restroom purging. The nurse knows that purging for a bulimic client serves which of the following purposes?
   1. An allergic reaction to the food served
   2. A method of getting approval from the staff
   3. An expression of anger against the client's parents
   4. Reduces the anxiety related to the guilt of overeating

6. A woman approaches a nurse regarding a problem she is having with her husband. The woman recently discovered that her husband secretly enjoys wearing women's clothing/undergarments. The

woman is distraught at the idea that her husband, in her words, "is gay and wants to be a woman." The nurse should explain that:
1. Transvestic Fetishism, in and of itself, does not guarantee that a man is homosexual or wishes to become a woman. Most men involved in transvestic behaviors are heterosexual and have no gender identity disorders.
2. While her husband may not wish to be a woman, he is obviously homosexual, and the wife should seek more information regarding initiating divorce proceedings.
3. The wife should behave less aggressively and domineering around her husband, so that he may comfortably revert back to his naturally masculine, dominant role in the relationship.
4. The husband does secretly wish to become a woman and his wife should help him by providing brochures and books to him regarding sex-reassignment surgery.

7. A 22-year-old man is brought in for a consultation by his mother. His mother explains that the man has repeatedly been caught covertly touching the buttocks or breasts of unsuspecting women while on the bus or in the subway. The nurse identifies the man's behaviors as which of the following?
1. Gender identity disorder
2. Sadism
3. Frotteurism
4. Voyeurism

8. A nurse sees a patient who complains of her difficulty becoming sexually aroused by her boyfriend during intercourse. Upon further discussion, the woman discloses that she only becomes extremely aroused if her partner demeans her during intercourse or if her partner tells her that she is worthless and dirty. The nurse identifies such behavior by the woman as indicative of which of the following?
1. Sadism
2. Masochism
3. Transvestic Fetishism
4. A normal and healthy sexual desire for a woman her age

9. The nursing assessment of a client with bulimia would most likely reveal which of the following?
1. Hoarseness and dental erosion
2. Elevated potassium level
3. Underweight for height
4. Clubbing of the fingers

10. Which of the following is a common assessment finding for a client with Anorexia Nervosa?
1. Overweight by 15%
2. Amenorrhea
3. Hypertension
4. Positive self-concept

LEARNING ACTIVITIES

1. How would you assess the adequacy of sleep/rest and activity for a person in a nursing home?

2. Present a sleep hygiene regimen for your 60-year-old home health client whom you are following for hypertension.

3. What are the day-to-day risks for a person suffering from Hypersomnia?

4. How would you tell the mother of four-year-old Joey to support him during the time he is experiencing night terrors?

5. What can you do as a nurse regarding primary prevention of Bulimia Nervosa and Anorexia Nervosa?

6. What nursing diagnosis/interventions are likely present/appropriate for clients with eating disorders?

7. How does a nurse balance her roles to "monitor food intake" and to build trust with an anorexic client?

8. Define *Altered sexuality patterns*, sexual dysfunction, and sexual disorder.

9. Examine your own feelings, attitudes, and beliefs about sexual expression and appropriate sexuality. What will you do when you encounter a client with views quite different from your own?

*Study*WARE™ CONNECTION

Using your *Study*WARE™ CD-ROM

1. Complete the Concentration activity for this chapter.
2. Complete the Quiz for this chapter in Test Mode.
3. Explore the other games and activities that support this chapter.

VIDEO LINK

Read and contemplate the following questions about Susan, the client experiencing Anorexia. Then watch the video "Eating Disorders: Anorexia Nervosa" on your *Study*WARE™ CD-ROM to observe Susan's interview with a psychiatrist. Consider these questions prior to listening to the psychiatrist's analysis:

1. What factors did Susan feel influenced her to develop her eating disorder?
2. At what age did she first experience her symptoms?
3. What did Susan family and friends do to encourage her to eat?
4. Did Susan lose her appetite?
5. How did she make the determination as to which form of weight control she was going to engage in depending on the situation?
6. How did she describe her mood at various points in her illness?
7. Which screening questions are important for persons suspected of having an eating disorder?
8. Do these questions usually elicit an accurate answer?
9. What are the manifestations that must be present for a person experiencing bulimia?
10. What is the treatment regime for a person experiencing bulimia?
11. What are the requirements that determine if a person has Anorexia Nervosa?
12. What symptoms did Susan display in order for her to fit the criteria for this diagnosis?
13. When Susan was at her lowest weight, was she at risk for mortality?
14. What nursing intervention is most important when an individual is out of control?
15. Develop a care plan for Susan at this acute phase in her illness.
16. Develop a care plan that considers her long-term treatment.
17. What community resources are available for clients and families?
18. The precise cause of eating disorders is unknown. What are some of the theories that have been put forward as a cause?
19. Is there a genetic propensity toward eating disorders?
20. Is treatment more successful in early or late-onset anorexia?
21. What is the prevalence among young adolescent and young adult females?
22. Consider the societal influences of Anorexia Nervosa and Bulimia Nervosa. What can you as a nurse do with regard to primary prevention?

REFERENCES

Agras, S. (1987). *Eating disorders.* New York: Pergamon.

Alessi, C. A., Martin, J. L., Webber, A. P, Cynthia Kim, E., Harker, J. O., & Josephson, K. R.(2005). Randomized, controlled trial of a nonpharmacological intervention to improve abnormal sleep/wake patterns in nursing home residents. *Journal of the American Geriatric Society, 53*(5), 803–810.

American Psychiatric Association. (2000). *Diagnostic and statistical manual* (Fourth Edition-Text Revision). Washington, DC: Author.

Anonymous. (1996). Pandora and the problem of evil. *Lancet, 347,* 1.

Anonymous (2007). Putting "sleepdriving" and new safety warning in perspective. *Johns Hopkins Medical Letter: Health after 50, 19*(6), 1–2.

Bancroft, J. (2002). The medicalization of female sexual dysfunction: The need for caution. *Archives of Sexual Behavior, 31*(5), 431–435.

Becker, J. V., & Kavoussi, R. J. (1994). Sexual and gender identity disorders. In R. E. Hales, S. C. Yudofsky, & J. A. Talbott (Eds.), *The American Psychiatric Press textbook of psychiatry* (2nd ed., pp. 666–667). Washington DC: American Psychiatric Association.

Berkman, N. D., Bulik, C. M., Brownley, K. A., Lohr, K. N., Sedway, J. A., Rooks, A., et al. (2006). Management of eating disorders. *Evidence Report/Technology Assessment* (Full Report; 135), 1–166.

Berkman, N. D., Lohr, K. N., & Bulik, C. M. (2007). Outcomes of eating disorders: A systematic review of the literature. *International Journal of Eating Disorders, 40*(4), 293–309.

Berman, J. R., Berman, L. A., Toler, S. M., Gill, J., Haughie, S., & Sildenafil Study Group. (2003). Safety and efficacy of sildenafil citrate for the treatment of female sexual arousal disorder: A double-blind, placebo controlled study. *Journal of Urology, 70*(6 Pt. 1), 2333–2338.

Bhat, A., & El Solh, A. A. (2008). Management of narcolepsy. *Expert Opinion on Pharmacotherapy, 9*(10), 1721–1733.

Bossuyt, P. M. (2008). Interpreting diagnostic test accuracy studies. *Seminars in Hematology, 45*(3), 189–195.

Braun, C. M., & Chouinard, M. J. (1992). Is anorexia nervosa a neuropsychological disease? *Neuropsychological Review, 3,* 171–212.

Bruch, H. (1973). *Eating disorders.* New York: Basic Books.

Bruch, H. (1978). *The golden cage: The enigma of anorexia nervosa.* Cambridge, MA: Harvard University Press.

Cahill, C. (1994). Implementing an inpatient eating disorders program. *Perspectives in Psychiatric Care, 30,* 26–29.

Cantor, J. M., Kabani, N., Christensen, B. K., Zipursky, R. B., Barbaree, H. E., Dickey, R., et al. (2008). Cerebral white matter deficiencies in pedophilic men. *Journal of Psychiatric Research, 42*(3), 167–183.

Chipkevitch, E. (1994). Brain tumors and anorexia nervosa syndrome. *Brain and Development, 16,* 175–179, 180–182.

Chitty, K. K. (1991). The primary prevention role of nurse in eating disorders. *Nursing Clinics of North America, 26*, 789–800.

Cohen, M. N. (1979). *Lewis Carroll, photography of children*. Philadelphia: Rosenbach Foundation and Clarkson W. Potter.

Coler, M., & Vincent, K. G. (1995). *Plans of care for specialty practice: Psychiatric mental health nursing*. Clifton Park, NY: Thomson Delmar Learning.

Crow, S. J., & Mitchell, J. E. (1994). Rational therapy of eating disorders. *Drugs, 48*, 372–379.

Crowther, J. H., Armey, M., Luce, K. H., Dalton, G. R., & Leahey, T. (2008). The point prevalence of bulimic disorders from 1990 to 2004. *International Journal of Eating Disorders, 41*, 491–497.

Davis, S., Papalia, M. A., Norman, R. J., O'Neill, S., Redelman, M., Williamson, M., et al. (2008). Safety and efficacy of a testosterone metered-dose transdermal spray for treating decreased sexual satisfaction in premenopausal women: A randomized trial. *Annals of Internal Medicine, 148*(8), 569–577.

Dierks, M. R., Jordan, J. K., & Sheehan, A. H. (2007). Prazosin treatment of nightmares related to posttraumatic stress disorder. *Annals of Pharmacotherapy, 41*(6), 1013–1017.

Eckert, E. D., Halmi, K. A., Marchi, P., Grove, W., & Crosby, R. (1994). Ten-year follow-up of anorexia nervosa: Clinical course and outcome. *Psychological Medicine, 25*, 143–156.

Edinger, J. D., & Sampson, W. S. (2003). A primary care "friendly" cognitive behavioral insomnia therapy. *Sleep, 26*(2), 177–182.

Emmelot-Vonk, M. H., Verhaar, H. J., Nakhai Pour, H. R., Aleman, A., Lock, T. M., Bosch, J. L., et al. (2008). Effect of testosterone supplementation on functional mobility, cognition, and other parameters in older men: A randomized controlled trial. *Journal of the American Medical Association, 299*(1), 39–52.

Fagan, P. J., Wise, T. N., Schmidt, C. W., Jr., & Berlin, F. S. (2002). Pedophilia. *Journal of the American Medical Association, 288*(19), 2458–2465.

Fedorowicz, V. J., Falissard, B., Foulon, C., Dardennes, R., Divac, S. M., Guelfi, J. D., et al. (2007). Factors associated with suicidal behaviors in a large French sample of inpatients with eating disorders. *International Journal of Eating Disorders, 40*(7), 589–595.

Fosnight, S. M., Holder, C. M., Allen, K. R., Hazelett, S. (2004). A strategy to decrease the use of risky drugs in the elderly. *Cleveland Clinic Journal of Medicine, 71*(7), 561–568.

Freund, K. M., Graham, S. M., Lesky, L. G., & Moskowitz, M. A. (1993). Detection of bulimia in a primary care setting. *Journal of General Internal Medicine, 8*, 236–242.

Fride, E., Bregman, T., & Kirkham, T. C. (2005). Endocannabinoids and food intake: Newborn suckling and appetite regulation in adulthood. *Experimental Biology and Medicine (Maywood), 230*(4), 225–234.

Goldstein, B. (1976). *Human sexuality*. New York: McGraw Hill.

Gruenewald, D. A., & Matsumoto, A. M. (2003). Testosterone supplementation therapy for older men: Potential benefits and risks. *Journal of the American Geriatric Society, 51*(1), 101–15; discussion 115.

Gull, W. W. (1868). The address in medicine delivered before the annual meeting of the British Medical Association, at Oxford. *Lancet, 2*, 171–176.

Hall, R. C.W., & Hall, R. C. W (2007) A profile of pedophilia: Definition, characteristics of offenders, recidivism, treatment outcomes, and forensic issues. *Mayo Clinic Proceedings, 82*(4), 57–71.

Harmat, L, Takas, J., & Bodzs, R. (2008). Music improves quality of sleep in students. *Journal of Advanced Nursing, 62*(3), 327–336.

Hauri, P. J., Silber, M. H., & Boeve, B. F. (2007). The treatment of parasomnias with hypnosis: A 5-year follow-up study. *Journal of Clinical Sleep Medicine, 3*(4), 369–373.

Herdman, H. (Ed). (2009). *Nursing diagnoses: Definitions and classifications, 2009–2011*. Oxford: Wiley Blackwell.

Hoek, H. W. (1991). The incidence and prevalence of anorexia nervosa and bulimia nervosa in primary care. *Psychological Medicine, 21*, 455–460.

Hoek, H. W., & van Hoeken, D. (2003). Review of the prevalence and incidence of eating disorders. *International Journal of Eating Disorders, 34*(4), 383–396.

Holbrook, A. M., Crowther, R., Lotter, A., Cheng, C., & King, D. (2000). Meta-analysis of benzodiazepine use in the treatment of insomnia. *Canadian Medical Association Journal, 162*(2), 225–233.

Hughes, J. R. (2007) Review of medical reports on pedophilia. *Clinical Pediatrics. 46*, 667–682.

Huppert, F. A., Van Niekork, J. K., & Herbert, J. (2000). Dihydroepiandrosterone (DHEA) supplementation for cognition and well-being. *Cochrane Database System Review.*

Irwin, E. G. (1993). A focused overview of anorexia and bulimia. *Archives of Psychiatric Nursing, 7*, 347–352.

Joughin, N. A., Crisp, A. H., Gowers, S. G., & Bhat, A. V. (1991). The clinical features of late onset anorexia nervosa. *Postgraduate Medical Journal, 67*, 973–977.

Kahan, S. E., Seftel, A. D., & Resnick, M. I. (2000). Sildenafil and the Internet. *Journal of Urology, 63*(3), 919–923.

Kawahara, S., Akashiba, T., Akahoshi, T., & Horie, T. (2005). Nasal CPAP improves the quality of life and lessens the depressive symptoms in patients with obstructive sleep apnea syndrome. *Internal Medicine, 44*(5), 422–427.

Kaye, W. H., Klump, K. L., Frank, G. K., & Strober, M. (2000). Anorexia and bulimia nervosa. *Annual Review of Medicine, 51*, 299–313.

Keel, P. K., Mitchell, J. E., Miller, K. B., Davis, T. L., & Crow, S. J. (1999). Long-term outcome of bulimia nervosa. *Archives of General Psychiatry, 56*(1), 63–69.

Kenworthy, T., Adams, C. E., Bilby, C., Brooks-Gordon, B., & Fenton, M.(2004). Psychological interventions for those who have sexually offended or are at risk of offending. *Cochrane Database of Systematic Reviews*, (3),CD004858.

Kim, S. W., & Paick, J. S. (1999). Short-term analysis of the effects of as needed use of sertraline at 5 P.M. for the treatment of premature ejaculation. *Urology, 54*(3), 544–547.

Kollai, M., Bonyhay, I., Jokkel, G., & Szonyi, L. (1994). Cardiac vagal hyperactivity in adolescent anorexia nervosa. *European Heart Journal, 15*, 1113–1118.

Kolton, D. J., Boer, A., Boer, D. P. (2001). A revision of the Abel and Becker Cognition Scale for intellectually disabled sexual offenders. *Sex Abuse, 13*(3), 217–219.

Krahn, L. E., Miller, B. W., & Bergstrom, L. R. (2008). Rapid resolution of intense suicidal ideation after treatment of severe obstructive sleep apnea. *Journal of Clinical Sleep Medicine, 4*(1), 64–65.

Kripke, D. F. (2007). Greater incidence of depression with hypnotic use than with placebo. *BMC Psychiatry, 7*, 42.

Krystal, A. D., Walsh, J. K., Lasha, E., Caron, J., Amato, D. A., Wessel, T. C., et al. (2003). Sustained efficacy of eszopicione over 6 months of nightly treatment: Results of a randomized, double-blind, placebo-controlled study in adults with chronic insomnia. *Sleep, 26*(7), 793–799.

Lamberg, L. (2005). Researchers seek roots of pedophilia. *Journal of the American Medical Association, 294*(5), 546–547.

Langer, L. M., Warheit, G. J., & Zimmerman, R. S. (1991). Epidemiological study of problem eating behaviors and related attitudes in the general population. *Addictive Behaviors, 16*, 67–73.

Lareau, R., Benson, L., Watcharotone, K., & Manguba, G. (2008). Examining the feasibility of implementing specific nursing interventions to promote sleep in hospitalized elderly patients. *Geriatric Nursing, 29*(3), 197–206.

Lawton, G. (2006) Get up and go. *New Scientist, 189*(2539), 34–38.

LeMone, P. (1993). Validation of the defining characteristics of altered sexuality patterns. *Nursing Diagnosis, 4*, 56–62.

LeMone, P., & Weber, J. (1995). Validating gender specific defining characteristics of altered sexuality. *Nursing Diagnosis, 6*, 61–69.

Lilly, R. A. (2003). Bulimia nervosa. *British Medical Journal, 327*, 380–381.

Love, C. C., & Seaton, H. (1991). Eating disorders: Highlights of nursing assessment and therapeutics. *Nursing Clinics of North America, 26*, 677–697.

Lubkin, I. (1990). *Chronic illness: Impact and interventions.* Boston: Jones and Bartlett.

Malesky, L. A., Jr. (2007). Predatory online behavior: Modus operandi of convicted sex offenders in identifying potential victims and contacting minors over the Internet. *Journal of Child Sexual Abuse, 16*(2), 23–32.

Marshall, W. L., Jones, R., Ward, T., Johnston, P., & Barbaree, R. E. (1991). Treatment outcome with sex offenders. *Clinical Psychology Review, 11*, 465–485.

Mayor, S. (2004). Pfizer will not apply for a license for sildenafil for women. *British Medical Journal, 328*(7439) 542.

Mehler, P. S. (2003). Clinical practice: Bulimia nervosa. *New England Journal of Medicine, 349*(9), 875–881.

Mond, J. M., Hay, P. J., Rodgers, B., Owen, C., & Beumont, P. J. (2004). Validity of the Eating Disorder Examination Questionnaire (EDE-Q) in screening for eating disorders in community samples. *Behavior Research and Therapy, 42*(5), 551–567.

Mond, J. M., Myers, T. C., Crosby, R. D., Hay, P. J., Rodgers, B., Morgan, J. F., et al. (2008). Screening for eating disorders in primary care: EDE-Q versus SCOFF. *Behaviour Research and Therapy, 46*(5), 612–622.

Montgomery, P., & Dennis, J. (2003). Cognitive behavioral interventions for sleep problems in adults aged 60+. *Cochrane Database Systematic Review, 1*, CD003161.

Morales, A., Barada, J., & Wyllie, M. G. (2007). A review of the current status of topical treatments for premature ejaculation. *BJU International, 100*(3), 493–501.

Morley, J. E., & Perry, H. M., III. (2003). Andropause: An old concept in new clothing. *Clinical Geriatric Medicine, 19*(3), 507–538.

Myer, S. A., & O'Brien, A. (1993). Multisystem complications of bulimia: A critical care case. *Dimensions of Critical Care Nursing, 12*, 194–203.

National Institutes of Health (NIH). (1990). *The treatment of sleep disorders of older people.* NIH Consensus Statement, March 26–28, 8(3), 1–22. Bethesda, MD: Author.

Okabe, K. (1993). Assessment of emaciation in relation to threat to life in anorexia nervosa. *Internal Medicine, 32*, 837–842.

Palmer, T. A. (1990). Anorexia nervosa, bulimia nervosa: Causal theories and treatment. *Nurse Practitioner, 15*, 12, 14–16, 18, 21.

Peate, I. (2003). Male menopause: Possible causes, symptoms and treatment. *British Journal of Nursing, 12*(2), 80–84.

Pope, H. G., & Hudson, J. I. (1989). Eating disorders. In H. I. Kaplan & B. J. Sadock (Eds.), *Comprehensive textbook of psychiatry* (20th ed., pp. 1854–1864). Baltimore: Williams & Wilkins.

Powers, P. S., Powers, H. P. (1984). Inpatient treatment of anorexia nervosa. *Psychosomatics, 25*, 512–527.

Pyle, R. L., Mitchell, J. E., Eckert, E. D., Hatsukami, D., Pomeroy, C., & Zimmerman, R. (1990). Maintenance treatment and 6-month outcome for bulimic patients who respond to initial treatment. *American Journal of Psychiatry, 147*, 871–887.

Rastam, M., & Gillberg, C. (1991). The family background in anorexia nervosa: A population-based study. *Journal of the American Academy of Child and Adolescent Psychiatry, 30*, 238–239.

Redmond, G. P. (1999). Hormones and sexual function. *International Journal of Fertility and Women's Medicine, 44*(4), 193–197.

Remschmidt, H., Wienand, F., & Wewetzer, C. (1990). The long-term course of anorexia nervosa. In H. Remschmidt & M. Schmidt (Eds.), *Anorexia nervosa* (pp. 127–136). Toronto: Hogrefe & Huber.

Roseborough, G. S., & Felix, W. A. (1994). Disseminated intravascular coagulation complicating gastric perforation in a bulimic woman. *Canadian Journal of Surgery, 37*, 55–58.

Ruggiero, J. S. (2003). Correlates of fatigue in critical care nurses. *Research in Nursing and Health, 26*, 434–444.

Ryan, V., Malson, A., Clarke, S., Anderson, G., & Kohn, M. (2006). Discursive constructions of "eating disorder nursing": An analysis of nurses' accounts of eating disorder patients. *European Eating Disorder Review, 14*(2), 125–135.

Salem, E. A., Wilson, S. K., Bissada, N. K., Delk, J. R., Hellstrom, W. J., & Cleves, M. A. (2008). Tramadol HCL has promise in on-demand use to treat premature ejaculation. *Journal of Sexual Medicine, 5*(1), 188–193.

Salisbury, J. J., & Mitchell, J. E. (1991). Bone mineral density and anorexia nervosa in women. *American Journal of Psychiatry, 148*, 768–777.

Sartorius, A., Ruf, M., Kief, C., Demirakca, T., Bailer, J, Ende, G. et al. (2008). Abnormal amygdale activation profile in pedophilia. *European Archives of Psychiatry and Clinical Neuroscience.* 258, 271–277.

Schenck, C. H., & Mahowald, M. W. (1996). Long-term, nightly benzodiazepine treatment of injurious parasomnias and other disorders of disrupted nocturnal sleep in 170 adults. *American Journal of Medicine, 100*(3), 333–337.

Segraves, R. T. (2003). Emerging therapies for female sexual dysfunction. *Expert Opinion in Emerging Drugs, 8*(2), 515–522.

Segraves, R. T., Croft, J., Kavoussi, R., Ascher, J. A., Batey, S. R., Foster, V. J., et al. (2001). Bupropion sustained release (SR) for the treatment of hypoactive sexual desire disorder (HSSC) in nondepressed women. *Journal of Sexual and Marital Therapy, 27*(3), 303–316.

Seto, M. C. (2004). Pedophilia and sexual offenses against children. *Annual Review of Sex Research, 15*, 321–361.

Sternbach, H. (1998). Age-associated testosterone decline in men: Clinical issues for psychiatry. *American Journal of Psychiatry, 155*(10), 1310–1318.

Strober, M. (1991). Family-genetic studies of eating disorders. *Journal of Clinical Psychiatry, 52*(Suppl.), 9–12.

Studer, L. H., & Aylwin, A. S. (2006) Pedophilia: The problem with diagnosis and limitations of CBT in treatment. *Medical Hypotheses, 67*(4), 774–781.

Study Group on Anorexia Nervosa. (1995). Anorexia nervosa: Directions for future research. *Journal of Eating Disorders, 17*, 235–241.

Sullivan, P. F. (1995). Mortality in anorexia nervosa. *American Journal of Psychiatry, 152*, 1073–1074.

Thiel, A., Broocks, A., Ohlmeier, M., Jacoby, G. I., & Schussler, G. (1995). Obsessive-compulsive disorder among patients with anorexia nervosa and bulimia nervosa. *American Journal of Psychiatry, 152*, 72–75.

Treasure, J., & Holland, A. (1990). Genetic vulnerability to eating disorders: Evidence from twin and family studies. In H. Remschmidt & M. H. Schmidt (Eds.), *Anorexia nervosa* (pp. 59–68). Toronto: Hogrefe & Huber.

Trotti, L. M., Bhadriraju, S., & Rye, D. B. (2008). An update on the pathophysiology and genetics of restless legs syndrome. *Current Neurology and Neuroscience Reports, 8*(4), 281–287.

Vanderycken, W., & Van Deth, R. (1994). *From fasting saints to anorexic girls.* New York: New York University Press.

Vestergaard, P., Emborg, C., Stoving, R. K., Hagen, C., Mosekilde, L., & Brixen, P. (2003). Patients with eating disorders. A high-risk group for fractures. *Orthopedic Nursing, 22*(5), 325–331.

Waldinger, M. D. (2007). Premature ejaculation: Definition and drug treatment. *Drugs, 67*(4), 547–568.

Walfish, S., Stenmark, D. E., Sarco, D., Shealy, J. S., & Krone, A. M. (1992). Incidence of bulimia in substance misusing women in residential treatment. *International Journal of the Addictions, 27,* 425–433.

Warheit, G. J., Langer, L. M., Zimmerman, R. S., & Biafora, F. A. (1993). Prevalence of bulimic behaviors and bulimia among a sample of the general population. *American Journal of Epidemiology, 137,* 569–576.

White, J. H. (1999). The development and clinical testing of an outpatient program for women with bulimia nervosa. *Archives of Psychiatric Nursing, 13*(4), 179–191.

Wilson, C. P., Hogan, C. C., & Mintz, I. L. (1985). *Fear of being fat: The treatment of anorexia nervosa and bulimia.* New York: Jason Aronson.

LITERARY REFERENCES

Benedict, R. (1974). *The chrysanthemum and the sword.* New York: Houghton Mifflin Company.

Bird, J. (1976). *Percy Grainger.* London: Paul Elek.

Byron, Lord. Don Juan, Canto 2, LXXX. Retrieved April 5, 2005, from http://website.lineone.net/~ssiggeman.donjuan2.html.

Calisher, H. (1982). The scream on Fifty-seventh Street. In J. C. Oates (Ed.), *Night walks: A bedside companion* (p. 40). Princeton: Ontario Review Press.

Dekker, T. (1982). On sleep. In J. C. Oates (Ed.), *Night walks: A bedside companion* (p. 138). Princeton: Ontario Review Press.

Dickens, C. (1969). *The posthumous papers of the Pickwick Club.* New York: Oxford University Press.

Dickens, C. (1982). Night walks. In J. C. Oates (Ed.), *Night walks: A bedside companion* (pp. 3–12). Princeton: Ontario Review Press.

Gillies, M., & Pear, D. (1994). *The all-round man: Selected papers of Percy Grainger, 1914–1961.* London: Clarendon Press.

Gray, R. (1994). *Nightmare of ecstasy: The life and art of Edward D. Wood, Jr.* Portland, OR: Feral House.

Hoppe, A. (1979). *The San Francisco Chronicle,* April 17, p. 35.

Mishkin, J. (1982). Insomnia. In J. C. Oates (Ed.), *Night walks: A bedside companion* (pp. 251–252). Princeton: Ontario Review Press.

Morton, B. (1992). To half fight nature: Percy Grainger. In T. P. Lewis (Ed.), *A source guide to the music of Percy Grainger* (pp. 32–37). White Plains, NY: ProAM Music Resources.

Sade, Marquis de. (1992). *The misfortune of virtue, and other early tales* (D. Coward, Trans./Ed.). Oxford: Oxford University Press.

Schonberg, H. C. (1992). Percy Grainger. In T. P. Lewis (Ed.), *A source guide to the music of Percy Grainger* (pp. 12–13). White Plains, NY: ProAM Music Resources.

Vanderycken, W., & Van Deth, R. (1994). *From fasting saints to anorexic girls.* New York: New York University Press.

SUGGESTED READINGS

Colton, H. R., & Altevogt, B. M. (Ed). (2006). *Sleep disorders and sleep deprivation: An unmet public health problem.* Washington, DC: National Academic Press.

Herrin, M. (2007). *The parents' guide to eating disorders: Supporting self esteem, healthy eating and positive body image at home* (2nd ed.). Carlsbad, CA: Gurze Books.

Leach, K. (1999). *In the shadow of the dreamchild.* London: Peter Owen.

Lee-Chaing, T. L. (Ed.). (2006). *Sleep: A comprehensive handbook.* Hoboken, NJ: Wiley-Liss.

Taylor R., Wakeling E., & Bunnell P. C. (2002). *Lewis Carroll, photographer.* Princeton, NJ: Princeton University Press.

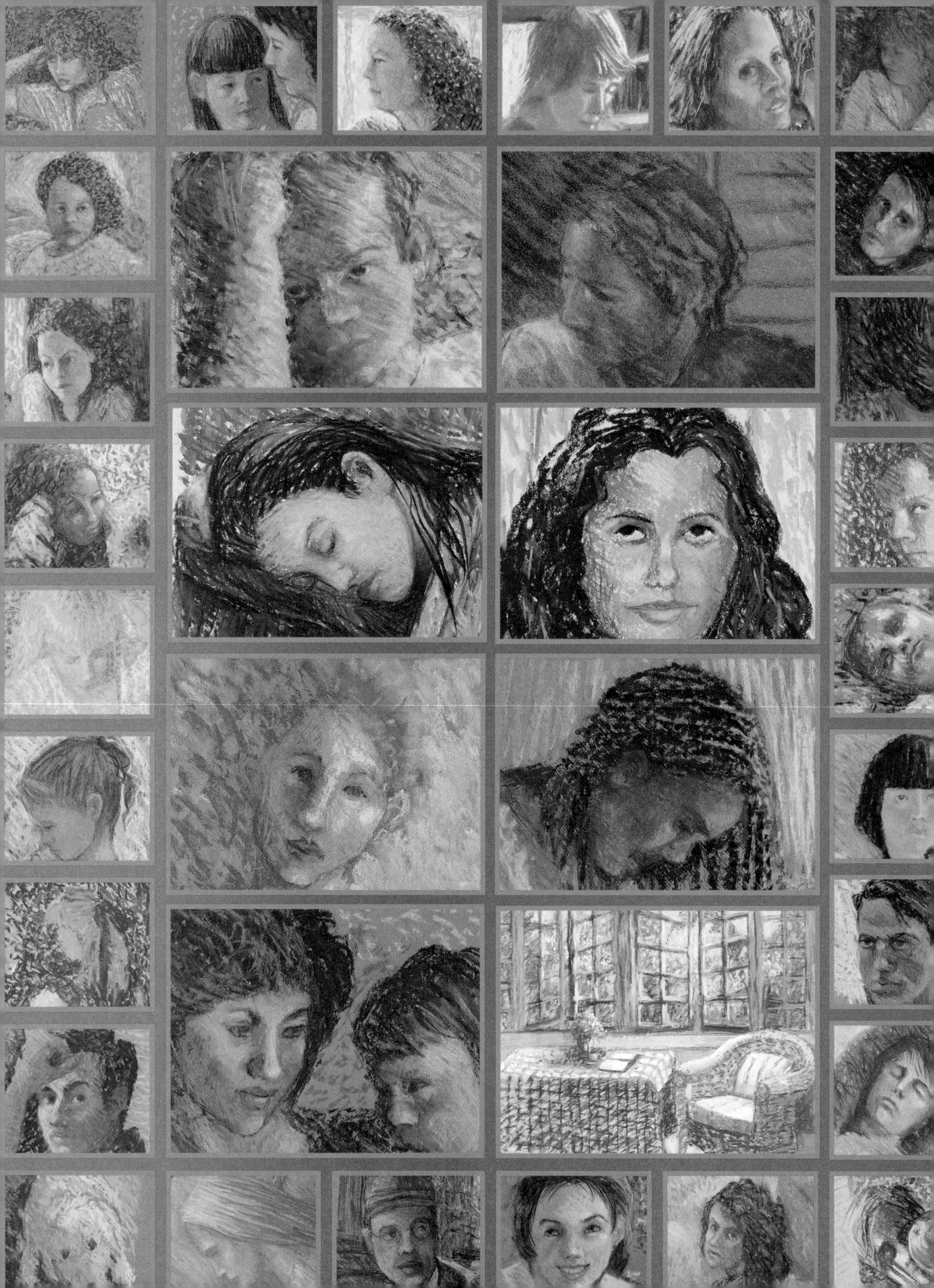

UNIT 3 Special Populations

What are the psychological challenges facing physically ill persons? Why should we be concerned about the mental health needs of persons in jail? Do children and adolescents have unique mental health concerns? How can the nurse recognize elderly people suffering from Alzheimer's disease? Violence continues to be a daily experience of many individuals, especially women and youth. What are the mental health implications of our culture of violence?

These questions reflect the content of the six chapters on *Special Populations*.

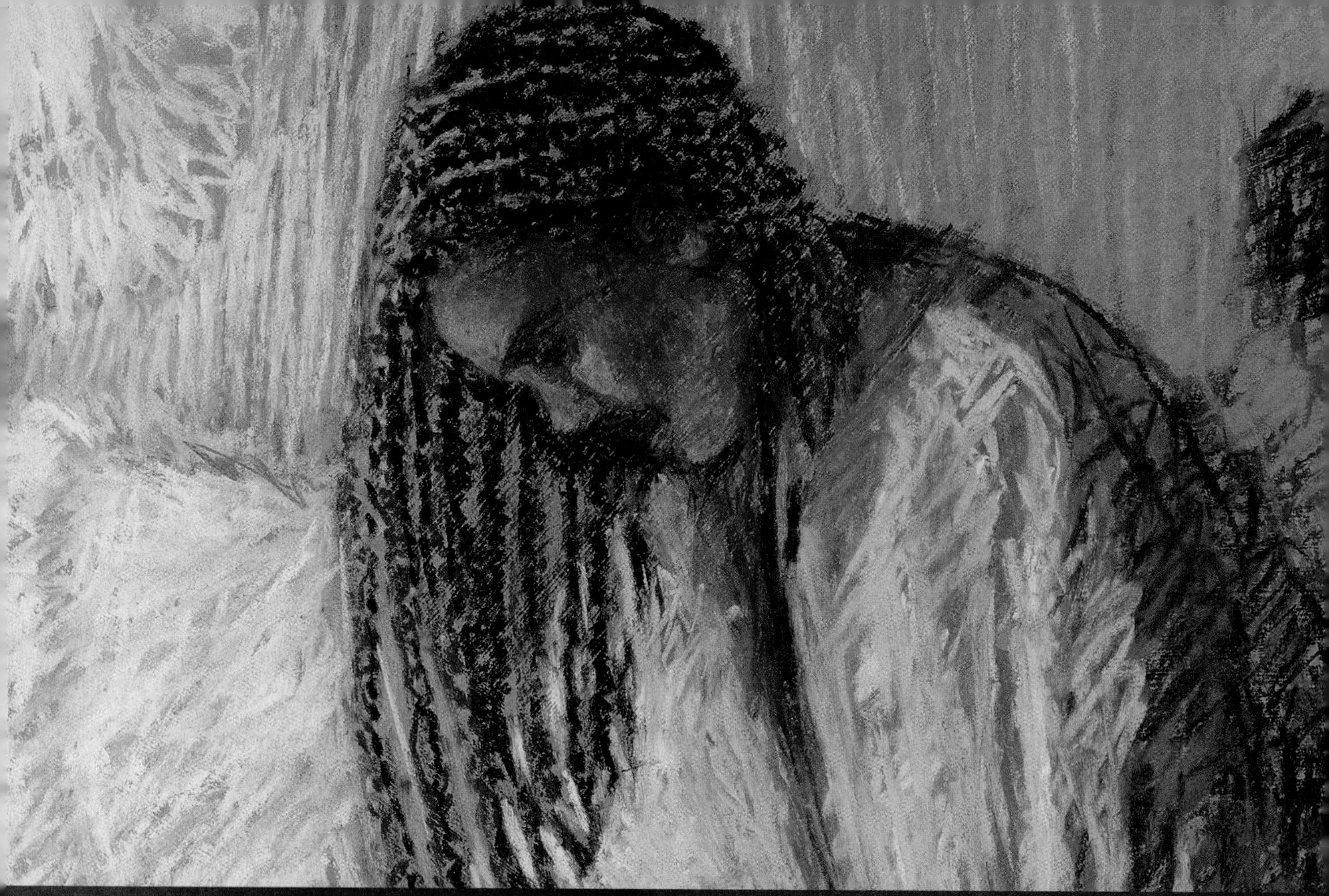

Future Tense

Physical Illness and Emotional Health

Think about a time when you were physically ill, particularly a time when your illness was serious or lasted a long time. How did your physical illness affect your emotions and mood?
Did you experience any of the following?

- ***Fear***
- ***Shame***
- ***Guilt***
- ***Depression***
- ***Anger***
- ***Loneliness***

Most nurses today recognize the connection between body and mind. When there is a physical illness, one can expect effects on emotions or mood, and these effects may have an impact on prognosis for recovery from the physical illness.

In this chapter, we will explore the sometimes dramatic emotional outcomes of physical illnesses to provide you with heightened awareness of your clients' needs for psychological support.

CHAPTER 21

The Physically Ill Client Experiencing Emotional Distress

NOREEN CAVAN FRISCH
LAWRENCE E. FRISCH

CHAPTER OUTLINE

COMPETENCIES

Upon completion of this chapter, the reader should be able to:

1. Identify those situations where a physical illness produces emotional stress to the point where a client may present with psychological symptoms.
2. Describe the common reactions clients have to cancer, heart disease, chronic pain, and neurological disorders that may require mental health and psychological adjustments.
3. Describe the role of the psychiatric liaison nurse.
4. Describe the role of the community mental health nurse in home care settings.
5. Describe the emerging field of body-mind medicine and its effects on holistic nursing care.
6. Utilize nursing theory to complete holistic nursing assessments and provide interventions in situations where the client is facing both physical and psychiatric symptoms.

KEY TERMS

Mind Modulation
Psychiatric Consultation-Liaison Nursing

There are important aspects of psychiatric mental health nursing practice involving clients with primarily somatic (or physical) illness. Somatic illness, particularly when chronic or life threatening, may often be a source of great stress. Individuals must call on all of their adaptive strengths to cope with the challenges of illness, and occasionally these strengths are insufficient to prevent the emergence of psychiatric symptoms. Anxiety, depression, or even psychosis may develop in individuals facing serious physical health problems. In such cases, it is usually clear that the physical illness preceded psychiatric symptoms. A major goal of this chapter is to increase nurses' sensitivity to psychological complications of physical illness so that timely—and sometimes life-saving—psychiatric care can be sought and provided.

IMPACT OF EMOTIONS ON HEALTH

The following excerpt is presented as a clear example of a case where emotional response to physical illness profoundly impacted the client's prognosis. The client is delusionally obsessed with death following a heart attack. Prior to his hospitalization for cardiac disease, this individual had no history of mental illness. His physician suspected depression when the client appeared to "give up" on rehabilitation. A consulting psychiatrist recognized the seriousness of the client's symptoms but was unable to offer help because of the family's resistance to intervention. This case is a striking example of a significant psychiatric disorder deriving from a physical illness:

THE KILLING FEAR OF DEATH

Julian Davies is a sixty-three-year-old architect who has suffered his second heart attack.... I was asked to see Julian Davies by his cardiologist, Samuel Medwar, because Dr. Medwar felt his patient had given up and was not participating in the program of rehabilitation, in spite of being in a stable physiological condition without serious aftereffects. I saw Mr. Davies three weeks after his heart attack.

A short, obese, bald man, reclining in his pajamas and silk bathrobe in a huge leather chair in his suburban home, Mr. Davies greeted me with a nod of the head and a downcast gaze. His wife hovered around him, straightening the blanket on his lap, refilling his water glass, offering him advice not to overexert himself, and regarding me with obvious suspicion.

I first asked Mr. Davies about his physical condition, and he assured me that he felt no pain or other serious symptoms. I then told him that he seemed to me somewhat depressed. He shrugged. I asked if he felt hopeless. He nodded. I asked if he had given up. He said, "Maybe." I asked why. Mr. Davies looked directly at me for the first time since I had entered the room. He told me that he knew he would die from his heart condition, and therefore he believed there was no good reason to follow the rehabilitation program. Mr. Davies reached out and grabbed my arm. His eyes were dilated, and his face was covered with perspiration. He seemed terrified....

Mr. Davies's mother had died in childbirth when he was eleven. He recalled his mother's death as a horrendous blow to the family, a crushing loss that had left him deeply wounded. His father had died a lingering death after a heart attack twenty years ago, weakening over the course of months, developing arrhythmia followed by heart failure, and finally dying from a pulmonary embolus. Mr. Davies confided to me that he felt helpless to prevent his condition from following the downhill course his father had taken. At night he awoke in terror that he would stop breathing or die in his sleep. He was obsessed with the fear.

Mr. Davies could not talk to his wife about his alarming thoughts. He accepted her deep concern and mothering as an additional sign that his condition was critical, or as he told me, "terminal." He could not accept the reassurance of his cardiologist, which he interpreted as professional dissembling. Before I left Mr. Davies, I asked him specifically if he were convinced he would die. He told me, again with horror in his gaze, that he was convinced....

After returning to my office, I called Dr. Medwar to express my concern that Mr. Davies had in fact given up and had a delusional conviction that he would die.... I recommended a brief psychiatric hospitalization, which I argued should be arranged as soon as possible. Dr. Medwar visited Mr. Davies but was unable to convince him either to enter a psychiatric hospital or to see me again. I called his home, but his wife refused to let me speak to him.

*Two weeks later, Dr. Medwar called to tell me Mr. Davies had died suddenly, without a clear-cut cause, a day after he had examined him and found his condition unchanged.... That same day Dr. Medwar had tried to talk Mrs. Davies into letting me or another psychiatrist visit the house.... Mrs. Davies had refused the request. Dr. Medwar was unable to change Mrs. Davies's mind, even though he reviewed the medical evidence with her and concluded that Mr. Davies was not in life-threatening ["physical"] danger but rather had developed an obsession.**

(Kleinman, 1988, pp. 149–150)

Depression is not uncommon after serious or life-threatening illness. The consulting psychiatrist recognized that this client's symptoms (such as expression of hopelessness, awakening at night in terror, and experiencing fear and anxiety) were not only those of depression. The psychiatrist recognized that Mr. Davies was profoundly convinced he would die from his illness. This kind of delusion can be so powerful that it leads, as here, to the client's death without any recognizable physical cause. Had Mr. and Mrs. Davies agreed to psychiatric hospitalization, it is possible that Mr. Davies could have overcome his delusional beliefs and survived his illness.

DSM-IV-TR AND PHYSICAL ILLNESS

As described in Chapter 4, the *Diagnostic and Statistical Manual of Mental Disorders*, Fourth Edition-Text Revision (DSM-IV-TR) uses the description Axis III to indicate a physical condition or physical illness. In the case of depression, DSM-IV-TR distinguishes two forms of depression occurring in the face of physical illness (American Psychiatric Association, 2000). The first is Mood Disorder Due to a General Medical Condition. These disorders are typically diagnosed when organic dysfunction directly influences the client's feelings, for example, poststroke, when it is thought that depression can be produced by a direct neurological effect as well as through the individual's recognition of loss of functioning. In the preceding excerpt, Mr. Davies does not have a Mood Disorder due to a general medical condition, for as DSM-IV-TR states, "When sadness, guilt, insomnia, or weight loss are present in a person with a recent myocardial infarction, each symptom would count toward a Major Depressive Episode because these are not clearly and fully accounted for by the physiological effects of a myocardial infarction" (American Psychiatric Association, 2000, p. 351). Individuals like Mr. Davies would be assigned an Axis III diagnosis along with the appropriate primary Axis I psychiatric diagnosis. For example, Mr. Davies could be assigned Major Depressive Disorder as an Axis I diagnosis and Diseases of the Circulatory System (Myocardial Infarction) as an Axis III diagnosis. While this notation may seem cumbersome, it calls attention to the fact that the management of psychiatric disorders complicating general medical illness is an important therapeutic role (American Psychiatric Association, 2000, p. 371):

> *Individuals with chronic or severe general medical conditions are at increased risk of developing a Major Depressive Disorder. Up to 20%–25% of individuals with certain general medical conditions (e.g., diabetes, myocardial infarction, carcinomas, stroke) will develop Major Depressive Disorder during the course of their general medical condition. The management of the general medical condition is more complex and the prognosis is less favorable if Major Depressive Disorder is present.*

*From *The Illness Narratives*, by Arthur Kleinman, Copyright © 1988. Reprinted with permission from BasicBooks, a member of Perseus Books, L.L.C.

PSYCHOLOGICAL RESPONSES TO PHYSICAL ILLNESS

As illustrated in the case of Mr. Davies, clients may have strong psychological responses to their physical illnesses. While any illness can trigger such responses, these responses are far more common when individuals are confronted with threats to life or to well-being. This section considers four common serious conditions: cancer, heart disease, chronic pain, and neurological disorders. Although the threats that each of these conditions present are similar—loss of autonomy, loss of livelihood, risk of death, and interference with social relationships—each is threatening in a different way and may lead to differing responses. Of course, every individual's illness and response is unique and must be approached individually and without preconception. The case examples provided through excerpts are given to help the nurse understand some of the many ways in which individuals may react to the stress of physical illness.

CANCER

A diagnosis of cancer can have a profound impact on a person's emotions and future life. Some clients describe receiving the diagnosis of cancer as a life-changing event, similar to the crisis events described in Chapter 11. From the day of diagnosis forward, these people become cancer survivors, and their diagnoses mark turning points in their lives. The reader may remember from Chapter 11 (focusing on crisis) the excerpt describing Stewart Alsop's experiences after being diagnosed with leukemia. Alsop had met Winston Churchill on two occasions and regarded him as a personal hero. Churchill led his country, England, through World War II partly through his great public speeches, which gave people courage despite the serious threat of defeat by Nazi Germany and the Axis Powers. In facing his own risk of death, Alsop tried to adopt Churchill's courageous attitude:

WE WILL FIGHT AMONGST THE PLATELETS

I wrote my letter as a takeoff on Winston's [Churchill] famous speech of defiance. "We will fight amongst the platelets," I wrote, "We will fight in the bone marrow. We will fight in the peripheral blood. We will never surrender."

*Having written this, I began, for the first time in about fifty years, to cry. I was utterly astonished, and also dismayed. I was brought up to believe that for a man to weep in public is the ultimate indignity, a proof of unmanliness. Only my elderly roommate was in the room, and he hadn't noticed. I ducked into our tiny shared bathroom, and closed the door, and sat down on the toilet, and turned on the bath water, so that nobody could hear me, and cried my heart out. Then I dried my eyes on the toilet paper and felt a good deal better.**

(Alsop, 1973, p. 68)

Early in his fight against cancer, Alsop tried to battle his own fears and depression by calling on his war memories, his youthful need for courage in the face of death, and his admiration for Churchill's coolness under severe threat. The nurse can recognize Alsop's behavior as his method of coping with significant stress. War memories, of the battles and the courage needed during these times, are a means many persons have to help them deal with fears, and Alsop predictably uses his past coping style to deal with his present situation. When these actions cannot make his situation better and alleviate his anxiety and fears, Alsop reverts to a heretofore unused coping method—he cries. Even though he acknowledges that he believes crying is unmanly, he does report that crying makes him feel better. The nurse must be aware of the fact that many clients in Alsop's situation feel overwhelmed by feelings of fear, depression, and powerlessness and find that their past coping patterns do not help.

The nurse has clues that privacy is more important to Alsop than interaction at the time he goes to the bathroom and cries in private. A caring nurse might approach him later in the evening when he is alone, and perhaps more stable emotionally, to spend time with him. Alsop is not in a position to meet demands that he behave in any particular way or that he talk. The nurse can offer self and express interest in his experience and feelings.

The following excerpt describes how another young client with cancer expressed his frustrations with the discomfort and perceived insensitivity he experienced during a long hospitalization for chemotherapy. He had brought a Halloween mask with him into the hospital and used it in a practical joke.

MY BREAKFAST NURSE

I awoke with the sun. Soon the breakfast carts began clanking down the hallway. Still tasting the remains of nausea, I nevertheless grinned as I stumbled towards the closet. I pulled out my Ape-Face.

REFLECTIVE THINKING 21-1

Supporting the Client without Hope

Consider Alsop's statements about his fight against cancer. He writes his letter of defiance and then begins to cry. His crying is an expression of hopelessness—unable to be manly and fearing inability to conquer his disease, he cries.

- **What do you think a caring nurse could do to assist and support this client?**
- **Is privacy more important to Alsop than support of another human being?**
- **Considering his need for privacy when crying, what would you do if you were the nurse?**

*From *Stay of Execution*, by Stewart Alsop, Copyright © 1973. Reprinted with permission from J. B. Lippincott.

Back in bed, I slipped the rubberband attachment over my head and then pulled the blue blanket over my head.... I could feel her getting closer and closer. Finally the magic moment as she pulled my blanket away.

*"Oh, shit. Oh, my God. Oh, no," she yelled and ran from the room. I smiled and lay back in bed. I had scored another victory against passivity and dependence.**

(Howe, 1982, pp. 147–148)

This highly sensitive young man somehow felt that his "breakfast nurse" perceived that chemotherapy had turned him into something ugly or frightening. He felt her to be "visibly nervous whenever I was around," and as a result, he decided to transform himself, if only for a few moments, into the monster that he thought she perceived him to be. Her response might have been laughter and a hug as she realized what he was trying to tell her with his "practical joke." Instead, she proved that he had correctly read her anxieties and insecurity.

While all nurses may try to give compassionate care to all clients, most nurses can identify situations in which they cannot give care to a particular client or to a client with a particular illness. It is important to know yourself and understand those situations in which you must seek help from other nurses to ensure that all clients receive the care they need.

Alsop and the young man in the other excerpt each found a means to surmount the threat of cancer and the fear and indignity that accompany its treatment. Only some persons achieve such success; for others, the diagnosis of cancer leads to significant depression. In the following excerpt, the novelist and poet May Sarton describes the weeks following her mastectomy. While she emphasizes that depression preceded her cancer diagnosis, her depression certainly was made worse by illness. It seems unlikely that the doctors and nurses who worked with her knew how depressed she was; very likely, her supportive network of friends and her strong love of nature allowed her to overcome depression and facilitate her own healing:

TUESDAY, JUNE 26TH

The operation was on the eighteenth and I came home yesterday welcomed by dear Martha and Marita who have been holding the fort here.

The York hospital, small, intimate, and kind, was an ideal place for me to be, especially as I was on their new plan, Joint Practice, where nurses are given unusual powers and work closely with the surgeon. The operation was not bad at all, a modified radical mastectomy ... modified meaning that they found no malignancy in the lymph glands. It looks as though I am in the clear.

I had a room of my own until the last night, and it was soon full of flowers, glorious flowers, among them a bunch of many sprays of delphinium, several blues, and white peonies. Another was a basket with six African violets of shades of pink and lavender. The first day Heidi brought a little bunch from her garden, and later on Martha and Marita brought me samples from my garden, one day two clematis, one deep purple and one white, another day, Siberian iris. The flowers were a constant joy. I opened my eyes to find them there, silent presences, and I slept a lot, grateful for the loss of consciousness.

The flowers helped, the visible sign of the love of many, many friends, and the great elm tree I looked at from the window helped too, its long branches waving gently in the wind. One evening an oriole came to rest there and sing. The changing skies and the admirable steadfast tree did me a lot of good. I needed it, for I had imagined that the loss of a breast would create catharsis, that I would emerge like a phoenix from the fire, reborn, with all things made new, especially the pain in my heart. I had imagined that real pain, physical pain, and physical loss would take the place of mental anguish and the loss of love. Not so. It is all to be begun again, the long excruciating journey through pain and rejection, through anger and not understanding, toward some regained sense of my self....

What I am fighting now is depression, but it is not, I think, wholly and perhaps at all, the result of the shock of a major operation on the body.... It is that I feel devalued and abandoned at the center of my being. I sometimes feel that everyone else manages to grow up and harden in the right way to survive, whereas I have remained a terribly vulnerable infant. When poetry is alive in me I can handle it, use it, feel worthy of being part of the universe. When I can't as now, when the source is all silted up by pain, I think I should have been done away with at birth....

One of the insights that has come to me through the operation is that physical disability rouses the will, so much so that extra power seems to be given in overcoming it, power beyond what is needed.... Whereas depression, mental anguish, destroy the will or numb it. So they are much harder to handle. I sometimes wonder whether I shall ever fully recover the sense of myself and of my powers as a writer and as a person after last year....

What the mastectomy does to each individual woman is, at least temporarily, to attack her womanhood at its most vulnerable, to devalue her in her own eyes as a woman. And each woman has to meet this and make herself whole again in her own way ... I would like to believe when I die that I have given myself away like a tree that

*From *Do Not Go Gentle*, by H. Howe, 1982. New York: W. W. Norton. Reprinted by permission of W. W. Norton and Herbert Howe.

REFLECTIVE THINKING 21-2

Exploring Your Reaction to Very Ill Clients

A young man expresses his own victory against passivity and dependence by playing a practical joke on the breakfast nurse. However, he believes that the nurse is uncomfortable around him. He does not feel good about himself, so he is particularly sensitive to the fact that the nurse is not comfortable in his presence.

- Are there clients with whom you are uncomfortable?
- Are there settings where you believe you cannot give care to clients?
- Can you give a specific example where you thought your feelings left you unable to care for a particular client?
- Are you able to discuss your feelings about clients with other nurses?

Psychiatric nursing is as much a practice of understanding as it is of providing care.

- How would you decide what methods of coping to suggest to a client?
- What if a client insists that none of these methods works for her?

Consider which of the coping methods listed here you might use if you were diagnosed with cancer.

*sows seeds every spring and never counts the loss, because it is not loss, it is adding to future life. It is the tree's way of being. Strongly rooted perhaps, but spilling out its treasure on the wind.**

(*Sarton, 1980, pp. 118–140*)

Sarton clearly exhibits depression; she expresses feeling depressed, devalued, abandoned, and being vulnerable. Further, she states, "I should have been done away with at birth," expressing that the cancer, its treatment, and the surgery have destroyed her will. It seems, though, that her depression never gave way to complete despair; she found joy in her flowers and recognized them as expressions of love and connectedness. In contrast to Sarton, some clients with cancer may be both depressed and suicidal (Schneider & Shenassa, 2008).

Perhaps nurses are more aware of the relationship between depression and cancer now than they were years ago. Nurses are alert to signs of hopelessness and depression and have come to value the role of support groups for both client and family. However, as noted in Chapter 14 (focusing

REFLECTIVE THINKING 21-3

How Clients Report Coping with Cancer

Clients describe several methods of coping with the diagnosis and treatment of cancer:

- Writing (a letter, journal, poem)
- Crying
- Laughing
- Using humor (practical jokes) for relief
- Taking control of treatment
- Regaining power
- Obtaining information
- Talking with others
- Receiving support from significant others

on depression), the suicide rate among cancer sufferers remains high. These excerpts illustrate that cancer provokes significant responses in individual clients. It is never adequate to treat the tumor alone; the client must be evaluated to uncover his response to the condition so that appropriate supportive interventions can be offered. Nurses should not forget, however, that sleep disturbance is associated with cancer diagnosis—even in the absence of depression (Sateia & Lang, 2008). Helping clients improve sleep can significantly raise quality of life. Box 21-1 provides examples of assessment questions around depression that can be used with clients. These questions are offered as examples that will help the nurse not only to initiate discussion and obtain information, but also to stimulate nurse-client discussion about issues of the client's support system, his knowledge of the disease, his beliefs, and his spiritual health. The questions thus constitute both assessment and intervention, as the nurse will be able to provide support by asking these questions and through the resulting conversations to explore the client's subjective experience of the cancer.

Cardiovascular and Pulmonary Disease

Clients are frequently depressed after a heart attack as they face the fear that resuming their preattack personal, vocational, and sexual activities may represent a physical risk of pain, breathing difficulty, or even sudden death. For many, preinfarction life patterns of eating, smoking, stress, and drinking may need to be changed if subsequent cardiac events are to be avoided. Such dramatic changes in lifestyle may provoke anxiety or depression. Some myocardial infarctions are truly life threatening in their severity, and studies show that depression is both a consequence and, in some circumstances a potential cause, of heart disease (Blumenthal, 2008). However, even in the absence of depression, the experience of life-threatening illness can be extraordinarily

BOX 21-1
ASSESSMENT QUESTIONS FOR CLIENTS UNDERGOING TREATMENT FOR CANCER

- Who are the significant people in your life?
- Do you have friends or family in town who are available to help you? Do you have someone you can call at any time?
- Do you belong to any groups?
- Can you ask others for help when you need it?
- What choices are available to you to enhance your healing?
- What information would you like to have about your cancer, its treatment, and recovery?
- How do your cancer and its treatment interfere with your life goals?
- How do your cancer and its treatment interfere with your family functioning?
- How hopeful are you about recovering?
- What is the most important or powerful thing in your life?
- How has your cancer influenced your faith or beliefs?

stressful. The following excerpt from a book by Martha Weinman Lear describes her husband's heart attack and hospitalization:

SHOULDN'T WE GET AN AMBULANCE?

He awoke at 7 A.M. with pain in his chest. The sort of pain that might cause panic if one were not a doctor, as he was, and did not know, as he knew, that it was heartburn.

He went into the kitchen to get some Coke, whose secret syrups often relieve heartburn. The refrigerator door seemed heavy, and he noted that he was having trouble unscrewing the bottle cap. Finally he wrenched it off, cursing the defective cap. He poured some liquid, took a sip. The pain did not go away. Another sip; still no relief.

Now he grew more attentive. He stood motionless, observing symptoms. His breath was coming hard. He felt faint. He was sweating, though the August morning was still cool. He put fingers to his pulse. It was rapid and weak. A powerful burning sensation was beginning to spread through his chest, radiating upward into his throat. Into his arm? No. But the pain was growing worse. Now it was crushing—"crushing," just as it is always described. And worse even than the pain was the sensation of losing all power, a terrifying seepage of strength. He could feel the entire degenerative process accelerating. He was growing fainter, faster. The pulse was growing weaker, faster. He was sweating much more profusely now—a heavy, clammy sweat. He felt that the life juices were draining from his body. He felt that he was about to die....

I'll be damned, he thought. I can't believe it....

He made his way back to the bedroom, clutching walls for support. He eased himself onto the bed, picked up the telephone receiver and, with fingers that felt like foreign objects, dialed the Manhattan emergency number.

A woman's voice, twangy: "This is 911. Can I help you?"

He spoke slowly, struggling to enunciate each word clearly:

"My name is Dr. Harold Lear. I live at ——. I am having a heart attack. My doctor's name is ——. I am too weak to look up his number. Please call him and tell him to come right away."

"Sir, I'm sorry. This is 911. I can't call your doctor.... This is strictly an emergency service.... I can't call your doctor. We don't do that."

Now he felt not panic, but a certain professional urgency. A familiar statistic plucked at his brain like an advertising slogan: 50 percent of all coronary victims die in the first ten minutes. "Thank you," he said to 911, and hung up.

Slowly he tugged on a robe, staggered back into the foyer and pressed for the elevator.... Suddenly he knew that if he did not lie down he would fall. He lowered himself to the floor. When the elevator door opened, he rolled out into the lobby and said to the startled doorman, "Get a wheelchair. Get me to the emergency room. I am having a heart attack."

"An ambulance, Doctor? Shouldn't we get an ambulance?"

"No. No time. A wheelchair." Then he lost clarity.

He was next aware of being in a wheelchair that was careening down the street. His head was way back, resting against a softness that seemed to be a belly. He did not know whose it was, but he was so pleased to have that belly for support.

The hospital—his hospital, where he was on staff—was nearby, a few blocks from his home. He felt the wheelchair take a corner with a wild side-to-side lurch and go rattling on toward the emergency room. Though his mind was floating and he could not keep his eyes open, that curiously disengaged observer within him reached automatically for the pulse. He could no longer detect any beat. He was very cold, very clammy, and he knew that he was in shock.

I am dying now, he thought. I am dying in a creaky wheelchair that is rattling down the avenue, half a block from the emergency room. Isn't this silly? And then: Well, if I am dying, why isn't my life flashing in front of me? Nothing is flashing. Where is my life?

The apartment-house doorman, who was steering the wheelchair, and a janitor, who was running alongside, recalled later that he was smiling. They wondered why....

Then, dimly, he felt himself being lifted onto a stretcher, sensed noise and light and a sudden commotion about him.... He understood that at this moment he was no more than a body with pathology. They were not treating a person; they were treating an acute coronary case in severe shock. They were racing, very quickly, against time. He himself had run this race so often, working in just this detached silent way on nameless, faceless bodies with pathologies. He did not resent the impersonality. He simply noted it. But one of the medical team, a young woman who was taking his blood pressure, seemed concerned about him. She patted him on the shoulder. She said, "How do you feel?" It was the only departure from this cool efficiency, and he felt achingly grateful for it....

(Later—he thought it was the same day, but it may have been the next—she came up to the coronary-care unit, and took his hand and said, "How are you doing, Dr. Lear?" and smiled at him. He never knew her name, and he never forgot her.)....

Now administrative forces descended upon him. They asked about next-of-kin.

His wife was out of the country, he said.

Where?

He wasn't sure.

Children?

His son was traveling too. He could not remember his daughter's married name.

Siblings? None. Parents? None. Finally he gave them the name of a friend....

He remembered thinking, just before he passed into a long, deep sleep, How can I get hold of Martha? I've got to get hold of Martha, because if I die without telling her, she will never forgive me.

*He knew this was the logic of a deranged mind. A nurse wondered, as his street escorts had wondered earlier, why he was smiling.**

(Lear, 1980, pp. 11–15)

In her book *Heartsounds*, Martha Weinman Lear describes her husband's heart attack. Dr. Lear suffers a severe heart attack and manages, despite an apparently unresponsive emergency system, to get himself transported to the nearby hospital in time to survive. Although in shock and nearly unconscious, he manages to stay in control of at least his means of transportation until he eventually finds his way to the hospital's emergency and intensive care units. Once under expert care, he seems willing to adopt a more passive role. Whether his chances of survival would have been less (as the narrative implies) had he asked 911 to send an ambulance, this certainly would have been a more conventional way to enter the hospital than the one he chose. Despite his surgeon's "take charge" attitude and behavior, this narrative emphasizes that Dr. Lear found great comfort in two episodes of human touch, mere physical contact with the "belly" of the doorman pushing his wheelchair and the kindness of one woman of the emergency department team.

Telling the story later, Dr. Lear's wife emphasizes his puzzling smile and offers some explanations for his behaviors. It would have been easy to misinterpret Dr. Lear's smile as a sign of complete self-control and detachment. In reality, his smile meant just the opposite: a sense of life—his life—being far more out of control than he was accustomed to. The smile expressed an ironic lack of trust in fate and the people on whom his life depended. Rather than an expression of self-confidence, Dr. Lear's smile was the nearest he could allow himself to a statement of fear and uncertainty. The nurse who saw his smile and wondered at it could perhaps best have responded by telling this brave, frightened, and lonely man something like, "You've fought hard for your life; give us your trust and let's get the healing of your heart started."

For some individuals who experience a heart attack, a smile observed by the nurse can most often be a sign of denial. Denial is a common response to life-threatening illness; indeed, Dr. Lear was in denial when he went to the refrigerator to treat his coronary ischemia with a soft drink. Denial, along with guilt and anger, are common emotional reactions that caregivers describe among patients who have experienced a significant cardiac event (Higgins, Murphy, Nicholas, Worcester, & Lindner, 2007). In describing a nursing study of adjustment following a heart attack, Johnson (1991) reported that "rather than face what had happened and the uncertainty of the future many of the informants continued to distance themselves by refusing to believe that the heart attack happened or by denying the diagnosis":

*Afterwards, it didn't seem like I had a heart attack. It didn't seem real. I thought, "Somebody else had it." It was funny.**

(Johnson, 1991, p. 25)

One of the important milestones in recovering from a heart attack, as with other severe physical illness, seems to be coming to terms with the question, "Why did it happen to me?" Johnson reports numerous similar comments from recovering cardiac clients:

I kept thinking about it for about the first month after I got home ... just going over in my mind "Why did this have to happen?" And then I'd sit and ponder over it....

*From *Heartsounds*, by Martha Weinman Lear. Reprinted by permission of Martha Lear and the Watkins/Loomis Agency.

*From "Learning to Live Again: The Process of Adjustment Following a Heart Attack," by J. Johnson, Copyright © 1991. In *The Illness Experience* (pp. 25–85), edited by J. M. Morse and J. L. Johnson. Reprinted with permission from Janice Morse, University of Utah College of Nursing.

*I felt mad because I did all the right things. I thought, "I walk up and down eight flights. I swim every day. I walk whenever I can." I'd been doing all the right things. I'd also been watching my diet like mad.... I've always been interested in nutrition.**

(Johnson, 1991, p. 31)

For some, this questioning turns to self-blame and guilt:

It's the old story I guess.... I've worked, I've put in long hours, lots of worry, frustration, lots of stress. I've worked for this heart attack, and I got it. I mean it's mine. I've worked for this, and I guess you could say I got what I deserved....

*I don't know how a person can opt out of not taking responsibility. And more so for a heart attack than cancer. I wouldn't feel the same way if I had cancer. I would say, "Hey, why me?" Or if I had been hit by a car, I could say, "Why me?" But I can't honestly say "Why me?" with a heart attack. I guess one could almost say I had it coming.**

(Johnson, 1991, p. 32)

There is a widespread belief that heart disease can be avoided via risk factor control; as a result, people who suffer heart attacks frequently do feel guilty, as if they "had it coming" or "got what they deserved" (Higgins et al., 2007). Through the questioning process of taking a nursing history, caretakers may contribute to this guilt instead of helping to dissipate it: "Some of the informants found the scrutiny of the health professionals distressing":

*There is a lot of finger pointing. You go along with them. And you start to think, "Something I did must have been wrong." Cause you're told this immediately. They tell you, "Well, let's see what you did that was wrong. Why did you get a heart attack?"**

(Johnson, 1991, p. 33)

Guilt is, of course, a major symptom of depression, and nurses need to be careful to avoid missing the presence of depression or adding to guilty feelings.

The nurse must understand that offering the client a chance to express the range of his feelings is extremely important and perhaps is the most valuable intervention the nurse has to offer. Often, fear is the hardest emotion to express. This may be truest for individuals like Dr. Lear, who have such a strong need to seem (and be) in control. Fear may arise at any time in the course of a heart attack, and the resulting adrenergic stimulation may put clients at increased risk for arrhythmia. Although the coronary care unit experience can be particularly fear provoking, leaving the hospital may be as traumatic for some heart attack sufferers as it was for Fitzhugh Mullan after his chemotherapy hospitalization:

I WAS AFRAID TO LEAVE

*I was afraid to leave. I thought, you know, "What if I have another heart attack?" At the hospital I'd be attended to right away.... I mean, they bring you your pills at a certain time, and you're looked after pretty good. And then you think, "Gee, when you go home, you're on your own. Am I going to make it? Am I going to manage?" Yes, it was a worry. Oh, the first week I think I was so scared at home. I was scared of having another heart attack and not getting to the hospital in time.**

(Johnson, 1991, p. 43)

In recent years, length of hospital stay for persons with myocardial infarction has been dropping significantly. It is unclear how shortening hospital stays will affect the fear and anxiety associated with leaving the hospital. Perhaps if clients have shorter hospital stays, they will be less likely to identify the hospital with safety. Nonetheless, returning home is often a time for anxiety and depression. This may be particularly true if there is nowhere to go outside the home:

SITTING AT HOME

*I find the worst part about it is sitting at home being idle. It is very frustrating. I guess I was a workaholic to a point. And to sit and not do anything, well. Like, when I was discharged I said, "Well, now I can go home. I can do some exercises." I was overweight. I knew that without having been told. I could do some exercises to strengthen, and as soon as I talked to my doctor, he says, "You don't do anything." I says, "Well, can't I?" He says, "You can go and you can walk, but you're not to leave the house." For the first week, I was housebound, I couldn't go anywhere.... I found it very frustrating to get up and not to have a purpose in life except to maybe exist until the next day.**

(Johnson, 1991, p. 44)

While today few, if any, patients would have their post-infarct activity controlled to such a degree, many clients must greatly restrict their own activities because of weakness

*From "Learning to Live Again: The Process of Adjustment Following a Heart Attack" by J. Johnson, Copyright © 1991. In *The Illness Experience* (pp. 25–85), edited by J. M. Morse and J. L. Johnson. Reprinted with permission from Janice Morse, University of Utah College of Nursing.

*From "Learning to Live Again: The Process of Adjustment Following a Heart Attack" by J. Johnson, Copyright © 1991. In *The Illness Experience* (pp. 25–85), edited by J. M. Morse and J. L. Johnson. Reprinted with permission from Janice Morse, University of Utah College of Nursing.

RESEARCH Highlight 21-1

An Examination of the Services Provided by Psychiatric Consultation Liaison Nurses in a General Hospital

STUDY PROBLEM/PURPOSE

Researchers sought to describe the extent and content of care provided by Psychiatric Consultation Liaison Nurses (PCLN) in a rural general hospital. Specifically, the researchers sought to document a profile of cases seen and to describe the outcomes and contributions of the PCLNs' work.

METHODS

The study used a descriptive survey design utilizing a questionnaire that had been used in prior studies. The tool was completed by the researcher and was used to record details of the patients assessed by the PCLN service and to record the depth of services provided. There were 66 cases reviewed and recorded over a three-month study period

FINDINGS

Seventy-seven percent of the patients referred were hospitalized for a medical condition such as shortness of breath or parasuicide attempt. The other 23% had an orthopedic, surgical, alcohol or other psychiatric problems. Forty-six percent of those referred were under 30 years of age and 53% had a past psychiatric history. However, 47% had no previous contact with mental health professionals. The PCLN nurses developed a plan of care for each client. In all, 46% of those seen were discharged to home within 24 hours, and only 9% were admitted to a psychiatric unit.

IMPLICATIONS

Provision of mental health services in the general hospital is challenging for all care providers. The work of a PCLN can provide support to other caregivers and assist nurses and physicians make appropriate choices in care provision. It is probable that the PCLNs serve mental health needs of clients while decreasing hospital length of stay.

Source: "An Examination of the Services Provided by Psychiatric Consultation Liaison Nurses in a General Hospital," by M. L. Johnston and S. Cowman, 2008, *Journal of Psychiatric and Mental Health Nursing*, *15*, 500–507.

or dyspnea. This sense of restriction, of being without "a purpose in life except to maybe exist," is also a part of depression. Depression becomes a greater risk when postinfarction heart failure or angina restricts physical activity:

NURSING TIP 21-1

Dealing with Client Guilt

1. Accept the client where he is; practice the art of unconditional acceptance.
2. Establish trust; demonstrate that you as the nurse are trustworthy by keeping appointments, doing everything you have promised to do, and letting the client know you have made time to be with him to meet his needs.
3. Ask yourself the following:
   - Do you really believe the client is at fault if he has had a heart attack?
   - How does your answer to the preceding question affect your ability to give care?

ONE DAY

*One day I started getting the angina. I mentioned it to them at the clinic. I had done, you know, the beds and tidied the bathrooms, and then in the afternoon, I went down, and I ironed, and they said, "Well, you know, you should iron maybe two pieces at a time to begin with." And here I stood there for half an hour. But I was so mad at myself. I kept on saying, "I'm sure I can do half an hour's ironing."**

(Johnson, 1991, pp. 48–49)

When a client is in recovery from a serious illness or physical crisis, such as the woman in the preceding example, the physiological limitations of recovery affect the client's autonomy. In the example, the client could no longer perform her household tasks without triggering her angina. She expressed anger and frustration at being unable to perform "half an hour's ironing" without feeling exhausted.

The nurse must explain that recovery often takes more time than both the client and nurse would like. It is important for the nurse to help the client pace activities. In this case, the nurse could state, "You have learned that the activity you tried doing was too much. How can you pace yourself to remain active without being at risk for angina? Let's look at a typical day together." When entering this conversation, the nurse must acknowledge the client's frustration and the risk of giving up. Sharing that many clients feel the same way is helpful. The nurse should remember to accept the client where she is and work together to maintain hope and establish a rehabilitation plan.

Some clients may simply be unable to cope. For one of the 14 participants in Johnson's study, depression proved overwhelming:

*From "Learning to Live Again: The Process of Adjustment Following a Heart Attack," by J. Johnson, Copyright © 1991. In *The Illness Experience* (pp. 25–85), edited by J. M. Morse and J. L. Johnson. Reprinted with permission from Janice Morse, University of Utah College of Nursing.

SHE GAVE UP

*She experienced numerous setbacks in the adjustment process and she was constantly setting goals and failing to meet them. Eventually she was no longer able to face perpetual disappointment. She stopped setting goals, refused to monitor her progress, and abandoned attempts.... Although ... by no means the most ill of the informants, she believed that she would not improve ... and at the time of the last interview she said she had given up.**

(Johnson, 1991, p. 85)

Johnson does not tell more about this informant's outcome and in particular whether a diagnosis of depression was formally made and treated.

The nurse's role in caring for clients with cardiovascular disease may be to ensure that the client is evaluated and treated holistically. Clearly, the life-threatening nature of the disease requires immediate and vigilant attention to the physiological state. However, recovery requires careful attention to the human response to both the illness and its treatment: caring for the emotions of depression, anxiety, guilt, and loneliness (as expressed by clients in the preceding excerpts) and assisting the client to make necessary changes in lifestyle that are conducive to continuing recovery and health. The nurse, in her role as a caring professional, can offer the client the chance to express emotions, examine the meaning of the illness and treatments, and provide support through establishment of a positive nurse-client relationship.

Severe shortness of breath, whether due to an intrinsic problem of the lungs (such as pneumonia, asthma, or emphysema) or to heart failure, can be an exceptionally frightening experience. Perhaps especially when accompanied by hypoxia, pulmonary disorders can lead to psychiatric disturbances, including anxiety, delirium, and even psychosis. Psychiatric care may sometimes be needed when symptoms related to severe dyspnea do not respond to reassurance and able medical-nursing management. The 2003 outbreak of severe acute respiratory syndrome (SARS) that affected hundreds of individuals in China led to a number of psychiatric disorders that required management through liaison care (Cheng, Tsang, Ku, Wong, & Ng, 2004). Many respiratory disorders result in clients being on ventilators for long periods of time, unable to talk or to communicate effectively with clinical staff or family members. This experience may be highly isolating and frightening and is sometimes referred to in nursing literature as the "ICU syndrome" (Granberg, Engberg, & Lundberg, 1999). Some individuals who survive lengthy periods of mechanical ventilation develop subsequent Post-Traumatic Stress Disorder, which may require treatment (Kapfhammer, Rothenhausler, Krauseneck, Stoll, & Schelling, 2004; Davydow, Gifford, Desai, Needham, & Bienvenu, 2008).

*From "Learning to Live Again: The Process of Adjustment Following a Heart Attack," by J. Johnson, Copyright © 1991. In *The Illness Experience* (pp. 25–85), edited by J. M. Morse and J. L. Johnson. Reprinted with permission from Janice Morse, University of Utah College of Nursing.

Chronic Pain

Those who experience significant pain have to make adjustments to daily living unlike any other group of clients. Often, the illness is not life-threatening, but it is ever present and impacts on virtually every one of the individual's social roles. The following is a description of a case being reviewed by a group of professionals in a chronic pain clinic. A psychiatrist is describing the case conference:

A CASE CONFERENCE

Helen Winthrop Bell is a twenty-nine-year-old minister's wife from a rural area in Georgia. She has had chronic pain in her arms for six years. She has undergone eight surgical procedures, has been treated with more than two dozen medications—two of them prescribed narcotics to which she briefly became addicted—and has been in the care of four different primary care physicians. She has already "failed" two local pain clinics. Mrs. Bell is at the end of her first week in the inpatient pain unit. The discussion of her case at the pain conference lasts thirty-six minutes. First, the anesthesiology resident reviews the past medical history and the results of X-rays, nerve and muscle tests, blood studies, and various physical examinations. Then one of the behavioral psychologists reads the results of the psychological test battery: depression, anxiety, bodily preoccupation, hysterical personality traits, and very substantial anger. Everyone shakes his head knowingly, and a few jokes are told to indicate what an extremely hostile and difficult patient Mrs. Bell is. It is noted that the pain seems to be an effective way for her to get angry at her husband. The social worker reports that Mrs. Bell is extremely difficult to interview. She denies all problems, even though there are reports in the medical records that she doesn't like her life as a minister's wife and has been on the verge of considering divorce.... The senior psychologist adds that the couple's sex life reportedly has come to a halt and that the patient's pain has been observed by the ward staff to worsen at the times her husband visits. He interprets this as evidence that the patient is "using" her pain to manipulate her marital relationship. The nurses jump in at this point with further impressions of the relationship between the Bells: evidence, it turns out, that is greatly contradictory. They have been observed arguing, but also holding hands and praying together....

The chief anesthesiologist admits that nothing has seemed to work, including the nerve blocks and analgesics.... The junior behavioral psychologist points out ... that the patient uses her anger to undermine the treatment program. [A] nurse breaks in, saying: "We all know what chronic pain patients are like: they are all angry and self-destructive. What's so special about Mrs. Bell?" The head nurse says she is special because she is so hostile and negative. Maybe we should discharge her before she causes a major problem on the unit, she suggests. "Do you psychiatrists have anything you want to add?" asks the chief anesthesiologist. "We only have a few minutes, because we have three other cases to get to," he cautions.

That's where I came in when I participated in this pain conference one spring afternoon in 1979. I could have told the group that Mrs. Bell satisfied the diagnostic criteria for major depressive disorder, a treatable psychiatric disorder. But she had met these criteria for three years and had been treated on numerous occasions with appropriate doses of antidepressant medication without significant effect on her depression or pain. I could have told them that I had also interviewed her husband and had found him to be even more profoundly depressed than his wife.... I could have told the group about my interview with Mrs. Bell, which was fairly typical of her interactions with the staff. Mrs. Bell did not want to speak to me. She told me that she did not have a psychiatric problem nor any other problem except for her pain.... I asked her how she had learned to deal with the anger "created by the pain," the rage that was so visible to me. Mrs. Bell shouted at me to leave the room, accusing me of provoking her and yelling that she was most definitely not angry....

I could also have reported a chat I had with Helen Bell's older sister, Agatha, who told me that Helen had been angry all her life; before the pain it was her relationship with their parents and with her that elicited Helen's anger. She also told me that anger was often expressed indirectly through chronic bodily complaints: first, headaches or backaches; later, her arm and shoulder pain. Agatha Winthrop told me that in their family no problems of a personal or family kind could be openly talked out.

I decided, given the very limited time, there was nothing further to be gained reviewing these problems. I told my colleagues, rather, that in my view we were part of the problem. I pointed out that the pain center itself had now been taken up in the angry, self-defeating relationships that characterized Mrs. Bell's life. We were now in the same situation as her many doctors, her husband, her sister, and other family members....

*I couldn't get any further. The chief anesthesiologist thanked me for my interventions, reminded me that time had run out, and asked if I didn't really want to see her receive the latest psychopharmacologic agent. He gently chided me for my utopian suggestion. Mrs. Bell was here on the ward and "something has to be done with her now."**

(Kleinman, 1988, pp. 175–180)

Pain is one of the fundamental responses to physiological dysfunction. All persons experience pain with injury, illness, surgery, childbirth, and sometimes for no discernible reason. For most persons, pain is a transient experience, sometimes requiring powerful medication for its alleviation. The pain of chronic disorders, such as arthritis or cancer, can frequently be controlled by appropriate interventions. One of the major achievements of health care in the last half of the twentieth century was the development of new forms of analgesia allowing most clients with severe somatic and visceral pain, even terminal cancer sufferers, to experience much pain relief. Nonetheless, there are individuals, like Mrs. Bell, whose agonizing pain seems to completely resist medical and psychological efforts at relief. While Mrs. Bell's narrative was recorded nearly 25 years ago, the condition of unalleviated chronic pain remains a significant health care problem today. Multidisciplinary "pain clinics" have been formed to bring the broadest scope of expertise to the problems of these individuals. Many of these clinics and their associated inpatient facilities function better as professional groups than does the one that Kleinman describes. While Kleinman is clearly annoyed at the chief anesthesiologist's domineering behavior, some readers may interpret Kleinman's description of nurses' "jumping in" and "breaking in" as a devaluing of nursing participation and as further evidence of this particular group's serious therapeutic dysfunction. But, of course, this dysfunction was precisely Kleinman's point: Mrs. Bell's pain is so tied up with her personal and social relationships that she draws everyone around her into her world of pain. An inpatient "pain unit" as torn by role and personal conflicts as this one is likely incapable of handling a client as tortured and complex as Mrs. Bell.

DSM-IV-TR includes a diagnosis of Pain Disorder in the category of Somatoform Disorder (see Chapter 19). This diagnosis recognizes that many clients, like Mrs. Bell, have no distinct physical condition that satisfactorily explains their pain. These individuals are given the DSM diagnosis Pain Disorder Associated with Psychological Factors, or, where physical diagnoses clearly contribute to the pain, Pain Disorder Associated with Both Psychological Factors and a General Medical Condition. The DSM-IV-TR diagnostic criteria for Pain Disorder are listed in Box 21-2.

As implied in Kleinman's description of Mrs. Bell's evaluation, treatment of individuals with Pain Disorder is difficult and complex. There is always a temptation to use yet another surgical procedure or "the latest psychopharmacologic agent." Even today, well-functioning multidisciplinary assessment and treatment teams are indispensable tools in

REFLECTIVE THINKING 21-4

Can the Treatment Team Be Part of the Problem?

Consider the case conference described in the preceding excerpt. The psychiatrist suggests that the treatment team is part of the client's continued difficulty, that the pain center staff had been taken up in the angry, self-defeating relationships that haunted the client's life.

Can you describe the difference between a treatment team that works to meet the client's needs and a treatment team that demands that the client receive treatment offered and get well?

Identify at least two examples of comments reportedly made by professionals at the case conference that were judgmental and uncaring. Restate each one in a manner that exemplifies human caring. What do you think the difference would be for the treatment team? For the client?

BOX 21-2
DIAGNOSTIC CRITERIA FOR PAIN DISORDER

- Pain in one or more anatomic sites is the predominant focus of the clinical presentation and is of sufficient severity to warrant clinical attention.
- The pain causes clinically significant distress or impairment in social, occupational, or other important areas of functioning.
- Psychological factors are judged to have an important role in the onset, severity, exacerbation, or maintenance of the pain.
- The symptom or deficit is not intentionally produced or feigned (as in Factitious Disorder or Malingering).
- The pain is not better accounted for by a mood, anxiety, or psychotic disorder. This disorder is not diagnosed if criteria for Somatoform Disorder are met.

From *Diagnostic and Statistical Manual of Mental Disorders*, Fourth Edition-Text Revision, 2000, Washington, DC: American Psychiatric Association.

the management of these seriously troubled clients and their families. These teams evaluate the meaning of the pain for the individuals. Interventions are planned that may not eliminate the pain but, rather, help the client to control the pain while having a life, as opposed to living in a situation where the pain controls every aspect of the individual's living. A nurse's role in management of chronic pain is, first and foremost, to provide a caring and compassionate response to the client's situation. Second, the nurse must work with others in a functional treatment team to help the client find interventions that allow the client to manage his life. Complementary treatments such as those described in Chapter 32 offer nonpharmacological interventions, such as hypnosis, guided relaxation, therapeutic touch, and acupuncture, that are helpful to some persons with chronic pain.

Nurses and social scientists have made scholarly contributions to understanding the way in which family dynamics, as in Mrs. Bell's story, influence the lived experience of chronic pain (Smith & Freidman, 1999; Werner, Isaksen, & Malterud, 2004). Smith and Friedman's work emphasized that in some families pain allows individuals to (dysfunctionally) regulate the intensity of their relationships with others. These psychodynamics, although very important, should not obscure the anesthesiologist's point in Kleinman's narrative. For many people, particularly those in pain from cancer, arthritis, AIDS, and degenerative disorders, current medications and medication delivery systems allow pain to be relieved effectively. Nurses are often intimately involved in the pharmacological care of such individuals. Effective pain management, whether "led" by doctors or nurses (Courtenay & Carey, 2008) requires a combination of pharmacological knowledge, psychological understanding, and mastery of the neurobiology of pain. Further, nurses recognize that it is necessary to adopt a holistic approach (Wilkes, Castro, Mohan, Sundaraj, & Noore, 2003)—often complemented by understandings from disciplines outside nursing (Afrell, Biguet, & Rudebeck, 2007; Steihaug, 2007) to improve health states of those with chronic pain. One group of nurse researchers has documented the application of a model to explain effects of chronic pain on the elderly and concluded that adequate treatment for pain address daily stressors and the accompanying depression seen so frequently in pain clients (Tsai, Tak, Moore, & Palencia, 2003). Nurses involved in pain programs also need political and administrative skills to assure that their clients receive the best possible care (Brown, 2000). Although the discussion is beyond the scope of this textbook, nurses involved in treating chronic pain frequently find themselves caught between an obligation to relieve pain and suffering and traditional social expectation that effective medications for nonmalignant pain (particularly opiates) should not be given to clients in order to avoid a perceived harm of creating physical and psychological dependency (Fontana, 2008). This conflict is very real, but may be lessening with time as it becomes more widely recognized that effective pain relief is appropriate for all persons, regardless of whether a "real" disease such as cancer or rheumatoid arthritis has caused their pain (Rosenblum, Marsch, Joseph, & Portenoy, 2008).

MOVEMENT AND NEUROLOGICAL DISORDERS

Movement and sensation are so much a part of everyday experience that impairment of these functions is felt as a particularly profound loss. Visual and hearing impairments pose a severe threat to full social and vocational participation. The following excerpt describes the experiences of progressive visual loss from the perspective of a man entering a rehabilitation program for the newly visually impaired.

ORDINARY DAYLIGHT

I had become incapable of dealing with my approaching blindness, and I signed up for a four-month residency with others also going blind. We all wanted to learn, with varying degrees of desperation, how to survive.... As difficult as the word rehabilitation was to handle, the word blind was worse. It was fraught with archetypal nightmares: beggars with tin cups, the useless, helpless, hopeless dregs of humanity. It was a word I still couldn't say, not to my friends or my family....

*I had been going downhill fast. Print looked as if it had been soaked in a bathtub. On my bad days, it looked eaten by acid. Sometimes, I could see headlines, but even they swam in and out of blind spots. Everything else appeared as in a dazzling snowstorm—gauzy and colorless. Already the blind areas, the scotomas, were widening considerably, like puddles in a heavy rain. I was frightened by the blanks, the no sights, which registered only by the notable absence of things I knew were there. Still, there was much I could see and do ... and because I was adept at hiding my impairment, I appeared ridiculously normal, especially at St. Paul's.**

(Potock, 1980, p. 55)

Potock vividly describes the experience of gradual visual loss—with some residual vision, he does not feel truly part of the blind world, but yet he finds himself unable to function usefully in the seeing world. The words he uses—*desperation, nightmares, hopeless, frightened*—reflect depression and are understandable responses to profound loss. Depression might be even more acute for Potock than others because prior to becoming blind he was an artist, a painter—he both lived and made his living through his eyes. Potock has come to St. Paul's Rehabilitation Center to begin to reconfigure his life for a future without sight. While at St. Paul's, he discovers that he is not alone in his loss, and he begins to take on a new identity as a blind adult.

Many neurological conditions, of which stroke is likely the most common, result in loss of motor function. This loss may be sudden (as in stroke) or gradual, such as occurs with multiple sclerosis. Postencephalitic parkinsonism is one of the rare causes of motor loss, but it can result in profound functional impairment that is nonetheless compatible with long survival. The following description of Rolando P., provided by Oliver Sacks, gives a sense of the tremendous grief and loss that can accompany a life impaired by neurological dysfunction. For Rolando, human support—initially his mother's and then a therapist's—was the thread that kept him from despair:

ROLANDO

Rolando P. was born in New York in 1917, the youngest son of a newly immigrated and very musical Italian family. He showed unusual vivacity and precocity as a child, acquiring speech and motor skills at an exceptionally early age. He was an active, inquisitive, affectionate and talkative child, until at thirty months of age his life was suddenly cut across by a virulent attack of encephalitis lethargica, which presented itself as an intense drowsiness lasting eighteen weeks, initially accompanied by high fever and influenzal symptoms.

As he awoke from the sleeping-sickness, it became evident that a profound change had occurred, for he now showed a completely masked and expressionless face, and had great difficulty in moving or talking.... He was generally taken to be mentally defective, except by his very observant and understanding mother, who would say: "My Rolando is no fool—he is as sharp and bright as he ever used to be. He has just come to a stop inside."....

"Rolando is not stupid," said a report in 1924. "He absorbs everything, but nothing can come out." This impression of him as purely absorptive, as a sort of unfathomable, black and hungry hole was to be echoed over the next forty years by all who observed him closely....

The next third of a century, in a back ward of the hospital, was completely eventless in the most literal sense of the word....

I examined Mr. P. and talked to him several times between 1965 and 1969. He was a powerfully built man at this time, who appeared far younger than his fifty-odd years; he would easily have passed for half his actual age. He would always be tied in his wheelchair, to prevent an otherwise irresistible tendency to fall forwards....

His voice was so soft as to be inaudible: sudden effort and excitement, however, rendered exclamatory speech possible for a few seconds. Thus, when I asked him whether his salivation disturbed him much, he exclaimed loudly: "You bet it does! It's one hell of a problem!" immediately afterwards relapsing into virtual aphonia [inability to speak]....

His best moods and functioning are brought out by his family, when they take him home for occasional weekends or holidays. In particular Mr. P. likes the hi-fi and swimming pool at his brother's country home. Very remarkable, Mr. P. can swim the length of the pool, and shows a great

*From *Ordinary Daylight*, by Andrew Potock, 1980, New York: Holt, Rinehart & Winston.

diminution of his Parkinsonism in the water; he apparently swims with an ease and fluency which he can never achieve when he moves on dry land.... But Mr. P.'s favourite occupation is to sit on the porch, watching the wild life which teems in the garden, or gazing at the wide prospects of upstate New York. Mr. P. is always intensely depressed when he returns from the country, and the sentiments he expresses are always the same: "What a goddamn relief to get out of this place! ... I've been shut up in places since the day I was born ... I've been shut up in this illness since the day I was born.... That's a hell of a life for someone to have.... Why the hell couldn't I have died as a kid? ..."

Despite progressive age and arthritis [Rolando's mother] would visit Rolando every Sunday without fail.... By the summer of 1972, however, Mrs. P. had become so disabled by arthritis that she was no longer able to come to the hospital. The cessation of her visits was followed by a severe emotional crisis in her son—two months of grief, pining, depression and rage, and during this period he lost twenty pounds. Mercifully, however, his loss was mitigated by a physiotherapist we had on the staff, a woman who combined the skills of her craft with an exceptionally warm and loving nature.... Under this benign and healing influence, Rolando's wound began to heal over—he became calmer and better-humoured, gained weight and slept well.

Unfortunately, at the start of February, his beloved physiotherapist was dismissed from her job (along with almost a third of the hospital staff) as a result of economies dictated by the recent Federal Budget.... Towards the end of February his state changed again, and he moved into a settled and almost inaccessible corpse-like apathy; he became profoundly Parkinsonian once again, but beneath the physiological Parkinsonian mask one could see a worse mask, of hopelessness and despair; he lost his appetite and ceased to eat; he ceased to express any hopes or regrets; he lay awake at nights, with wide-open, dull eyes. It was evident that he was dying, and had lost the will to live....

*A single episode (in early March) sticks in my mind: the medical staff, extremely alert for "organic disease" (but seemingly blind to despairs of the soul), arranged for Rolando to have a battery of "tests," and I was on the ward, that morning, when the diagnostic trolley came up, laden with syringes and tubes for blood, and accompanied by a brisk, white-coated technician. At first, passively, apathetically, Rolando let his arm be taken for blood, but then he suddenly burst out in an unforgettable, white-hot passion of outrage. He pushed the trolley and the technician violently away, and yelled: ... "Don't you have eyes and ears in your head? Can't you see I'm dying of grief? For Chrissake let me die in peace!" These were the last words which Rolando ever spoke. He died in his sleep, or his stupor, just four days later.**

(*Sacks, 1983, pp. 105–118*)

Detaillierte Passion: ein Gestalter

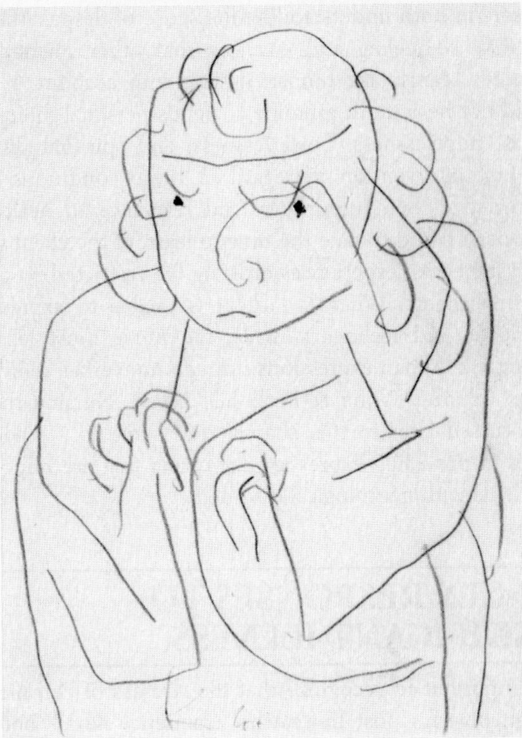

This cartoonlike figure looks with a mixture of anger and disbelief at deformed hands and fingers. This drawing was made only a few months before Klee's death from scleroderma, a collagen vascular disorder associated with severe arthritis and loss of mobility. Prior to being struck by this disorder in 1935, Klee's paintings and drawings were full of exuberant and inventive line and color. Here is one of the most beloved of modern artists contemplating his own disability—and imminent death.

While Rolando's tragic story involves a rare disorder, his grief, desperation, and loss of will to live are not uncommon among persons devastated by neurological disease. Oliver Sacks, the neurologist who described Rolando's life and death, wrote tellingly of despairs of the soul. As Sacks implies, Rolando's death was due to more than just depression: Cut off from the few persons who truly mattered to

*From *Awakenings*, by O. Sacks, 1983, New York: Dutton (Obelisk paperback).

him, Rolando entered into spiritual impoverishment. Without extraordinary nursing intervention to restore his will to live, Rolando's death was inevitable. A nurse has an important role in both understanding the sense of despair that clients may be feeling and ensuring that other members of treatment teams take human despair into account. Nurses should not hesitate to examine a client's personal interpretation of hopelessness, powerlessness, and spiritual distress. The first intervention in regard to these conditions is to acknowledge their importance and relevance to health for every person and to take the time to learn of the client's personal, subjective experiences of living life restricted by physical impairments. When the client is unable to express his experience and feelings verbally, the nurse must learn to understand human expressions through nonverbal, individual means (Tuffrey-Wijne & McEnhill, 2008). Nursing theory, as discussed later in this chapter, can serve as a guide for nurses in providing expressions of caring that are important for clients with neurological disorders.

FAMILY RESPONSES TO SIGNIFICANT ILLNESS

It is important to recognize that the stresses of chronic disease involve not just those who experience illness but also family members whose lives are affected through their roles as the caretakers for ill family members. Spouses and parents are most often greatly affected by illness in a close family member, and these persons may feel particularly vulnerable when attention is given to the involved individual but not to their own needs or to the adjustments required of the family accommodating the needs of one very ill person. In the next excerpt, a woman describes the profound impact the illness of her son had on the family:

THE WILLIAMS FAMILY

Mavis Williams is a forty-nine-year-old architect and mother of three. She is a single head of household; eight years ago she and her husband of fifteen years divorced. Her oldest child, Andrew, age twenty-three, suffers from inherited muscular dystrophy. Now in a wheelchair, he is progressively losing control of his speech, arms, and upper body. The disorder first appeared when he was nine years old, but it seriously accelerated when he was twelve. It is incurable. His neurologist's prognosis is a slow decline of motor activity over three to five years, with subsequent mental deterioration and death. I met Mrs. Williams not through clinical consultation but in the course of a field research project. I had administered several questionnaires to her to ascertain her reaction to her son's illness and to obtain her evaluation of its effect on their family.

"Dr. Kleinman, I hope you don't mind me saying this to you, but I found the questions ridiculous. I filled in all the little boxes, but I think the questions are superficial. You really want to know what impact my son's illness has had? All right then, you need to get at the way it has torn us apart, divided me from my husband, affected each and every one of us and our plans and dreams. When the questionnaire says, "Has the effect on your relationships with your spouse or your children been minimal, moderate, serious," or whatever it says—you know the question I mean—what does that have to do with a family turned into a cauldron? With explosions of rage, with a daily grief that sucks your eyes dry, with turning away hurt and empty? It is the totality of its effects, its all-encompassingness that you should study. And especially its deep currents of desperation and failure. There is a little voice in me which, if I knew you better, would scream at you: Doctor, it has murdered this family.

There is no stability; we can't work it through. Andrew's illness doesn't end. It tortures him, it does the same to us. John, my husband, blamed me. It seems to come from my side of the family. John collapsed, literally collapsed. He couldn't handle it or do anything for any of us, even himself. He ran away and drank. He was no help, no help at all. But I can't really blame him. Who can expect to meet a test like this? It is the daily struggle to stay on top of it. I blame me for being absolutely, totally incapable of separating any part of me from Andrew's suffering. I have no free space, no private and protected place to get away and call my own. It has taken all of me. What is a mother to do? Between this horror and working to support the family I have, I really have, no—no—time! Zero time for me.

Look at Barbara and Kim [her other children]. What have their lives been like? Guilt because they are normal. Anger, intense anger because Andrew has required so much of my time and energy. I have had, I'll admit, precious little left over for them. But they can't express any of this. How can you, when the person responsible is dying slowly, day by day, in front of your eyes? So they can't express it to him; they take it out on me! Like John does, like Andrew does, like I want to also—since there is no one else strong enough to take it.

OK, tell me. How do you convert this into a +3 or −3 answer, to a decimal? How do you compare it with other people's reactions? I insist it is illegitimate to make comparisons. We are not things. This is not an "interpersonal problem," a "family stress"—this is a calamity! I do not exaggerate. Before Andrew's disaster we were like everyone else: some days good, some bad. Then we had problems. But looking back, that was a kind of paradise I can hardly believe was real. Now we are burning up. I sometimes

Talk to Her

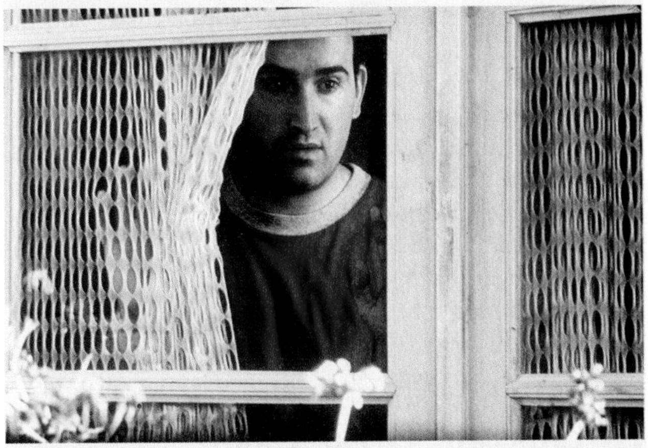

Courtesy: El Deseo/The Kobal Collection/Bracho, Miguel

In this clip from *Talk to Her* the character Benigno is obsessively watching a neighbor who eventually comes under his nursing care when a brain injury leads to a "persistent vegetative state." While Benigno's nursing interventions are not all benign, viewers will sympathize fully with his devotion to treating each coma victim as a living being needing both physical and emotional care.

*think we are all dying, not just Andy. Even my parents and brothers and sisters have been more than "affected," Dr. Kleinman. You look around you—you look! This, what you see, this tomb, our family's tomb.**

(Kleinman, 1988, pp. 183–184)

Nurses are familiar with the nursing diagnoses of *Interrupted family processes* and *Compromised family coping. Interrupted family processes* is the diagnosis used when a family that is functioning well encounters an event or situation requiring an adjustment. Significant illness of any family member requires adjustment of those who are to provide care. If the illness is chronic, no matter how well the family attempts to adjust and cope, the problem may be so overwhelming that the family's coping is ineffective.

The diagnosis of *Caregiver role strain* was added to the NANDA International (NANDA-I) taxonomy to identify the difficult roles family members experience when providing care over time. The difficulty in identifying the diagnosis of *Caregiver role strain* is that the nurse may have difficulty following through as a nurse may not be in a position to provide or arrange for respite care. The nurse may be able to identify the problem, but without well- developed community resources, there may be little the nurse can provide to an individual other than understanding and validation of the difficult situation and problem solving to help the caregiver look for alternatives of action. On the community level, however, the nurse can advocate for appropriate support services for families caring for chronically ill individuals, such as support groups, respite care, and volunteer programs to help meet needs of family members.

*From *The Illness Narratives*, by Arthur Kleinman, Copyright © 1988. Reprinted with permission from BasicBooks, a member of Perseus Books, L.L.C.

NURSING ROLES

There are two nursing roles in regard to assisting clients with physical illness who have strong emotional reactions. The first is liaison psychiatric nursing, a field that developed in the 1960s in which psychiatric professionals serve as consultants to health care providers in the general medical settings. The second, more recent role is that of the psychiatric nurse specialist in home care. Each is discussed following.

PSYCHIATRIC CONSULTATION-LIAISON NURSING

Over the past several decades the subspecialty of the **Psychiatric Consultation-Liaison Nursing** (PCLN) has arisen in response to the increased recognition of the importance of psychophysiological interrelationships and their impact on physical illness, recovery, and wellness (Minarik & Neese, 2002; Broom, Shirk, Pehrson, & Peterson, 2008). One of the early roles of the subspecialty was consultation with nonpsychiatric health care providers, particularly those working in general hospitals, about clients whose problems involved both physical and psychological symptoms. Early on, liaison psychiatry was defined as being concerned with the study, diagnosis, treatment, and prevention of psychiatric illness in the physically ill and of the psychological factors affecting physical conditions (Pasnau, 1982). Consultation-liaison nursing seems to have begun at Duke University in the 1960s when psychiatric nurses made their skills and expertise available to assist nurses working on other hospital units (Johnson, 1963). In a classic book describing the speciality in the 1980s, Lewis and Levy (1982) described the major goals of psychiatric liaison nursing: to demonstrate and teach mental health nursing concepts and their application to practice, to effect an appropriate psychiatric and nursing intervention for individual clients, to support nurses providing quality nursing care, to promote and develop the professional self-esteem of the nurse, and to encourage tolerance among members of the nursing staff in situations where immediate or effective resolution of issues is unattainable.

Today the American Nurses Association has recognized the PCLN as a subspecialty and as a role for an advanced practice nurse. The PCLN is prepared to take on several tasks, including case consultation and administrative consultation, professional development of staff, and unit liaison (Sharrock & Happell, 2002). Box 21-3 lists the characteristics of a PCLN in today's practice. The PCLN may be called on to consult about a particular client case or regarding an administrative organizational issue impacting client care. One author describes the use of holistic assessments on a cardiac

BOX 21-3
ROLES AND KNOWLEDGE/EXPERTISE OF THE PCLN

ROLES

1. Consultation to nursing staff and administration
2. Education of client care team
3. Direct, specialized care to clients and their families

KNOWLEDGE AND EXPERTISE

1. Expertise in psychiatric problems, normal and abnormal responses to illness, and adaptation responses
2. Knowledge of interrelationships between physical and psychological states
3. Knowledge of systems theory and group process, nursing and psychological/ psychiatric theories
4. Ability to provide liaison between and among disciplines

service that provide a means for the PCLN to uncover cases of client depression as well as issues of substance abuse, client and family resources, and characteristics of resiliency among family members (Ragaisis, 2007). Thus, the PCLN can focus on client and family strengths at a time where the acute illness directs most to focus on weaknesses. The liaison role is distinct from pure "consultation" in that it requires regular interactions and close associations between the PCLN and the nonpsychiatric service. This liaison activity may also have strong focus on staff education and development. One author emphasizes that the PCLN must be a nurse with good knowledge and background in physical illness in order to understands its impact on emotional and interpersonal functioning (Ragaisis, 2005). She writes that the PCLN must herself possess "strong emotional competencies" (p 197).

As nurses in the general hospital, clinic, and home care settings continue to encounter clients with emotional and psychiatric symptoms and reactions that impede recovery from physical disease, the work of the PCLN becomes increasingly important (Chase, Gage, Stanley, & Bonadonna, 2000). Further, as nurses more readily identify the holistic needs of their clients, the PCLN may be called to assist in areas of perceived weaknesses (Johnston & Cowman, 2008). Indeed, several studies have indicated that nurses tend to be unsure of their knowledge base in meeting their clients' psychiatric and psychological needs and lack confidence in their ability to do so. The PCLN interventions have been shown to increase nurses' confidence to accomplish this work and to have a positive impact on client care outcomes (Sharrock & Happell, 2000). In our current era of evidence-based practice, recent commentaries about the role of the PCLN have called for increasing attention to documentation and evaluation of outcomes of the role. Limited data are collected on several parameters that could document outcomes and the actual practice of the role (Yakimo, 2006). Authors have suggested that the PCLN can impact care on three levels: (1) the client/family level, where the outcome of the role may be, for example, a decrease in psychiatric symptom distress, increased treatment adherence, and positive caregiver interaction; (2) the hospital unit level, where the outcome may be increased staff satisfaction and improved communication with clients; and (3) at the institutional level, where the outcome could be decreased length of stay (Yakimo, Kurlowicz, & Murray, 2004).

Psychiatric Home Care Behavioral Health

Psychiatric liaison nursing roles originally evolved in the general hospital setting at a time during which relatively lengthy hospitalizations for general medical conditions were not uncommon. In today's economic climate, diagnostic evaluations often take place outside hospitals, and clients move rapidly in and out of the inpatient setting. While there is little doubt that the psychiatric nurse has an important contribution to make to an increasingly ambulatory model of patient care, new roles are developing in the field of community psychiatric care and for psychiatric nursing in home health care (see also Chapter 31).

The psychiatric clinical nurse specialist in home care takes responsibility to monitor and follow clients who are chronically mentally ill, as well as those clients and families who are dealing with psychosocial crises (Mellon, 1994). Particularly during times when early hospital discharge leaves clients and families feeling vulnerable, the nurse with psychiatric experience has much to offer in areas of prevention and wellness care. In some settings, psychiatric nurses have defined specialized populations with whom they work; for example, some provide mental health services to the elderly in their homes (Harper, 1989; Thobaben & Kozlak, 1990) or long-term care facilities (Craig & Pham, 2006); others develop programs to support persons with acquired immunodeficiency syndrome (AIDS; Frey, Oman, Robins, & Smith, 1991); while others accept referrals from accident and emergency units (Wand & White, 2007).

NURSING THEORY

All nursing theories call on nurses to view the client holistically. Adaptation theories, such as those of Callista Roy or Helen Erickson and colleagues, directly address the need for the client to react to stress in some way that returns the self to a state of homeostasis. This thinking fits well with the notion that any client adapts to physical disease and that his adaptation includes changes on both an emotional and a physical level. Understanding the connections between mind and body will assist a nurse in making holistic assessments and providing interventions that meet the client's need for peace and harmony. The Modeling and Role-Modeling theory (see Chapter 3) specifically calls on nurses to assess the client's physical state and to further assess the client's needs, worries, and wants to facilitate the nurse's evaluation of the client's emotional reactions to physical illness and events surrounding treatment. The numerous case examples in this chapter emphasize the great need to evaluate the client's emotional, physical, and attitudinal states in working with clients for whom somatic illness is the primary factor in seeking care. Table 21-1 summarizes the nursing process for clients with emotional responses to physical illness using the Modeling and Role-Modeling theory.

Further, the nursing theories that emphasize human caring are also relevant to the nurse providing care to clients with physical illness. The case examples in this chapter emphasize client feelings of abandonment, loneliness, rejection, and depression. These feelings are rather common human responses to life's situations that the clients believe no one else can really understand. The presence of a caring nurse—the therapeutic presence of another human being who provides connection—is an intervention all too often lacking in current health care settings. The nurse using theories of human caring can validate that caring in and of itself is an important and worthy activity. The case example of Rolando exemplifies the need for human care and may help the reader to remember how crucial care can be for health and, ultimately, for survival.

PSYCHIATRIC NURSING AND MIND-BODY MEDICINE

In a chapter focusing on mental health nursing involving clients with somatic illness, it is important to acknowledge the emerging research on mind-body medicine—the connection between thought, emotion, and physical functioning. While there is strong emerging evidence that stress is associated with cardiovascular disease (Brotman, Golden, & Wittstein, 2007) and other serious illness, nurses have long intuited that the mind and body function as one in a way such that factors influencing the mind have profound effects on physiological processes. However, only in the late 1980s did a new field of scientific inquiry emerge to study and evaluate how the mind can affect physiology.

Rossi used the term **mind modulation** to refer to those processes by which thoughts, feelings, attitudes, and emotions are converted by the brain into neurohormonal messenger molecules (Rossi, 1986). Thus, Rossi provided explanations for how the mind modulates biochemical functions through several of the body's systems. For example, the mind affects the autonomic nervous system in the following ways: Images and thoughts are generated in the frontal cortex; these images and thoughts are transmitted through areas of the limbic-hypothalamic system to the neurotransmitters that regulate the autonomic nervous system branches; and the neurotransmitters (norepinephrine and acetylcholine) initiate the biochemical changes within different tissues down to the cellular level, resulting in either sympathetic or

TABLE 21-1 Summary of Nursing Process for Clients with Physical Illness, with Emotional Responses Using Modeling and Role-Modeling Theory

NURSING PROCESS STEP	NURSING ACTION BASED ON MODELING AND ROLE-MODELING THEORY
Assessment	What is the meaning of the illness to the client? What are the client's needs, worries, and wants? What does the client want the nurse to do? Is the client able to cope with the illness and treatment? What support does the client need?
Diagnosis	Nursing diagnoses written based on preceding assessment. *Examples: Ineffective coping*, related to feeling overwhelmed by the demands of treatment; *fear* of disease and treatment regime; *hopelessness*, related to lack of sense of future/belief that recovery is not Possible.
Outcomes	The client will be able to cope effectively with illness; the client will receive treatment and move toward recovery or the ability to live with illness as part of his life.
Interventions (begin with the five aims)	1. Build trust 2. Promote positive orientation. 3. Promote perceived control. 4. Promote strengths. 5. Set mutual goals that are health related.
Evaluation	Mutual evaluation of client's condition.

parasympathetic responses. Further, neurotransmitters act as messenger molecules, crossing nerve cell junctional gaps and fitting onto receptors in the cell walls, changing the receptor molecular structure (Dossey, 1995). These explanations began to help nurses to understand why interventions such as imagery, relaxation, music therapy, and hypnosis produce effects in that the interventions permit calming influences of the client's parasympathetic system to take over in situations that would otherwise be stress inducing (Dossey, 1995).

Data from others' work continued to suggest profound mind-body connections. Dossey reports that state of mind is statistically associated with morbidity and mortality. The "Black Monday" syndrome is a powerful example. In the United States, more persons died of heart attacks on Mondays than any other day of the week (Rabkin, Mathewson, & Tate, 1980); and more persons had heart attacks between the hours of 8:00 A.M. and 9:00 A.M. than at any other time (Kolata, 1986). These observations led others to study and conclude that one factor—job satisfaction—is the single most important risk factor in predicting (or perhaps preventing) heart attack (Dossey, 1991). While at least one investigation has not concluded that job satisfaction has such a predictive risk (Hlatky, Lam, Lee, Clapp-Channing, Williams, Pryor, et al., 1995), other research continued to suggest that the client's faith in the treatment, perception of support, and sense of hope can, indeed, affect clinical outcome (Dossey, 1991).

Psychoneuroimmunology

Psychoneuroimmunology (PNI) is a branch of scientific study that "seeks to understand the mind-body connection" (Schwartz, 1994, p. 4), and "strives to show the connections among psychology, neuroendocrinology, and immunology" (Bartol & Courts, 2009, p. 601). Psychoneuroimmunology is based on a theoretical model of the relationships between psychological factors and immune function via the hypothalamic pituitary axis of the sympathetic nervous system. Based on Selye's General Adaptation (or Stress) Syndrome, the model suggests that psychosocial stressors influence health via the hypothalamic pituitary axis by affecting the secretions of glucocorticoids, which can suppress immune function (Schwartz, 1994). While the field of study is evolving and there are significant methodological problems with the design and conduct of related work, PNI has led many to rethink traditional ideas that the mind and body are separate. Indeed, as early as 1986, Pert, of the National Institutes of Health, wrote: "The more we know about neuropeptides, the harder it is to think in the traditional terms of a mind and a body. It makes more sense to speak of a single integrated entity, a '*bodymind*'" (Pert, 1986, p. 9).

Nurses must take into account the meaning of a body-mind connection in all aspects of nursing care. There are many ways to do so, but the authors suggest that nurses begin with the following:

1. Examine how attitudes—such as feelings of hope or despair, love or fear, perceptions of an event as a crisis or a challenge, feelings of personal control or powerlessness—can influence an individual client's recovery.
2. Treat every client in a holistic manner, that is, ensure that the nursing assessment not only is of the client's physical state and mental status but also includes an understanding of the client's attitudes, fears, challenges, and supports.
3. When the client has physical disease that affects emotions, take time to understand the emotions. Accept the client as he is, never judging that one reaction is appropriate or is better than another.

RESEARCH Highlight 21–2

Psychoneuroimmunology and Related Mechanisms in Understanding Health Disparities in Vulnerable Populations

STUDY PURPOSE

In an annual review of nursing research, the author set out to provide a review of how neuroendocrine and immune functions are affected in factors that impact vulnerability.

METHOD

The researcher reviewed original databased articles published over a five-year period retrieved through a PubMed search.

FINDINGS

Of particular impact to nurses are the findings that both aging and stress have documented negative impact on immune functioning. Moreover, the effects of stress are influenced by three factors: magnitude of the stress, duration, and the individual's response. Strategies that modulate the stress response (relaxation therapies, hypnosis, and exercise) have positive effects on the endocrine and immune functioning. Lastly, cytokine-induced symptoms are adaptive in nature.

IMPLICATIONS

Specific considerations for the elderly must be taken and they have increased risk for infection. Stress assessment should certainly be incorporated in caring for the elderly, as well as others thought to be facing stress. Stress modulation techniques can appropriately be incorporated into nursing care.

Source: "Psychoneuroimmunology and Related Mechanisms in Understanding Health Disparities in Vulnerable Populations," by T. Briones, *Annual Review of Nursing Research*, *25*, 219–256.

FUTURE DIRECTIONS

Every nurse who is caring for a client in a holistic manner recognizes that the body and the mind are, indeed, one and that any illness in the physical body affects the client's psychoemotional state, and that the psychoemotional state in turn affects the recovery and healing of a physical problem.

Today more than ever, professional nurses are playing a key role in the understanding and care of clients experiencing emotional distress in relation to physical conditions. A nursing intervention in psychiatric nursing can sometimes be as elementary as a hug and a smile or as complex as performing one of the complementary modalities described in Chapter 32, such as guided imagery. The growing field of PNI is changing the way health professionals look at and treat clients. As the body of evidence that physical health can be influenced and seriously affected by mental and emotional health grows, nurses will need to be more sensitive to the psychological complications of physical illness in order to arrange for and, if appropriate, provide timely psychiatric care. Nurses in psychiatric liaison services will be called on to assess clients in the general medical setting and to assist other nurses in establishing the appropriate approach to care. Over the next few years, the number of psychiatric nurses working in home care is expected to grow. These nurses will play a critical role in bringing the awareness of the body-mind relationship to others working to support client care.

KEY CONCEPTS

- Persons must call on their adaptive strengths when facing chronic or life-threatening illnesses. Occasionally, these strengths are insufficient to prevent the emergence of psychiatric symptoms.
- It has been clearly documented that clients with certain physical illnesses face serious emotional adjustments. These conditions are cancer, heart disease, chronic pain, and neurological disorders.
- Liaison psychiatric nursing has emerged as a means for psychiatric professionals to provide consultation in general medical settings regarding clients whose problems involve both physical and psychological symptoms.
- Community psychiatric nursing is a developing role within home care to provide mental health services to clients with primarily physical conditions.
- Nursing theory serves to guide nurses in providing holistic care that addresses the connections between body, mind, and emotions.
- Body-mind medicine is an emerging area of scientific study of the connections and relationships between thoughts, emotions, and physical conditions.

REVIEW QUESTIONS

1. A client has been admitted for surgical removal of a benign tumor. The nurse assesses that the client is anxious and fearful about the impending surgery. The most therapeutic action that the nurse can take would be which of the following?
   1. Ask a family member to stay with the client until she goes to surgery
   2. Allow the client to express her fears and concerns regarding the surgery
   3. Contact the client's physician and request that the surgery be postponed
   4. Request that the physician meet with the client and discuss details of the surgery

2. A teen-aged boy was brought to the hospital after an accident on the school football field. The client is in stable condition. When the family arrives at the hospital, the mother is hysterical and the father is cursing the football coach and demanding to see his son. Which approach by the nurse would be most therapeutic?
   1. Take the parents to their son's room so they can talk with him
   2. Contact the physician and request a sedative for the boy's mother
   3. Ask the hospital security to escort the parents off of the unit until they are calmer
   4. Take the parents to a quiet room so they can calm down before seeing their son

3. A client has been admitted to a hospice unit as a result of terminal cancer. The nurse recognizes that the priority intervention is:
   1. Nutritional needs
   2. Rest and social needs
   3. Elimination needs
   4. Comfort and hygienic needs

4. A client is diagnosed with a terminal condition. Which nursing intervention would provide spiritual support to the client?
   1. Assisting the client to develop skills for self-care
   2. Problem solving for the client to facilitate growth

3. Helping the client to search for meaning in their experience
4. Teaching the client techniques of relaxation and guided imagery

5. A client is admitted to the hospital with complaints of severe back pain. During the initial interview the client states to the nurse, "The pain is constant. I've tried everything, but nothing seems to help. It's difficult for me to play with my children or make love to my wife. I have not been to work in weeks because the pain is so bad." The nurse understands that the priority is to further assess which of the following problems identified by the client:
1. Level of pain
2. Coping strategies
3. Possible future unemployment
4. Altered family role performance

6. A client is admitted to the hospice program after diagnosis of terminal cancer. The client states to the nurse, "I've tried to live a good life. I have always worked hard and tried to be helpful to individuals less fortunate. Why is God punishing me?" The nurse recognizes that the client's statement is an indication of which of the following?
1. Ineffective coping
2. Spiritual distress
3. Altered body image
4. Fear of the unknown

LEARNING ACTIVITIES

1. Describe the reaction of a client you have known who was facing a life-threatening illness. What nursing supports did this client require? What kind of services would you provide?

2. What are the means you have as a nurse to meet the emotional needs of clients in the general medical setting?

3. Consider the case presented in this chapter of Mrs. Bell, attending a clinic for clients with chronic pain. What could you do as a nurse to address the dysfunctional work of the team attending to her pain?

4. Describe the clues apparent in assessing that a client who presents with psychological symptoms has a physical disorder.

5. What nursing theories assist you in your assessment of the client with psychological and physical symptoms?

6. How is the field of body-mind medicine reflected in your work as a holistic nurse?

*Study*WARE™ CONNECTION

Using your *Study*WARE™ CD-ROM

1. Review the audio glossary for key terms in this chapter.
2. Explore the other games and activities that support this chapter.

REFERENCES

Afrell, M., Biguet, G., & Rudebeck, C. E. (2007). Living with a body in pain—between acceptance and denial. *Scandinavian Journal of Caring Sciences, 21*(3), 291–296.

American Nurses Association. (1990). *Standards of psychiatric consultation and liaison nursing*. Kansas City, MO: Author.

American Psychiatric Association. (2000). *Diagnostic and statistical manual of mental disorders* (Fourth Edition-Text Revision). Washington, DC: Author.

Bartol, G., & Courts, N. (2009). The psychophysiology of body-mind healing. In B. Dossey and L. Keegan (Eds). *Holistic nursing: A handbook for practice* (5th ed. pp. 601–615). Jones & Bartlett: Boston.

Blumenthal, J.A. (2008). Depression and coronary heart disease: Association and implications for treatment. *Cleveland Clinic Medicine, 75*(*Suppl 2*), 838–852.

Broom, C., Shirk, M. J., Pehrson, K. M., & Peterson, K. (2008). Perspectives on psychiatric consultation liaison nursing: Psychiatric-mental health—advanced practice nurses: Transforming nursing practice. *Perspectives in Psychiatric Care, 44*(2), 131–134.

Brotman, D., Golden, S., & Wittstein, I. (2007). The cardiovascular toll of stress. *Lancet 370*(9592), 1089–1100.

Brown, S. T. (2000). Outcomes analysis of a pain management project. *Journal of Nursing Care Quality, 14*(4), 28–34.

Chase, P., Gage, J., Stanley, K. M., & Bonadonna, J. R. (2000). The psychiatric consultation/liaison nurse role in case management. *Nursing Case Management, 5*(2), 73–77.

Cheng, S. K., Tsang, J. S., Ku, K., Wong, C. W., & Ng, Y. K. (2004). Psychiatric complications in patients with severe acute respiratory syndrome (SARS) during the acute treatment phase: A series of cases. *British Journal of Psychiatry, 184*, 359–360.

Courtenay, M., & Carey, N. (2008). The impact and effectiveness of nurse-led care in the management of acute and chronic pain: A review of the literature. *Journal of Clinical Nursing, 17*(15), 2001–2013.

Craig, E., & Pham, H. (2006). Consultation-liaison psychiatry services to nursing homes. *Australasian Psychiatry, 14*(1), 46–48.

Davydow, D. S., Gifford, J. M., Desai, S. V., Needham, D. M., & Bienvenu, O. J. (2008). Posttraumatic stress disorder in general intensive care unit survivors: A systematic review. *General Hospital Psychiatry, 30*(5), 421–434.

Dossey, B. (1995). The psychophysiology of bodymind healing. In B. Dossey, L. Keegan, C. Guzzetta, & L. Kolkmeier (Eds.), *Holistic nursing: A handbook for practice* (pp. 77–95). Rockville, MD: Aspen.

Dossey, L. (1991). *Meaning and medicine.* New York: Bantam Books.

Fontana, J. S. (2008). The social and political forces affecting prescribing practices for chronic pain. *Journal of Professional Nursing, 24*(1), 30–35.

Frey, D., Oman, K., Robins, J., & Smith, E. J. (1991). Psychiatric home care with AIDS patients. *Journal of Home Health Care Practice, 3,* 34–45.

Granberg, A., Engberg, I. B., & Lundberg, D. (1999). Acute confusion and unreal experiences in intensive care patients in relation to the DCU syndrome Part II. *Intensive Critical Care Nursing, 15*(1), 19–33.

Harper, M. S. (1989). Providing mental health services in the homes of the elderly. *Caring, 8,* 4–6, 8–9, 52–53.

Higgins, R. O., Murphy, B. M., Nicholas, A., Worcester, M. U., & Lindner, H. (2007). Emotional and adjustment issues faced by cardiac patients seen in clinical practice: A qualitative survey of experienced clinicians. *Journal of Cardiopulmonary Rehabilitation and Prevention, 27*(5), 291–297.

Hlatky, M. A., Lam, L. C., Lee, K. L., Clapp-Channing, N. E., Williams, R. B., Pryor, R. B., et al. (1995). Job strain and the prevalence and outcome of coronary artery disease. *Circulation, 92,* 327–333.

Johnson, B. S. (1963). Psychiatric nurse consultant in a general hospital. *Nursing Outlook, 11,* 728–729.

Johnson, J. (1991). Learning to live again: The process of adjustment following a heart attack. In J. M. Morse & J. L. Johnson (pp. 25–85), *The illness experience.* Newbury Park, CA: Sage.

Johnston, M. L., & Cowman, S. (2008). An examination of the services provided by Psychiatric Consultation Liaison Nurses in a general hospital. *Journal of Psychiatric and Mental Health Nursing, 15*(6), 500–507.

Kapfhammer, H. P., Rothenhausler, H. B., Krauseneck, T., Stoll, C., & Schelling, G. (2004). Posttraumatic stress disorder and health-related quality of life in long-term survivors of acute respiratory distress syndrome. *American Journal of Psychiatry, 161*(1), 45–52.

Kee, C. C. (2003). Older adults with osteoarthritis: Psychological status and physical function. *Journal of Gerontological Nursing, 29*(12), 26–34, 50–51.

Kolata, G. (1986, July). Heart attacks at 9:00 A.M. *Science,* 417–418.

Lewis, A., & Levy, J. (1982). *Psychiatric liaison nursing.* Reston, VA: Reston.

Mellon, S. K. (1994). Mental health clinical nurse specialists in home care for the 90s. *Issues in Mental Health Nursing, 15,* 220–237.

Minarik, P. A., & Neese, J. B. (2002). Essential educational content for advanced practice nurses in psychiatric consultation liaison nursing. *Archives of Psychiatric Nursing, 19*(1), 3–15.

Pasnau, R. O. (1982). Consultation-liaison psychiatry at the crossroads: In search of a definition for the 1980s. *Hospital & Community Psychiatry, 33,* 989–995.

Pert, C. (1986). The wisdom of the receptors: Neuropeptides, the emotions, and bodymind. *Advances, 3,* 8–16.

Rabkin, S. W., Mathewson, A. L., & Tate, R. B. (1980). Chronobiology of cardiac sudden death in men. *Journal of the American Medical Association, 244,* 1357–1358.

Ragaisis, K., (2007). A Place for the PCLN in Cardiac Rehabilitation. *Perspectives in Psychiatric Care, 43*(3), 154–156.

Ragaisis, K. (2005). Perspectives in Psychiatric Consultation Liaison Nursing: Bridging the Gap. *Perspectives in Psychiatric Care, 41*(4), 197–198.

Rosenblum, A., Marsch, L. A., Joseph, H., & Portenoy, R. K. (2008). Opioids and the treatment of chronic pain: Controversies, current status, and future directions. *Experimental and Clinical Psychopharmacology, 16*(5), 405–416.

Rossi, E. (1986). *The psychobiology of mind-body healing.* New York: Norton.

Sateia, M. J., & Lang, B. J. (2008). Sleep and cancer: Recent developments. *Current Oncology Reports, 10*(4), 309–318.

Schneider, K. L., & Shenassa, E. (2008). Correlates of suicide ideation in a population-based sample of cancer patients. *Journal of Psychosocial Oncology, 26*(2), 49–62.

Schwartz, C. E. (1994). New directions in psychoneuroimmunology, introduction: Old methodological challenges and new mind-body link in psychoneuroimmunology. *Advances, 10,* 4–7.

Sharrock, J., & Happell, B. (2000). The role of the psychiatric consultation-liaison nurse in the general hospital. *Australian Journal of Advanced Nursing, 18*(1), 34–39.

Smith, A. A., & Friedman, M. L. (1999). Perceived family dynamics of persons with chronic pain. *Journal of Advanced Nursing, 30*(3), 543–551.

Steihaug, S. (2007). Women's strategies for handling chronic muscle pain: A qualitative study. *Scandinavian Journal of Primary Health Care, 25*(1), 44–48.

Storer, D., Whitworth, R., Salkovskis, P., & Atha, C. (1987). Community and psychiatric nursing intervention in an accident and emergency department: A clinical pilot study. *Journal of Advanced Nursing, 12,* 215–222.

Thobaben, M., & Kozlak, J. (1990). Home health care's unique role in serving the elderly mentally ill. *Home Healthcare Nurse, 8,* 37–39.

Tsai, P. F., Tak, Moore, C., & Palencia, I. (2003). Testing a theory of chronic pain. *Journal of Advanced Nursing, 43*(2), 158–169.

Tuffrey-Wijne, I., & McEnhill, L. (2008). Communication difficulties and intellectual disability in end-of-life care. *International Journal of Palliative Nursing, 14*(4), 189–194.

Wand, T., & White, K. (2007). Examining models of mental health service delivery in the emergency department. *Australian and New Zealand Journal of Psychiatry, 41*(10), 784–791.

Werner, A., Isaksen, L. W., & Malterud, K. (2004). "I am not the kind of woman who complains of everything": Illness stories on self and shame in women with chronic pain. *Social Sciences and Medicine, 59*(5), 1035–1045.

Wilkes, L. M., Castro, M., Mohan, S., Sundaraj, S. R., & Noore, F. (2003). Health status of patients with chronic pain attending a pain center. *Pain Management Nursing, 4*(2), 70–76.

Yakimo, R. (2006). Outcomes in Psychiatric Consultation-Liaison Nursing. *Perspectives in Psychiatric Care, 42*(1), 59–62.

Yakimo, R., Kurlowicz, L., & Murray, R. (2004). Evaluation of Outcomes of PCLN Practice. *Archives of Psychiatric Nursing, 18*(6), 215–227.

LITERARY REFERENCES

Alsop, S. (1973). *Stay of execution.* New York HarperCollins.

Howe, H. (1982). *Do not go gentle.* New York W. W. Norton.

Johnson, J. (1991). Learning to live again: The process of adjustment following a heart attack. In J. M. Morse & J. L. Johnson (pp. 25–85), *The illness experience.* Newbury Park, CA: Sage.

Kleinman, A. (1988). *The illness narratives: Suffering, healing, and the human condition.* New York BasicBooks.

Lear, M. W. (1980). *Heartsound.* New York Simon & Schuster.

Potock, A. (1980). *Ordinary daylight.* New York: Holt, Rinehart & Winston.

Sacks, O. (1983). *Awakenings.* New York: Dutton (Obelisk paperback).

Sarton, M. (1980). *Recovering, a journal.* New York: Norton.

SUGGESTED READINGS

Cassell, E. J. (2004). *The nature of suffering and the goals of medicine* (2nd ed.). New York: Oxford and Oxford University Press.

Drench, M. E. (2003). *Psychosocial aspects of health care.* Upper Saddle River, NJ: Prentice Hall.

Ferrell, B. R. (1996). *Suffering.* Boston: Jones and Bartlett.

Kleinman, A. (1988). *The illness narratives: Suffering, healing, and the human condition.* New York: BasicBooks.

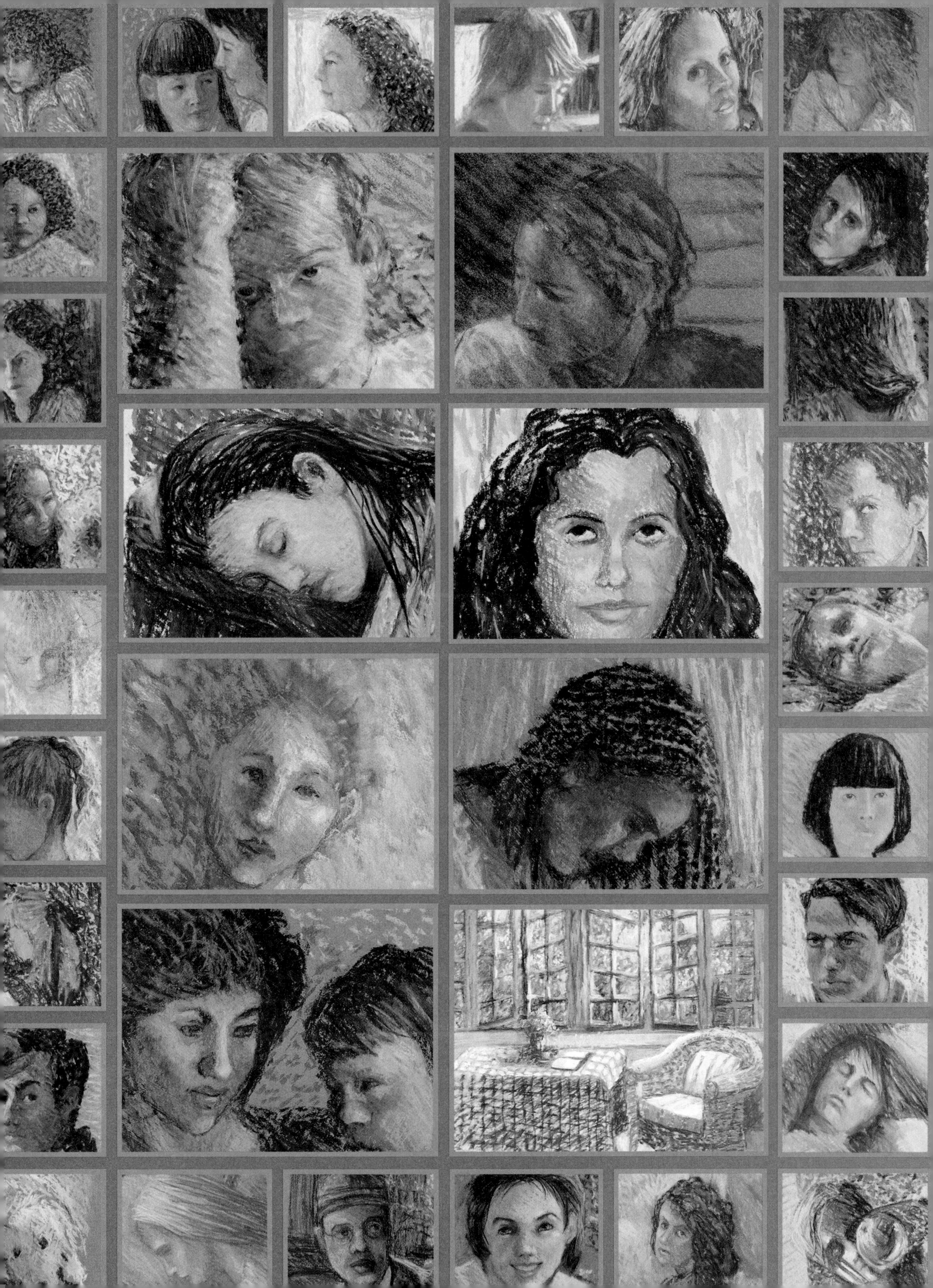

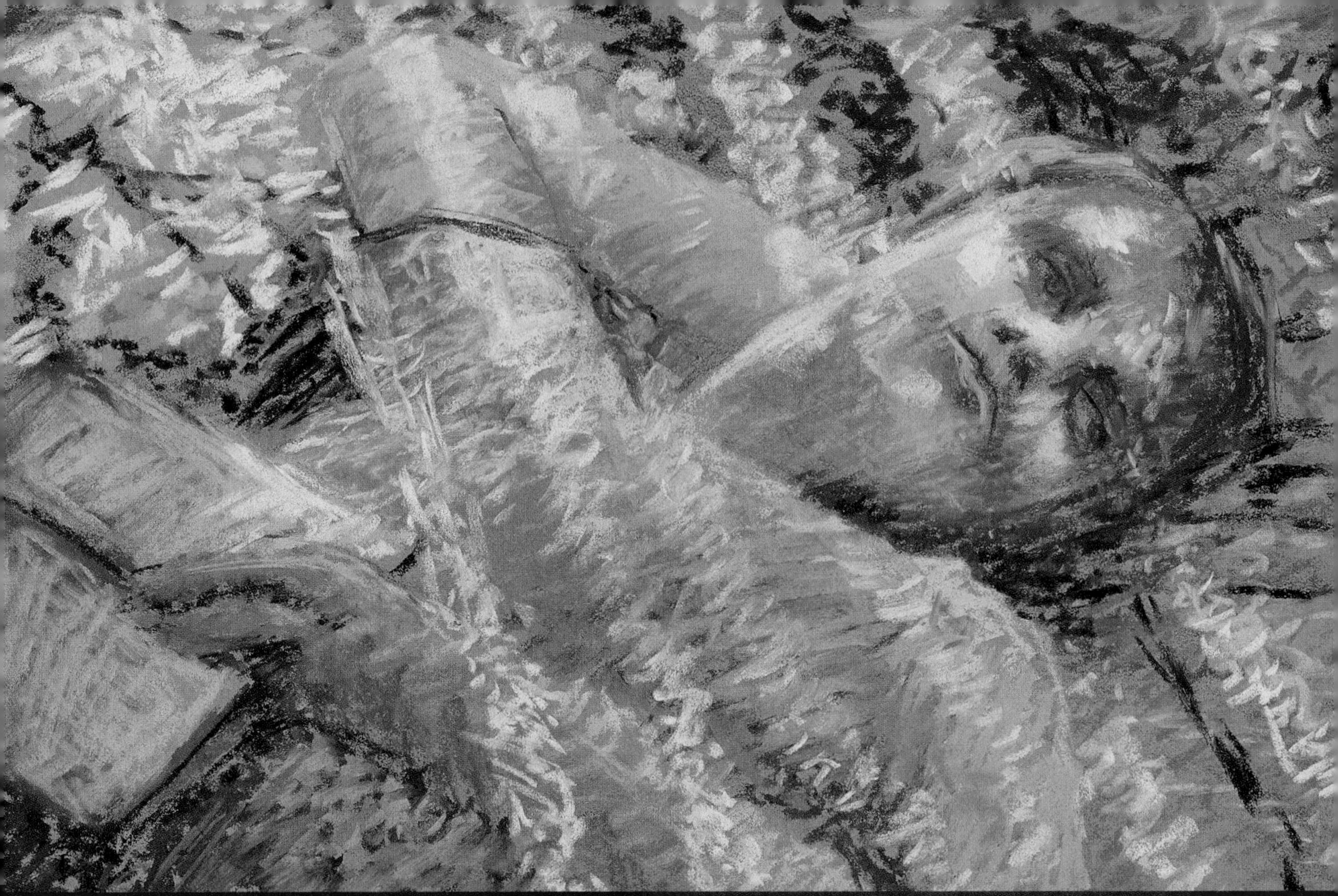

Nothing but Time

Walking Down the Street

Walk down the street in any major U.S. city and notice the persons sitting in doorways, sleeping in subway stations, and asking for food. Consider what you know, what you feel, and what you believe about your encounters with these persons.

What you know

- ***Where do these homeless persons come from?***
- ***How did they become "down and out"?***
- ***What are their day-to-day lives like?***

What you feel

- ***Do you feel any of the following: anger, fear, repulsion, sadness, and/or annoyance?***

Walking down the same city street, notice the construction of a new prison (a very common sight now in the United States). Reflect on the following:

- ***Why did the United States become the world leader in incarceration?***
- ***Who are the persons in jails?***
- ***Are you prepared to provide nursing services to the incarcerated?***
- ***What needs do you think the incarcerated have for care, safety, and rehabilitation?***

What you believe

- ***Examine your own beliefs about individual and societal responsibilities regarding the homeless and the prison population. Before reading on, reflect on your beliefs and feelings regarding both the homeless and the incarcerated. In order to provide nursing care, one must be able and willing to see the world from the perspective of one's own clients. Information in this chapter may help you to be aware of a new perspective.***

CHAPTER 22

Forgotten Populations

The Homeless and the Incarcerated

NOREEN CAVAN FRISCH
LAWRENCE E. FRISCH

CHAPTER OUTLINE

THE HOMELESS
- Mental Illness
- Physical Illness
- Health Care Needs

APPLICATION OF THE NURSING PROCESS

THE INCARCERATED
- The Prison Population
- Mental Health Needs
- Mental Health Services
  - Risk of Suicide
  - Substance Abuse/Addiction

APPLICATION OF THE NURSING PROCESS

MENTAL HEALTH OF TORTURE VICTIMS AND THOSE FLEEING FROM TORTURE

ADVOCACY FOR FORGOTTEN POPULATIONS
- Prevention

COMPETENCIES

Upon completion of this chapter, the reader should be able to:

1. Describe the economic and social factors leading to the number of homeless persons currently in the United States.
2. Assess the basic needs of the homeless population.
3. Describe nursing services and interventions helpful in meeting the needs of the homeless from an individual and a community nursing perspective.
4. Describe the changing and growing population of prisoners in the United States.
5. Identify the major mental health needs and risks of the prison population.
6. Describe the nursing services and interventions helpful in meeting the needs of the incarcerated.

KEY TERMS

Deinstitutionalization
Homelessness
Incarcerated
NIMBY Syndrome

The purpose of this chapter is to discuss some issues related to the care of persons in two very specific environments: (1) the streets, shelters, and other locales of the homeless, and (2) the prison system. The homeless and prisoners are similar in a number of ways—both groups have a prevalence of psychiatric disorders, particularly substance abuse, much higher than that of the population at large. In addition, there is a significant degree of overlap between the homeless and the incarcerated. It is not unusual to find homeless individuals who have spent time in prison and prisoners who have a history of homelessness. There are, however, important differences between the two groups, perhaps the most important being that society mandates basic health services for prisoners, but such services are often unavailable (and virtually never legally mandated) to the majority of the homeless.

While many nurses may encounter neither the homeless nor the incarcerated in their professional careers, others will build careers working with one or the other of these groups. Despite major problems of health care access, the homeless do receive services from a variety of public and private agencies. Nurses working in these agencies and in various health care facilities, including emergency rooms, inpatient units, and mental health programs, are likely to encounter the homeless on a regular basis. The growing U.S. investment in prison construction means that increasing numbers of nurses will find employment serving the health care needs of prisoners. This chapter does not attempt to provide exhaustive information about the health needs of either the homeless or the incarcerated; it offers a basic overview of the special characteristics and needs of these populations.

THE HOMELESS

The following excerpt from an article by sociologist Christopher Jencks (1994a) offers a vivid introduction to the mental health developments that contributed to the origins of today's view of the homeless:

> *Late in the 1970s Americans began noticing more people sleeping in public places, wandering the streets with their possessions in shopping bags, rooting through garbage bins in search of food or cans, and asking for handouts. By January 1981 when Ronald Reagan took office, a small group of activists led by Robert Hayes and Mitch Snyder had given these people a new name—"the homeless"—and had begun to convince the public that their plight was a serious one. Later that year America entered its worst recession in half a century, and the homeless became far more numerous. At the time, many people saw this as a temporary problem that would vanish once the economy recovered, but they were wrong.*
>
> *Clinicians who examine the homeless typically conclude that about a third have "severe" mental disorders. The homeless seem to share this view of their mental health. A third of [one] Chicago sample said they could not work because of "mental illness" or "nervous problems." [These same] homeless adults [were asked] whether they had had any of the following experiences within the past year:*
>
> *Hearing noises or voices that others cannot hear.*

Having visions or seeing things that others cannot see.

Feeling you have special powers that other people don't have.

Feeling your mind has been taken over by forces you can't control.

About a third of the Chicago homeless reported having had at least one of these experiences at a time when they were neither drunk nor taking drugs. While no symptom is ever definitive, [hallucinations and] delusions of this kind are usually linked to schizophrenia. The homeless are also more likely than other people to be depressed, confused, angry, paranoid....

My guess is that more than a third of today's homeless would have been in hospitals during the 1950s. Sleeping in public places was then illegal, and few shelters accepted applicants who appeared crazy. People who were homeless and showed signs of mental illness had frequent run-ins with the police. If they had no place to go, the police routinely took them to a mental hospital for evaluation. Psychiatrists, in turn, treated homelessness as evidence that a patient could not cope with the stresses of everyday life and needed professional care. As a result, the homeless were likely to be hospitalized even when their symptoms were relatively mild. Dismantling this system has, I think, played a major part in the spread of homelessness.

Those who advance this argument must, however, answer at least one obvious objection. The fraction of the adult population sleeping in state mental hospitals fell from 0.47% in 1955 to 0.12% in 1975 without any apparent increase in homelessness. Why, then, should deinstitutionalization have suddenly begun to produce widespread homelessness after 1975? The answer is that deinstitutionalizing was not a single policy. Rather, it was a series of quite different policies, all of which sought to reduce the number of patients in state mental hospitals, but each of which moved these patients to a different place. The policies introduced before 1975 worked quite well. Those introduced after 1975 worked very badly....

By the mid 1970s most state mental hospitals had discharged almost everyone whom they could get someone else to care for. Their remaining inmates were either chronic patients whom nobody else wanted or short term patients getting acute care. But advocates of deinstitutionalization were far from satisfied. During the 1960s a group of civil-libertarians inspired by Thomas Szasz had argued that states should not be allowed to lock up the mentally ill unless they broke the law. By the early 1970s a number of judges had accepted this argument and had begun issuing orders restricting involuntary commitment. The Supreme Court encouraged this trend throughout the decade. In 1975, for example, it ruled in O'Connor v. Donaldson that mental illness alone was insufficient justification for involuntary commitment. By 1980 almost every state had rules that prevented hospitals from locking up patients for more than a few days unless they posed a clear danger to themselves or others.

Once these rules were in place, seriously disturbed patients began leaving state hospitals even when they had nowhere else to live. When their mental condition deteriorated, as it periodically did, many broke off contact with the mental health system and with the friends or relatives who had helped them deal with other public agencies. As a result, many lost the disability benefits to which they were theoretically entitled. In due course these lost souls often ended up not only friendless but penniless and homeless.

By the end of the 1970s, slow economic growth and a nationwide tax revolt were putting enormous pressure on states to cut their outlays. Meanwhile, federal regulations were forcing states to improve conditions in their hospitals. So instead of trying to persuade chronic patients with nowhere else to live that they should remain in a hospital, state mental health systems began encouraging such patients to leave. Once the courts broke the taboo against discharging patients to the streets, states found the practice very appealing, and it spread rapidly. By 1990 only 0.05% of the adult population was sleeping in a state hospital on an average night.

*States could have kept many of these people off the streets by finding them a rented room and paying the rent directly to the landlord. But once civil libertarians endowed the mentally ill with the same legal rights as everyone else, state politicians felt free to endow them with the same legal responsibilities as everyone else, including responsibility for paying their own rent. Not surprisingly, many ended up on the streets. States compounded the problem by cutting their cash payments to the mentally ill. Most states had supplemented federal SSI benefits for the disabled during the 1970s. Almost all states let these supplements lag behind inflation during the 1980s. While most states spent more on subsidized housing for the mentally ill, no state guaranteed the mentally ill a place to live.... No other affluent country has abandoned its mentally ill to this extent.**

(Jencks, 1994a, pp. 20–27)

*From "The Homeless," by Christopher Jencks, 1994a, *New York Review of Books, 41*, 20–27.

Jencks does not claim that the entire problem of **homelessness** can be attributed to "deinstitutionalization" of mental health care. In a book that expands on the previous comments, Jencks (1994b) concludes that at least four factors explain the recent rise in homelessness. These include **deinstitutionalization**, the loss of American opportunities for casual nonskilled employment, the closing of commercial single-room housing structures, and the availability of crack cocaine.

The nature of casual employment allows persons with substance dependence or other fluctuating mental health conditions to work when they feel well and to remain out of the workforce during days of illness or inebriation. Many cities once had labor markets to which individuals (primarily men) would go to look for a single day's employment. These markets have shrunk dramatically and in most cities have disappeared altogether. As a result, there are few, if any, work opportunities for marginally employable individuals. The major factor in such loss of casual labor opportunity is probably the increasing mechanization of unskilled work. Powered lawnmowers, "weed-eaters," hedge trimmers, car washes, and the like have significantly decreased the need for human labor. And while mechanization plays a major role, in many cases, particularly in the public sector, jobs involving cleaning or maintenance are simply not being done or are done less thoroughly than they were a generation ago (Jencks, 1994b).

Short-term housing for the very poor has become more costly, in large part because municipal inspection and regulation have closed many of the cheap hotels previously used by individuals without steady sources of income. Rezoning and urban redevelopment have also resulted in the conversion of many such hotel facilities to other, more upscale (and profitable) enterprises. Fewer of the poor today can afford even the cheapest and least pleasant forms of private accommodations than in the past, and only the streets or public shelters remain as alternatives.

Cost increases are, however, only one factor in the shortage of housing for the poorest Americans who, like their more affluent peers, must choose how to allocate their scarce funds among competing priorities. While food, clothing, and housing are major needs for everyone, some of the poorest surely do spend a significant proportion (or even all) of their available income on intoxicants. Nonetheless, when researchers ask substance-dependent persons to choose among food, drugs, or housing, the majority of individuals *report* spending their money preferentially on food and shelter, with whatever is left going to drugs (Petry, 2001). In this study, some heroin users and those substance misusers with a significant past history of homelessness did acknowledge choosing drugs over shelter; however, while clearly associated with being homeless, neither drugs nor mental illness have been convincingly shown to be primary causes of homelessness (Sullivan, Burnam, & Koegel, 2000).

Even though it likely has not directly caused America's current homeless problem, the availability of cocaine as a relatively inexpensive mood-enhancing stimulant has unquestionably had a huge impact on the lives of many poor people. Whatever the cause-and-effect relationship might be, crack cocaine usage is clearly correlated with homelessness and other social marginalization (Fischer et al., 2006). Drug and alcohol dependency—both have been prominent features of American poverty life for generations—continue to be part of the cause of today's burden of homelessness.

Although the preceding discussion accurately reflects many aspects of homelessness, it fails to recognize that the homeless population is quite diverse. Many people, even those with a history of psychiatric disorders, move in and out of homelessness or are only briefly homeless. Even at the time Jencks was writing, others observed that homeless people were only modestly more likely to have a history of psychiatric illness than were controls (Winkleby, Rockhill, Jabolis, & Fortmann, 1992). Other writers suggested that biased sampling may overestimate the relationship between mental illness and the homelessness (Phelan & Link, 1999). In working with the homeless, a group of nurse researchers used previously homeless "peer educators" to work with homeless clients in an effort to restore the dignity and self-confidence needed to leave the homeless subculture (Connor, Ling, Tultle, & Brown-Tezera, 1999). Recognizing that the longer a person stays homeless the more difficult it is to remove them from that subculture, O'Toole and colleagues have more recently tried to assess what services persons seek out when they first become homeless (O'Toole, Conde-Martel, Gibbon, Hanusa, Freyder, & Fine, 2007). If we know what these services are, the authors postulate that we might focus early intervention activities on decreasing the likelihood of chronic homelessness. While results depended on underlying mental and physical health (those with illness were likely to seek medical or psychiatric care), soup kitchens were a "first stop" for nearly half of the individuals interviewed. Studies suggest that these sites can be a useful place for interventions in the lives of the homeless (Rosenblum, Magura, Kayman, & Fong, 2005). Others have reported successful nursing interventions to reduce the risk that persons will be discharged to shelters—or even to the streets—after stays in inpatient psychiatric facilities (Forchuk, Joplin, Schofield, Csiernik, Gorlick, & Turner, 2007).

REFLECTIVE THINKING 22-1

Cost of Housing/Cost of Drugs

In many cities it has become cheaper to buy cocaine than to purchase a room for the night.

- Has this knowledge affected planning for services in your community?
- Consider discussing this issue with those providing social services to the homeless in your community.

Mental Illness

While not all of the homeless are mentally ill, mental illness is common and widespread in the homeless population. Not surprisingly, given the immediately preceding discussion, substance-related disorders and depression are among the most common diagnoses that affect the homeless. Urine screening of New York City homeless showed positive tests for cocaine in 66% and for all tested substances combined in 80% (Cuomo, 1993). Further, another study reported a 26.6% prevalence of Major Depressive Disorder, more than five times higher than that found in the general population (Kales, Barone, Bixler, Miljkovic, & Kales, 1995). The few reported studies of smaller, more rural areas have also suggested high rates of substance-related disorders. Relatively few studies have focused on homeless women, but those that have been reported suggest that psychiatric disorders are not uncommon among this group. Random interviews with women in St. Louis shelters found substance abuse diagnoses in a third. Post-Traumatic Stress Disorder was equally common. In contrast, Bipolar Disorder and Schizophrenia were decidedly uncommon (Smith, North, & Spitznagel, 1993). The women in these St. Louis shelters were relatively young and frequently had young children living with them. While Schizophrenia was not common among the women in the St. Louis study, individuals with schizophrenia may frequently find themselves homeless. An epidemiologic study of schizophrenic women found that these women were more likely to be homeless if they had inadequate family support, had associated substance abuse problems, or had an additional diagnosis of Antisocial Personality Disorder (Caton, Shrout, Dominguez, Eagle, Opler, & Cournos, 1995).

Homelessness is a problem outside the United States as well, but comparable studies from other countries have shown somewhat differing findings. For example, a British study researched an estimated 80% to 90% of the homeless in one moderate-sized community. Only 34% of this population admitted to substance abuse problems (compared to 66% to 80% of individuals in U.S. studies), but many had previously been residents of psychiatric hospitals, prisons, or both (Shanks, George, Westlake, & al-Kalai, 1994). In one Australian study, neither substance abuse nor significant mental illness was found among homeless youth—suggesting an opportunity for early interventions to reduce the risk of subsequent chronic morbidity in this high-risk population (Rosenthal, Mallett, Gurrin, Milburn, & Rotheram-Borus, 2007). However, an Austrian study showing that both substance abuse and psychiatric illness were highly prevalent among homeless youth in that country suggests that the Australian experience might be atypical (Aichhorn, Santeler, Stelzig-Schoeler, Kemmler, Steinmayr-Gensluckner, & Hinterhuber, 2008). There is little doubt, however, that homeless youth are an important target for interventions to prevent serious risks to their well-being (Slesnick, Kang, Bonomi, & Prestopnik, 2008; Gwadz, Gostnell, Smolenski, Willis, Nish, Nolan, et al., 2008).

Another interesting study compared homelessness in Amsterdam (the Netherlands) and New York City. In contrast to New York, the homeless in Amsterdam nearly all receive some kind of government assistance and have access to subsidized housing, so that neither lack of funds nor housing availability is a fundamental cause of homelessness in the Netherlands. Mentally ill persons and chronic heroin users are found frequently among the homeless in Amsterdam and appear to account for a significant proportion of Dutch homelessness. Amsterdam has a smaller proportion of homeless people than New York City (Sleegers, 2000). Many Europeans seem threatened by the homeless but are sympathetic to their plight (Brandon, Khoo, Maglajlic, & Abuel-Egleh, 2000).

REFLECTIVE THINKING 22-2

Services for the Homeless

As you review statistics on the homeless, inquire about the services that are available in your own community:

- **Are there mental health services for the homeless? Where?**
- **Is there someone to do screening and mental health evaluations for the homeless?**

Physical Illness

Some of the homeless have significant chronic medical conditions, including alcoholic liver disease, tuberculosis, and acquired immunodeficiency syndrome (AIDS; Strehlow & Amos-Jones, 1999). Not surprisingly, homeless individuals also suffer from conditions (asthma, back pain, diabetes, and hypertension) similar to those affecting persons who live in more fortunate circumstances (Savage, Lindsell, Gillespie, Dempsey, Lee, & Corbin, 2006). These conditions require ongoing medical care, but that care often requires development of therapeutic relationships with health care providers—particularly nurses (Savage, Lindsell, Gillespie, Lee, & Corbin, 2008). Many homeless individuals have great difficulty maintaining any sort of ongoing relationship, and as a result, both their physical and mental health may suffer seriously:

> *The homeless have almost as much trouble maintaining relationships with loved ones as with employers. More than half the Chicago homeless told Rossi that they had no good friends, and 36 percent reported no friends at all. A third also said they had no contact with their relatives, even though they almost all had kin in the Chicago area.**
>
> *(Jencks, 1994a, p. 22)*

*From "The Homeless," by Christopher Jencks, 1994a, *New York Review of Books, 41*, 20–27.

The combination of ill health and social isolation can be particularly debilitating. Marked psychological distress, sometimes manifested by suicidal ideation, is not unusual among the homeless and is made much worse by social isolation (Schutt, Meschede, & Rierdan, 1994).

Health Care Needs

Whereas 65% of one homeless population in England had a source of primary health care (Shanks et al., 1994), American homeless are more likely to use public hospital emergency rooms for health care. This reliance on emergency rooms prevents any continuity of care and limits opportunities for preventive intervention. Access to care for the mentally ill homeless has probably not improved recently in Britain where overdependence on emergency facilities has also been noted (Woollcott, 2008). There have been some efforts to develop programs to meet the special physical health care needs of homeless populations as well as programs specifically focused on mental health needs. One such program emphasizing mental health services reported in a one-year follow-up evaluation that program completers (48% of the total) were able to find secure housing and remain off the streets (Murray, Baier, North, Lato, & Eskew, 1995). Another program worked primarily with inner city chemically dependent homeless clients (Bennett & Scholler-Jaquish, 1994). Although outcome measures were less clearly defined for this program, the authors observed that innovative and caring efforts can at least connect the homeless to sources of primary health care, allowing some to overcome substance dependency and homelessness. Carling reported on the efforts of the Center for Community Change Through Housing and Support in Vermont, a state with a strong reputation for innovative community-based management of mental illness (Carling, 1993). The center described efforts to develop housing for mentally ill individuals through various community actions, efforts often frustrated by the **NIMBY syndrome** (not in my backyard). Jencks observes, "most Americans want the homeless off the streets, but no one wants them next door" (Jencks, 1994b, p. 117). The relatively high prevalence of substance misuse among the homeless—nearly 50% in some studies (Glasser & Zywiak, 2003)—makes these individuals and their plight less attractive to many who would otherwise provide help and services. Mobile street clinics for the homeless have been established in many communities, and while evidence for their effectiveness in reducing morbidity and the very significant premature mortality suffered by homeless persons remains incomplete, these clinics offer a mechanism for the homeless to have access to care and community resources (MacReady, 2008).

Comprehensively addressing the mental health needs of the homeless is an enormous challenge. Over many decades, Americans have tended to view the poor as either "worthy" or "unworthy" of public support. Children and their mothers have generally been regarded as worthy, whereas their fathers, the elderly, criminals, the mentally ill, and substance abusers have frequently been regarded as unworthy—those who are regarded as chiefly having themselves to blame for misfortune. Through the 1970s and 1980s, Americans remained relatively generous in providing programs for the worthy poor, however, more recent attitudes supporting reduced governmental roles in civic life have made it unlikely that current programs for either the

REFLECTIVE THINKING 22-3

Not in My Backyard Syndrome

Although most compassionate Americans want services for homeless individuals, many persons do not want such services provided in their own neighborhoods.

- **Provide at least three reasons why a person might reject a plan to provide services next to his own home.**
- **How do you assess the validity of the reasons you provided in response to the preceding item?**
- **What do you believe is the best direction for your community to take in developing services for the homeless?**

The Lovers on the Bridge

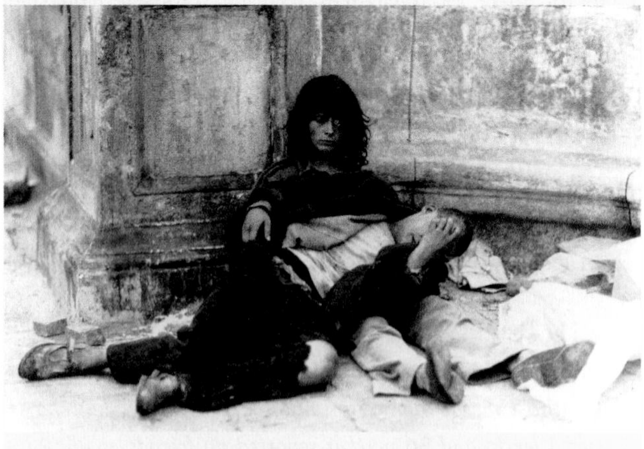

Courtesy: Films Christian Fechner/The Kobal Collection

Homeless in Paris, the great Juliette Binoche and her down-and-out lover played by Denis Levant create a stunning film experience about love and loss that manages to escape full-blown tragedy without avoiding the bitter realities of poverty.

NURSING TIP 22-1

The Clubhouse Model—One Approach to Caring for the Homeless

To avoid the revolving door of hospital admissions, and to decrease the number of mentally ill persons living on the streets, programs to assist and support these persons in the community are needed everywhere in the country. A specific model, the Clubhouse Model, is a form of rehabilitative service available in many communities throughout the country. The Clubhouse Model provides housing, employment, and job and social skills to those who wish to participate. A voluntary program, it is based on the philosophy that recovery from a mental illness must involve the person in a community offering respect, hope, and opportunity to access work, housing, education, and the friendship of others. Such a philosophy has become a "clubhouse culture"—a way of viewing mental illness and a framework for dealing with the human and social costs of caring for those disabled with mental illness. The model was established to counter the societal barriers that keep mentally ill persons segregated from everyday life. The isolation many mentally ill persons experience is believed to exacerbate disability. In contrast, the Clubhouse Model serves to minimize disability and help people with recovery and rehabilitation.

The model has existed for more than 50 years. The first facility based on this model is called Fountain House and is located in New York City. Established in 1948, the program was set up as a club where people with mental illness could belong as members. The clubhouse culture that evolved is based on the notion that persons could participate in self-help activities and learn to live, work, and socialize in the larger community. The director of Fountain House, James Beard, developed a "therapy" over time that encouraged mentally ill persons to participate in work activities—both at the clubhouse and eventually out in society. Fountain House staff negotiated with employers for jobs in the community. The staff guaranteed employers that the job would get done, either by the Fountain House club members or by the staff. The program differed significantly from traditional rehabilitation programs in which clients participate in training programs or work in sheltered workshops. Work done through Fountain House was real—in the community for pay. Mentally ill persons boosted their self-esteem and readiness to contribute to society. Workers learned job skills and habits required to keep their jobs. By the late 1970s, others in the mental health field sought to replicate the Fountain House program. Through a National Institute of Mental Health (NIMH) grant, many across the country received training. The terms "clubhouse model" and "transitional employment" were used to describe such programs. In 1994, an International Center for Clubhouse Development (ICCD) was established to provide a network of programs throughout the world.

Attitudes that underpin clubhouse programs are that members should be made to feel that their presence is expected and their participation makes a difference to someone. Programs are to be set up so that each member becomes a wanted and needed contributor, and all clubhouse activities should be carried out jointly by staff and members working together—meeting the basic human desire to be needed. Other beliefs that pervade every aspect of these programs are that even the most disabled psychiatric client has potential for productivity; and work and participation in gainful employment is a "generative and reintegrative force" for each person. Nurses have commented that the "hope of recovery, and living, working, and loving in a community, is a significant advance from previous notions of how to care for persons with mental illness" (Farrell & Deeds, 1997, p. 27).

worthy or the unworthy will be maintained, much less expanded. It is unlikely that any society can eliminate poverty, much less mental illness, substance abuse, and homelessness. However, it seems unlikely that American society can continue to ignore the plight of the homeless. Jencks comments,

> *our dilemma, both as individuals and as a society, is to reconcile the claims of compassion and prudence. When I ponder that problem I often think of a homeless woman whom Elliot Liebow quotes at the end of Tell Them Who I Am: "I'm 53 years old," Shirley says. "I failed at two marriages and I failed at every job I ever had. Is that any reason I have to live on the street?"**
>
> *(Jencks, 1994b, p. 122)*

Most nurses, the authors of this textbook hope, would say to Shirley, "No, that is no reason you should have to live on the street." Surely, a just and civil society can provide more for its poor—even its "unworthy" poor—than ours has provided in recent years.

*From *The Homeless*, by Christopher Jencks, 1994b. Cambridge, MA: Harvard University Press Copyright © 1994 NYREV, Inc. Reprinted with permission from New York Review of Books.

APPLICATION OF THE NURSING PROCESS 22-1

Nursing interventions for the homeless may be directed toward either the individual person or the community as a whole. Individual assessments and care plans are made as with any client; however, the client's condition of homelessness and poverty poses obvious challenges when choosing acceptable and realistic interventions and providing follow-up care. The homeless have seen their needs in concrete terms—jobs, food, and shelter (Mulkern & Bradley, 1986)—and this perspective remains a very reasonable perspective that must be taken into account. Many nurses view the nursing role with the homeless as one of advocacy for the homeless population, and here the nurse works with the community as a client in efforts to establish appropriate services and support for the population. The following sections on the nursing process include the community perspective (see also Chapter 31).

ASSESSMENT

It is important for nurses to evaluate both individual clients and the homeless population as a group in their own communities. The homeless are not a homogeneous group. Early studies estimated the prevalence of alcoholism and/or chemical dependency among the homeless is 50% to 70% (Fischer & Breakey, 1992). Other early studies indicated that the severely and persistently mentally ill are highly represented among the homeless, with over half the individuals in one study carrying diagnoses of Schizophrenia or Bipolar Disorder (Murray, Baier, North, Lato, & Eskew, 1995). Recent data confirms the estimates and show that a relationship between homelessness and drug abuse persists (Greenberg & Rosenheck, 2008; Kemp, Neale, & Robertson, 2006; Kim & Ford, 2006). In addition, current research presents a profile of conditions that lead to homelessness. Among these are: violence and experience of trauma (Kim & Ford, 2006); unemployment and having little education/job skills (Greenberg & Rosenberg, 2006; Kim & Ford, 2006); loss of mobility and physical functioning, death of a partner, and history of disputes with co-tenants and/or neighbors (Crane, Warnes, & Fu, 2006). Of concern, as well, is the data that 25.6% of patients discharged from a large public hospital in the United States were homeless at the time of discharge and an additional 19.4% were marginally housed at the time of discharge (Tsai, Weintraub, Gee, & Kuschel, 2005). Each homeless person should be evaluated at a point of care (shelter, soup kitchen, or any other setting where the nurse may encounter clients receiving social services). Nursing assessment usually begins with evaluation of physical health related to basic needs for food or clothing, and evaluation of communicable disease, chronic conditions, and skin problems. Psychiatric assessment should include questions regarding any previous hospitalizations, diagnoses, or recommended treatments. Further, the nurse may ask questions to determine if there have been psychiatric symptoms, such as: "Have you ever heard voices that

RESEARCH Highlight 22–1

Powerlessness and Social Disaffiliation in Homeless Men

STUDY PROBLEM/PURPOSE

The purpose of this research was to explore the meanings of powerlessness and social disaffiliation in homeless men and the effects of these conditions on their health.

METHODS

The researcher conducted a qualitative, phenomenological investigation of 10 homeless men. Data were collected through semistructured interviews that were tape-recorded and analyzed according to Girogi's method.

FINDINGS

The homeless respondents described their lived experiences as uncertainty, self-rejection, depersonalization, discrimination, and isolation.

IMPLICATIONS

These homeless individuals are at risk for both physical and psychosocial health problems. Many of these problems will be unresolved as long as the men continue living on the streets. Interventions that strive to decrease barriers to social integration would be appropriate for this vulnerable population.

Source: "Powerlessness and Disaffiliation in Homeless Men," by C. R. Lafuente, 2003, *Journal of Multicultural Nursing and Health*, 9(1), 46–54.

(*Continues*)

APPLICATION OF THE NURSING PROCESS 22-1 (Continued)

RESEARCH Highlight 22–2

Prevalence of Human Immunodeficiency Virus, Hepatitis B, and Hepatitis C among Homeless Persons with Co-occurring Severe Mental Illness and Substance Use Disorders

STUDY PROBLEM/PURPOSE

To determine the prevalence of human immunodeficiency virus (HIV), hepatitits B virus (HBV), and hepatitis C virus (HCV) among homeless persons with co-occurring severe mental illness and substance use disorders and to determine associated risks.

METHOD

As part of a longitudinal study of this population, researchers from the Missouri Institute of Mental Health performed serological testing of 114 homeless individuals previously diagnosed with severe mental illness.

FINDINGS

About 6% of the participants were HIV positive, nearly one-third had evidence test for either HBV or HBC, and such results were strongly associated with prior exposure to HBV, and 30% were antibody positive for HCV. About 44% had a reactive with substance abuse and injection drug use.

IMPLICATIONS

High prevalence of bloodborne pathogens represent a significant health threat to homeless individuals. Mental health professionals should take a proactive role in identification of these conditions and in initiation of treatments.

Source: "Prevalence of Human Immunodeficiency Virus, Hepatitis B, and Hepatitis C among Homeless Persons with Co-occurring Severe Mental Illness," by D. Klinkenberg, Caslyn, Morse, Yonker, McCudden, Keterna, et al., 2003, *Comprehensive Psychiatry*, *44*(4), 293–302.

others cannot hear?" "Have you ever had visions and seen things others could not see?" "Do you believe you have special powers others do not have?" "Have you ever felt that your mind is out of your control?" If a nurse works in a community facility for the homeless, over time, that nurse will be able to document the population the facility is serving.

NURSING DIAGNOSIS

There are several nursing diagnoses that apply to the mental health and social needs of the homeless. *Ineffective coping: alcoholism or chemical dependency* is a diagnosis that will be made for any person whose homeless life is being complicated by drugs. Those with psychoses or diagnosable psychiatric disease could be given a DSM-IV-TR (American Psychiatric Association, 2000) diagnosis as well as nursing diagnoses of *Disturbed thought processes* or *Disturbed sensory perceptions: hallucinations*. For many homeless persons, the nursing diagnoses of *Social isolation*, *Hopelessness*, and *Powerlessness* can be made as well.

OUTCOME IDENTIFICATION

Outcomes of nursing care will be individualized and depend on the diagnosis made. A priority for each person may be that the individual receive services dealing with his or her primary problem; for example, as a result of nursing assessment and intervention, client A will receive services for alcoholism and client B will receive services for untreated schizophrenia. Given that the homeless as a group do not have access to services, an outcome of nursing assessment and diagnosis may be that nurses work with other community workers and mental health workers to develop services for this population.

(*Continues*)

APPLICATION OF THE NURSING PROCESS 22-1 (Continued)

PLANNING/INTERVENTIONS

Several successful interventions have been reported by nurses in their work and advocacy with the homeless. Nurses dealing with the severely and persistently mentally ill who are homeless recognize that transitional residential programs are needed to stabilize the client's mental illness and to teach living skills.

Homeless clients benefit from knowledge of how to negotiate the system, since some persons are eligible for services and assistance but have been unable to apply for aid. Providing knowledge of how to apply for services, job retraining, and transitional living programs is important.

Lastly, nursing care that treats the client with respect and dignity and offers authentic person-to-person interactions is an intervention that addresses the diagnoses of *social isolation* and *chronic or situational low self-esteem*. The nurse must always remember that the homeless are shunned by most of society and that a relationship with a caring nurse may be the first step for some in caring about self.

Clearly, other nursing interventions for the homeless are the range of activities within any community to advocate for services such as shelters, food, and health care. Nurses throughout the country are participating in community activities that aim to assist those in greatest need.

EVALUATION

Nursing evaluation is always done based on stated outcomes. Individuals may begin to receive needed care and treatment because of nursing assessment and referral. Community services can be improved and have been due to the efforts of many caring individuals. The following two Research Highlights illustrate successful nursing interventions with this population.

THE INCARCERATED

Another significant forgotten population in the United States is the **incarcerated**, or what some see as the most unworthy of the unworthy poor. While jail life is far from pleasant for most, Jencks (1994b) astutely observes that a 1980 survey "found that those who had spent time in both [homeless] shelters and jails rated the jails superior to the shelters on cleanliness, safety, privacy, and food quality" (p. 45). The irony of these findings is that, like homeless shelters, jails are rarely clean, safe, or private. As Columbia University's David Rothman emphasized, they are also far from cheap:

> *"It was once commonplace to observe that a year in jail was as expensive as a year at Harvard, and by the 1990s the jail costs in many cities were even higher" (Rothman, 1994, p.34). At present, researchers estimate that the costs of housing an inmate in a medium security facility are $65,000 per year (Pew Center on the States, 2008); "still considerably higher than the tuition and living expenses at a private university" (Rothman, 1994, p. 34).*

A complete accounting for the reasons behind such very high costs is beyond the scope of this discussion. Clearly, the need for close supervision of inmates plays a role, as does the legal requirement to provide health care. As Rothman (1994) observed, New York City spent over $50 million a year on court-ordered treatment for inmates with AIDS, some of whom must be housed in special isolation cells, each of which costs $450,000 to construct.

THE PRISON POPULATION

In recent years, the United States has invested enormously in providing incarceration for a remarkably high percentage of its population. Between 1980 and 1990, the number of adults on probation or parole more than doubled, and it continues to rise today. The U.S. federal and state prison population has almost tripled in the same period and now likely numbers a million or more. This significant growth in the prison population has affected black Americans far more than whites; for example, 57% of young black men in Baltimore are in prison, on probation, on parole, or under a warrant for arrest. Black women are 41/2 times more likely to be in prison than are white women (Hatton, Kleffel, & Fisher, 2006). Some believe that the extraordinary growth of the prison and postprison population is a factor in the decreasing urban incidence of violent crime, but this growth has above all had a huge impact on the nation's prisons themselves. Overcrowding, poor services, and outdated facilities have given rise to numerous court orders for improvements, new services, and new construction. The eventual result will likely be a better equipped, better staffed prison system. Court-imposed requirements to deliver health and mental health services will provide opportunities and challenges to health care professionals, including nurses. Whether or not history will regard America's decision to become the world's leader in imprisonment to be wise social policy, it is a decision that will affect nursing and nurses in the twenty-first century.

Mental Health Needs

Although there have been some studies of mental health needs among prison residents, there is limited definitive data on psychiatric diagnoses and needs in prisoners. Literature reviews focusing on incarcerated adults (Fazel & Danesh, 2002) and youth (Fazel, Doll, & Langstrom, 2008) confirm the importance of mental illness in the prison system (see Figure 22-1). Psychosis, depression, and especially a variety of personality disorders are found more commonly among the imprisoned than in the general population (Fazel & Danesh, 2002). Substance abuse disorders are, of course, common among incarcerated persons worldwide, though it should probably come as no surprise that the prevalence of substance abuse diagnoses is high in American prisons, with more than 90% of one recent sample having a lifetime or current diagnosis of a substance or mental health disorder (Gunter, Arndt, Wenman, Allen, Loveless, Sieleni, et al., 2008). Since one of the major causes for recent increases in the jail population has been an increased emphasis on mandatory sentences for possession and selling of illegal substances, particularly crack cocaine, the correlation between imprisonment and mental health/addictions diagnosis should not be a surprise. Other diagnoses seen among prisoners include psychoses, personality disorders, and organic disorders (Gunn, Maden, & Swinton, 1991) with mood disorders, psychosis, and suicidal risk highly prevalent in some studies (Gunter et al., 2008), and nonsubstance-related mental disorders occurring in well over half of incarcerated Australian women (Tye & Mullen, 2006). An early study suggested that up to 15% of prisoners had not only a diagnosable psychiatric condition, but also severe or significant functional impairment (Steadman, Holohan, & Dvoskin, 1991). Currently, several authors report that other mental health issues of depression, risk for suicide, stress, anxiety, and drug/alcohol abuse are common among prison populations (Meeks, Sublett, Kostiwa, Rodgers, & Haddiz, 2008; Fazel, Hope, O'Donnell, & Jacoby, 2004; Hatton, Kleffel, & Fisher, 2006; Anthony & McFadyen, 2005). Individuals accused of committing crimes but unable to stand trial because of legal insanity may be treated in high-security forensic units within the mental health system. Other psychotic individuals may be judged competent to stand trial and after conviction may be sent to prisons. The psychiatric needs of both of these groups may be extensive. Another group of prisoners with potentially unique mental health needs is the developmentally disabled, some of whom are in prison and others of whom may, like some psychotic defendants, be judged incompetent to stand trial. Many of these individuals are dually diagnosed with both developmental and psychiatric disorders. In addition, a probably unanticipated phenomenon currently is the advancing age of prisoners, rendering issues of both physical and mental health and illness more challenging as prisoners face conditions of cardiovascular, endocrine, and musculoskeletal disorders, as well as mental illness (Fazel et al., 2004).

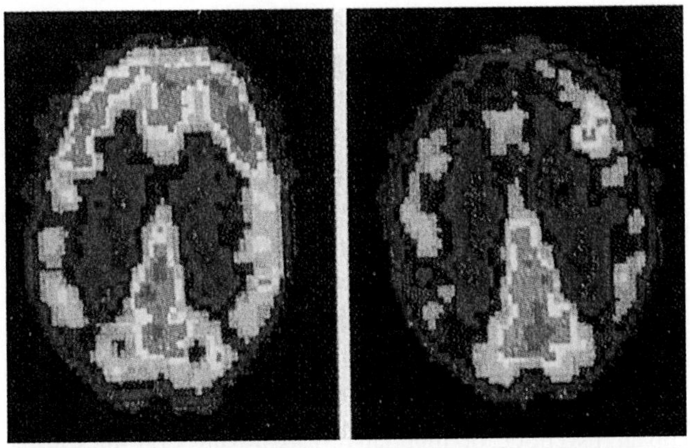

Figure 22-1 Persons who commit murder make up only a small percentage of inmates, but most murders spend many years in prison. Neurophysiologists have studied murderers using PET scanning. These PET scan images show less activity in the frontal cortex (top one-third of the image) when a murderer (right) is compared with a control subject (left). Decreased frontal lobe activity may reflect impaired regulation of aggressive impulses. (COURTESY OF DRS. ADRIAN RAINE AND MONTE S. BUCHSBAUM. FROM "SEEKING THE CRIMINAL ELEMENT," BY W. WAYT GIBBS. 1995, *SCIENTIFIC AMERICAN*, MARCH, P. 103.)

Although jails may be required by law or court ruling to provide mental health care to psychotic inmates, such severely ill persons are relatively rare in prison populations (as they are in the population at large). Only 5% to 8% of California inmates were judged psychotic in one survey, and others have described prevalences not much different from those of the community at large (Lamb & Grant, 1982; Jerrell & Komisaruk, 1991). Care of these individuals, however, may be problematic. A more recent study indicated that prison staff feel far better able to hand physical than mental health issues for those under their charge (Mead & Moseley, 2004). In addition, a study in the United Kingdom found that only 18% of prisoners with psychiatric disorders were prescribed psychotropic medications, while the prisoners with physical health problems were far more likely to have appropriate medication prescribed (Fazel et al., 2004). Indeed, mental health services ranked thirteenth on a list of prison deficiencies that have gave rise to court orders for change in the 1990s with far more common concerns of overcrowding, fire hazard, inadequate medical care, and poor food (Kerle, 1991), all of which remain concerns today. Still, two of the major mental health challenges in prison care are providing care to those who are psychotic and preventing in-prison suicide.

Mental Health Services

Prior to deinstitutionalization, prisons could often readily transfer inmates to nearby mental institutions for evaluation and treatment. Rules governing committal apply to prisoners as well as to the population at large—there must be a strong presumption of potential harm to self or others. Today, in most settings, such transfers are not feasible, and as a result,

NURSINGALERT 22-1

Suicide Risk among Prison Inmates

Indicators that suicide risk is high include:

- History of alcoholism or drug abuse, or both, intoxication
- Young age with diagnoses of Conduct Disorder, depression, and substance abuse
- Being under the influence of drugs or alcohol
- Being held for the short term in a high-turnover holding facility

prisons must provide their own procedures for internal psychiatric evaluation and treatment. Large state and federal prisons can (and do) employ psychiatric staff, including psychiatric nurses, psychologists, and psychiatrists. City and county jails may have much more difficulty dealing with psychotic inmates because these individuals, while mentally ill, may not be judged to be any danger to themselves and, being in jail, may pose little risk to others. Resources for in-prison mental health services are very limited in some facilities. When psychiatric care can be provided, prisoners do not lose their civil rights protections so that in the absence of risk to themselves or others, they cannot be medicated without their express consent. Nurses who work in a correctional setting face many personal and ethical challenges.

Risk of Suicide

Suicide is among the most important mental health concerns in the prison population. In one study nearly a third of inmates were judged to be at significant suicidal risk (Gunter et al., 2008). Another study reported that 72% of prisoners who completed suicide in prison were identified on reception to the prison as having at least one psychiatric diagnosis (Anthony & McFayden, 2005). City and county jails have higher risk of attempted and completed inmate suicide because they have much higher turnover than do federal or state penitentiaries. Many inmates are brought to local jails immediately after arrest, often under the influence of various substances and with relatively unknown psychiatric histories. Such "pass-through" inmates often come at night, when staffing needs for close supervision may be stretched and personnel for psychiatric assessment may be unavailable. Adolescents held in adult jails may be particularly susceptible to suicide. While not inconsequential in larger, more stable prison populations, studies have suggested that suicide risk is greatest in facilities with rapid inmate turnover (Winfree & Wooldredge, 1991). The subject of suicide in prison is discussed in more detail in Chapter 16.

Suicide is a major source of legal liability for prison administrators and health care workers. Nurses working in prisons must maintain a high index of suspicion for suicide risk. Close supervision, especially of recently arrived inmates, those with histories of psychiatric disorders, or those who appear psychotic or inebriated, can usually prevent suicide attempts.

RESEARCH Highlight 22-3

Prisoners' Perceptions of Their Health Problems and Healthcare in a U.S. Women's Jail

STUDY PROBLEM/PURPOSE

To describe the perceptions of female prisoners regarding their health and health care needs.

METHOD

The researchers interviewed women who were incarcerated, analyzed data, and reported issues that served as barriers for the women to secure health services.

FINDINGS

Female prisoners reported that the prison health system was not set up to serve gender-specific diseases, specifically STDs, breast lumps, lack of menses, endometriosis, and miscarriages. The women often did not seek treatment for potentially serious problems because of concerns related to lack of privacy, lack of dignity, long waiting times, and the need for co-payments, Additionally, some women sought to conceal health problems to obtain work opportunities. Of particular concern to the women was the fact that the health providers were male and the women perceived they were not being treated with compassion or respect.

IMPLICATIONS

The authors caution that prior to arrest, many of the women prisoners have faced serious health issues: STDs, history of violence and victimization, attempted suicide, depression, and mental illness. Since these women may be suffering from potentially serious health problems, the prison health system providers should take measures to provide adequate care, recognizing that the rate of incarceration of women is increasing steadily.

Source: "Prisoners' Perceptions of Their Health Problems and Healthcare in a U.S. Women's Jail," by D. C. Hatton, D. Kleffel, & A. Fisher. 2006. *Women and health*, *44*(1), 119–124.

Substance Abuse/Addiction

Since substance-related disorders are a major cause of arrest, many incarcerated individuals are at significant risk of undergoing withdrawal while in jail. Alcohol and opioids (separately or together) are the most likely substances to produce withdrawal. The management of withdrawal syndromes is

APPLICATION OF THE NURSING PROCESS 22-2

Nurses working within the penal system will provide direct care to clients, the major nursing role being provision of primary care and direct screening services. Nurses working in corrections will be guided by the ANA Standards of Practice for this specialized area. In addition, the emerging field of psychiatric forensic nursing brings advanced-level competencies to the practice of care for individuals who are mentally ill and who have been perpetrators or victims of crime, or both. Client needs, both physical and mental, should be assessed, and appropriate nursing interventions initiated. The American Nurses Association (ANA, 2007) has published Standards of Nursing Practice for nurses working in correctional facilities. A nurse working in the prison must demonstrate basic standards of professional nursing in a practice setting where health care is not the primary mandate. Nurses in prison settings will apply the nursing process to complete assessments and make diagnoses and will follow up care based on outcome identification. The following sections provide guidelines for application of the nursing process in correctional facilities.

ASSESSMENT

Priority data collected are determined by the client's immediate needs. Nurses will assess physical conditions and emotional state. Data collection involves the client, significant others, health care providers, and other criminal justice system personnel.

NURSING DIAGNOSIS

The nurse makes diagnoses based on assessment data collected. These diagnoses are documented so that a plan of care may be developed. Emotional and social diagnoses that are relatively common in the prison population include *Ineffective coping, Hopelessness, Risk for suicide, Risk for violence, Chronic or situational low self-esteem*, and *Social isolation*.

DISCHARGE PLANNING

Evidence suggests that mentally ill homeless individuals with a history of previous incarceration in excess of six months may have a poorer prognosis than those who serve shorter sentences (McGuire & Rosenheck, 2004). This difference in outcomes may reflect more severe underlying mental illness with or without associated Axis II (personality) disorders. It also might reflect lack of planning at the time of leaving jail. Nurses who provide mental health care within the justice system may need to be particularly assertive in ensuring that mentally ill clients are released into services that can provide both shelter and mental health treatment. Such programs can improve the lives of mentally ill inmates who end up on the streets because there is evidence that well-designed services can significantly decrease the likelihood of continuing homelessness (Tsemberis, Moram, Shinn, Asmussen, & Shern, 2003).

OUTCOME IDENTIFICATION

Outcomes are based on unique factors of the individual as well as the setting. For example, length of stay, overall safety, and lack of information about prior health needs will affect the nurse's ability to provide care. Nonetheless, the nurse will identify outcomes that are realistic within the setting and include a time estimate for attainment.

PLANNING/INTERVENTIONS

Appropriate nursing interventions and actions for clients within the prison system will be quite similar to those for clients outside the prison system. For example, the client who is addicted to alcohol will need medical services during the withdrawal period and follow-up care that will support sobriety. Attendance at Alco-

(*Continues*)

APPLICATION OF THE NURSING PROCESS 22-2 (Continued)

holics Anonymous meetings is possible in many prison settings, as is individual counseling from an addictions worker. For the client who is depressed, particularly the client at risk for suicide, the nurse should request mental health services and initiate careful monitoring with the correctional facility staff to prevent suicide.

EVALUATION

Evaluation of nursing services is based on initial outcomes. The nurse should gather data and monitor outcomes systematically. Revisions in diagnoses and in care plans are made during evaluation.

discussed in Chapter 17. In many prison settings, withdrawal may be managed by transfer to an acute-care medical setting, but the nurse needs to be able to recognize signs of impending withdrawal so that the inmate's condition can be monitored and the need for transfer assessed in a timely manner.

MENTAL HEALTH OF TORTURE VICTIMS AND THOSE FLEEING FROM TORTURE

Many repressive governments in the world still practice torture as a means of gathering information from dissidents and as a form of social control, recent experiences in Iraq notwithstanding. Torture may end in death, but when the victim escapes, he or she may attempt to reenter his or her own society or flee the country of origin to make a new life. It is without question that those who have experienced torture while incarcerated experience post-traumatic stress and are at high risk for depression, suicidal ideation, and other stress-related conditions. Such disorders are greatly complicated by language and cultural barriers, as in situations where the torture/imprisonment is perpetrated by an occupying force.

Individuals fleeing torture and other abuses may attempt immigration to the United States or another country. These persons are often held in detention pending status hearings while they request asylum. While their treatment in detention may not be brutal, it is often greatly different from what the torture victim would expect from reading the famous poem on the Statue of Liberty:

Not like the brazen giant of Greek fame,
With conquering limbs astride from land to land;
Here at our sea-washed, sunset gates shall stand
A mighty woman with a torch, whose flame
Is the imprisoned lightning, and her name,
Mother of Exiles. From her beacon-hand
Glows world-wide welcome; her mild eyes command
The air-bridged harbor that twin cities frame.
"Keep, ancient lands, your storied pomp!" cries she
With silent lips. "Give me your tired, your poor,
Your huddled masses yearning to breathe free,
The wretched refuse of your teeming shore.
Send these, the homeless, tempest-tost to me,
I lift my lamp beside the golden door!"

Potential immigrants in detention do not know whether and when they will be deported to their home country, and they will likely be returned unless they can prove to a judge that they are in imminent danger of being killed or tortured again on return. Needless to say, the combination of uncertainty and previous injury potentially leads to a variety of stress and psychiatric disorders among these individuals, which are complicated by the separation that detention imposes between immigrants and any family or friends they have who are currently living in the United States. Immigrants from northern Africa (Ethiopia and Somalia) may be particularly likely to have experienced torture and would need services in response (Jaranson, Butcher, Halcon, Johnson, Robertson, Savik, et al., 2004). Torture victims, especially from these countries, often include women as well as men. There is some evidence from nursing literature that while mental health needs are great among all refugees from war-torn countries, torture in itself may not increase the risk for subsequent mental illness (Hermansson, Timpka, & Thyberg, 2003). The uncertainty, delays, and incarceration associated with asylum seekers has been associated with significant suicide risks in this group in a variety of countries (Cohen, 2008; Hallas, Hansen, Staehr, Munk-Andersen, & Jorgensen, 2007); Silove, Austin, & Steel, 2007; Procter, 2005). Whether the absence of similar reports from the United States reflects better mental health care for asylum seekers or a failure to report this outcome remains to be determined.

ADVOCACY FOR FORGOTTEN POPULATIONS

With either population, the homeless or the incarcerated, nurses will find themselves in the role of client advocate. The nurse will often be the first person to discover that the basic needs of the client are not being met within the system designed to provide care. Advocacy may take on several roles, and these may include working within the system to provide additional services, working to shift funds from one service to another, and overt political action demanding that community and social services be developed. Additionally, nurses in such advocacy roles may expand their practices by becoming dually credentialed, such as by becoming an RN/correctional officer, an RN/social worker, or an RN/judge.

PREVENTION

One approach to nursing services for both the homeless and the incarcerated is to consider these "forgotten" populations within the context of society as a whole. Many believe that the considerable increase in the numbers among both groups is a direct result of social ills—poverty, powerlessness, and the individual's inability to take a place in society. Nurses have suggested that any nursing diagnosis could be considered at the level of the individual, family, or community such that diagnoses such as *Powerlessness* or *Ineffective coping* could be attributed to a community at large (Warren, 1991) and a nursing role in serving communities could be described and validated. If this idea of community diagnoses is developed, nurses can consider interventions aimed at improving the community's ability to meet the needs of its members. For example, nurses have suggested a new nursing diagnosis of "impaired ability to participate in workforce" as a potential diagnosis (Coler, 1996), relating to the problems faced by unemployed and underemployed youth, who frequently choose a lifestyle of drugs and crime when they perceive they have no option of being productive, employed members of a community. Nursing in the community may take on roles that overlap with the community developer or social worker.

KEY CONCEPTS

- At least four factors have contributed to the increased numbers of homeless persons in the United States: deinstitutionalization, loss of jobs for unskilled workers, loss of low-cost housing, and crack cocaine.
- Mental illness, most specifically chemical addiction, major depression, Bipolar Disorder, and schizophrenia, is found in higher prevalence among the homeless than among the population at large.
- Physical illness among the homeless includes liver disease, tuberculosis, and AIDS.
- Health care for the homeless is often sporadic and provided only through emergency rooms.
- Health care is mandated for prisoners in most settings, but is not mandated for the homeless.
- Mental illness seen in the prison population includes chemical dependency, psychoses, personality disorders, and organic disorders.
- Suicide potential is high among prisoners, particularly in "pass-through," or holding, jails.
- Nurses working with these "forgotten" populations take on roles of assessment, referral, direct service, advocacy, and prevention.

REVIEW QUESTIONS

1. A nurse is dealing with a homeless person with chronic mental illness and recognizes that an important approach to stabilizing the client's mental illness would be which of the following?
   1. Giving the client $500 and a list of possible job openings
   2. Referring the client to a transitional residential program for the mentally ill
   3. Contacting local law enforcement agencies to provide extra monitoring of the homeless client
   4. Telling the client's family that if they do not take him in, he will most likely die on the streets in a few years

2. A key benefit that a nurse can provide a homeless client that is not strictly of a medical nature includes which of the following?
   1. A few hundred dollars to help the person get back on his feet
   2. Case studies of the negative outcomes for other clients who failed to heed the nurse's advice
   3. Advocating for the client in order to force family members to show more compassion
   4. Assisting the client with negotiating the system in order to apply for services, job training, and transitional living programs

3. A nurse working in a detention facility frequently encounters a homeless client who has been incarcerated. Upon release from the facility, the nurse always provides the client with a list of local homeless shelters. Yet the client consistently winds up back in jail, especially during cold winter nights. The nurse understands this behavior is based on which of the following facts?
   1. The client is a pathological criminal, who will always be in and out of jail
   2. The client prefers being incarcerated over living in a homeless shelter
   3. The client is obviously severely mentally ill and cannot grasp the reality of how much better a homeless shelter would be to jail

4. The client uses this as his only means of seeing the nurse, whom he is quite fond of, on a regular basis

4. A nurse starting work in a prison environment, after previously working in a community mental health center, will assess that the environments are different in which of the following ways?
1. There is a higher instance of substance abuse problems in the prisons
2. There is a dramatically lower incidence of mental illness and substance abuse in the prison system
3. Because of government funding, prison systems provide better access to mental health treatment than that provided to the average citizen who is not incarcerated
4. The percentage of severely psychotic and schizophrenic individuals is higher in the prisons

5. A nurse working in an immigration detention center meets a female detainee from northern Africa. The nursing assessment reveals that the client is experiencing a high degree of anxiety and other psychiatric disorders. The nurse hypothesizes that the client's current mental status is NOT likely associated with which of the following?
1. Post-Traumatic Stress Disorder (PTSD) as a result of being tortured in her home country
2. Fear that she may not be united with family that is currently living in the United States
3. Uncertainty over whether or not she will be sent back to her home country
4. A lack of understanding of the freedoms she will have in the United States if she is allowed to stay

LEARNING ACTIVITIES

1. Learn about the homeless population in your own community.
a. Where do the homeless persons come from?
b. Where and how do these people receive health care?
c. Are there shelters? Who uses them?
d. Are there nurses working with the homeless in your community?

2. Examine what is known about the prison population in your state.
a. What is the number of prisoners?
b. How are health care and mental health care being provided?

3. What role do you believe professional nursing has in addressing major societal problems?

*Study*WARE™ CONNECTION

Using your *Study*WARE™ CD-ROM

1. Complete the Concentration activity for this chapter.
2. Review the audio glossary for key terms in this chapter.
3. Explore the other games and activities that support this chapter.

REFERENCES

Aichhorn, W., Santeler, S., Stelzig-Schoeler, R., Kemmler, G., Steinmayr-Gensluckner, M., & Hinterhuber, H. (2008). Prevalence of psychiatric disorders among homeless adolescents. *Neuropsychiatry, 22*(3), 180–188.

American Nurses Association. (2007). *Scope and standards of nursing practice in correctional facilities.* Washington, DC: Author.

American Psychiatric Association. (2000). *Diagnostic and statistical manual of mental disorders* (Fourth Edition-Text Revision). Washington, DC: Author.

Anthony, D., & McFayden, J. (2005). Mental health needs assessment of prisoners. *Clinical Effectiveness in Nursing, 9,* 26–36.

Bennet, J. B., & Scholler-Jaquish, A. (1994). The winner's group: A self-help group for homeless chemically-dependent persons. *Journal of Psychosocial Nursing and Mental Health Services, 33,* 14–19.

Brandon, D., Khoo, R., Maglajlic, R., & Abuel-Egleh, M. (2000). European snapshot homeless survey: Results of questions asked of passers-by in European cities. *International Journal of Nurse Practitioners, 6*(1), 39–45.

Carling, P. J. (1993). Housing and supports for persons with mental illness: Emerging approaches to research and practice. *Hospital and Community Psychiatry, 44,* 439–449.

Caton, C. L., Shrout, P. E., Dominguez, B., Eagle, P. F., Opler, L. A., & Cournos, F. (1995). Risk factors for homelessness among women with schizophrenia. *American Journal of Public Health, 84,* 1153–1156.

Cohen, J. (2008). Safe in our hands?: A study of suicide and self-harm in asylum seekers. *Journal of Forensic and Legal Medicine, 15*(4), 235–244.

Coler, M. (1996). *Community diagnoses.* Presentation at the 12th conference on nursing diagnoses, Pittsburgh, PA .

Connor, A., Ling, C. G., Tuttle, J., & Brown-Tezera, B. (1999). A peer education project with persons who have experienced homelessness. *Public Health Nursing, 16*(5), 367–373.

Crane, M., Warnes, A.M., & Fu, R. (2006). Developing homelessness prevention practice: Combining research evidence and professional knowledge. *Health and Social Care in the Community, 14*(2), 156–166.

Cuomo, A. (Ed.) (1993). *The way home: A new direction in social policy.* New York: New York City Commission on the Homeless.

Doherty, J., & Stuttaford, M. (2007). Preventing homelessness among substance users in Europe. *Journal of Primary Prevention, 28*(3–4), 245–263.

Farrell, S. P., & Deeds, E. S. (1997). The clubhouse model as exemplar: Merging psychiatric nursing and psychosocial rehabilitation. *Journal of Psychosocial Nursing and Mental Health Services, 35*(1), 27–34.

Fazel, S., & Danesh, J. (2002). Serious mental disorder in 23,000 prisoners: A systematic review of 62 surveys. *Lancet, 359*(9306), 545–550.

Fazel, S., Doll, H., & Langstrom, N. (2008). Mental disorders among adolescents in juvenile detention and correctional facilities: A systematic review and meta-regression analysis of 25 surveys. *Journal of the American Academy of Child Adolescent Psychiatry, 47*(9), 1010–1019.

Fazel, S., Hope, T., O'Donnell, I, & Jacoby, R. (2004). Unmet needs of older prisoners: A primary care survey. *Age and Ageing, 33*(4), 396–398.

Fischer, B., Rehm, J., Patra, J., Kulousek, K., Haydon, E., Tyndall, M., & El-Guebuly, N. (2006). Crack Across Canada: Comparing crack users and crack non-users in a Canadian multi-city cohort of illicit opoid users. *Addiction, 101*(12), 1760–1770.

Fischer, P. J., & Breakey, W. R. (1992). The epidemiology of alcohol, drug and mental disorders among homeless persons. *American Psychologist, 46*, 1115–1128.

Folsom, D. P., Hawthorne, W., Lindamer, L., Gilmer, T., Bailey, A., Golshan, S., et al. (2005). Prevalence and risk factors for homelessness and utilization of mental health services among 10,340 patients with serious mental illness in a large public mental health system. *American Journal of Psychiatry, 162*(2), 370–376.

Forchuk, C., Joplin, L., Schofield, R., Csiernik, R., Gorlick, C., & Turner, K. (2007). Housing, income support and mental health: Points of disconnection. *Health Research Policy and Systems, 5*, 14.

Forchuk, C., MacClure, S. K., Van Beers, M., Smith, C., Csiernik, R., Hoch, J., et al. (2008). Developing and testing an intervention to prevent homelessness among individuals discharged from psychiatric wards to shelters and 'No Fixed Address.' *Journal of Psychiatric and Mental Health Nursing, 15*(7), 569–575.

Glasser, I., & Zywiak, W. H. (2003). Homelessness and substance misuse: A tale of two cities. *Substance Use and Misuse, 38*(3–6), 551–576.

Greenberg, G. A., & Rosenheck, R. A. (2008). Jail, incarceration, homelessness and mental health: A national study. *Psychiatric Services, 59*, 170–177.

Gunn, J., Maden, A., & Swinton, M. (1991). Treatment needs of prisoners with psychiatric disorders. *British Medical Journal, 303*, 338–341.

Gunter, T. D., Arndt, S., Wenman, G., Allen, J., Loveless, P., Sieleni, B., et al. (2008). Frequency of mental and addictive disorders among 320 men and women entering the Iowa prison system: Use of the MINI-Plus. *Journal of the American Academy of Psychiatry and the Law, 36*(1), 27–34.

Gwadz, M. V., Gostnell, K., Smolenski, C., Willis, B., Nish, D., Nolan, T. C., et al. (2008). The initiation of homeless youth into the street economy. *Journal of Adolescence*. Epub Aug 8.

Hallas, P., Hansen, A. R., Staehr, M. A., Munk-Andersen, E., & Jorgensen, H. L. (2007). Length of stay in asylum centers and mental health in asylum seekers: A retrospective study from Denmark. *BMC Public Health, 7*, 288.

Hatton, D. C., Kleffel, D., & Fisher, A. (2006). Prisoner's perceptions of their health problems and healthcare in a U.S. women's jail. *Women and Health, 44*(1), 119–136.

Hermansson, A. C., Timpka, T., & Thyberg, M. (2003). The long-term impact of torture on the mental health of war-wounded refugees: Findings and implications for nursing programmes. *Scandinavian Journal of Nursing Science, 17*(4), 317–324.

Jahn Moses, D., Kresky-Wolff, M., Bassuk, E. L., & Brounstein, P. (2007). Guest editorial: The promise of homelessness prevention. *Journal of Primary Prevention, 28* (3–4), 191–197.

Jaranson, J. M., Butcher, J. I., Halcon, I., Johnson D. R., Robertson, C., Savik, et al. (2004). Somali and Oromo refugees: Correlates of torture and trauma history. *American Journal of Public Health, 94*(4), 591–598.

Jencks, C. (1994a). The homeless. *New York Review of Books, 41*, 20–27.

Jencks, C. (1994b). *The homeless*. Cambridge, MA: Harvard University Press.

Jerrell, J. M., & Komisaruk, R. (1991). Public policy issues in the delivery of mental health services in a jail setting. In J. A. Thompson & G. L. Mays (Eds.), *American jails: Public policy issues* (pp. 100–115). Chicago: Nelson-Hall.

Johnson, T. P., & Fendrich, M. (2007). Homelessness and drug use: Evidence from a community sample. *American Journal of Preventive Medicine, 32*(6 Suppl), S211–218.

Kales, J. P., Barone, M. A., Bixler, E. O., Miljkovic, M. M., & Kales, J. D. (1995). Mental illness and substance abuse among sheltered homeless persons in lower-density population areas. *Psychiatric Services, 46*, 592–595.

Kemp, P., Neale, J., & Robertson, M. (2006). Homelessness among problem drug users: Prevalence, risk factors and trigger events. *Health and Social Care in the Community, 14*(4), 319–328.

Kerle, K. E. (1991). Introduction. In J. A. Thompson & G. L. Mays (Eds.), *American jails: Public policy issues* (p. x). Chicago: Nelson-Hall.

Kim, M. M., & Ford, J. D. (2006). Trauma and post-traumatic stress among homeless men: A review of current research. *Journal of Aggression, Maltreatment and Trauma, 13*(2), 1–22.

Klinkenberg, D., Caslyn, R. J., Morse, G. A., Yonker, R. D., McCudden, S., Keterna, R., et al. (2003). Prevalence of human immunodeficiency virus, hepatitis B, and hepatitis C among homeless persons with co-occurring severe mental illness. *Comprehensive Psychiatry, 44*(4), 293–302.

Lafuente, C. R. (2003). Powerlessness and disaffiliation in homeless men. *Journal of Multicultural Nursing and Health, 9*(1), 46–54.

Lamb, H. R., & Grant, R. W. (1982). The mentally ill in an urban county jail. *Archives of General Psychiatry, 39*, 17–22.

MacReady, N. (2008). House calls for homeless people in the USA. *Lancet, 371*(9627), 1827–1828.

Massing, M. (2000). *The fix*. Berkley: The University of California Press.

McGuire, J. F., & Rosenheck, R. A. (2004). Criminal history as a prognostic indicator in the treatment of homeless people with severe mental illness. *Journal of Psychiatric Services, 55*(1), 42–48.

Mead, D., & Moseley, L. (2004). Awareness of the health needs of prisoners. *NT Research, 9*(3), 194–207.

Meeks, S., Sublett, R., Kostiwa, I., Rodgers, J., & Haddiz, J. (2008). Treating depression in the prison nursing home. *Clinical Case Studies, 7*(6), 555–574.

Mulkern, V., & Bradley, V. (1986). Service utilization and service preference of homeless persons. *Psychosocial Rehabilitation Journal, 10*, 23–31.

Murray, R., Baier, M., North, C., Lato, M., & Eskew, C. (1995). Components of an effective transitional residential program for homeless mentally ill clients. *Archives of Psychiatric Nursing, 9*, 152–157.

O'Toole, T. P., Conde-Martel, A., Gibbon, J. L., Hanusa, B. H., Freyder, P. J., & Fine, M. J. (2007). Where do people go when they first become homeless? A survey of homeless adults in the USA. *Health and Social Care in the Community, 15*(5), 446–453.

Petry, N. M. (2001). The effects of housing costs on polydrug abuse patterns: A comparion of heroin, cocaine and alcohol abuse. *Experiments in Clinical Psychopharmacology, 9*(1), 47–58.

Pew Center on the States, (2008). One in 100: Behind bars in America 2008. Washington, DC: Author. Available at: www.pewcenteronthestates.org (retrieved January, 11, 2008).

Phelan, J. C., & Link, B. G. (1999). Who are the homeless? Reconsidering the stability and composition of the homeless population. *American Journal of Public Health, 89*(9), 1334–1335.

Procter, N. G. (2005). "They first killed his heart (then) he took his own life." Part 1: A review of the context and literature on mental health issues for refugees and asylum seekers. *International Journal of Nurse Practitioners, 11*(6), 286–291.

Rosenblum, A., Magura, S., Kayman, D. J., & Fong, C. (2005). Motivationally enhanced group counseling for substance users in a soup kitchen: A randomized clinical trial. *Drug and Alcohol Dependence, 80*(1), 91–103.

Rosenthal, D., Mallett, S., Gurrin, L., Milburn, N., & Rotheram-Borus, M. J. (2007). Changes over time among homeless young people in drug dependency, mental illness and their co-morbidity. *Psychology, Health, & Medicine, 12*(1), 70–80.

Rothman, D. J. (1994, February 17). The crime of punishment. *New York Review of Books, 41*, 34–38.

Savage, C. L., Lindsell, C. J., Gillespie, G. L., Dempsey, A., Lee, R. J., & Corbin, A. (2006). Health care needs of homeless adults at a nurse-managed clinic. *Journal of Community Health Nursing, 23*(4), 225–234.

Savage, C. L., Lindsell, C. J., Gillespie, G. L., Lee, R. J., & Corbin, A. (2008). Improving health status of homeless patients at a nurse-managed clinic in the Midwest USA. *Health & Social Care in the Community, 16*(5), 469–475.

Schutt, R. K., Meschede, T., & Rierdan, J. (1994). Distress, suicidal thoughts, and social support among homeless adults. *Journal of Health and Social Behavior, 35*, 134–142.

Shanks, N. J., George, S. L., Westlake, L., & al-Kalai, D. (1994). Who are the homeless? *Public Health, 108*, 11–19.

Silove, D., Austin, P., & Steel, Z. (2007). No refuge from terror: The impact of detention on the mental health of trauma-affected refugees seeking asylum in Australia. *Transcultural Psychiatry, 44*(3), 359–393.

Sleegers, S. (2000). Similarities and differences in homelessness in Amsterdam and New York City. *Psychiatric Services, 51*(1), 100–104.

Slesnick, N., Kang, M. J., Bonomi, A. E., & Prestopnik, J. L. (2008). Six- and twelve-month outcomes among homeless youth accessing therapy and case management services through an urban drop-in center. *Health Services Research, 43*(1 Pt 1), 211–229.

Smith, E. M., North, C. S., & Spitznagel, E. L. (1993). Alcohol, drugs, and psychiatric comorbidity among homeless women: An epidemiologic study. *Journal of Clinical Psychiatry, 54*, 82–87.

Steadman, H. J., Holohan, E. J., Jr., & Dvoskin, J. (1991). Estimating mental health needs and service utilization among prison inmates. *Bulletin of the American Academy of Psychiatry Law, 19*, 297–307.

Story, A., Murad, S., Roberts, W., Verheyen, M., & Hayward, A. C. (2007). Tuberculosis in London: The importance of homelessness, problem drug use and prison. *Thorax, 62*(8), 667–671.

Strehlow, A. J., & Amos-Jones, T. (1999). The homeless as a vulnerable population. *Nursing Clinics of North America, 34*(2), 261–174.

Sullivan, G., Burnam, A., & Koegel, P. (2000). Pathways to homelessness among the mentally ill. *Social Psychiatry and Psychiatric Epidemiology, 35*(10), 444–450.

Tsai, M., Weintraub, R., Gee, L., & Kushel, M. (2005). Identifying homeless at an urban public hospital: A moving target? *Journal of Health Care for the Poor and Underserved, 16*(2), 297–307.

Tsemberis, S. J., Moran, L., Shinn, M., Asmussen, S. M., & Shern, D. L. (2003). Consumer preference programs for individuals who are homeless and have psychiatric disabilities: A drop-in center and a support hoursing program. *American Journal of Community Psychology, 32*(3–4), 305–317.

Tye, C. S., & Mullen, P. E. (2006). Mental disorders in female prisoners. *Australian and New Zealand Journal of Psychiatry, 40*(3), 266–271.

Warren, J. (1991). Implications of introducing axes into a classification system. In R. M. Carroll-Johnson (Ed.), *Classification of nursing diagnoses: Proceedings of the 9th conference* (pp. 38–44). Philadelphia: Lippincott.

Winfree, L. T., Jr., & Wooldredge, J. D. (1991). Exploring suicides and deaths by natural causes in America's large jails. In J. A. Thompson & G. L. Mays (Eds.), *American jails: Public policy issues*. Chicago: Nelson-Hall.

Winkleby, M. A., Rockhill, B., Jabolis, D., & Fortmann, S. P. (1992). The medical origins of homelessness. *American Journal of Public Health, 82*(10), 1394–1398.

Woollcott, M. (2008). Access to primary care services for homeless mentally ill people. *Nursing Standard, 22*(35), 40–44.

SUGGESTED READINGS

Elsner, A. (2004). *Gates of injustice: The crisis of American prisons*. Upper Saddle River, NJ: Prentice Hall.

Gottschalk, M. (2006). *The prison and the gallows: The politics of mass incarceration in the United States*. Cambridge: Cambridge University Press.

Klofus, S., & Stojkovic, S. (1995). *Crime and justice in the year 2010*. Belmont, CA: Wadsworth.

Roberts, J. J. (2004). *How to increase homelessness: Real solutions to the absurdity of homelessness in America*. Bend, OR: Loyal Publishing.

Thompson, J. A., & Mays, G. L. (1991). *American jails: Public policy issues*. Chicago: Nelson-Hall.

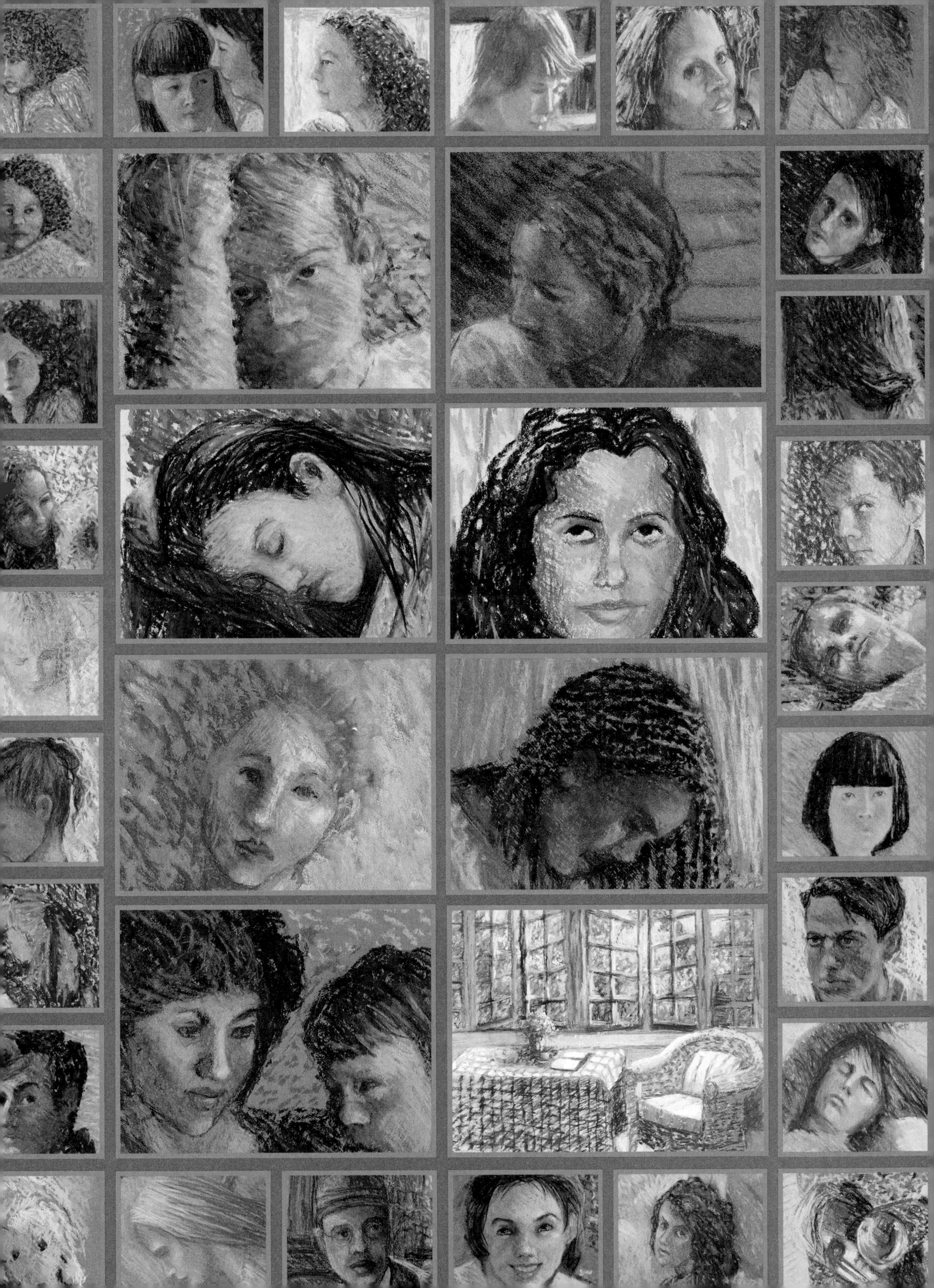

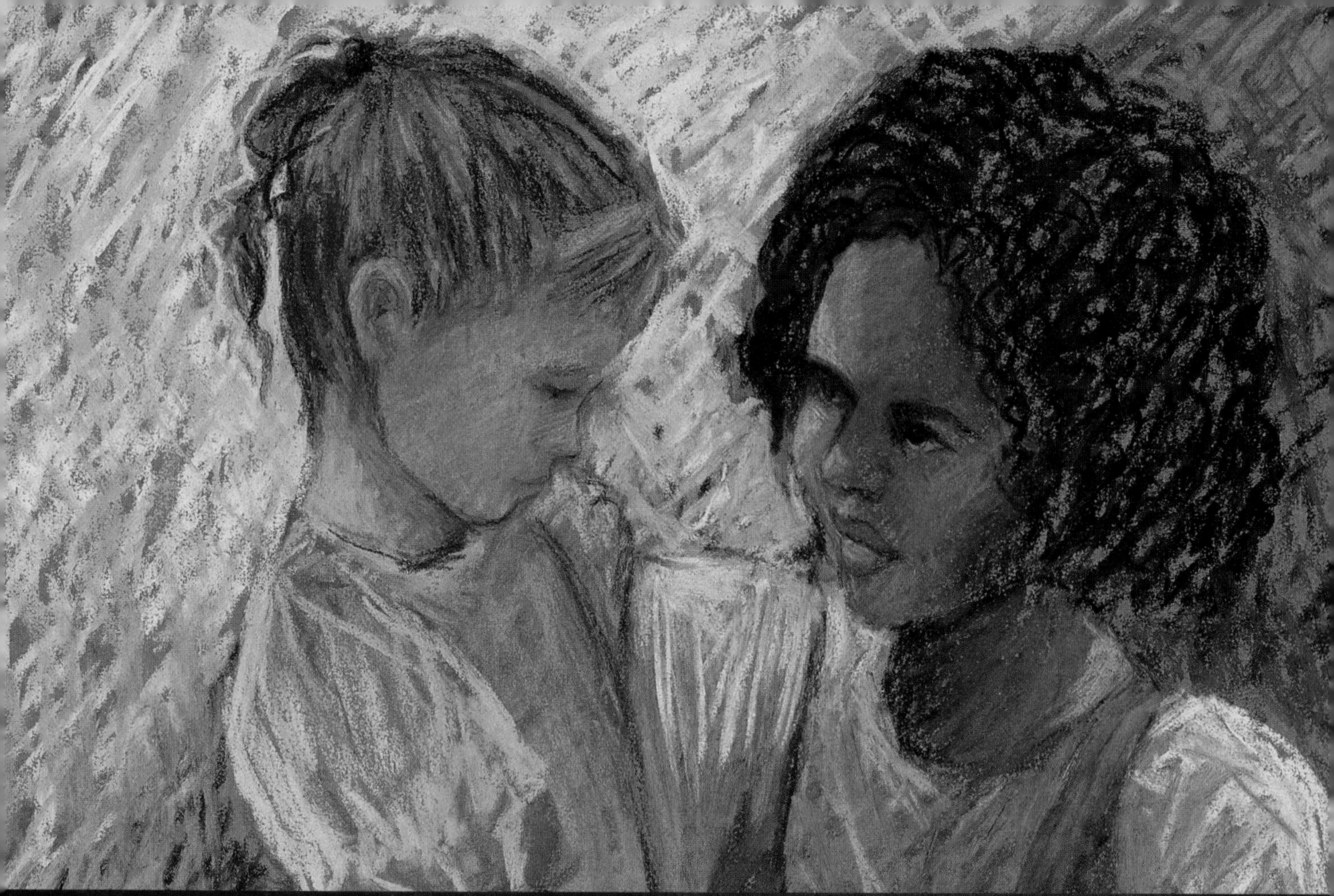

We'll Make it Together

Working with Children Who Have Emotional Disorders

Working with children who have mental health or emotional disorders is challenging and requires you to be self-aware. Use the following questions to examine your personal feelings:

- *How do I feel toward caregivers who seem to neglect or abuse or who are over coercive or over permissive with their children?*
- *What are my feelings about children who lie, steal, act aggressively toward others or animals, withdraw from others, or set fires?*
- *Have I ever been in the presence of a depressed child? How did I feel?*
- *How do I feel when caring for a hyperactive child?*
- *How do I feel about physical abuse of children? Verbal abuse? Sexual abuse?*
- *Have I ever been in the presence of an autistic child? How did I feel during the encounter? After the encounter?*

CHAPTER 23

The Child

Lawrence E. Frisch
Noreen Frisch

CHAPTER OUTLINE

COMPETENCIES

Upon completion of this chapter, the reader should be able to:

1. Discuss the prevalence of and risk factors for psychiatric disorders in children.
2. Explain how to assess the emotional, social, and educational needs and problems of children and their families.
3. Describe the common psychiatric disorders of childhood.
4. Apply the nursing process to children with psychiatric disorders through assessment, diagnosis, outcome identification, planning individualized care, and evaluating care based on outcomes.
5. Describe various treatment modalities relevant to the care of children with these disorders.

KEY TERMS

Asperger's Syndrome
Autism
Conduct Disorder
Dysthymia
Oppositional Defiant Disorder
Reactive Depression
Separation Anxiety
Social Phobia

If one looks at paintings created in the late Middle Ages and early Renaissance, the children depicted often look remarkably like adults, smaller of course, but proportioned as if they are fully grown. We know that children don't *really* look that way, and we wonder why so many artists of that period seemed to replace accurate depictions of children with miniature adults. Perhaps in the same way, we understand that in psychological terms children are not just small adults. We know that the processes of growth and development begin in utero and extend throughout adolescence. We expect children to behave differently than adults, to reason differently, and to respond somewhat differently to stress and illness. It should not come as a surprise that the psychiatric and mental health problems of children are not the same as those of adults. Many adult disorders are given the same names when they occur in children, but children are affected differently by them. While the manifestations of disorders may differ when they first occur in childhood, we have come to recognize that the majority of adult mental illness has its first manifestations in childhood (Kessler & Wang, 2008). This reality makes the understanding, recognition, and treatment of childhood mental illness exceptionally important if our goal is to prevent or minimize adult disability due to psychiatric disorders—a goal that remains tantalizing but elusive (Kessler, Amminger, Aguilar-Gaxiola, Alonso, Lee, & Ustun, 2007). At the same time, we must continue to recognize the special characteristics of children's lives that determine how mental illness is experienced in childhood. As we see from the discussion that follows, a long depressive episode (which would truly only be an unpleasant *episode* in an adult's life) can occupy most of a child's lifetime. And, since we know from our own recollections that the experience of time is itself much different in childhood (a day for a child can seem unending, whereas for an adult it often passes very quickly), even briefer psychologically charged events can seem longer and perhaps more intense to a child. Many of the experiences of mental illness—anxiety, depression, suicidal thoughts, hallucinations—are very frightening to adults. Surely these same experiences must be even more frightening to children whose language and reasoning skills are as yet incompletely developed and for whom, even normally, the distinction between dream and reality is sometimes difficult to make. The major psychiatric symptoms and illnesses—depression, mania, anxiety, psychosis, somatization, substance abuse, suicidality, and disorders of appetite and sleep—all occur in children. In addition, some disorders are seen almost exclusively in children and adolescents. For these important reasons, this book includes this chapter on psychiatric and mental health problems of children and the following chapter on adolescence. In writing this chapter, we have not attempted to be exhaustive. For example, schizophrenia, though rare, is increasingly recognized in the very young. The nurse who has read Chapter 13 should have an adequate understanding of schizophrenia, including its effect on other family members, even if childhood schizophrenia is not explicitly discussed. In contrast, depression in childhood is common and may present differently in children than in adults. This chapter on children's mental illness does consider depression and mood disorders in general. In contrast, attention deficit/hyperactivity disorder (ADHD) is increasingly recognized in adults, but it is primarily a disorder of childhood. Consequently, ADHD is discussed in this chapter, but it is not treated elsewhere in the text as an adult disease.

Such distinctions are necessarily arbitrary, but our goal is to ensure that nurses reading this chapter understand two concepts: (1) that some disorders occur only or primarily in childhood and are explicitly *psychiatric/mental health disorders of childhood*, and (2) adult disorders that occur in children are experienced by the child's still-developing mind. Children may develop adult disorders, but they experience them as children. Many of the literary examples in this chapter come from books written for children or by adults trying very hard to remember how they felt as children. We hope that, as in other chapters, these readings will help you understand both the illness described and the way it is filtered through the child's view of our frequently confusing adult world.

ATTENTION-DEFICIT/ HYPERACTIVITY DISORDER

LENORA, YOU ARE A GOOD GIRL

"Lenora you are a good girl and if you only put your head to the books you can get a scholarship and go to high school and even teacher college and be a credit to all of us but this last year you havent even tried."

And I confuse confuse because one mind in me say that I should study and pass exam so that I can go to high school and speak good and wear pretty dress and high heel shoes like Miss Martin the other teacher and Teacher Wife who is also a teacher and I think it would really grieve Dulcie to see me succeed like that because she is always fas'ing with me head and I have to wear her old dress and she tell everybody is ol bruck I wear but is only because she is stupid and cant pass anything at all and even though she older than me Teacher put us in the same class .... And I confuse because another voice say that MeMa will vex and she wont give me any encouragement even if I pass scholarship and Pa say he don't business. And she might send me back to my mother who I don't even know and who I hear have more children since she have me and she never once send me a Paradise Plum or come to see how I grow. So maybe I should learn sewing or how to be postmistress and stay round here so I can take care of Pa and MeMa in their old age because even if I go high school and study ... suppose I don't want teach I don't know if I could get work anywhere else.

*O Lord I confuse confuse.**

(Senior, 1986, p. 111)

Lenora is a young girl growing up in rural Jamaica, and her dialect doesn't make for easy reading. She has been adopted by her stepmother "MeMa," who, she thinks, is fonder of her real children and merely tolerates Lenora. Lenora's closest friend, an old woman who intuitively recognized and supported Lenora's estrangements, has recently died, and her one other friend—a soulful musician—seems to have wandered away. Lenora's troubles in school surely derive in part from these losses in her life. But even despite being told in an unfamiliar (to us) Jamaican dialect, Lenora's story seems to jump erratically from idea to idea: school, hairdo, dress, hair, MeMa, real mother, sewing, work, and confusion. Lenora may just be distracted and confused by a world falling to pieces around her, but her narrative has the rapid-fire changes of focus characteristic of attention-deficit/hyperactivity disorder. As its name implies, ADHD is diagnosed when children display signs of either inattention, hyperactivity, or both. Children who suffer from inattention have difficulty paying attention to

*From *Summer Lightening and Other Stories*, by O. Senior, 1986, Essex, England: Longman Group Limited.

RESEARCH Highlight 23-1

Unintentional Injury in Children with ADHD

STUDY PROBLEM/PURPOSE

To determine if children with attention deficit/hyperactivity disorder (ADHD) and oppositional defiant disorder (ODD) are more likely to present to an emergency room with accidental injuries than are other children.

METHODS

A sample of 47 children 25–60 months of age presenting with unintentional (accidental) injuries to an emergency room at one children's hospital was matched with 46 control children who presented to the same emergency room with non-injury related complaints. Parents were asked to complete two standardized questionnaires, one assessing injury risk based on reported behavior, and the other based on DSM-IV diagnostic criteria for ADHD and ODD. The injury behavior questionnaire included questions about both behavior (e.g., jumping down stairs) and history of minor injuries. Logistic regression was used to assess which factors related to behavior or ADHD/ODD were related to the occurrence of injury.

FINDINGS

Not surprisingly, injured children were reported to be more likely to engage in "high injury risk-taking behavior" than children who were not injured. Overall, about 17% of children met criteria for ADHD. ADHD and ODD were both more common among children who had been injured, but for neither diagnosis was the difference statistically significant. On the other hand, children with either of these diagnoses had significantly more reported behaviors that might have led to injury.

IMPLICATIONS

Case control studies provide only a relatively "weak" form of evidence best suited for testing hypotheses. In this case the study did not support others' findings that children with ADHA and ODD are at enhanced risk of injury. However, there were relatively few such children among the injured (only six with ADHD and, perhaps surprisingly, 15 with ODD—32% of the sample). Further studies might be of interest, perhaps involving a larger number of children so that the overall finding of higher, but not statistically significant, injury risk associated with this diagnosis might be further explored.

Source: "Do Attention Deficit/Hyperactivity Disorder and Oppositional Defiant Disorder Influence Preschool Unintentional Injury Risk?" by D. L. Garzon, H. Huang, and R. D. Todd, 2008, *Archives of Psychiatric Nursing*, 22(5), 288–296.

details and are easily distracted by classroom events. As a result, they almost always have serious difficulties in school, and are often mistakenly thought by teachers or parents to be purposefully ignoring spoken instructions or assigned tasks. They suffer from disorganization, often losing their school books and assignments and frequently making careless errors in their work. Although inattention and hyperactivity—the two core symptoms of ADHD—both interfere seriously with success in school and similar activities requiring concentration, each of the two manifests in different ways.

Inattention is manifested by rapid shifts in attention from topic to topic, as in Lenora's narrative. Even when not physically moving quickly from place to place, inattentive children have difficulty keeping their concentration on one idea. They may not listen, remember, or follow through on tasks. Because of these behaviors, they may fall behind in learning and as a result become frustrated or even depressed. They may not say it the same way Lenora does, "I confuse confuse," but surely they must often feel that way.

Hyperactivity generally results in difficulty with remaining in one place for an age-appropriate period of time. Hyperactive children tend to fidget and squirm; they may be disruptive in class by moving out of their seats and interfering with teaching activities for other students. Hyperactivity may be apparent even in very young preschoolers, though separating this behavior from normal preschool responses takes considerable experience and judgment. Even in school-aged children, hyperactivity-like symptoms do occur normally, but in children with ADHD, such symptoms are frequent, recur in a variety of school settings, and cause both academic and social difficulties. Children with ADHD may appear socially immature because of their tendency to interrupt and volunteer answers to class questions without being called on. This behavior, not surprisingly, is unpopular both with fellow students and with teachers. Although the school setting usually provokes the most difficulties for ADHD children, many of them have significant difficulties with behavior and attention at home as well.

Even though awareness of ADHD and its symptoms has increased in recent years, these children often provoke anger, and their behaviors often subject them to disciplinary corrections at home and at school. DSM-IV-TR requires that children display a number of symptoms in order to receive a diagnosis of ADHD. These symptoms are listed in Table 23-1.

In addition to the symptoms in Table 23-1, DSM-IV-TR requires that some hyperactive-impulsive or inattentive symptoms that cause impairment must be present before age seven, and some impairment from the symptoms should be present in two or more settings (e.g., at school [or work] and at home). Further, there must be clear evidence of clinically significant impairment in social, academic, or occupational functioning, and these symptoms should not be part of some other psychiatric diagnosis.

Anyone who has spent much time around young children will recognize that many of these symptoms occur from time to time in unaffected children. However, in children with ADHD they occur very frequently and in several settings, at home and at school, or when visiting with friends, *and* they interfere with the child's functioning. It should be noted that the criteria allow a diagnosis of ADHD to be made regardless of the presence or absence of specific learning problems such as dyslexia or developmental disorders. Many children with ADHD do have associated learning difficulties, but ADHD can be seen in very bright and academically successful students. Since many parents and teachers think ADHD only occurs in children with learning disabilities, bright ADHD children may be labeled as behavior problems rather than given the appropriate diagnosis. Whether or not they have an associated learning disorder, children suffering from ADHD may perform poorly at school; they may be unpopular with their peers if other children perceive them as being unusual or a nuisance; and their behavior can present significant challenges for parents (American Psychiatric Association, 2000). For unknown reasons, there is a significant association between hyperactive behavior and the development of other disruptive disorders, particularly conduct and oppositional-defiant disorder (discussed later). Some experts think that the impulsivity attention deficits associated with ADHD interfere with social learning or with attachment to parents in a way that predisposes to the development of behavior disorders (Barkley, 1998). There is also emerging genetic data suggesting that ADHD and conduct disorder may be part of the same diagnostic spectrum (Anney, Lasky-Su, O'Dushlaine, Kenny, Neale, Mulligan, et al., 2008).

One of the challenges in managing children with ADHD is the absence of any specific test for the disorder. While such tests are lacking for most disorders in psychiatric mental health nursing, many parents, teachers, and occasionally psychologists think that psychological testing or the use of standardized scales for documenting school behavior can lead to a diagnosis of ADHD, which is not the case. Nurses should be aware that ADHD can only be diagnosed by matching children's observed and reported behavior against DSM-IV-TR criteria. *No other test exists to establish the diagnosis.*

DSM-IV-TR offers fairly specific but quite complex criteria for the diagnosis of ADHD. Many health care practitioners probably make ADHD diagnoses in children who may fail to meet some aspects of the DSM-IV-TR criteria, which makes it difficult to be certain of the precise prevalence of ADHD, but a variety of early studies suggested that it occurs in 3% to 5% of school-age children (Anderson, Williams, McGee, & Silva, 1987; Esser, Schmidt, & Woerner, 1990; Wolraich, Hannah, Pinnock, Baumgaertel, & Brown, 1996). More recently, studies have been completed indicating that boys are four times more likely to have the illness than are girls (Scahill & Schwab-Stone, 2000). The disorder is found in all cultures, although prevalences differ; whether these differences reflect real biopsychological variation or merely reflect variable diagnostic criteria is unclear (American Psychiatric Association, 2000). It is probable that ADHD is the most common psychiatric diagnosis in children.

Etiology of ADHD

Because stimulant drugs (the mainstay of treatment for ADHD—see next section) increase the availability of the neurotransmitter dopamine, the "dopamine hypothesis" of ADHD causation has gained a wide following. This hypothesis

TABLE 23-1 Symptoms of Attention Deficit/Hyperactivity Disorder

INATTENTION

Must have six or more of the following difficulties with attention or concentration present for 6 months or more and of a degree that is age-inappropriate:

- Fails to pay close attention to details or makes careless mistakes in schoolwork, work, or other activities
- Cannot sustain attention in tasks or play activities
- Does not seem to listen when spoken to directly
- Does not follow through on instructions and fails to finish schoolwork, chores, or duties in the workplace (not due to oppositional behavior or failure to understand instructions)
- Has difficulty organizing tasks and activities
- Avoids, dislikes, or is reluctant to engage in tasks that require sustained mental effort (such as schoolwork or homework)
- Loses things necessary for tasks or activities (e.g., toys, school assignments, pencils, books, or tools)
- Is easily distracted by extraneous stimuli
- Is forgetful in daily activities

HYPERACTIVITY

Six (or more) of the following symptoms of hyperactivity-impulsivity must also be present and have persisted for at least 6 months to a degree that is maladaptive and inconsistent with developmental level:

- Fidgets with hands or feet or squirms in seat
- Leaves seat in classroom or in other situations in which remaining seated is expected
- Runs about or climbs excessively in situations in which it is inappropriate (in adolescents or adults, may be limited to subjective feelings of restlessness)
- Has difficulty playing or engaging in leisure activities quietly
- Is often "on the go" or acts as if "driven by a motor"
- Talks excessively

IMPULSIVITY

- Blurts out answers before questions have been completed
- Has difficulty awaiting turn
- Interrupts or intrudes on others (e.g., butts into conversations or games)

Source: Diagnostic and Statistical Manual of Mental Disorders (Fourth Edition-Text Revision; p. 92), 2000, Washington, DC: American Psychiatric Association.

suggests that ADHD is due to inadequate availability of dopamine in the central nervous system. The neurotransmitter dopamine plays a key role in initiating purposive movement, increasing motivation and alertness, reducing appetite, and inducing insomnia; all these effects are often seen when a child with ADHD is given stimulant drugs. As in schizophrenia (in which the "dopamine hypothesis" has also been important), most experts feel that dopamine is only part of the explanation for this complex set of behaviors and symptoms.

The role of genetics in ADHD is also complicated. ADHD runs in families, and in fact many parents go through their childhood and early adulthood with undiagnosed ADHD, only to discover their own diagnosis when a child's symptoms bring him or her to clinical attention (Faraone & Doyle, 2000). Between 10% and 35% of children with ADHD have a first-degree relative with past or present ADHD. Approximately one-half of parents who themselves had ADHD as children have a child with the disorder. Twin studies in ADHD have shown that when ADHD is present in one twin, it is significantly more likely to occur in the other twin if the relationship is identical (monozygotic) rather than fraternal (dizygotic). As with a variety of other psychiatric disorders, genomic studies have produced interesting results of uncertain practical relevance. Genetic mapping studies have attempted to link ADHD to genes on two chromosomes: DRD on chromosome 11 and the dopamine-transporter gene (DAT1) on chromosome 5 (Swanson, Posne, Fusella, Wasdell, Sommer, & Fan, 2001). Other studies have found evidence for abnormalities of the dopamine-transporter gene (DAT1) in children with very severe forms of ADHD (Waldman, Rowe, Abramowitz, Kozel, Mohr, Sherman, et al., 1998). Highly complex searches to establish genetic links between areas of chromosomal variation (single nucleotide polymorphisms) and ADHD have started to appear in the clinical literature (Lasky-Su, Neale, Franke, Anney, Zhou, Maller, et al., 2008).

While scientists are working hard to unravel the genetic contributors to ADHD, nongenetic factors are also of potential importance. The nature of these factors remains obscure, though much popular attention has focused on children's diet and food additives. It seems likely that for a small number of children the consumption of food additives, and perhaps sucrose and other simple sugars, can increase the symptoms of inattention or hyperactivity. Most experts feel that such effects are neither common nor consistent, and that ADHD is neither caused by nor generally worsened by diet or food additives. In contrast, there is some suggestion that maternal use of stimulants, in particular cocaine, may influence the development of ADHD in offspring (Weiss & Landrigan, 2000). Tobacco smoking during pregnancy has been shown in several studies to be associated with excess risk for ADHD (Milberger, Biederman, Faraone, & Jones, 1998). Curiously, perhaps, nicotine usage is common among children with ADHD, who have much higher rates of smoking than do children without ADHD. The link between ADHD and smoking is particularly strong in girls, and there is some evidence for a genetic association between the two (Monateaux, Faraone, Hammerness, Wilens, Fraire, & Biederman, J. et al, 2008). Studies suggest that nicotine may have significant benefit in controlling symptoms of ADHD, although its therapeutic use for this purpose has not been proposed or accepted (Potter & Newhouse, 2004). On the other hand, alternative substances that act on nicotinic receptors are currently being considered as potential treatments for ADHD (Weisler, 2007). One of the most interesting recent findings in ADHD research is the recognition that closed head injury in children may result in ADHD-like symptoms or exacerbation of ADHD in children with preexisting ADHD (Levin, Hanten, Max, Li, Swank, Ewing-Cobbs, et al., 2007). Many of these children have traumatic injury to the right side of their brain involving the putamen (Herskovits, Megalooikonomou, Davatzikos, Chen, Bryan, & Gerring, 1999), a part of the basal ganglia of the brain that is probably more involved in learning than movement (movement disorders such as Parkinsonism are often associated with abnormalities in the basal ganglia). Intriguingly, MRI studies increasingly show right putamen lesions in children with ADHD who do not have a history of known brain injury (Ellison-Wright, Ellison-Wright, & Bullmore, 2008). These studies suggest that at least in some children ADHD may be due to a local defect in the area of the right basal ganglia. Further studies are needed to confirm these findings and to establish whether the observed basal gangliar changes are due to genetic or environmental factors.

Pharmacological Treatment of ADHD

Treatment for ADHD has been greatly influenced by the Multi-Modal Treatment (MTA) study of ADHD, an ongoing evaluation of ADHD treatment (Shaywitz, Fletcher, & Shaywitz, 2001). Based on randomized controlled study design, the MTA data shows clearly that treatment with psychoactive drugs is effective for ADHD, and that this effectiveness is maintained for at least 14 months, but with some decrease in the benefit compared to cognitive behavior therapy and "usual community care" over the final 10 study months (MTA Cooperative Group, 2004a). At least four separate psychostimulant medications (methylphenidate, dextroamphetamine, pemoline, and a mixture of amphetamine salts) consistently improve the symptoms of ADHD in the majority of children treated (Shaywitz et al., 2001). Methylphenidate (Ritalin) remains the most commonly used; others are typically employed if Ritalin produces unacceptable side effects or inadequate response. Although longer-acting forms including a transdermal skin patch are available and now FDA-approved (Cormier, 2008), the MTA study primarily employed short-acting formulations given frequently (three times daily) each day of the week—in and out of school. Common side effects of these stimulant drugs include insomnia, decreased appetite, abdominal pain, headaches, and jitteriness. Some children may develop tics, often viewed as troublesome by parents and children alike, but at least one study suggests that these may disappear with continued treatment (Gadow, Sverd, Sprafkin, Nolan, & Grossman, 1999). Most other side effects are mild, recede over time, and respond to dose changes, though mild impairment in growth appears to persist in some children during the entire treatment period (MTA Cooperative Group, 2004b). Even though the MTA study addressed only short-acting medications, it is likely that many children are now being treated with forms of stimulant drugs that can be given once daily (Leung & Lemay, 2003). Whether these drugs will be as effective as their shorter-acting forms remains to be established, as does the long-term effectiveness of stimulant treatment. If no benefit has been shown from either of several stimulant medications properly employed, or if side effects are unacceptable to parents or children, other medications may have value. Well-controlled trials have shown tricyclic antidepressants to be superior to placebo but less effective than stimulants (Elia, 1991). Antidepressants are not infrequently used to treat adult ADHD, but are not FDA-approved for use in children as treatment for ADHD.

Recently, atomoxetine (Strattera) has become widely used for ADHD. Atomoxetine is a norepinephrine reuptake inhibitor that, like tricyclic antidepressants such as desipramine, increases brain norepinephrine levels. Despite its effect on norepinephrine, atomoxetine is neither primarily an antidepressant nor is it classified as a controlled substance. This freedom from being stigmatized as a controlled substance, along with once- or twice-daily dosing, has made it attractive for both doctors and parents. Atomoxetine now caries FDA warnings of liver toxicity and the development of suicidal ideation. It also appears to be somewhat less effective than either dextroamphetamine or methylphenidate, and is probably best used as a "second line" treatment when other medications are ineffective or otherwise unacceptable (Gibson, Bettinger, Patel, & Crismon, 2006). Clonidine and guanfacine, while not currently FDA approved, are antidepressant medications that have shown some efficacy in "off label" treatment of ADHD (Posey & McDougle, 2007).

Psychosocial Treatment of ADHD

The MTA study also demonstrated some benefit for psychosocial/behavioral treatments, though such treatments appeared to work best in conjunction with drug therapy (Kaiser, Hoza, & Hurt, 2008). Helpful behavioral techniques typically employ "time-out," point systems, and positive reinforcement for appropriate home and school behavior. Often, children who are disruptive receive the most attention in class when they behave unacceptably. Although ADHD behavior is not primarily attention-seeking, if the only attention children get in class is negative, this may reinforce their undesired behaviors. Daly and colleagues provide an excellent review of psychosocial treatments (Daly, Creed, Xanthopoulos, & Brown, 2007). Parent training has become more commonly used as a relatively short (typically under 20 sessions) approach to giving families skills needed to help children learn more effective behaviors.

ADHD and Schools

ADHD is regarded as a developmental disability, and schools are mandated to provide an Individual Educational Plan (IEP) for each student with this disorder. Many children with ADHD are mainstreamed in normal classrooms. When disruptive behavior is severe, there is pressure to place children in more controlled settings, but this often means children who already have difficulties with peer relationships are placed in classes with children who have other serious psychiatric morbidity. Many parents are reluctant to agree to such placements out of concern for their children's safety and emotional development. The general topic of schools and children with psychiatric mental health disorders is discussed later in this chapter.

Safety of Long-Term Stimulant Use

Even though the MTA study found no evidence for health risks of stimulant medication over a 14-month period, concerns have been raised about the longer-term safety of stimulant treatment. Two specific concerns have been raised: (1) potential effects on appetite and growth, and (2) potential for subsequent substance misuse or abuse. Despite reason for worry (stimulant drugs are used to promote weight loss in obese adults), there is little evidence that stimulant use greatly affects either weight or normal childhood growth (Spencer, Biederman, & Wilens, 1998). In one study, childhood use of stimulant drugs *reduced* by 85% the likelihood of later substance abuse (Biederman, Wilens, Mick, Spencer, & Faraone, 1999), and these finding have been generally accepted by pediatric psychiatric practitioners (Upadhyaya, 2008). Some children or their family members may sell or otherwise misuse prescribed stimulants. Many of these children have comorbid Conduct Disorder and may be candidates for atomoxetine—a drug that has no recognized abuse potential and may actually reduce Conduct Disorder-associated behaviors. The patch form of methylphenidate may be particularly useful for children who might divert their medications because the patch cannot be reapplied after it has been removed (Cormier, 2008).

Prognosis of ADHD

In many children the symptoms of ADHD (particularly hyperactivity) decrease with time. Impulsivity may persist into adulthood, and many children retain all of the symptoms of ADHD throughout adolescence and into their adult years. Increasingly, ADHD is being diagnosed—sometimes for the first time—in adults. Whether or not ADHD *symptoms* persist past childhood, the effects of childhood ADHD may still be felt in adult years. Recent studies suggest that it may be useful to divide ADHD into two subsets based on predominant symptoms: inattentive ADHD and impulsive/hyperactive ADHD (American Psychiatric Association, 2000). There is considerable evidence that the inattentive variety (and also a combined type with both inattention and impulsivity/hyperactivity) has a worse academic outcome with more long-term learning difficulties. In contrast, children with primarily impulsive/hyperactive symptoms have reasonably good academic outcomes. These children, however, have more problems with interpersonal relationships. They also experience more physical injuries, presumably as a result of their impulsive behavior patterns.

DEPRESSION AND SUICIDE IN CHILDREN

SOMEWHERE—I LOST WHAT IT WAS TO BE HAPPY

Somewhere between the repetition of Sunday School lessons and the broken doll which the lady sent me one Christmas I lost what it was to be happy. But I didn't know it then even though in dreams I would lie with my face broken like the doll's in the pink tissue of a shoebox coffin. For I was at the age where no one asked me for commitment and I had a phrase which I used like a talisman. When strangers came or lightning flashed, I would lie in the dust under my grandfather's vast bed and hug the dog, whispering "our worlds wait outside" and be happy.

I knew all about death then because in dreams I had been there. I also knew a great deal about love. Love, I thought, was like an orange, a fixed and sharply defined amount, limited, finite. Each person had this amount of love to distribute as he may. If one had many people to love then the segments for each person would be smaller and eventually love, like patience, would be exhausted. That is why I preferred to live with my grandparents then since they had fewer people to love than my parents and so my portion of their love-orange would be larger.

TABLE 23-2 Age-Specific Symptoms of Depression

AGE	SYMPTOMS
Preschoolers: 2.5–5 years	Less exuberance in play Lower assertiveness than peers Frequent complaints of stomachaches Increased clinginess and whiny behavior around primary caregiver Greater fearfulness than peers about separating from caregiver Fear of abandonment
School-age children: 5–10 years	Complaints of not having friends Picked on by peers Deeply sad facial expressions and unwillingness to talk about sad feelings Frequent complaints of headaches Frequent tantrums with caregivers Unusual combativeness and argumentativeness Frequent fights with peers Inappropriate behavior in school, that is, class clown, bad guy
Preteens: 10–13 years	Excessive self-recrimination and expressions of low self-esteem Persistent sadness, inhibition Isolation from peers Isolation from family Inability to sleep Excessive sleep Eating disorders

*My own love-orange I jealously guarded. Whenever I thought of love I could feel it in my hand, large and round and brightly coloured, intact and spotless. I had moments of indecision when I wanted to distribute the orange but each time I would grow afraid of the audacity of such commitment. Sometimes I would extend the orange to the dog or my grandmother but would quickly withdraw my hand each time.**

(Senior, 1986, p. 11)

This excerpt is from another short story about growing up in rural Jamaica by the author of Lenora's narrative. For this child, who feels she has "lost what it was to be happy," any concept of happiness lies far away where "our worlds wait outside." Her inner world and her dreams are occupied by thoughts of death symbolized by a voodoo-like doll with "half a face and a finger missing" lying "in the pink tissue of a shoebox coffin." The child narrator sees herself to be mutilated like the doll, but her loss is happiness and the capacity to love freely, not just the side of a face or a finger. This story provides a glimpse of the experience of depression for children. Several presentations of depression are discussed in the following paragraphs, and Table 23-2 lists age-specific symptoms of depression.

*From *Summer Lightening and Other Stories*, by O. Senior, 1986, Essex, England: Longman Group Limited.

REACTIVE DEPRESSION

Reactive depression, or "adjustment disorder with depressed mood," is probably the most common form of mood problem in children. Depressed feelings are short-lived in children suffering from reactive depression, and usually occur in response to some adverse experience, such as a rejection, a slight, a letdown, or a loss. Mood tends to improve with a change in activity or an interesting or pleasant event. Such transient mood swings in reaction to minor environmental adversities are not regarded as a form of mental disorder, but if severe may require some form of psychotherapeutic treatment.

MAJOR DEPRESSIVE DISORDER

Major Depressive Disorder, Dysthymic Disorder, and Bipolar Disorder are DSM-defined psychological conditions increasingly

NURSING ALERT 23-1

Incidence of suicide attempts in children peaks in midadolescence.

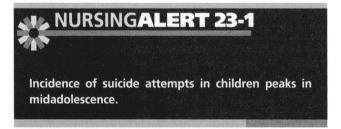

diagnosed in children who have "lost what it was to be happy." Mood disorders lead to great suffering on the part of children and their families. Normal developmental tasks, including developing stable family ties and interpersonal relationships, are greatly complicated by depressive illness. Only recently has depression come to be recognized and treated in children; in the past, children could spend many years in severe depression without their symptoms being acknowledged, diagnosed, or treated. Children with untreated depression may look back on childhood years with a sense of unhappiness and unfulfillment, as if the pleasures of growing up had been denied them. Such a sense of loss may adversely color adult life and perhaps contribute to later depression or even suicidal ideation. Because mood disorders do increase the risk of suicide, any suicidal behavior associated with depressed mood is a matter of serious concern. Although completed suicide is relatively rare in children, the incidence of suicide attempts reaches a peak during the midadolescent years, and mortality from suicide, which increases steadily through the teens, is the third leading cause of death at that age (NIMH 2009).

As in adults, Major Depressive Disorder in children is characterized by one or more major depressive episodes lasting on average from seven to nine months unless treated. Depressed children appear sad; they lose interest in activities that used to please them, and they criticize themselves and feel that others criticize them. They sleep poorly and may have changes in appetite, often eating less than normal, but sometimes overeating. They feel pessimistic or even hopeless about the future; they may come to think that life is not worth living. More so than adults, depressed children and adolescents are often irritable, and their irritability may lead to aggressive behavior. In addition to being irritable, depressed children may be indecisive or have problems concentrating, and they may lack energy and motivation. As with adults, they may neglect their appearance and hygiene (American Psychiatric Association, 2000). Psychotic features are less common in depressed children than they are in adults, and when they occur, auditory hallucinations have been thought to be more common than delusions (Birmaher, Ryan, Williamson, Brent, & Kaufman, 1996; Birmaher, Ryan, Williamson, Brent, Kaufman, Dahl, et al., 1996). Compared to adults, depressed children may be more likely to express symptoms of anxiety (such as school or social phobia) or of somatization (nonlocalized pain, stomachaches, and headaches) having obvious implications for school nurses (Davis, 2005). Although some of these symptoms may be "depressive equivalents" and may disappear with treatment of the depression, others may be specific comorbidities (anxiety disorders, migraine, or peptic ulcer disease) that need targeted psychological or medical treatment. For this reason, most children with depression need careful medical assessment as well as psychological care. Nurses caring for children with depression and somatization should be very careful to assess for the possibility of serious family pathology as an underlying cause. Child abuse, domestic violence, sexual abuse, eating disorders, or substance abuse (by family members or the child herself) may be important comorbidities that can be missed if not specifically sought.

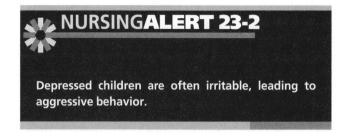

NURSINGALERT 23-2

Depressed children are often irritable, leading to aggressive behavior.

Dysthymia in Children

Dysthymia, considered in detail earlier in this text as an adult disorder, is also felt to occur in children. Because of its persistent nature, this disorder is particularly likely to interfere with normal psychosocial development. As in adult cases, an affected child is depressed for most of the day, on most days, and symptoms continue for several years. Such prolonged mood depression in a very young child can have a profound effect on self-image. The following anecdote about a well-known blues refrain and book/movie title may illustrate the effects of prolonged Dysthymia in the young. In 1966, the Grateful Dead sang a traditional blues song "Been Down so Long" in a San Francisco concert. One of the stanzas of this song was:

I can't stand moving but I don't like standing still.
The hole that I've been in looks more and more like a hill ...
I been down so long it looks like up to me.

In the same year, Richard Farina published a very successful "coming of age in the 1960s" novel with the title *Been Down So Long It Looks Like Up to Me,* followed in 1971 by a (forgettable) movie with the same memorable title. Although neither book nor movie are about Dysthymia, "I've been down so long it looks like up to me" and "the hole that I've been in looks more and more like a hill" would seem to be accurate poetic descriptions of the feelings that many dysthymic children experience during the course of their illness. While major depressive episodes last from two weeks to several months, it is not unusual for Dysthymia in children to last three or four years. A child of eight who has been depressed for a month can easily remember happier times, but when that mood depression extends to half a lifetime, any past happiness may recede beyond the ability to recall. Children with Dysthymia can truly be depressed so long that they do not even recognize their mood as abnormal; as a result, they may not complain of feeling depressed when directly asked. They have been down so long it seems normal for them to feel that way.

Bipolar Disorder

Bipolar Disorder is a mood disorder in which episodes of depression alternate with episodes of mania. In adults and adolescents, mania manifests as intensive purposive behavior that often leads to self-harm: overeating, sexual indiscretion,

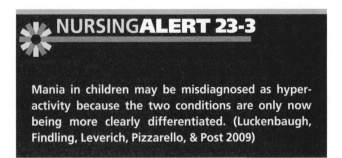

> **NURSINGALERT 23-3**
>
> Mania in children may be misdiagnosed as hyperactivity because the two conditions are only now being more clearly differentiated. (Luckenbaugh, Findling, Leverich, Pizzarello, & Post 2009)

or buying sprees. Bipolar Disorder frequently begins in adolescence, but in recent years there has been increasing recognition that mania, and hence Bipolar Disorder, may also occur in children. Mania in older children and adolescents is often associated with high levels of energy and activity: multiple projects begun but not finished, markedly increased talkativeness, decreased need for sleep, and expansive mood. Because children do not have the independence or the developmental level of adults or adolescents, mania presents differently in the very young and is often misdiagnosed as hyperactivity and ADHD. Experts suggest that the two conditions can be differentiated when hyperactive symptoms are episodic with intervening normal behavior (more common in mania than in ADHD) and when school performance is overall good (more common in mania).

Unfortunately, ADHD and Bipolar Disorder may coexist frequently in the same child, making accurate diagnosis particularly difficult. The lack of high-quality studies identifying the best treatments for Bipolar Disorder in children further complicates the diagnosis and treatment of this condition (Wolf & Wagner, 2003). Despite side effects, including, in some cases, considerable weight gain, atypical antipsychotics such as risperidone have been used with increasing frequency in children with a variety of childhood psychiatric conditions, including Bipolar Disorder (Simeon, Milin, & Walker, 2002). Among these conditions are Asperger's syndrome, autism, pervasive developmental disorder, anxiety, depression, schizophrenia, and Obsessive-Compulsive Disorder. Many of these disorders are discussed elsewhere in this chapter.

DEPRESSION

Depression is relatively common in childhood. Population studies show that at any one time between 10% and 15% of the child and adolescent population has some symptoms of depression, though not necessarily a disorder diagnosable under DSM. Depression has been diagnosed in preschoolers, and current evidence is that from 0.3% to 1.4% of preschoolers experience depression, while 1.0% to 2.0% of prepubertial children experience depression (Kapornai & Vetro, 2008). Rates of depression vary with ethnicity, with American Indian and Hispanic children having higher rates than whites and African American children (Davis, 2005).

Depression tends in children, as in adults, to be a chronic illness characterized by recurrences. The age of first onset of depression appears to play a role in its course. Children who first become depressed before puberty seem to be at higher risk for developing some form of mental disorder in adulthood than are those who first become depressed after puberty.

Causes and Prevention of Depression

The precise causes of depression in children are not known, partly because less research has been performed on children than on adults. Most experts assume that, as in adults, childhood depression has both biological and psychosocial causation. Children of depressed parents are more than three times as likely as children with nondepressed parents to experience a depressive disorder. Experts can't yet say how much of this tendency of depression to run in families is genetic and how much is environmental.

Some of the core symptoms of depression, such as changes in appetite and sleep patterns, are related to the functions of the hypothalamus. The hypothalamus is, in turn, closely tied to the function of the pituitary gland, and both of these brain regions are closely tied to the processes of growth and pubertal development. Abnormalities of pituitary function, such as increased rates of circulating cortisol and hypo- or hyperthyroidism, are well established (if incompletely understood) features of depression in adults (Goodwin & Jamison, 1990). There has been considerable interest in the relationship between an individual's "mindset" or approach to perceiving external events and a predisposition to depression. Persons who have a tendency toward what is called a pessimistic "attribution bias" (Hops, Lewinsohn, Andrews, & Roberts, 1990) tend to have increased likelihood of becoming depressed. There is evidence that children and adolescents who previously have been depressed may learn, during their depression, to interpret events pessimistically, and so develop a "pessimistic attribution bias," which may predispose them to future episodes of depression (Nolen-Hoeksema, Morrow, & Fredrickson, 1993).

Psychological Treatment of Depression

Although both cognitive-behavioral therapy and antidepressant medications have been shown to be effective in treating acute depression in adults, equivalent proof of efficacy in children has been slower to emerge. Over the years, there has been strong expert opinion that some kinds of cognitive-behavioral interventions can be effective in children (Kaslow & Thompson, 1998), and studies have recently shown that cognitive behavioral therapy is of significant value for children and adolescents with depression, Generalized Anxiety Disorder, Obsessive-Compulsive Disorder, and Post-Traumatic Stress Disorder (Muñoz-Solomando, Kendall, & Whittington, 2008). One apparently helpful treatment involves "self-control" therapy that assists children to exert control over thoughts and behaviors.

Pharmacological Treatment of Depression

Numerous clinical trials in children and adolescents have failed to demonstrate efficacy for tricyclic antidepressants in younger children. In contrast, in the 1990s selective serotonin reuptake inhibitors (SSRIs) were thought to have efficacy, though the number of studies at that time was small (Kutcher, 1998; Eisenberg, 1996; Emslie, Weinberg, Kowatch, Hughes, Carmody, & Rush, 1997; Strober, DeAntonio, Schmidt-Lackner, Pataki, Freeman, Rigali, et al., 1999).

The use of SSRIs has become an increasingly controversial topic in children and adolescents. There is mounting evidence that many of these medications may cause an increase in suicidal ideation and suicide among children and adolescents (Whittington, Kendall, Fonagy, Cottrell, Cotgrove, & Buddington, 2004). The Food and Drug Administration (FDA) has instructed manufacturers to strengthen warnings about suicide risk with SSRI antidepressants, and European regulators have recommended that paroxetine not be given to children or adolescents. In late 2004, an FDA expert panel recommended a prominent "black box" warning label on the medications concerning use in children (Vedantam, 2004). Since most data (Whittington et al., 2004) suggest that fluoxetine (Prozac) has a lower risk of suicidal ideation than do other related medications, this drug continues to be used for depression in both the United States and Europe and may be more efficacious than are other drugs—especially for adolescents (Tsapakis, Soldani, Tondo, & Baldessarini, 2008). Some experts have expressed concern that "antagonism to drug treatment" might deprive the estimated 2% to 4% of children who suffer from depression of receiving potentially beneficial treatment (Hazell, 2002). The FDA has now placed "black box" warnings on antidepressants about potential increased risk of suicidal ideation or suicide. These warnings have proven controversial because of observational studies that show that suicide rates decreased steadily during the years that increasing numbers of children and adolescents were treated with antidepressants. While uncertainty remains about the risk of antidepressants, there is accumulating evidence that black box warnings *have* decreased the use of antidepressants among children and adolescents (Olfson, Marcus, & Druss, 2008). Whether such decreased usage will decrease or increase risk of suicide remains to be seen.

Knowledge of treatment effectiveness is much less for Bipolar Disorder and Dysthymia in children than for Major Depressive Disorder (or for any of these disorders in adults). Uncontrolled studies and case series support the use of valproic acid, lithium, and carbamazepine in children—much as in adults (Kowatch, Suppes, Carmody, Bucci, Hum, Kromelis, et al., 2000). Each of these drugs has potential safety risks in this age group (Geller & Luby, 1997), and treatment should be supervised by individuals with considerable experience in diagnosis and therapy. Atypical antipsychotics are often used for mania and mixed mania/depression involving children and adolescents, even though evidence for efficacy remains incomplete (Chang, 2008). Dysthymia in children is treated with SSRI medications and psychotherapy, and at least two preliminary descriptive studies suggest benefit from this course of treatment (Rabe-Jablonska, 2000; Waslick, Walsh, Greenhill, Eilenberg, Capasso, & Lieber, 1999).

ANXIETY DISORDERS

Although no single anxiety disorder occurs as frequently in children as does ADHD, collectively the prevalence of the anxiety disorders (13%) is higher than that of other mental disorders of childhood and adolescence (Costello, Angold, Burns, Stangl, Tweed, Erkanli, et al., 1996). Anxiety disorders not infrequently diagnosed in children include Separation Anxiety Disorder, Generalized Anxiety Disorder, Social Phobia, and Obsessive-Compulsive Disorder. Of these, only Separation Anxiety Disorder is unique to children.

SEPARATION ANXIETY DISORDER

Separation anxiety is a term used to describe symptoms that occur when children are forced to separate from a parent, usually their mother. In practice, most cases of separation anxiety occur during ordinary daily separations such as when the parent goes to work or the child goes to school or to a babysitter's. Separation anxiety may occasionally manifest at bedtime when a child is required to sleep in his or her own room away from the parent. Separation anxiety is commonly seen in infants and toddlers and is regarded as part of normal development at an early age. Somewhere between the ages of two and four most children develop the ability to separate from their parents without severe anxiety, especially if they are going to a familiar environment. When separation anxiety occurs in older children, a diagnosis of Separation Anxiety Disorder may be made if the anxiety lasts longer than a month and clearly causes distress or affects social, academic, or job functioning (American Psychiatric Association, 2000). Children with separation anxiety may insist on sleeping with a parent and have difficulty falling asleep by themselves at night. When separated, they may express fear that their parent will be involved in an accident or taken ill, or in some other way be permanently "lost." Separation anxiety affects children's ability to attend school or camp, stay at friends' houses, or be in a room by themselves. Children may express anxiety through somatization; symptoms may include dizziness, nausea, or palpitations (American Psychiatric Association, 2000). Nightmares are common, but frequently occur in normal children and are not by themselves indicative of separation anxiety. Separation anxiety is often associated with symptoms of depression and fear that they or a family member might die. Separation anxiety is quite common and occurs in about 4% of children and young adolescents (American Psychiatric Association, 2000). It is important that nurses seeing children with this disorder explore the symptoms realistically from the child's point of view. Some children live in neighborhoods or attend schools that are sufficiently dangerous that fear of leaving the house is appropriate. These children may have seen peers or siblings injured or even killed in their own neighborhoods. Such children have important needs for safety, and some may meet criteria for post-traumatic distress syndrome, but they do not have Separation Anxiety Disorder if their fears are reasonable. Separation Anxiety Disorder does tend to improve with time and may have a fluctuating course. The symptoms resemble a childhood form of Agoraphobia, and indeed in some children the condition may last for years or actually be a precursor to Panic Disorder with Agoraphobia. Little is known about the cause of Separation Anxiety Disorder, although there are a number of theories based on case studies (Goenjian, Pynoos, Steinberg, Najarian, Asarnow, Karayan, et al., 1995). As with many other anxiety disorders, separation anxiety sometimes runs in families, but the significance of genetic and environmental factors has not been established.

Generalized Anxiety Disorder

When it occurs in children, Generalized Anxiety Disorder is sometimes termed "overanxious disorder of childhood." Children with this condition are very much like their adult counterparts. They worry excessively about a variety of events and occurrences such as academic or athletic performance, being on time, or natural disasters such as earthquakes. The worry persists even when school and social successes demonstrate that the child has nothing substantive to worry about. The frequency with which this disorder occurs in childhood is incompletely understood, but many adults seeking treatment for this disorder report that it began in childhood or adolescence.

Social Phobia

Children with **social phobia** (also called Social Anxiety Disorder) have a persistent fear of being embarrassed in social situations, or under circumstances in which they perceive (often correctly) that their performance is being judged by others as during a speech, class recitation, or musical recital. For some children symptoms can be provoked by nonjudgmental situations such as simple conversation or even eating in public. Feelings of anxiety in these situations can often produce physical reactions such as palpitations, tremors, sweating, diarrhea, and blushing. Social phobia can be harder to recognize in children than in adults, who may have less difficulty in describing symptoms of anxiety. Especially when it occurs in childhood, social phobia may be hard to distinguish from Avoidant Personality Disorder (see Chapter 18).

Obsessive-Compulsive Disorder

Obsessive-Compulsive Disorder (OCD) is characterized by recurrent, time-consuming thoughts (obsessions) and repetitive behaviors such as hand washing or counting rituals that act to reduce the anxiety caused by obsessive thoughts (American Psychiatric Association, 2000). In her novel *The Cuckoo's Child,* Suzanne Freeman tells the story of Mia, a preadolescent girl whose parents mysteriously disappear on a sailing trip in the Mediterranean after their small boat deviates from its planned course. Mia's mother was the navigator, and Mia comes to suspect she may have impulsively altered their course: "With my mom, I thought, it could have been almost anything that made her shift course—a school of dolphins swimming by, an island on the horizon, whatever path the moonlight made across the water." In the novel, Mia's life comes to be dominated by internal compulsions that at times similarly controls where and how far she ventures into the unknown:

IT WAS MY ONLY HOPE

Just ahead of me was the narrow space between the garage and the wooden fence. It wasn't night yet. There was still the low gloomy light of the end of the day, but in that space it was already black, the deepest black that could swallow you. I shivered, already knowing. The command was coming.

It came. Go in there. Go on in that space.

I had to. You didn't argue. You didn't bargain. I turned sideways and squeezed through the narrow opening. Cobwebs were everywhere. I pushed them away from my face, and they stuck to my fingers. The darkness was like a cloth thrown over your head. You could feel its weight. More than anything I wanted to move my eyes to look back out at the everyday world with its fading light and the smell of fried meat from the houses and the dull clatter of the dinner pans being scrubbed in the sinks. But it wasn't allowed. Just for thinking of it, I had to move five steps deeper into the dark space, five steps farther away from the world.

*I stood there, counting to a hundred. Twice I had to start over for counting too fast, for rushing through it. Something shifted in the dry leaves, some little animal close to my feet, but I counted on. It was my only hope, just to follow these orders, the harder the better. It was what I could do. Fifty-seven. Wait. Fifty-eight. Wait. Fifty-nine. More slowly than my heart could ever beat, I counted.**

(Freeman, 1997, p. 215)

In reading Mia's story, one can't help wondering whether some similar obsession drove her mother's ship off its course to an unknown fate, but we never really learn whether it was whim or obsession that led Mia's mother to her doom. Instead, the passage quoted here captures brilliantly the power that obsessive thoughts can have over a child with OCD. Mia periodically finds herself obsessed with dark or dangerous places, an obsession manifested by an irresistible command to walk into a fearful deathlike darkness. She cannot disobey the command; she is able to control her fear by a compulsive behavior—a slow counting that protects her from panic when cobwebs brush her face and unknown creatures slither at her feet.

OCD is increasingly recognized to be a relatively common disorder in children (Geller, 2006), and as a consequence, many children share Mia's experience of suffering its symptoms without diagnosis or treatment. As implied in Mia's story, there is a strong familial component to OCD (Gilbert & Maalouf, 2008), best seen in twin studies. OCD

*From *The Cuckoo's Child,* by Suzanne Freeman, Copyright © 1996. Reprinted with permission from HarperCollins Children's Books.

is increased among first-degree relatives of children with OCD. An affected child is likely to have an affected parent, although it is more likely to be a father than a mother (Lenane, Swedo, Leonard, Pauls, Sceery, & Rapoport, 1990). Interestingly, children and their parents may share this disorder, but the actual symptoms of OCD frequently differ between involved relatives. This difference implies that the child is not merely mimicking behaviors that he or she observes in an involved parent (Leonard, Rapoport, & Swedo, 1997). Many adults with either childhood- or adolescent-onset OCD show evidence of abnormalities in a neural network known as the orbitofrontalstriatal area (Rauch & Savage, 1997; Grachev, Breiter, Rauch, Savage, Baer, Shera, et al., 1998). Fascinating data suggest that in some children a streptococcal infection may immediately precede the abrupt onset or worsening of symptoms (Swedo, Pleeter, Richter, Hoffman, Allen, Hamburger, et al., 1995). Researchers believe that this form of OCD—termed PANDAS for *Pediatric Autoimmune Neuropsychiatric Disorders Associated with Streptococcal* infections—occurs through an immunological cross-reaction between brain tissue and streptococcal bacterial antigens. While the concept of PANDAS remains controversial (Murphy, Sajid, & Goodman, 2006), some experts think that PANDAS may explain up to 10% of childhood cases of OCD (Trifiletti & Packard, 1999).

Psychotherapy Treatment of Anxiety

Although anxiety disorders are relatively common in children, there has been relatively limited research on the efficacy of psychotherapy (Kendall, Flannery-Schroeder, Panichelli-Mindel, Southam-Gerow, Henin, & Warman, 1997). Childhood phobias have been shown to respond well to the technique of contingency management (Ollendick & King, 1998), as well as to desensitization. At least one pilot study shows efficacy of cognitive-behavioral approaches to social phobia in female adolescents (Hayward, Varady, Albano, Thienemann, Henderson, & Schatzberg, 2000), but while there has been considerable use of cognitive-behavioral approaches to managing anxiety in children (Ollendick & King, 1998; Kendall, Chansky, Kane, Kim, Kortlander, Ronan, et al., 1992; Morgan, Singer-Harris, Bernstein, & Waber, 2000; Barrett, Dadds, & Rapee, 1996), a large recent study of children with separation anxiety, Generalized Anxiety Disorder, or social phobia clearly showed the effectiveness of cognitive-behavioral therapy (Walkup, Albano, Piacentini, Birmaher, Compton, Sherrill, et al., 2008). This study also demonstrated that higher response rates were obtained when cognitive-behavioral approaches were combined with use of the antidepressant sertraline.

Pharmacotherapy Treatment of Anxiety

Research suggests that selective serotonin reuptake inhibitors (SSRIs) generally provide effective treatment of Separation Anxiety Disorder and other anxiety disorders of childhood and adolescence (Reinblatt & Riddle, 2007), and as noted previously, their combination with cognitive-behavioral therapy may increase the likelihood of favorable response (Walkup et al., 2008). SSRIs appear to be effective in reducing symptoms of OCD in children, although efficacy is perhaps better established for adults (Flament, Rapoport, Berg, Sceery, Kilts, Mellstrom, et al., 1985; DeVeaugh-Geiss, Moroz, Biederman, Cantwell, Fontaine, Greist, et al., 1992). As noted in the section on depression, some European countries have restricted the use of some SSRI drugs for treatment of children and adolescents because of worries about a possible increase in suicidal ideation and suicide. Similar concerns in the United States have led the FDA to mandate a significant strengthening of manufacturers' warnings. While risk of suicide may be higher in depression than in anxiety, it seems very likely that concerns about use of SSRI medications apply equally when the drugs are employed to treat anxiety or depression. At the time of writing, the best evidence is that fluoxetine (Prozac) is relatively free of suicidal risk (Whittington et al., 2004), although fluoxetine is among the drugs singled out by the FDA for stronger warnings. Despite warnings, worsening anxiety is among the symptoms that the FDA has cited as potentially signaling enhanced suicidal risk in children (or adults) taking antidepressants. Anxiolytic drugs such as benzodiazepines have no established role in the management of childhood anxiety disorders.

OTHER MENTAL DISORDERS IN CHILDREN AND ADOLESCENTS

Developmental Disorders

A thorough understanding of normal child development is one of the key competencies for nursing practice. Many well-characterized factors can interfere with development, but in the majority of situations in which developmental delay occurs, no specific causal factor can be identified. This is very much true of the two conditions to be discussed next: **autism** and **Asperger's syndrome**. These relatively uncommon disorders are so striking in their presentation that they are generally given more attention in psychiatric texts than are more frequently seen forms of developmental delay such as Down syndrome, fragile X syndrome, and cerebral palsy.

Autism

Autism has a prevalence of about 3 in 1,000 children over the age of three years (Yeargin-Allsopp, Rice, Karapurkar, Doernberg, Boyle, & Murphy 2003) and is characterized by profound lack of interest in social interactions. The more inclusive diagnosis of "Autism Spectrum Disorders" appears to be significantly more common and may involve as many as one in every 150 children (1% in the population; Rapin & Tuchman, 2008). The "must-see" film *Rain Man*, starring Tom Cruise and Dustin Hoffman, describes two brothers, one autistic, who strive to reach each other across the divide that

Autism imposes. How hard it is to cross that divide is emphasized in the following passage written by Donna Williams who relates a dream that takes her back to an autistic childhood. Few other persons recover sufficiently from this pervasive developmental disorder to write of their experiences.

NOBODY NOWHERE

I would face the light shining through the window and rub my eyes furiously. There they were. The bright fluffy colors moving through the white. I discovered the air was full of spots. People would walk by, obstructing my magical view of nothingness. I'd move past them. They'd gabble. My attention would be firmly set on my desire to lose myself in the spots, and I'd ignore the gabble. I learned eventually to lose myself in anything I desired—the patterns on the wallpaper or carpet. Even people became no problem. Their words became a mumbling jumble. I could look through them until I wasn't there, and then, later, I learned to lose myself in them. Other people's expectations for me to respond to them was a problem. This would have required my understanding what was said, but I was too happy losing myself to want to be dragged back by something as two-dimensional as understanding. For the first three and a half years of my life ... my language consisted of repeating what others said, complete with intonation and inflection of those I came to think of as "the world." The world seemed to be impatient, annoying, callous and unrelenting. I learned to respond to it as such, crying, squealing, ignoring it, and running away. The more I became aware of the world around me, the more I became afraid. Other people were my enemies, and reaching out to me was their weapon.

*I never hugged either of my caregivers; neither was I hugged. I didn't like anyone coming too close to me, let alone touching me. I felt that all touching was pain, and I was frightened. For many years I played with, touched, and chewed on my own hair. Touching other children's hair was the only friendly physical contact I would make.**

(Williams, 1992, pp. 3–5, 8–9)

Children with Autism remain emotionally detached from others. They resist eye contact, touch, and most kinds of interpersonal contact. This aversion to human contact is often evident in very young infants who are often perceived by their parents as unusual, uncuddly, and unresponsive babies. As children get older, many develop a fascination with inanimate objects, particularly those that rotate. Autistic children will often engage in strikingly repetitive behaviors. More characteristic behaviors include rocking back and forth for long periods and spinning in circles. Most are severely delayed in acquiring language, but some do develop verbal skills, and others can be helped to establish interpersonal relationships. Many children with Autism do not respond to physical illnesses; their caregivers must, therefore, be observant, and when something is wrong, take action to initiate health care treatments.

Intensive, sustained special education programs and behavior therapy early in life can increase the ability of the child with Autism to acquire language and ability to learn. It is difficult to study outcomes of rare disorders rigorously because of the small numbers available for investigation, but it appears that special education programs in highly structured environments can help affected children acquire self-care, social, educational, and even job skills. Myers and colleagues have reviewed evidence and current expert opinion on effective psychological and educational interventions for Autism Spectrum Disorder (Myers & Johnson, 2007).

A number of medications have been tried in managing autistic children. The antipsychotic drug haloperidol has been shown to be superior to placebo in the treatment of autism (Perry, Campbell, Adams, Lynch, Spencer, Curren, et al., 1989), although a significant number of children develop dyskinesias as a side effect. As noted in Chapter 27, such side effects may be both permanent and disabling. The newer atypical neuroleptics are generally less likely to produce such extrapyramidal side effects, and preliminary studies suggest that these drugs may also be somewhat effective in treating autistic children. The FDA has approved the atypical antipsychotic risperidone for controlling irritability and aggressive behavior in Autism (Myers et al., 2007). Since many autistic behaviors appear ritualistic, drugs effective in inhibiting ritualistic behavior in OCD have been tried. Two of the SSRIs, clomipramine (Gordon, State, Nelson, Hamburger, & Rapoport, 1993) and fluoxetine (McDougle, Naylor, Cohen, Volkmar, Heninger, & Price, 1996), have been shown to have benefit, at least in older children (Sanchez, Campbell, Small, Cueva, Armenteros, & Adams, 1996).

Children with Autism have been studied with a variety of imaging techniques such as computerized tomography (CT), magnetic resonance imaging (MRI), and positron emission tomography (PET) scans, but while no breakthrough understanding has emerged (Rapin & Katzman, 1998; Piven, 1997; Zilbovicius, Garreau, Samson, Remy, Barthelemy, Syrota, et al., 1995), research has begun to yield interesting findings. Serotonin synthesis is decreased in autistic children compared to normal children, and the decrease is localized to certain brain areas—mostly the left hemisphere and the right cerebellum (Wallace & Treffert, 2004). Data summarized by these authors also show remarkable differences in brain and head growth in very young autistic children. Many of these children begin life with relatively small heads and then undergo unusually rapid growth of the head and the underlying brain. As a result, many autistic children have unusually large heads and brains in early childhood. Since nurses typically measure head size at routine visits during the first two years of life, they may be among the first professionals to recognize this abnormal growth and ask questions

*From *Nobody Nowhere*, by D. Williams, 1992. Reprinted with permission of the author.

about development that can lead to early diagnosis of autism. However, head enlargement is temporary because brain growth then slows, so that by adolescence most autistic children have quite normal measurements. These changes in brain and skull growth seem, at least in some cases, to be linked to abnormalities of a gene known as hoxI, which is associated with the rate of brain growth. While no definite genetic causation has been proven, evidence for genetic influences derives in part from twin studies showing that identical twins are more likely to share this disorder than are fraternal twins (Cook, 1998). More recent MRI studies show that the rapid head growth is associated with significant proliferation of brain white matter (Hughes, 2007), which is followed by disturbed brain connections between association areas—including the corpus callosum connecting the left and right sides of the brain (Minshew & Williams, 2007). This disturbed brain connectivity undoubtedly underlies the behavioral characteristics of Autism Spectrum Disorders.

Asperger's Syndrome

I AM **REALLY** INTERESTED IN THE WEATHER

I know that everyone talks about the weather but not like me. I am really, really, REALLY interested in the weather.

My dad got me some information from the weather office and it was neat. There were maps and all sorts of numbers. The first thing I do in the morning when I wake up is turn on my radio and listen to the forecast. Once I missed it and once it did not come on until twenty-two minutes after seven. When it is not on time, it upsets me but I am learning to be patient and wait. Once I'm up, I dress really quickly so that I can go downstairs and see the weather maps on TV. I also check the thermometer outside the kitchen and the barometer.

*I must learn not to talk about the weather all the time. Then maybe the other kids won't call me the "Weather Weebie." At first I thought it was a good name. But then they started making jokes about the weather that I didn't understand. Once at school, they told me it was raining when it was supposed to be sunny so I rushed to the window to look and then the whole class laughed.**

(Schnurr, 1999, pp. 23–25)

The narrator in Rosina Schnurr's book *Asperger's Huh?* is a 10-year-old with recently diagnosed Asperger's syndrome. He is beginning to understand how his odd behavior comes across to others (though this is hard because he lacks normal intuitions of how others "read" and react to what he says and does.) "I must learn not to talk about the weather all the time" is probably an idea he has learned from his parents and therapist, rather than deduced from his classroom reception as a "Weather Weebie." The purpose of Dr. Schnurr's wonderful book is to help children with Asperger's syndrome see that others share their predicament and understand some of the changes they must make in their lives in order to adapt to a world in which they don't easily fit.

Another marvelous evocation of the world of Asperger's syndrome is a novel by Mark Haddon entitled *The Curious Incident of the Dog in the Night-Time* (2003). This is a detective story written in the voice of a young man with Asperger's syndrome whose life is as controlled by logic, mathematical formulas, and the absence of emotion as it is disturbed by the brutal murder of the neighbor's dog.

*From *Asperger's Huh? A Child's Perspective*, by Rosina G. Schnurr, 2000, Gloucester, Ontario, Canada: Anisor Publishing.

RESEARCH Highlight 23-2

Measuring the Effect of Mothers' Negative Thinking on Their Children's Behavior

STUDY PROBLEM/PURPOSE

Negative thoughts are common in depression, and reducing these thoughts is one of the targets of cognitive behavioral therapy. The present study sought to identify negative thoughts in single mothers with children between two and six years of age, and to correlate these thoughts with reported child behavior as measured on a standardized checklist.

METHODS

Two hundred and five women, most never married, were given a variety of standard measures of depression and stress as well as the "Crandall Cognitions Inventory," which assesses frequency of negative thoughts. Mothers rated their children's behavior on the Child Behavior Checklist, and this instrument provided measures of both internalizing (anxiety, depression, and somatization) and externalizing (aggression, disruptiveness, and impulsivity) in the children.

FINDINGS

There was a relationship between both internalizing and externalizing negative child behaviors and mothers' stressors and depressive symptoms. Stress and depressive symptoms in mothers explained 21% to 27% of the variability in children's behavior in mothers and were associated with maternal negative thoughts. The authors conclude by hypothesizing that helping mothers to reduce negative thinking could allow them to perceive fewer behavior problems in their children.

Source: "Maternal Factors Associated with Child Behavior," by L. A. Hall, M. K. Rayens, & A. R. Peden, 2008, *Journal of Nursing Scholarship*, *40*(2), 124–130.

Christopher, the narrator, is accused of the crime, but undeterred by this accusation he proceeds in his obsessively logical way to solve the crime.

Children with Asperger's share many of the characteristics of Autism, but are far less severely affected. Asperger's syndrome is characterized by the combination of severe impairments in social interaction with highly repetitive patterns of interests and behaviors. These interests are often highly limited, but children with Asperger's frequently gain a great deal of knowledge about a relatively narrow range of topics. Weather is a typical example; another child with Asperger's syndrome has an encyclopedic knowledge of movies, directors, and actors. Unlike Autism, where communication skills are severely impaired, children with Asperger's have normal receptive and expressive language. Their overall intellectual abilities are generally normal, and may be exceptionally high. The main deficit in Asperger's syndrome is a consistent inability to regulate social interactions by responding to verbal and especially nonverbal cues. Children with this disorder may not seek out friendships, and in school ages and adolescence they may lack the ability to establish friendships, even when desired. They may talk at length about their topic of special interest (weather, movies, etc.) when others are clearly uninterested in hearing more. This behavior contrasts with that of autistic children who typically prefer to avoid social interaction entirely. Children with Asperger's syndrome have no specific neurological abnormalities, though they are often clumsy when participating in sports activities. Seizures may occasionally occur, though no specific association has been established with epilepsy.

NURSINGTIP 23-1

Helping Children Who Exhibit Unacceptable Behavior

- Praise accomplishments through touch, verbal affection, or small rewards such as stickers or stars on an activity calendar.
- Model desirable traits, such as sharing and honesty.
- Acknowledge positive or desirable behaviors.
- Correct unacceptable or undesirable behaviors immediately and calmly.
- Communicate that the behavior, not the child, is unacceptable.
- Have the child help determine acceptable behavior parameters.
- Explain expectations in clear terms.
- Ensure that the child understands expectations by asking the child to repeat instructions.
- Be certain that expectations are within the child's developmental parameters.
- Clearly outline consequences for unacceptable behaviors, and follow through on their implementation.

In many ways, Asperger's syndrome resembles one of the "odd" personality disorders such as schizoid or avoidant, but most child psychiatrists feel that the condition is distinctive enough to require its own diagnostic label. This syndrome was only defined in the 1980s, so it is one of the newest in DSM-IV-TR. The prevalence of Asperger's syndrome is uncertain, but it is not exceptionally rare. There is no specific treatment unless comorbidities such as mood disorder or anxiety disorder (social phobia, OCD) are diagnosed. Psychotherapy can help children better understand how others see them and make changes in their behavior to compensate for their lack of intuition about such matters. Children with Asperger's may remain undiagnosed until early adolescence because their overall normal abilities do not cause any educational handicap, and their social disabilities may be overlooked in primary and middle school.

Disruptive Disorders

Disruptive disorders, such as **Oppositional Defiant Disorder** and **Conduct Disorder**, are characterized by antisocial behavior and as a result seem to be more a collection of socially deviant behaviors than a diagnostic pattern of mental dysfunction. These behaviors are not infrequently precursors to the development of Antisocial Personality Disorder (see Chapter 18), and may also be associated with ADHD, discussed earlier in this chapter. In some children, ADHD progresses to Conduct Disorder and then to Antisocial Personality Disorder, though this progression is seen in only a minority of children with ADHD.

Oppositional Defiant Disorder

Oppositional defiant disorder (ODD) is diagnosed when there is a consistent pattern of rejecting adult authority. ODD is characterized by behaviors such as persistent fighting and arguing, being easily annoyed, and deliberately annoying or being vindictive to other people (Hamilton & Armando, 2008). Children with ODD may repeatedly lose their temper, argue with adults, deliberately refuse to comply with requests or rules of adults, and blame others for their own mistakes. They are stubborn and often test adult limits (American Psychiatric Association, 2000; Weiner, 1997). ODD is sometimes a precursor to conduct disorder, which is discussed in the following section.

ODD is not rare, and studies suggest a population prevalence in childhood ranging from 1% to 6%, depending on the population studied and on whether interviews are conducted with children alone or with children, teachers, and parents (Rapoport, Inoff-Germain, Weissman, Greenwald, Narrow, & Jensen et al. 2000). Before puberty, the condition is more common in boys, but after puberty this difference disappears. In preschool boys, high reactivity, difficulty being soothed, and high motor activity may indicate risk for the disorder. Although it is common for very young children to snatch something they want from another child, this kind of behavior may suggest risk for emerging ODD if it persists to the age of four or five and later.

Conduct Disorder

Conduct Disorder is one of the most serious conditions of childhood; children with Conduct Disorder show a pattern of cruelty and disrespect for the rights of others and are capable of severe violence and murder. Recent episodes of school shootings have made identification and management of children with this disorder an important priority for schools, though by no means do all children who commit acts of lethal violence have Conduct Disorder. Similarly, neither are all children with Conduct Disorder dangerously violent. Many children or adolescents with Conduct Disorder also have symptoms of ODD. In addition, they behave aggressively by fighting, bullying, intimidating, physically assaulting, sexually coercing, or being cruel to people or animals. Vandalism with deliberate destruction of property, such as setting fires or smashing windows, is common, as are theft and truancy; other manifestations include early substance use and precocious sexual activity that may involve coercion. Gang affiliations and involvement with prostitution are not unusual for either sex. These behaviors usually interfere substantially with school performance, such that even individuals with very high potential rarely perform at a level consistent with their abilities. Perhaps not surprisingly, depression, suicidal thoughts, suicide attempts, and completed suicide are not unusual in children diagnosed with Conduct Disorder The prevalence of Conduct Disorder is estimated to be 0.4% to 3.3%, with males being two to three times more likely than females to carry the diagnosis (Braun, Froehlick, Daniels, Dietrick, Hornung, Auinger, & Lanphear, 2008). Overall, between a quarter and a half of highly antisocial children become antisocial adults and have persistent problems with jobs, marital stability, and the law.

The known social risk factors for Conduct Disorder include early maternal abandonment, early institutionalization, family neglect, abuse or violence, parents' psychiatric illness, parental marital discord, large family size, crowding, and poverty (Loeber & Stouthamer-Loeber, 1986; Sampson & Laub, 1993). There is some suggestion that children with certain physical and neurological characteristics, such as diminished perception of pain, may be at increased risk of developing Conduct Disorder (Raine, Reynolds, Venables, Mednick, & Farrington, 1998). As with ODD, there appears to be a correlation between aggressive behavior at preschool ages with subsequent preadolescent aggression (Raine et al., 1998; Sampson & Laub, 1993). Although it is unlikely that all aggressive three-year-olds will develop Conduct Disorder, the recognition that traits of aggressiveness are relatively stable through childhood offers an opportunity to help some children learn to moderate their aggression (Johnson & Breckenridge, 1982). Very recent work suggests that environmental factors and exposure to toxins such as lead is a risk factor for conduct disorder (Braun et al., 2008).

Treatment Perhaps some children with Conduct Disorder can be helped by relatively small classes and caring, talented teaching. Most severely disturbed children need intensive interventions with both psychosocial methods and, often, psychoactive drugs. There is some evidence that behavior-shaping programs can be effective for children with Conduct Disorder (Brestan & Eyberg, 1998). The most effective programs involved parents in efforts to modify their children's behavior.

Drug Treatment Conduct-disordered children are frequently treated with a variety of psychoactive medications, but none has been uniformly effective. Four drugs are commonly used to treat this disorder: lithium, methylphenidate (Ritalin), carbamazepine, and clonidine (Campbell & Cueva, 1995; Klein, Abikoff, Klass, Ganeles, Seese, & Pollack, 1997; Kafantaris, Campbell, Padron-Gayol, Small, Locascio, & Rosenberg, 1992; Kemph, DeVane, Levin, Jarecke, & Miller, 1993). These drugs all have significant side effects, and need to be monitored carefully to avoid serious or even fatal outcomes. Conduct Disorder is nearly always associated with ADHD, Oppositional Defiant Disorder, or—less commonly—anxiety or depression (Turgay, 2005). Medication treatment is often directed more at one of these disorders rather than conduct disorder itself.

APPLICATION OF THE NURSING PROCESS 23-1

ASSESSMENT

There are many levels of mental health assessment, the earliest of which is screening for risk. Screening involves understanding the forces or factors that put children at risk for poor outcomes.

When a child is referred for psychological services, both the child and family are assessed. Assessment of the family should occur before assessment of the child. This focus on the family rather than the child initially gives the message that everyone is involved in the problem and its solutions, and decreases some of the pressure placed on the child. The assessment process varies depending on the age and developmental level of the child, the nurse's skills, and the clinical setting. Assessment data should be gathered from multiple sources, including interviews with the child and with members of the nuclear and extended families,

(*Continues*)

APPLICATION OF THE NURSING PROCESS 23-1 (Continued)

NURSINGALERT 23-4

Risk Factors for Childhood Emotional Disorders

- Poverty
- Minority status
- Homelessness
- Severe caregiver conflicts or divorce
- Caregiver psychopathology or substance abuse
- Physical or sexual abuse
- Chronic illness or disability of caregivers

observations of the child in interactions with others, caregivers' reports of the child's behavior, data gathered from questionnaires or behavior checklists, and interviews with teachers.

The nurse gathers in-depth information about the nature and extent of the child's problem in order to generate nursing diagnoses and a plan of care. A framework for data collection has been used for many years, using three means for collecting data: (1) the nurse's therapeutic use of self, (2) gathering information from the child and family, and (3) use of specific techniques or tools (Bumbalo & Siemon, 1983). The nurse's use of self may be the most important communication method, because establishment of trust and rapport are necessary for obtaining complete and valid data. A child and family are more likely to be open and honest if trust and mutual respect have been established with the nurse and the nurse is viewed as one who will understand and can help resolve the child's and family's concerns.

The child and family are also an important source of information. They can provide an invaluable history of the problem as well as information about school performance, relationships with peers, and family relationships. It is sometimes more productive to interview the older child without the caregivers present, because the child might be angry with them for being referred to treatment or may not be willing to disclose certain information in front of caregivers. Because the child is part of a family system, observations of the child should also be made in the family context. This can be accomplished by seeing the child with the caregivers and having an interview with the extended family, including the siblings, grandparents, other caretakers, and so on. Although there are no truly unique skills necessary to assess a child, the usual methods of observation and history taking need to be adapted for the child's age and developmental level. Assessment of the young child requires a nurse who is comfortable with play techniques and is able to use concrete language skills. The school-age child is better able to verbalize than the younger child; however, he may still feel more comfortable engaged in an activity such as a board game or clay modeling as he talks. This aged child often reveals his personality, conflicts, and feelings through play, drawings, and stories.

The third method for collecting data involves specific techniques and tools. The child's drawings, games, puppet and doll play, standardized tests, and various rating scales, questionnaires, and checklists provide additional data. Standardized measures should be used to augment other data collection methods, not to stand alone as a source of information (Bumbalo & Siemon, 1983).

Throughout the assessment interview, the nurse gathers information in the following areas:

- Presenting problem: onset, severity, duration, impact
- Health history: birth history, allergies, illnesses, past medical problems, surgeries, current health problems, previous and current medications
- School and social history: school performance; relationships with peers, teachers, and family; living arrangements; play activities
- Developmental history and status of child and family
- Psychiatric history: history of psychiatric disorders, substance abuse problems, organic mental disorders in the child and family members
- Physical assessment and exam
- Mental status exam: appearance, motor behavior and coordination, thought process and content, speech and language, emotional status, manner of relating to examiner

(Continues)

APPLICATION OF THE NURSING PROCESS 23-1 (Continued)

Ideally, the assessment of the child and family culminates in the formation of both nursing and medical diagnoses. The validity of the nursing diagnosis depends on the accuracy of the information obtained in the assessment. Once the assessment data have been gathered, the next step is to determine if the behavior and symptoms are maladaptive. When assessing a child's behavior, it is important to remember that it should be measured against the usual developmental responses characteristic of a certain age and a child's unique temperament and personality. For example, a temper tantrum may express the normal negativism of a toddler; on the other hand, temper tantrums on slight provocation in a six-year-old child may indicate psychological disturbance.

Several characteristics of behaviors are used to define serious emotional disorders. First, is that the disordered behaviors extend beyond age appropriateness for either the type or frequency of the behavior. Many behaviors that appear dysfunctional are normal behaviors for certain periods of development. Second, the disordered behaviors are of such intensity that they become detrimental to the child's functioning. Most acting-out behaviors do not seriously impair the child's functioning, even though the child may experience consequences of his behavior. However, behaviors that are self or other destructive create a situation in which the child's or another's safety becomes a reason for seeking treatment. The third characteristic is that the behaviors often deviate from social or cultural norms. Hearing voices, vandalism, cruelty to animals, fire setting, and similar behaviors are deviant in that they defy socially or culturally acceptable norms. These three criteria are not exhaustive; yet, they provide an initial guideline to distinguish behaviors indicative of normal development from those reflecting more serious disorders.

Mermaids

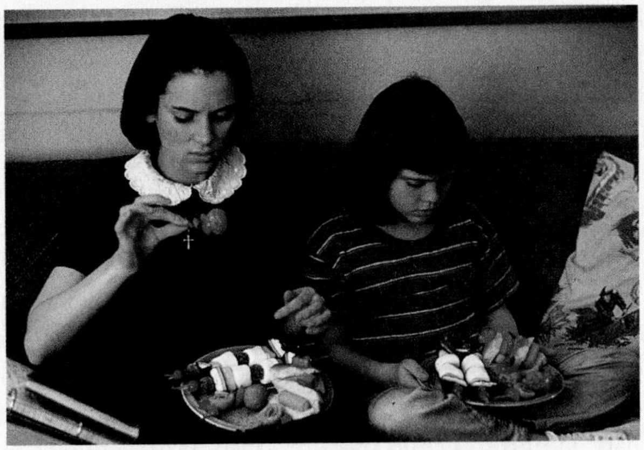

Source: Orion Pictures (Courtesy: The Kobal Collection)

Among the most poignant of human truths is that children cannot choose the families or the life circumstances into which they are born. In the film *Mermaids*, Charlotte and Kate live with a personality-disordered mother whose fear of close relationships results in numerous precipitous moves from one town to the next. *Mermaids* paints a realistic, if at times overly optimistic and humorous, picture of children's lives in a profoundly dysfunctional family.

NURSING DIAGNOSIS

The following are several common diagnoses that deal with issues and problems facing children.

ANXIETY

Children who are anxious may appear very active. Gentle touch and redirection is often helpful to reduce anxiety and restore self-control. When this does not work, the child may have to be placed in a less-stimulating environment. Children may experience anxiety because of fear of separation from their caregivers. Explore the child's fear of separation from the caregiver as well as the caregiver's possible fears of separation from the child. Caregivers may be so frustrated with the child's clinging and demanding behaviors that they need assistance in problem solving.

(Continues)

APPLICATION OF THE NURSING PROCESS 23-1 (Continued)

IMPAIRED SOCIAL INTERACTION

The behavior of some children is intrusive and immature. Conveying acceptance of the child separate from the behavior increases feelings of self-worth. The child must know which behaviors are and are not acceptable and the consequences of unacceptable behavior. Children can learn appropriate social skills in their relationships with nurses, in group therapy, and by role playing. For the child with an anxiety disorder, social interactions can be impaired because of excessive self-consciousness and inability to interact with unfamiliar people.

INEFFECTIVE COPING

Ineffective coping involves the inability to utilize an adaptive problem-solving approach when confronted by anticipated and unanticipated life events. Children must develop effective coping strategies appropriate to each phase of development. For example, a young child may withdraw from unsatisfactory play situations. The child's ability to use effective coping strategies grows in direct relation to developmental progress. When the child has not learned effective coping skills, dysfunctional behaviors may develop.

RISK FOR VIOLENCE

Children need to learn ways of handling conflict without becoming aggressive toward self or others. However, most children in inpatient psychiatric units have a limited notion of feelings, usually only identifying anger, and an equally limited way to express themselves. Risk for violence is highest when children are not able to express feelings through other than physical means or react in a manner inconsistent with their developmental age and the severity of the situation.

LOW SELF-ESTEEM

Decreased self-esteem underlies many dysfunctional behaviors. How a child feels about himself is largely determined by how he is regarded by others. A child develops positive self-esteem through positive relationships with others, beginning in infancy with attachment to caregivers and broadening throughout childhood. When a child is confronted with consistent negative or rejecting communication, his perception of self-worth is diminished. The child can eventually adopt behaviors indicative of low self-esteem: excessive need for reassurance from caregivers, poor eye contact, self-derogatory verbalizations, lack of initiative, somatic complaints such as stomach- and headaches, withdrawal from friends or family, depression, and aggressive or attention-getting behavior.

OUTCOME IDENTIFICATION

The nurse can help the caregivers and child to establish realistic and achievable goals that take into account the child's developmental level and family situation. Areas of concentration can include having the child focus on learning effective coping strategies for developmental age, learning appropriate means for expressing self and getting needs met, and beginning to identify own strengths as opposed to concentrating on weaknesses. For children experiencing anxiety, short-term outcomes can include steps such as the child staying with the sitter for two hours with minimal distress. For children needing help with social interactions, caregivers should be taught to gradually encourage small contributions from the child in social settings until the child is able to participate more fully. Focusing on and praising small, intermediate successes will increase the child's self-confidence while decreasing self-consciousness.

In inpatient units, outcomes need to be targeted to tasks that the child can achieve within the boundaries of the setting. To help reduce anxiety, for instance, an attachment object such as a favorite doll or blanket

(*Continues*)

APPLICATION OF THE NURSING PROCESS 23-1 (Continued)

can be offered to reduce fears about separation. To realize improved social interaction, the child can attend groups with the nurse and other children, where the nurse can facilitate and support the child's efforts to interact with others.

Identifying adaptive coping skills that the child can use in the face of anxiety is another important outcome. This can be achieved through practice via role play, which facilitates the use of adaptive behaviors in the face of stressful situations. Caregivers can to be taught to give positive reinforcement for appropriate, desired behaviors.

PLANNING/INTERVENTIONS

When working with children with emotional problems, the nurse may react as if the child were part of her family of origin or her current family. In this situation, the nurse needs help to identify personal experiences that limit her perception of the child. In working with the family, the nurse should avoid taking a critical position, but should attempt to establish a collaborative relationship in problem solving and intervention. The nurse's capacity for empathy is limited by reacting to the child and family from her own beliefs, values, and stereotypes. When working with families from different cultural backgrounds, the nurse must guard against imposing her own cultural assumptions about child rearing. When helping caregivers to alter their child-rearing behaviors, it is important to remember that these behaviors are usually based on the child-rearing practices that the caregivers experienced as children. Because their beliefs about child rearing tend to be based on long-standing experiences, simply teaching new approaches is not adequate. They need to talk about their reactions to these new ideas. Nurses may need help to deal with their feelings toward caregivers who seem to neglect or abuse or who are over coercive or over permissive with their children. However, in most cases, we need to remember that caregivers are doing the best job they can with their children. Additionally, they often describe feelings of guilt, anxiety, denial, and embarrassment when confronted with the decision to obtain psychiatric services for their child. Thus, support and understanding are essential to establishing a trusting relationship with the family.

Once the assessment has been completed and nursing diagnoses formulated, a plan of care is developed. Intervention is optimally aimed at two levels, the family and the child. The family members, especially the caregivers, need assistance in changing their responses to the child. The child needs to learn more-adaptive coping skills. A variety of treatment modalities exist that are effective in caring for a child with an emotional problem.

A continuum of options exists for managing behavior that is escalating or getting out of control. The least restrictive is teaching and encouraging acceptable ways for children to express themselves and to get their needs met. Then, procedures such as time-outs (quiet time spent alone in a nonstimulating environment) can be used if needed. As a last resort, holding and seclusion may be used. When behavior has been out of control, the child can be encouraged to review the situation in order to gain insight into what happened, why it happened, and how to avoid this loss of control in the future.

One of the most important nursing interventions to improve self-esteem is to help the child identify and promote his strengths rather than weaknesses. Caregivers need to identify methods they can use to help their child gain a more positive self-esteem, such as listening to their child, having realistic expectations, offering praise for accomplishments, and the like. The nurse can encourage the child to engage in activities in which he is likely to succeed and to focus on aspects of his life for which positive feelings exist.

PLAY THERAPY

Most younger children find it difficult to express themselves verbally. Their limited vocabularies restrict the ability to identify feelings and concerns. Play therapy is one of the most useful techniques for expressing feelings, exploring relationships, and attempting new solutions to problems. Play provides an opportunity for developing a therapeutic relationship between the nurse and child. Therapeutic play provides the

(Continues)

APPLICATION OF THE NURSING PROCESS 23-1 (Continued)

opportunity for hidden and threatening content to be presented. Play can serve additional functions. The child can learn basic skills and social skills, explore the environment, release excess energy, and imitate and acquire adult roles. Toys that are imaginative and age appropriate should be offered to the child, such as blocks, a play house, dolls that represent family members, trucks, cars, and soldiers. The child is urged to play without any directions from the nurse. The nurse should not guide the play or make interpretations that link the play to the child's life experiences.

INDIVIDUAL THERAPY

A child enters therapy with a different perspective than does an adult. Many adults enter therapy willingly because they realize they have problems for which they need help. Children tend not to see themselves as having problems; therefore, the need for therapy may not be recognized. Often the child believes that he has been forced into treatment against his will by his caregivers. The nurse is seen as having allied herself with the caregivers, so the child may distrust her also. In order to develop a trusting relationship with the child, the nurse needs to avoid taking sides. Communicating a sense of acceptance of the child separate from his unacceptable behavior is essential.

Another characteristic of children in therapy is that they often perceive the nurse as an all-powerful, all-knowing adult to whom they look for direction. Thus, the nurse becomes a powerful role model whose verbal and nonverbal behaviors must be consistent to gain the child's respect. Additionally, a child's cognitive level and language abilities necessitate the need to act out feelings and situations. The nurse must use methods that provide the vehicle for the safe acting out of feelings, such as role playing, games, and journals.

FAMILY THERAPY

Family therapy is an especially important treatment for children with psychiatric disorders. Child disorders cannot be fully understood without exploring the family context. Family therapy is based on the premise that the behavior of one person cannot be changed without bringing about change in the entire family. Studies have shown that treating the family system produces more rapid and enduring changes. For additional information on family therapy, refer to Chapter 28.

PSYCHOPHARMACOLOGY

Psychopharmacology is one aspect of a treatment program for children. The use of psychotropic medications in this population often arouses controversy about efficacy, side effects, and long-term impact on growth and development. Several issues are important to consider when discussing pediatric psychopharmacology. One issue is the risk-to-benefit ratio: The benefit to the child must outweigh the risks. The possibility of toxicity, the possibility of paradoxical reactions, and the possibility of adverse effects on the child's cognitive and social development must be considered when assessing the risks. Ideally, medication should either not impair learning or should improve a child's ability to benefit from learning experiences.

The fact that a child is growing and developing makes any period of less-than-optimal functioning of greater importance than in an adult. For an adult to be "zonked" for a few weeks due to medications is not good, but usually does not have grave implications. For a child, however, to be excessively sedated or socially unresponsive for a period of weeks or even months may have severe implications for the child's development. Another issue is that children, whose metabolic and neurological systems are still developing, react differently to medications than do adults. Dosages of medications for children should be based on research with children, rather than extrapolated from standard doses for adults. Unfortunately, such data are often not available. Finally, legal issues must be considered in the use of psychotropic medications. It is

(Continues)

APPLICATION OF THE NURSING PROCESS 23-1 (Continued)

important to have the informed consent and informed cooperation of both the child and caregivers in any medication trial. Caregivers often have extremely strong feelings about the use of psychoactive medications in their children; therefore, it is essential that they be well informed about the risks and benefits and about their right to accept or reject the recommendation for medication, and that they truly give informed consent. The child and caregivers should also have an opportunity to discuss their feelings about medications. It must be remembered that medication is not the sole treatment indicated. The complexity of emotional problems demands an integrated approach involving various therapies: psychodynamic (individual, family, or group), behavioral, milieu, medication, and resources in the family and school.

EVALUATION

Evaluation of the effectiveness of the interventions and care plan should include not only the child's progress toward achieving targeted outcomes but also the family unit's progress toward a more healthy, supportive, and interactive relationship with the child. Progress in many instances may be slow, requiring weeks or months or even years to realize, so it is important for the nurse to help the family view their successes in increments and to maintain realistic expectations of the outcomes they will see. It is also critical for the family and child to view together their successes and failures, so they can mutually agree on what tactics are most effective and those that should be changed.

NURSING CARE PLAN: NURSING PROCESS FORMAT 23-1

Jean, 10 years old, was admitted to a child and adolescent inpatient psychiatric unit. Her admission was part of a court evaluation for stealing cigarettes from a convenience store, her second infraction with the law in a year. Jean's caregivers divorced when she was 3 years old, after many years of conflict and fighting. Jean now lives with her mother and 6-year-old brother because her father, with whom she lived for the past 7 years, was sentenced to prison for robbery. She no longer attends public school, having been expelled for threatening her teacher with a knife, and smoking and drinking alcohol on school premises. Jean's mother reports that at home Jean frequently fights with her brother, has threatened him, and has stayed out all night for several nights at a time.

ASSESSMENT

Jean has had a continued pattern of antisocial behaviors, including violation of rules, theft, bullying, and aggression with a weapon toward others, and she lacks feelings of guilt or remorse. She has used tobacco and alcohol earlier than her peer group's expected age. Low self-esteem is manifested by a "tough girl" demeanor. Her level of academic achievement is low in relation to her age and IQ. She exhibits the following characteristics: poor impulse control, poor frustration tolerance, irritability, and frequent temper outbursts.

NURSING DIAGNOSIS 1 *Risk for self-directed violence* and *Risk for other-directed violence*, related to negative caregiver role models and dysfunctional family dynamics, as evidenced by poor impulse control.

(Continues)

NURSING CARE PLAN: NURSING PROCESS FORMAT 23-1 (Continued)

OUTCOMES	NIC	NURSING ACTIONS	EVALUATION
• Jean will not harm herself, others, or others' property. • Jean will learn to express anger appropriately.	• Behavior management • Anger control assistance	• Communicate expected behavior to Jean; state limits firmly; offer substitute behaviors. • Explain the consequences of unacceptable behaviors • Set limits that are not negotiable to ensure safety. • State the reasons for limits. • Give positive reinforcement for appropriate behaviors and observation of limits. • Ignore misbehavior every time it occurs. • Redirect violent behavior with physical outlets. • Use time-outs for unacceptable behaviors.	Many conduct-disordered clients are adept at becoming socialized to the milieu and may show rapid "improvement." Because of shortened hospital stays, it may be necessary to evaluate short-term goals as opposed to intermediate or long-term goals. Evaluation is made of the behavioral changes in the client. This is accomplished by determining if the goals of treatment have been achieved. Evaluate the following areas for improvement: prevention of harm to self, others, or others' property; ability to express anger in an appropriate manner; development of more adaptive coping strategies to deal with anger and feelings of aggression.

NURSING DIAGNOSIS 2 *Chronic low self-esteem*, related to lack of positive feedback and unsatisfactory caregiver/child relationship, as evidenced by "tough girl" demeanor, denial of problems, and projection of responsibility.

OUTCOMES	NIC	NURSING ACTIONS	EVALUATION
• Jean will demonstrate increased feelings of self-worth by verbalizing positive statements about self and exhibiting more appropriate, behaviors.	• Self-esteem enhancement	• Plan activities that allow for success. • Praise appropriate behaviors in front of others • Identify Jean's perceptions of any strengths or special qualities she values • Assist her in developing more effective social skills.	Evaluate the following for improvement: ability to verbalize positive statements about self; ability to interact with others without engaging in manipulation; less blaming of others.

NURSING DIAGNOSIS 3 *Ineffective coping*, related to maturational crises, as evidenced by use of manipulative behaviors to express emotions and to get needs met.

(*Continues*)

NURSING CARE PLAN: NURSING PROCESS FORMAT 23-1 (Continued)

OUTCOMES	NIC	NURSING ACTIONS	EVALUATION
• Jean will verbalize those behaviors that are self-defeating. • She will connect her manipulative behaviors to particular feelings or family situations. • She will ask directly for need needs to be met.	• Coping enhancement	• When observing manipulative behaviors, confront Jean with these behaviors. • Explore the self-defeating nature of these behaviors. • Explore what she accomplishes when using these behaviors, that is, the need to control her environment. • Explore ways to promote a more positive sense of control at home, at school, and with peers.	Evaluate progress by looking to Jean's new ability to accept responsibility for own behavior and her ability to accept feedback without becoming manipulative.

REFLECTIVE QUESTIONS

1. **ASSESSMENT**
   Do you think that interviewing Jean's teachers or peers might provide additional insight into her troubled behaviors? What environmental factors could you evaluate that might also affect her demeanor?
2. **NURSING DIAGNOSIS**
   What other nursing diagnoses are applicable to this case?
3. **OUTCOMES**
   Do you agree with the nurse's goals for Jean? What other goals would you select?
4. **NURSING ACTIONS**
   If the nursing actions directed toward managing Jean's aggressive and manipulative behaviors have been ineffective, what other interventions might be appropriate?
5. **EVALUATION**
   What behavioral changes do you think are realistic over a two-week period? One month? Six months? Should you include changes in caregiver attitudes when evaluating Jean's progress? How would you do this?

SCHOOLS AND SPECIAL-NEEDS CHILDREN

This chapter discusses only a small number of the disorders that interfere with children's normal physical, psychological, and emotional development. It is estimated that more than 5,000,000 American children have a disability, and most of these children need some sort of accommodation from schools to support their progress. The Individuals with Disabilities Education Act (IDEA) was passed in 1975 and sets requirements that public schools must follow in providing for handicapped children. According to IDEA, schools must provide each child, whatever his or her handicap, with an "appropriate" education that meets individual needs. Those needs may dictate a variety of services in varying amounts, restricted class size, and specific peer composition of the class. IDEA gives a variety of rights to parents and children: to have the child assessed, to examine the child's school records (at least under certain conditions), to attend school educational planning meetings, to participate in developing the child's educational plan, and to resolve any disputes through a specified legal process. The laws do not specify any explicit educational requirements for children with disabilities, nor do they state specifically that children with similar diagnoses need to be managed equivalently; all planning is supposed to be negotiated between parents and school—ideally with the individual child's best interests as the primary consideration. Central to IDEA is the Individual Educational Plan (IEP) that must be completed for each child and reviewed yearly. Parents participate actively in the three steps of the IEP process: the primary IEP eligibility meeting, the creation of an initial written educational plan for the child, and the yearly review of the IEP. Parents frequently come to IEP meetings with independent psychological or educational evaluations of their children, and they may seek help from other consultants, including attorneys specializing in this area of children's rights. Although the IEP process often moves smoothly with close cooperation between school and parents, there frequently may be significant differences between what schools, constrained by their budgets and staffing, are able to offer, and what parents perceive is required for their children's education. Sometimes these disputes are resolved by IEP-level negotiation, but at times they are resolved only by court action.

IDEA requires that a child's disability fall into one of the following categories:

- Mental retardation
- Hearing, speech, or language impairment
- Visual impairment
- Orthopedic impairment or traumatic brain injury
- Specific learning disability
- Autism
- Serious emotional disturbance

Under IDEA, emotional disturbances qualify for special education if they have been present for a significant time and cause learning impairment. In general, children can qualify under IDEA if emotional disturbance includes significant relationship problems (as in Asperger's syndrome or similar conditions), difficulties with behaviors or feelings (as with ODD or conduct disorders), pervasive unhappiness (as with mood disorders), or school-related physical symptoms or fears (as with separation anxiety or school phobia). In principle, most children with one of the conditions discussed in this chapter should be found eligible under the IEP process. ADHD has recently been explicitly included as a disability that qualifies a child under IDEA.

Establishing eligibility requires evidence that the condition has had an adverse impact on the child's school performance, an issue over which schools and parents may substantially disagree. Assessment begins with an IEP prepared by the school and presented to the parents. This IEP typically outlines the proposed assessment and describes what will be done and by whom. Parents are given the opportunity to approve and/or modify the assessment plan and then to meet with the individual responsible for the assessment. Assessments vary in their depth and content. Most will include some degree of formal psychological testing as well as teacher and parent reports. Some will include additional data such as pediatric or psychiatric evaluations (either arranged by the school or submitted by the parents). Parents may supplement these official assessments with other expert consultation, though school districts will rarely pay for these. Following the assessment, an IEP meeting is scheduled to assess eligibility and create an official IEP report that parents may either accept or reject.

The initial IEP process may go smoothly or may be a very difficult one for parents (and for the school). Assessments can reflect school budgetary constraints as well as the child's actual best interests. Parents' information or concerns may not be reflected in the final assessment, and parents may sometimes feel that they are treated bureaucratically by the IEP process. Parents are sometimes very upset at discovering that their child has a serious problem and may bring these emotions with them to the assessment process, complicating the school's interest in moving easily to an approved IEP plan.

Areas for disagreement between parents and schools may include any or all of the following:

- Does the child actually have a handicap?
- Does the child have a handicap that actually qualifies for special educational services under IDEA?
- Is the handicap accompanied by academic impairment?
- Are the proposed remedial plans enough to help the child?
- Will the proposed remedial plans expose the child to added physical or emotional risk—as from placement with violent or disturbed children in a special classroom?

For many parents the IEP process goes smoothly from beginning to end and provides their children with valuable special education. For others the process ends up in legal and administrative hearings that proceed slowly and often at considerable financial (and emotional) cost to the parents, who may be required to fund extensive alternative evaluations and seek expensive legal advice. Many parents benefit greatly from affiliating with parents' organizations whose members can often provide support and offer stories of successful (and unsuccessful) IEP efforts. Most of these organizations have a presence on the Internet:

- Family.com
- Federation for Children with Special Needs: Parent Training and Information Centers (PTI Centers are also located in each state.)
- National Information Center for Children and Youth with Disabilities
- National Parent Network on Disabilities
- Center for Law and Education
- Children and Adults with Attention Deficit Disorder (CHADD)
- Autism Society of America
- National Tourette Syndrome Association
- National Association of Psychiatric Treatment Centers for Children
- Federation of Families for Children's Mental Health

KEY CONCEPTS

- Some psychiatric disorders occur only in children; other adult psychiatric disorders occur in children, but are experienced by children differently than by adults.
- ADHD is the most common psychiatric disorder in children.
- Diagnosis of ADHD is done by matching the child's observed/reported behavior against DSM diagnostic criteria; there is no psychological test for ADHD.
- The role of dopamine and the role of genetics are complicated but are thought to contribute to the behaviors seen in ADHD.
- Psychoactive drugs, particularly stimulants, have been shown to be effective in managing the symptoms of ADHD.
- Only recently has depression in childhood been recognized and treated.
- Depressed children feel sad, lose interest in activities, criticize themselves, and eat poorly; they also may be irritable and exhibit hyperactivity.
- Bipolar Disorder, a disorder in which depression and manic episodes alternate, does occur in children.
- It is believed that depression in childhood has both biological and environmental determinants.
- Cognitive-behavioral therapy and drug treatment have been effective in treating childhood depression.
- No single anxiety disorder occurs as frequently in children as does ADHD, but collectively the prevalence of anxiety disorders is higher than that of other mental disorders.
- Anxiety disorders diagnosed frequently in children include: Separation Anxiety Disorder, Generalized Anxiety Disorder, Social Phobia Disorder, and Obsessive-Compulsive Disorder.
- Autism is a disorder in which children remain emotionally detached.
- Intensive, sustained special educational programs and behavior therapy in early life can be helpful in assisting the child with Autism to learn and to acquire language.
- Children with Asperger's syndrome share some of the characteristics of those with Autism, but are far less affected.
- Children with Asperger's syndrome have normal receptive and expressive language and may be very bright, but demonstrate a consistent inability to regulate social interactions and do not respond appropriately to verbal and nonverbal cues in interactions.
- Children with Oppositional Defiant Disorder reject adult authority; children with Conduct Disorder exhibit disruptive behaviors with aggression, bullying, and assaultive behavior.
- Children with disruptive disorders are treated with a combination of small classes, talented teaching, psychosocial methods (such as behavior shaping), and drugs.

REVIEW QUESTIONS

1. A nurse assigned to a behavioral unit for children with emotional problems should base nursing interventions on which of the following principles?
   1. Children should be praised and approval shown for desirable behaviors
   2. The nurse and staff should be very permissive
   3. Appropriate punishment should be initiated for bad behavior
   4. Children need consistency on the part of all staff members

2. A child is brought to a residential treatment facility by his mother who informs the nurse that the child was diagnosed as having Autism. Which of the following behaviors would the nurse anticipate assessing?
   1. Rocking, spinning, and poorly developed speech
   2. Enuresis, encopresis, apathy, and irritability
   3. Friendliness, sociable, and very attentive
   4. Angry, crying, and easily distracted

3. Health teaching for the parents of a child with ADHD who is prescribed Ritalin would include which of the following?
   1. The child's weight should be measured every week
   2. If the child misses a dose of methylphenidate (Ritalin), the next dose should be doubled
   3. The child should be placed on a low-sodium, high-caloric diet
   4. Punish the child if he breaks any rules at school or home

4. A child with ADHD is running around chasing the other children on the unit. The nurse's initial response would be to say which of the following?
   1. "Stop running right now."
   2. "If you don't stop I will give you a shot."
   3. "Why are you chasing those other children?"
   4. Aren't you tired? I think you need a nap."

5. A five-year-old child diagnosed with ADHD is placed on methylphenidate (Ritalin). The mother asks, "Are there any side effects of this medication?" The nurse would be accurate in responding with which of the following?
   1. There are no side effects from Ritalin
   2. The side effects are not important; your child needs the medication
   3. Common side effects of Ritalin include: insomnia, decreased appetite, and headaches
   4. Common side effects of Ritalin include: nausea, vomiting, and elevated temperature
6. The nurse working in a mental health facility for children would understand that which of the following is the most common mood disorder in children?
   1. Dysthymia
   2. Reactive Depression
   3. Major Depression
   4. Bipolar Disorder

LEARNING ACTIVITIES

1. Describe how a child's experience of depression or anxiety might be different than that of an adult.
2. Consider how a family would alter its patterns to accommodate a child with ADHD, and describe the changes in family processes.
3. How would a child with ADHD be treated in your neighborhood school? Consider the role of the school nurse in treatment and management of ADHD children. If you can, interview a school nurse on this subject.
4. Describe the behaviors of a child with OCD, and evaluate how this might be different from an adult.
5. How would you approach a child at an acute care hospital who was having separation anxiety?
6. What would be an appropriate approach at a youth camp for a child with social phobia?
7. Describe the similarities and differences between Autism and Asperger's syndrome.
8. What are the roles of parents, teachers, and society at large in treating children with disruptive disorders?
9. What are the primary nursing roles in child mental health?

*Study*WARE™ CONNECTION

Using your *Study*WARE™ CD-ROM

1. Complete the Flashcard activity for this chapter.
2. Review the audio glossary for key terms in this chapter.
3. Explore the other games and activities that support this chapter.

VIDEO LINK

Attention-Deficit/Hyperactivity Disorder

Read and contemplate the questions below about Shawn, the client experiencing Attention Deficit Hyperactivity Disorder. Then watch the video "Attention Deficit Hyperactivity Disorder" on your *Study*WARE™ CD-ROM to observe Shawn's interview with a psychiatrist. Consider these questions prior to listening to the psychiatrist's analysis.

1. How does the researcher who is commentating describe ADHD?
2. Define ADHD as per the criteria in the DSM-IV-TR.
3. How many of these symptoms are required to make a diagnosis?
4. What are the two subtypes of ADHD? What type does Shawn have?
5. By what age must these symptoms be present?
6. How does Shawn's mother describe his behavior?
7. Were his schools equipped to deal with this diagnosis?
8. What is the concern with a bright child being diagnosed with ADHD?
9. What was Shawn's relationship with his peers?
10. What change occurred when Shawn started at UCI?
11. What behavioral treatment worked especially well?
12. Describe the pharmacological treatment of ADHD.
13. Describe Shawn's pharmacological treatment. What were the challenging side effects?
14. How does genetics play a role in ADHD?

15. What is the "dopamine hypotheses"?
16. Describe "executive function" and the neuroanatomy in ADHD.
17. Do food additives play a role?
18. What are the effects of tobacco?
19. How did Shawn's mother describe the combination therapy of psychosocial behavioral treatment and pharmacological treatment?
20. What is the prognosis of ADHD as children age into adulthood?
21. Consider the family implications.

Autism

View the video on Autism located on your *Study*WARE™ CD, and answer the following questions.

1. What are the two main areas of research in Autism and what do they reveal?
2. What is the prevalence of Autism in children?
3. How is it characterized?
4. How does the child in this clip reveal such symptoms?
5. Are autistic children self-aware?
6. Describe the "theory of mind."
7. Describe the behavioral work they are doing with the child in this DVD.
8. What pharmacological treatments are being used?
9. What are the concerns with regard to the side effects of these medications?
10. Do autistic children respond to physical illnesses?
11. What is significant about the head growth of autistic children?
12. What community supports are available for families with children experiencing Autism?

REFERENCES

American Psychiatric Association. (2000). *Diagnostic and statistical manual of mental disorders* (Fourth Edition-Text Revision). Washington, DC: Author.

Anderson, J. C., Williams, S., McGee, R., & Silva P. A. (1987). DSM-III disorders in preadolescent children: Prevalence in a large sample from the general population. *Archives of General Psychiatry, 44*(1), 69–76.

Anney, R. J., Lasky-Su, J., O'Dushlaine, C., Kenny, E., Neale, B. M., Mulligan, A., et al. (2008). Conduct disorder and ADHD: Evaluation of conduct problems as a categorical and quantitative trait in the international multicentre ADHD genetics study. *American Journal of Medical Genetics B Neuropsychiatry and Genetics. 147B*(8), 1369–1378

Barkley, R. A. (1998). Attention-deficit hyperactivity disorder. *Scientific American, 279*(3), 66–71.

Barrett, P. M., Dadds, M. R., & Rapee, R. M. (1996). Family treatment of childhood anxiety: A controlled trial. *Journal of Consulting and Clinical Psychology, 64*, 333–342.

Biederman, J., Wilens, T., Mick, E., Spencer, T., & Faraone, S. V. (1999). Pharmacotherapy of attention deficit/hyperactivity disorder reduces risk for substance use disorder. *Pediatrics, 104*, e20.

Birmaher, B., Ryan, N. D., Williamson, D. E., Brent, D. A., & Kaufman, J. (1996). Childhood and adolescent depression: A review of the past 10 years. Part II. *Journal of the American Academy of Child and Adolescent Psychiatry, 35*, 1575–1583.

Birmaher, B., Ryan, N. D., Williamson, D. E., Brent, D. A., Kaufman, J., Dahl, R. E., et al. (1996). Childhood and adolescent depression: A review of the past 10 years. Part I. *Journal of the American Academy of Child and Adolescent Psychiatry, 35*, 1427–1439.

Brestan, E. V., & Eyberg, S. M. (1998). Effective psychosocial treatments of conduct-disordered children and adolescents: 29 years, 82 studies, and 5,272 kids. *Journal of Clinical Child Psychology, 27*, 180–189.

Braun, J. M., Froehlick, T. E., Daniels, J., Dietrick, K. N., Hornung, R., Auinger, P., & Lanphear, B.P. (2008). Association of environmental toxicants and conduct disorder in U.S. children. *Environmental health Perspectives, 116*(7), 956–962.

Bryson, S. E., & Smith, I. M. (1998). Epidemiology of autism: Prevalence, associated characteristics, and service delivery. *Mental Retardation and Developmental Disabilities Research Reviews, 4*, 97–103.

Bumbalo, J. A., & Siemon, M. K. (1983). Nursing assessment and diagnosis: Mental health problems of children. *Topics in Clinical Nursing, 5*(1), 41–54.

Campbell, M., & Cueva, J. E. (1995). Psychopharmacology in child and adolescent psychiatry: A review of the past seven years. Part II. *Journal of the American Academy of Child and Adolescent Psychiatry, 34*, 1262–1272.

Chang, K. D. (2008). The use of atypical antipsychotics in pediatric bipolar disorder. *Journal of Clinical Psychiatry, 69*(Suppl. 4), 4–8.

Cook, E. H., Jr. (1998). Genetics of autism. *Mental Retardation and Developmental Disabilities Research Reviews, 4*, 113–120.

Cormier, E. (2008). Attention deficit/hyperactivity disorder: A review and update. *Journal of Pediatric Nursing, 23*(5), 345–357.

Costello, E. J., Angold, A., Burns, B. J., Stangl, D. K., Tweed, D. L., Erkanli, A., et al., (1996). The Great Smoky Mountains Study of Youth: Goals, design, methods, and the prevalence of DSM-III-R disorders. *Archives of General Psychiatry, 53*, 1129–1136.

Daly, B. P., Creed, T., Xanthopoulos, M., & Brown, R. T. (2007). Psychosocial treatments for children with attention deficit/hyperactivity disorder. *Neuropsychiatry Review, 17*, 73–89.

Davis, N. (2005). Depression and Children and Adolescents. *Journal of School Nursing, 21*(5), 311–317.

DeVeaugh-Geiss, J., Moroz, G., Biederman, J., Cantwell, D., Fontaine, R., Greist, J. H., et al., (1992). Clomipramine hydrochloride childhood and adolescent obsessive-compulsive disorder: A multicenter trial. *Journal of the Academy of Child and Adolescent Psychiatry, 31*, 45–49.

Eisenberg, L. (1996). Commentary. What should doctors do in the face of negative evidence? *Journal of Nervous and Mental Disease, 184*, 103–105.

Elia, J. (1991). Stimulants and antidepressant pharmokinetics in hyperactive children. *Psychopharmacology Bulletin, 27*, 411–415.

Ellison-Wright, I., Ellison-Wright, Z., & Bullmore, E. (2008). Structural brain change in Attention Deficit Hyperactivity Disorder identified by meta-analysis. *BMC Psychiatry, 8*, 51.

Emslie, G. J., Weinberg, W. A., Kowatch, R. A., Hughes, C. W., Carmody, T. J., & Rush, A. J. (1997). Fluoxetine treatment of depressed children and adolescents. *Archives of General Psychiatry, 54*, 1031–1037.

Esser, G., Schmidt, M. H., & Woerner, W. (1990). Epidemiology and course of psychiatric disorders in school-age children—results of a longitudinal study. *Journal of Child Psychology Psychiatry, 31*(2), 243–263.

Faraone, S. V., & Doyle, A. E. (2000). Genetic influences on attention deficit hyperactivity disorder. *Current Psychiatry Report, 2*(2), 143–146.

Flament, M. F., Rapoport, J. L., Berg, C. J., Sceery, W., Kilts, C., Mellstrom, B., et al., (1985). Clomipramine treatment of childhood obsessive-compulsive disorder: A double-blind controlled study. *Archives of General Psychiatry, 42*, 977–983.

Gadow, K. D., Sverd, J., Sprafkin, J., Nolan, E. E., & Grossman, S. (1999). Long-term methylphenidate therapy in children with comorbid attention-deficit disorder and chronic multiple tic disorder. *Archives of General Psychiatry, 56*, 330–336.

Geller, B., & Luby, J. (1997). Child and adolescent bipolar disorder: A review of the past 10 years. *Journal of the American Academy of Child and Adolescent Psychiatry, 36*, 1168–1176.

Geller, D. A. (2006). Obsessive-compulsive and spectrum disorders in children and adolescents. *Psychiatric Clinics of North America, 29*(2), 353–370.

Gibson, A. P., Bettinger, T. L., Patel, N. C., & Crismon, M. L. (2006). Atomoxetine versus stimulants for treatment of attention deficit/hyperactivity disorder. *Annals of Pharmacotherapeutics, 40*(6), 1134–1142.

Gilbert, A. R., & Maalouf, F. T. (2008). Pediatric obsessive-compulsive disorder: Management priorities in primary care. *Current Opinions in Pediatrics, 20*(5), 544–550.

Goenjian, A. K., Pynoos, R. S., Steinberg, A. M., Najarian, L. M., Asarnow, J. R., Karayan, I., et al., (1995). Psychiatric comorbidity in children after the 1988 earthquake in Armenia. *Journal of the American Academy of Child and Adolescent Psychiatry, 34*, 1174–1184.

Goodwin, F., & Jamison, K. (1990). *Manic-depressive illness*. London/New York: Oxford University Press.

Gordon, C. T., State, R. C., Nelson, J. E., Hamburger, S. D., & Rapoport, J. L. (1993). A double-blind comparison of clomipramine, desipramine, and placebo in the treatment of autistic disorder. *Archives of General Psychiatry, 50*, 441–447.

Grachev, I. D., Breiter, H. C., Rauch, S. L., Savage, C. R., Baer, L., Shera, D. M., et al., (1998). Structural abnormalities of frontal neocortex in obsessive-compulsive disorder [Letter]. *Archives of General Psychiatry, 55*, 181–182.

Haddon, M. (2003). *The curious incident of a dog in the night-time*. Doubleday New York:.

Hamilton, S. S., & Armando, J. (2008). Oppositional defiant disorder. *American Family Physician, 78*(7), 861–866.

Hayward, C., Varady, S., Albano, A. M., Thienemann, M., Henderson, L., & Schatzberg, A. (2000). Cognitive behavioral therapy for social phobia in female adolescents: Results of a pilot study. *Journal of the American Academy of Child and Adolescent Psychiatry, 39*(6), 721–726.

Hazell, P. (2002). Depression in children and adolescents. *Clinical Evidence, 9*, 356–366.

Herskovits, E. H., Megalooikonomou, V., Davatzikos, C., Chen, A., Bryan, R. N., & Gerring, J. P. (1999). Is the spatial distribution of brain lesions associated with closed-head injury predictive of subsequent development of attention-deficit/hyperactivity disorder? Analysis with brain-image database. *Radiology, 213*(2), 389–394.

Hops, H., Lewinsohn, P. M., Andrews, J. A., & Roberts, R. E. (1990). Psychosocial correlates of depressive symptomatology among high school students. *Journal of Clinical and Child Psychology, 19*, 211–220.

Hughes, J. R. (2007). Autism: The first firm finding = underconnectivity? *Epilepsy & Behavior, 11*(1), 20–24.

Johnson, D. L., & Breckenridge, J. N. (1982). The Houston Parent-Child Development Center and the primary prevention of behavior problems in young children. *American Journal of Community Psychology, 10*, 305–316.

Kafantaris, V., Campbell, M., Padron-Gayol, M. V., Small, A. M., Locascio, J. J., & Rosenberg, C. R. (1992). Carbamazepine in hospitalized aggressive conduct disorder children: An open pilot study. *Psychopharmacology Bulletin, 28*, 193–199.

Kaiser, N. M., Hoza, B., & Hurt, E. A. (2008). Multimodal treatment for childhood attention-deficit/hyperactivity disorder. *Expert Reviews in Neurotherapeutics, 8*(10), 1573–1583.

Kapornai, K., & Vetro, A. (2008). Depression in children. *Current Opinion in Psychiatry, 21*(91), 1–7.

Kaslow, N. J., & Thompson, M. P. (1998). Applying the criteria for empirically supported treatments to studies of psychosocial interventions for child and adolescent depression. *Journal of Clinical Child Psychology, 27*, 146–155.

Kemph, J. P., DeVane, C. L., Levin, G. M., Jarecke, R., & Miller, R. L. (1993). Treatment of aggressive children with clonidine: Results of an open pilot study. *Journal of the American Academy of Child and Adolescent Psychiatry, 32*, 577–581.

Kendall, P. C., Chansky, T. E., Kane, M. T., Kim, R., Kortlander, E., Ronan, K. R., et al., (1992). Anxiety disorders in youth: Cognitive-behavioral interventions. Needham Heights, MA: Allyn & Bacon.

Kendall, P. C., Flannery-Schroeder, E., Panichelli-Mindel, S. M., Southam-Gerow, M., Henin, A., & Warman, M. (1997). Therapy for youths with anxiety disorders: A second randomized clinical trial. *Journal of Consulting and Clinical Psychology, 65*, 366–380.

Kessler, R. C., Amminger, G. P., Aguilar-Gaxiola, S., Alonso, J., Lee, S., & Ustun, T. B. (2007). Age of onset of mental disorders: A review of recent literature. *Current Opinions in Psychiatry, 20*(4), 359–364.

Kessler, R. C., & Wang, P. S. (2008). The descriptive epidemiology of commonly occurring mental disorders in the United States. *Annual Review of Public Health, 29*, 115–129.

Klein, R. G., Abikoff, H., Klass, E., Ganeles, D., Seese, L. M., & Pollack, S. (1997). Clinical efficacy of methylphenidate in conduct disorder with and without attention deficit hyperactivity disorder. *Archives of General Psychiatry, 54*, 1073–1080.

Kolvin, I., Barrett, M. L., Bhate, S. R., Berney, T. P., Fumuyiwa, O. O., Fundudis, T., et al., (1991). *British Journal of Psychiatry* (Suppl.), 9–21.

Kowatch, R. A., Suppes, T., Carmody, T. J., Bucci, J. P., Hum, J. H., Kromelis, M., et al. (2000). Effect size of lithium, divalproex sodium, and carbamazepine in children and adolescents with bipolar disorder. *Journal of the American Academy of Child and Adolescent Psychiatry, 39*(6), 713–720.

Kutcher, S. (1998). Affective disorders in children and adolescents: A critical clinically relevant review. In B. T. Walsh (Ed.), *Child psychopharmacology* (pp. 91–109). Washington, DC: American Psychiatric Association Press.

Lasky-Su, J., Neale, B. M., Franke, B., Anney, R. J., Zhou, K., Maller, J. B., et al. (2008). Genome-wide association scan of quantitative traits for attention deficit hyperactivity disorder identifies novel associations and confirms candidate gene associations. *American Journal of Medical Genetics Part B: Neuropsychiatry and Genetics. 147B*(8):1337–1344.

Lenane, M. C., Swedo, S. E., Leonard, H., Pauls, D. L., Sceery, W., & Rapoport, J. L. (1990). Psychiatric disorders in first degree relatives of children and adolescents with obsessive-compulsive disorder. *Journal of the American Academy of Child and Adolescent Psychiatry*, 29, 407–412.

Leonard, H. L., Rapoport, J. L., & Swedo, S. E. (1997). Obsessive-compulsive disorder. In J. M. Weiner (Ed.), *Textbook of child and adolescent psychiatry* (2nd ed., pp. 481–490). Washington, DC: American Academy of Child and Adolescent Psychiatry, American Psychiatric Press.

Leung, A. K., & Lemay, J. F. (2003). Attention deficit hyperactivity disorder: An update. *Advances in Therapy*, 20(6) 305–318.

Levin, H., Hanten, G., Max, J., Li, X., Swank, P., Ewing-Cobbs, L., et al. (2007). Symptoms of attention-deficit/hyperactivity disorder following traumatic brain injury in children. *Journal of Developmental and Behavioral Pediatrics*, *28*(2), 108–118.

Loeber, R., & Stouthamer-Loeber, M. (1986). Family factors as correlates and predictors of juvenile conduct problems and delinquency. In M. Tonry & N. Morris (Eds.), *Crime and justice* (Vol. 7). Chicago: University of Chicago Press.

Luckenbaugh, D. A., Findling, R. L., Leverich, G. S., Pizzarello, S. M., Post, R. M. (2009) Earliest symptoms discriminating juvenile-onset bipolar illness from ADHD. *Bipolar Disorders*, *11*(4), 441–451.

McDougle, C. J., Naylor, S. T., Cohen, D. J., Volkmar, F. R., Heninger, G. R., & Price, L. H. (1996). A double-blind, placebo-controlled study of fluvoxamine in adults with autistic disorder. *Archives of General Psychiatry*, 53, 1001–1008.

Melnyk, B. M., Foinstein, N. F., Tuttle, J., Moldenhauer, Z., Herendeen, P., Veenema, T. G., et al., (2002). Mental health worries, communication, and needs in the year of the U.S. terrorist attack: National KySS survey findings. *Journal of Pediatric Health Care*, *16*(4), 222–234.

Milberger, S., Biederman, J., Faraone, S. V., & Jones, J. (1998). Further evidence of an association between maternal smoking during pregnancy and attention deficit hyperactivity disorder: Findings from a high-risk sample of siblings. *Journal of Clinical Child Psychology*, 27(3), 352–358.

Minshew, N. J., & Williams, D. L. (2007). The new neurobiology of autism: Cortex, connectivity, and neuronal organization. *Archives of Neurology*, *64*(7), 945–950.

Monuteaux, M. C., Faraone, S. V., Hammerness, P., Wilens, T. E., Fraire, M., & Biederman, J. (2008). The familial association between cigarette smoking and ADHD: A study of clinically referred girls with and without ADHD, and their families. *Nicotine and Tobacco Research*, *10*(10), 1549–1558.

Morgan, A. E., Singer-Harris, N., Bernstein, J. H., & Waber, D. P. (2000). Characteristics for children referred for evaluation of school difficulties who have adequate achievement scores. *Journal of Learning Difficulties*, *33*(5), 489–501.

MTA Cooperative Group. (2004a). National Institute of Mental Health Multimodal Treatment Study of ADHD follow-up: 24-month outcomes of treatment strategies for attention-deficit/hyperactivity disorder. *Pediatrics*, *113*(4), 754–761.

MTA Cooperative Group. (2004b). National Institute of Mental Health Multimodal Treatment Study of ADHD follow-up: Changes in effectiveness and growth after the end of treatment. *Pediatrics*, *113*(4), 762–769.

Muñoz-Solomando, A., Kendall, T., & Whittington, C. J. (2008). Cognitive behavioural therapy for children and adolescents. *Current Opinions in Psychiatry*, *21*(4), 332–337.

Murphy, T. K., Sajid, M. W., & Goodman, W. K. (2006). Immunology of obsessive-compulsive disorder. *Psychiatric Clinics of North America*, *29*(2), 445–469.

Myers, S. M., Johnson, C. P; The American Academy of Pediatrics Council on Children With Disabilities. (2007). Management of children with autism spectrum disorders. *Pediatrics*, *120*(5), 1162–1182.

Neff, N. A., & Dale, J. (1996). Worries of school-age children. *Journal of the Society of Pediatric Nurses*, *1*(1), 27–32.

NIMH, (2009) Suicide in the U.S. Statistics and Prevention. http://www.nimh.nih.gov/health/publications/suicide-in-the-us-statistics-and-prevention/index.shtml#children, Retrieved August 13, 2009.

Nolen-Hoeksema, S., Morrow, J., & Fredrickson, B. L. (1993). Response styles and the duration of episodes of depressed mood. *Journal of Abnormal Psychology*, 102, 20–28.

Olfson, M., Marcus, S. C., & Druss, B. G. (2008). Effects of Food and Drug Administration warnings on antidepressant use in a national sample. *Archives of General Psychiatry*, *65*(1), 94–101.

Ollendick, T. H., & King, N. J. (1998). Empirically supported treatments for children with phobic and anxiety disorders: Current status. *Journal of Clinical Child Psychology*, *27*, 156–167.

Perry, R., Campbell, M., Adams, P., Lynch, N., Spencer, E. K., Curren, E. L., et al., (1989). Long-term efficacy of haloperidol in autistic children: Continuous versus discontinuous drug administration. *Journal of the American Academy of Child and Adolescent Psychiatry*, 28, 87–92.

Piven, J. (1997). The biological basis of autism. *Current Opinions in Neurobiology*, 7, 708–712.

Posey, D. J., & McDougle, C. J. (2007). Guanfacine and guanfacine extended release: Treatment for ADHD and related disorders. *CNS Drug Reviews*, *13*(4), 465–474.

Potter, A. S., & Newhouse, P. A. (2004). Effects of acute nicotine administration on behavioral inhibition in adolescents with attention-deficit/hyperactivity disorder. *Psychopharmacology* (E-pub ahead of print) April 9.

Rabe-Jablonska J. (2000). Therapeutic effects and tolerability of fluvoxamine treatment in adolescents with dysthymia. *Child and Adolescent Psychopharmacology*, 10, 9–18.

Raine, A., Reynolds, C., Venables, P. H., Mednick, S. A., & Farrington, D. P. (1998). Fearlessness, stimulation-seeking, and large body size at age 3 years as early predispositions to childhood aggression at age 11 years. *Archives of General Psychiatry*, 55, 745–751.

Rapin, I., & Katzman, R. (1998). Neurobiology of autism. *Annals of Neurology*, 43, 7–14.

Rapin, I., & Tuchman, R. F. (2008). Autism: Definition, neurobiology, screening, diagnosis. *Pediatric Clinics of North America*, *55*(5), 1129–1146.

Rapoport, J. L., Inoff-Germain, G., Weissman, M. M., Greenwald, S., Narrow, W. E., Jensen, P. S., et al. (2000) Childhood obsessive-compulsive disorder in the NIMH MECA study: Parent versus child identification of cases. Methods for the Epidemiology of child and adolescent mental disorders. *Journal of Anxiety Disorders*, *14*(6), 535–48.

Rauch, S. L., & Savage, C. R. (1997). Neuroimaging and neuropsychology of the striatum. Bridging basic science and clinical practice. *Psychiatric Clinics of North America*, 20, 741–768.

Reinblatt, S. P., & Riddle, M. A. (2007). The pharmacological management of childhood anxiety disorders: A review. *Psychopharmacology (Berlin)*, *191*(1), 67–86.

Sampson, R. J., & Laub, J. H. (1993). *Crime in the making: Pathways and turning points through life*. Cambridge, MA: Harvard University Press.

Sanchez, L., Campbell, M., Small, A., Cueva, J., Armenteros, J., & Adams, A. (1996). A pilot study of clomipramine in young autistic children. *Journal of the American Academy of Child and Adolescent Psychiatry*, 35(4), 537–544.

Scahill, L., & Schwab-Stone, M. (2000). Epidemiology of ADHD in school-age children. *Child and Adolescent Psychiatric Clinics of North America 2000*, *9*(3), 541–555, vii.

Shaywitz, B. A., Fletcher, J. M., Shaywitz, S. E. (2001). Attention deficit hyperactivity disorder. *Current Treatment Options in Neurology*, 3, 229–236.

Simeon, J., Milin, R., & Walker, S. (2002). A retrospective chart review of risperidone use in treatment-resistant children and adolescents with psychiatric disorders. *Progress in Neuropsychopharmacological and Biological Psychiatry, 26*(2), 267–275.

Spencer, T., Biederman, J., & Wilens, T. (1998). Growth deficits in children with attention deficit disorder. *Pediatrics, 102,* 501–506.

Strober, M., DeAntonio, M., Schmidt-Lackner, S., Pataki, C., Freeman, R., Rigali, J., et al., (1999). The pharmacotherapy of depressive illness in adolescents: An open-label comparison of fluoxetine with imipramine-treated historical controls. *Journal of Clinical Psychiatry, 60*(3), 164–169.

Swanson, J., Posne, M., Fusella, J., Wasdell, M., Sommer, T., & Fan, J. (2001). Genes and attention deficit hyperactivity disorder. *Current Psychiatry Report, 3*(2), 92–100.

Swedo, S. E., Pleeter, J. D., Richter, D. M., Hoffman, C. L., Allen, A. J., Hamburger, S. D., et al. (1995). Rates of seasonal affective disorder in children and adolescents. *American Journal of Psychiatry, 152,* 1016–1019.

Trifiletti, R. R., & Packard, A. M. (1999). Immune mechanisms in pediatric neuropsychiatric disorders: Tourette's syndrome, OCD, and PANDAS. *Child and Adolescent Psychiatric Clinics of North America,* 8, 767–775.

Tsapakis, E. M., Soldani, F., Tondo, L., & Baldessarini, R. J. (2008). Efficacy of antidepressants in juvenile depression: Meta-analysis. *British Journal of Psychiatry, 193*(1), 10–17.

Turgay, A. (2005). Treatment of comorbidity in conduct disorder with attention-deficit hyperactivity disorder (ADHD). *Essential Psychopharmacology, 6*(5), 277–290.

Upadhyaya, H. P. (2008). Substance use disorders in children and adolescents with attention-deficit/hyperactivity disorder: Implications for treatment and the role of the primary care physician. *Primary Care Companion to the Journal of Clinical Psychiatry, 10*(3), 211–221.

Vedantam, S., (2004). Child antidepressant warning is urged. *Washington Post,* September 15, 2004, p. A02. Retrieved January 12, 2005 form http:www.washington post.com/wp-dyn/articles/A21780-2004Sep14,html.

Waldman, I. D., Rowe, D. C., Abramowitz, A., Kozel, S. T., Mohr, J. H., Sherman, S. L., et al., (1998). Association and linkage of the dopamine transporter gene and attention-deficit hyperactivity disorder in children: Heterogeneity owing to diagnostic subtype and severity. *American Journal of Human Genetics, 63*(6), 1767–1776.

Walkup, J. T., Albano, A. M., Piacentini, J., Birmaher, B., Compton, S. N., Sherrill, J. T., et al. (2008). Cognitive Behavioral Therapy, Sertraline, or a Combination in Childhood Anxiety. *New England Journal of Medicine, 359*(26), 2753–2766.

Wallace, G. L., & Treffert, D. A. (2004). Head size and autism. *Lancet, 363,* 1003–1004.

Waslick, B. D., Walsh, B. T., Greenhill, L. L., Eilenberg, M., Capasso, L., & Lieber, D. (1999). Open trial of fluoxetine in children and adolescents with dysthymic disorder or double depression. *Journal of Affective Disorders, 56,* 117–136.

Weiner, J. M. (1997). Oppositional defiant disorder. In J. M. Weiner (Ed.), *Textbook of child and adolescent psychiatry* (2nd ed., pp. 459–463). Washington, DC: American Academy of Child and Adolescent Psychiatry, American Psychiatric Press.

Weisler, R. H. (2007). Emerging drugs for attention-deficit/hyperactivity disorder. *Expert Opinions on Emerging Drugs, 12*(3), 423–434.

Weiss, B., & Landrigan, P. J. (2000). The developing brain and the environment: An introduction. *Environmental Health Perspective, 108*(Suppl. 3), 373–374.

Whittington, C. J., Kendall, T., Fonagy, P., Cottrell, D., Cotgrove, A., & Buddington, E. (2004). Selective serotonin reuptake inhibitors in childhood depression: Systematic review of published versus unpublished reports. *Lancet 363*(9418), 1341–1345.

Wolf, D. V., & Wagner, K. D. (2003). Bipolar disorder in children and adolescents. *CNS Spectrums, 8*(12), 954–959.

Wolraich, M. L., Hannah, J. N., Pinnock, T. Y., Baumgaertel, A., & Brown, J. (1996). Comparison of diagnostic criteria for attention-deficit hyperactivity disorder in a county-wide sample. *Journal of the American Academy of Child and Adolescent Psychiatry, 35*(3), 319–324.

Yeargin-Allsopp, M., Rice, C., Karapurkar, T., Doernberg, N., Boyle, C., & Murphy, C. (2003). Prevalence of Autism in a U.S. Metropolitan Area. *Journal of the American Medical Association, 289,* 49–55.

Zilbovicius, M., Garreau, B., Samson, Y., Remy, P., Barthelemy, C., Syrota, A., et al. (1995). Delayed maturation of the frontal cortex in childhood autism. *American Journal of Psychiatry, 152,* 248–252.

SUGGESTED READINGS

Hadden, M. (2003). *The curious incident of a dog in the night-time.* New York: Doubleday.

James L. (2008). *Tigger on the couch: The neuroses, psychoses, disorders and maladies of our favourite children's characters.* Glasgow: Harper Collins.

Jensen, P., & Hoagland, K. (2008). *Improving children's mental health through parent empowerment: A guide to assisting families.* New York: Oxford University Press.

Storch, E. A., & Elder, J. H. (2009). Introduction to the special series on child and adolescent mental health. *Journal of Pediatric Nursing, 24*(1), 1–2.

LITERARY REFERENCES

Freeman, S. (1997). *The cuckoo's child.* New York: Hyperion Paperbacks for Children.

Schnurr, R. G. (2000). *Asperger's huh? A child's perspective.* Gloucester, Ontario, Canada: Anisor Publishing.

Senior, O. (1986). *Summer lightening and other stories.* Essex, England: Longman Group Limited.

Williams, D. (1992). *Nobody nowhere.* New York: Avon Books.

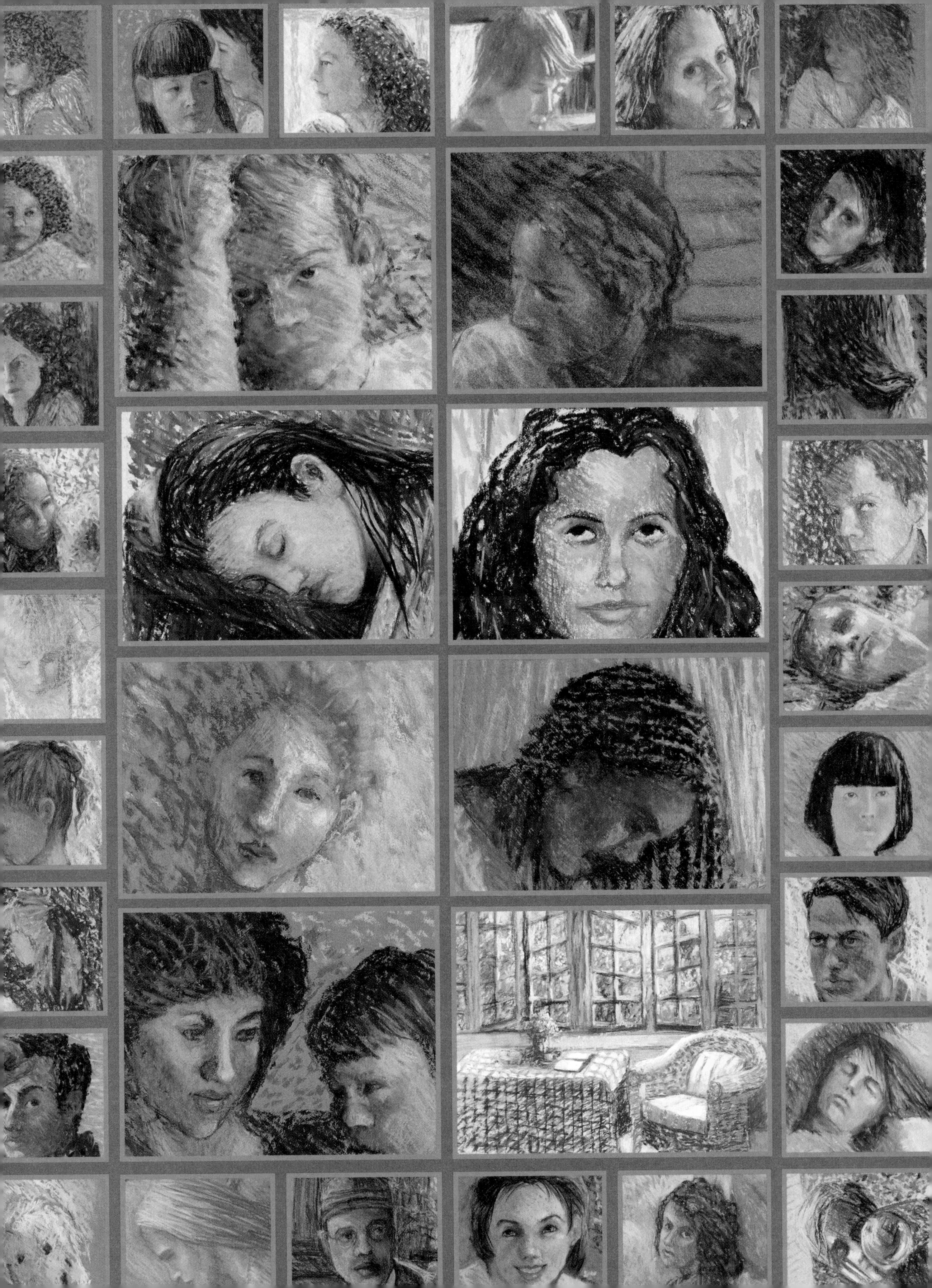

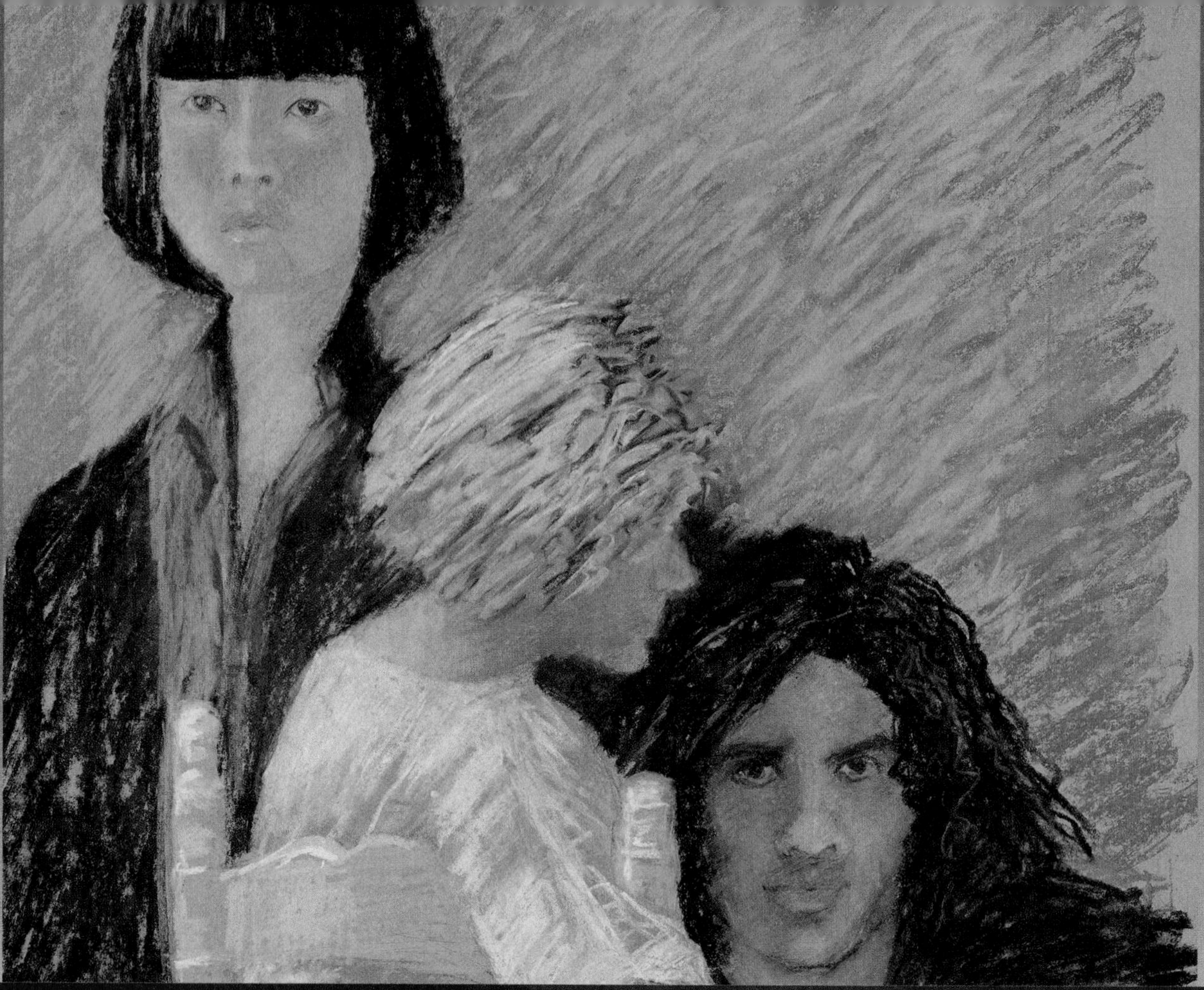

One for All and All for One

Transitions in Adolescence

Remember your own transition from childhood to adulthood:

- ***What were the significant changes you experienced?***
- ***What emotions did you experience with these changes?***
- ***How did your friends and family members respond to these changes?***
- ***How did this transition affect your sense of personal identity?***
- ***How did this transition affect your sense of competence and responsibility as an adult?***

Keep these experiences in mind as you read this chapter.

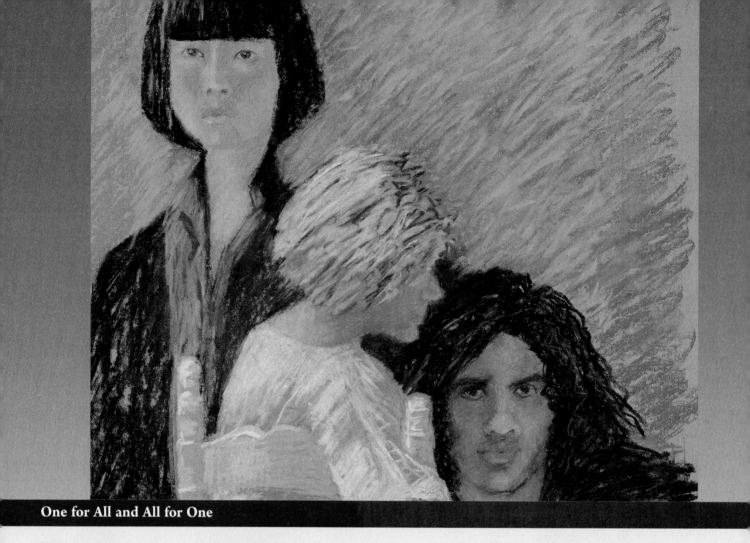

CHAPTER 24

The Adolescent

LYNN REW

CHAPTER OUTLINE

COMPETENCIES

Upon completion of this chapter, the reader should be able to:

1. Differentiate various definitions of adolescent mental health.
2. Identify the physical, cognitive, emotional, and social transitions of adolescence.
3. Examine concepts and theories about identity formation and social competence.
4. Reflect on your own sense of personal identity and social competence.
5. Identify major mental health needs and concerns of adolescents.
6. Apply the nursing process to the care of adolescent clients.
7. Integrate nursing theories into planning care for the adolescent in need of mental health services.

KEY TERMS

Foreclosure
Gender Identity
Gender Role
Identity Achievement
Identity Diffusion
Identity Formation
Identity Status
Moratorium
Presence
Self-Awareness
Self-Efficacy
Sexual Orientation
Social Competence
Suicidal Ideation
Transgender

Adolescence, the period of transition from childhood to adulthood, is a decade filled with profound and often confusing changes. Dramatic physical and psychological development is typically accompanied by cognitive, emotional, and social changes; decreasing levels of adult supervision; increasing experimentation with adult behaviors and responsibilities; and changes in the social milieu of school and work. All of these can upset an individual's sense of identity and social competence. The purposes of this chapter are threefold: (1) to identify various ways to define mental health during the developmental phase of adolescence, (2) to examine the many ways in which the transitions experienced by adolescents create a need for mental health care, and (3) to demonstrate the application of nursing theories to the care of adolescents with mental health concerns.

ADOLESCENCE DEFINED

In the current American culture, adolescents are viewed as neither children nor adults. The decade of adolescence, conceptualized as the ages of 11 to 21 years, is composed of three arbitrary subphases: early adolescence (ages 11 to 14), middle adolescence (ages 15 to 17), and late adolescence (ages 18 to 21; American Academy of Pediatrics, 2008). Early adolescence is evident with the onset of puberty, which involves many biological changes such as height and weight spurts, development of internal and external genitalia, and hair growth. Middle adolescence is characterized by increasing focus on peers and the pressures of conforming to a normative group on the basis of how one dresses, speaks, and acts. Late adolescence is marked by the final shift from preoccupation with appearances and conformity to commitment to roles and responsibilities within the adult society. The transitions from childhood to adolescence can create internal and interpersonal conflict as the adolescent struggles for a concrete personal identity, skills of social competence, and a commitment to play a particular role as an adult within the community.

The central developmental task of adolescence, according to Erikson (1950, 1968), is **identity formation**. The issue of identity concerns finding a place for oneself in the larger society beyond one's family (Figure 24-1). Adolescents are challenged with finding out who they are and what part they will play in society as responsible adults.

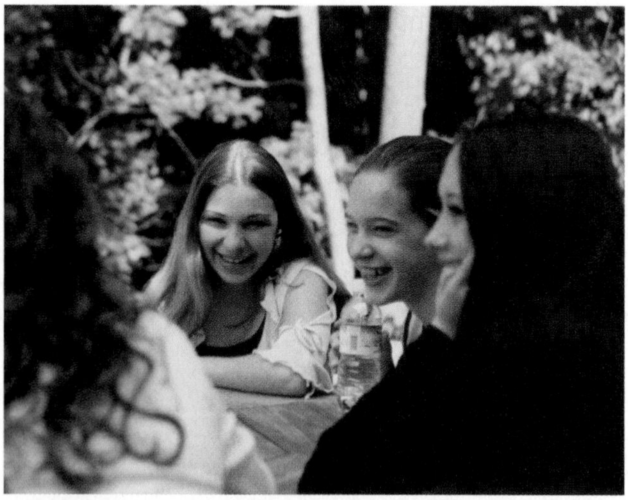

FIGURE 24-1 According to Erikson, adolescence is a time of identity formation. (DELMAR/CENGAGE LEARNING.)

Identity formation begins with an understanding of the self, which starts in early childhood. Early life experiences shape one's development of a personality complete with attitudes and beliefs, talents, capacities, and limitations. Experiences alone and with other people help the child form an awareness of one's separateness as well as relatedness within a social order. As Erikson (1950) conceptualizes it, early childhood allows the individual to tackle the tasks of developing trust, autonomy, initiative, and industry by overcoming mistrust in infancy, shame and doubt as a toddler, and guilt and inferiority during school age. The child who successfully masters these psychosocial tasks and incorporates these qualities into a personality structure is well equipped to face the complexities of adolescent identity formation.

The adolescent whose childhood has been characterized by positive interactions with a loving and supportive family and community and who has developed a strong sense of self-worth and self-esteem experiences this period of transition with some confusion and self-doubt. Emotions go up and down like the proverbial roller coaster. New challenges and problems are stressors that must be met with new coping and problem-solving skills. On the other hand, the adolescent whose childhood has been marred by neglect; emotional, physical, and/or sexual abuse; or some other type of trauma faces even greater confusion and self-doubt during this time of profound change. Scars from a wounded childhood can make the adolescent vulnerable to identity problems and **suicidal ideation**, or thoughts about killing oneself. Others may have to face this time of transition with a diagnosable mental illness carried over from childhood or one that finally erupts full blown with adolescence.

Many adolescents feel confusion and conflict as they resolve the developmental task of identity formation. Emotions swing from wanting to remain within the safety and security of childhood to wanting to experiment with new freedoms associated with being an adult. Behaviors and beliefs that were initially formed and approved by the nuclear family are now exposed to the approval of peers in the larger community. The period of adolescence is necessarily lengthy in our society so that the individual has ample time to explore and incorporate the sense of mastery of psychosocial tasks, including identity formation, into a repertoire of attitudes, beliefs, values, behaviors, and skills that will serve society in a responsible manner. In other societies in which less emphasis is placed on individual identity, the transitional phase of adolescence is less lengthy and less associated with conflict and confusion. At the conclusion of the adolescent phase of development, the individual essentially makes a commitment or statement to society about what he stands for and about his role in the society.

Physical Transitions

The onset of puberty signals the beginning of physical maturation that transforms the child into a sexually mature adult. The physical changes of puberty are set in motion by the production of hormones that direct the development of secondary sexual characteristics and physical functions that permit reproduction. These physical and biochemical alterations occur within the social context of family and community and within a personal framework of personality and previous experiences.

The physical changes in early adolescence are accompanied by an increasing interest in sexual attractiveness. Those individuals who mature early may experience situations in which older adolescents find them sexually attractive (Auslander, Rosenthal, & Blythe, 2005). Yet, the young adolescent is cognitively and socially unprepared for the risks associated with early sexual activity and is at special risk for unwanted pregnancy and sexually transmitted diseases. Middle (ages 15 to 17) and late (ages 18 to 21) adolescents, on the other hand, are cognitively more mature and better able to make decisions about the consequences of their behaviors in social settings with little adult supervision.

Recent developments in neuroimaging and genetics suggest that development of the brain is not complete by the end of adolescence as it is defined here. Moreover, these studies indicate that changes in the brain are different for males and females and have implications not only for cognition, but also for emotions and behavior (Giedd, 2008). Because the frontal lobes undergo significant changes during adolescence, many youth face challenges regarding impulse control and decision-making that make them vulnerable to adverse effects of alcohol, nicotine, and other substances (Joffe & Morris, 2008).

Cognitive Transitions

The cognitive, or intellectual, changes that occur in adolescence point to the need for mental health prevention and intervention strategies. In particular, adolescents are often characterized by impulsivity and high risk taking in an attempt to feel good, to be accepted by a peer group, and to experiment with adult behaviors. Decisions about being sexually active, driving motor vehicles without seatbelts or helmets, and using alcohol and other drugs are often made with little thought to the consequences of such behaviors (Byrnes, 2002). These high-risk behaviors are potentially destructive not only to the individual but to his or her family and society. For example, females who become pregnant in early or middle adolescence are at high risk for dropping out of school. This has enormous economic implications for them and their children, as a large percentage remain on welfare as adults.

School-based prevention programs, such as sex education that focus on consequences of behaviors rather than on moral dictums, have been successful. The nurse can assist in acknowledging that adolescents have a need to be accepted by a peer group and to feel good, but at the same time must have visions for the future so that decisions that may affect the rest of their lives are not left to sudden whims of desire and passion.

Emotional Transitions

The emotional changes that accompany puberty are often characterized by feelings of anxiety and depression. Anxiety about physical changes is related to eating disorders, sleeping problems, and the inability to pay attention in school with subsequent poor performance. Anxiety is also aroused as the adolescent strives to become part of a normative peer group and may face conflicts with expected behaviors that are different from those approved of by caregivers. Increases in anxiety may lead the adolescent to engage in other high-risk behavior such as alcohol and drug abuse, gang involvement, or sexual promiscuity.

The lengthy period of adolescence and identity formation is one of exploration, in which the adolescent "tries on" various ways of being alone and with groups. Some individuals adopt identities without exploration, simply hanging on to childhood beliefs and coping strategies, whereas others remain adrift, making no effort to explore or resolve the issue of identity formation (Josselson, 1994). The complex process of identity formation is addressed in myriad ways in the mental health needs and concerns of adolescents.

Social Transitions

The social milieu of the adolescent includes the family, peer, school, and working environments. This social world contains the opportunities and barriers for the individual to explore various roles and responsibilities associated with being a responsible member of the community (Perry, Kelder, & Komro, 1993). As the child moves into adolescence, he may experience changes within the family structure and function as caregivers and siblings also mature. Stereotypically, adolescents begin to spend more time away from their caregivers and other supervisory adults. They seek out peers who are also engaging in more activities with less adult supervision. Thus they begin to experiment with more adult-like behaviors including working part-time jobs, making their own decisions about spending money and leisure time, driving motorized vehicles, using alcohol, tobacco, and other drugs, and initiating sexual activities. Engaging in these behaviors may have a variety of consequences for the adolescent, including poor performance at school and work as well as an increase in other risky and violent behavior. According to Jessor (1991), most of these risky behaviors are purposeful and goal oriented. They help adolescents to cope with anxiety and frustration and to gain peer respect and acceptance, and are significant in establishing a break with the status of being a child.

Behaviors during early adolescence (ages 11 to 14) are often erratic and impulsive as these youngsters shift their primary role models from caregivers to peers. As they spend more time with peers, they are more susceptible to making risky decisions and engaging in risky behaviors. However, their ability to resist peer pressure and, consequently, to make less risky decisions and engage in fewer risky behaviors increases through late adolescence (Gardner & Steinberg, 2005).

Adolescents and their caregivers experience increasing conflicts around issues such as appropriate attire, school work, curfews, and use of leisure time. Caregiving style has been shown to be related to high-risk behaviors among adolescents. Authoritative caregivers provide clear boundaries and expectations for their children. As a result, the children of such caregivers, in general, engage in less substance abuse, display greater psychosocial maturity, and perform better in school than children whose caregivers are indifferent or uninvolved (Meschke & Patterson, 2003). As depicted in the following excerpt, misunderstanding between caregivers and children can be even more trying when the adolescent has a bona fide need for mental health intervention:

LISA, BRIGHT AND DARK

"Listen to me!" Lisa shouted.

Everyone did.

"I think I'm going crazy," Lisa said again. "I think I'm going out of my mind. Could we get some help or something?"

"Like what?" her mother asked. "You've mentioned this before, but you never say what you want to do about it."

M. N. [Mary Nell] was startled. This was the first time she'd ever heard Lisa say anything about this.

"Besides," Mrs. Shilling went on, "I think it's very rude of you to discuss this sort of thing when we have guests."

"Oh," M. N. smiled sheepishly, "don't mind me. Really."

"Since you don't pay any attention to me when we're alone," Lisa protested, "I thought you might with other people around."

"All right, all right," Mrs. Shilling sighed. "What is it you think you need?"

"Well," said Lisa, calmer, quiet but not hopeful, "maybe a psychiatrist or someone. I mean," she added quickly, "it wouldn't have to be an expensive one. Just someone who would understand and know what to do."

"You've seen too many movies," Mr. Shilling said.

"Who else has a psychiatrist, Lisa, in your class?" her mother wanted to know.

*"How should I know?" Lisa said, clenching her teeth, trying to smile politely.**

(Neufeld, 1970, p. 10)

Lisa and her caregivers illustrate some of the common communication patterns that develop between adolescents and their caregivers. Lisa shouts and deliberately brings up an emotionally laden topic in front of her friend to get her caregivers' attention. This pattern of communication does not necessarily indicate the need for mental health intervention, but in this case, it is a drastic attempt by Lisa to let her caregivers know that she really feels something is wrong with her mental health.

*From *Lisa Bright and Dark*, by J. Neufeld, 1970, New York: Penguin Books. Reprinted with permission from S.G. Phillips, Inc.

Juno

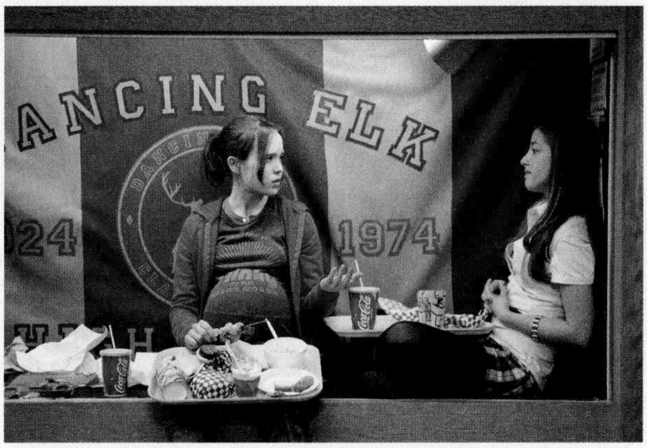

Courtesy: Fox Searchlight/The Kobal Collection/Gregory, Doane.

Outrageously nonchalant about her pregnancy at age 16, Juno MacGuff (Ellen Page) moves steadily toward adulthood in this funny and attractive film about growing up.

Lisa's mother feels embarrassed about her daughter's outburst in front of one of her friends and does not pass up the opportunity to discipline Lisa in front of Mary Nell by telling her how rude she thinks this type of communication is. Lisa, on the other hand, is trying to be honest and forthright with her caregivers by telling them directly that she thinks she needs to visit a psychiatrist. She adds that the doctor does not need to "be an expensive one," possibly reflecting other previous conflicts with her caregivers over the cost of other requests (not an uncommon area of conflict between caregivers and youth).

Lisa's caregivers continue to either deny that Lisa has a mental health problem or fail to sense her pain and frustration in their last responses. Lisa's father dismisses her request by commenting that she has simply seen too many movies (suggesting that watching movies about people who visit psychiatrists puts "ideas" into her young head). Lisa's mother dismisses her request by asking who else in her class has seen a psychiatrist (suggesting that her outburst and request for help are simply mimicry of some teenaged idol). The story of Lisa's mental illness (schizophrenia) exemplifies the importance of communication between caregivers and teens as well as the suffering that results when that communication is perceived as a source of caregiver-child conflict.

Transitions from elementary to middle to high school create new opportunities and social stresses for the adolescent. With each transition comes a new set of rules and expectations, creating the need for great adaptability within the individual. Often, adolescents find themselves not only in a new physical environment, but also with peers and upperclassmen who were unknown to them in the previous school. Those whose families move from one location to another also experience increased stress in adjusting to new locations and peers. Loneliness may become an everyday experience for the adolescent who feels misunderstood or rejected from the normative group in the new school (Brage, Meredith, & Woodward, 1993). Such social exclusion has been shown to have a significant negative impact on the development of prosocial behavior and moral reasoning later in life (Twenge, Baumeister, DeWall, Ciarocco, & Bartels, 2007).

THEORIES OF ADOLESCENT DEVELOPMENT

Several theoretical approaches can help to clarify the unique phase of life known as adolescence. Two approaches that are of particular relevance to the mental health of adolescents are theories of identity formation and social competence. The concepts central to these theories blend well with nursing approaches to the adolescent client.

Identity Formation

Identity formation is a central concept in the developmental theory of Erikson (1950, 1968). Erikson's theory is related to, but different from, classical, or Freudian, psychoanalytic theory. Rather than having a focus on psychopathology rooted in one's libido, this psychosocial theory focuses on adaptation and interaction between the individual and the environment or society (Marcia, 1994). According to Erikson, adolescence is the phase in life in which previous childhood tasks of development are revisited and integrated. The first developmental stage of learning to trust oneself and others must be integrated as the adolescent questions what people and which ideas should be trusted and how trustworthy the adolescent himself is. Ultimately, this is a question of identity whose roots extend far back into infancy.

The second developmental stage of autonomy also centers around identity, an identity that is to be revisited in adolescence. The maturing individual, much like the toddler, must face issues of independence and making decisions based on free will. A sense of pride in one's choices and shameless approval of one's peers are important in settling the issue of identity in the second decade of life. Similarly, as the school-age child displays initiative and industry in learning the skills that enable problem solving and coping with the stresses of living, so too does the adolescent resolve again to express initiative and industry in determining an identity and role to which to be committed within the larger society (Erikson, 1968).

Marcia (1994) extended the psychosocial development theory of Erikson by conducting extensive research on the stage of adolescence, in which the crisis of identity versus identity confusion is generally resolved. Marcia believed that identity is a process by which adolescents decide how to take a place in the world as responsible adults who are committed to a particular way of being. The process is characterized by exploration of alternatives. While much of identity formation takes place in adolescence, significant life changes—such as the birth of a child, marriage, or death of a loved one—call for identity reformulation throughout the life span.

Marcia identified four categories of styles used by adolescents to resolve the issue of identity. These four styles, termed **identity statuses**, are outlined in Table 24-1. The first status is called **foreclosure**. These individuals have not thoroughly explored the possibilities of identity before making a commitment about adult status. They are closely tied to their families because to question caregiver values would be too threatening and would make them feel guilty. Their families are generally warm, but this is contingent on the child's decision to follow the family's rules and adhere to their values and beliefs. The second status is characterized by exploring alternatives in search of an adult-sized identity and suffering the crisis and consequences of this exploration. This status is called **moratorium** and represents an expected period of delay in making a final decision about identity. The third status is **identity achievement** and involves making a commitment to a specific identity after a period of exploration. Finally, the fourth status, **identity diffusion**, refers to avoiding making commitments and may indicate a need for mental health services. Some of these individuals are socially skilled but are not reaching their intellectual or physical potentials. They may have some or all of the characteristics of individuals with Schizoid Personality Disorder, which is a pattern of restricted emotional expression and detachment from other people (American Psychiatric Association, 2000). Still others may suffer from a more severe type of psychiatric disorder such as Borderline Personality (Marcia, 1994). Individuals with Borderline Personality are impulsive in ways that are potentially self-damaging (e.g., diagnostic criteria include impulsivity in at least two of the following: spending money, reckless driving, sex, substance abuse, and binge eating), display frantic activity to avoid feelings of abandonment, experience unstable interpersonal relationships with others, and suffer from identity disturbance, recurrent suicidal or self-mutilating behaviors, unstable affect, chronic feelings of emptiness, inappropriate anger, and transient paranoid ideas (American Psychiatric Association, 2000).

The majority of adolescents behave as if their status were that of moratorium. That is, adolescence is a time for

TABLE 24-1 Four Adolescent Identity Statuses

STATUS	CHARACTERISTICS	EXAMPLES
Foreclosure	Identity decision made before options explored	Mary Ellen decides to live at home and work in the family dry-cleaning business rather than apply to a college. Her parents show strong approval of this decision even though Mary Ellen has previously expressed an interest in studying music at a nearby university.
Moratorium	Identity decision delayed until options explored	Jeffrey is feeling ambivalent about what to do after high school. His father encourages him to think about medical school and, thus, follow in his father's footsteps. His mother encourages him to do whatever he wants to do. Jeffrey considers going to a community college for a year or two until "I can find myself."
Identity diffusion	Identity decision avoided	Lindsey is a charming 16-year-old. He easily finds an after-school job at a fast-food restaurant, but maintains a poor work record and soon leaves to pursue employment at a bakery. His interpersonal relationships lack commitment as he flits from one new girlfriend to another in a few weeks' time. His teachers and parents often lament that Lindsey is just not "living up to his potential."
Identity achievement	Identity decision made after options explored	Jill has explored many alternatives when considering what to do after graduating from high achievement school. She recognizes that she has many different interests, including sports, music, and writing. She has been active in a variety of extracurricular activities in high school and won a letter in the Senior Debate Team. This experience taught her to examine issues critically, solve problems creatively, and display self-confidence.

Source: Adapted from *Interventions for Adolescent Identity Development*, edited by S. L. Archer, 1994, Thousand Oaks: Sage Publications.

experimenting with how one might want to be as an adult. These adolescents show wide variety in their experimentation and are sensitive to the responses of others. As a group, they do not necessarily require help for mental health problems related to identity. These individuals may exhibit experimental behaviors such as wearing dramatic makeup, changing hairstyles (e.g., the 14-year-old boy who shaves his head on a dare from his friends is merely experimenting with autonomy and self-expression), and donning particular fashion styles (e.g., jeans with ragged knees). The behavior represents an honest search for what "fits" and is not indicative of outright rebellion or confusion. After a variable period of moratorium, most adolescents determine who they are, what they like, and what they want to do in the future. Thus, they arrive at the status of identity achievement after a period of exploration. Again, these youngsters seldom need specific mental health interventions directly related to achieving this status, although caregivers may need some direction on appropriate responses to behaviors.

Youth who attain a status of foreclosure or identity diffusion, on the other hand, may well be in need of specific mental health interventions. For example, the child who has been seriously abused or expected to take on adult-like responsibilities throughout childhood may arrive in adolescence holding the belief that he or she is to put self-interests aside and continue to attend to the needs of others. Such an individual may foreclose on an identity or occupation when he really has neither the aptitude nor healthy motivation to pursue such a path. Mental health interventions such as group counseling may be helpful for such a teen to sort out what is part of his or her identity and what is emotional trauma or baggage left over from a wounded childhood. The school nurse may identify such individuals through their consistent serious attitude about the needs of others, often at the expense of their own needs and wishes.

Similarly, the individual who experiences identity diffusion may need specific psychiatric intervention to deal with a serious personality disorder such as one of those identified previously. Again, the school nurse or clinic nurse giving routine physicals should be alert to signs of a more serious underlying condition. For example, an adolescent with disturbed diffusion may exhibit signs of social isolation or feeling empty inside.

Social Competence

Social learning theory is based on the premise that human behavior is motivated and regulated to some degree within the context of social structure. People learn to act in ways that they perceive as rewarding from either their own personal experiences or observing the experiences of others within the social setting. An individual's behaviors are both internally and externally motivated, evaluated, and regulated. Self-efficacy is a central concept in the social learning theory developed by Bandura (1997). Competence in responding to demands from the environment is not attained once and for all nor is it simply a matter of following a prescribed set of rules or instructions. **Self-efficacy**, or competence in managing one's personal response to the environment, involves forming intentions, setting goals, monitoring, and regulating behavior (Bandura & Locke, 2003). **Self-awareness**, or a perception of one's competence, influences the types of choices or judgments the individual makes in facing demands from the larger society.

Positive mental health in adolescence has been associated with the construct of **social competence**, or "the degree to which significant others rate an individual as successful in solving and completing relevant social tasks" (Compas, 1993, p. 164). Specific skills or competencies that are mastered for positive mental health include understanding how to decode social cues and interpreting these in meaningful ways. Other skills consist of initiating behavioral responses to these cues from a set of alternatives and monitoring the effects of displaying the chosen responses. These skills are complex and related to previous experiences in social interactions and problem solving. These skills also vary with the social context in which the adolescent is acting. For example, decoding, interpreting, and responding to social cues within the adolescent's home may be very different from doing so in school or at a party.

MENTAL HEALTH IN ADOLESCENCE

From a broad psychosocial point of view, mental health can be defined as the absence of psychosocial and behavioral dysfunction and the presence of optimal psychosocial functioning or well-being. Mental health in adolescence is defined differently by mental health professionals, caregivers, society at large, and adolescents themselves. The perspective of mental health professionals, including nurses, is usually based on a theoretical framework such as a theory of personality development, motivation for human behavior, or psychopathology. Caregivers and society at large, in contrast, tend to conceive of adolescent mental health in terms of stable and predictable behaviors and conformity with the rules of social conduct. For example, caregivers and teachers expect youngsters to display increasing self-responsibility in going to school and doing their homework. Adolescents themselves view mental health more subjectively, in terms of their individual well-being and feelings of contentment and happiness (Compas, 1993). For example, an adolescent who spends his time in the company of several friends, is included in social activities, and perceives little intrusion from caregivers and teachers on what he thinks and how he acts may consider himself to be happy and content. On the other hand, when an adolescent does not have peers as a frame of reference for what he is feeling or experiencing, he may feel quite unhappy and even "crazy." The following example of positive mental health comes from an eighth-grader who wants more information about what is "normal." *Deenie* by Judy Blume provides many such examples through the main character of the same name:

DEENIE

We're starting a new program in gym. Once a month we're going to have a discussion group with Mrs. Rappoport. It sounds very interesting because Mrs. Rappoport asked us each to write down a question and drop it into a box on her desk. The question could be about anything, she said, especially anything we need to know about sex. She told us not to put our names on the paper. She doesn't want to know who's asking what. It's a good thing too, because I'd never have asked my question if I had to sign my name. I wrote:

Do normal people touch their bodies before they go to sleep and is it all right to do that?

On Tuesday, when we walked into gym, Mrs. Rappoport told us to sit in a circle so we could talk easily. The first questions she discussed were all about menstruation. But I already knew most everything from my booklet. After that she said, "Okay, now I think we can move on to another subject. Here's an interesting question." She read it to us. "Do normal people touch their bodies before they go to sleep and is it all right to do that?"

*I almost died! I glanced around, then smiled a little, because some of the other girls did, and hoped the expression on my face looked like I was trying to figure out who had asked such a thing.**

(Blume, 1973, pp. 82–83)

Positive mental health consists of two fundamental dimensions. The first of these dimensions is to develop skills that enable the individual to handle stress, manage emotions, and solve problems effectively. The second dimension is to develop skills that enable the individual to be involved in activities that are purposeful and meaningful. These skills are based on obtaining accurate information. As illustrated in the previous excerpt, Deenie exhibits a healthy curiosity about her body. She also expresses a social sensitivity to the normative behavior of her peers by smiling and looking around. She has both the courage to ask an important question and the desire to be accepted by her friends. Once developed, such skills enhance feelings of self-esteem and social competence. They are developed within the context of family and other sociocultural factors such as community (e.g., school), ethnicity, and race. Thus, positive mental health, which consists of these two dimensions, can be evaluated from several perspectives: coping skills; level of involvement in meaningful activities; perspectives of different groups such as caregivers, health professionals, and the adolescents themselves; developmental factors; and sociocultural factors (Compas, 1993).

Because the definitions of mental health differ among health professionals, caregivers, and adolescents themselves, misunderstanding and conflict may arise when describing problems and planning for solutions. Mental health professionals may label an adolescent's behavior in a specific way that reflects a theoretical understanding of the complexity of motivation, emotion, and behavior. Such a label may have adverse effects on the adolescent and his family. For example, to label an adolescent as "suicidal" may unleash a host of fears and expectations that are difficult to overcome. The same individual may be viewed by caregivers and teachers as "a loner, lazy, or an underachiever." In terms of the adolescent's personal and subjective view, he may simply feel lonely, sad, confused, and helpless.

Mental Health Care Needs

Adolescents face considerable changes and pressures that are among the most complex of the life cycle (Ferguson, 1993). These changes and pressures converge in ways that challenge the stability and mental health of many, but not all, adolescents (see Figure 24-2). Adolescents who may benefit from mental health care services include those with diagnosable mental illnesses such as Conduct Disorder, mood disorders (including major depression), schizophrenia, Obsessive-Compulsive Disorder, and Adjustment Disorder, as well as those adolescents who engage in high-risk behaviors that make them vulnerable to mental health problems, such as substance use and abuse, irresponsible use of motor vehicles, and early initiation of sexual activity.

The Centers for Disease Control and Prevention (CDC, 2008) notes that approximately one in five children and

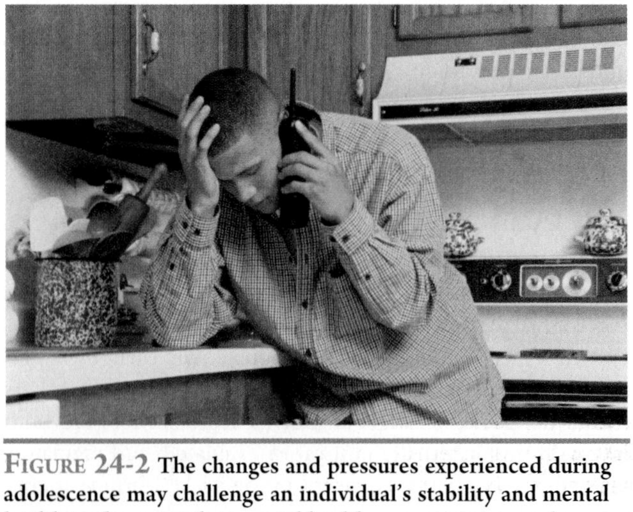

Figure 24-2 The changes and pressures experienced during adolescence may challenge an individual's stability and mental health to the point that mental health care services may be beneficial. (DELMAR/CENGAGE LEARNING.)

*Reprinted with permission of the Atheneum Books for Young Readers, an imprint of Simon & Schuster Children's Publishing Division from *DEENIE* by Judy Blume. Copyright © 1973 Judy Blume.

adolescents in the United States between the ages of 9 and 17 has a diagnosable behavioral or emotional health disorder, and less than one in three actually receives help. In a school-based survey of 17,193 adolescents, nearly 25% identified themselves as having a serious problem such as emotional distress or suicidal ideation, and those who decided they needed professional help had a history of abuse, physical health problems, and suicidal ideation (Saunders, Resnick, Hoberman, & Blum, 1994).

Many disorders that originate and are diagnosed first in childhood (e.g., Autism, Conduct Disorder, and Attention-Deficit/Hyperactivity Disorder) continue into adolescence and adulthood (Kazdin, 1993). Conduct Disorder, for example, is one of the most frequently diagnosed psychiatric conditions in children and adolescents. Prevalence rates range from less than 1% to more than 10% in general population studies (American Psychiatric Association, 2000). Conduct Disorder is characterized in childhood by aggression toward one's peers. In the adolescent-onset type (absence of diagnosis before age 10), aggression is less common, but the individual may engage in delinquent behaviors such as lying, stealing, and truancy from school, usually with little expression of guilt or remorse. Conduct Disorder is often associated with other risk-taking behaviors such as those noted previously.

Other disorders, such as Anorexia Nervosa and Bulimia Nervosa, may be diagnosed first in adolescence. The average age of onset of Anorexia Nervosa is 17, often associated with stressful life events such as leaving home to attend college (American Psychiatric Association, 2000). This disorder is characterized by an intense fear of gaining weight, refusal to maintain acceptable minimum body weight, disturbed body image, and amenorrhea. Anorexia is diagnosable in approximately 0.5% of females and occurs more frequently (90%) in females than in males. Bulimia Nervosa, on the other hand, is characterized by recurrence of concern about body shape and weight, binge eating, misuse of laxatives and diuretics, and, often, purging through self-induced vomiting. Bulimia is diagnosable in 1% to 3% of the population and occurs more frequently (90%) in females than in males (American Psychiatric Association, 2000).

Depressive disorders are relatively common among adolescents. The National Institute of Mental Health (NIMH) estimates that 8.3% of all adolescents currently suffer from some form of depression and approximately 7% of these commit suicide (http://www.nimh.nih.gov; NIMH, 2001b). Depression is often difficult to diagnose, particularly in adolescence, because the symptoms are frequently on a continuum with normal behavior and do not lead to functional impairment (Kutcher & Chehil, 2008). However, it occurs in at least 10% of adolescents and is diagnosed more frequently in girls than in boys. Moodiness in the form of pervasive and persistent sadness is seen in less than 50% of cases, while the majority with the diagnosis have symptoms of anhedonia (that is, they lack enjoyment in or pleasure from the usual activities of daily living), anger, or irritability (Hoberman, 1995). The majority go untreated in spite of other symptoms, including sleep disturbance, weight change, and thoughts of death or suicide.

RESEARCH Highlight 24-1

High School Youth and Suicide Risk: Exploring Protection Provided through Physical Activity and Sport Participation

STUDY PROBLEM/PURPOSE

To evaluate if participation in physical activity or sports has an association with hopelessness or suicidality in youth. Specifically, the researchers sought to: (1) evaluate if youth (both males and females) who engage in physical activity have lower risk of hopelessness and suicidal behaviors than those who do not engage in physical activity, and (2) evaluate if those who participate in sports have reduced risk.

METHODS

Researchers evaluated data from the Center for Disease Control and Prevention's (CDC) Youth Risk Behavior survey, for a sample of more than 13,000 high school students, grades 9 through 12, who were a representative sample of the U.S. youth population. Suicidal risk was determined by students' self-report (answers to specific questions on the survey tool). The researchers analyzed data through a logistic regression model to assess associations between/among variables and relative risk.

FINDINGS

For both males and females, there was a lower risk of suicidality among athletes compared to nonathletes. Frequent vigorous physical activity reduced the risk of hopelessness and suicidality for males. Lack of physical activity increased the risk of hopelessness and suiciality for females.

IMPLICATIONS

Findings suggest that involvement in sports may produce psychosocial benefits for many adolescents, and that physical activity may have direct impact or association with positive feelings about self and may have direct mental health benefits. Nurses should use this information to encourage participation in extra-curricular activities and physical activities.

Source: "High School Youth and Suicide Risk: Exploring Protection Provided through Physical Activity and Sport Participation," by L. A. Taliaferro, B. A. Rienzo, M. D. Miller, R. M. Pigg, and V. J. Dodd, 2008, *Journal of School Health*, *78*, 545–553.

Suicide is among the leading causes of death among adolescents between the ages of 10 and 24 (CDC, 2008). Suicidal ideation, which includes thinking about the reasons for and ways of killing oneself, and suicide attempts are related to a variety of life events in childhood and adolescence. In general, adolescents who attempt or complete suicide have experienced more turmoil in their families, sexual abuse during adolescence, frequent changes in residence, and having to repeat a grade in school (De Wilde, Kienhorst, Diekstra, & Wolters, 1992). There are significant gender differences in rates of adolescent suicide. Whereas more females admit to having suicidal ideation and make more attempts at suicide, more males actually succeed in completing suicide. These differences have been found to be related to greater feelings of loneliness and experiences of substance abuse in males than in females (Rich, Kirkpatrick-Smith, Bonner, & Jans, 1992). Researchers also found that males express greater fear of social disapproval for having suicidal thoughts while females express more fear of injury.

Expression of suicidal ideation should always be taken seriously. Unfortunately, it is not always easy to identify signs of suicidal ideation. Troubled adolescents who are contemplating suicide rarely ask directly for help. Males, in particular, may ask for help only indirectly by acting out or by withdrawing from usual activities (Dumont, 1991). Preventing suicide in adolescents depends to some extent on identifying those individuals at highest risk. These include those who (1) have other psychiatric problems (particularly substance abuse or depression), (2) have a history of suicide within the family, (3) are experiencing high levels of stress (particularly related to achievement or sexuality), and (4) are experiencing parental rejection, family conflict, or family disruption (Steinberg, 1996).

Needs Related to Physical Transitions

As sexual maturation continues, issues related to gender identity, gender role, and sexual preference increase. Gender Identity Disorder is characterized by two major indicators: (1) a persistent and strong identification of self as the other sex, and (2) persistent discomfort with being one's assigned sex (American Psychiatric Association, 1994). **Gender identity** refers to the individual's subjective or private experience of gender, whereas **gender role** is the public recognition of one's gender assignment as biological male or female and the expression of appropriate social behaviors related to that assignment. **Sexual orientation** is an expression of one's attraction to members of the opposite or same sex and represents a continuum rather than dichotomous categories. **Transgender** individuals refers to a person whose sex assignment at birth does not match his or her gender identity (Meininger & Remafedi, 2008). Confusion and frustration in coming to terms with gender identity, gender role, and sexual orientation may lead to feelings of depression and suicidal ideation that require professional intervention.

Other mental health problems are related to the physical transitions of adolescence. Skin problems such as acne may lead to diminished self-esteem and social isolation and loneliness. Eating disorders become more prevalent, particularly among females. Adolescents (both males and females) who participate in sports that require weight limits may develop eating disorders in an effort to meet weight requirements. Adolescents, both males and females, who participate in specific sports associated with strength training may also suffer from mental health problems related to use of anabolic steroids in addition to other substances (Taylor, 2002).

Other physical problems that may result from accidental injury or illness are of great concern to the adolescent because they are often perceived as a threat to body image

Blue Boy by Picasso

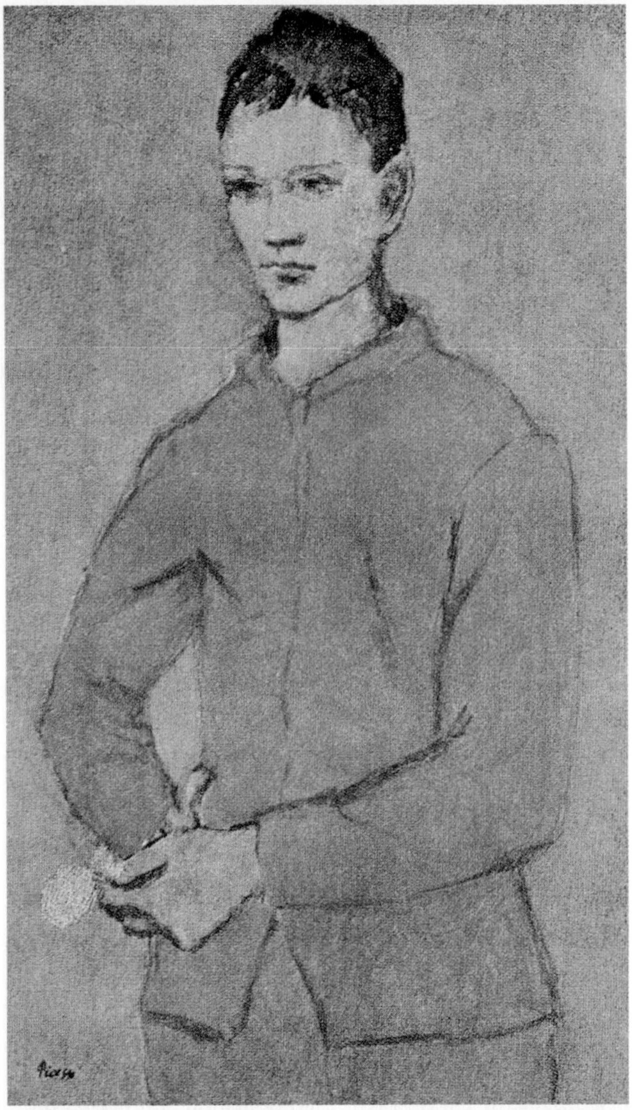

Blue Boy by Picasso. Source: Copyright © 2011 Estate of Pablo Picasso/ Artists Rights Society (ARS) New York

Picasso's *Blue Boy* depicts a somber young man posed awkwardly as if to represent the state of adolescence. The young man is pensive and thoughtful, at the door of adulthood, yet holding back. While we often think of adolescence in terms of violence or frivolous and uninhibited behavior, *Blue Boy* presents a differing perspective.

and identity. For example, the adolescent who sustains a spinal cord injury resulting from a recreational sport, such as skiing or climbing, faces enormous mental health concerns related to loss of function and the perception that he no longer has a future or would be a desirable companion for peers. Issues of sexuality and reproduction require much sensitivity on the part of health care professionals who counsel these youngsters during rehabilitation.

Needs Related to Cognitive Transitions

Cognitive limitations that the adolescent may have experienced in childhood may continue to be problematic during the many transitions of adolescence. The individual with Attention-Deficit/Hyperactivity Disorder (ADHD) will continue to need mental health assistance during this phase of life. Such limitations will become an essential dimension for the adolescent to integrate into an adult identity, and the young person should be encouraged to ask for assistance with learning disabilities during each new transition.

Academic achievement may continue to be impaired in the adolescent with ADHD and is often a source of conflict with caregivers and teachers. The risk for dropping out of school is high, and subsequent ability to find meaningful work decreases. The tendency toward impulsivity and inappropriate social behavior interferes with the adolescent's development of self-efficacy related to skills needed for satisfying social relationships.

Needs Related to Emotional Transitions

The adolescent often experiences transient periods of depression. With the loss of childhood and the associated security of childhood routines and expectations, the adolescent must engage in some normal grieving. However, depression that is marked by increasing withdrawal from social contact and declining feelings of self-worth may require professional intervention. Such feelings of depression can lead to self-destructive behaviors including suicide. Depression in adolescents may be difficult to spot because these young people often avoid intimacy and are at a stage in life where they spend increasingly smaller amounts of time with family members. Caregivers and teachers should be alert to the possibility of depression as a response to perceived trauma, regardless of its source, in the adolescent. Perceived inadequacy in social relationships, such as dating, or in social competency, such as making the football team or cheerleading squad, can trigger an intense emotional response that, to an adult, may not seem proportional to the stimulus. However, in the life of an adolescent, such disappointments are of paramount importance. Nursing Alert 24-1 identifies some of the life events that place an adolescent at risk for suicide. The adolescent's response to such life events depends on the internal and external assets or resources available. Internal assets include a commitment to learning, positive values, social competencies, and a positive identity. External assets include social support such as satisfying relationships with friends and family members, feeling safe and valued by adults, boundaries and expectations, and constructive use of time (Search Institute, 2002).

Depression may also result from more traumatic events, such as the loss of a caregiver or friend. When a change in behavioral patterns that is marked by withdrawal from usual activities, excessive sleeping, poor appetite, and sudden outbursts of anger is noted, depression may be the adolescent's problem and he needs professional assistance. The adolescent whose caregiver commits suicide is also at higher risk for suicide when depressed. Such individuals should be encouraged to seek help (see Chapters 13 and 15).

It is important not to ignore the warning signs of depression and suicide in the adolescent client. Nurses who work with adolescents must be comfortable in talking with them about the possibility of suicide and in responding seriously to any indications that the adolescent might give. It is a mistake to reassure the individual that everything will turn out all right. What is important is to ask direct questions in a calm manner, refer the person to a professional skilled in crisis intervention, and continue to provide support even after the crisis is past (Sherer, 2008).

Needs Related to Social Transitions

All of the previously discussed transitions occur within the context of social interactions within the family, school, and community. These interactions are characterized by patterns of communication that can lead to mental health problems. During the drastic and rapid transitions of adolescence, communication within the family, between student and teacher, among friends, and with members of the community at large is essential to the mental health and well-being of all. Nurses should bear in mind that adolescents from minority racial and ethnic groups may also experience mental health concerns related to their immigration and acculturation status.

NURSING**ALERT** 24-1

Risk Factors for Adolescent Suicide

- Loss of significant relationship with friend, family member, or pet
- Feelings of hopelessness or emptiness
- Giving away prized possessions
- Suicide of a friend, relative, or public figure
- Homophobic response of family members to an adolescent's sexual preference (e.g., rejection)
- Divorce of parents
- Break-up with a girl- or boyfriend
- Unattainment of a significant goal (e.g., acceptance at a particular college)
- Dropped out of school
- Only child in family
- Previous conduct disorder
- Previous suicide attempt

NURSINGALERT 24-2

Warning Signs of Potential Adolescent Suicide

- Drastic changes in behavior (e.g., sudden withdrawal in an otherwise socially active person or sudden gregariousness in an otherwise shy person)
- Stated feelings of sadness, loneliness, hopelessness, or despair
- Increased impulsive risk-taking behaviors (e.g., disregard for safety by not wearing seatbelt)
- Alienating behaviors (e.g., withdrawal or aggression)
- Giving away possessions (especially those with special meanings)
- Preoccupation with death or dying
- Sudden changes in personal appearance and hygiene
- Previous suicide attempt or gesture
- Direct suicidal comments such as "I wish I were dead"

NURSINGALERT 24-3

Nursing Interventions for the Suicidal Adolescent

- Always take seriously the expression of a wish to die.
- Provide a safe environment.
- Obtain a verbal contract that the individual will not do anything to harm himself without talking to you or another responsible adult.
- Check on the adolescent's feelings of safety and control at frequent intervals.

Statistically, adolescents at highest risk for mental health problems are those from single-caregiver homes and homes in which one or more caregivers have a history of alcoholism or drug use, suicide attempts, or antisocial behaviors (Vernon, 1991). Moreover, the adolescent may have grown up in a violent atmosphere with caregivers who fight or batter one another. As they become older and more independent, many adolescents who are the victims of violent homes or abusive families may take matters into their own hands and run away from home to escape the pain of abuse and violence. These youth may become homeless, fall in with gangs, or resort to prostitution, all of which will introduce additional mental and physical health risks. Although the exact number of homeless youth is unknown, a national representative sample of adolescents indicated that about 6% of children in grades 7–12 run away from home each year (Sanchez, Waller, & Greene, 2006). Homeless adolescents include not only those who run away from home to escape abuse and neglect, but also those who are thrown out of their homes; many of these are youth with long-standing psychiatric and conduct problems, including Post-Traumatic Stress Disorder (Tyler, Cauce, & Whitbeck, 2004; Whitbeck, Johnson, Hoyt, & Cauce, 2004). Homeless youth are at increased risk for further sexual abuse, sexually transmitted diseases including acquired immune deficiency syndrome (AIDS), injury, violence, substance abuse, and a lifestyle characterized by poverty. Drug addiction or prostitution may lead these youth to encounters with the law. Nurses working in public health settings or detention institutions such as jails and prisons are instrumental in assessing the need for mental health services.

Poverty places the adolescent at risk for mental health problems. Poverty and crowding in inner cities contribute to what Schorr (1998) refers to as "rotten outcomes." For example, by the time many youngsters growing up in crowded cities reach the eighth grade, they have lost hope for meaningful employment in the future. Many have dropped out of school and have turned to the streets for identity and for seeking a way out of the downward spiral of poverty. As adolescents spend more time away from caregivers and family and more time with peers, opportunities to become involved with groups who exhibit high-risk behaviors for violent activity, such as gangs, increases. Gangs are most likely to develop in youth who are unsuccessful in school and are rejected by peers (Dishion, Nelson, & Yasui, 2005). Homicide may be a standard for acceptance within the peer group and may also be associated with other risky behaviors such as dealing in illicit drugs.

A growing number of adolescents, particularly African Americans, are living in single-caregiver households. The greatest impact of this trend is economic: 75% of African American families who are not in metropolitan areas live below the poverty line (Millstein, Irwin, & Brindis, 1991). In addition, an increasing number of adolescents have been raised as "latchkey children," returning home after school to no adult supervision.

Adolescents are at risk for specific health-related problems, such as early initiation of sexual intercourse, teen-age pregnancy, violence and sexual victimization. Adolescents are at particularly high risk for date or acquaintance rape. This is the most common type of sexual assault among adolescents and is defined as sexual intercourse involving threat of force or actual force from a perpetrator known to the victim and without the person's consent (Rickert, Ryan, & Chacko, 2008). Health care providers should screen for this type of victimization when treating adolescents for other health-related concerns. Nurses working with adolescents in schools or other clinical settings should provide educational information on ways to prevent the occurrence of sexual assault (see Nursing Tip 24-1).

Because sexuality is a major developmental task for adolescents, their naiveté and inexperience may increase their vulnerability to nonconsensual sexual activity and reduce their ability to cope with its consequences. In a study of young adolescents (those aged 12–15), researchers found that males more than females agreed that forcing a dating partner to have sex was acceptable. Moreover, they found that having parents who weren't involved in their children's lives and, among males, watching music videos and pro wrestling, were significantly associated with thinking forced sex was acceptable (Kaestle, Halpern, & Brown, 2007).

In a study of secondary school students, Telljohann and colleagues (1995) found that females more than males correctly identified behaviors that indicated nonconsensual sex. For example, 81% of the females and only 64% of the males in the sample of 588 youth agreed that an uncle was at fault for touching the private parts of his niece. Adolescents who run away from home, or who are thrown out of their homes and become homeless, are at greatest risk for nonconsensual sexual activity, especially females. In a study of 240 such youth in the Midwest, Terrell (1997) found that homeless adolescents were at high risk for aggravated sexual assault because of aggressive and abusive parents (e.g., 67% reported being hit with an object by their parents) and were further victimized after retreating to the streets (i.e., 21% sexually assaulted, 35% assaulted with a weapon, and 50% threatened with a weapon).

NURSING TIP 24-1

Addressing Sexual Concerns with Adolescents

- Explore the adolescent's sexual preference (self-identity as homosexual, bisexual, or heterosexual).
- Ask open-ended questions about their worries or concerns (e.g., what concerns do you have about your sexual preferences?).
- Use correct anatomical and socially accepted terms for genitalia and sexual expression (e.g., penis and vagina; gay and lesbian).
- Provide accurate and factual information when possible (use books, pamphlets, fact sheets, hotlines).
- Refer adolescents to community resources when appropriate (Planned Parenthood for contraceptive options, Caregivers & Friends of Lesbian and Gays [PFLAG] for support of sexual orientation, etc.).
- Encourage contact with school resources (counselors and nurses).

C.R.A.Z.Y

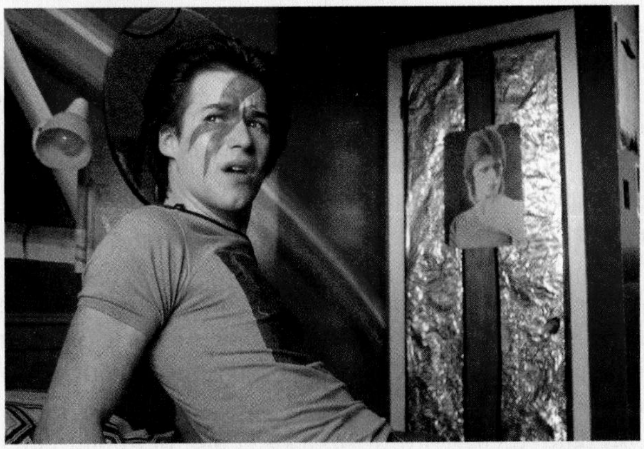

Cirus (Courtesy: The Kobal Collection)

Growing up gay in Quebec in the 1980s rock music world of long hair and sexual ambiguity, Zac can't meet all of his father's expectations. But this warm film—with lots of great period music—does chart Zac's maturing into acceptance of the person he is.

The role of communities in providing support for adolescent development was studied by Blyth and Leffert (1995). These researchers found that youth in the ninth to twelfth grades experienced different types of community strengths. Youth who were vulnerable benefited more from living in communities where other youth engaged in few problem behaviors than from living in communities where youth engaged in more problem behaviors. Healthier communities included those where families were caring and supportive and provided monitoring and discipline to their youth. Such communities also included schools that were perceived as caring and supportive, where a high percentage of youth were committed and motivated to continue to learn, and where a high percentage of caregivers were involved. Other strengths within the healthiest communities were the percentage of youth involved in religious services and structured activities, such as sports or music, and the peer norms related to personal values and responsibility.

In a recent survey study of more than 12,000 adolescents in grades 7–12, Resnick and colleagues (1997) found that the main threats to the health and well-being of adolescents are risk behaviors that they choose for themselves. The two most important factors that protected these youth from experiencing emotional stress, suicidal thoughts and behaviors, violence, early sexual behavior, and the use of, alcohol, cigarettes, and marijuana were connectedness with parents and family and with their schools. Among high school students, appearing to be older than one's peers

NURSINGTIP 24-2

Guidelines for Avoiding Sexual Assault/Rape

Help adolescents prevent sexual assault or rape by offering the following guidelines:

- Avoid hitchhiking or giving rides to hitchhikers/strangers.
- Avoid taking walks (or shopping) alone; go with a friend.
- Walk confidently; avoid looking uncertain about your destination.
- Keep one arm free to defend yourself against an attacker.
- When getting into your car, check backseat for intruders.
- Keep car locked when driving and lock it at your destination.
- Be sure car has sufficient gas to get you to your destination.
- If being followed in your car, drive to a business or the police station.
- Do not open door of house to strangers.
- Do not go to a secluded location on a first date.

was significantly associated with emotional distress and suicidal thinking and behavior. Among both junior and senior high students, repeating a grade in school was associated with emotional distress. Low-risk behaviors were also associated with high parental expectations concerning school achievement.

NURSING THEORIES

As the following nursing theories will demonstrate, communication and caring are important components of all successful interventions, regardless of setting. These theories emphasize the importance of the relationship between nurse and client.

Humanistic Nursing

The Humanistic Nursing Theory of Paterson and Zderad (1988) began in 1960 when these two nurses engaged in discussions with other nurses about their experiences in caring for clients (Decker-Brown, 2003). They were not impressed with the objective nature of empirical science that viewed human beings objectively and as predictable objects. Rather, they believed that their work as nurses would be facilitated by understanding how people experience their existence. Thus, they were led to literature concerning existential philosophy. Humanistic and existential philosophy assert a broad view of human beings and their potential.

Paterson and Zderad stated, "Nursing is an experience lived between human beings" (1988, p. 3). It is a transactional relationship based on an awareness of both nurse and client of self and of each other. A major assumption of this definition of nursing is that human beings are unique and capable of making choices. This philosophical framework is appropriate for understanding the adolescent's struggles with making choices and forging a unique identity for self in society. This perspective also assumes that one person's presence is of value to another person. Nursing is a caring and nurturing response of one human being toward another with the aim of developing more well-being (Praeger & Hogarth, 1985). Within this context, nursing focuses on the whole person rather than on reducing the person to components such as a mind, behavior, or body parts. Such an approach can be very encouraging to the adolescent and can help to consolidate identity.

The goal of humanistic nursing is attainment not of mere health or well-being but as a state of dynamic "more-being." The objective is for the nurse to assist the client to become *more,* to realize a potential not yet attained in the present moment of their interaction. Health is conceptualized as a process of becoming whatever is possible for the human being. Again, this approach is very appropriate for working with adolescents in various settings. Adolescents often resist a concrete set of rules from adults in authority but need the support of adults who understand their developmental phases and who can offer empathic support that encourages the unique development of the individual.

Nursing phenomena, those things that nurses think are important and to which they must pay close attention, are experienced as nurturing, being nurtured, or the process between these two reference points: "It is a quality of being that is expressed in the doing" (Paterson & Zderad, 1988, p. 13). While other theories of nursing may focus on what the nurse does *to* or *for* the client, humanistic nursing focuses on the intersubjective experience. The most important activity for the nurse to engage in may be the use of self, or presence with the client. **Presence** is the activity of being physically present with another person that begins with the nurse's genuine commitment to caring and nurturing the potential of the client. The nurse must hold the belief that an authentic interaction between nurse and client is a valuable opportunity to develop human potential. Communicating caring is the essence of nursing based on this belief and theory. From an existential viewpoint, every action that a nurse takes in relation to the client is a unique event. It is shaped by the experiences and expectations of the individuals relating to one another within the context of nurturing and being nurtured. The physical needs of the client are of basic concern to the nurse. How the client experiences his body, its functioning, and its relationship with the environment are of fundamental importance to the nursing relationship. The nurse is concerned with the client's

BOX 24-1
HUMANISTIC NURSING BEHAVIORS

1. The nurse introduces herself to the client and refers to the client by name. The use of names supports the dignity, worth, and individual identity of the client and is essential for an authentic subject-subject relationship.
2. The nurse provides information about the client's situation as it is sought by the client or when the nurse perceives the client is puzzled about what is happening. This action on the part of the nurse is based on the existential belief that the client has the right to know and make choices about his own life, and such choices are shaped by honest information.
3. The nurse accepts the client's expression of feelings by verbalizing this acceptance when appropriate. This also validates that the client has a right to feelings and can learn appropriate ways to express feelings.
4. The nurse accepts the client's expression of feelings by staying with the client or doing something for the client when a verbal expression of acceptance by the nurse is not appropriate. The message conveyed here is that the feeling the client is experiencing is valid, but a better method of expressing the feeling is socially desirable. By remaining with the client, the nurse validates the feeling and may model a more appropriate behavioral expression.
5. The nurse expresses authentic positive feelings for the client when appropriate. The purpose of this action is to refute negative self-concepts that the client may hold.
6. The nurse supports the client's rights to have loving relationships with family members, staff, and other clients.
7. The nurse shows respect for clients as persons who have rights to make choices as their capabilities permit.
8. The nurse helps clients consider current expression of feelings and behaviors in the light of previous life experiences. This behavior enables clients to formulate self-understanding by recognition of patterns that may be helpful or unhelpful to their healing.
9. The nurse encourages clients to express themselves openly so that the nurse can respond in a helpful and therapeutic manner.
10. The nurse verifies the intuitive grasp of how the client experiences events by asking questions and making comments to the client, and then observing the client's response.
11. The nurse encourages realistic (not false) hope through discussing the positive outcomes that might occur if the client were to engage in a therapeutic opportunity.
12. The nurse supports the client's self-image with concrete examples.

Adapted from *Humanistic Nursing*, by J. G. Paterson and L. T. Zderad, 1988, New York: National League of Nursing.

unique expression of the body related to its position in time and space.

When the nurse goes beyond being an object within the perceptual field of the client, there is an opportunity for the nurse to express authentic presence. The nurse must maintain the commitment to care and to be open to experience the dialogue with the client. The commitment to care and to nurture is accompanied by "a sense of responsibility or regard for what is seen as the patient's vulnerability" (Paterson & Zderad, 1988, p. 28). The dialogue that unfolds between client and nurse represents what Paterson and Zderad refer to as a "call and response" (p. 29). The client calls for nursing care with an expectation that care will be provided or an unmet need will be satisfied. The nurse responds with the intention of providing the care or satisfying the unmet need.

Paterson and Zderad (1988) outline 12 behaviors that nurses perform in providing comfort to a client. These are directly applicable to the nursing care of the adolescent with a psychiatric mental health problem and are outlined in Box 24-1.

Case Example 24-1 an application of these 12 behaviors in providing nursing care for Juanita, a 14-year-old Hispanic girl who was hospitalized in an adolescent psychiatric hospital for an eating disorder, Anorexia Nervosa. Juanita's primary nurse exhibited these behaviors on Juanita's admission to the unit.

Health as Expanding Consciousness

The nursing theory of Margaret Newman (1994), offers a similar view of the relationship between client and nurse. This theory may be of special relevance for the adolescent who suffers from a diagnosed mental illness such as depression or Conduct Disorder. Rather than viewing disease as an objective entity, Newman conceptualizes disease within the whole person and focuses on the pattern that the individual expresses within the environment. Human health is an experience of consciousness that follows a rhythmic pattern of order and disorder. Disease is not something to get rid of, but something to incorporate into one's understanding of self.

Nursing care given within Newman's framework focuses on helping the client to experience congruence between emotional and physical feelings. As in humanistic nursing, the nurse offers *presence* to the client by being physically and emotionally committed to the client through an authentic relationship. When working with a hospitalized adolescent, the focus of nursing is not on treatment of the disease but on helping the client understand the meaning of his pattern of health and how it fits into the scheme of the universe. Nursing is an expression of caring for the client, whatever manifestation of health is present.

The adolescent client who is depressed is manifesting a particular pattern or expression of how she fits into the world. Through a caring relationship, the nurse helps the client to expand her consciousness about this unique experience. By listening to the client's words and nonverbal communication, the nurse can help the adolescent to connect

CASE EXAMPLE 24-1

Juanita

Introduction

"Hi, Juanita, may I call you that? My name is Ann and I will be your nurse until 11 o'clock tonight."

Information

"I would like to show you around the unit and tell you about our routines here. We think it is important for you to know about us as we also try to learn what can be helpful to you. I hope you understand that any time you have questions about what is happening here, you can ask me or any of the other nurses."

Accepting Feelings

After Ann makes the previous statements, Juanita stomps her feet, pulls her hair, and says, "I don't want to know anything about this place and I don't want to be here!" Ann responds, "Juanita, I understand that you are frustrated and angry about being in the hospital. I hope you will continue to tell us how you feel about yourself and your treatment here. We will help you find more ways to express your feelings directly so you won't have to feel like pulling your hair and stomping your feet so hard."

Staying with the Client

Ann points to two chairs and a sofa in the recreation room and says to Juanita, "I would like to spend a few more minutes with you. Would you care to sit in a chair or on the sofa?"

Authentic Positive Feelings

Juanita shrugs her shoulders, then flops down on the sofa, looking at the floor and folding her arms across her chest. Ann responds, "Thank you for taking the time to be with me. It really helps me to do my job if I can get to know you a little better. I think you have a beautiful name. Is there a story behind it?"

Support Loving Relationships

Juanita is silent for a few seconds, then shrugs her shoulders again and says softly, "I was named after my grandmother." Ann says, "You must feel very special to have a family with such traditions. Tell me more about your grandmother."

Respect for Choices

Juanita's posture relaxes a little. She begins to confide slowly, "Yeah, I like my grandmother, but she lives in Mexico. I wish I could live with her instead of with my mom and step-dad." Ann responds, "It sounds

(Continues)

CASE EXAMPLE 24-1 (Continued)

as if you have given this some thought. What do you think would be best about living with your grandmother?"

Previous Life Experiences

Juanita says, "She doesn't hassle me. My folks just hassle me all the time. Grandmother just likes me the way I am." Ann replies, "It sounds as if some things have happened with your family that make you feel frustrated and angry."

Encourages Open Expression

Juanita unfolds her arms and pounds her fists firmly into the sofa cushions. "No kidding! Sometimes I just wish I could hit them [parents], they make me so mad. They just nag at me all the time and they won't listen. They will never understand me the way Grandmother does."

Intuitive Grasp

Ann replies, "It seems like you feel misunderstood by your parents and unable to find safe ways to please them."

Encourages Realistic Hope

Ann continues, "I hope we can help you find some new ways to tell your parents how strongly you feel about how they treat you and what you would like for them to change. We have several people on staff here who are pretty good about that. Tell me about some of the ways you have already tried to tell your parents about how they hassle and nag at you."

Encourages Self-image

Juanita begins to glance occasionally at Ann and to list ways in which she has fallen short of pleasing her parents. Ann identifies the strengths in this list of complaints and states, "Juanita, what you are telling me is that you are a good student even though you don't make straight A's and that you are also a fine musician even though you didn't make first violin in the orchestra. While you are here I hope we can help you see that these are real positive skills that you have already developed and that you don't have to be so hard on yourself by trying to be perfect."

the emotional feelings to thoughts about self-identity and self-worth. Through mere presence, staying quietly and securely with the client, the nurse affirms the client's right to feel depressed. Through continued interaction, the nurse also assists the adolescent in connecting physical distress, such as inability to sleep or eat, with the emotions and thoughts that may seem disordered and threatening. Throughout the nurse-client interaction, the focus is on the rights of the client to express himself through appropriate feelings and behaviors without the nurse judging them as sick or crazy or wrong. As the client becomes more consciously aware of the connections between emotions, thoughts, and behaviors, the client begins to experience health in a different, and perhaps better, way.

APPLICATION OF THE NURSING PROCESS 24-1

ASSESSMENT

Transitions are of central importance to nursing intervention and care and are therefore necessarily a focus in the assessment of adolescents. Nurses interact frequently with clients during periods of transition, not only in the developmental phase of adolescence but also in transitional situations such as acute illness or death, which may occur at any stage of life. In a comprehensive review of nursing literature on the topic of transitions, Schumacher and Meleis (1994) and Meleis, Sawyer, Im, Messias, & Schumacher, (2000), identified three types of indicators of healthy transitions that can be useful to nurses during the assessment process: subjective well-being, role mastery, and well-being of relationships. In addition, these researchers also identified three nursing measures to assist clients with transitions: assessment of readiness, preparation for transition, and role supplementation. Assessment of readiness includes identifying the meaning of the transitional experience to the client. In the adolescent, for example, the transition from junior high to high school may be desirable or dreaded. Similarly, expectations about the transition may vary from those that are realistic to those that are extremely unrealistic. The adolescent whose expectations are unrealistic is poorly prepared for such a transition. Preparation for the transition includes education and skill development. The developmental phase of adolescence is filled with opportunities to learn and master skills for adult living. Role supplementation provides additional experience in mastering skills required for a healthy transition.

NURSINGTIP 24-3

Assessing Mental Health of Adolescents

The following should be assessed when planning nursing care for the adolescent with a history of physical, emotional, or sexual abuse:

- Experience of flashbacks. These are fragments of memory that may appear suddenly with no conscious forethought.
- Feelings of anger or hostility that are expressed in self-mutilation or threat of injury to others.
- Ability to concentrate on tasks at hand.
- Experiences of amnesia in past or present. These may indicate lack of coherent identity formation due to severe abuse.
- Body memories that interfere with physical examination or development of intimacy with others (e.g., nervous twitches, nausea, pain with no stimuli).
- Withdrawal from social situations, especially those involving close interpersonal contact.
- Lack of appropriate affect (e.g., numb response to painful stimuli).
- Ability to maintain eye contact with another person.
- Feelings of safety and control in social situations.
- Strategies for coping with anxiety-producing situations and memories.

NURSINGTIP 24-4

Working with Adolescents

A nurse working in an alcohol treatment center may be viewed with more credibility if he wears jeans and a sport shirt rather than a suit and tie and introduces himself to his client(s) as Jim rather than as Mr. Brown. Similarly, a sincere effort to understand and use the jargon of adolescents in conversations with clients can convey acceptance. However, the nurse should proceed cautiously so he does not come across to the client as mocking the language or mannerisms of youth. Also, if the nurse is clearly not comfortable with narrowing the gap between age and professional status in this way, the adolescent will quickly recognize this, and credibility will be lost.

(Continues)

APPLICATION OF THE NURSING PROCESS 24-1 (Continued)

Nurses have opportunities to work with adolescents in many settings. For example, the school nurse is in an optimum position to provide education and guidance in promoting positive mental health. The school nurse has the advantage of observing and listening to adolescents in one of their usual social settings and can thus plan and intervene with groups as well as individuals. Nurses may also work with adolescents in health care facilities such as drug treatment and rehabilitation centers, psychiatric hospitals, and general hospitals and clinics. Again, nurses should be well prepared to identify the usual, as well as the more serious, mental health needs of adolescents.

REFLECTIVE THINKING 24-1

The Role of the School Nurse

Imagine that you are the school nurse responsible for maintaining the health records and responding to the health care needs of a suburban middle school. This school is located in a fairly affluent neighborhood and has students who are predominantly Caucasian, Asian, Mexican American, and African American (in decreasing order of prevalence).

- Which transitions of adolescence are you most likely to encounter with these students?
- What mental health care concerns would you be most likely to encounter on a daily basis in this setting?
- What kinds of mental health programs would be appropriate for students in this school?

NURSING DIAGNOSIS

The most common nursing diagnoses seen in adolescents relate to the effects of the developmental changes that the adolescent is experiencing. *Disturbed body image* and *Ineffective role performance* can be common responses from individuals who are struggling to cope with the often overwhelming transitions that occur in the few short years of adolescence. Clients who have suffered abuse may be diagnosed with *Chronic low self-esteem* if they harbor lingering feelings of shame or blame themselves for their past experiences; such a teen will need assistance in exploring the past in an effort to effectively move forward in the present and in developing or realizing a self-concept that is acceptable to his current state of mind. Teens who have been victims of abuse or violence may also exhibit related symptoms, such as *Insomnia* related to memories of abuse as evidenced by anxiety, restlessness, and flashbacks and *Disturbed thought processes* related to past experiences as evidenced by lack of concentration or fear of being victimized.

Adolescents are also particularly vulnerable to experiencing *Social isolation* or *Impaired social interaction* related to past experiences, comfort level with peers, and self-perception of abilities in social contexts. These individuals will need interventions designed to focus on their positive qualities while developing skills that will help them achieve their desired level of social integration.

OUTCOME IDENTIFICATION

Identifying outcomes for adolescents receiving mental health care is critical for developing an attainable and realistic plan of care. The first step typically involves having the adolescent acknowledge the need for care and agreeing to be a partner in that care. Mutually outlining targeted outcomes respects the adolescent's independence while providing needed guidance; it also ensures that the adolescent's expectations of progress and success will be realistic and in line with what is likely to occur.

The nurse must be careful to ensure that outcomes are realizable in terms of the targeted mental health state that the client is capable of achieving and that appropriate time frames are identified. Goals that are realistic and attainable ensure success, while goals that are long term and ambiguous may contribute to greater anxiety and confusion.

PLANNING/INTERVENTIONS

Nursing science remains in a state of infancy concerning which interventions work and which do not for many mental health needs of adolescents. In general, however, interventions that are based on a sincere

(*Continues*)

APPLICATION OF THE NURSING PROCESS 24-1 (Continued)

interest in and respect for the adolescent as an individual and adolescence as a genuine phase of development will be most helpful. When working with young adolescents in particular, the nurse should be as concrete as possible in providing information about treatment plans and in communicating expectations about behavior. To enhance the chances of success, the nurse should find out about the adolescent's interests and favorite activities when planning interventions. Activities that are managed by the adolescent, such as keeping a journal, listening to music, and practicing guided imagery, may be most appropriate for individuals who need to maintain a feeling of control. Adolescents needing assistance in role identity and self-confidence may find reassurance with a nurse and family who help set limits and offer guidance.

Meeting the mental health needs of children and adolescents provides a unique challenge to nursing and other health care professions. As society becomes more complex with rapid changes in technology, the adolescent faces an increasingly difficult crisis in forging an identity that incorporates skills for survival and for finding meaning and purpose in life. Research is needed to identify the genetic and environmental influences on adolescent development and behavior. Strategies must be developed to strengthen the family, school, and community interactions with youth in assisting them with the crisis of identity formation. Multidisciplinary interventions that are culturally appropriate must be investigated to promote optimum physical and mental health for youth in the second decade of life.

Longitudinal studies need to be done to explore how cognitive, emotional, and social transitions are experienced relative to health (National Institute of Nursing Research, 1993). The influence of peers in developing health-promoting lifestyles and in reducing high-risk behaviors also needs to be studied. Nurses in school- and community-based clinics have a tremendous responsibility for identifying the mental health care problems and needs of adolescents and in proposing innovative ways to provide useful services.

EVALUATION

When evaluating the success of the nursing care plan and the effectiveness of the interventions, the nurse should look at the progress the teen has made toward realizing the targeted outcomes that were mutually agreed on. Successes can be judged in increments and should be shared with the adolescent and family so that all can feel a sense of accomplishment. If certain goals are not met, the nurse, adolescent, and family should jointly review what the expectations were at the outset of care and reassess how realistic the targeted goals were. An evaluation of resources available and family support may also indicate additional areas that could be called on to increase chances of success in reaching goals.

NURSING CARE PLAN: NURSING PROCESS FORMAT 24-1

The following case study is based on a fictionalized account of an adolescent client who presents with a history of emotional, physical and sexual abuse.

ASSESSMENT

Sally is a 15-year-old high school junior who was sexually abused by her stepfather between the ages of 6 and 14 years. Last year her mother and stepfather were divorced, and the abuse came to an end. Since that time, Sally has had difficulty sleeping. She awakens nearly every night with nightmares, and sometimes during the day she experiences flashbacks to those nights when her sleep was interrupted by her stepfather's sexual advances. These flashbacks interfere with her school work and she is having increasing difficulty paying attention in school. Sally startles easily when other students move around the classroom, and she avoids talking with boys between classes and after school.

(Continues)

NURSING CARE PLAN: NURSING PROCESS FORMAT 24-1 (Continued)

NURSING DIAGNOSIS 1 *Insomnia*, related to psychological stress, as evidenced by interrupted sleep and nightmares.

OUTCOMES	NIC	NURSING ACTIONS	EVALUATION
• The client will acknowledge that her sleep pattern is disturbed. • The client will verbalize her anxiety and fear about sexual abuse. • The client will identify the daytime flashbacks as memories of childhood sexual abuse. • The client will identify at least two relaxation strategies that will enhance her ability to sleep at night. • The client will practice at least two relaxation strategies.	• Sleep enhancement • Simple relaxation therapy	The nurse will assist the client in acknowledging that her nightmares frighten her and remind her of the past by: • Being present with Sally when she talks about the nightmares and flashbacks. • Using active and empathetic listening. • Communicating her acceptance of Sally regardless of the content of her nightmares. • Teaching Sally two relaxation techniques: (1) using music that she enjoys, and (2) using a mental image she describes as peaceful to her.	At the end of 4 weeks Sally was able to state that she understood the relationship between her nightmares and flashbacks and her memories of sexual abuse as a child. She gradually began to trust the nurse and provided more details of the abuse, which were similar to the images in her nightmares and flashbacks. At first she had difficulty relaxing with music before going to bed, but after 3 weeks she found a recording of flute music that helped her feel calm. Sally also practiced using a mental image of herself resting on a warm beach and reported that this helped her to relax and fall asleep.

NURSING DIAGNOSIS 2 *Social isolation*, related to inability to engage in satisfying personal relationships, as evidenced by insecurity and fear of being alone with others.

OUTCOMES	NIC	NURSING ACTIONS	EVALUATION
• The client will acknowledge her fear of being alone with boys. • The client will state how her current behavior around boys is related to early experiences of abuse. • The client will identify goals for future relationships with boys. • The client will demonstrate at least two ways in which she can feel safe around male peers.	• Socialization enhancement • Hope inspiration	• The nurse supports the client's right to have loving relationships. • The nurse helps Sally consider how her current behavior is related to previous experiences. • The nurse encourages realistic hope for developing healthy relationships outside her family. • The nurse demonstrates two ways in which Sally can feel safe in the company of boys: (1) by	During the first week of treatment, Sally refused to talk about going out with boys, but gradually she began to trust the nurse and to say that she was afraid to be alone with boys but she didn't really know why. During the second week of treatment, the nurse encouraged Sally to identify things about boys that scared her. After making a short list, Sally began to say that she

(Continues)

NURSING CARE PLAN: NURSING PROCESS FORMAT 24-1 (Continued)

OUTCOMES	NIC	NURSING ACTIONS	EVALUATION
		writing self-affirmative statements such as "I am respectable and have a right to say no about anything that makes me uncomfortable," and (2) by role playing a situation in which she will say to a boy, "I do not want to be alone with you right now, I feel uncomfortable." • The nurse facilitates Sally's self-understanding by describing the pattern of current behavior as it relates to fear of childhood abuse.	thought she was afraid they would harm her the way her stepfather had. During the third and fourth weeks, Sally began talking daily with the nurse about her fear of boys and how they might harm her. She also wrote self-affirmations daily and reported that this made her feel stronger and more secure. She role-played affirmations with the female nurse, and at the end of 4 weeks asked if she could role-play with a male nurse or doctor.

NURSING DIAGNOSIS 3 *Disturbed thought processes*, related to previous experiences of abuse, as evidenced by distractibility.

OUTCOMES	NIC	NURSING ACTIONS	EVALUATION
• The client will state how difficult it is for her to feel safe in the classroom. • The client will identify how her lack of concentration is related to her fear of being victimized. • The client will demonstrate at least two ways in which she can concentrate on material presented in the classroom. • The client will feel more relaxed in a classroom setting.	• Emotional support • Anxiety reduction • Calming technique	• The nurse will encourage Sally to verbalize her feelings about paying attention in the classroom through the nurse's presence and active listening. • The nurse will assist Sally in connecting her feelings to past experiences of abuse and her need to be vigilant. • The nurse will assist Sally in increasing her concentration through meditation and relaxation exercises.	During the first week, Sally had difficulty paying attention to what the nurse was saying to her. As the nurse continued to remain with her, Sally began to tell the nurse that she was confused about what she should be doing at school. In the second week of treatment, the nurse taught Sally progressive relaxation exercise, and while she was relaxed, Sally began to relate her thoughts about being a bad person and deserving the abuse. By the end of the fourth week, she was able to practice progressive relaxtion on her own and was able to sit for a period of 30 minutes and read without being startled.

(Continues)

NURSING CARE PLAN: NURSING PROCESS FORMAT 24-1 (Continued)

NURSING DIAGNOSIS 4 *Chronic low self-esteem*, related to sexual abuse, as evidenced by feelings of shame/guilt.

OUTCOMES	NIC	NURSING ACTIONS	EVALUATION
• The client will verbalize her feelings about the sexual abuse. • The client will state with conviction that she was not to blame for the abuse. • The client will identify at least two ways in which she can share her feelings with her mother. • The client will demonstrate at least two behaviors that reflect a positive self-image.	• Self-esteem enhancement • Coping enhancement • Counseling	• The nurse will encourage the client to express her feelings orally (through the nurse's active listening), in writing (in a daily journal), and by sculpting clay. • The nurse will acknowledge that the client's feelings are appropriate and will not judge her. • The nurse will role-play with the client ways in which she can tell her mother about her feelings about the abuse and about herself. • The nurse will reflect to the client the client's ability to express herself appropriately in writing, speaking, and sculpting.	At the end of the first week of treatment, Ms. Ivanhoe was writing in her journal daily and beginning to state how she felt about herself and her responsibility for allowing her stepfather to abuse her. By the end of the third week, she had made six clay sculptures of her as a small helpless child and increasing in size and strength to portray herself as a mature and capable young woman. Ms. Ivanhoe role-played with the nurse how to talk to her mother, and at the end of 4 weeks asked the nurse to help her confront her mother with her feelings.

REFLECTIVE QUESTIONS

1. **ASSESSMENT**
   What additional information might the nurse need to plan more comprehensive and holistic care for this client? What other health care team members should be brought into the assessment loop?
2. **NURSING DIAGNOSIS**
   What other nursing diagnoses might be made in this situation?
3. **OUTCOMES**
   How realistic are these outcomes? What would the nurse do if the client could not concentrate or trust the nurse enough to participate in setting goals for nursing care? What additional outcomes might be met as the client began to respond to the nurse? How would the outcomes change if the client did not feel that she could trust the nurse?
4. **NURSING ACTIONS**
   What specific skills does the nurse need to care for this client? How can previous experiences of the nurse help or hinder her ability to care for this client? What kind of environment will facilitate these nursing interventions?
5. **EVALUATION**
   What kind of outcomes might have been achieved if the nurse had only a few days to work with this client? How might the outcomes have been different if the primary nurse had gone on a two-week vacation in the middle of Ms. Ivanhoe's treatment? What can the nurse do to reinforce her care plan after the client leaves the treatment facility?

KEY CONCEPTS

- Adolescence is a transitional phase of development, with significant changes occurring in physical, emotional, cognitive, and social dimensions.
- Identity formation is a major developmental task for the adolescent.
- Positive mental health is optimal psychosocial competence or well-being.
- Mental health concerns in adolescence include diagnosable problems such as depression and Conduct Disorder, as well as distress related to cognitive, emotional, and social transitions.
- Adolescents at highest risk for mental health problems are from families in which at least one parent has a history of alcoholism, drug use, suicide attempts, antisocial behavior, and/or violence.
- Poverty also places adolescents at risk for mental health problems including dropping out of school, gang involvement, and substance abuse.
- Sexual development, identity, and orientation are issues central to the mental health of adolescents.
- Suicidal ideation and behavior are the most serious outcomes related to adolescent mental health problems and may be related to childhood abuse, neglect, and homelessness.
- Nursing interventions for adolescents with mental health problems are based on developing an authentic caring relationship between nurse and client, and on increasing the adolescent's conscious awareness of connections between experiences, feelings, and behaviors.

REVIEW QUESTIONS

1. A 16-year-old admitted with a diagnosis of Conduct Disorder is watching television in the dayroom when the night nurse comes on duty. When questioned about this behavior, the adolescent states, "The other nurse let's me stay up as long as I want." The most appropriate response by the nurse is which of the following?
1. I know you must be lying about that nurse
2. Well, unfortunately I'm not the other nurse
3. Watching television in the dayroom after 9 P.M. is against the rules
4. That nurse is new and she doesn't understand the rules for this unit

2. An adolescent is admitted to the unit for treatment. He has been referred by his high school counselor because of truancy, stealing, bullying other students, and smoking marijuana on school grounds. Once admitted to the unit, the client begins to agitate the staff and other clients with his behavior. The most appropriate action for the nurse is which of the following:
1. Discuss the unit rules and consequences for breaking unit rules
2. Place the teen in seclusion so he won't upset others on the unit
3. Tell the client that if he cannot control his behavior, he will be placed in restraints
4. Ignore the behavior and tell the staff "kids will be kids"

3. The nursing care plan for an adolescent admitted to a psychiatric unit should include which of the following?
1. The nurse should do all of the planning
2. Allow the adolescent to decide what should be done
3. Include the adolescent and parents in the planning process
4. Allow the parents to formulate the plan because they know what is best

4. A teenager is admitted to the hospital after inhaling glue with his classmates. Which of the following would the nurse expect to uncover during the assessment?
1. Nausea, vomiting, and slurred speech, and delusions
2. Aggressiveness, apathy, poor judgment, and hallucinations
3. Unsteady gait, diaphoresis, tachycardia, and hallucinations
4. Diaphoresis, nausea, headaches, vomiting, and hallucinations

5. A 15-year-old boy is hospitalized on a psychiatric unit after experiencing severe depression. During a one-to-one session with the boy, he states to the nurse, "I don't want anyone to know I'm here. It is embarrassing to be considered a nut case." Understanding the boy's developmental stage, the nurse would be correct that the boy is most likely referring to which of the following individuals?
1. Parents
2. Peer group
3. Teachers
4. Church members

6. A 13-year-old is admitted to the behavioral unit in a local mental health facility. The girl refuses to bathe and participate in any unit activities. The priority response by the nurse would be which of the following?

1. Set firm limits on the client's behavior
2. Place the client in restraints until she cooperates
3. Tell other clients to invite the girl to a group meeting
4. Contact the girl's parents and inform them of her behavior

7. A 16-year-old male client is in his bed masturbating. The nurse who entered the room without knocking observes the activity. What should the nurse do next?
1. Refer the client to a sex therapist
2. Leave the room without saying anything
3. Inform the parents of the client's behavior
4. Warn the client that his behavior is inappropriate

8. The mother of a 14-year-old calls the mental health clinic because she found pornographic pictures on his computer and several *Playboy* magazines under his bed. The mother states to the nurse, "I don't want my son to become a sex addict. I don't know why he is looking at such trash. Can someone at the clinic talk to him?" Which response by the nurse would be most therapeutic?
1. Coach the mother on ways to discuss the issue with her son
2. Schedule the mother and her son for an appointment in the clinic
3. The nurse should state, "Did you provide sex education for your son?"
4. Tell the mother to ask the school health teacher to meet with the son

LEARNING ACTIVITIES

1. How might the difference between an adolescent's subjective feeling of mental health and a mental health professional's (e.g., school counselor) definition of mental health lead to conflict between these two individuals?
2. What effect could an adolescent's relocation from Texas to New Jersey during high school have on that person's identity formation?
3. How might a person's experiences with emotional abuse in childhood affect his feelings of self-efficacy or competence as an adolescent?
4. How did your personal experiences with peers' evaluations during adolescence contribute to your role as an adult?
5. What are the effects of loneliness on the adolescent?
6. How can Paterson and Zderad's theory of humanistic nursing help you plan your interactions with adolescent clients?
7. How can Newman's theory of health as expanding consciousness help you to understand mental health in adolescents?
8. List the various nursing interventions that might be helpful to an adolescent who is struggling with identity formation.

*Study*WARE™ CONNECTION

Using your *Study*WARE™ CD-ROM

1. Complete the Concentration activity for this chapter.
2. Review the audio glossary for key terms in this chapter.
3. Explore the other games and activities that support this chapter.

REFERENCES

American Academy of Pediatrics. *Bright futures guidelines* (3rd ed.). Retrieved August 1, 2009, from: http://brightfutures.aap.org/pdfs/Health_Promotion_Information_Sheets/mentalhealth.pdf.

American Psychiatric Association. (2000). *Diagnostic and statistical manual of mental disorders* (Fourth Edition-Text Revision). Washington, DC: Author.

Auslander, B. A., Rosenthal, S. L., & Blythe, M. J. (2005). Sexual development and behaviors of adolescents. *Pediatric Annals, 34*, 785–793.

Bandura, A. (1997). *Self-efficacy: The exercise of control.* New York: W. H. Freeman.

Bandura, A., & Locke, E. A. (2003). Negative self-efficacy and goal effects revisited. *Journal of Applied Psychology, 88*(1), 87–99.

Blyth, D. A., & Leffert, N. (1995). Communities as contexts for adolescent development: An empirical analysis. *Journal of Adolescent Research, 10*(1), 64–87.

Brage, D., Meredith, W., & Woodward, J. (1993). Correlates of loneliness among Midwestern adolescents. *Adolescence, 28*, 685–693.

Byrnes, J. P. (2002). The development of decision-making. *Journal of Adolescent Health, 31*(6S), 208–215.

Centers for Disease Control and Prevention. (2008). Healthy youth! August 16, 2008, from: http://www.cdc.gov/HealthyYouth/health topics/index.htm on August 16, 2008.

Compas, B. E. (1993). Promoting positive mental health during adolescence. In S. G. Millstein, A. C. Petersen, & E. O. Nightingale (Eds.), *Promoting the health of adolescents* (pp. 159–179). New York: Oxford University Press.

De Wilde, E. J., Kienhorst, C. W. M., Diekstra, R. F. W., & Wolters, W. H. G. (1992). The relationship between adolescent suicidal behavior and life events in childhood and adolescence. *American Journal of Psychiatry, 149*(1), 45–51.

Decker-Brown, K. (2003) Humanistic theory information website. http://www.humanisticnursingtheory.com/. Accessed August 13, 2009.

Dishion, T. J., Nelson, S. E., & Yasui, M. (2005). Predicting early adolescent gang involvement from middle school adaptation. *Journal of Clinical Child and Adolescent Psychology, 34*(1), 62–73.

Dumont, L. (1991). *Surviving adolescence: Helping your child through the struggle to adulthood.* New York: Villard Books.

Erikson, E. (1950). *Childhood and society.* New York: W. W. Norton.

Erikson, E. (1968). *Identity: Youth and crisis.* New York: W. W. Norton.

Ferguson, J. (1993). Youth at the threshold of the 21st century: The demographic situation. *Journal of Adolescent Health, 14,* 638–644.

Gardner, M., & Steinberg, L. (2005). Peer influence on risk taking, risk preference, and risky decision making in adolescence and adulthood: An experimental study. *Developmental Psychology, 41,* 625–635.

Giedd, J. N. (2008). The teen brain: Insights from neuroimaging. *Journal of Adolescent Health, 42,* 335–343.

Hoberman, H. M. (1995). *Suicide and depression in children and adolescents: Clinical characteristics, assessment, and intervention approaches.* Lecture in Child and Adolescent Psychiatry, University of Minnesota School of Medicine,, September 23, 1995.

Jessor, R. (1991). Risk behavior in adolescence: A psychosocial framework for understanding and action. *Journal of Adolescent Health Care, 12,* 597–605.

Joffe, A., & Morris, R.E. (2008). Adolescent substance use and abuse. In L. S. Neinstein (Ed.), *Adolescent health care: A practical guide* (5th ed., pp. 863–877). Philadelphia: Wolters Kluwer/Lippincott Williams & Wilkins.

Josselson, R. (1994). The theory of identity development and the question of intervention. In S. L. Archer (Ed.), *Interventions for adolescent identity development* (pp. 12–25). Thousand Oaks, CA: Sage Publications.

Kaestle, C. E., Halpern, C. T., & Brown, J. D. (2007). Music videos, pro wrestling, and acceptance of date rape among middle school males and females: An exploratory analysis. *Journal of Adolescent Health, 40,* 185–187.

Kazdin, A. E. (1993). Adolescent mental health: Prevention and treatment programs. *American Psychologist, 48,* 127–141.

Kutcher, S., & Chehil, S. (2008). Adolescent depression and anxiety disorders. In L. S. Neinstein (Ed.), *Adolescent health care: A practical guide* (5th ed., pp. 994–1017). Philadelphia: Wolters Kluwer/Lippincott Williams & Wilkins.

Marcia, J. E. (1994). Identity and psychotherapy. In S. L. Archer (Ed.), *Interventions for adolescent identity development* (pp. 29–46). Thousand Oaks, CA: Sage Publications.

Meininger, E., & Remafedi, G. (2008). Gay, lesbian, bisexual and transgender adolescents. In L. S. Neinstein (Ed.), *Adolescent health care: A practical guide* (5th ed., pp. 554–561). Philadelphia: Wolters Kluwer/Lippincott Williams & Wilkins.

Meleis, A. I., Sawyer, L. M., Im, E-O., Messias, D. K. H., & Schumacher, K. (2000). Experiencing transitions: An emerging middle-range theory. *Advances in Nursing Science, 23*(1), 12–28.

Meschke, L. L., & Patterson, J. M. (2003). Resilience as a theoretical basis for substance abuse prevention. *Journal of Primary Prevention, 23,* 483–514.

Millstein, S. G., Irwin, C. E., & Brindis, C. D. (1991). Sociodemographic trends and projections in the adolescent population. In W. R. Hendee (Ed.), *The health of adolescents* (pp. 1–15). San Francisco: Jossey-Bass.

National Institute of Mental Health. (2001a). *Prevalence of mental disorders in children and adolescents.* http://www.nimh.nih.gov/publicat/childqa/cfm.

National Institute of Mental Health. (2001b). *NIMH Fact Sheet.* http://www.nimh.nih.gov/publicat/depchidresfact.cfm.

National Institute of Nursing Research. (1993). *Health promotion for older children and adolescents.* Report of the NINR Priority Expert Panel on Health Promotion. Bethesda, MD: U.S. Department of Health and Human Services.

Newman, M. A. (1994). *Health as expanding consciousness* (2nd ed.). New York: National League for Nursing Press. Retrieved September 9, 2008 from, http://www.healthasexppandingconsciousness.org/home/retrieved9/.

Paterson, J. G., & Zderad, L. T. (1988). *Humanistic nursing.* New York: National League for Nursing.

Perry, C. L., Kelder, S. H., & Komro, K. A. (1993). The social world of adolescents: Family, peers, schools, and the community. In S. G. Millstein, A. C. Petersen, & E. O. Nightingale (Eds.), *Promoting the health of adolescents* (pp. 73–96). New York: Oxford University Press.

Praeger, S. G., & Hogarth, C. R. (1985). Josephine E. Paterson and Loretta T. Zderad. In J. B. George (Ed.), *Nursing theories* (2nd ed., pp. 287–299). Englewood Cliffs, NJ: Prentice-Hall.

Resnick, M. D., Bearman, P. S., Blum, R. W., Bauman, K. E., Harris, K. M., Jones, J., et al. (1997). Protecting adolescents from harm: Findings from the National Longitudinal Study on Adolescent Health. *Journal of the American Medical Association, 178,* 823–832.

Rich, A. R., Kirkpatrick-Smith, J., Bonner, R. L., & Jans, F. (1992). Gender differences in the psychosocial correlates of suicidal ideation among adolescents. *Suicide and Life-Threatening Behavior, 22,* 364–373.

Rickert, V. I., Ryan, O., & Chacko, M. R. (2008). Sexual assault and victimization. In L. S. Neinstein (Ed.), *Adolescent health care: A practical guide* (5th ed., pp. 1042–1055). Philadelphia: Wolters Kluwer/Lippincott Williams & Wilkins.

Sanchez, R. B., Waller, M. W., Green, J. M. (2006). Who runs? A demographic profile of runaway youth in the United States. *Journal of Adolescent Health, 39*(5), 778–781

Saunders, S. M., Resnick, M. D., Hoberman, H. M., & Blum, R. W. (1994). Formal help-seeking behavior of adolescents identifying themselves as having mental health problems. *Journal of the American Academy of Child and Adolescent Psychiatry, 33,* 718–728.

Schorr, L. B. (1998). *Within our reach: Breaking the cycle of disadvantage.* New York: Anchor/Doubleday.

Schumacher, K. L., & Meleis, A. I. (1994). Transitions: A central concept in nursing. *IMAGE: Journal of Nursing Scholarship, 26,* 119–127.

Search Institute (2002). *The asset approach.* Minneapolis, MN: Search Institute.

Sherer, S. (2008). Suicide. In L. S. Neinstein (Ed.), *Adolescent health care: A practical guide* (5th ed., pp. 1018–026). Philadelphia: Wolters Kluwer/Lippincott Williams & Wilkins.

Steinberg, L. (1996) *Adolescence* (4th ed.). New York: McGraw-Hill.

Taylor, W. N.(2002) *Anabolic Steroids and the Athlete* (2nd ed.) Jefferson, NC: McFarland.

Telljohann, S. K., Price, J. H., Summers, J., Everett, S. A., & Casler, S. (1995). High school students' perceptions of nonconsensual sexual activity. *Journal of School Health, 65,* 107–112.

Terrell, N. E. (1997). Street life: Aggravated and sexual assaults among homeless and runaway adolescents. *Youth & Society, 28,* 267–290.

Thatcher, W. G., Reininger, B. M., & Drane, J. W. (2002). Using path analysis to examine adolescent suicide attempts, life satisfaction, and health risk behavior. *Journal of School Health, 72*(2), 71–77.

Treadway, L., & Yoakam, J. (1992). Creating a safer school environment for lesbian and gay students. *Journal of School Health, 62,* 352–357.

Twenge, J. M., Baumeister, R. F., DeWall, C. N., Ciarocco, N. J., & Bartels, J. M. (2007). Social exclusion decreases prosocial behavior. *Journal of Personality and Social Psychology, 92*(1), 56–66.

Tyler, K. A., Cauce, A. M., & Whitbeck, L. (2004). Family risk factors and prevalence of dissociative symptoms among homeless and runaway youth. *Child Abuse & Neglect, 28,* 355–366.

Vandemark, L. M. (2006). Awareness of self and expanding consciousness: Using nursing theories to prepare nurse-therapists. *Issues in Mental Health Nursing, 27,* 605–615.

Vernon, M. E. L. (1991). Life-style, risk taking, and out-of-control behavior. In W. R. Hendee (Ed.), *The health of adolescents* (pp. 162–185). San Francisco: Jossey-Bass.

Whitbeck, L. B., Johnson, K. D., Hoyt, D. R., & Cauce, M. A. (2004). Mental disorder and comorbidity among runaway and homeless adolescents. *Journal of Adolescent Health, 35,* 132–140.

LITERARY REFERENCES

Blume, J. (1973). *Deenie.* New York: Dell.

Neufeld, J. (1970). *Lisa, bright and dark.* New York: Penguin Books.

SUGGESTED READINGS

Abram, K. M., Choe, J. Y., Washburn, J. J., Teplin, L. A., King, D. C., & Dulcan, M. K. (2008). Suicidal ideation and behaviors among youths in juvenile detention. *Journal of the Academy of Child and Adolescent Psychiatry, 47,* 291–300.

Atkins, R. (2007). The association of personality type in childhood with violence in adolescence. *Research in Nursing & Health, 30,* 308–319.

Belfer, M. L. (2008). Child and adolescent mental disorders: The magnitude of the problem across the globe. *Journal of Child Psychology and Psychiatry, 49,* 226–236.

Bossarte, R. M., Simon, T. R., & Swahn, M. H. (2008). Clustering of adolescent dating violence, peer violence, and suicidal behavior. *Journal of Interpersonal Violence, 23,* 815–833.

Fothergill, K. E., & Ensminger, M. E. (2006). Childhood and adolescent antecedents of drug and alcohol problems: A longitudinal study. *Drug and Alcohol Dependence, 82,* 61–76.

Gwadz, M. V., Nish, D., Leonard, N. R., & Strauss, S. M. (2007). Gender differences in traumatic events and rates of post-traumatic stress disorder among homeless youth. *Journal of Adolescence, 30,* 117–129.

Klomek, A. B., Marrocco, F., Kleinman, M., Schonfeld, I. S., & Gould M. S. (2008). Peer victimization, depression, and suicidality in adolescents. *Suicide and Life-threatening Behavior, 38,* 166–180.

Levy, S., & Woolf, A. D. (2008). Psychoactive substances of abuse used by adolescents. In L. S. Neinstein (Ed.), *Adolescent health care: A practical guide* (5th ed., pp. 908–940). Philadelphia: Wolters Kluwer/Lippincott Williams & Wilkins.

Measelle, J. R., Stice, E., & Hogansen, J. M. (2006). Developmental trajectories of co-occurring depressive, eating, antisocial, and substance abuse problems in female adolescents. *Journal of Abnormal Psychology, 115,* 524–538.

Rew, L. (2007). What's so special about adolescence? *Issues in Mental Health Nursing, 28,* 3–5.

Rew, L., & Bowman, K. (2008). Protecting youth from early and abusive sexual experiences. *Pediatric Nursing, 34*(1), 19–25.

Schinke, S. P., Fang, L., & Cole, K. C. A. (2008). Substance use among early adolescent girls: Risk and protective factors. *Journal of Adolescent Health, 43,* 191–194.

U.S. Department of Health and Human Services, Centers for Disease Control and Prevention. (2008). *Adolescent health in the United States, 2007.* DHHS Pub. No. (PHS) 2008-1034. Hyattsville, MD: National Center for Health Statistics.

U.S. Department of Health and Human Services, Center for Mental Health Services (2004). *Building bridges: Co-occurring mental illness and addiction: Consumers and service providers, policymakers, and researchers in dialogue.* DHHS Pub. No. (SMA) 04-3892. Rockville, MD: Substance Abuse and Mental Health Services Administration.

Witte, T. K., Merrill, K. A., Stellrecht, N. E., Bernert, R. A., Hollar, D. L., Schatschneider, C., & Joiner, T. E. Jr. (2008). "Impulsive" youth suicide attempters are not necessarily all that impulsive. *Journal of Affective Disorders, 107,* 107–116.

RESOURCES FOR ADOLESCENTS WITH MENTAL HEALTH CONCERNS

Academy of Child & Adolescent Psychiatry: http://www.aacap.org/

AIDS Hotline: 1-800-235-2331

Boys Town National Hotline (for teens dealing with stress): 1-800-448-1833.

National Gay and Lesbian Task Force (NGLTF): www.thetaskforce.org

Suicide Hotline: 1-800-SUICIDE

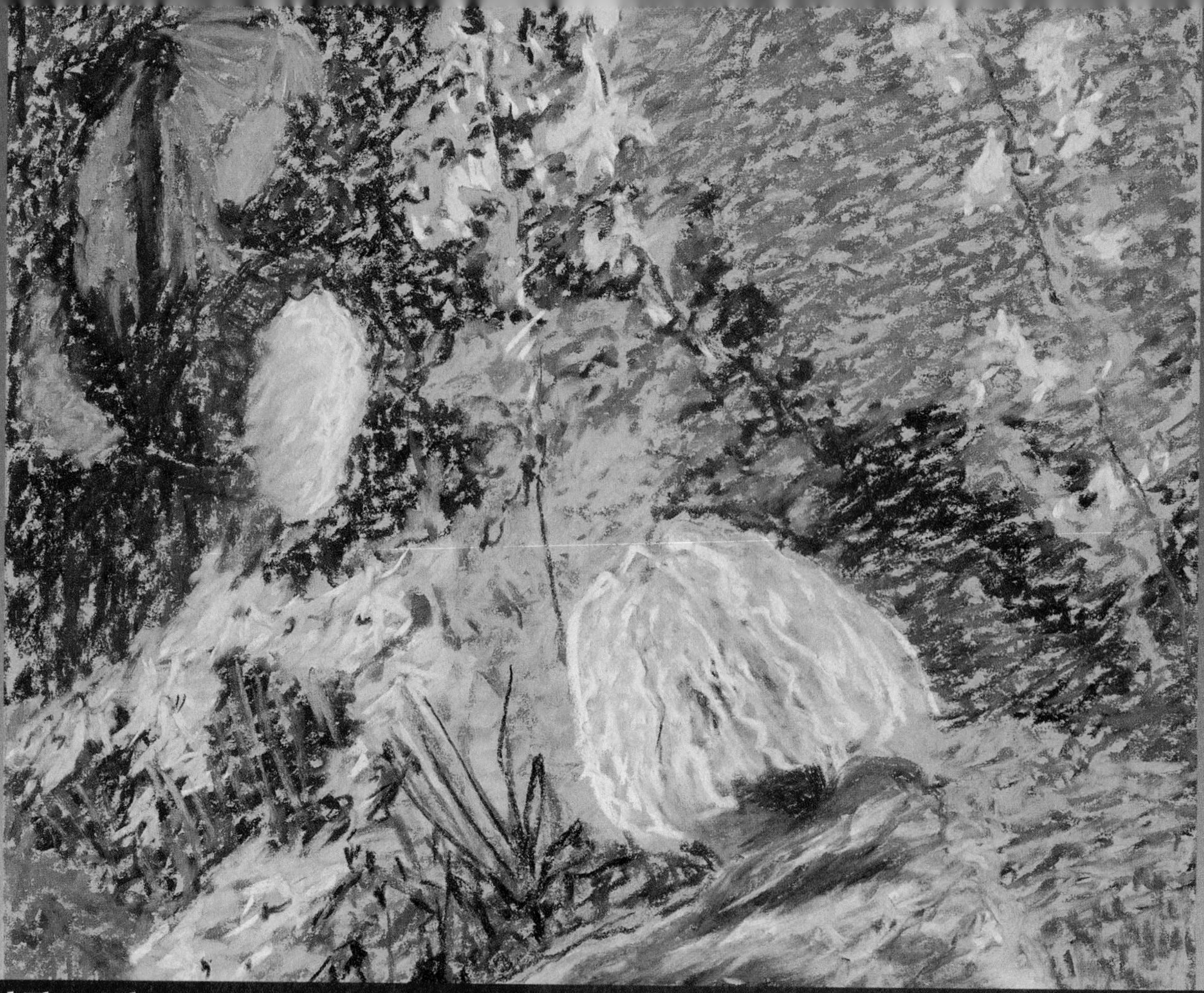

The Person Within

Consider the following situations and how they might change your perception of who you are:

- ***How would you feel if you woke up tomorrow and realized that no one was still alive who had known you as a child?***
- ***Choose a residence, three favorite possessions, and three characteristics that you would like to have into your old age. Now imagine that these are all suddenly taken away from you; how would you feel?***
- ***Suppose you gradually start losing things several times a day at home, at school, or at work. Your friends and family tell you it must just be stress but you feel that something else is wrong. Your doctor tells you that you need to "get more rest." Your mental function continues to deteriorate until you are totally dependent on someone else for dressing, bathing, and eating. You do not recognize any of your friends or family and are only able to mumble "Take me home ... I don't live here ... I need to go home." What would your emotional response be?***

Many individuals find themselves in such situations as they age; reflect on these as you read this chapter.

CHAPTER 25

The Elderly

Brenda P. Johnson

CHAPTER OUTLINE

COMPETENCIES

Upon completion of this chapter, the reader should be able to:

1. Recognize the interconnected role that physical health and family support systems play in the mental health of older adults.
2. Identify pathological processes that are responsible for the disorders of cognition and affect most commonly seen in the older adult.
3. Analyze how ageist stereotypes and socioeconomic factors affect the occurrence of mental illness in the elderly.
4. Describe the most common physiological causes of delirium in the elderly.
5. Envision and describe ways in which severe memory loss poses a challenge to self-concept and human dignity.
6. Propose nursing interventions for demented elders and their caregivers that are derived from a caring framework.
7. Identify environmental and physiological risk factors for depression in the elderly.
8. Explain the basis for treatment modalities of depression in older adults.

KEY TERMS

Agnosia
Aphasia
Apraxia
Catastrophic Reaction
Cognition
Confabulation
Confusion
Delirium
Dementia
Mutuality

History has given us countless examples of powerful, creative, and productive elders. Michelangelo was appointed chief architect of St. Peter's Cathedral in Rome at the age of 71, and over the next 18 years, until his death at 89, he personally supervised the creation of the vast main body of the church. Picasso was painting until the day he died, at the age of 91. And Mary Baker Eddy, at the age of 89, was still the leader of the Christian Science Church (Dychtwald, 1989).

The "elderly" are often characterized as anyone over the age of 65. However, life as experienced by an 85-year-old is often as different from the experience of a 65-year-old as is an adolescent's from a child's. The significance of differentiating the "old-old" from the "young-old" is heightened by the growing numbers of the very old. Persons 85 years of age and older (old-old) constitute the fastest growing segment of the U.S. population. While the percentage of those over 65 has more than tripled since 1900, the 85 and older group was over 35 times larger in 2000 than in 1900. The number of centenarians also is steadily growing. There were 50,545 persons over 100 years old in 2000, a 35% increase from the number in 1900 (Administration on Aging [AOA], 2002b). In many respects, the oldest old are quite different from younger old people in that they have outlived the life expectancy of their generation.

While old age is not synonymous with illness and disability, the number of chronic illnesses grows steadily with age. Most older persons have at least one chronic illness, such as arthritis, hypertension and heart disease, diabetes, or a hearing or visual impairment. Almost three-fourths of those aged 80 and over report at least one disability, and over half of these individuals report severe disability. Nearly 35% need assistance as a result of disability. There is a strong correlation between disability and self-reported health status. Among those 65 and older with a severe disability, over half report their health as fair or poor. Among those over the age of 65 with no disability, only approximately 1 out of 10 persons reports fair or poor health (Administration on Aging, 2002a). In the presence of slight disability, the majority of older adults rate their health as good. Although less than 5% of the over-65 age group is institutionalized at any given time, about one in four adults will spend some time in a nursing home in the last years of his or her life. The percentage living in nursing homes increases dramatically with age, reaching over 18% for persons over the age of 85 (AOA, 2002a). When the disability from multiple chronic illnesses and failing health results in the inability to care for oneself or to be the primary caregiver for a life partner, self-worth and personal identity can be greatly affected. This change is made worse by stereotypical attitudes of those who do not look beyond the physical decline to see the person inside the failing body.

The following poem was found in a bedside table in a geriatric ward in a hospital in Ireland. It was written by an anonymous "Crabbit Old Woman" and first appeared in the Christmas issue of *Beacon House News*, the magazine of the Northern Ireland Association for Mental Health.

A CRABBIT OLD WOMAN

What do you see nurses, what do you see?
Are you thinking when you are looking at me?
A crabbit old woman, not very wise,
Uncertain of habit, with far-away eyes;
Who dribbles her food and makes no reply
When you say in a loud voice "I do wish you'd try."
Who seems not to notice the things that you do,
And forever is losing a stocking or shoe.
Who, unresisting or not, lets you do as you will
When bathing and feeding the long day to fill.
Is that what you are thinking, is that what you see?
Then open your eyes, nurse, you are not looking at me!
I'll tell you who I am as I sit here so still,
As I wee at your bidding, as I eat at your will.
I'm a child of ten with a father and mother,
Brothers and sisters who love one another.
A young girl of sixteen with wings on her feet,
Dreaming that soon now a lover she'll meet.
A bride soon at twenty, my heart gives a leap,
Remembering the vows that I promised to keep.
At twenty-five now I have young of my own,
Who need me to build a secure, happy home.
A woman of thirty, my young now grow fast,
Bound to each other with ties that should last.
At forty my young ones now grown and will be gone,
But my man stays beside me to see I don't mourn.
At fifty once more babies play round my knee,
Again we know children, my loved ones and me.
Dark days are upon me, my husband is dead.
My young ones are all busy rearing young of their own,
And I think of the years and the love that I've known.
I'm an old woman now, and nature is cruel—
Tis her jest to make old age look like a fool.
The body it crumbles, grace and vigor depart.
There now is a stone where I once had a heart.
But inside this carcass a young girl still dwells,
And now and again my battered heart swells.
I remember the joys, I remember the pain,
And I'm loving and living life over again.
I think of the years all too few; gone too fast ...
I accept the stark fact that nothing can last.
So open your eyes, nurses, open and see
*Not a crabbit old woman; look closer—see me!**

Anonymous

MENTAL HEALTH IN THE AGED

The elderly are a very heterogeneous group. The influence of an individual's work and home environments and cultural and economic conditions combine to make each person's life experience grow more different from every other with each passing day. Physical health, financial resources, family support, and living conditions vary greatly among the elderly. A change in any one of these can significantly impact quality of life. For example, the death of a spouse may not only mean the loss of a life partner, but also the loss of a primary caregiver and, thus, the loss of home, independence, and even financial security. The proportion of older adults living with their spouse decreases with age, especially for women. In 2003, 41% of older women lived with their spouse, compared with 78% of older men (He, Sengupta, Velkoff, & DeBarros, 2005). Only 13% of women over the age of 85 are married, and there are 241 women for every 100 men (American Association for Geriatric Psychiatry [AAGP], 2004). Related, in 2003, 78% of women over the age of 85 years were widowed, compared to 35% of men (He et al., 2005).

The most common mental health problems of the elderly are anxiety, severe cognitive impairment, and depression or depressive symptoms. Clinically significant symptoms of depression are evident in approximately 15% of community dwelling elders (AAGP, 2004) and nearly 50% of nursing home residents. Just as with physical disorders, the signs and symptoms of mental disease are also different in the elderly. In a study of 30 elderly women diagnosed with depression, fatigue and weakness were identified as more troubling symptoms than were the more commonly associated depressive symptoms of weight loss, suicidal ideation, and feelings of guilt and worthlessness seen in younger adults (Ugarriza, 2002). When depression occurs for the first time late in life, it is often attributed to poor physical health, disability, bereavement, and inadequate social support. It has been suggested that the higher rates of depression for women in old age may be largely related to bereavement and financial problems from the loss of a spouse (Ugarriza, 2002). Milder depressive symptoms are often associated with the losses that frequently accompany old age. Death, retirement, and physical frailty change the pattern of one's life dramatically. The milder symptoms of late-life depression, however, must not overshadow the sad reality that the rate of suicide is higher among older adults than any other age group. The suicide rate for persons 85 years and older is the highest of all—twice the overall national rate.

*Courtesy of Northern Ireland Association for Mental Health.

Clinically relevant symptoms of anxiety and depression are often comorbid with physical health problems. Recent studies of agitation among the cognitively impaired have shown that many of the behaviors that have been identified as "abusive" or as "catastrophic reactions" may, in, fact, be the result of untreated pain (Douzjian, Wilson, Shultz, Berger, Tapnio, Blanton, 2002). When chronic illness results in disability and chronic pain, anxious and depressive symptoms may be a barometer of the discomfort rather than a mental disorder.

The issue of substance abuse, notably alcohol, tobacco, and prescription drugs and the elderly is a complex one. Medication and alcohol are less efficiently metabolized in advanced age. An amount that may once have been socially and physically acceptable may now cause problems. For example, recommendations for safe alcohol use in late life are no more than one standard drink per day for men and slightly less for women (Evans, 2007). Since the chance of developing one or more chronic illnesses greatly increases in old age, the number of prescription drugs also greatly increases. Unfortunately, the body's ability to detoxify and excrete drugs also decreases in old age. Drugs with long half-lives and anticholinergic side effects are especially problematic. Although the use of illicit drugs, such as cocaine and heroine, has been less common among the elderly, it may become more prevalent as the baby boomer cohort begins to reach old age.

Major mental health disorders such as schizophrenia, major depression, and psychosis are less likely to occur for the first time in old age. However, persons with life-long mental illness have special needs as they age, including coping with new chronic illnesses, disability, and losses commonly associated with aging. Because of their likely isolation, they are at greater risk of receiving no or poorer health care (Bartels, Miles, Dums, & Pratt, 2003). They are more likely to pose particular challenges on admission to hospitals or long-term care units because of paranoid behavior or difficulty communicating their needs.

The most profound and significant effect on the mental health of an older adult may be related to the physiology of the brain. Due in part to its high metabolic rate, brain tissue is particularly susceptible to the damaging effects of trauma or biochemical abnormalities. If temporary and reversible, a disorder in thought and level of alertness is called **delirium**. If chronic and mainly a disorder of memory, cognition, and behavior, the disorder is called **dementia**. Depression in the elderly is sometimes referred to as "pseudodementia" because it often results in a significant impairment in cognition and is very often mistaken for dementia.

It is important to understand that mental illness in the elderly is a complex multifactoral problem. Mental health decline is not an inevitable part of aging, and there is some evidence that mental illness occurs less frequently in older adults than in younger persons. When it does arise, the symptoms and manifestations are often different, and physical illness is often present. The complex interaction of mental and medical illness in late life leads to excessive disability and poor rates of recovery from acute illness or injury. Interdisciplinary models of care that coordinate the physical, mental, and social needs of the elderly in a culturally appropriate, affordable, and accessible way are needed across the array of settings for geriatric health care (e.g., hospitals, outpatient clinics, nursing homes, assisted living, hospice, and home care). Models of care such as the Eden Alternative (Thomas, 1996) are based on the belief that life can be fulfilling at any age if lived within an environment that supports a balance of interaction with nature and other human beings in a milieu of mutuality, diversity, and spontaneity (Barba, Tesh, & Courts, 2002). Children, pets, plants, and a management system that values and nurtures the staff who care for a population of frail, elderly residents are the hallmarks of the Eden Alternative to long-term care. Promoting mental health for an older adult often involves addressing the mental and physical health of the caregiver and providing the resources needed to maintain a safe, comfortable, and familiar home environment for those experiencing mental and physical frailty.

> **NURSINGTIP 25-1**
>
> **Caring for the Elderly**
>
> Remember the following when caring for elderly clients:
>
> - Common disorders may affect cognition, which in turn may affect personhood.
> - A primary goal of nursing care must be to ensure that the dignity and personhood of the elderly client are preserved to the fullest extent possible.
> - Needs of caregivers must be addressed as important to preserving the pattern, integrity, and dignity of family life.

COGNITION IN THE ELDERLY

The latter part of the twentieth century is known as the Information Age. Just as a computer relies on stored memory to function, so does the cognitive aspect of the human brain rely on memory to make decisions. **Cognition** is generally described as the process by which a person "knows the world" and interacts with it. The human brain is far more complex, however, than even the most sophisticated computer circuitry. The linking of geographical areas of the cerebral cortex with specific human functions such as speech and sight provided the map for twentieth-century neurology. However, it has become all too evident that such a map can only be a guide and does little to help us actually understand the highly complex interactions, images, and capabilities of the human mind.

Intellectual capacity does not diminish with advancing age. However, the brain as it ages is more susceptible to injury from a variety of external and internal environmental factors. Factors such as drugs, electrolyte imbalances, and ischemia diminish the supply of oxygen and nutrients or alter the chemical or electrical environment needed to sustain adequate brain function. Common symptoms of temporary cognitive dysfunction include a limited attention span, sensory misperceptions (illusions), hallucinations, distorted thoughts, and disturbances of activity patterns and the sleep-wake cycle. Unfortunately, although these symptoms are the result of temporary injury to brain tissue, unless this trauma can be reversed, permanent brain injury can result. For the elderly, this is a situation that happens all too frequently when changes in orientation, alterations in attention, or agitation is seen not as symptomatic of a physical illness, but as the untreatable consequence of old age or "senility."

Cognitive disorders are divided into four diagnostic categories according to the specific symptoms observed and the disorder causing the impairment: delirium, dementia, amnestic disorders, and other cognitive disorders (American Psychiatric Association, 2000). In general, delirium is an acute change in a person's level of consciousness and cognition that develops over a short period of time. Delirium is not usually due to nervous system abnormalities but, rather, to potentially reversible medical abnormalities such as infection, dehydration, or drug toxicities. Dementia is a broad diagnostic category that includes multiple physical disorders characterized by alterations in memory, abstract thinking, judgment, and perception; dementia often results in a progressive decline in intellectual functioning and decreased capacity to perform daily activities. Unlike delirium, dementias are more typically characterized by gradual onset, usually over months or years. The common factor in all of the dementing disorders is a significant degree of memory loss and a progressive decline in intellectual functioning to the extent that daily function is affected. Although forgetfulness is a very common complaint of older adults, memory problems severe enough to cause decreased abilities to function in everyday family and social life are not normal at any age. The diagnosis of mood disorder in elderly persons is made on the same diagnostic criteria, such as feelings of depression, hopelessness, and despair, is that apply to younger individuals. However, among the elderly clinical depression is more likely to cause functionally important impairment of cognition than is the case in a younger population (Figure 25-1).

To care for an older adult experiencing a change in cognitive abilities, the nurse must understand as much as possible about the basis for these impairments. In order to maximize quality of life, the nurse must differentiate between the reversible cognitive impairments for which medical intervention is warranted and those that cannot be reversed and for which assistance with managing the deficits is indicated. Outcomes will be determined mainly by the extent to which the impairment in cognition may be arrested or reversed. After all attempts have been made to correct physiological abnormalities and treat cognitive impairments resulting from depression, nursing care must be directed toward preserving the dignity and integrity of a person's self-hood and the well-being of the family structure to the fullest extent possible.

DELIRIUM

Characteristics and Diagnosis

Delirium is characterized by a disturbance of consciousness and a change in cognition that develops over a short period of time, usually hours or days (American Psychiatric Association, 2000). It is an abnormality in the physiology of the central nervous system that clouds consciousness and causes a person's level of alertness to fluctuate from lethargy to agitation within a 24-hour period of time. Visual hallucinations are common and delirium can be mistaken for psychosis (Muller, 2002). For example, the person may be coherent and calm in the morning and by the evening be agitated, pulling out any tubes or intravenous lines and seeing spiders crawling all over the walls. Delirious persons often continuously shift attention from one stimulus to another. Their speech is often difficult to understand because they shift abruptly and inappropriately from one thought to another. It is difficult to engage such persons in conversation because of their inability to focus or sustain attention on any certain stimulus. Disorientation is more often to time and place rather than to self. Emotions may also fluctuate from fear and irritability to apathy and anger. Although memory impairment is common to both a delirium and a dementia, the person with a dementia alone does not have the extreme fluctuations in alertness that is seen in delirium. The sudden way in which the symptoms present is also very helpful in distinguishing between delirium and dementia. Misdiagnosis of delirium can have serious and even fatal consequences. If delirium is not properly diagnosed and the underlying pathology responsible for the symptoms reversed, the damage

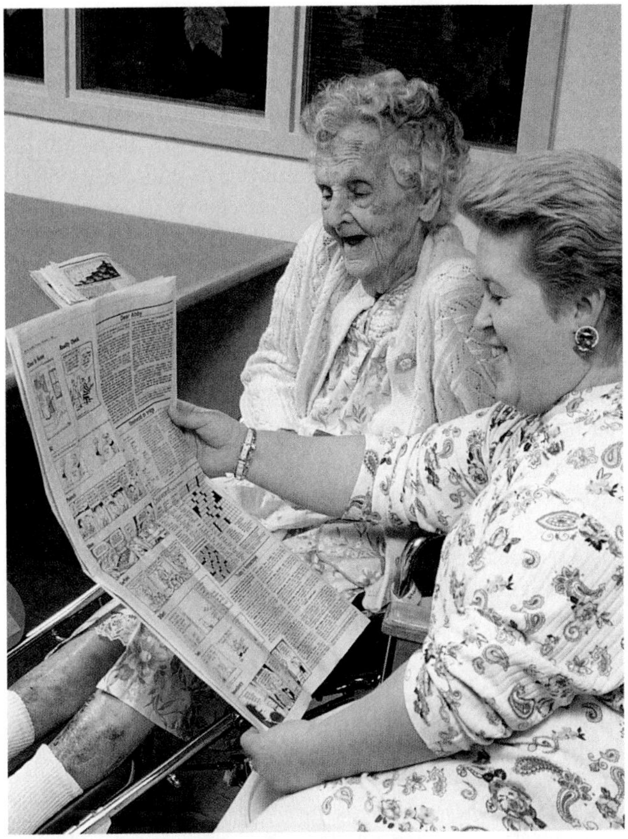

Figure 25-1 A shared laugh or discussion of current events can provide a welcome respite from the confinements of a wheelchair or hospital bed. (DELMAR/CENGAGE LEARNING.)

to the brain can be permanent. However, if diagnosed and treated in a timely fashion, delirium is a potentially reversible condition with no permanent sequelae. Unfortunately, the failure to identify and correct delirium in the older adult adversely affects many outcomes such as increased length of stay for the hospitalized elder, morbidity and mortality, and quality of life (Holmes & House, 2000). Delirious clients are also at high risk for incontinence, immobility, and falls.

Common causes of delirium are infections, dehydration, adverse drug reactions, electrolyte imbalances, hypoglycemia, and hypoxia. Any condition, however, that results in an impairment in the physiological function of the central nervous system, especially brain or neurotransmitter function, can be a cause of delirium. Elders with dementia are also at increased risk of delirium, and the development of delirium in persons with dementia may lead to irreversible functional decline or even death (Givens, Jones, & Inouye 2009).

Recognizing delirium is occasionally difficult in someone with dementia. Doing so, however, is crucial since acute confusion is often the first symptom of serious illness (e.g., pneumonia, myocardial infarction, heart failure) and if ignored, will lead to unnecessary morbidity, disability, and mortality.

NURSINGALERT 25-1

Warning Signs of Delirium

- Rapid fluctuation in level of consciousness (agitated to lethargic)
- Difficulty in maintaining attention span
- Illusions or hallucinations
- Unfocused speech and disorganized thinking
- Disorientation to place or time
- Strong emotional reactions
- Memory problems

BOX 25-1

PATHOLOGIES THAT MAY CAUSE DELIRIUM

I – Infection: encephalitis, meningitis, syphilis, HIV, sepsis

W – Withdrawal: alcohol, barbiturate, sedative-hypnotic

A – Acute metabolic: acidosis, alkalosis, electrolyte disturbances, hepatic failure, renal failure

T – Trauma: closed-head injury, heat stroke, postoperative, severe burns

C – CNS pathology: abscess, hemorrhage, hydrocephalus, subdural hematoma, infections, seizures, stroke, tumors, metastases, vasculitis

H – Hypoxia: anemia, carbon monoxide poisoning, hypotension, pulmonary or cardiac failure

D – Deficiencies: vitamin B12, folate, niacin, thiamine

E – Endocrinopathies: hyper/hypoadrenocorticoidism, hyper/hypoglycemia, myxedema, hyperparathyroidism

A – Acute vascular: hypertensive encephalopathy, stroke, arrhythmia, shock

T – Toxins or drugs: prescription drugs, illicit drugs, pesticides, solvents

H – Heavy metals: lead, manganese, mercury

From "Delirium," by O. Gleason, 2003, *American Family Physician*, 67, 1027–1035.

APPLICATION OF THE NURSING PROCESS 25-1

ASSESSMENT

Acute confusional states (ACS) is the term often used by nurses to describe the behavioral and cognitive manifestations of delirium. Nurses are often the first to identify sudden changes in behavior or cognition, which are harbingers of medical pathology. Although the term *confused and disoriented* has been a common one used by clinicians in both acute and long-term care, confusion was for some time a largely undefined, undescribed behavioral phenomenon. Wolanin's (1977) groundbreaking work was among the first to attempt to define the phenomenon of confusion. A major implication of this study was the finding that sensory deficits (loss of hearing and vision) accounted for much of the changes in behavior and cognition being labeled as confusion.

(*Continues*)

APPLICATION OF THE NURSING PROCESS 25-1 (Continued)

Subsequent nursing studies have attempted to define and explore ACS from a holistic perspective and to identify risk factors that are amenable to manipulation by nurses. **Confusion** can generally be viewed as a multidimensional phenomenon incorporating changes in both cognition and behavior.

Assessment of risk factors for acute confusion places the nurse in a proactive role of preventing rather than merely identifying delirium. Delirium is a diagnostic term with specific objective criteria that reflect a pathophysiological basis. Acute confusional states may not be the same phenomenon as delirium, although it may incorporate some aspects of that phenomenon. Confusion is more than just cognitive changes. Acute confusional states is a multidimensional phenomenon that incorporates a variety of cognitive and behavioral responses. Older clients are at high risk for becoming confused during hospitalization. In one study, nearly three out of every four older adults in a medical intensive care unit experienced delirium (Peterson, Pun, Dittus, Thomason, Jackson, Shintani, et al., 2006). As many as 60% of elderly clients become delirious prior to or during a hospitalization, but it is not diagnosed 70% of the time (Waszynski, 2001).

Delirium assessment protocols that include multifactorial interventions, staff education, and caregiver-patient interventions significantly reduce the duration of delirium, length of hospital stay, and mortality in delirious patients (Inouye, Bogardus, Charpentier, Leo-Summers, Acamporo, Holford, et al., 1999; Lundstrom, Edlund, Karlsson, Brannstrom, Bucht, & Gustafson, 2005). The detection and management of ACS/delirium is essential to improving the outcomes for acutely ill elderly. There are a variety of tools that can be used to quickly identify delirium, as well as those that have also been found to be useful for monitoring the progression of delirium (Table 25-1).

Delirium is a medical emergency that is best treated through an interdisciplinary approach. Medical management involves treating pathological conditions and adjusting or discontinuing medication that is contributing to the problem. Nursing management involves reducing background sensory stimulation such as buzzers, alarms, television noise, and glaring lights that may be misperceived by a delirious mind to be voices or images.

When the term *confusion* is used to label client behaviors rather than to describe and investigate the basis for them, the term is being used in error. Implications of research findings suggest a holistic approach to

TABLE 25-1 Assessment Tools for ACS/Delirium

TOOL	PROPERTIES	SOURCE
Delirium Rating Scale (DRS)	10-item scale that indicates severity and allows for monitoring improvement or deterioration over time	Trzepacz, Baker, & Greenhouse (1988)
Memorial Delirium Scale	10-item, 4-point scale; quantifies severity in medically ill clients	Breitbart, Rosenfeld, Roth, Smith, Cohen, & Passik (1997)
Mini-Mental State Exam (MMSE)	Widespread use for baseline mental status; also valid for delirium	Folstein, Folstein, & McHugh (1975)
NEECHAM Confusion Scale	Specific for ACS and identifies "at-risk" clients as well as those exhibiting signs	Neelon, Champagne, Carlson, & Funk (1996)
The Confusion Assessment Method (CAM)	2-part; distinguishes delirium from nonreversible cognitive disorders	Inouye et al. (1990)
The Confusion Assessment	Adaptation of the CAM; designed specifically for mechanically ventilated patients; Rapid (2 min.) administration	Ely, Inouye, Barnard, Gordon, Francis, May, et al. (2001)

(Continues)

APPLICATION OF THE NURSING PROCESS 25-1 (Continued)

prevention and management of the confused client. Prevention involves nursing interventions aimed at avoiding adverse medication effects, immobilization, inadequate treatment of pain, malnutrition, urinary incontinence, sleep deprivation, inadequate use of visual or hearing aids, and meaningless sensory overstimulation.

NURSING DIAGNOSIS

Identification of pathophysiological risk factors for delirium can be described by collaborative nursing diagnoses (Table 25-2). Pathophysiological responses are those resulting from dehydration, electrolyte disturbances, drug toxicities, metabolic disturbances, and musculoskeletal conditions or any disorder that causes pain. The inability to attend appropriately to environmental stimuli and to communicate needs and feelings poses a serious threat to dignity and safety. The inability to focus and attend to anything for any length of time results in some degree of inability to care for one's bodily needs.

TABLE 25-2 Nursing Diagnoses often Associated with Acute Confusional States

COLLABORATIVE PATHOPHYSIOLOGICAL RESPONSES	RESPONSES TO BRAIN DYSFUNCTION	THREATS TO DIGNITY AND SAFETY
Cardiac output, Decreased	Sensory perception, Disturbed	Fear
Electrolyte imbalances	Communication, Verbal, Impaired	Powerlessness
Fluid volume, Deficient	Thought processes, Disturbed	Falls, Risk for
Gas Exchange, Impaired	Disturbed sleep pattern	Injury, Risk for
Hypothermia/hyperthermia		Self-care Deficit
Infection		Urinary Incontinence, Functional/Urge
Nutrition: Imbalanced less than body requirements		Post-trauma Syndrome, Risk for
Pain, Acute/Chronic		Anxiety
Sleep, Deprivation		Physical mobility, impaired
Tissue perfusion, altered cerebral		

OUTCOME IDENTIFICATION

One desired outcome is to diminish the risk of precipitating an acute confusional state by correcting any potential environmental stimulant, such as sensory overstimulation or understimulation for a bedridden client. Another is to correct pathophysiological causes of delirium via collaborative interventions. The desired outcomes will depend on the physiological abnormality. For example, if dehydration is present, adequate urine output and serum osmolality are desirable outcome criteria. The prevention or reversal of delirious symptoms is evidenced by the client's maintenance or return to his or her usual level of alertness and cognitive function. This includes a predelirious pattern of sleep, alertness, and function.

PLANNING/INTERVENTIONS

Preventing sensory overstimulation and understimulation is a major factor in preventing or diminishing the severity of acute confusional states in the elderly. Family members may be able to help reduce the severity of confusion seen in acutely ill clients by reading and talking about events and matters going on outside the

(Continues)

APPLICATION OF THE NURSING PROCESS 25-1 (Continued)

hospital. Playing familiar music is also a soothing and therapeutic action to take. The research, however, is contradictory in regard to how effective attempts at reorientation are in acute confusional states (Foreman, 1989).

Sleep deprivation is a frequent confounding variable in acute confusional states. In hospitals nurses can control how frequently clients are interrupted during the night. In the great majority of cases this can be accomplished by timing medication administration, vital signs, and other planned aspects of care at the beginning and end of the night shift. Turning off nonessential equipment and intentionally lowering the decibel level of the voice can make a significant contribution toward creating an environment conducive to sleep.

Hallucinations and memory loss pose a very clear threat to personhood and self-esteem. In order to protect the integrity of an individual's self-concept during acute confusional states, the nurse has a responsibility to explain the physical basis of the delirium to the greatest degree possible to the person experiencing it. Oftentimes simple reassurances that such experiences are not the result of a "psychiatric problem" and that they do not mean that the person is "losing his mind" but rather are the result of the physical illness or drug treatment for which the person is being hospitalized are helpful and comforting.

Impairments in judgment, communication, motor strength, and agility pose grave threats to the independence and dignity of an older adult experiencing an acute confusional state. Anticipating the person's need for food and water, elimination, and communication in as private and dignified a manner as possible is a fundamental caring action.

When hospitalized clients become restless during acute confusional states, one concern is that tubes will be dislodged or pulled out. Another is that the client will not have the cognitive capacity to call for assistance before attempting to ambulate (usually to the bathroom) and will be at risk for falling. These concerns about the potential for physical injury as well as the responsibility for carrying out the medical regimen have been the major reasons nurses have given for using restraints on hospitalized clients.

The nurse's privilege to confine or restrict a client's movement by chemical or physical means is legal only within carefully prescribed limitations. The particular setting (nursing home, hospital, or mental health facility) will largely determine the legal parameters. In general, there must be significant threats to an individual's safety, no other alternative for control of the behavior putting the person at risk, and evidence that the least restrictive measures are being used. Sedation should not be used as a first-line intervention. However, when the agitation, delusions, and hallucinations of delirium are posing a serious threat to the patient's safety or comfort, a low-dose antipsychotic may be necessary. There is a greater risk in the elderly of extrapyramidal symptoms (EPS) from even low doses of neuroleptics such as haloperidol that have traditionally been used as a first-line therapy in the treatment of delirium. Newer antipsychotics such as olanzapine and risperidone, with a lower incidence of EPS, may be better tolerated and a useful alternative to haloperidol in the treatment of delirium (Parellada, Baez, dePablo, & Martinez, 2004). Benzodiazepines, such as lorazepam, are recommended for delirium associated with alcohol withdrawal, but must be monitored very carefully if used in cases of nonalcohol withdrawal delirium (Evans, 2007).The use of restraints in nursing homes is controlled by the Nursing Home Reform Law, which is a part of the Omnibus Budget Reconciliation Act (OBRA) of 1987. The influence of OBRA in limiting or preventing the use of restraints is beginning to be reflected in the policies of acute-care hospitals.

REFLECTIVE THINKING 25-1

The Experience of Being Restrained

- **What questions would you have if you were to awaken in a hospital room, have no memory of how or why you are there, and find yourself tied to the bed frame via a vest restraint?**
- **What fears would you have if you were sick, tied down to a bed or chair, and completely dependent upon strangers for your every need?**

(*Continues*)

APPLICATION OF THE NURSING PROCESS 25-1 (Continued)

Restraint use poses very serious threats to an elderly person's physical well-being. The increased incidence of pneumonia, urinary incontinence, urinary tract infections, and venous thrombosis from immobility is well documented. Older adults have described being physically restrained as a traumatic event outside of the usual range of human experience—feelings of being jailed or of feeling like a caged animal without an escape—and have stated, "I felt like a dog and cried all night" (Strumpf & Evans, 1988). Feelings of being threatened, fear, and helplessness may be exaggerated since the restrained person expects to be safe and protected in the hospital and yet is being restrained over protests and usually cannot understand the rationale for the restraints. Depending on the person's interpretation, it is even conceivable that the experience may lead to the development of Post-Traumatic Stress Disorder (Sullivan-Marx, 1995). The trauma of the emotional response may be made worse when nurses offer no opportunity for the client to discuss the assault on their personal integrity by ignoring the experience once the person has recovered from the delirious state. Helping the older person to understand the basis for the delirious symptoms (e.g., hallucinations, inability to concentrate or focus, etc.) and reflect upon the frightening experience and loss of control may be therapeutic.

Rather than triggering the response to restrain, behavior associated with delirium and acute confusional states should elicit in-depth assessment, medical consultation, environmental manipulation, and collaborative interventions to reverse physical pathophysiology. The risk of permanent brain damage can only be decreased if there is a timely and competent response to confusion as a symptom of pathology.

EVALUATION

Successful intervention for preventing or reversing delirium or an acute confusional state must be based on the client's baseline level of everyday cognitive and social function. A variety of models of specialized (acute care units for the elderly, geriatric resource nurses) geriatric care have been shown to improve outcomes, including a decrease in delirium for older adults (Asplund, Gustafson, Jacobsson, Bucht, Wahlin, Peterson, et al., 2000; Guteri, Edinger, & Schumacher, 2003; and Saltvedt, Opdahl, Fayers, Kaasa, & Sletvold, 2002).

DEPRESSION

Depression affects approximately 15% of all adults over the age of 65. It affects a much higher percentage of the elderly in hospitals and nursing homes (Task Force on Aging Research Funding, 2003). The suicide rate for the elderly is higher than for any other age group and for those over the age of 85 is nearly twice the national rate. *Depression* is defined as a loss of pleasure in one's usual activities. Old age, on the other hand, is not depressing! Overall, life satisfaction is good among the elderly, even those with one or more functional impairments. The elderly tend to rate their health according to how much the disorder affects their daily function. In general, they rate their own health higher than health professionals rank it. The elderly often compensate for quite severe impairment to the point that it affects function very little and is not seen, personally, as a major detriment to their overall health and well-being.

The same factors that are associated with life satisfaction in younger years hold true for old age: an adequate income, security, a variety of adequate relationships, good health, and a sense of control over one's life. The prevailing myth that vitality and zest for life naturally wane with advancing years is perhaps the biggest barrier to the appropriate recognition and treatment of depression in the elderly. The widespread belief in this myth of waning vitality in combination with the intermingling of physical illness and multiple losses experienced by the elderly makes the diagnosis and treatment of depression in the elderly particularly challenging.

Theories of Depression

Biological theories attempt to explain the association among neurotransmitters, cortisol levels, physical illness, and depression. There is some evidence that the concentration of the neurotransmitters norepinephrine and serotonin is decreased in old age. However, it is thought that it is not so much the decrease in concentration as it is the decreased sensitivity of the postsynaptic cell receptors to the neurotransmitters that is responsible for the physiological effect on mood. It is by restoring this decreased receptor sensitivity (also referred to as "down regulation") back to normal that the effectiveness of electroconvulsive therapy and many antidepressant drugs is explained. The disregulation of the hypothalamus-pituitary-adrenal feedback loop found more commonly in the elderly is a purported mechanism by which chronic stress is responsible for depression. Chronic stress leads to elevated cortisol levels. Since the normal feedback mechanism that would lower the output of cortisol is thought to diminish in all people as they age, the increasing concentration of cortisol is thought to contribute to depression. One aspect of stress that may make the elderly particularly vulnerable is that chronic stress is thought to have more harmful psychological and physiological consequences than do sporadic stressful events. Many of the stressful situations that the elderly experience, such as caregiving for a dependent spouse, financial worries, or pain, are chronic daily stressors.

Psychosocial theories also exist to explain the increasing prevalence of depression in old age. Erickson, Erickson, and Kibnick (1987) speculate that depression in the elderly may result from unfulfilled desires or accomplishments. According to this theory, the inability to acquire a sense of integrity in regard to the evaluation of their lives can result in a sense of despair and depression for older adults. It is important, however, to resist the temptation to oversimplify the emotional response to aging to that of "successful aging" by staying active, socially engaged, and busy. This so-called "busy ethic" is being challenged by recent studies that suggest that a few well-chosen and personally meaningful activities may have a greater impact on well-being than many activities engaged in for the main purpose of filling the hours in a day (Everard, 1999). In fact, when physical problems make it difficult to stay socially involved, the oldest old usually welcome the freedom that can come by detachment from bothersome and demanding responsibilities and stressful relationships (Johnson & Barer, 1997).

The effect of the sociocultural environment on depression in the elderly is somewhat complex. A supportive social environment has certainly been found to be a buffer for most older adults in protecting them from the multiplicity of environmental stressors and losses that occur with increasing frequency in old age. In fact, some would argue that issues such as poverty, isolation, the loss of role and status, and their effect on the emotional and physical well-being of the aged have been largely ignored. However, the health of an aged population is greatly affected by the cultural, political, and physical environments as is health at *any* age.

While financial strain is associated with higher rates of depressive symptomatology in both men and women, social support significantly modifies this effect. However, the elderly may actually be more resistant to social stressors as they anticipate and "rehearse" some of these stressors. For example, it is a well-known fact that most women outlive their husbands. Many women, therefore, have already done some mental preparation as they experience widowhood through other women friends. The Theory of Thriving (Haight, Barba, Tesh, & Courts, 2002) attempts to identify critical attributes for living life fully across the life span. Although some people seem to thrive more easily than others because of an internal strength described as resilience (Haight & Hendrix, 1998), social connectedness, the ability to find meaning in life, and the ability to attach and adapt to one's changing environment and physical disabilities are critical attributes of thriving. In the case of a frail older person who has moved to a nursing home, the professional caregivers, fellow residents, and way in which the physical environment fosters interaction with nature (sunlight, plants, and pets) and children may be the key variables from a Thriving Framework. The Eden Alternative is based on the Theory of Thriving and is an attempt to change the nursing home environment from that of a sterile, medical institution to a "human habitat," where resident animals, daily children's activities, plants, and staff empowerment are key elements of the transformation (Barba, Tesh, & Courts, 2002).

Characteristics and Diagnoses

The difficulty of correctly identifying depression in the elderly is similar in complexity to the identification and diagnosis of delirium. Depression may be a symptom of certain physical disorders, especially endocrine disorders such as hypothyroidism, pancreatic, and adrenal disorders. Drugs that may cause depression, such as certain antihypertensives, antianxiety drugs, narcotics, and hormones, are often prescribed for disorders that occur with greater frequency in the elderly. Nutritional deficiencies and the use of alcohol are associated with depressive symptoms as well as delirium. Depression affects approximately 25% of those with chronic illness and is particularly common in older adults with arthritis, Alzheimer's disease, Parkinson's disease, cancer, chronic lung diseases, heart failure, and diabetes (AAGP, 2004; Arthur, 2006). Depressive symptomatology is present in almost half of older adults with dementia or Parkinson's disease (Serby & Yu, 2003).

Because of the likelihood of physical disease and disability, depressed mood is often not as reliable nor as prominent a sign of depression in elders as it is in younger adults. Physical complaints often mask the change in function, depressed mood, and feelings of hopelessness and worthlessness that characterize the depression of a younger person. Common manifestations of depression in older adults include paranoia, pessimism, sadness, self-degradation, difficulty in concentrating and thinking, and disturbances of appetite and sleep. Sleep difficulties are among the most common and severe symptoms of depression in the elderly along with disturbances in cognition.

Without recognition and treatment, there are serious negative consequences for elderly clients, such as cognitive impairments, physical disability, social isolation, substance abuse, and suicide. The term *amplification* has been applied to the effect that depression often has in old age as it can "turn up the volume" and accelerate both the course of a medical illness as well as the negative impact that illness can have on functional capacity and well-being in everyday life (Butcher & McGonigal-Kenney, 2005; Katz, Streim, & Parmalee, 1994). The good news is that depression can be very successfully treated in late life—as good as 60% to 80% of the time with approximately 80% of the elders remaining relapse free with medication maintenance for 6 to 18 months. However, since depression is so closely linked with acute and chronic illness, early treatment with relapses and longer-term maintenance is especially important. Thus, the key to adequate treatment and referral is often the responsibility of nurses in both acute and long-term care who can identify and refer for treatment all ranges of depression, major or minor, that interfere with the day-to-day functioning of the older client.

Subtypes of Depression

Major Clinical Depression

Major clinical depression manifests as a broad range of symptoms in the elderly. These range from psychotic, life-threatening ones to a significant impairment of enjoyment while maintaining the ability to function on a day-to-day basis. Not all elderly with clinically significant symptoms will meet the criteria for a diagnosis of major depression as defined by the American Psychiatric Association (2000). This criteria requires a sad, depressed mood or a loss of interest or pleasure in usual activities over at least a two-week period, along with a minimum of five other symptoms that may include weight loss or a change in appetite; fatigue or loss of energy; feelings of worthlessness or excessive guilt; diminished ability to think, concentrate, or make decisions; or recurrent thoughts of death or plans regarding suicide (APA, 2000).The prevalence of major depression among those elderly residing in the community is lower in late life than in midlife. It is estimated that 20% to 25% of clients with Alzheimer's disease suffer from major depression (National Institute on Aging [NIA], National Institutes of Health [NIH], 1999). Bipolar depression with alternating periods of manic and depressive symptoms occurs less commonly in the elderly. When it does occur, the expansive, euphoric mania is found to be expressed more often than in younger adults as angry outbursts or irritability. Antidepressant medication is the mainstay of treating major depression. The American Association for Geriatric Psychiatry (2008) published recommended guidelines for referring elderly depressed patients to a geriatric psychiatrist. They include failure of patient response to one or two 8–12 week trials of antidepressants, difficulty with medication side effects, worsening of symptoms, or the need for evaluation regarding electroconvulsive therapy (ECT). For those elderly who do not respond favorably to drug treatment or who are experiencing severe, psychotic symptoms, electroconvulsive therapy has been thought by some experts to be particularly effective, though the quality of scientific evidence supporting the safety and efficacy of geriatric ECT is not high (Salzman, Wong, & Wright, 2002; Van der Wurff, et al., 2003). Although dementia clients may be more prone to an ECT-induced delirium and may possibly experience further memory loss from ECT, dementia is not considered a contraindication to ECT in severe or life-threatening depression (van der Wurff, et al., 2003)

Dysthymic Disorder

Chronic, milder forms of depression are called Dysthymic Disorder and are more common among older persons than is major depression. Symptoms must occur for at least two weeks and be present the majority of the time during those two weeks. Since psychosocial factors are thought to be greatly responsible for this type of depression, counseling often focuses on a restructuring and greater involvement in social activities with an emphasis on the "here and now" rather than on past disappointments or abilities. Reminiscence therapy and life review, however, may also be considered beneficial in helping the elderly feel more positive about themselves and their lives. Comorbid chronic illness that results in a degree of disability, loss of independence, and, in many cases, chronic pain is frequently a major factor. About 25% to 30% of persons with Alzheimer's disease are also suffering with minor depression (NIA, NIH, 1999). Certain populations of older adults with severe or chronic disabling conditions have significant rates for a combination of major and minor depression.

Adjustment Disorder with a Depressed Mood

This type of depression is distinguished from the other types in that the symptoms are linked to a specific physical or environmental stressor. Among the elderly, physical illness is the most common stressor. Retirement, financial difficulties, and a change in residence are other frequent precipitants. Within one year of moving into a nursing home, 13% of residents develop a new episode of major depression and 18% develop new depressive symptoms (Lebowitz, 2004). Loneliness is a frequent and serious problem among elderly residing in institutional settings. Factors that have been implicated in this problem are lack of intimate relationships, increased dependency, and the loss of friends, home, independence, and self-identity (Hicks, 2000). By definition, the condition is self-limiting. However, because most illness and disability in the elderly are chronic, symptoms may be sporadic, in keeping with the remissions and exacerbations of the physical illness. Education plays a big role in treating this type of depression. Family members must usually be closely involved in order to recognize the behaviors as depressive symptoms rather than hostility or a worsening of the physical condition. Empathetic family members who can encourage positive thoughts while validating the depressed symptoms can have a very therapeutic effect. Nurses in long-term care also play key roles in identifying those persons who are lonely and in need of more meaningful contact with family, nature, pets, or children.

Grief and Depression

Since death and loss are such close companions to the aged, the topic of grief and depression is a complex one. Grief is not considered a mood disorder in the elderly, just as it is not in a younger population. However, more depressive symptomatology is often associated with bereavement in the elderly. In fact, grief may be quite different for the man or woman who has lost a spouse of 50+ years and for whom there was such a complete intertwining of their lives as to make a separation of identities virtually impossible. The same is true for an older adult who loses the last remaining immediate family member or the last remaining person who knew him or her as a child.

It has been said that as long as one still has a parent, one is still a child! Many older adults who have lost a spouse had been witness to a slow decline in their spouse's health and have even had to move their loved one into a nursing home when the demands of caregiving became too great. Thus, death is sometimes seen as freedom from suffering. In some ways the anticipatory grieving has allowed time for the spouse to work through feelings in advance and resolve unfinished business. In others, the ill health and strain of caregiving has caused what many spouses perceive to be a significant decline in the marital relationship in the last few months or years. It is not uncommon for the death of a spouse in late life to be accompanied by some degree of depression as the enormity of the loss is fully realized. The grieving person may have difficulty imagining the future or seeing any purpose in life. It is usually very difficult and ill-advised for individuals to make major decisions that can be deferred during at least the first year following the death. In response to a profound sense of loneliness, some widows find comfort in keeping busy and relying on family and friends for support, whereas others find comfort in more solitary activities such as meditation, prayer, and reflecting on memories (Moneyham & Scott, 1995). Elderly widows are at great risk for disorientation and confusion related to nutritional and sleep deprivation, and nurses should be alert to the danger of such grief reactions being mislabeled as a dementia (Hegge & Fischer, 2000). Widowhood is also a possible risk factor for alcohol abuse—especially in older women (Figure 25-2).

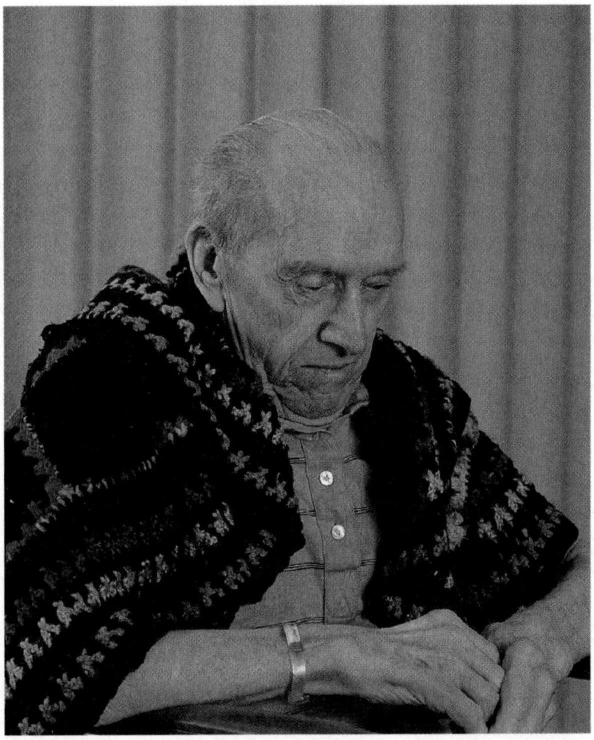

FIGURE 25-2 **Older adults may be particularly saddened by losses of people or situations that have been a part of their lives for many years. Nurses can be supportive of these emotions by showing empathy and taking the time to listen to the client's stories and reminiscences.** (DELMAR/CENGAGE LEARNING.)

SURVIVED BY HIS WIFE

Margaret Flanagan
Eyes swollen she lay in their bed—
head covered, legs drawn up,
cold though her forehead was damp—
who had warmed herself on his warm flesh.
Now his absence was a constant companion:
his hairbrushes, his keys,
his clothes still smelling of him
in his closet, covered, like a museum
She shuddered, remembering the shoes he wore
Were still beneath the bed
exactly as he left them,
as if covered by a glass case.
All of the things he had handled,
used, inhabited, and finally left
were covered or lying about
*like the frames of stolen paintings left behind.**

(Flanagan, 1987, p. 103)

*From "Survived by His Wife," by M. Flanagan Eicher, 2003. In *When I Am an Old Woman I Shall Wear Purple* (p. 103), Watsonville, CA: Papier-Mache Press. Reprinted with permission.

APPLICATION OF THE NURSING PROCESS 25-2

ASSESSMENT

Nurses hold a privileged position because of the unique access they have to the very personal and private parts of people's lives. Knowing the details of an individual's abilities and difficulties with such personal activities as bathing, eating, drinking, and toileting oftentimes provides the bridge by which the symptoms

APPLICATION OF THE NURSING PROCESS 25-2 (Continued)

NURSINGALERT 25-2

Warning Signs of Depression in the Older Adult

Sudden or progressive change in appearance, speech, movement, behaviors, or cognition, as evidenced by:

- Self-neglect and poor hygiene
- Weight loss and anorexia
- Avoidance of liquids
- Unwillingness to socialize with family or friends
- Lack of attention to finances (e.g., paying bills)
- Complaints of memory loss or difficulty concentrating
- Repetitive health concerns or expressions of unrealistic fears
- Disruptive vocalizations such as screaming or shouting (seen mainly in those who are cognitively impaired)

Iris

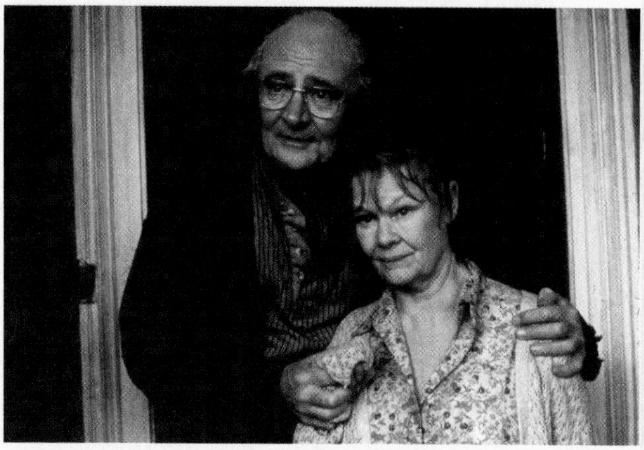

Miramax/Mirage (Courtesy: The Kobal Collection)

The novelist and one-time philosophy professor Iris Murdoch succumbed to Alzheimer's disease in 1999, ending a 40+ year and oddly matched marriage with her bookish husband, John Bayley. Judi Dench plays Iris (who is also portrayed as a younger woman by Kate Winslet) in the years when Alzheimer's began to take its dreadful toll on her personal and creative life.

of depression can be assessed. Along with privilege comes the responsibility of acting on this information with compassion and informed knowledge. There are several key elements that may help unmask the symptoms of depression in the stories of older adults.

The onset and pattern of symptoms may provide clues as to the etiology of the symptoms. These causes could range from the possibility of a dementia rather than a depressive disorder, chronic illness with significant functional impairment and severe pain, or a severe grief response. Regardless of the cause or particular symptoms being displayed, the key to recognizing depression is that it represents a change from a previous level of function and satisfaction with life. The nurse must also listen closely to the client's story for possible links of the symptoms to a reversible cause such as a concomitant physical illness or adverse drug reaction. Family history may help determine specific types of depression for which the individual may be at particularly high risk. For example, if someone has a reported history of bipolar depression, the risk of this specific type of depression may be also greater for his or her siblings. Open-ended questions will generally yield the most beneficial information when screening for depression in the elderly. However, when time is limited or whenever warning signs of depression are noted, a screening instrument should be used for further validation.

One such popular instrument designed specifically for screening for depression in the elderly is the Geriatric Depression Scale (Yesavage & Brink, 1983). The complete scale has 30 items, and there is a shorter version that contains 15 items (see Box 25-2). Each item can be responded to with "yes" or "no" answers.

As stated previously, screening instruments do not confirm a diagnosis, but, rather, merely point out the need for a more in-depth assessment or referral. An often relied upon assessment instrument for depression in nursing homes, the Minimum Data Set (MDS) should not be used alone for detection of depression in this population (Kerber, Dyck, Culp, & Buckwalter, 2005).The nurse must also keep in mind that many elderly clients may downplay their emotional feelings

(Continues)

APPLICATION OF THE NURSING PROCESS 25-2 (Continued)

BOX 25-2
GERIATRIC DEPRESSION SCALE

1. Are you basically satisfied with your life? (no)
2. Have you dropped many of your activities and interests? (yes)
3. Do you feel that your life is empty? (yes)
4. Do you often get bored? (yes)
5. Are you in good spirits most of the time? (no)
6. Are you afraid that something bad is going to happen to you? (yes)
7. Do you feel happy most of the time? (no)
8. Do you often feel helpless? (yes)
9. Do you prefer to stay home at night, rather than go out and do new things? (yes)
10. Do you feel that you have more problems with memory than most? (yes)
11. Do you think it is wonderful to be alive now? (no)
12. Do you feel pretty worthless the way you are now? (yes)
13. Do you feel full of energy? (no)
14. Do you feel that your situation is hopeless? (yes)
15. Do you think that most persons are better off than you are? (yes)

Score 1 point for each response that matches the "yes" or "no" answer after each question.

From "Development and Validation of a Geriatric Depression Screening Scale," by J. A. Yesavage and T. L. Brink, 1983, *Journal of Psychiatric Research*, *17*, 37–49. Reprinted with permission from Elsevier.

due to fear of stigma; careful questioning and observation by the nurse will help uncover true feelings and their impact.

Symptoms of depression in the elderly more commonly manifest as changes in cognition (memory deficits, paranoia, and agitation) and physical symptoms (muscle aches, joint pains, gastrointestinal disturbances, and headache) than they do in younger adults. Symptoms of anxiety are also frequently seen in depressed older adults. Weight loss and nutritional deficits are also common symptoms of depression in the elderly.

Nurses must also understand the basis for certain laboratory studies. Physiological indicators of depression may be measured with a Dexamethasone Suppression Test or assay of neurotransmitter metabolites. Reported hallucinations and delusions will usually call for a computed tomography (CT) scan, magnetic resonance imaging (MRI), and an electroencephalogram (EEG) in order to rule out the possibility of organic brain disorders such as brain tumors, hematomas, or hydrocephalus. Laboratory studies such as serum drug levels, complete blood counts, and thyroid function studies are often done to rule out a physical pathological basis for the symptoms. Educating the client about the strong connection between physical illness and depression plays an important role in prevention as well as treatment.

Assessing the risk of suicide should be a high priority. The elderly have the highest rate of suicide of any age group. Since cognitive impairments are a common symptom of depression in the elderly, the risk of suicide by drug overdose or gunshot may be greater when judgment and inhibitions are impaired.

NURSING DIAGNOSIS

The dependency brought on by chronic physical illness or a cognitive impairment can lead to feelings of helplessness and despair, as characterized by the nursing diagnoses *Hopelessness, Situational or Chronic Low Self-Esteem*. These feelings are often compounded by multiple losses brought about by physical frailty or death. A barrage of losses within a short period of time often causes a "spiraling-down" effect that can lead to depressive symptoms. The combination of personality, isolation, and cognitive impairments can also put the elderly person at high *Risk for self-directed violence*, *Risk for suicide*, *Ineffective Coping*, and *Spirit-*

(*Continues*)

APPLICATION OF THE NURSING PROCESS 25-2 (Continued)

ual Distress. Just as with younger individuals, the importance of validating these responses with the depressed older individual and family cannot be overemphasized.

OUTCOME IDENTIFICATION

The yardstick by which success is measured in treating depression in the elderly is by nature a highly individual one. A severely depressed individual is not usually capable of setting goals at the onset of treatment. Realistic outcomes for the initial stages of treatment may merely be an increase in food intake or some degree of participation in self-care activities. The final outcome may be to see the depressed older adult return to a level of independence and social interaction that makes life more meaningful for him as well as for his family and loved ones. Consideration must often be given to the effect that irreversible chronic physical or cognitive disorders may have on the individual's capacity for independence and level of activity.

PLANNING/INTERVENTIONS

The need to reinforce that depression is an illness is one that presents itself in a multitude of ways. Caregivers often look to nurses for assistance with the physical complaints and needs of the elder with chronic mental or physical impairments. The nurse must help the caregiver and the depressed elder to recognize the effect that depression can have on physical symptoms such as insomnia, appetite, and memory loss. Living with chronic illness often makes an older person more resigned to the unavailability of effective medical treatment. This attitude, in turn, often carries over to an acceptance that things must just be "the way they are" in emotional health as well. Nurses have the responsibility to inform the elderly that not only should they expect the treatment of depression to work, but also that they have the right to demand adequate treatment. Recurrence, however, is a common problem, especially after acute exacerbation of a chronic illness and hospitalization. Treatment for late-life depression must include a collaborative approach with geropsychiatrists, pharmacists, gerontological nurse specialists, social workers, psychologists, occupational therapists, and physical therapists. Evans (2007) notes that the treatment of choice for mild depression is, at least, initially nonpharmacological, which may be any combination of interpersonal, cognitive, reminiscence therapy (Hill & Brettle, 2005; Puentes, 2004; Woods, 2004), exercise (Fitzsimmons, 2001), or light therapy (Sumaya, Rianzi, Deegan, & Moss, 2001). Adequately treating pain, enhancing physical function and social support, and maximizing independence in daily activities are an important part of both pharmacotherapy and psychosocial therapies.

Drug therapy for depression in the elderly presents a special challenge. While it is often very effective in relieving the depressive symptoms, drug therapy is associated with a high incidence of adverse side effects. Monoamine oxidase inhibitors (MAOIs) are infrequently used because of their risk profile in the elderly. Although tricyclics have a long track record of use in the elderly for major depressive disorders, anticholinergic side effects are a significant concern with their use, especially postural hypotension and the potential for falls. Thus, fall risk assessment, as well as informing patients and families of the risk of falls as a side effect and measures that can be taken to reduce the risk of injury while maintaining mobility, are important, especially when drug therapy is being initiated. Prescribers must select a particular drug based on its desired side effect profile (e.g., more or less sedating) in keeping with the distressing symptoms (e.g., lethargy vs. agitation) being experienced by the elderly person with the depression. Selective serotonin reuptake inhibitors (SSRIs) are generally preferred as a first-line pharmacological treatment because of their low risk of adverse effects (American Geriatrics Society & American Association for Geriatric Psychiatry, 2003). Since nurses play a primary role in monitoring for adverse effects, understanding the risk profile of different types of antidepressants is essential to being a competent patient advocate. In general, it is necessary to start antidepressant medication at low doses in elderly clients and to closely monitor for a therapeutic effect and whether a dose adjustment is warranted. For example, a drug such as bupropion may have fewer anticholinergic side effects, while another such as nefazodone may be useful for bedtime sedation but may cause daytime drowsiness (Serby & Yu, 2003). In general, it is the anticholinergic and sedating side effects that must be most closely regulated.

(*Continues*)

APPLICATION OF THE NURSING PROCESS 25-2 (Continued)

NURSINGALERT 25-3

Risk Factor Assessment for Suicide

Self-transcendence is thought to be specific to the success of older adults in meeting the multiple changes of later life. Two questions addressing self-transcendence are:

1. Who is most meaningful (important) to you now?
2. What is most meaningful (important) to you now?

The inability to answer these questions warrants further assessment regarding the client's risk of suicide during any type of major transition or crisis.

From "Suicidal Thought and Self-Transcendence in Older Adults," by D. Buchanon, C. Farran, and D. Clark, 1995, *Journal of Psychosocial Nursing and Mental Health Services*, *33*(10), 31–34.

Safety issues are especially high priorities in cases of irreversible dementias or whenever memory loss is present as a symptom of depression. Nurses must often collaborate with family members in managing behaviors that may threaten the lives of not only the depressed elder but others as well. Driving, leaving the stove on, or smoking in bed may become issues that will require creative strategies for each unique set of circumstances. Regardless of the interventions, focusing on maximizing control and choices plays a central and primary role in the management of depression for older adults. Kivnick (1993) speaks of the importance of the reinforcement and nurturance of the "vital spirit"—those things in life (no matter how seemingly small) that give meaning and pleasure. By helping the depressed person identify those activities and special habits that have given them pleasure through the years and that they can still participate in, the focus is on the positive and not the negative. These pleasures can be anything from drinking coffee out of a favorite mug to reading a newspaper first thing in the morning, cooking a favorite dish, attending religious services, or listening to favorite music while sitting in a warm, sunny spot in a favorite chair. Nightingale (1969) recognized the importance of environmental influences (light, color, movement, and touch) on healing nearly a century ago. Recent studies are reinforcing the validity and importance of these techniques.

EVALUATION

Pharmacotherapy and psychotherapy have been found to be very effective in treating depression in the elderly. The chronic nature of depressive symptomatology and presence of physical illness, however, may be a complicating factor. Outcomes include a decrease in such depressive symptoms as anxiety and memory loss and an improved level of function in activities of daily living. Self-perceptions of control and well-being may also be useful indicators of treatment effectiveness.

NURSING CARE PLAN: NURSING PROCESS FORMAT 25-1

The Parkers' son and daughter were very concerned about the health status and living conditions of their parents, 78-year-old Viola Parker and 82-year-old Ernest Parker. Their parents had lived in the same home for the past 35 years. Five years ago Mr. Parker had two myocardial infarctions and Mrs. Parker took over management of the household duties.

The Parkers' children lived in other cities and visited their parents once or twice a year. The Parkers' daughter had noticed that her mother had been sounding very tired and "down" over the telephone for about a month. However, it was not until a long time neighbor called her to express concern about the trash and papers piling up in the yard that she began to realize what a virtual recluse her mother had become. She immediately called her brother and they made arrangements to visit their parents.

(Continues)

NURSING CARE PLAN: NURSING PROCESS FORMAT 25-1 (Continued)

They were shocked at the disheveled appearance of both parents and the cluttered and dirty house (their mother had always been an immaculate housekeeper). After much resistance, they were able to convince both parents to make an appointment with their family doctor. Diagnostics indicated that Mr. Parker was anemic and hypoxic secondary to an exacerbation of his congestive heart failure and malnutrition. He was admitted to the hospital for further diagnostics and treatment. The history and physical for Mrs. Parker revealed no acute physical abnormalities, only a gradual worsening of her osteoarthritis. However, she was admitted to the geriatric inpatient mental health unit because of noted hallucinations, change in mental status, and an obviously debilitated physical condition.

A multidisciplinary team evaluation found that Mrs. Parker could not perform any activities of daily living (ADL) without assistance. She would eat only a few bites of food at mealtimes and only if someone else put them in her mouth. She had a very flat affect and would answer most questions with "I don't know" or no response at all. She had no interest in visiting her husband three floors away. Based on the multidisciplinary team assessment and thorough medical evaluation, Mrs. Parker was diagnosed with a psychotic major depression that had presented in her case as a pseudodementia. The psychiatrist decided to treat Mrs. Parker with ECT rather than antidepressants due to the severity of her symptoms.

ASSESSMENT

Both Mr. and Mrs. Parker were exhibiting changes in cognition that had been developing over a relatively short period of time (weeks to a month or two). In Mr. Parker the cognitive impairment was manifested as lack of interest in ADL such as bathing, shaving, and dressing, and a lack of judgment and perception that anything was wrong with himself or his wife. Mrs. Parker's symptoms manifested as a pseudodementia, with her social withdrawal and complete lack of interest in her own appearance and hygiene as well as in maintaining even basic sanitary conditions in their home. Open-ended questions revealed that Mrs. Parker's long time friend and confidante had died eight months before. In the previous few weeks, Mrs. Parker had not been sleeping more than three hours at a time and often awakened with joint pain. Mrs. Parker had been taking the nonsteroidal anti-inflammatory drug (NSAID) prescribed for her arthritic pain only in the middle of the night, when she would awaken in pain because she did not like to take "too much medicine."

(NOTE: Care must be planned individually for Mr. and Mrs. Parker during the acute phase. Discharge plans will obviously be dependent on the outcome in health and level of independence in self-care for *both* husband and wife and must include consideration of Mr. Parker's condition.) The following care plan is for Mrs. Parker.

NURSING DIAGNOSIS 1 *Imbalanced Nutrition: Less than Body Requirements,* related to inability to ingest nutrients, as evidenced by inadequate food intake and need for assistance with feedings.

OUTCOMES	NIC	NURSING ACTIONS	EVALUATION
• The client will feed herself at least one-half of the meals served her within 1 week.	• Nutrition management	• The nurse will assist her in eating and sit with her during mealtime until she is able to eat without help. If son or daughter is available, they will be encouraged to eat with their mother.	Mrs. Parker responded immediately to ECT therapy by eating two-thirds of her meal.

(Continues)

NURSING CARE PLAN: NURSING PROCESS FORMAT 25-1 (Continued)

NURSING DIAGNOSIS 2 *Self-care deficit: Bathing/Hygiene,* related to depression and activity intolerance, as evidenced by disheveled appearance.

OUTCOMES	NIC	NURSING ACTIONS	EVALUATION
• The client will be bathing and dressing herself within 1 week.	• Self-care assistance	• The nurse will encourage client to choose time of day for bathing and assist with preparing tub and clothes for her. Nurse will ask daughter to bring in one of her mother's favorite pictures to guide makeup and hair care, and nurse will encourage daughter's participation in mother's care.	It took nearly a week and a half for the medication to decrease her joint discomfort, which increased her independence in ADL.

NURSING DIAGNOSIS 3 *Impaired Social Interaction, related to depressed mood, as evidenced by anhedonia and withdrawal*

OUTCOMES	NIC	NURSING ACTIONS	EVALUATION
• *Short-term goal:* Client will show interest in husband's condition and will engage in brief conversation within 1 week. *Long-term goal:* By discharge, client will identify one outside activity (e.g., church choir or Bible study, craft group, volunteering, or exercise group) that she would like to attend on a regular basis. Nurse will attempt to engage client in conversations in day room and during mealtimes.	• Socialization enhancement	• Nurse will take client to visit husband in adjoining hospital unit and client will be assisted as desired to call husband on the phone.	After beginning ECT treatment, client greeted husband with a hug and exclaimed, "I've been so worried about you." She reluctantly (only on her son's and daughter's insistence and a visit from two women friends) agreed to begin attending a weekly Bible study at her church. Mrs. Parker's daughter decided to start telephoning 3 to 4 times a week in order to encourage her mother's social interaction.

REFLECTIVE QUESTIONS

1. **ASSESSMENT**
   What factors of Mr. Parker's care should you consider that will have a direct impact on Mrs. Parker's status and progress? What questions might you ask the Parkers' daughter?

(Continues)

NURSING CARE PLAN: NURSING PROCESS FORMAT 25-1 (Continued)

2. **NURSING DIAGNOSIS**
   Which (if any) of the nursing diagnoses are life threatening? How would you prioritize them?
3. **OUTCOMES**
   What outcomes will be evidence of Mrs. Parker's renewed interest in her role as caregiver and household manager?
4. **NURSING ACTIONS**
   What is the nurse's role in discharge planning for Mrs. Parker's return to her home and the stress of caregiving?
5. **EVALUATION**
   What avenues exist for follow-up of Mrs. Parker's physical and emotional conditions and her ongoing ability to cope with the chronic stress of caregiving?

DEMENTIA

The essential characteristics of a dementia are the development of multiple cognitive deficits that include an impairment of memory and at least one of the following cognitive disturbances: **aphasia**, **apraxia**, **agnosia**, or a disturbance in executive functioning. This impairment must be significant enough to cause a disturbance in everyday functioning and it must be a decline from a previously higher level of functioning (American Psychiatric Association, 2000). At least half of nursing home and assisted living facility residents have dementia (Rosenblatt, Samus, Steele, Baker, Harper, Brandt, et al., 2004). Although a variety of disorders are responsible for the development of a dementia, they all share similarities in the way in which symptoms present.

Poor judgment and poor insight are common in dementia. Although affected persons are often aware of their declining abilities, they are generally not able to judge the consequences of the loss of memory and cognition. This presents a great challenge to family members or caregivers faced with figuring out how to curtail activities such as driving or the control of banking and finances for an older individual who is completely unaware of the risks involved (and who is accustomed to independence in such matters for nearly a lifetime).

ALZHEIMER'S DISEASE

Characteristics and Prevalence

Alzheimer's is the cause of dementia the majority of time in persons over age 65. Alois Alzheimer has been credited with the first known description of the disease in 1907. Alzheimer's disease (AD) is now often cited as the number one mental health problem among our rapidly increasing aging population. Alzheimer's disease is a progressive disorder characterized by stages of increasing impairments and dependency. Although memory impairment is generally characterized as the key diagnostic criteria for AD, the earliest objective signs of the disease may often be changes in behavior or mood. These may include behaviors such as suspiciousness and paranoia, irritability, aggression or angry outbursts, hoarding, withdrawal, or a report from others of poor performance at work. As the disease progresses, gait and motor disturbances may appear along with severe cognitive impairments. Up to 90% of persons with AD will be affected by other neuropsychiatric symptoms including agitation, aggression, delusions, wandering, and repetitive vocalization (Lyketrsos, Colenda, Beck, Blank, Doraiswamy, Kalunian, et al., 2006) and nearly 50% will experience depression. In the latter stages, the person may become bedridden and nonverbal. Although a person with Alzheimer's may live as many as 20 years or more from the onset of symptoms, the average duration of the illness is eight years. Approximately 4 million Americans currently have Alzheimer's disease, and, in the absence of a cure, this number will rise to an estimated 14 million within the next 50 years (AAGP, 2004).

Diagnosis and Pathophysiology

The cause of AD is still unknown, although numerous genetic, viral, environmental, nutritional, and immunologic factors are being explored. The pathological brain lesions associated with the disease are beta-amyloid plaques and neurofibrillary tangles. The role of plaques and tangles in interfering with the normal processes of neuronal repair and the function of the neurotransmitter acetylcholine that has been identified as an essential component of cognition and memory is a fertile area of research.

Genetic and Environmental Risk Factors

The genetic versus environmental factors for AD also have been a topic of much debate and research. The genetic basis for AD that occurs during middle age (thirties to sixties) has been linked to different genes and chromosomes than that of late-onset disease. Early-onset AD is rare (about 10% of cases) and is more likely to follow a single-gene inheritance pattern.

BOX 25-3
PATHOLOGIES THAT MAY CAUSE DEMENTIA

INFECTIONS
- Human immunodeficiency virus (HIV)
- Syphilis

DEGENERATIVE NEUROLOGICAL DISORDERS
- Alzheimer's disease
- Creutzfeldt-Jakob disease
- Dementia with Lewy bodies
- Huntington's disease
- Parkinson's disease
- Pick's disease

VASCULAR DISORDERS
- Ministrokes (cardiovascular accidents)

STRUCTURAL DISORDERS OF BRAIN TISSUE
- Normal-pressure hydrocephalus
- Subdural hematoma
- Head injury
- Tumors

Early-onset AD also often progresses faster than the more common late-onset form. As much as 50% of familial AD is now known to be caused by defects in three genes located on three different chromosomes. There are mutations in the amyloid precursor protein (APP) gene, a protein essential for nerve growth and development on chromosome 21; mutations in a gene on chromosome 14 called presenilin 1; and a mutation in a gene on chromosome 1 called presenilin 2. Mutations in presenilin 1 are found in about 40% of people with early onset familial AD (NIA, NIH, 1999). All three mutations have been associated with either the formation of beta-amyloid plaque or an acceleration of the rate at which nerve cells are targeted for death. The role that genetics and the environment plays in late-onset AD is slightly less clear than in early onset AD. Although there is clearly an association with the gene that controls lipoprotein (APOE) production, several other genes have been implicated in the accumulation of the beta-amyloid plaque.

Whether plaque initiates the inflammatory response or whether some other more direct mechanism stimulates both is still unknown. However, it has become quite clear that chronic inflammation and the production of free radicals may play a role in the damaging effects seen on autopsy in the brain tissue of those having been diagnosed with AD. Free radicals may destroy neurons by making an abnormal form of the protein tau. The normal form of tau lends shape to the neuronal cell by binding tightly to microtubules. The abnormal tau causes the nerve cells to fall apart and is the chief component of twisted fibers called neurofibrillary tangles.

Diagnosis and Treatment

Although it is very important to diagnose and treat any reversible condition that may be causing the memory or cognitive impairment, in the absence of a treatable condition, an early diagnosis of AD is also important because it gives affected individuals a greater chance of benefiting from existing treatments. The diagnostic certainty can be quite high when a systematic evaluation is done that includes a thorough history, cognitive tests, neurological and physical exams, and neuroimaging studies. A review of medications and laboratory tests is an important part of identifying reversible causes for the presenting symptoms. In general, cognitive enhancing drugs are mainly effective in slowing down the progression of the disease or for facilitating a slight improvement in self-care for some individuals with mild to moderate deficits, but only for a period of time. Current drug treatment, therefore, must be used before severe cognitive impairment has ensued if it is to have any beneficial effect. The mainstays of cognitive-enhancing drugs are the Cholinesterase Inhibitors (CEIs) such as domepezil (Aricept), galantimime, and rivastigmine. Unlike these drugs which act by increasing brain acetylcholine levels, the newer agent Namenda (memantine) acts on dopamine receptors. Some evidence suggests a trial combining a CEI with memantine for treating mild to moderate AD (Gauthier, Wirth, & Mobius, 2005; Lyketsas, et al., 2006). Vitamin E, nonsteroidal inflammatories (NSAIDS), and estrogen have shown some promise in delaying the onset of disease, which is especially important as a whole new diagnostic category is being used to describe individuals who have a memory problem but who do not meet the generally accepted clinical criteria for AD. It is now known that 40% of these individuals with mild cognitive impairment (MCI) will develop AD within three years. Although there is no clear evidence, there is hope that anti-inflammatory and free-radical scavenger drug treatments will someday be beneficial in preventing or delaying the onset of AD among those individuals who are at risk as identified by genetic markers, neuroimaging, and/or neuropsychological testing. At the present time, there is sufficient evidence supporting the use of some cholinesterase inhibitors in mild to moderate dementia to justify their use for slowing the progression of cognitive decline (Birks, Grimley, Iakovidou, & Holt 2009).

VASCULAR DEMENTIAS

Characteristics and Prevalence

The second most common dementia, often coexisting with AD, is vascular dementia. This type of dementia, often referred to as multi-infarct dementia, accounts for 10% to 20% of all dementias. Vascular dementia typically results from the occurrence of multiple small strokes over a period of time. A gradual occlusion and blockage of arteries to the brain usually leads to such a gradual decline in function that each event is not noticed. However, a more severe disruption of cerebral perfusion may result in immediate neurological symptoms, usually including one-sided weakness, focal neurological signs, or language disturbances. Although the

BOX 25-4
DIAGNOSTIC CRITERIA FOR DEMENTIA OF THE ALZHEIMER'S TYPE

A. The development of multiple cognitive deficits manifested by both:
   1. Memory impairment (impaired ability to learn new information or to recall previously learned information)
   2. One (or more) of the following cognitive disturbances:
      a. Aphasia (language disturbance)
      b. Apraxia (impaired ability to carry out motor activities despite intact motor function)
      c. Agnosia (failure to recognize or identify objects despite intact sensory function)
      d. Disturbance in executive functioning (i.e., planning, organizing, sequencing, or abstracting)
B. The cognitive deficits in criteria A1 and A2 each causes significant impairment in social or occupational functioning and represents a significant decline from a previous level of functioning.
C. The course is characterized by gradual onset and continuing cognitive decline.
D. The cognitive deficits in criteria A1 and A2 are not due to any of the following:
   1. Other central nervous system conditions that cause progressive deficits in memory and cognition (e.g., cerebrovascular disease, Parkinson's disease, Huntington's disease, subdural hematoma, normal-pressure hydrocephalus, brain tumors)
   2. Systemic conditions that are known to cause dementia (e.g., hypothyroidism, vitamin B12 or folic acid deficiency, niacin deficiency, hypercalcemia, neurosyphilis, HIV infection)
   3. Substance-induced conditions
E. The deficits do not occur exclusively during the course of a delirium.
F. The disturbance is not better accounted for by another axis I disorder (e.g., Major Depressive Disorder, schizophrenia).

From *Diagnostic and Statistical Manual of Mental Disorders, Fourth Edition-Text Revision*, 2000, Washington, DC: American Psychiatric Association. Reprinted with permission.

symptoms are similar to those of AD, the course of vascular dementia tends to be more sporadic and with less memory impairment and more specific cognitive losses. The person may appear to be completely normal for a few hours or days and then suddenly, without warning, become very inappropriately suspicious, belligerent, or forgetful. Signs and symptoms of damage to specific areas of the brain, such as weakness of an extremity or gait abnormalities, often coincide with the behavioral and memory changes. The unpredictability of the person's behavior and impairment in cognition create a "roller coaster" effect on the emotions and coping abilities of the person's loved ones and caregivers.

Diagnosis and Pathophysiology

Causes include atherosclerosis, dysrythmias, and spasms of blood vessels. Contributing risk factors include diabetes mellitus, obesity, smoking, and hypertension. Destruction of brain tissue resulting from the small emboli or strokes may be localized or diffuse. Evidence of both new and old infarctions may be detected by CT and MRI. Diagnosis is typically based on a history of cardiovascular disease, reported episodic decline in function, and physical examination of neurological abnormalities.

Relationship between Alzheimer's and Vascular Dementia

Numerous studies and collaborative efforts by institutes are being undertaken to explore the interrelationships among age-related cognitive decline, dementia, cerebrovascular disease, and cardiovascular disease. Results form the NUN study (Snowdon, Greiner, Mortimer, Riley, Greiner, Markesbery, 1997) found that patients with AD who also had evidence of a brain infarction at autopsy had more severe clinical dementia and poorer performance on specific tests of language and cognitive function and higher frequency of dementia than did those with AD alone. High levels of homocysteine, which have been found to be a risk factor for atherosclerosis, have also been implicated as a risk factor for AD (Clarke, Smith, Jobst, Refsum, Sutton, Ueland, 1998). Findings from the NUN study also suggest a link between folate and brain dysfunction. This process may be linked to homocysteine since one of folate's functions, along with vitamins B_6 and B_{12}, is to convert homocysteine to the more useful amino acid methionine.

Other Dementias

A variety of other neurological, metabolic, and infectious disorders are responsible for the remaining types of dementias. Since many of these disorders arise at a younger age, it is not only the elderly who may be affected. These disorders include alcoholic dementia (Korsakoff's syndrome), a condition of unknown etiology called Creutzfeldt-Jakob disease (CJD), the human immunodeficiency virus causing acquired immunodeficiency syndrome (AIDS), a dementia associated with the spirochete causing Lyme's disease, and a dementia associated with the neurological disorders Parkinson's and Huntington's diseases. All of these dementias share similar damage to memory and intellectual function. However, the balance and degree to which behaviors, memory, and judgment or cognition are affected may vary slightly from one disorder to another. For example, there tends to be a blunting of emotion (or at least the ability to display emotion) in Parkinson's disease as contrasted with the often exaggerated and explosive emotions of vascular dementia. Cerebellar and

BOX 25-5
DIAGNOSTIC CRITERIA FOR VASCULAR DEMENTIA

A. The development of multiple cognitive deficits manifested by both:
   1. Memory impairment (impaired ability to learn new information or to recall previously learned information)
   2. One (or more) of the following cognitive disturbances:
      a. Aphasia (language disturbance)
      b. Apraxia (impaired ability to carry out motor activities despite intact motor function)
      c. Agnosia (failure to recognize or identify objects despite intact sensory function)
      d. Disturbance in executive functioning (i.e., planning, organizing, sequencing, and abstracting)
B. The cognitive deficits in criteria A1 and A2 each cause significant impairment in social or occupational functioning and represent a significant decline from a previous level of functioning.
C. Focal neurological signs and symptoms (e.g., exaggeration of deep tendon reflexes, extensor plantar response, pseudobulbar palsy, gait abnormalities, or weakness of an extremity) or laboratory evidence indicative of cerebrovascular disease (e.g., multiple infarctions involving cortex and underlying white matter) that are judged to be etiologically related to the disturbance.
D. The deficits do not occur exclusively during the course of a delirium.

From *Diagnostic and Statistical Manual of Mental Disorders, Fourth Edition-Text Revision*, 2000, Washington, DC: American Psychiatric Association. Reprinted with permission.

extrapyramidal deficits with myoclonus and other involuntary movements often occur in Creutzfeldt-Jakob disease, along with a rapidly progressive course of dementing symptoms. The time span from onset of symptoms to death of 6 to 12 months is much shorter in CJD than in most other forms of dementia. Many treatable disorders in the elderly will cause permanent brain damage if not treated in a timely fashion. Thus, when symptoms suggestive of a dementia appear, the most important step is a thorough medical assessment to determine whether these symptoms are caused by a reversible condition such as an infection, adverse effect of medication, vitamin or protein deficiency, thyroid problem, minor head trauma, brain tumor, or hydrocephalus.

Symptoms and Sequelae

How a particular dementia manifests as specific changes in mood, personality, and behavior is probably a combination of the physiology of the condition and the unique personality of the individual. Understanding the basis for the expected behaviors as well as the peculiarities and typical pattern for the individual person are essential for planning safe, individualized care that honors the dignity and personhood of the person living with dementia. All behavior has meaning and it is the nurse's responsibility to make sense of the behavior for the purpose of meeting the person's physical, emotional, and spiritual needs. Current models such as the Progressively Lowered Stress Threshold and Need-Driven Dementia Compromised Behavior explain the behaviors commonly seen in dementia as the best way that the person has to express unmet needs and the stress of living with the condition (Remington, Gerdner, & Buckwalter, 2005).

Memory Loss

Even in the absence of disease, some memory loss does seem to occur with advancing age. For example, an older man may forget the name of his best friend's daughter. He is acutely aware of and frustrated by his memory loss and searches his memory until he eventually remembers again. In contrast, however, the demented adult may be completely unaware that he has forgotten—"forgets that he forgets"—or may frequently try to cover up his memory loss. This **confabulation**, or intentional filling in of memory gaps, is not so unlike the tricks we have all used at one time or another when we forget an acquaintance's name on a chance meeting and attempt to cover it up with conversation that does not require us to speak the person's name. However, in a dementia the extensiveness and frequency with which confabulation is used far exceeds the occasional use made of it during normal, everyday life. Family members are often surprised by the details that their loved one with dementia can remember about weddings, vacations, or events from 30 or 40 years before while having no recollection about going to church or the movies two days before.

In a rare personal account of what it is like to be immersed in the early throes of a dementia, Reverend Robert Davis describes his experience with memory loss in the early stages of this disease:

MY JOURNEY INTO ALZHEIMER'S DISEASE

I still have the aggravations of daily living. For instance, it is annoying to be unable to remember information such as my license tag. It is embarrassing and irritating to go to a service station and have to make two trips back to the car to check the license plate because I forgot the number between the pump and the cash register. How frightening it is to go into a large, familiar shopping center with crowds and blinking lights and become totally lost! How humiliating it is to be unable to make the right change and ask the cashier to pick the correct coins from my hand!

It is still sometimes terrifying at night. When I let my mind go in order to go to sleep, my mind still slips into blankness and moonlight. However, this is all just surface frustration, brought on by the constant process of losing

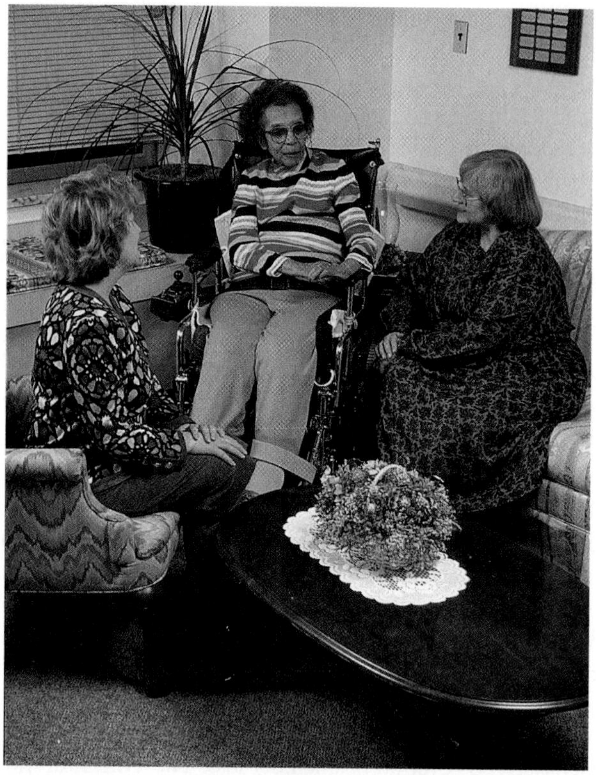

FIGURE 25-3 **Spending time with family and friends helps the older client feel valued and enjoy days that might otherwise be lonely.** (DELMAR/CENGAGE LEARNING.)

*control at the daily living level. I can either struggle angrily and uselessly against the inevitable, or else I can admit my inadequacy and humbly ask for help. I choose to do the latter and keep a calmer and more peaceful mind. Fortunately, I can still make this choice, but it is possible with the progress of the brain damage that I will lose this ability.**

(*Davis, 1989, pp. 56, 57*)

As Reverend Davis points out, the ability to choose a response and find a peaceful way to cope with the frustration of memory loss is often lost as the disease progresses. This lack of control in combination with unique personality factors gives life to a broad range of behaviors commonly associated with dementia.

Just as significant as the effect that memory loss may have on behavior, but even more difficult to understand, is the way in which severe memory loss affects self-identity. Self-concept is the identity each person has acquired of himself over a lifetime. Self-concept is fashioned out of how well persons believe that they have reached their potentials, along with the nature and satisfaction of their relationships to both other persons and their environments. This enduring aspect of self is at least partially dependent on memory. The extent to which varying degrees of memory loss destroy an individual's identity and self-concept is almost

REFLECTIVE THINKING 25-2

Early Stages of a Dementia

Liz was 68 years old when she first complained of feeling "funny in the head" and a tingling sensation in her arm. Hypertension with possible transient ischemic attacks (TIAs) was diagnosed in the emergency room, and she was prescribed antihypertensives and told to follow up with her family doctor. Liz's blood pressure kept fluctuating over the next few weeks, and she felt "hazy and tired" as different medications were tried.

Liz and her husband ran a drapery business out of their home. Her husband noticed that Liz was beginning to have difficulty with calculations. A calculator solved this problem for several months, until one day her husband noticed that Liz was completely disregarding any fractions and adding only whole numbers. Liz had always taken pride in her attention to detail, and this kind of oversight was very uncharacteristic of her. Liz's husband, however, attributed this change to her being more tired. She had been having some difficulty sleeping at night and some angry outbursts that her husband also attributed to lack of sleep. One day Bill walked in while Liz was attempting to charge a customer $500 for a $50 job.

Several months later, Liz had to be rushed once more to the emergency room, this time because of slurred speech and numbness of her entire left side. She was diagnosed with a cerebrovascular accident (stroke).

- What were the first signs of a cognitive impairment being exhibited by Liz?
- What possible reversible causes needed to be investigated?
- How will you answer Bill's question, "Will my wife continue to have mental problems? What can I do to help?"

solely a matter for conjecture and speculation. If memory and identity are purely subjective states, one can only learn about them through personal accounts made possible by self-reflection. However, the pathologies that result in severe memory loss also hinder the ability for self-reflection and to communicate the personal meaning of such loss. Oliver Sacks (1987) explores the possible ramifications of an extraordinary case of near-complete recent memory loss in a young man in his forties. The medical diagnosis was completely unknown.

THE MAN WHO MISTOOK HIS WIFE FOR A HAT

I found an extreme and extraordinary loss of recent memory—so that whatever was said or shown to him was apt to be forgotten in a few seconds' time. Thus I laid out my watch, my tie, and my glasses on the desk, covered

*From *My Journey into Alzheimer's Disease*, by Robert Davis, Copyright © 1989. Reprinted with permission from Tyndale House Publishers, Inc. All rights reserved.

*them, and asked him to remember these. Then, after a minute's chat, I asked him what I had put under the cover. He remembered none of them—or indeed that I had even asked him to remember.**

(Sacks, 1987, p. 27)

*I wrote in my notes, "isolated in a single moment of being, with a moat or lacuna of forgetting all round him.... He is a man without a past (or future), stuck in a constantly changing, meaningless moment." ... I kept wondering, in this and later notes—unscientifically—about "a lost soul," and how one might establish some continuity, some roots, for he was a man without roots, or rooted only in the remote past.**

(Sacks, 1987, p. 29)

Aphasia

The person with dementia commonly has difficulty with the recall of words. This condition is called aphasia. For example, in the midst of a conversation, the individual may not be able to recall the word "car" and will attempt to get the message across by describing the car's purpose, such as "the box that goes everywhere" or "the machine with wheels."

Delayed Response Time

Simple calculations may be impossible for the person to perform within a reasonable time frame. Being confronted with figuring out the right amount of money at the grocery store, for example, may be distressing. Not only mental response time but physical response time may often be affected. Driving becomes a hazardous situation when the person with dementia cannot react quickly enough—not to mention getting lost! Such individuals are usually attempting to conduct a familiar autonomic behavior but become confused and over stimulated.

Paranoia

Suspiciousness and paranoia also frequently accompany dementia. When items are "lost" because the person cannot remember where they were last placed, loved ones are often blamed for "stealing" them. This can progress to a rather persistent paranoia that becomes very emotionally draining on family members who are being suspected of wishing to harm their loved one when they are so desperately trying in vain to help. These paranoid ideations may be accompanied by delusions and hallucinations. A daughter describes the sequelae of door keys lost by her demented mother:

WHEN I GROW TOO OLD TO DREAM

*She would take all the keys out of the doors, even the wardrobe keys, and they would be stowed away anywhere. She lost the backdoor key, then attacked the lock with a hammer. She then called to say someone had broken into the house and there was no peace until we were able to get up there to do the necessary repairs. After that we attached the key by a chain to each appropriate door. The wardrobe-door keys were removed altogether. Then there were the bricks piled up at the back door to be put against it at night. There were pieces of wood and long sticks beside the bed, a whistle (which didn't work) was under her pillow. Again, looking back, I realize she must have felt very insecure which was not like Mom at all.**

(Naughtin, 1992, p. 126)

REFLECTIVE THINKING 25-3

Understanding the Aphasic Client

A frustrating and common dilemma that caregivers must often face on a daily basis is interpreting the sometimes garbled sentences of their aphasic loved ones. Would you be able to figure out what the aphasic individual is attempting to say in the following situation?

You are in a crowded mall with an individual who has AD. Suddenly, this person becomes slightly agitated and begins to repeat the phrase "I want . . . box with a top . . . people here . . . I want . . . box with a top . . . people, people, people."

- **How would you respond?**
- **How would you go about trying to determine what the aphasic person is trying to say?**

This may be the person's way of trying to tell you that he wants to go home. Asking simple yes or no questions such as "Are you tired?" and "Do you want to stop at another store?" or finding a quiet spot and saying, "Let's sit here and rest for a minute," may be an appropriate response.

Alterations in Perception

Some of the most unusual of responses to dementia and the most complex to comprehend are the perceptual problems. These alterations in interpretation of images and sounds take many forms. A husband describes the difficulty his wife, Joyce, had in bathing herself:

The order of washing up and any cleaning became affected by the inability to remember the normal sequence. She was unable to mop the floor unless she cleaned ahead of herself, which meant she walked over the wet floor as she cleaned. The reason for this was simply that she could see what was ahead of her, but not what was behind. Her mind's eye could no longer perceive and recall what was behind. For Joyce, "behind" no longer existed. Her range of vision became the limit of her ability. This then began to affect her ability to shower.

She would go into the shower and wash her hair first. She could put the shampoo into her hands and lift them to her head to apply shampoo, but, not being able to see the soap in her hair, she didn't rinse it out.

She kept the spray of water in front of her running from her breasts and down. She didn't wash her back or up between her legs and she didn't dry the parts she couldn't see.

It seemed as if she were unable to feel that she was wet. She used to come out of the shower and put on her cotton dressing gown. Then it would be very noticeable that she hadn't dried herself because the back of the gown was wet and her hair was still soapy.

*"Come here darling, let's go back into the shower and I'll help you." I would say with a kiss.**

(Naughtin, 1992, p. 110)

Wandering

A serious safety issue for caregivers arises when the demented person begins to wander. At times, the wandering may merely be from one room to another as the person is looking for something or someone. It may even be an attempt to combat frustration and boredom. Joyce's wandering is described by her husband and caregiver:

Joyce also frequently realised that something was wrong, and her frustration and anger led her to the wandering off into the bush. Our home is surrounded on three sides by forested bushland. There are tracks along which we had walked many hundreds of kilometers together, but always together. The wandering became a daily looking for her, but usually the wrong way, and there was always the danger that she would return while I was searching in the wrong place.

*In a strange way, her dementia was a blessing in disguise. After some time, she would forget that she was running away and her mind would simply revert to having a normal walk. She was not lost as the area was very familiar to her. She would return with no idea that anything was wrong. The initial wanderings were of about one to one and a half hours duration, but this slowly decreased in time, because she began to forget her original anger and frustration much more quickly. Eventually she reached a stage where she would go out of the back door, walk up the path, reach the edge of the forest, immediately forget what she was doing, and walk back into the house all in about thirty seconds.**

(Naughtin, 1992, pp. 106, 107)

Disinhibition

Personality is always a major determinant of the way in which physical or emotional problems present and progress in the older adult. Dementia does not change this fact altogether. As pathology worsens, however, there is often a general loss of inhibition that may take a variety of forms. Spontaneous undressing without regard for privacy may occur. Inappropriate sexual overtures to friends or family are not uncommon and can be particularly distressing to caregivers. Episodes of physical or verbal aggressiveness may also occur. A mother describes the effect of her husband's, Les's, disinhibitions and aggressions on both her and her daughter:

Les went through a stage of total rejection of any conversation between my daughter and any males of her age. She was seventeen, at school, making her debut, and she's quite attractive. Kids of that age just talk to one another without it having any particular meaning to it.

I knew he was in one of those moods one day when she was coming home. A boy she knew rode past, came back, and rode with her. It was very hot, so Les only had his underpants on. He got tangled up getting his shorts on, and I had enough time to get out in the street and warn them.

Aggression—physical, verbal and psychological—was a big problem for Les, one I found hard to deal with. We had to hide the gun, because we were a bit worried that he'd either take it to himself or he'd get too aggressive towards others.

It seemed to involve an exaggeration of his basic prejudices. If you look at his life as a child, and the fears and the prejudices he developed then, what you see now are those same prejudices just accentuated, without the social damper that he would normally put on them.

*The problems with my daughter and the general aggressiveness are examples of how his inhibitions began to diminish. Sometimes he becomes totally uninhibited and totally unreasonable. Alzheimer's disease obviously strips away socialization and social understanding.**

(Naughtin, 1992, pp. 160, 166)

Catastrophic Reactions

Agitation and angry outbursts may build to the point of a **catastrophic reaction**, or severe overreaction out of proportion to the stimulus. As the disease progresses, the individual may have great difficulty completing even the simplest of tasks. For example, it is not uncommon for the person to jump up every few minutes from the dinner table with no apparent purpose but to pace around the room or walk into another. Impulsiveness also takes the form of angry outbursts—often in response to questions that the person may have difficulty in answering because of memory loss.

Thankfully, the outburst is usually short-lived and the anger easily forgotten if the individual can be distracted. However, this is not always the case, and a very volatile situation with verbal and physical outbursts may result in a catastrophic reaction. The emotional outbursts are often precipitated by fatigue and overstimulation. Providing a quiet and more soothing environment or taking the person away from the stimulation may distract the person and prevent or halt the overreaction. A calm tone of voice and soothing touch may also somewhat alleviate the catastrophic response.

Distraction, however, is not always the correct response to increasing agitation. Behaviors that get classified as "resistive," "agitated," or "aggressive" and that occur more often may be the result of insensitive or depersonalized care. Lack of privacy, exposure to cold air or water, or pain due to movement of painful arthritic joints are examples of circumstances that may lead to agitated behavior in the cognitively-impaired elderly. An empathetic and sensitive caring approach that ensures comfort and that respects privacy has been shown to result in more "cooperation" than less "aggression" (Rader, Barrick, Boeffer, Sloane, McKenzie, Talerico, et al., 2006).

MY JOURNEY INTO ALZHEIMER'S DISEASE

Just because a person is incontinent or requires feeding does not give some eighteen-year-old twit the right to call them "dearie," or "sweetie."

Watching some of the Alzheimer's day care centers featured on television gives me the "willies." I could never bear to be talked to and treated like a child at summer camp. "All right boys and girls, let's all stretch our arms to the music; let's dance the hokey pokey."

I am repulsed by activity directors on cruise ships, much less some twenty-year-old trying to get me to play childish exercises to rock music. I'm sure I would try to get back to my room and if stopped in this attempt I would become churlish and belligerent. If the insensitive director continued to push or become condescending and began to pat my arm, I would probably explode with all the violence pent up in my six-foot-seven frame. If I were then restrained or tied in my chair, my fury would take me right out of my mind.

*Why? Is this a result of Alzheimer's disease? No, this is how I would react now in my best state of mind. I cannot stand the beat of rock music or the bouncing around of even senior citizen aerobic exercise classes. Human dignity demands that I have the right of refusal for any activity or entertainment that I do not perceive as entertaining. I deserve the right to withdraw from any situation and to go to a place of quiet and calm that I have appreciated over the years.**

(Davis, 1989, p. 102)

The Straight Story

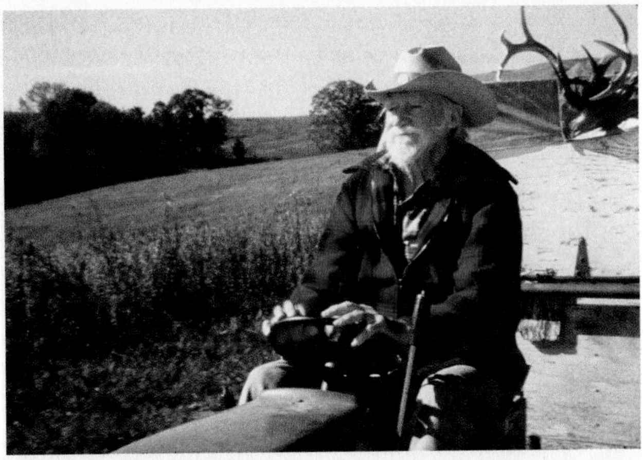

Source: Straight Story INC (Courtesy: The Kobal Collection)

What do you do in rural America when your estranged brother is dying and you're too infirm to have a driver's license (or a car)? If you're Alvin Straight, you hitch a trailer on your riding lawnmower and head for the open road. *Straight Story* puts actor Richard Farnsworth on Alvin's John Deere and sets out across Iowa for a series of unforgettable senior adventures.

*Reprinted with permission. From *My Journey into Alzheimer's Disease*, by Robert Davis,

APPLICATION OF THE NURSING PROCESS 25-3

ASSESSMENT

The older person experiencing significant short-term memory loss and impairments in reasoning, judgment, and overall intellectual ability is nearly always very resistant to acknowledging his or her difficulties and to seeking help. If the individual lives alone, it is often neighbors who first recognize changes in the person's behavior (e.g., leaving garbage to pile up or walking outside only partially dressed). Once family members are involved and start to look more closely into personal and financial matters, a pattern of gradual decline

(Continues)

APPLICATION OF THE NURSING PROCESS 25-3 (Continued)

over months and even years in the individual's ability to manage household, financial, and personal affairs usually emerges. The changes noted may be as subtle as gradual withdrawal from social activities (dining out or regular attendance at religious services) or as dramatic as writing checks for household repairs that were never done or a $10,000 check for a $10.95 bill.

The struggle to remain an independent and competent, respectable adult is a very normal and expected response to the mental decline. However, the family's concerns for the person's safety and needs for assistance in personal, household, and financial matters require some type of recognition and identification of the problem. Generally, it is a plea from family that first reaches the ears of a health professional (nurse, physician, or social worker). Often, the story emerges when the person with a dementia is seeking health care for another physical problem in a clinic or hospital setting.

From a medical perspective, the diagnosis of dementia is one of exclusion. When symptoms of a gradual cognitive decline similar to the pattern previously described occur, a thorough medical workup is indicated. It includes a battery of tests to rule out a reversible cause for these impairments. Nurses may be the first to recognize risk factors such as nutritional intake or poor management of diabetes as a reversible type of impairment and be responsible for medical consultation.

Common reversible conditions that may be causing the symptoms of dementia include depression or any of the pathophysiological disorders that may cause a delirium.

Completing this first step in assessment usually takes at least 3 to 4 weeks. If a drug toxicity is suspected, it generally takes this long for drugs to be cleared from the older adult, who has diminished renal function and slower excretion rates. If no treatable condition can be identified, an interdisciplinary assessment is required for the diagnosis of dementia.

A complete interdisciplinary assessment is usually performed at a geriatric mental health facility on either an outpatient or inpatient basis. An interdisciplinary assessment has a twofold purpose: validation of an irreversible dementia and identification of the level of care required to meet the individual's functional deficits or behavioral manifestations.

Many different screening instruments can be used to measure the various degrees of impairment in at least 12 categories of cognitive function and mental status (McDougall, 1990). Different screening instruments focus on different domains, with few covering all 12.

Precise differentiation of delirium, dementia, or depression is difficult since the presenting symptoms often overlap. Often a combination of screening instruments will be used in an assessment. The difficulty in selecting any one instrument for any one specific purpose is that each instrument measures a different blend of affective function, cognitive function, functional ability, and mental status. Two commonly used tests to differentiate Alzheimer's from other types of dementia are the Brief Cognitive Rating Scale (BCRS) (Reisberg & Ferris, 1988) and the Dementia of the Alzheimer Type Inventory (DAT) (Cummings & Benson, 1986). In a retrospective study of 50 patients, the DAT correctly identified 100% of those individuals with AD and 94% of those individuals without it (Cummings & Benson, 1986). The "Clock drawing test" has been

NURSING**ALERT** 25-4

Warning Signs of Dementia

- Withdrawal from usual social activities
- Financial misappropriations
- Neglect of household repairs or maintenance
- Unusual or bizarre behaviors in dress, personal contacts, business contacts, or correspondence

BOX 25-6
CATEGORIES OF COGNITIVE FUNCTION

- Attention span
- Concentration
- Intelligence
- Judgment
- Learning ability
- Memory
- Orientation
- Perception
- Problem solving
- Psychomotor ability
- Reaction time
- Social intactness

(Continues)

APPLICATION OF THE NURSING PROCESS 25-3 (Continued)

shown to correlate highly with MMSE and other neuropsychological test scores as an indicator of constructional apraxia, which is often seen early in dementia (Moretti, Torre, Antonella, Cozzato, & Bova, 2002). Although this should be merely a screening test, it is an easily used one in a variety of settings. A psychologist is usually responsible for administering the battery of neuropsychological tests used to differentiate types of cognitive impairments and rule out depression as the cause or exacerbating condition.

Nurses and occupational therapists contribute to an evaluation of the individual's abilities and difficulties in the performance of activities of daily living (ADL). Nurses are usually best able to assess personal self-care activities such as bathing, dressing, eating, toileting, and walking. Occupational therapists usually assess the instrumental activities of daily living (IADL) such as shopping, using a telephone, food preparation, housekeeping, doing laundry, and handling finances.

Conclusions derived from the interdisciplinary assessment can have a variety of meanings for the demented individual and his family. Being labeled with a progressively deteriorating condition for which there is no cure is a difficult experience. A spouse describes her feelings as she first shares her husband's diagnosis of Alzheimer's with others:

BOX 25-7
MEDICAL SCREENING FOR PATHOPHYSIOLOGICAL CAUSES OF COGNITIVE IMPAIRMENT

DIAGNOSTICS

- CT/MRI scan of brain to rule out tumor, hematoma, or hydrocephalus
- EEG/positron emission tomography scans
- Fasting serum glucose to rule out hypoglycemia
- Serum calcium, $K+$, and $Na+$ to identify electrolyte deficits that can cause a change in mental status
- Serum B_{12} and folate to identify vitamin deficiencies
- Thyroid and renal function studies to identify hyper/hypothyroidism or renal failure
- Urinalysis to rule out infection
- Complete blood count with differential to rule out anemia and septicemia
- Serum drug levels to rule out drug toxicities

MEDICAL INTERVENTIONS

- Withdrawal from all nonessential medications to eliminate toxicities or drug interactions (usually takes 2 to 4 weeks for all drugs to be cleared from body tissues)
- Administer antibiotics and hydrate (as needed) for infectious disorders
- Correct medical disorders and electrolyte imbalances
- Surgery for structural abnormalities of brain tissue, such as tumor, hematoma, or hydrocephalus

OUTCOMES

The prognosis will be determined by the cause of the condition. In general, the earlier that treatment is initiated in the course of the abnormality, the better the prognosis. When aggressive interventions are needed to reverse severe alterations in homeostasis, the chances of iatrogenic complications become more likely. Irreversible physiological abnormalities may result in a permanent cognitive impairment.

(*Continues*)

APPLICATION OF THE NURSING PROCESS 25-3 (Continued)

CATCH A FALLING STAR

Reactions, once the news is out, are interesting. Our neighbor Veron says, "Hank could not have lost all his expertise unless something was drastically wrong. Alzheimer's explains his present condition."

Others, good friends included, seem to have a father, mother or ancient aunt to whom they compare Hank. Some divulge useful, helpful information.

*Mostly, though, it's hard to take. This is not someone from another era we're talking about. This is a contemporary. This is my HUSBAND! I feel we are being put into some antique category. This really hurts.**

(*Spohr & Bullard, 1995, p. 52*)

On the other hand, a definitive diagnosis can also be somewhat of a relief for both the individual experiencing these changes as well as the caregiver unable to make any long-term plans until a diagnosis is made. Joyce's husband said:

WHEN I GROW TOO OLD TO DREAM

In my opinion, the best thing that any medical practitioner can do, if he or she suspects possible dementia, is to advise the carer immediately. Do not wait to be sure, for by that time the patient will be on the autopsy table. Tell the carer there is a possibility that the patient could have an irreversible disease of the brain. Further tests and observations may disprove that. I wish I had known earlier about how the deterioration of memory might affect the patient.

Taking into consideration the carer's condition or attitude as a reason for not telling them is not really helpful. If it is true that the patient has progressive dementia, the carer is going to find out in any case, the hard way. If the possible diagnosis is later disproved, then the carer will be happy. If not, then the carer will be prepared.

For me, understanding had to come first. Then, there was acceptance and finally the ability to cope. I feel it would be the same for most people.†

(*Naughtin, 1992, p. 113*)

NURSING DIAGNOSIS

The level of dependence and specific behaviors that result from the unique blend of personality traits and physical and cognitive impairments will determine the nursing diagnosis profile for the person with chronic dementias. Self-care deficits, altered nutrition, incontinence, fear, and anxiety are common responses.

Chronic dementias not only affect an individual, but also generally change the entire family process. Because of the intense and heavy demands such conditions place on caregivers, the profound effect of caregiving on daily life has been termed "the 36-hour day" (Mace, 1983). Common nursing diagnoses for the family and caregiver, therefore, reflect the physical and emotional stresses of caring for every physical need, as well as coping with difficult behavioral responses and the safety risk imposed by a person who may wander off at any given moment of the day or night.

Another major factor influencing caregiving needs is the extended period of time for which care will be required. Given the average span of 10 to 15 years for AD, the caregiver must make many decisions regarding future financial, legal, and ethical issues. Emotional adjustments to the role changes brought about by the caregiving relationship and dependent position of the demented loved one will be required. In order to make these adjustments, family members need a great deal of information regarding the usual progression of the disease and types of services available for respite care as well as assistance in the home. *Deficient knowledge* is, therefore, a common nursing diagnosis for families caring for a demented loved one.

*From *Catch a Falling Star: Living with Alzheimer's*, by Betty Spohr and Jean Bullard, 1995, Seattle: Sirpos Press. Reprinted with permission.

†From *When I Grow Too Old to Dream*, by G. Naughtin and T. Laidler, Copyright © 1992. Reprinted with permission from HarperCollins Religious, Melbourne, Australia.

(*Continues*)

APPLICATION OF THE NURSING PROCESS 25-3 (Continued)

OUTCOME IDENTIFICATION

From a strictly biomedical perspective, maintaining the independence and function of the demented older adult is the major therapeutic goal. However, limiting nursing care to the biomedical model is more akin to the maintenance of a machine than to the care of a human being. In contrast, nursing care from a human caring theory perspective is more strongly focused on methods and ways of intuiting how dignity and selfhood can be preserved. While this may certainly include attention to independence in daily functions and activities to the fullest extent possible, it is not the only purpose or even the major purpose of nursing care. Many human conditions exist for which there is vulnerability and the threat to autonomy and selfhood. Although dementia may be only one such condition, it is a particularly poignant one since there is usually only the rare possibility of a cure and the prognosis generally involves years of gradual decline in the cognitive abilities associated with independence, self-control, and self-identity.

PLANNING/INTERVENTIONS

Watson's (1988) theory of human care nursing can provide a foundation for practice with demented adults that responds to the spiritual and emotional needs as well as the physical ones. As discussed in Chapter 3, Watson views caring as the substance of nursing. The transpersonal exchange of energy between nurse and client is based on the nurse's genuine commitment to dignity, support, warmth, and comfort. This commitment involves both the art and science of nursing.

The art of nursing involves a transcendence or interpretation in order to appreciate the essence of the individual's state of being. The importance to Watson of **mutuality**, or client involvement in the therapeutic relationship, does not rule out the importance of intuition in the art of nursing. This process of "being with" is often referred to as empathy. The intuitive knowing that enables nurses to step inside another's reality even when that person cannot verbalize all his thoughts and feelings has also been called the "art/act" (Chinn & Kramer, 1991). According to Chinn and Kramer, it is this "comprehension of meaning in a singular particular, subjective expression" (p. 10) called the art/act that enables nurses to know what is significant in the moment and to "envision what is possible but not yet real" (p. 10). The art of nursing when combined with the science of nursing allows for judgments to be made about specific caring behaviors that will promote health and dignity for the person with a cognitive impairment in any given situation, experience, or moment.

VIEWING COGNITIVE IMPAIRMENTS FROM A CARING FRAMEWORK

The person with memory loss is disconnected from his or her past. In being robbed of the past, the person is stripped of much of his identity, at least identity as others have known it. In order to plan nursing care from the perspective of Watson's (1988) human care theory, the nurse must first understand what it is like for a human being to live in a manner where he is denied of his past and a sense of self-control and identity.

Promoting self-identity in the presence of severe cognitive impairments requires an ongoing collaboration between the nurse and family caregivers. Personal history and experience guides creative problem-solving approaches to managing behaviors, identifying physical needs, and meeting those needs in a way that honors a lifetime of habits and preferences. Several general principles, however, may be useful guides for planning individualized care.

When loss of memory and judgment makes even the most minor of decisions a major obstacle, simplification of the environment and consistency in daily routines may lessen the stress. Identifying lifelong habits in preparing for bedtime, mealtimes, or morning rituals and consistently adhering to them seems to ease the daily frustrations for the person with the impairment as well as for the caregiver. Caregivers have also discovered that simplifying the environment by removing mirrors and any unnecessary clutter or background

(*Continues*)

APPLICATION OF THE NURSING PROCESS 25-3 (Continued)

BOX 25-8
NURSING DIAGNOSES FOR THE INDIVIDUAL AND FAMILY EXPERIENCING CHRONIC IMPAIRMENTS IN COGNITION

CLIENT

- Self-Care Deficit: Bathing/Hygiene/Dressing/Grooming/Feeding/Toileting
- Imbalanced Nutrition: Less than Body Requirements
- Functional Urinary Incontinence
- Anxiety
- Fear
- Risk for Injury
- Situational Low Self-Esteem
- Ineffective Role Performance
- Impaired Social Interaction
- Impaired Physical Mobility
- Spiritual distress

CAREGIVER/FAMILY

- Deficient Knowledge
- Fatigue
- Interrupted Family Processes
- Caregiver role strain
- Ineffective Role Performance
- Compromised Family Coping
- Disabled Family Coping

noises such as television or radio may have a calming influence on the person frustrated by memory loss and alterations in perception. Displaying familiar pictures or objects imbued with meaning may serve as orienting cues. Subtle methods such as these are preferable to more direct attempts at reality orientation, such as correcting or bombarding the person with facts and figures. The latter type of approach relies on short-term memory, which is the first to go in various forms of dementias. Constant reminders of memory failure result in little or no significant improvement in functional status and may do harm by assaulting the already fragile identity and self-esteem of the older adult with cognitive impairments.

Making the most of remaining abilities is a key element in a healthy and meaningful existence for both the cognitively impaired and their caregivers. The ability to respond and express emotion seems to remain intact after other cognitive abilities have been lost. Emphasizing the affective component of communication (e.g., eye contact, tone of voice, and touch) is generally best received by the demented person. When instructions or specific messages must be conveyed, using language that is simple and direct in structure is usually most effective and least frustrating. Expressing a message in a statement format such as "Let's sit down here" is usually preferable to a question such as "Where would you like to sit when you get tired?" Validation therapy has grown in popularity in recent years as a technique that focuses on the interpersonal aspects of communicating with the individual who is cognitively impaired (Feil, 1989). The primary purpose of this therapy is the validation of feelings rather than reorientation with current facts.

Plenty of exercise is important for overall general health. Many caregivers have found that they can manage to keep a daily walk in the person's routine long after other activities have become unmanageable, so long as the walk is done at the same time of day and over the same route. Maintaining as much social interaction as possible is important for an overall sense of well-being for most individuals. In the institutional setting, exterior spaces for walking, homelike settings with small groups of patients, and inclusion of nature (plants, animals, outdoors, and nature sounds) are all ways to enhance a sense of well-being and health (Cohen-Mansfield & Bester, 2006). Once again, individuality and life-long preferences must be taken into consideration. Reminiscence therapy is frequently used in long-term care facilities to promote social involvement and self-identity not only among the cognitively impaired but also among the nonimpaired healthy elderly. Familiar items such as articles of clothing, newspaper headlines, old songs, or photographs are used to elicit past memories. A sharing of personal stories associated with these memories is encouraged for the purpose of social interaction and validation of self-worth.

(*Continues*)

APPLICATION OF THE NURSING PROCESS 25-3 (Continued)

Regardless of communication techniques utilized, as cognition declines there is a significant decline in the ability of persons with cognitive impairments to express their physical needs or discomforts. Subtle changes in behavior, such as agitation or restlessness, may be anything from an expression of physical discomfort such as a shoe rubbing a callous, or a full bladder, to a life-threatening medical problem such as impaction, sepsis, or dehydration. Knowing the individual and using the process of elimination is often the best way for a caregiver to determine the reason for the change in behavior. Use of a behavioral observation log over a two- to three-day period can help track when and under what circumstances the behavior occurs (Smith & Buckwalter, 2005) and in identifying unmet needs that warrant intervention (Evans, 2007). At other times, however, agitation may be a more direct response to the daily frustration of living with a cognitive impairment, and distraction may be the most useful way to prevent the behavior from escalating into a catastrophic reaction.

Nonpharmacologic interventions previously discussed such as environmental modification (familiar objects, reduced clutter and noise, incorporating nature, homelike setting, and exercise), interpersonal approaches (eye contact, soothing and respectful tone of voice, simplified language, and use/avoidance of touch) and cognitive interventions (subtle reminders such as clocks, and reminiscence prompts and cues) should be first-line therapy for maintaining function and improving quality of life. When psychotic symptoms such as hallucinations and extreme paranoia become frightening to the person or regularly result in aggressive behavior toward others, referral to a geriatric psychiatrist for pharmacological therapy may be indicated. Although there is some evidence that psychotic symptoms may occur at some time in close to 50% of patients with Alzheimer's (Ropacki & Jeste, 2005), not all symptoms are troubling to the person, and usually the psychotic symptoms become less prominent after one year. In recognition of the high risk of adverse effects of neuroleptics such as haloperidol and antipsychotics, the American Geriatrics Society and the American Association of Geriatric Psychiatrists (2003) recommend that all drugs used to manage behavioral symptoms in the person with dementia should be tapered and discontinued after six months of treatment (Evans, 2007).

EVALUATION

The progressively declining nature of various dementias makes improvements in function an unlikely goal of nursing care. Therefore, the effectiveness of care must be evaluated from a different perspective. If dignity and comfort are the major goals, listening to the stories of elders and caregivers gives us insight into the fears of those with dementia. A caregiver for persons with dementia noted the following of many of the individuals for whom she had cared: "None of us enjoys being organised and pushed around faster than we can personally manage and not one of us likes to feel that we do not have control over our own lives" (Naughtin & Laidler, 1992, p. 214). Such stories tell us that fear of loss of dignity and ultimately of control and personality weigh heavily on the person with dementia.

Evaluation within a caring framework, therefore, must include the degree to which persons with dementia maintain control and dignity over their lives. The degree to which they remain functional and independent in ADL is one aspect of control and dignity. Since loss of control and resulting frustration may be manifested as a catastrophic reaction, the degree to which such reactions are reduced may be another reflection of how well control and dignity are being maintained. An even more direct evaluative approach may be undertaken in partnership with the demented elder and his primary caregivers. This partnership is formed for the purpose of designing and evaluating care that honors the elder's pattern of habits, lifestyle, and personality traits that have developed over a lifetime and are now threatened by disease. The plan of care will be a continually evolving one as cognitive abilities decline. However, all outcomes will be judged against the degree to which the individual's established pattern is being maintained in the presence of declining cognitive abilities.

CARING FOR THE CAREGIVERS

The "graying of America" is changing the composition of the American family. Most families have members in four generations and some have members in five or six.

Unlike the familiar rearing of children in which family caregivers are typically young and healthy parents, the caregivers of older persons are often spouses or adult children, many in their sixties, seventies, and older, who may also be struggling with chronic illness. Women still provide the bulk of caregiving in our society. In fact, a woman today can expect to spend 18 years of her life caring for aging parents (the average amount of time spent caring for children is 17 years!). These women are often referred to as the "sandwich generation" or "the women in the middle," as they try to juggle the needs of adult children, a household, their own personal and career needs, and the physical and emotional needs of a dependent parent or spouse. The mental and physical stresses of caregiving may include isolation and alienation from friends, sleep disturbances, fatigue, and more frequent complaints of stress-related illnesses such as headaches and gastrointestinal disturbances.

Approximately 22 million households have a family member with Alzheimer's and the number of people with Alzheimer's is expected to nearly triple by the year 2050 (Alzheimer's Association, 2008). People with Alzheimer's tend to live with their families until the disease is in advanced stages. The average amount of time an Alzheimer's caregiver spends is 17.6 hours/week. Approximately 60% of caregivers state that they make some type of out-of-pocket contribution to care (e.g., medications, in-home services; Alzheimer's Association, 2008). The needs of caregivers are a growing responsibility for geropsychiatric nurses both today and in the future.

The changes in roles and relationships established over a lifetime and the practical, legal, financial, and everyday demands of caregiving for a demented loved one exact an emotional and physical toll. Certain themes are expressed repeatedly as caregivers tell their stories of caring for cognitively impaired loved ones (Naughtin & Laidler, 1992). These themes, presented in what follows, provide much-needed insight for nurses providing care to the caregiver.

Honesty with the Diagnosis

A direct approach when informing a person of his diagnosis early in the course of the disease helps both the individual and the family to recognize that they are not going "mad." Caregivers also say that once the diagnosis is made, they benefit from a clear statement regarding the nature of the illness, the likely process of its development, and information about resources that will help them cope both emotionally with role and relationship changes as well as with the practical day-to-day problems.

Relationship Tensions

The insidious onset and delay in diagnosis lead often to much tension between the person with dementia and the primary caregiver when the caregiver holds the demented loved one responsible for personality changes and problem behaviors. Caregivers need reinforcement from professionals and friends and family that these behaviors are not intentional and truly are typical of the disease.

Financial and Legal Affairs

Decisions about legal matters such as wills and powers of attorney are best handled in the early stages of dementia, when the person with dementia can still participate in the decision-making process.

Use of Community Resources

There seems to be a general reluctance to use community support services. Caregivers seem often to feel that this is an admission of failure or see such services as "welfare." Or they may be simply unaware of them. Caregivers do acknowledge the importance of knowing all the variety of options of support available to them. One form of service that is overwhelmingly well received by caregivers is respite or day care. While there often is some initial reluctance to use respite caregivers and persons with dementia struggle with admitting that they are like "all those other people," there is general acceptance once a pattern is established. Caregivers find it vital as pressure mounts.

Psychoeducational programs and support groups are growing in popularity. One advantage of these programs over psychotherapy or personal counseling is that their educational nature takes away the stigma or feelings of failure often attached to the more traditional types of mental health services. There is also usually no cost associated with self-help groups (except for small donations for refreshments or minor associated costs). All groups involve a mutual sharing of emotional support as well as practical tips on everyday problems encountered during caregiving. A recent development is computer "online" support groups. An advantage of this type of service is that caregivers may join in the discussion at any time (day or night) from the convenience of their own homes. Nurses serve as moderators for some of these groups.

Guilt over Nursing Home Placement

Placing a loved one in permanent residential care is one of the most difficult decisions caregivers must make. The caregiver often experiences much guilt when coaxing the loved one into the ambulance or car that will take the loved one to the facility. Moments of agony often follow as the caregiver must walk away from a loved one pleading not to be left. This is often a scene replayed over and over again in the caregiver's mind. After spending years attending to the loved one's every need, the caregiver often finds the care provided by a nursing home to be very unsatisfactory. This feeling, however, can change over time as the loved one adapts to the new environment and the caregiver begins to recognize the dedication of the staff and the quality of care being given.

Humor

Caregivers often talk about the benefit of being able to see humor in the absurd and of being able to laugh with their loved ones over the uncontrollable.

The Positive Aspects

Caregiving is not only about stress and negative consequences. Caregivers also relate the experience of joyful moments. Of no minor significance is the satisfaction of love, affection, and commitment expressed by the act of caregiving!

FUTURE DIRECTIONS

For the foreseeable future, mental health and aging can be characterized by the balance between cure and care. New advances in gene mapping and discoveries in neurophysiology are giving hope of a cure for Alzheimer's disease. Pharmacological advances have made successes possible in the delay of onset as well as the management of symptoms of Alzheimer's. For at least the near future, however, these new technologies will not take away the need for social support as families care for loved ones with dementia.

Historically, geropsychiatry owes its recognition and growth to the burgeoning interest in AD some 25 years ago. The study of cognitive impairments has received the "lion's share" of attention in this field. The prevalence of and need for research into other mental illnesses experienced by older adults, such as schizophrenia, substance abuse, and anxiety disorders, will be expanding areas of study.

Lastly, much attention to date has been given to mental illness and aging. There is a recognized need for a greater emphasis to be placed on the essence of mental health in old age. Questions are being raised as to how we as a society can nurture, support, and fuel the "vital spirit" of old age. Much more needs to be learned, not only about the factors and forces that allow certain individuals to resist the stresses of aging, but also about those characteristics that contribute to the wisdom and hardiness of old age.

The future holds promise for a more in-depth and broader understanding of both mental health and mental illness in old age. In order to be a part of this future, nurses will need to become active participants in the political and economic issues that will influence the success of this endeavor.

KEY CONCEPTS

- There is a strong association between physical illness and mental illness in the elderly.
- Ageist myths and stereotypes are major barriers to the identification and treatment of mental illness in the elderly.
- Impairments in cognition can be the result of a dementia, delirium, or depression. An incorrect diagnosis can lead to much needless suffering, permanent impairment, and even death.
- Dementia is generally an irreversible condition characterized by memory loss. Delirium is a harbinger of an acute medical condition and is characterized by a clouding of consciousness. Dementia is slow in onset; delirium is rapid.
- Intellectual function does not diminish with age. However, the aging brain is more susceptible to injury.
- Memory deficits pose a serious threat to self-esteem and identity.
- An interdisciplinary assessment is essential for the diagnosis and management of delirium, depression, and dementia in the older adult.
- Severe memory deficits are not the result of normal aging. The first priority is to look for an acute, reversible cause.
- Confusion is an important phenomenon for nursing research. Confusion should not be used as a label for the behavioral manifestations of impairments in cognition or memory loss.
- Old age is not depressing. However, multiple losses, financial strain, and poor health are risk factors for depression in old age.
- Insomnia and physical complaints are frequent symptoms of depression among an aged population.
- Pharmacotherapy and psychotherapy have good success rates in treating depression in the elderly.
- The risk of suicide is high among the elderly.
- Maximizing control and the opportunity for choices should be a major goal of nursing care for the depressed older adult.

REVIEW QUESTIONS

1. A family brings a grandparent to the hospital because he is demonstrating signs of dementia. The son asks the nurse, "Why does my father get so confused in the evening?" The nurse's assessment of the situation indicates that the client's behavior is an example of which of the following?

1. Confabulation
2. Confusion
3. Dementia
4. Sundown syndrome

2. The nurse working in a nursing home for the elderly would most likely find which of the following laboratory results for clients diagnosed with Alzheimer's disease?
1. Increased levels of acetylcholine
2. Decreased levels of acetylcholine
3. Normal levels of acetylcholine

3. The elderly client lacerated her hand while carving a turkey at the family's Christmas dinner. The client was taken to the emergency department for treatment. The community nurse has scheduled a follow-up visit with the client to determine whether the wound is healing as expected. Which of the following findings would alert the nurse to the possibility of infection?
1. Change in mental status
2. Difficulty with mobility
3. Loose fitting dentures
4. Change in elimination diet

4. An elderly client with dementia frequently roams the halls of the nursing home looking for his mother who died 20 years earlier. An appropriate nursing diagnosis for this behavior would be which of the following?
1. Thought process disorder related to psychosis
2. Insomnia related to new environment
3. Alteration in mobility related to aging process
4. Confusion related to dementia

5. Nursing intervention to address confusion in an elderly client would include which of the following?
1. Keep the client restrained at all times
2. Keep environment free of excess stimulation
3. Leave the television or radio turned on continuously
4. Wake client several times in evening to check orientation

6. The son of a client with stage II of Alzheimer's disease visits his mother three times a week. As the nurse enters the room the son states, "My mother doesn't even know who I am." What is the best therapeutic response the nurse can make at this time?
1. "I'm sure she is just joking with you."
2. "Do you want to come out to the station and talk about it?"
3. "I will page the doctor so he can examine her."
4. "Memory loss is very common in individuals with Alzheimer's disease."

LEARNING ACTIVITIES

1. Describe the physiological basis for at least three disorders that result in an irreversible dementia. List one type of dementia that is potentially reversible.
2. Describe three common symptoms of dementia. Explain how the symptoms may affect self-esteem and dignity.
3. Describe the major differences in caring for an older adult with dementia between Watson's caring framework and care from a strictly biomedical perspective.
4. List the components of an interdisciplinary assessment of dementia.
5. What are the distinguishing symptoms that characterize a delirium from a dementia?
6. Describe at least two therapeutic modalities used with cognitively impaired individuals in long-term care.
7. State the common variables associated with acute confusional states.
8. What is confusion? Why can its use as a label for patient behaviors hamper treatment goals?
9. Explain the mechanism of action of antidepressant drugs and anticonvulsant therapy in the treatment of depression in the aged.
10. Identify at least three sociocultural stressors that increase the risk of depression in the elderly.
11. What are some symptoms that characterize depression in the older adult?
12. Describe the adverse effects of antidepressant drugs most commonly experienced by the older adult.

*Study*WARE™ CONNECTION

Using your *Study*WARE™ CD-ROM

1. Complete the Crossword activity for this chapter.
2. Review the audio glossary for key terms in this chapter.
3. Explore the other games and activities that support this chapter.

REFERENCES

Administration on Aging. (2002a). *A profile of older Americans: 2002: Living arrangements.* Retrieved May 20, 2004, from http://www.aoa.gov/prof/Statistics/profile/4.asp

Administration on Aging. (2002b). *A profile of older Americans: 2002: The older population.* Retrieved May 20, 2004, from http://www.aoa.gov/prof/Statistics/statistics.asp.

Alzheimer's Association (2008). 2008 Alzheimer's Disease Facts and Figures, pp. 1–41. Retrieved October 10, 2008, from http://www.alz.org.

American Association for Geriatric Psychiatry. (2004). Geriatrics and mental health–The facts. Retrieved May 20, 2004, from http://www.aagpgpa.org/prof/facts-mh.asp.

American Association for Geriatric Psychiatry. (2008). When to refer depressed elderly patients to a geriatric psychiatrist. Retrieved September 21, from http://www.aagpgponline.org/prof/facts-referral.asp.

American Geriatrics Society & American Association for Geriatric Psychiatry (2003). Consensus statement on improving the quality of mental health care in U.S. nursing homes: Management of depression and behavioral symptoms associated with dementia. *Journal of the American Geriatrics Society,* 51, 1286–1298.

American Psychiatric Association. (2000). *Diagnostic and Statistical Manual of Mental Disorders* (Fourth Edition-Text Revision). Washington, DC: Author.

Arthur, H. M. (2006). Depression, isolation, social support and cardiovascular disease in older adults. *Journal of Cardiovascular Nursing, 21*(55), 52–57.

Asplund, K., Gustafson, Y., Jacobsson, C., Bucht, G., Wahlin, A., Peterson, J., Blom, J. O., & Angquist, K. A. (2000). Geriatric-based versus general wards for older acute medical patients: A randomized comparison of outcomes and use of resources. *Journal of the American Geriatric Society, 48*(11), 1381–1388.

Barba, B. E., Tesh, A. S., & Courts, N. F. (2002). Promoting thriving in nursing homes: The Eden Alternative. *Journal of Gerontological Nursing, 28*(3), 7–13.

Bartels, S. J. (2003). Improving system of care for older adults with mental illness in the United States: Findings and recommendations for the President's New Freedom Commission on Mental Health. *American Journal of Geriatric Psychiatry, 11,* 486–497.

Bartels, S. J., Miles, K. M., Dums, A. R., & Pratt, S. I. (2003) Factors associated with community mental health service use by older adults with severe mental illness. *Journal of Mental Health and Aging, 9,* 123–135.

Birks, J., Grimley, E., Iakividou, V., & Holt, F. E. (2009). Rivastigmine for alzheimer's disease. *Cochrane Database of Systematic Reviews,* April *15*(2), CD 001191.

Blacker, D., Wilcox, M. A., Laird, N. M., Rodes, L., Horvath, S. M., Go, R. C., et al. (1998). Alpha-2 macroglobulin is genetically associated with Alzheimer disease. *Nature Genetics, 19,* 357–360.

Breitbart, W., Rosenfeld, B., Roth, A., Smith, M. J., Cohen, K., & Passik, S. (1997). The memorial delirium assessment scale. *Journal of Pain and Symptom Management, 13,* 128–137.

Buchanon, D., Farran, C., & Clark, D. (1995). Suicidal thought and self-transcendence in older adults. *Journal of Psychosocial Nursing and Mental Health Services, 33*(10), 31–34.

Butcher, H. K., & McGonigal-Kenney, M. (2005). Depression and dispiritedness in later life. *American Journal of Nursing, 105*(12), 52–62.

Chinn, P. L., & Kramer, M. K. (1991). Nursing's pattern of knowing. In P. L. Chinn & M. K. Kramer (Eds.), *Theory and nursing: A systematic approach* (3rd ed., pp. 1–18). St. Louis: Mosby.

Clarke, R., Smith, A. D., Jobst, K. A., Refsum, H., Sutton, L., Ueland, P. M. (1998). Folate, vitamin B_{12}, and serum total homocysteine levels in confirmed Alzheimer disease. *Archives of Neurology, 55*(11), 1449–1455.

Cohen-Mansfield, J., & Bester, A. (2006). Flexibility as a management principle in dementia care: The Adards example. *Gerontologist, 46*(4), 540–544.

Cummings, J. L., & Benson, F. (1986). Dementia of the Alzheimer type: An inventory of diagnostic clinical features. *Journal of the American Geriatrics Society, 32*(1), 12–19.

Douzjian, M., Wilson, C., Shultz, M., Berger, J., Tapnio, J., Blanton, V. (2002). A program to use pain control medication to reduce psychotropic drug use in residents with difficult behavior. *Nursing Home Medicine: The Annals of Long-Term Care,* 1–7. Retrieved May 20, 2004, from http://www.mmhc.com/nhm/articles/NHM9804/Douzjian.html.

Dychtwald, K. (1989). Conversation with ... interview by Richard Peck. *Geriatrics 44*(3), 117–119.

Ely, E. W., Inouye, S. K., Bernard, G. R., Gordon, S., Francis, J., May, L., et al. (2001). Delirium in mechanically ventilated patients: Validity and reliability of the confusion assessment method for the intensive care unit (CAM-ICU). *JAMA,* 286(21), 2703–2710.

Erickson, E. H., Erickson, J. M., & Kibnick, H. Q. (1987). *Vital involvement in old age.* New York: W. W. Norton.

Evans, L. K. (2007). Module VIII. Mental health issues in aging (pp. 1–15). Enhancing Gerontology Content in Senior-level Baccalaureate Courses, Portland, Oregon American Association of Colleges of Nursing, Geriatric Nursing Education Consortium Faculty Development Institute, June 27–29.

Everard, K. M. (1999). The relationship between reasons for activity and older adult well-being. *Journal of Applied Gerontology, 18*(3), 325–340.

Feil, N. (1989). *Validation: The Feil method.* Cleveland, OH: Edward Feil Production.

Fitzsimmons, S. (2001). Easy riderwheelchairbiking: A nursing-recreation therapy clinical trial for the treatment of depression. *Journal of Gerontological Nursing,* 27(5), 14–23.

Folstein, M., Folstein, S., & McHugh, P. (1975). Mini-mental state: A practical method for grading the cognitive state of patients for the clinician. *Journal of Psychiatric Research, 12,* 189–198.

Foreman, M. (1989). Confusion in the hospitalized elderly: Incidence, onset, and associated factors. *Research in Nursing and Health, 12,* 21–29.

Gauthier, K. S., Wirth, U., & Mobius, H. J. (2005). Effects of memantine on behavioral symptoms in Alzheimer's disease patients: An analysis of the neuropsychiatric inventory data of two randomized, controlled studies. *International Journal of Geriatric Psychiatry,* 20(5), 459–464.

Givens, J. L., Jones, R. N., Inouye, S. K. (2009) The Overlap Syndrome of Depression and Delirium in Older Hospitalized Patients. *Journal of the American Geriatrics Society.* 57(8), Published Online: Jun 3 2009 10:45AM DOI: 10.1111/j.1532-415.2009.02342.x.

Gleason, O. (2003). Delirium. *American Family Physician, 67,* 1027–1035.

Guteri, P. F, Edinger, G., & Schumacher, S. (2003). TWICE: A NICHE program at North Memorial Healthcare. *Geriatric Nursing* , *23*(3), 133–138.

Haight, B. K., Barba, B. E., Tesh, A. S., & Courts, N. F. (2002). Thriving: A life span theory. *Journal of Gerontological Nursing, 28*(3), 14–22.

Haight, B. K., & Hendrix, S. (1998). Suicidal intent/life satisfaction: Comparing the life stories of older women. *Suicide and Life-Threatening Behavior, 28*(3), 272–284.

He, W., Sengupta, M., Velkoff, V., & DeBarros, K. (2005). *65+ in the United States: Current population reports.* Washington, DC: U.S. Government Printing Office.

Hegge, M., & Fischer, C. (2000). Grief responses of senior and elderly widows. *Journal of Gerontological Nursing, 26*(2), 35–43.

Hicks, T. J. (2000). What is your life like now? Loneliness and elderly individuals residing in nursing homes. *Journal of Gerontological Nursing, 26*(8), 15–19.

Hill, A., & Brettle, A. (2005). The effectiveness of counseling with older people: Results of a systematic review. *Counseling and Psychotherapy Research, 5*(6), 265–272.

Holmes, J. D., & House, A. O. (2000). Psychiatric illness predicts poor outcome after surgery for hip fracture: A prospective cohort study. *Psychological Medicine, 30*(4), 921–929.

Inouye, S., van Dyck, C., Alessi, C., Balkin, S., Siegal, A. I., & Horwitz, R. (1990). Clarifying confusion: The confusion assessment method. *Annals of Internal Medicine, 113*(12), 941–948.

Inouye, S. K., Bogardus, S. T., Charpentier, P. A., Leo-Summers, L., Acamporo, D., Holford, et al. (1999). A multicomponent intervention to prevent delirium in hospitalized older patients. *New England Journal of Medicine, 340*(9), 669–676.

Johnson, C. L., & Barer, B. M. (1997). *Life beyond 85 years.* New York: Springer Publishing Company.

Katz, I. R., Streim, J., & Parmalee, P. (1994). Prevention of depression, recurrences, and complications in late life. *Preventive Medicine, 23*, 743–750.

Kerber, C. S., Dyck, M. J., Culp, K. R., & Buckwalter, K. (2005). Comparing the Geriatric Depression Scale, Minimum Data Set, and primary care provider diagnosis for depression in rural nursing home residents. *Journal of the American Psychiatric Nurses Association, 11*(5), 269–275.

Kivnick, H. (1993, Winter/Spring). Everyday mental health: A guide to assessing life strengths. *Generations, 17*(1), 13–20.

Koenig, H. (1999). Late-life depression: How to treat patients with comorbid chronic illness. *Geriatrics, 54*(5), 56–61.

Kurlowicz, L. (1997). Nursing standard of practice protocol: Depression in elderly patients. *Geriatric Nursing, 18*(5), 192–199.

Lebowitz, B. (2004). Trends in mental illness among nursing home patients. *Long-term Care Forum, 1*(2), 3–5. Retrieved May 20, 2004, from http://www.aagpgpa.org/prof/LTCvlissue2.pdf.

Lundstrom, M., Edlund, A., Karlsson, S., Brannstrom, B., Bucht, G., & Gustafson, Y. (2005). A multifactorial intervention program reduces the duration of delirium, lengths of hospitalization, and mortality in delirious patients. *Journal of the American Geriatrics Society, 53*(4), 622–628.

Lyketsos, C. G., Colenda, C. C., Beck, C., Blank, K., Doraiswamy, M.P., Kalunian, D.A., et al. (2006). Position statement of the American Association for Geriatric Psychiatry regarding principles of care for patients with dementia resulting from Alzheimer Disease. *American Journal of Geriatric Psychiatry, 14*(7), 561–573.

Mace, N. (1983). *The 36-hour day: A family's guide to caring for persons with Alzheimer disease, related dementing illnesses, and memory loss in later life.* Baltimore: Johns Hopkins University Press.

McDougall, G. (1990). Review of screening instruments for assessing cognitive and mental status in older adults. *Nurse Practitioner, 15*(11), 18–28.

Moneyham, L., & Scott, C. (1995). Anticipatory grieving in the elderly. *Journal of Gerontological Nursing, 21*(7), 23–28.

Moretti, R., Torre, P., Antonella, R., Cozzato, G., & Bova, A. (2002). Ten Point Clock Test: A correlation analysis with other neuropsychological tests in dementia. *International Journal of Geriatric Psychiatry, 17*(4), 347–353.

Muller, R. J. (2002, December). Delirium missed as the cause of psychotic symptoms in the E. R. *Psychiatric Times, 19*(2), 68–75.

National Institute on Aging, National Institutes of Health. (1999). *Progress Report on Alzheimer's Disease.* Bethesda, MD: Author.

Naughtin, G., & Laidler, T. (1992). *When I grow too old to dream.* North Blackburn, Australia: Harper Collins *Religious.*

Neelon, V., Champagne, M., Carlson, J., & Funk, S. (1996). The NEECHAM confusion scale: Construction, validation and clinical testing. *Nursing Research, 45*, 324–330.

Nightingale, F. (1969). *Notes on nursing.* Unabridged republication of 1st American edition, 1860, by D. Appleton & Company. New York: Dover Publications.

O'Keefe, S. T., Mulkerrin, E. C., Nayeem, K., Varughese, M., & Pillay, I. (2005). Use of serial MMSE to diagnose and monitor delirium in elderly hospitalized patients. *Journal of the American Geriatrics Society, 53*(5), 867–870.

Osgood, N. (1992). *Suicide in later life.* New York: Lexington Books.

Parellada, E., Baez, I., dePablo, J., & Martinez, G. (2004). Risperidone in the treatment of patients with delirium. *Journal of Clinical Psychiatry, 65*, 348–353.

Peterson, J. F., Pun, B. T., Dittus, R. S., Thomason, J. W., Jackson, J. C., Shintani, A. K., et al. (2006). Delirium and its motoric subtypes: A study of 614 critically ill patients. *Journal of the American Geriatrics Society, 54*(3), 479–484.

Puentes, W. J. (2004). Cognitive therapy integrated with life review techniques: An eclectic treatment approach for affective symptoms in older adults. *Journal of Clinical Nursing, 13*, 84–89.

Rader, J., Barrick, A. L., Boeffer, B., Sloane, P. D., McKenzie, D., Talerico, K. A., et al. (2006). The bathing of older adults with dementia. *American Journal of Nursing, 106*(4), 40–49.

Rapp, C., Wakefield, B., Kundrat, M., Mentes, J., Tripp-Reimer, T., Culp, K. et al. (2000). Acute confusion assessment instruments: Clinical versus research usability. *Applied Nursing Research, 13*(1), 37–45.

Reisberg, B., & Ferris, S. (1988). Brief cognitive rating scale (BCRS). *Psychopharmacology Bulletin, 24*(4), 629–636.

Remington, R., Gerdner, L. A., & Buckwalter, K. (2005). Nursing management of clients experiencing dementias of late life: Care environments, clients and caregivers. In K. D. Melillo & S. C. Houde (Eds.), *Geropsychiatric and Mental Health Nursing*, 267–286. Boston: Jones & Bartlett Publishers.

Ropacki, S. A., & Jeste, D.V. (2005). Epidemiology of and risk factors for psychosis of AD: A review of 55 studies published from 1990 to 2003. *American Journal of Psychiatry, 162*(11), 2022–2030.

Rosenblatt, A., Samus, Q. M., Steele, C. D., Baker, A. S., Harper, M. G., Brandt, J., et al. (2004). The Maryland Assisted Living Study: Prevalence, recognition, and treatment of dementia and other psychiatric disorders in the assisted living population of central Maryland. *Journal of the American Geriatrics Society, 52*(10), 1618–1625.

Ryff, C. D., & Singer, B. H. (2005). Social environments and the genetics of aging: Advancing knowledge of protective health mechanisms. *The Journals of Gerontology: Series B: Psychological Sciences and Social Sciences, 60B* (Special Issue I), 12–23.

Saltvedt, I., Opdahl, E. S., Fayers, P., Kaasa, S., & Sletvold, O. (2002). Reduced mortality in treating acutely sick frail older patients in a geriatric evaluation and management unit. *Journal of the American Geriatrics Society, 50*, 792–98.

Salzman, C., Wong, E., & Wright, C. (2002). Drug and ECT treatment of depression in older adults, 1996–2001: A literature review. *Biological Psychiatry, 52*(3), 265–284.

Serby, M., & Yu, M. (2003, September). There's good news about depression in the elderly. *The Clinical Advisor,* 64–75.

Smith, M., & Buckwalter, K. (2005). Behaviors associated with dementia. *American Journal of Nursing, 105*(7), 40–53.

Snowdon, D. A., Greiner, L. H., Mortimer, J. A., Riley, K. P., Greiner, P. A., & Markesbery, W. R. (1997). Brain infarction and the clinical expression of Alzheimer disease: The NUN study. *Journal of the American Medical Association, 277*(10), 813–817.

Strumpf, N. E., & Evans, L. K. (1988). Physical restraint of the hospitalized elderly: Perceptions of patients and nurses. *Nursing Research, 37,* 132–137.

Sullivan-Marx, E. M. (1995). Psychological responses to physical restraint use in older adults. *Journal of Psychosocial Nursing and Mental Health Services, 33*(6), 20–25.

Sumaya, I. C., Rienzi, B. M., Deegan, J. F., & Moss, D. E. (2001). Bright light treatment decreases depression in institutionalized older adults: A placebo-controlled crossover study. *The Journals of Gerontology Series A, Biological Sciences and Medical Sciences, 56*(6), M356–M360.

Task Force on Aging Research Funding. (2003). *Sustaining the commitment.* Retrieved May 20, 2004, from http://www.agingresearch.org/brochure/taskforce/index.html.

Thomas, W. (1996). *Life worth living: How someone you love can still enjoy life in a nursing home.* Acton, MA: VanderWyk & Burnham.

Trice, L. B. (1990). Meaningful life experience to the elderly. *Image: The Journal of Nursing Scholarship, 22,* 248–251.

Trzepacz, P. T., Baker, R. W., & Greenhouse, J. (1988). A symptom rating scale for delirium. *Psychiatry Research, 23,* 89–97.

Ugarriza, D. (2002). Elderly women's explanation of depression. *Journal of Gerontological Nursing, 28*(5), 22–29.

Van der Wurff, G. B., Stek, M. L., Hoogendijk, W. J. G., & Beekman, A. T. F. (2003). Electroconvulsive therapy for the depressed elderly. *The Cochrane Library,* CD003593.

Wagnild, G., & Young, M. (1990). Resilience among older women. *Image: The Journal of Nursing Scholarship, 22*(4), 252–253.

Waszynski, C. (2001). Confusion assessment method. *Hartford Foundation Institute for Geriatric Nursing, 2*(13) 1.

Watson, J. (1988). *Nursing: Human science and human care: A theory of nursing.* New York: National League for Nursing.

Wolanin, M. O. (1977). Confusion study: Use of grounded theory as methodology. In Western Interstate Commission for Higher Education. *Communicating Nursing Research, 8,* 68–75.

Woods, B. (2004). Review: Reminiscence and life review are effective therapies for depression in the elderly. *Evidence-Based Mental Health, 7*(3), 81

Wykle, M. L. (1994). The physical and mental health of women caregivers of older adults. *Journal of Psychosocial Nursing, 32*(3), 41–42.

Yesavage, J. A., & Brink, T. L. (1983). Development and validation of a geriatric depression screening scale: A preliminary report. *Journal of Psychiatric Research, 17,* 37–49.

LITERARY REFERENCES

Anonymous. *A crabbit old woman.* Northern Ireland Association for Mental Health.

Davis, R. (1989). *My journey into Alzheimer's disease.* Wheaton, IL: Tyndale House.

Naughtin, G., & Laidler, T. (1992). *When I grow too old to dream.* North Blackburn, Australia: Harper Collins *Religious.*

Flanagan Eicher, M. (1987). Survived by his wife. In *When I am an old woman I shall wear purple* (p. 103). Watsonville, CA: Papier-Mache Press.

Sacks, O. (1987). *The man who mistook his wife for a hat.* New York: Harper Perennial.

Spohr, B., & Bullard, J. (1995). *Catch a falling star: Living with Alzheimer's.* Seattle, WA: Storm Peak Press.

SUGGESTED READINGS

Administration on Aging. (2003). *A profile of older Americans: Disability and activity limitations.* Retrieved May 20, 2004, from http://www.aoa.ahhs.gov/prof/Statistics/profile/2003/15.asp.

Administration on Aging. (2002b). *A profile of older Americans: The older population.* Retrieved May 20, 2004, from http://www.aoa.ahhs.gov/prof/Statistics/statistics.asp.

Bayley, J. (1999). *Elegy for Iris.* New York: St. Martin's Press.

Daniel, J. (1996). *Looking after: A son's memoir.* Washington, DC: Counterpoint.

Dyer, J. (1996). *In a tangled wood: An Alzheimer's journey.* Dallas: Southern Methodist University Press.

Naughtin, G., & Laidler, T. (1992). *When I grow too old to dream.* North Blackburn, Australia: HarperCollins *Religious.*

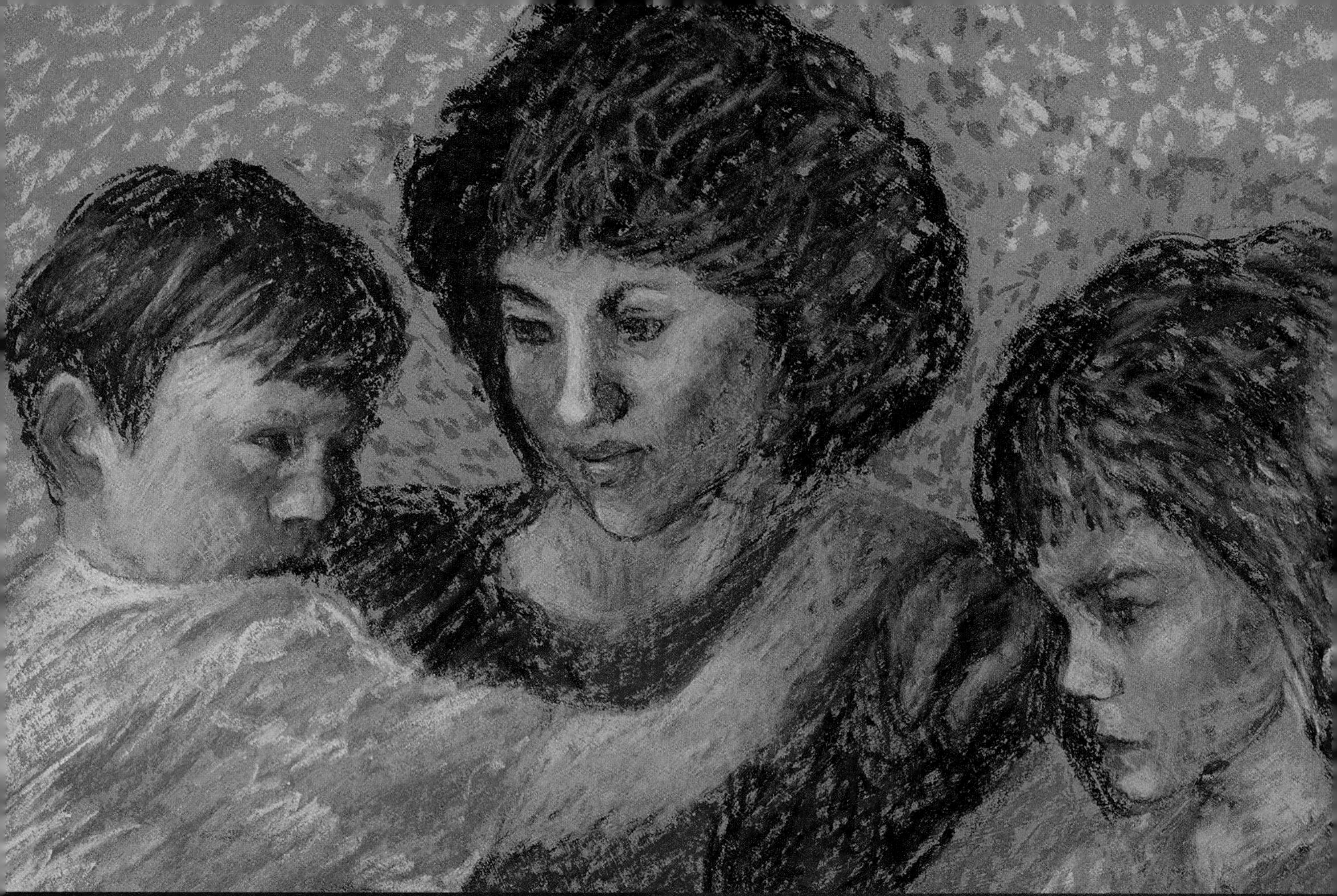

All in the Family

Reflections on Abuse

Wherever one looks in the oral and written literature of humanity, violence seems an inescapable part of the human experience—think about Cain's murder of Abel in the Old Testament, *the Trojan war in the* Iliad, *Krishna's endorsement of war in the* Bhagavad Gita, *Sun Tzu's sixth century B.C.E.* Art of War, *and the "sword verses" in the* Koran. *While one can surely find exhortations to nonviolence in each of these sources and in the cultures that gave rise to them, societal or philosophical interest in nonviolence often derives from the recognition that violence is either self-defeating or runs counter to human values perceived to be of a "higher" or nobler order. Since violence is too complex a topic to treat exhaustively in a single chapter, the discussion here can only be introductory. From a perspective of psychiatric mental health nursing, consider the following:*

- *What is violence?*
- *Are violent people born violent, or is their behavior primarily learned?*
- *What effect does the media have on violence?*
- *What roles do mental illness or substance abuse play in violence?*
- *Where does violence occur?*
- *Who are the victims of violence?*

These questions will be addressed in the chapter to provide some answers.

CHAPTER 26

Violence: An Issue for Psychiatric Mental Health Nursing

LAWRENCE E. FRISCH
with contributions on nursing care/nursing process by
MARSHELLE THOBABEN

CHAPTER OUTLINE

COMPETENCIES

After reading this chapter, the reader should be able to:

1. Understand some of the basic issues surrounding human violence.
2. Identify some of the factors that cause individuals to commit violent acts.
3. Identify the types of domestic violence.
4. Describe issues related to violence in workplaces or schools.
5. Describe issues related to street violence.
6. Understand the violent results of war and political violence.
7. Understand issues related to violence against women.
8. Apply the nursing process to clients who are victims of violence.

KEY TERMS

Battery
Bullying
Child Abuse
Child Molestation
Child Neglect
Child Pornography
Child Soldiers
Domestic Violence
Elder Abuse
Elder Neglect
Incest
Intimate Partner Violence (IPV)
Mental Injury
Negligent Treatment
Physical Injury
Rape Refugee
Severe Violence
Sexual Abuse
Sexually Explicit Conduct
Sexual Exploitation
Stranger Violence
Structural Violence
Suicide
Severe Violence
Trafficking
Violence

Note to the readers: Violence is so prevalent in our world (in books, newspapers, media, and the Internet) that the authors have chosen to omit literary references and descriptions of violent acts from this chapter.

WHAT IS VIOLENCE?

While there is some evidence that the worldwide incidence of violence has decreased in recent years, violence remains very much a reality for many people and is one of the most important topics for nurses to understand. Because cultures and eras define violence differently, a universal definition or description is difficult to construct (Muehlenhard & Kimes, 1999). Practices that may be normative in some cultures (genital cutting of young girls may be a prime example) have come to be viewed internationally as repressive and violent. Given the nature of human diversity, cross-cultural standards for all behaviors are highly unlikely to develop, but an understanding of violence does require that we achieve some degree of shared definition. In 2002, the World Health Organization (WHO) released its *World Report on Violence and Health* (WHO, 2002) which has subsequently been translated into multiple languages. The report created both a definition of **violence**:

The intentional use of physical force or power, threatened or actual, against oneself, another person, or against a group or community, that either results in or has a high likelihood of resulting in injury, death, psychological harm, maldevelopment, or deprivation

and a classification schema for types of violence. The WHO's first category (self-directed violence) is addressed in Chapter 16. The other two categories are "interpersonal" and "collective." Interpersonal violence is in turn subcategorized into "family or partner" (further divided into "child," "partner," and "elder") and "community" (also further divided into "acquaintance" and "stranger"). The discussion in this chapter is organized somewhat differently, but it is consistent with the WHO typology.

The WHO definition prominently includes the concept of "intention." By this definition, violence occurs when the perpetrator *intends to use force,* regardless of whether the intention also included harming. According to the WHO definition, persons may be regarded as acting violently even if they themselves (or the culture to which they belong) do not recognize a given act as inherently violent. And of course, according to the WHO definition, violence need not be solely physical. Sexual violence, psychological violence, and even neglect of dependent persons (most prominently children and the elderly) are classified as violent by the report. Including such a broad range of human experience in the definition may lead to considerable variability in how individuals see violence, especially when they are the victims. This variability of viewpoint occurs especially with respect to sexual violence both in North America (Zeitler, Paine, Breitbart, Rickert, Olson, Stevens, et al., 2006) and internationally (Wood, Lambert, & Jewkes, 2007). Also, despite the WHO definition, some ambiguity may still exist in deciding whether a given event is or is not termed violent. Consequently, some experts have chosen to focus attention on **severe violence** (Tyrer, Cooper, Herbert, Duggan, Crawford, Joyce, et al., 2007). Since severe violence is more likely to result in injury or death, much of our understanding of the epidemiology of violence is based on analysis of severe violent events.

Worldwide, **suicide** is the most common cause of death from violence (14.5 deaths yearly per 100,000 persons), compared to homicide (8.8/100,000) and war-related injury (5.2/100,000). Some readers may be surprised to learn that of the 1.6 million deaths due to suicide, homicide, and war, 90% occur in low- or middle-income countries. Violence and its consequences have a strong relationship to poverty and economic underdevelopment: In poorer countries the age-adjusted mortality rate from violence is more than twice that of high income countries (WHO, 2002). This relationship between violence and poverty holds both between and within countries. For example, in the United States there are major disparities in homicide rates between black and white youth that correlate well with indicators of poverty (Jones-Webb & Wall, 2008).

While we know a fair amount about homicide and suicide, it is far more difficult to assess the incidence of nonfatal violence. Much intimate partner abuse, child abuse, and sexual assault remain unreported. A five-country study of adolescent violent behavior suggested that, except for bullying (lowest in Sweden), reported rates of fighting, fight-related injury, and weapon carrying were quite comparable among the countries (Smith-Khuri, Iachan, Scheidt, Overpeck, Gabhainn, Pickett, et al., 2004). In this study, about 40% of adolescents reported fighting, 15% reported fight-related injuries, and 10% reported carrying weapons. This study did include U.S. adolescents, but did not survey youths in Great Britain where knife carrying has recently been recognized as a risk for more serious violence outcomes (Leyland, 2006). There is also some evidence of increasing weapon carrying among young women in several other countries (Erickson, Butters, Cousineau, Harrison, & Korf, 2006).

Paul Farmer (Farmer & Sen, 2003), describing pathologies of power, and others (Gilligan, 1997) have proposed that any understanding of violence that is based solely on the WHO definition is too narrow because it ignores "**structural violence**." This concept recognizes that most poor people have little control over social, political, and economic conditions in their lives that—in the words of the WHO violence definition—"result in or ha[ve] a high likelihood of resulting in injury, death, psychological harm, maldevelopment, or deprivation." Since Gilligan, Farmer, and others argue that these social, economic, and political arrangements are neither accidental nor unintended, the harm that occurs as a result clearly meets the WHO definition of violence. One might respond that those who create (or allow to persist) the social and economic circumstances leading to poverty don't intend that harm comes to poor people. But, as the authors of the WHO report say, intention to cause harm is not required for violence to be defined if "the use of ... power ... has a high likelihood of resulting in ... harm." As an explanatory example, the authors of the WHO report observe that "a parent may vigorously shake a crying infant with the intent to quieten it. Such an action may instead cause brain damage.... without the intention of causing an injury (WHO, 2002)." Structural violence causes immense harm and suffering worldwide, especially among the most disenfranchised members of society, some of whom may also suffer from significant mental illness related to their deprivation.

WHAT CAUSES PEOPLE TO BE VIOLENT?

Many researchers on violence support an "ecological" view of the causes of violent behavior (WHO, 2002). In this commonsense model, behavior is influenced by interactions among personal predisposition, relationships, community, and society. Each of these factors is additive, and violence occurs when together they interact in a way that facilitates violent expression. According to this theory, persons who might behave violently in some contexts may find themselves in relationships, communities, or societies that effectively keep violent behavior from occurring. In contrast, the theory also suggests that persons who might *not* act violently under normal circumstances may do so when conditions in society, the community, or their relationships facilitate this behavior. Both of these circumstances correspond to our commonsense views—most of us feel ourselves capable of violence at times, but are held back by social controls; and there is reason to believe that "normal" people can behave violently under a variety of social stimuli.

In the famous 1960s Milgram experiments, subjects were instructed to administer a series of electric shocks to persons who scored incorrect answers on a memory test (Blass, 2004). Unknown to the subjects, their victims were actors who feigned pain on receiving the imaginary electric shocks and also purposefully failed to learn the words required in the memory task—hence leading the experimental subjects to feel expected to administer increasing levels of what they believed to be electric shock. As the voltages apparently increased, the victims would scream and bang on the wall separating them from the subjects who thought they were administering the shocks. Most of the subjects followed instructions and administered what they believed to be increasing levels of electric shock, despite their victims' screams and protestations about heart ailments. Those who expressed qualms were told that they were not personally responsible for any adverse outcomes. In this experiment and multiple subsequent repeats, more than half of the subjects were willing to administer what they thought to be potentially dangerous voltages despite expressing serious concerns to the experimenter.

The Milgram experiments have raised many ethical concerns and today would not be allowed to proceed except with imaginary or "virtual" victims (Slater, Antley, Davison, Swapp, Guger, et al., 2006). These experiments were done in many more variations than can be described here and were intended to assess to what degree normal persons might behave cruelly in obedience to authority. Milgram's work has been thought relevant to the behavior of individuals in settings such as Nazi Germany or the Iraq Abu Ghraib prison—both circumstances in which social expectations seem to have increased the likelihood of cruel and violent behavior or at least acquiescence to suffering (Waller, 2002; Fiske, Harris, & Cuddy, 2004).

Ecological Model of Violence

The ecological model is a useful way to organize thinking around how violence occurs, especially under coercive or authoritarian societal conditions. It is certainly helpful for understanding violence in wartime when citizens are required or coerced into violent activities in support of political aims. The model may also help us to understand some of the constraints on violent behavior that our normal social structures create. Above all, the model reinforces the strong Western belief in free will and responsibility by assuming that the individual's conscience is a "first-line" defense against violent behavior, whereas the consciences of other individuals ("bystanders") and of society act as second-line inhibitors of violence (Banyard, 2008).

The model, however, potentially simplifies a number of important questions. Perhaps the most important of these might be phrased as "What personal characteristics lead to potentially violent behavior?" Some individuals, especially those who commit violence against strangers, often have a life-long pattern of violent expression originating with childhood conduct disorder and leading to adult Antisocial Personality Disorder (Hill & Nathan, 2008; Simonof, Elander, Holmshaw, Pickles, Murray, & Rutter, 2004). Further, in some families the tendency for extreme violence is passed from generation to generation (Butterfield, 1996), though whether that passage is due to genetics (Baschetti, 2008) or social imprinting remains in dispute. While some find the genetic "bad seed" explanation persuasive, the literature favoring familial social factors in the intergenerational passage of violent traits is quite strong. There is, for example, considerable evidence that abuse during childhood is associated with violent adult behavior (a reflection of what some call "the cycle of violence"; Volavka, 2004). Interestingly, recalling that suicide is the commonest fatal violent outcome in the WHO typology, childhood abuse may not only increase the risk of suicide attempts in that individual (Brodsky & Stanley, 2008), but in their own children as well (Melhem, Brent, Ziegler, Iyengar, Kolko, Oquendo, et al., 2007). Evidence from these last two studies suggests that at least some forms of violence occurring in childhood may have a significant intergenerational effect. Prenatal exposure to alcohol is associated with subsequent violent behavior in some individuals, though how much of any relationship is due to alcohol-related effects on brain development and how much to postnatal influences remains unclear. Exposure to lead and perhaps other pollutants during critical postnatal periods of brain growth may be linked to subsequent violent behavior (Hwang, 2007).

Violence among the Mentally Ill

Even though the majority of mentally ill persons do not behave violently, a small number of psychiatric disorders are associated with violence. Among these are substance abuse, pathological gambling, unipolar and bipolar depressive disorders, several anxiety disorders (Panic Disorder without Agoraphobia and specific phobia) and several personality disorders (paranoid, schizoid, histrionic, and obsessive-compulsive; Pulay, Dawson, Hasin, Goldstein, Ruan, Pickering, et al., 2008). Readers may find some surprises in this list—both in the disorders associated with violence risk and those, such as Antisocial Personality Disorder and schizophrenia, that do not make an appearance.

It should, however, come as no surprise that the strongest associations found were with alcohol and drug-related disorders. Much evidence supports a link between **stranger violence** (violence perpetrated on someone unknown to the assailant) and alcohol/substance abuse (Shaw, Amos, Hunt, Flynn, Turnbull, Kapur, et al., 2004). In one British study, alcohol or substance misuse played some role in the majority of 1,600 homicides, even though in only 68 cases (just over 4% of the total) was the role judged to have been critical (Shaw, Hunt, Flynn, Amos, Meehan, Robinson, et al., 2006). Interviews with U.S. perpetrators of homicide suggested that a significant proportion of these murders was alcohol related (Spunt, Brownstein, Goldstein, Fendrich, & Liberty, 1995). **Intimate partner violence** (to be discussed in more detail later in this chapter) is strongly associated with substance misuse—particularly for alcohol, marijuana, cocaine, and methamphetamine (Ernst, Weiss, Enright-Smith, Hilton, & Byrd, 2008; Stuart, Temple, Follansbee, Bucossi, Hellmuth, & Moore, 2008). Opiate dependence substantially increases the likelihood of being both a perpetrator and a victim of domestic violence (El-Bassel, Gilbert, Wu, Go, & Hill, 2005). As noted before, pathological gambling (itself highly associated with substance abuse) is linked to violence, and despite movie stereotypes (Richards & Richards, 1997), probably more to intimate partner abuse than to stranger violence (Korman, Collins, Dutton, Dhayananthan, Littman-Sharp, & Skinner, 2008).

Schizophrenia—perhaps surprisingly—is absent from the list of disorders linked to violent behavior in the epidemiological survey reported by Pulay and coworkers (Pulay et al., 2008). While the majority of individuals with Schizophrenia are not violent toward others, some clearly do have a risk for outwardly directed violent behavior (Hodgins, 2008).

Violent behavior may precede the diagnosis of schizophrenia by years, suggesting that in some persons conduct disorders and antisocial personality might be antecedents of schizophrenia. In others, violent behavior occurs only after the diagnosis of schizophrenia. In these individuals a pattern of violence may emerge soon after diagnosis, or violence (often directed at caretakers) may occur only many years after diagnosis. While schizophrenia is relatively uncommon among convicted murderers, persons with this diagnosis do commit murder. Even though some persons with schizophrenia experience auditory command hallucinations in which voices tell them to act violently, murders committed by schizophrenic individuals may not be a direct consequence of their psychosis—or at least may not be due to command hallucinations or the specific content of delusions (Laajasalo & Häkkänen, 2006). Nonetheless, the risk of violent behavior in response to command hallucinations seems to increase with age (Shawyer, Mackinnon, Farhall, Sims, Blaney, Yardley, et al., 2008). Such late emergence of violence in some schizophrenic individuals suggests either that violence is a random event whose probability increases with duration of illness or that disease progression might decrease the effectiveness of brain pathways that inhibit patterns of fear and rage generated within the limbic system (see Chapter 4). In support of this second possibility, there is evidence that persons with schizophrenia do have excessive activation of the amygdala under a variety of circumstances (Hall, Whalley, McKirdy, Romaniuk, McGonigle, McIntosh, et al., 2008; Gur, Loughead, Kohler, Elliott, Lesko, Ruparel, et al., 2007). The amygdala seems likely to be the source of fear and rage emotions, and if this brain organ is activated or disinhibited, then violent behaviors might be expected to emerge.

When mental illness is associated with serious or lethal violent behavior, both juries and mental health professionals may have considerable difficulty determining whether or not the perpetrator of violence was mentally competent at the time of the crime. Since it is widely held that individuals freely choose to engage in substance use, being "under the influence" is rarely a successful defense in criminal cases involving violent behavior. Some of the most perplexing cases occur when persons seem to suffer "temporary insanity" not directly attributable to substance use. At least two cases of murder apparently committed while sleepwalking have been reported and compellingly analyzed (Cartwright, 2004). There have been suggestions that violence may occur as part of complex partial seizures, but while violent-seeming gestures may occur during seizure activities, little evidence supports a relationship between seizures and actual violent behavior. In contrast, psychosis *following* a seizure is not uncommon and may rarely be associated with violent behavior—including suicide and murder (Devinsky, 2008).

Violence and the Media

A significant proportion of persons who act violently are not diagnosably mentally ill, are not under the influence of substances, do not have personality disorders, have not been abused as children, and are not engaged in sleepwalking. Why do these people behave violently? While the answer to this question remains unknown, researchers have explored links between observing or hearing/reading about violent behavior in the media and perpetrating violence. Most studies have been short-term in nature and have sought changes in aggressiveness following a variety of media exposures. There is good evidence that exposure to violence in television, movies, and perhaps video games increases both short and long-term aggressiveness among viewers. Even television news presentations can influence violent behavior (Huesmann & Taylor, 2006). As identified in the ecological model of violence (WHO, 2002), most people have personal, relationship, community, or societal impediments to acting out violently even in the face of media exposures or other risks to violent incitement. Nonetheless, some people may be uniquely susceptible to media influences, and this susceptibility may explain occasional suicide clusters following reports of adolescent suicide (Huesmann & Taylor, 2006; Insel & Gould, 2008). School shootings, while quite rare, may be another form of violence that is potentially influenced by media coverage.

WHERE DOES VIOLENCE HAPPEN?

While many people think of "mean streets" or "the hood" as the primary settings for violence, for most individuals, home and worksite are the places of highest risk.

Violence at Home

Violence in the home, or **domestic violence**, is highly prevalent, though accurate assessments of its frequency are hard to come by. Domestic violence encompasses at least three types of occurrences: child abuse/neglect, intimate partner violence, and elder abuse/neglect. Each is a complex topic deserving more lengthy discussion than this chapter can provide, and each is of great importance to nurses practicing in any area of healthcare. Any nurse who works with either children or elders will encounter instances of abuse during his or her career. Victims of intimate partner abuse are commonly seen in all healthcare settings, but the abuse is frequently overlooked by healthcare providers who do not ask important screening questions such as "Do you feel safe in your current relationship?" or "Is there a partner from a previous relationship who is making you feel unsafe now?" Neither nurses nor doctors are immune from intimate partner abuse in their own personal lives. Child abuse, elder abuse, and intimate partner abuse will each be discussed separately in the sections that follow.

Child Abuse and Neglect

While children have surely been abused for centuries, child abuse was effectively brought to North American public and medical attention in the 1960s by the pediatrician C. Henry Kempe and psychiatrist Brandt Steele. Not long after this,

> **NURSING TIP 26-1**
>
> Wearing a button that says, "It's OK to talk to me about family violence and abuse" makes a difference in what clients may choose to share with nurses during routine visits.

the child psychiatrist Ruth Kempe recognized the importance of child neglect when she and others described the syndrome of "non-organic failure to thrive." There is, sadly, little evidence that either abuse or neglect has decreased in prevalence in the nearly half-century since the Kempes and others raised professional awareness. In the United States, the most recent national incidence study (NIS-3) found significant increases in child abuse and neglect incidence over the preceding 10-year period (Sedlak & Broadhurst, 1996). NIS-4 is scheduled for completion in December, 2008, and when released should help us know whether this trend of increasing incidence has persisted.

Definitions of **child abuse** and **child neglect** differ somewhat from region to region, though there is still modest variability between countries as documented in the *World Perspectives on Child Abuse* (Daro, 2006). There appears to be widespread agreement that each of the following constitutes child abuse or neglect: sexual abuse, physical abuse, children living on the streets, and child prostitution. In the United States, the Child Abuse Prevention and Treatment Act (CAPTA) has created a definition of child abuse as: "Any recent act or failure to act on the part of a parent or caretaker, which results in death, serious physical or emotional harm, sexual abuse, or exploitation, or an act or failure to act which presents an imminent risk of serious harm." (CAPTA, 2003, [Section 111, 42 US.C 5106g])

CAPTA sets minimum standards so that states are free to adopt more inclusive definitions. The Centers for Disease Control and Prevention (CDC) has created a set of standard definitions and needed data elements to enable effective surveillance for child abuse and neglect (http://www.cdc.gov/ncipc/dvp/CM_Surveillance.pdf). These definitions are important for research standardization and data collection, but may not be as useful in clinical practice.

The following definitions of child abuse and neglect have been adopted from the Victims of Child Abuse Act:

- **Child abuse** is any physical or mental injury, sexual exploitation, negligent treatment, or maltreatment of a child under the age of 18 (or the age specified by the child protection law of the state in question) by a parent or parent substitute.
- **Negligent treatment** is the failure of a parent or parent substitute to provide, for reasons other than poverty, adequate food, shelter, or medical care to seriously endanger the physical health of a child.
- **Physical injury** includes, but is not limited to, lacerations, fractured bones, burns, internal injuries, severe bruising, or serious bodily harm.
- **Mental injury** is harm to a child's psychological or intellectual functioning. It may be exhibited by severe anxiety, depression, withdrawal, or outward aggressive behavior or a combination of those behaviors, which may be demonstrated by a change in behavior, emotional response, or cognition.
- **Sexual abuse (child)** includes the employment, use, persuasion, inducement, enticement, or coercion of a child to engage in or assist another person to engage in sexually explicit conduct. It is the rape, molestation, prostitution, or other forms of sexual exploitation of children or incest with children.
- **Sexually explicit conduct** is actual or simulated sexual intercourse whether with persons of the same sex or of the opposite sex, bestiality, masturbation, lascivious exhibition of the genital or pubic area of a person or animal, or sadistic or masochistic abuse.
- **Child molestation** is sexual involvement such as oral-genital contact, genital fondling, and viewing, or masturbation.
- **Sexual exploitation** is child pornography, sexually explict reproduction of a child's image, or child prostitution (US Code Annotated, Title 42, 1990, PL 104, pp 4806 – 4807).
- **Incest** is sexual relations between children and blood relatives or surrogate family member.

Prevalence of Child Abuse

Much reported child abuse in the United States does not involve life-threatening injury. According to the 1996 NIS-3 study, over 1.5 million U.S. children were harmed by child abuse during that year. Of these, about 15% were sexually abused, 25% emotionally neglected, and the remaining 60% were either physically neglected or abused (with slightly more children abused than neglected). The risk of serious injury, however, is very much higher if the child is under a year of age or if shaking is the mechanism of injury. Shaking of babies can result in brain and retinal bleeding that can leave a child severely damaged or lead to fatal outcomes.

Although in each case there was a perpetrator—often one or both natural parents—the relationship of abuse to poverty is striking. Children from households well below the poverty level and those from large families are many times more likely to be abused than are children whose family incomes are at or just above poverty and who are in single child families. While deaths from child abuse are relatively rare, children living in extreme poverty are 60 times more likely to die from abuse than are children whose family incomes are closer to or somewhat above the poverty line. It is important to recognize that this striking comparison is with *less poor* children, not with wealthy children. Abuse does occur among the well-off, but because

Mysterious Skin

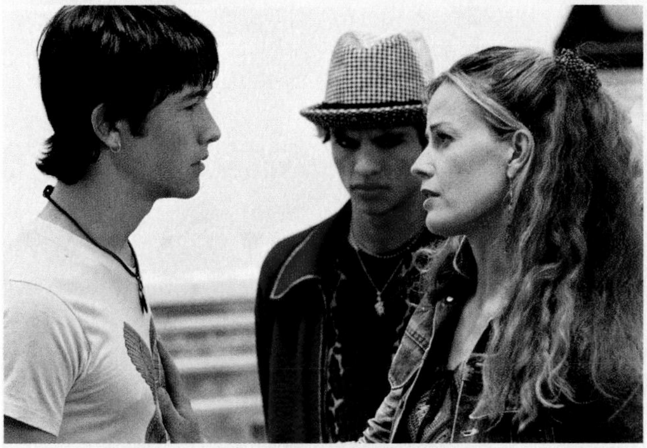

Desperate Films (Courtesy: The Kobal Collection)

Child sexual abuse by a baseball coach has very different impacts on two boys from differing but dysfunctional family backgrounds. Neil and Brian eventually find each other to explore what has happened to them and what the experience of abuse has meant for their lives.

of its strong linkage to the stresses and deprivations of poverty, some might consider child abuse a form of structural violence.

Boys are more likely to be severely physically injured by abuse and to be emotionally neglected than are girls, but by age three, girls are three times more likely to be sexually abused. In contrast to physical abuse and neglect, only about a quarter of sexually abused children are abused by a birth parent. About half of sexual abuse perpetrators were abused by someone other than a parent, with the remainder divided between birth parents and other caretakers. Nearly all the perpetrators of sexual abuse were male—in contrast to physical abuse and neglect where a parent of either sex was equally likely to cause harm. Sexual abuse is perhaps less strongly associated with poverty than physical abuse, but NIS-3 reported that children from extremely poor homes were still 18 times more likely to be sexually abused than those from more privileged backgrounds. Boxes 26-1 and 26-2 provide characteristics of child abuse and neglect and the caregivers who abuse or neglect their children.

Reporting Laws

In order to meet the requirements of CAPTA, all states have enacted child abuse statutes that include mandatory reporting by many professionals (registered nurses are likely mandated reporters in all states, but are not listed explicitly in the laws of a handful—most of these states designate health care professionals as reporters without further specifics). In 18 states and Puerto Rico, all members of the public who suspect child abuse are required to report their concerns, though only in Wyoming is there no additional assignment of reporting obligation to professionals, such as doctors, nurses, teachers, police, or clergy (Child Welfare Information Gateway, 2007). Persons who report abuse are generally protected from any liability in the event evidence of abuse is not found, and their names cannot be released to the alleged perpetrator. In most states, penalties can be invoked if a mandated reporter fails to report, though the application of such penalties is likely rare, particularly because less than 30% of reported cases receive any investigation according to the NIS-3 study.

Assessment and Treatment of Child Abuse

The ideal management of a case of child abuse or neglect would begin with reporting, followed by a rapid investigation (preferably within 24 hours). In most cases a child should be seen by a physician or nurse practitioner to document whether there is objective evidence of physical injury on physical examination or, where indicated, diagnostic imaging.

Allegations of sexual abuse require examination by a health care professional trained in forensic evaluations but also able to carry out highly sensitive genital examinations with extreme gentleness. When a child is old enough to potentially describe physical or sexual abuse—this description is important for subsequent proceedings—it is important that only one highly skilled interviewer conduct the interview so as to minimize trauma and reduce the risk of suggesting

NURSING TIP 26-2

Child Abuse Reports

The report should carefully document the physical evidence of abuse and neglect without making judgments about the family. Child abuse reports should include the following:

- The name of the victim
- Current location of the victim
- Type of abuse you are reporting
- Types of injuries you observed and how severe
- Parent's or caregiver's account of the injuries
- When possible, children's account of their injuries
- Why you suspect the child is being abused or neglected
- In the client's record, chart your observations and your report to the child protective agency

BOX 26-1
CHARACTERISTICS OF CAREGIVERS WHO ABUSE OR NEGLECT THEIR CHILDREN

- Has history of abuse or neglect as a child, reveals concern about having been abandoned and punished by own parents
- Uses harsh discipline inappropriate to the child's age
- Believes that violence is a way to reduce tension, exhibits violent feelings and behavior, has a low tolerance for frustration, has poor impulse control
- Never mentions any good qualities in the child
- Fails to respond to the child or responds inappropriately
- Is extremely protective or jealous toward the child
- Is critical of the child and angry with the child for being injured or sick, shows no concern about the child's injury, treatment, prognosis, or follow-up care, often disappears from the hospital shortly after the child is admitted, and tends not to visit the child
- Leaves small children alone or abandons them
- Significantly misperceives the child, distrusts the child, falsely accuses the child of sexual promiscuity
- Has marital difficulties, lives in a chaotic home life
- Is insulated from the influence of others, is socially isolated
- Has feelings of hopelessness and helplessness
- Has personality disorders, misuses alcohol or other drugs
- Lacks knowledge of childhood developmental issues
- Often neglects own physical health
- Attempts to conceal the child's injury, is evasive or contradicts self about the child's injury or illness, protects the identity of person responsible for the child's injuries
- Is unable to admit the need for help
- Lives in unsanitary or unsafe living conditions
- Encourages the child to engage in prostitution or sexual acts in the presence of parent

events that may not have happened. If a crime has likely been committed (in most states physical and sexual abuse are criminal offenses) police officers may need to be present during some interviews or examinations or they may be required to conduct interviews with the child and any other potential witnesses.

During the time it takes for this evaluation to take place, it is essential that the child be held in a safe environment. In many cases that may be a hospital emergency room, but hospital admission is often the ideal way to ensure a child's safety and obtain the testing and interviewing needed. If the purported abuse or neglect has led to harm to the child, social service workers might choose to place the child in foster care until a full investigation has established the certainty of abuse/neglect, the likely perpetrator, the severity of injury, and the risk to the child of returning to their environment. Ideally, with serious or recurrent abuse/neglect, states or district attorneys should be involved early in the course of evaluation in case it appears that termination of parental rights is the best option.

Mental health evaluation of parents by a psychiatric nurse, social worker, or psychiatrist/psychologist may assist in estimating recurrence risk and may help determine whether therapy for parents (for example, treating depression or substance abuse or helping with anger management) might be of use. A variety of social services may be needed, especially if families are stressed by economic deprivation. Many parents could benefit from parenting classes to help them cope with normal childhood behavior or an unusually difficult child. Especially if the child has been traumatized sexually or over a long period of time, a therapeutic school placement or other therapy arrangement may be desirable. In the event of serious physical injury from physical or sexual abuse, ongoing medical treatment may be necessary. In any case, close follow up by a pediatrician, nurse practitioner, or other professional is critical to observe the child's progress and to monitor for further abuse in either home or foster care.

The scenario just described represents the authors' preferred approach to management of abuse and neglect, but it is not representative of the real-life practice of child welfare agencies in many states. Once again, the best information available is the National Incidence Study (NIS-3). According to NIS-3, protective services workers investigated only 26% of cases in which a child was severely or "moderately" injured. During the 10 years between NIS-2 and

BOX 26-2
CHARACTERISTICS OF CHILD ABUSE AND NEGLECT

CHILD'S SYMPTOMS OF PHYSICAL ABUSE

- Bruises and welts in various stages of healing showing the shape of the items used—belt marks, shoe prints—in unusual patterns or clustered
- Human bite marks
- Burns: on the dorsal surface of the hand (if children burn their hand by accident, they usually burn the palm), by an iron or cigarettes or immersion in scalding liquid (glove or doughnut-shaped burns on the buttocks or genitalia)
- Fractures: spiral fractures of upper extremities, skull, jaw, or nasal bones; x-ray of healed or healing bones with no history of treatment, or multiple fractures
- Malnutrition, failure to thrive
- Lacerations and abrasions: injury to the oral mucosa or frontal dental ridge (from having a bottle jabbed into the mouth), or to external genitalia
- Shaken-baby (whiplash) syndrome or retinal hemorrhage (from being shaken too hard or cuffed about the head) in infants and toddlers
- Repeated injuries, always explained as accidental
- Chunks of hair missing from the scalp

CHILD'S SYMPTOMS OF NEGLECT

- Malnourished, comes to school hungry; often does not have lunch money
- Poor skin care, consistently dirty
- Tired, no energy
- Clothes dirty or wrong for weather
- Lacks needed medical care, glasses, or dental care
- Lacks emotional care or attention
- Unsupervised for extended periods of time, especially when engaged in dangerous activities
- Has been abandoned

CHILD'S BEHAVIOR

- Frequently absent, late, or comes to school much too early; hangs around after school is dismissed, causes trouble in school; often has not done homework
- Acts unpleasant and demanding, causes trouble or interferes with others, or is unusually shy, avoids other people including children, seems exceptionally fearful of adult authority (or lack of it)
- Often does not obey
- Behaves wary when in the presence of adults, avoids physical contact with adults, or seeks affection from any adult
- Appears too anxious to please, seems too ready to let other people say and do things to him or her without protest
- Frequently breaks or damages things
- Begs or steals food
- Uses alcohol or drugs
- Engages in vandalism
- Engages in sexual misconduct
- Resists physical examination/assessment
- Wears long sleeves or other concealing clothing to hide injuries
- Child's or adolescent's story of how an injury occurred is not believable; it does not fit the type or seriousness of the injury
- Seems frightened of parents, shows little or no distress at being separated from parents
- Reports injury by parents

BOX 26-3
CHILD'S SYMPTOMS OF SEXUAL ABUSE

VERBAL

- Reports to a friend, a teacher, or the authorities that sexual activity with adults has occurred
- Physical complaints
- Indirect comments or statements about the abuse or statements about being sexually assaulted by parent/parent substitute

PHYSICAL

- Itching, bruises, bleeding or pain in the external genitalia, vagina, or anal area, edema of the cervix, vulva, or perineum, or stretched hymen at a very young age
- Pain or injury to the mouth
- Vaginal or penile discharges: semen or evidence of a sexually transmitted disease (STD)
- Bladder infections
- Pregnancy in an older child
- STDs

BEHAVIORAL

- Reluctance or fear of a person or of certain places, such as showers or bathrooms
- Torn, stained, or bloody undergarments
- Regression to babyish habits, such as thumb sucking or bed wetting
- Temper tantrums, aggressive behavior, running away, or engaging in delinquent acts
- Acting out sexual or abusive behavior with toys, animals, or people
- Preoccupation with sexual organs of self or others with younger children
- Sexual promiscuity or prostitution in older children
- Change in sleeping patterns, nightmares, or sudden fear of falling asleep
- Poor peer relationships, reluctance to participate in sport or other recreational activities
- Feelings of guilt, fear, anger, shame, confusion, or isolation
- Delinquency, truancy, acting out, or runaway behavior
- Use of alcohol and other drugs
- Phobias or avoidance behavior
- Depression or suicidal behavior
- Evidence of child pornography

NIS-3, the percentage of abused or neglected children whose case had a child protective investigation fell nearly 40% in the face of a comparable rise in reported incidence. Overall, the same *number* of cases were investigated, but the percentage decreased significantly. Hopefully, NIS-4 will show a reversal of this trend because unless case management proceeds at least somewhat as sketched in the previous paragraph, abuse is likely to be recurrent, may result in serious injury or death, and may lead to the intergenerational perpetuation of violence described earlier in this chapter.

While NIS-3 suggests shortcomings in management of child abuse still occur, progress has been made in understanding prevention of abuse and neglect. Work in the 1970s at the Hawaii Family Stress Center suggested the value of risk factor screening of all hospital births with a follow-up home visit for all willing new mothers with social risks. Ongoing nurse home visiting ("Nurse-Family Partnerships") was also established by David Olds and shown to have significant benefit in reducing abuse and neglect, child behavior problems, child substance use, and in improving school performance (Olds, 2002). Olds' work has been replicated in various communities throughout the United States, and Nurse-Family Partnerships have been created in 25 states. The program operates on a very strictly followed 18-element model illustrated on the Partnership's Web site at http://www.nursefamilypartnership.org (accessed July 31, 2008). The model defines eligibility, nurse staffing, underlying theoretical assumptions, and evaluation processes, and assures consistent reproducibility in national implementations. A nurse-family partnership program focused on reducing child health disparities has recently been established in 20 British sites as well with plans for further expansion. Somewhat similar home visiting programs entitled "Healthy Start" and, in Scotland, "Starting Well" were based on the Hawaii model and have also been replicated widely under the leadership of pediatrician Calvin Sia and others.

Realities of Child Abuse

Child abuse statistics only partially reflect the true incidence of child maltreatment since a vast number remain underreported. Some unsubstantiated reports of child maltreatment may be actual cases of abuse, and many abuse cases are never reported. The decision to report child abuse is often subjective and depends on the beliefs and observations of the potential reporter. Few family members are willing to admit they have abused or neglected their child because they are afraid of criminal prosecution, being exposed as unfit parents, or having their children removed from their home. Abused or neglected children generally do not reveal that they have been mistreated, even when they have been badly brutalized. Children who have lived with being abused their whole lives may think it is normal or that they deserve the abuse because they have done something wrong. They may be scared that their parents will retaliate against them or desert them. They may feel loyalty to their parents or believe that they will be removed from their parents. They may be too young to report or understand what has happened to them.

Child abuse is important to the field of psychiatric nursing for many reasons. Perhaps above all it reflects a need—worldwide—to remove the conditions that inhibit full human development for so many children. Each abused or neglected child has one or more identifiable "perpetrators" who bear responsibility for his or her maltreatment. But given the powerful association of abuse and poverty, child abuse is best seen as a critical form of structural violence: the hazards that our current social order creates for the least empowered among us. While the link between childhood abuse and adult violence is highly influenced by other protective factors in the ecological model (e.g., societal expectations that children will *not* be abused), for some the scars of abuse lead to unfulfilled lives in which violence continues to play a life-long role. In psychiatric mental health nursing, you will encounter many survivors of child abuse who have not fared well. There are few areas in public health practice where prevention is more needed or potentially more welcome.

Elder Abuse and Neglect

Violence is almost always perpetrated by the strong against the weak, and it may derive either from newly provoked rage or, not infrequently, from smoldering resentments based on perceived past slights or injustices.

> *In many ways the famous "riddle of the Sphinx" encapsulates the reality of elder abuse. In ancient Greece, the monster "Sphinx" positioned herself outside the gates of the city of Thebes. The word sphinx comes from a Greek language root that relates to strangling, and despite being depicted as part lion strangling was the sphinx's preferred method of violence. A highly sociopathic monster, she would give passers-by a simple alternative to being brutally killed: they could give a correct answer to the following now-famous riddle: "What goes on four legs in the morning, two legs at noon, and three legs in the evening?" If anyone could provide an answer to that question, not only would the Sphinx spare their lives, but she would immediately self-destruct – hence freeing the city from a serious impediment to tourism and commerce. Oedipus, whom you may recall had experienced serious child abuse in infancy, having been left in the wilderness to die soon after birth because the Oracle forewarned that he would kill his father and marry his mother, had just returned to Thebes. Having unwittingly killed his father in a swordfight over who had the right-of-way he was anxious to get on with the rest of his tragedy and readily provided the answer to the Sphinx's riddle: "Man crawls on four legs as a baby, walks on two legs during his adult life, and walks with a cane in his elder years." That was the end of the Sphinx and the beginning of one of the great human stories of guilt and self destruction.*

The riddle of the Sphinx reminds us that the human condition starts with infantile dependency and ends with decline. It also serves as a reminder that victims of childhood violence may enact violence on their own parents when the latter become weakened and in need of support. (Of course a history of child abuse is neither necessary nor sufficient to be a perpetrator of elder abuse—but more of this shortly.) Finally, the Sphinx—the monster at our walls devouring citizens who cannot give what she demands of them—is surely an embodiment of Gilligan's concept of structural violence. There is no Sphinx at the walls of our cities, but in most countries the poor find their life prospects strangled by social realities that the physician/anthropologist Paul Farmer has termed "pathologies of power."

Prevalence of Elder Abuse

As relevant as this myth might be to our understanding of elder abuse, the facts of elder abuse are far from myths. Much remains unknown about elder abuse, but the best U.S. estimates are that more than a million persons over 65 have been injured or exploited. Between 2% and 10% of Americans suffer some form of elder abuse during their lifetime. In the year 2000, nearly half a million reports of elder abuse are received by state authorities—a number somewhat lower than for child abuse. However, it is estimated that no more than one case in five is ever reported, even in states with mandatory reporting statutes (Anonymous, 2005).

Elder abuse comprises physical abuse, psychological abuse, sexual abuse, neglect, exploitation (often including financial exploitation). Some experts include self neglect as a form of elder abuse because other responsible individuals fail to recognize or prevent self-induced harm. As noted previously, while the realities of child maltreatment have been recognized for centuries, it was only in the 1960s that concerted efforts were made to identify, categorize, and prevent the harm that comes to children from abuse and neglect. Similarly, maltreatment of elders has likely occurred in human society since before recorded history, but only since the 1970s have professionals tried to take steps to increase recognition of abuse and neglect and restore some measure of dignity and safety to the lives of those who suffer from maltreatment. Not surprisingly, perhaps, those seeking better approaches to the management of elder abuse have been strongly influenced by the approaches taken to bring child abuse to professional and public recognition. Just as the NIS studies for child abuse have brought increased understanding of the realities and management of this disorder, so the 1998 National Elder Abuse Incidence Study (NEAIS; National Center on Elder Abuse, 1998) added to a limited knowledge base about elder abuse. One major limitation of the study is that only "free living" elders were considered: there was no attempt to include those living in nursing homes or other assisted living arrangements. Among the important findings of NEAIS were that 90% of perpetrators in elder abuse are family members, with two-thirds being either spouses or children; females are abused more often than males even when reports are adjusted for the relative proportion of males and females in the population; and those over 80 are more likely to be abused than are younger individuals. While the NEAIS study identified over 500,000 cases of abuse or neglect during the year studied (1996), a significant percentage of these were self neglect. Investigations established that abuse or neglect had truly taken place in over 100,000 cases. Of these, 40% had self-neglected, while the remaining 60% were mistreated by someone else—usually a family member. In this latter group (about 70,000 cases), neglect was most common—occurring in about half of all cases—followed by emotional abuse, financial abuse, and physical abuse. About 15% of the total had been physically abused, but many individuals appear to have suffered more than one kind of abuse or neglect. Financial and emotional abuse had roughly equal numbers of reports, with the latter occurring slightly more commonly.

While no equally comprehensive study has been done since 1996, the National Research Council report estimated the incidence of elder abuse as up to 2 million cases yearly (Bonnie & Wallace, 2002). The authors observed that several risk factors have been identified for elder abuse. These include living with family members (other than a spouse) and low levels of social support for families. Some studies have found that dementia increases the risk for abuse, but this has not been substantiated in all studies. Mental illness, including alcohol or substance abuse, in caretakers increases abuse risk. Alcohol misuse and depression in caretakers have been the two most clearly documented risk factors for abuse. Since reporting of abuse is a prerequisite for social intervention, all but six states have mandatory reporting laws, and where mandatory reporting is required, registered nurses and mental health personnel are generally required to report. Since laws and regulations may change without notice, readers should regularly confirm which regulations for elder and child abuse reporting apply in their jurisdiction.

Neither the United States nor Canada currently has federal legislation related to elder abuse. In 2003, the U.S. Senate Finance Committee approved the Elder National Justice Act, which would, among other provisions, have created a national elder abuse advisory council and would have directed more research money toward the problem of elder abuse. The bill was never brought to a vote, and since then, there has been no further action taken at the federal level on elder abuse initiatives.

All states have developed Adult Protective Services (APS) modeled on the Child Protective Services required under federal CAPTA legislation. In most cases a report to APS leads to an investigation—ideally within 24 hours. In many jurisdictions investigations are carried out jointly by social services and the police to determine whether an abuse complaint is substantiated. If the elder appears to be at immediate risk, then medical care or out-of-home placement may be arranged. In the event that abuse or neglect has occurred, most Adult Protective Services require that workers complete a plan for intervention to prevent re-abuse. In many states this plan includes placing caretakers' names on an "abuse registry" to more easily recognize future problems and to prevent other individuals from coming under the care of an abusive caretaker. While fairly routine in practice, the effectiveness of these commonsense measures in preventing re-abuse or serious harm to elders has never been validated.

Since elder abuse is relatively common, most nurses will encounter this problem during their career. Fractures and bruises remain the most common manifestations of abuse in both elders and children. Evaluation in elders is complicated by the presence of osteoporosis in many and the frequent use of aspirin and other drugs that may make bruising after minor trauma more likely. Nonetheless, elder abuse should be considered when clients present with broken bones or bruises. Fractures for which no satisfactory explanation can be given are serious "red flags" for abuse. X-rays can help determine whether osteoporosis or a bony tumor could be the cause of a fracture as fractures due to osteoporosis typically occur in the hip, wrist, and spine. Fractures at other sites—especially spiral fractures of long bones—should especially generate suspicion of abuse (Bitondo-Dyer, Connolly, & McFeely, 2000). Bruises and (less often) lacerations on extensor surfaces are common in the elderly, but bruises on the face, ears, and genitals rarely occur from falls and are common in abusive situations. Multiple cuts, bruises and scars should raise the suspicion of elder abuse.

Screening for Elder Abuse

Researchers in Canada have developed an "Elder Abuse Suspicion Index" (EASI) that can help clinicians assess the likelihood or risk of abuse in a given situation (Yaffe, Weiss, Wolfson, & Lithwick, 2007). This index is completed during a private interview with the elder client, and in conducting the interview, the clinician asks the client to provide answers to five questions, such as "In the last 12 months, have you relied on people for any of the following: bathing, dressing, shopping, banking, or meals? If yes, have problems been common between these people and you?" The areas questioned on the tool are: neglect; verbal, psychological, and emotional abuse; financial exploitation; and physical and/or sexual abuse. There is opportunity for the clinician to observe factors that could indicate elder abuse, such as those listed in the Box 26-4. This tool is the first of its kind and, while its use is only for screening for risk, may prove helpful in determining those situations needing further assessments or home visits. While the items on the tool are not complex, they do require the client to have a relatively intact cognition, thus its use is limited to those situations where the elder can respond.

Treatment for Elder Abuse

In 2006, the American Bar Association published a set of recommendations concerning the diagnosis and legal prosecution of elder abuse (Stiegel, 2006). Dyer and colleagues have created a framework for the understanding of risk factors for

BOX 26-4
OBSERVABLE FINDINGS ASSOCIATED WITH ELDER ABUSE

- Poor eye contact
- Withdrawn nature
- Malnourishment
- Hygiene issues
- Cuts, bruises
- Inappropriate clothing
- Medication compliance issues

self neglect that should prove useful in subsequent empirical studies of this important topic (Dyer, Goodwin, Pickens-Pace, Burnett, & Kelly, 2007). As the population ages, stresses on caretakers will increase, and the number of dependent older adults will also increase substantially. Nurses in all fields of health care will need to recognize and manage situations in which abuse has occurred or is at significant risk for occurrence.

Intimate Partner Violence

The third major form of domestic violence, already touched on in an earlier section of this chapter, is currently best referred to as **intimate partner violence (IPV)** or, sometimes, intimate partner abuse. Intimate partner violence is likely the most prevalent form of domestic violence, though comprehensive statistics are lacking. It is important not to forget that there is strong overlap of IPV with both child abuse and elder abuse—since anger control is a major factor in IPV perpetrators and victims may be more likely to strike out at children, and as noted in the previous section, many elders report experiencing violence at the hand of intimate partner caretakers. The majority of IPV involves female victims and male perpetrators, but there is also a considerable literature (Reid, Bonomi, Rivara, Anderson, Fishman, Carrell, et al., 2008; Houston & McKirnan, 2007) on same sex violence (predominantly describing IPV in male relationships).

A variety of forms of violence are included in the definition of IPV. In the World Report on Violence and Health (WHO, 2002) the authors define as IPV any behavior that causes physical, psychological or sexual harm to a person in an intimate relationship. Among the forms of IPV are slapping, hitting, kicking, and beating; psychological abuse such as humiliation or belittling; unwanted sexual relations (currently regarded as rape, even in the context of marriage); and what the authors term "various controlling behaviors" including "isolating a person from their family and friends, monitoring their movements, and restricting their access to information or assistance" (Krug, Dahlberg, Mercy, Zwi, & Lozano, 2002, p. 89). Stalking is yet another a form of IPV, effectively illustrated in films such *Play Misty for Me* (1971) or *Fatal Attraction* (1987). In both of these films, the stalker is a woman, but real-life stalking (portrayed more accurately in *Sleeping with the Enemy* starring Patrick Bergin and Julia Roberts) much more commonly involves a male monitoring the movements of or otherwise interfering in the life of a female who has attempted to end a previous relationship through separation or divorce. Stalking may occasionally occur quite apart from an intimate partner relationship as portrayed by the actor Robin Williams in *One Hour Photo*. As in that film, when stalking is combined with harassment, the experience may be highly destructive to the personal and family life of victims (McEwan, Mullen, & Mackenzie, 2008).

The severity of IPV clearly varies with the relationship, and its effect on health or well-being may be dependent on qualities of resilience in victims. Nonetheless, it is important to remember that death and permanent disability or disfigurement are consequences of IPV. The U.S. Surveillance for Violent Deaths in 16 states for 2005 reported a total of 594 deaths related to IPV (Karch, Lubell, Friday, Patel, & Williams, 2008). These deaths comprised 15% of all single homicides during this period. The majority of victims (65%) were female, and the majority of perpetrators (78%) male. Deaths occurred at all ages, but were most common among persons aged 35–44, with the second highest incidence in the 45–44 age range. The perpetrator age ranges followed a similar pattern, though other studies suggest that a couple age gap (greater than 15 years if the man is older or greater than 10 years if the woman is older) is associated with an increased homicide risk (Breitman, Shackelford, & Block, 2004). Studies in other countries (perhaps where community levels of stranger violence are lower) have found that 40%–70% of female homicide victims are murdered within an abusive intimate relationship, the comparable rate for males being about 4%–9% (Krug, Dahlberg, Mercy, Zwi, & Lozano, 2002). The Violent Deaths Surveillance Study (Ernst, et al., 2008) reported that 65% of IPV homicide victims had significantly elevated blood alcohol levels, and 15%–20% had detectable cocaine or other drugs. These data emphasize the important link between serious IPV and substance abuse for victims, but also for perpetrators, whose reported use of alcohol and drugs typically exceeds that of victims.

Prevalence of IPV

As with child and elder abuse, the prevalence of IPV is difficult to ascertain. Telephone surveys using standardized questionnaires have been used in some studies, though this limits respondents to those who have non-cellular telephones and to those (often about 50%) who agree to cooperate. Given these limits (and also assuming that those who have remained enrolled in a large HMO for three years or more are representative of others in American society), Thompson and colleagues found that about 15% of women reported IPV to have occurred in the preceding five years, and 44% reported being victims of IPV at some time in their adult life (Thompson, Bonomi, Anderson, Reid, Dimer, Carrell, et al., 2006). The duration differed among reported types of violence, but a significant minority of women reported IPV extending over 20 years or more. IPV is significantly linked to pregnancy—women are more likely to suffer abuse while pregnant, with consequent risk of injury to themselves or the fetus. Abuse frequently continues into the postpartum period and may significantly interfere with the well-being of both mother and baby (Chambliss, 2008).

While IPV may sometimes result in murder, for most victims the experience is of repeated violence occurring over long periods of time—sometimes in association with several consecutive partners. There is emerging evidence that IPV is associated with poorer than expected physical health. On the U.S. Behavioral Risk Factor Surveillance Survey, IPV victims report higher smoking prevalence, more asthma, more pain symptoms, more limitations to physical activity, more alcohol use, and less likelihood of having seen a physician for needed health care in the preceding year (Breiding, Black, & Ryan, 2008). Since pregnancy is a significant risk factor for physical abuse, adverse reproductive outcomes such as prematurity and pregnancy loss are more common among women who experience IPV (Sarkar, 2008). Adverse mental health outcomes have also been reported, especially depression and symptoms of Post-Traumatic Stress Disorder. Psychological abuse and stalking seemed in one study to be most closely related to adverse mental health outcomes (Mechanic, Weaver, & Resick, 2008). Other studies have also associated physical violence with symptoms of PTSD (Basile, Arias, Desai, & Thompson, 2004).

Patterns of IPV: Common Couple Violence and Battering

There is some evidence that IPV occurs in two distinct patterns (Krug, Dahlberg, Mercy, Zwi, & Lozano, 2002). The first, often termed "common couple violence," describes an on-going pattern of frustration and anger periodically erupting into violence. The pattern reflects relationship challenges often seen among couples in what are sometimes called "toxic marriages," but with more severe expression of verbal and physical hostility such as slapping, pushing, or throwing something at the other individual. Women may sometimes be both victims and perpetrators in common couple violence, and while the likelihood of severe physical injury may be low in many such relationships, many of these dysfunctional violent relationships continue for years without recognition or therapy. The second pattern, sometimes referred to as battering, describes much more intense physical violence with a very much higher risk of serious injury or death. In this pattern, the perpetrator—almost always a male—typically engages in a cyclical accelerating pattern of physical abuse. Abuse tends to increase in frequency and severity until an injury occurs, often requiring medical attention. The injury is often accompanied by profuse apologies, expressions of love, and promises to reform behavior. Even when seeking medical care for injuries, victims may disguise the cause, often out of fear of reprisal, but sometimes believing that the perpetrator's apparent remorse is genuine and will be followed by a change in behavior. This pattern of abuse is often associated with alcohol and substance use, and may frequently result in serious injury. In addition to physical violence, batterers typically use threats and other means of

RESEARCH Highlight 26–1

Through the Eyes of Women: Cultural Insights into Living as a Battered Woman in Hawaii

STUDY PROBLEM/PURPOSE

To explore the meaning of living in a violent relationship for women in Hawaii.

METHODS

Through a phenomenological investigation, the researchers interviewed 10 women who were victims of intimate partner violence and who were willing to talk about their experiences. The sample included a multiethnic group: two women were part-Hawaiian, three were Japanese, one was Korean, one was Filipina, and three were Caucasian. Six of the women had children, five were single, three were divorced, one was married, and one was separated. Half reported family incomes of less that $15,000 per year; three reported family incomes of over $60,000 per year.

FINDINGS

Using Colaizzi's method of phenomenological data analysis, the researchers uncovered three clusters of themes that described the experience of living in violence. The themes were: (1) *Living in misery.* The women described being anxious, helpless, and fearful; (2) *Enduring terror and sadness.* The women provided details of the abuser and the abuse; and (3) *No happy ending.* The women reached a realization that they could not continue to live in violence and be safe.

IMPLICATIONS

Given that Hawaii is the most ethnically diverse state in the United States, it is interesting to note that the study participants represented quite differing cultures, yet the women experienced very similar emotions and fears. The findings from the study show that hopelessness and hope can co-exist for these women. The researchers comments that "it is possible for women to grow beyond an overwhelming negative situation" to take actions to live safe lives.

Nurses should understand that the lived experiences women feel in relation to a violent relationship will be unique to each person, however, there seems a universal instinctive personal response to the abusive situation.

Source: "Through the Eyes of Women: Cultural Insights into Living as a Battered Woman in Hawaii" by Lois Magnussen, Mary Jane Amundson, and Nancy Smith. 2008. *Nursing and Health Sciences, 10*(2), 125–130.

controlling behavior and restricting contact with others outside the relationship. They are likely to attend any medical encounters with the victim and may attempt to dominate discussion with a nurse or other provider. When weapons are threatened or actually used within either pattern of IPV, or when victims are choked or hit repeatedly about the head, the likelihood of abuse accelerating to a fatal outcome is greatly increased.

Treatment of IPV

The clinical management of IPV is important but can be quite complex. The first challenge is recognizing the occurrence of domestic violence. As with child and elder abuse, inadequately explained physical injuries should raise suspicion. Persons with unexplained physical symptoms may have an increased likelihood of unrecognized IPV. Depression and various anxiety symptoms are also not uncommon presentations in victims of IPV. The link between substance use disorders and IPV is strong, and each should be looked for when the other is uncovered during a clinical encounter. As noted earlier in this chapter, many nurses choose to wear a button stating "It is OK to talk to me about family violence and abuse." Buttons or office signs may increase the likelihood that patients will share their experiences of domestic violence. Once the nurse recognizes that his or her client is involved in a violent relationship, choices of action become more difficult (Walton-Moss & Campbell, 2002).

Most states have no mandatory reporting for IPV unless a purposeful injury was caused by a knife or gun. Police jurisdictions vary in the effectiveness with which they intervene in IPV. Some police forces have highly developed skills and resources in IPV management that can be very effective when coupled with a legal system able to combine protection for the victim and treatment for the abuser (Danis, 2003; Erez, 2002), but in some instances, police intervention can increase the risk of harm to the victim. The nurse's goal in assisting a victim of IPV should be to maximize the client's safety. Especially when the nature of IPV is battering, it is important to be sure that the victim knows how to reach a place of safety such as a local women's shelter. Having clothing and other necessities packed in advance (and for children, as well, if they need to accompany the victim in an escape) can be lifesaving. The nurse should be very cautious about offering written materials, including cards with shelter telephone numbers, because their discovery may precipitate severe abuse. At the same time, nothing is more important for victims of severe violence than being aware of potential paths to safety.

Nurses attempting to help victims of IPV must be aware of two frequent complicating factors. The first is that perpetrators will often "hover" during any clinical encounter such that it may be very difficult to have contact with a potential victim in privacy. Any discussion of IPV with the perpetrator present may risk escalating the level of abuse, or might even precipitate violence toward the nurse. A major challenge in responding to the needs of IPV victims is manipulating the clinical encounter so that provider and client can have an opportunity to discuss matters out of earshot of the perpetrator. A second complicating factor is that many victims of IPV deny risk—even in the face of serious injuries—and will not initially accept help. The nurse should not be surprised if offers of assistance or support are rejected and should work to build an ongoing supportive relationship that the victim can rely on when circumstances worsen to the point of intolerability. When abuse is less serious, as in common couple violence, there may be less likelihood of such complications, and both members of the couple may be willing to be referred for counseling and other mental health assistance (for example, management of depression or substance use disorders).

Intimate partner violence is common in all settings, including those in which psychiatric mental health nurses work. Some studies suggest that 20% or more of women visiting an emergency room have been abused, but few have their plight recognized during their visit. Nurses in any field of work can greatly enhance their ability to help by being aware of the risk of IPV when providing care to any adult—of any age and either sex.

> **NURSING TIP 26-3**
>
> **Exit Plan for Battered Women**
>
> A battered woman should have a carefully planned exit plan when she anticipates leaving a violent relationship. Advise her to do the following ahead of time:
>
> - If injured, go to the emergency department or call the police.
> - Know exactly where to go, how to get there, and arrange for transportation.
> - Take house, car, and office keys.
> - Obtain copies of medical records to help when filing charges with the district attorney's office (restraining orders, assault charges).
> - Store clothes, toilet articles, medications, children's favorite toys, and so on, at a family member's or friend's house.
> - Take identification, divorce papers, insurance papers, and any other legal papers that might be needed.
> - Take the children's birth certificates, Social Security cards, and school records.
> - Bring money, bank records, credit cards, and other important financial records.
>
> From *Domestic Violence: The Facts*, by Peace At Home, Inc., 2000, Jamaica Plain, MA: Author.

VIOLENCE IN THE WORKPLACE AND AT SCHOOLS

During most of their lives, people spend eight or more hours daily in school or at a worksite. Many individuals find both school and work to be stressful, and conflicts are not unusual in either location. On occasion these conflicts erupt into violence, or unexpected violence occurs that may cause injury or death.

NURSING TIP 26-4

Reasons Women Remain in Abusive Relationships

Women may not leave battering immediately because they:

- Have insufficient financial resources to provide for basic needs for self or children
- Lack educational and employment skills
- Have immigrant status and are fearful of being deported
- Are threatened by the batterer to harm or kill her or their children if she leaves
- Fear losing their children because the batterer tells them he will report them to Child Protective Services or take the children out of the country
- Lack support from friends and family
- Love the batterer and believe that the battering behavior will change
- Have psychological problems such as depression and anxiety
- Do not know about or have access to community resources
- Have religious and cultural beliefs toward marriage and the role of women that prevents them from leaving
- Believe that children need their father

From: University of California Davis Extension: The Center for Human Services, 2004.

Bullying in school and comparable practices at work (Hutchinson, Vickers, Jackson, & Wilkes, 2006) are forms of violence that can cause great distress for those who experience them. Bullying has been defined several ways, but there is agreement that bullying is an intentional act causing harm to another. The harm is frequently inflicted through verbal harassment, physical assault, or other more subtle methods of manipulation or coercion. While school mass shootings capture public attention, chronic lower levels of violence (such as bullying) are endemic in some schools. Similarly, many work sites maintain unpleasant power dynamics that result in psychological harm even when physical violence does not occur. Physical violence, however, does occur in some worksites. Nurses may work in settings (hospitals, emergency rooms, and some mental health facilities) where there is real risk of violent injury. Some nurses choose to work in the field of occupational health, providing care to persons who have experienced workplace violence, or promoting programs to reduce the incidence and impact of violence at the worksite.

Violence in the Workplace

Violence in the workplace includes physical assault, murder, verbal abuse, psychological abuse, and sexual abuse/assault. Murder is the easiest of these events to track, and studies suggest that overall occupational homicide has declined at a rate of about 6% per year. During the same period, homicides in all categories declined in the United States, but somewhat less rapidly than did occupational homicides (Hendricks, Jenkins, & Anderson, 2007). Taxi drivers have the highest risk for homicide of any major occupation, with police and corrections officers in second and third place. Perhaps surprisingly, the fatality rate for taxi drivers in the 1990s was more than three times that of these other two occupations (National Institute of Occupational Safety and Health, [1996]. Violence in the workplace: Risk factors and prevention strategies. CIB #57.) The overall annual decline in deaths is largely attributable to fewer robbery-associated murders of taxi drivers and chauffeurs due to concerted efforts to make this dangerous occupation safer, but there has not been an equally significant fall in homicides in other at-risk occupations. Service industries, especially those involving exchange of money, account for the majority of workplace homicides and 85% of nonfatal violent injuries. Gas station and convenience store workers are at particular risk of homicide, and as noted before, their safety has not improved greatly in recent years. The most effective intervention for reducing risk in these occupations has been to close facilities earlier in the evening. This, however, reduces profit, job availability, and services to the public. Among the efforts that seem to have helped reduce taxi homicides have been isolating taxicab drivers from their customers by "assault-proof" barriers, reducing the amount of cash carried, using surveillance cameras, and installing geographic positioning systems with "panic buttons." At the time of this writing, very little evidence supports the value of any of these innovations except perhaps for partitions.

According to NIOSH reports, *each week* 20 U.S. workers are killed at work and 18,000 are assaulted (NIOSH [1995], Violence in the workplace: Risk factors and prevention strategies. CIB #57.) Workplace homicides differ significantly

REFLECTIVE THINKING 26-1

Dangerous Occupation

The U.S. National Institute of Occupational Safety and Health (NIOSH) has a very interesting Taxi Safety Blog where you can read what taxi drivers and others have to say about various safety-related interventions for this very dangerous occupation (available at http://www.cdc.gov/niosh/blog/nsb061608_taxiviolence.html, as accessed August 3, 2008).

Read the blog and consider what it means day to day to be a worker in this job. Does the public appreciate the risks these drivers take? What impact do you think the risk has on families? What about other occupations for which risk is real?

from the other 85% of U.S. homicides in being 10 times more likely to be associated with robbery, and in being perpetrated by an individual unknown to the victim. Hospitals, especially emergency rooms, are worksites with relatively high levels of violence toward staff. Gates and colleagues report on the experience of one urban emergency service where in a convenience sample, over 60% of ER workers reported that they had been harassed or assaulted by patients in the preceding six months. Most of these episodes had not been reported to hospital administration (Gates, Ross, & McQueen, 2006). A study from an inner city hospital in Vancouver, British Columbia, Canada, found that 57% of staff had been physically assaulted by a patient or patient's accompanying visitor/family member in the preceding year, and most had witnessed coworkers receiving similar verbal abuse along with either physical assault or threats of assault (Fernandes, Bouthillette, Raboud, Bullock, Moore, Christenson, et al., 1999). Focus group studies by a nurse researcher in Vancouver confirmed nearly daily threats and verbal assaults from patients and family members (Henderson, 2003). Additional Canadian studies confirmed these findings and also documented significant emotional and sexual harassment perpetrated by coworkers (Hesketh, Duncan, Estabrooks, Reimer, Giovannetti, Hyndman, et al., 2003). Sadly (since we hope many of you will seriously consider careers in psychiatric mental health nursing), working in mental health confers no protection from such threats and violent behavior. New Zealand nurses experienced levels of largely verbal violence similar to those of Canadian colleagues during their first year in mental health practice (McKenna, Poole, Smith, Coverdale, & Gale, 2003). These authors also reported that some nurses experienced stalking by patients, a disconcerting form of harassment/violence also described by other New Zealand researchers (Hughes, Thom, & Dixon, 2007). While we know you will find nursing to be among the most personally rewarding of all occupations, some settings of care do expose nurses to violence or to behaviors that many nurses find uncomfortable. Most experienced nurses find that the benefits of bringing comfort and care to many persons strongly outweigh the risks of abuse or even violence from a few.

Bullying and Workplace Incivility

Once regarded as annoying but acceptable childhood behavior, bullying in schools has come under intense scrutiny in recent years because it may lead to subsequent victimization in work and other relationships, depression, and suicide (Williams & Guerr, 2007). Being a victim of bullying more than doubles the (very low) odds of engaging in a school shooting incident (Anderson et al., 2002). While bullying is harmful to its victims, bullies themselves are also at significant risk of a variety of subsequent problems in relationships, work, health, substance use, and criminal justice (Nansel et al., 2004). The worst long-term outcomes seem to occur among individuals who are both bullied themselves and then subsequently engage in bullying behavior. As suggested earlier, bullying may carry over into the workplace. Many nurses describe bullying behavior (often termed "workplace incivility") occurring in hospital settings, perpetrated either by patients/family members, other nurses, or physicians (Simons, 2008).

There has been considerable interest in reducing the incidence of bullying in schools. Programs have been developed to change school culture so that bullying becomes less socially acceptable and other students are encouraged to intervene in bullying situations. Several Belgian studies have shown reductions in bullying behavior in elementary schools. The researchers found evidence for persistence of improved bullying attitudes and behaviors after the study's completion (Stevens, De Bourdeaudhuij, & Van Oost, 2000), but there is as yet no certainty that the intervention will have long-lasting effects lasting into the secondary school years. The same authors were unable to show reduction of bullying when programs were offered in

RESEARCH Highlight 26–2

Peer Victimization of Children with Attention-Deficit Hyperactivity Disorder

STUDY PROBLEM/PURPOSE

The researchers studied the factors that correlated psychosocial adjustment with victimization through bullying for children with Attention Deficit Disorder.

METHODS

The researchers did an analysis of data collected through a psycho-educational assessment of children through the state of Florida's Division of Child and Adolescent Psychiatry. Of those who were assessed, more than one-third (116 children) had a diagnosis of ADHD. Standardized tools were used to evaluate behavior, anxiety, depression, and parental ratings.

FINDINGS

Findings indicated that peer victimization or bullying was correlated with parent reports of anxiety, depression, social problems, delinquent behavior, and aggressive behavior. Children with ADHD have a higher rate of peer victimization than those without.

IMPLICATIONS

School nurses, pediatric nurses, as well as teachers and social workers have a role in identifying those children whose behaviors seem to invite bullying from their peers. Every professional has a role in creating school cultures where bullying is not accepted. The nurse roles of education and advocacy are of critical importance.

Source: J. L. Humphrey, E. A. Storch, and G. R. Geeken. (2007). Peer victimization in children with attention-deficit hyperactivity disorder. *Journal of Child Health Care, 11*(3), 248–260.

BOX 26-5
STANDARDS FOR A HEALTHY CLINICAL WORKPLACE

The American Association of Critical-Care Nurses has proposed six commonsense standards for improving clinical workplaces:

- Skilled Communication
- True Collaboration
- Effective Decision Making
- Appropriate Staffing
- Meaningful Recognition
- Authentic Leadership

AACN, 2005. AACN standards for establishing and sustaining healthy work environments: A journey to excellence. *American Journal of Critical Care, 14,* 187–197.

secondary schools (Stevens, Van Oost, & De Bourdeaudhuij, 2000). A similar mixed evaluation was reported from Seattle where a standardized anti-bullying program implementation had no overall measureable effect on either physical bullying or more subtle forms such as spreading rumors about other students, but the program was associated with reduction in the incidence of physical bullying behavior among some subsets of students (Bauer, Lozano, & Rivara, 2007).

There is a similar need for programs to improve working environments, including those in health care where a variety of coercive practices creates the potential for workplace violence (St-Pierre & Holmes, 2008). Nurse leaders have proposed the creation of "healthy work environments" and have advanced guidelines for implementation of workplace improvement.

While none of these appears to directly address workplace civility, several of the clinical examples given to support these standards illustrate incivility and call for changes in professional behavior (AACN, 2005). Researchers have confirmed that nurses in high-performing units recognize values closely related to these standards and in particular value collaborative interdisciplinary practice and a "communication-rich culture" (Kramer & Schmalebnerg, 2008). Even in hospitals achieving high performance "magnet status," these authors also identify considerable differences among units in the degree to which these values are supported (Schmalenberg & Kramer, 2008). It would appear that in both schools and workplaces we have a preliminary understanding of what is needed to reduce the prevalence of harassment and violence. However, there remains considerable uncertainty as to which precise steps are needed to reach these desired ends.

Violence on the Street

Perhaps because of movie and television portrayals, many people equate violence with robbery or assault by strangers. As we have seen, the majority of violence, particularly violence resulting in severe injury or death, occurs among people who know each other—often in families. Still, according to the National Violent Death Reporting System (Karch, Lubell, Friday, Patel, Williams, 2008), about a third of homicides occur in association with other crimes—with robberies being the most common association and assault (not as uniformly a stranger crime) the second most common. However, it may be surprising to learn that a quarter of robberies of men and over half of robberies of women are perpetrated by persons known to the victim (U.S. Department of Justice. *Crime Statistics.* Available at http://www.ojp.usdoj.gov, as accessed August 4, 2008). While the perpetrator of some murders is never identified, U.S. Department of Justice data state that only 14% of *known* murderers in 2002 were strangers to the victim (U.S. Department of Justice. *Crime Statistics.* Available at http://www.ojp.usdoj.gov, as accessed August 4, 2008). While **stranger violence** (violence perpetrated by one unknown to the victim) is clearly less common than violence involving persons who know one another, it remains a public health concern in nearly all countries.

As with other forms of violence, the poor are more likely to be victims of stranger violence, and with the exception of sexual violence (discussed later in this chapter), men are affected more than are women. Poor youth, especially of Hispanic ethnicity, are also more likely to be involved with gangs. Victim reports indicate that about 6% of all crimes are gang related, but a significant portion of victims who survive violent crimes are either unable or unwilling to tell authorities whether they believe gang members were responsible for the crime they experienced. One of the major unanswerable questions about stranger violence is the degree to which it is linked to illicit drug distribution. About 3% of homicides are related to "drug trade" (Karch et al., 2008), but it is difficult to ascertain how many other crimes are committed either in relationship to drug use or under the influence of illicit substances.

Stranger Crime as a Public Concern

Reducing stranger crime is a desirable social and public health outcome with little available evidence to point the way to success. Britain has invested heavily in public surveillance cameras, and there is some very limited evidence of reduced severity and incidence of violent crime in areas where these are deployed (Sivarajasingam, Shepherd, & Matthews, 2003). Through the 1990s, there was much emphasis on community policing in the United States and elsewhere (Palmiotto, 2008). Community policing is an effort to take police out of offices and automobiles and put them on foot in troubled communities where they can get to know community members, help mediate disputes, and assist the community in solving problems that lead to major crimes. There is much logic behind community policing, and it still receives considerable encouragement from the U.S. Department of Justice. While there was a highly significant decline in crime of all kinds from the 1980s through 2005—a time in which community policing was widely utilized—little evidence was produced that this policing model was responsible for the improvements in public safety. In recent years emphasis has been shifted from community policing to a "zero tolerance" model that reestablishes police officers as figures of authority and punishment rather than as community mediators. While police deployment in either of the two quite different roles currently proposed—community policing or zero tolerance—may have some impact on crime, it also seems highly likely that stranger crime is greatly influenced by community economic opportunities and by the abuse of crack cocaine and perhaps methamphetamine as well (Kirk, 2008; Blumstein, Rivara, & Rosenfeld, 2000). Policing policies may have less influence on street crime than do policies that improve the economic lot of the least advantaged among us.

Violence of Politics and War

With the incessant media coverage of violence all over the world, it is not easy to recognize that political violence is lower now than at any time in recent history (Mack, 2007). Political violence and war were responsible for millions of deaths during the last 100 years, including many millions from genocide among Armenians, and in Germany, former Yugoslavia, and Rwanda. Despite the optimism expressed previously, violence and even genocide still continue in North Africa. Two fundamental questions have troubled philosophers for generations: What are the roots of human violence in war and other politically motivated aggressive activities, and when is war justified? Both of these questions are too complex to address in the limited space available here, but interested readers should find some useful discussions in the suggested readings at the end of this chapter.

Refugees—The Escape from Violence

The victims of modern war are often the civilians around whom battles are fought. Not only may they be killed or maimed during those battles, but they may suffer post-traumatic stress disorders as a result of their experiences. Not only does conflict frequently take place in countries with low levels of economic development, but war seriously damages agricultural and economic infrastructure necessary for human well-being. Civilians are often inadvertently injured during conflicts, but they also not infrequently suffer persecution, physical abuse, rape, torture, and death because of real or perceived loyalties in those conflicts. As a result of these factors, there has been unprecedented movement of refugees in the past decades. Some of these individuals have spent literally all of their lives trapped in "temporary" refugee camps. Others have managed to migrate to safe havens in Europe or North America. Still others have died in the process of migration, been forced into bondage through trafficking (more on trafficking later in this chapter), or reached potential havens after perilous journeys only to be turned back by local authorities. While refugees from civil conflicts comprised a "first migrant wave" and have sometimes (but not always) found an open door in the European and North American countries to which they turn, poor people escaping economic injustice and "pathologies of power" currently comprise a second and important group of migrants worldwide. These refugees are much more likely to meet closed borders, to enter countries illegally without access to health care or social services, and to suffer discrimination and ill health. Migration in response to violence, whether its roots are in war, economic injustice, or both, is among the most important public health problems faced in the world today.

Child Refugees

A particularly poignant subset of refugee migration involves children. Some refugee children are orphans of war or human immunodeficiency virus (HIV), others may be decommissioned child soldiers who potentially face hardships or revenge in their own countries, some have been sent by family members (or chosen their own path) to seek economic opportunities unlikely to become available in home countries during their lifetimes. The system for admitting political refugees into the United States is exceptionally complex for adults (Silove, Steel, & Mollica, 2001), but it is particularly ill-equipped to accommodate child refugees (Newman & Steel, 2008). Refugees, many of whom have had harrowing war and torture experiences and are at risk of being murdered if they return to their native countries, are placed into detention centers until they can receive a hearing before an administrative judge. The outcome of that hearing is unpredictable, a source of severe anxiety for some, and the hearing process may take months or even years during which time needed mental health support or treatment is often limited or unavailable (Keller, Ford, Sachs, Rosenfeld, Trinh-Shevrin, Meserve, et al., 2003). Even purely economic refugees may have survived harrowing experiences during their travel to highly developed countries and may have serious physical and mental health problems that need to be addressed (Brymer, Steinberg, Sornborger, Layne, Pynoos, 2008).

The use of children as combatants in civil conflicts has become more widespread in recent years. Many of these **child soldiers** are forced into military involvement, so this problem overlaps considerably with child trafficking (discussed next). In addition to the serious physical injuries that war inflicts, children are at greater risk from heat illness, malaria, and other infectious diseases than are adults. There is accumulating evidence of significant mental health problems among persons who have been child soldiers (Kohrt, Jordans, Tol, Speckman, Maharjan, Worthman et al., 2008). Readers of this chapter are encouraged to read Singer's 2006 book *Child Soldiers* which is referenced in the Suggested Readings list at the chapter's end.

Human Trafficking

One of the most devastating realities in today's very large movements of migrants about the world is the prevalence of **trafficking**—especially for women and children. Trafficking is a form of bondage in which people are moved from one country to another and in the process incur "debts" to those who facilitated their passage that are so large that they may take years to discharge—or they may never be discharged. Some persons voluntarily enter into these financial arrangements to receive "safe" passage into the United States or a European country. But many victims of trafficking are sold

Voces Inocents (Innocent Voices)

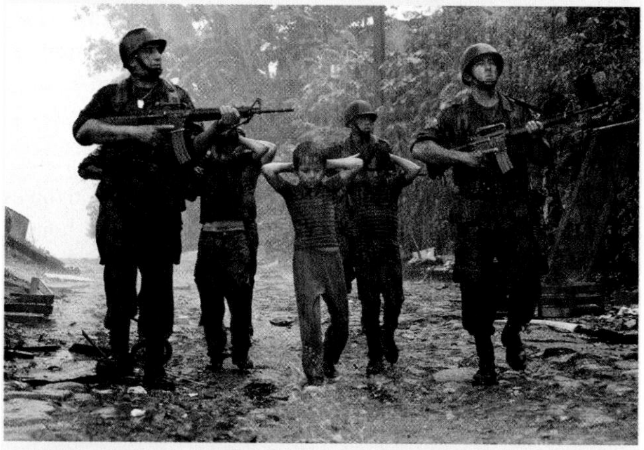

Lawrence Bender Productions (Courtesy: The Kobal Collection)

Voces Inocents is one of several affecting films about child soldiers in Africa and, as in this film, South America. Thousands of children worldwide have been directly affected by violence in this way. Rehabilitation for these children is often underfunded or completely lacking.

into bondage or kidnapped. Most of these are women or young girls, and most of them find their way into commercial sex work in the country to which they are taken. Their families may sell them to avoid paying a dowry for marriage, or families may falsely believe that they have arranged a better life for these children.

Trafficking, especially when sexual bondage is involved, is one of today's most serious public health problems because of the large numbers of persons involved, and because many end up with HIV, abortion-related septic death, substance addictions, or other risks associated with commercial sex. A large percentage of children are trafficked into brothels in their early teens (the mean age of trafficked girls in one 1994 study was 14 years), and these girls are often turned out onto the street after their "debt" is repaid, replaced by younger victims, and then either live in extreme poverty or return to rejection, starvation, or murder in their home of origin (Human Rights Watch, 1995). Much has been written about trafficking within Asia, but many trafficked women and girls end up in the United States or Europe. Influenced by a variety of non-governmental organizations (NGO), the United States has been quite proactive in creating legislation to combat trafficking. As President George W. Bush said:

> *Human trafficking is an offense against human dignity, a crime in which human beings, many of them teenagers and young children, are bought and sold and often sexually abused by violent criminals. Our nation is determined to fight and end this modern form of slavery (Anonymous, 2007).*

In its report prefaced by President Bush's quotation, the government sketched four areas of focus for 2006: (1) improving coordination of services to victims; (2) monitoring and combating labor trafficking; (3) achieving better data on the size of the trafficking problem; and (4) doing a better job of identifying victims within the United States. Women who are confirmed to have been trafficked into the United States are potentially eligible to receive refugee visas. This is in contrast to some other countries, where entering the country illegally or having worked in prostitution both result in automatic denials of immigration status—apparently without regard to whether either the illegal entry or sex work was done under bondage (Stewart & Gajic-Veljanoski, 2005). The reader should recognize that trafficking—whether for sex work or for physical labor—is a form of slavery and hence prohibited under the Bill of Rights of the U.S. Constitution. While the numbers of women, children, or men trafficked yearly cannot be known, it is likely that more people have today been trafficked into slavery than were slaves in the United States at the time of the Civil War (Barrows & Finger, 2008). One older estimate puts the number of persons illegally trafficked yearly at up to 4,000,000, with at least 700,000 of these being women and children. Of these latter, an estimated 50,000 find their way into the United States each year (Gushulak & MacPherson, 2000). Others, recognizing the uncertainty of estimates, suggest that the number of women and girls trafficked may reach 600,000–800,000 (Stewart & Gajic-Veljanoski, 2005).

The U.S. Congress requires that the Attorney General make an annual report on efforts made to combat trafficking. In addition to many international grants to study trafficking worldwide, the report describes a network of centers created with the United States to identify and provide services to victims of trafficking. Figure 26-1 is a map of the location of these centers taken from the 2007 report (Department of Justice, 2008).

While U.S. government efforts have undoubtedly had some effect both in this country and abroad, the prestigious NGO Human Rights Watch has urged the government to eliminate its requirement that any organization receiving U.S. funding officially pledge opposition to prostitution. Human Rights Watch argues that to reach and help women who have been trafficked, organizations must be able to work closely with sex workers, their clients, and the infrastructure that supports and maintains them. An organization viewed widely as opposed to prostitution is unlikely, they believe, to be able to create the kinds of relationships that allow trafficking to be better understood and—ultimately—eliminated. Human Rights Watch has also expressed criticism of some of the U.S. reports on trafficking that commend anti-trafficking

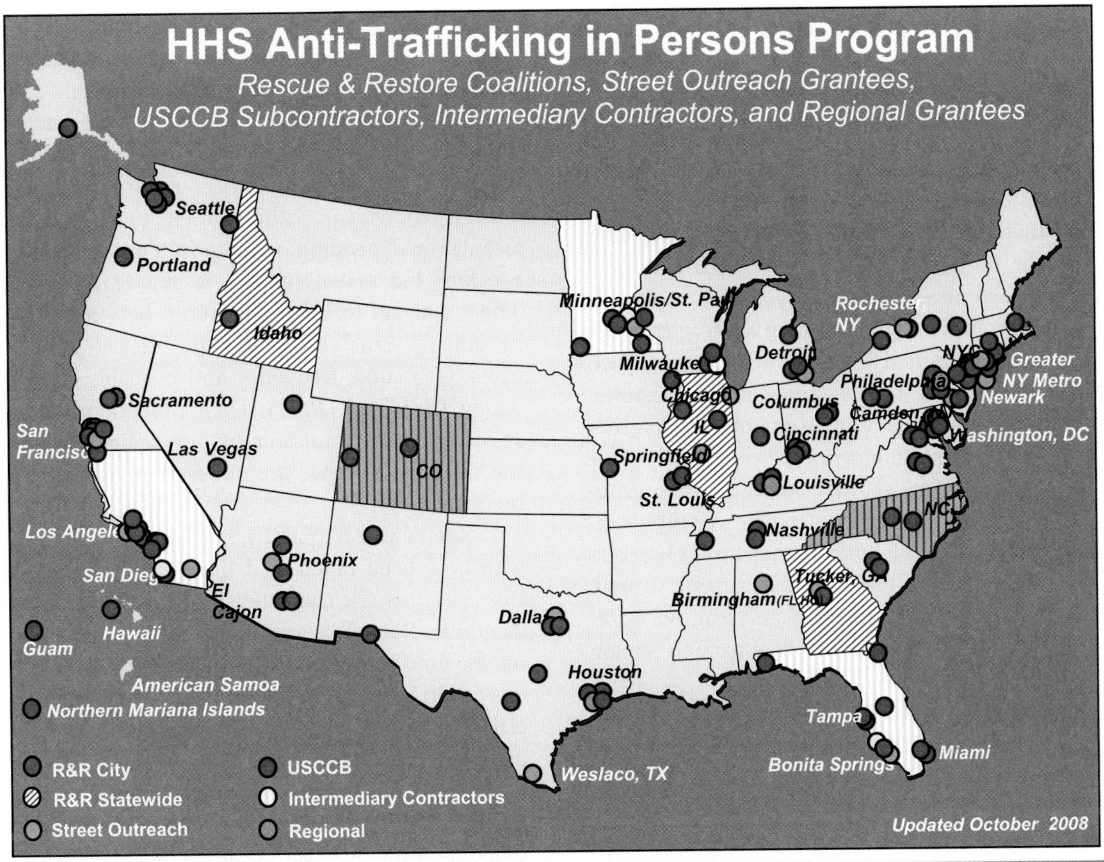

FIGURE 26-1 **Map of the location of centers to identify and provide services to victims of human trafficking. (Taken from the 2007 report, Department of Justice, (2008) Attorney General's Annual Report to Congress and Assessment of the U.S. Government Activities to Combat Trafficking in Persons Fiscal Year 2007 available at URL: http://www.usdoj.gov, as accessed on August 5, 2008).**

activities of countries who summarily deport trafficked women and children rescued from bondage by local NGOs or identified by police. Such deportation "rescues" women from bondage only to return them without resources or support, and sometimes ill with HIV, to the very environment in which they were originally sold into slavery. As Human Rights Watch notes, trafficking is a serious rights and public health problem demanding sensitive and thoughtful international attention:

> *Trafficking in persons—the illegal and highly profitable recruitment, transport, or sale of human beings for the purpose of exploiting their labor—is a slavery-like practice that must be eliminated. The trafficking of women and children into bonded sweatshop labor, forced marriage, forced prostitution, domestic servitude, and other kinds of work is a global phenomenon. Traffickers use coercive tactics including deception, fraud, intimidation, isolation, threat and use of physical force, and/or debt bondage to control their victims. Women are typically recruited with promises of good jobs in other countries or provinces, and, lacking better options at home, agree to migrate. Through agents and brokers who arrange the travel and job placements, women are escorted to their destinations and delivered to the employers. Upon reaching their destinations, some women learn that they have been deceived about the nature of the work they will do; most have been lied to about the financial arrangements and conditions of their employment; and all find themselves in coercive and abusive situations from which escape is both difficult and dangerous.* (Human Rights Watch)

Despite the large numbers of persons involved in trafficking within the United States, few have access to health care, and it is likely that few have the freedom to seek care even where it is potentially available to poor immigrant populations. Nurses should remain alert to the possibility that women for whom they provide care, or their children—especially those whose country of origin is outside the United States—may be victims of trafficking.

VIOLENCE AGAINST WOMEN

Even though they are less often victims of homicide and stranger crimes then are men, women are not spared the experience of violence. Most sexual violence is directed toward women; women are more frequently harassed and have their movements and other social choices controlled or constrained than is the case for men. Women are more commonly caught in trafficking and other activities that obligate them to have unwanted sexual activities or engage in commercial sex work; and some women are tragically the victims of culturally sanctioned violence such as genital cutting and honor killing. As noted earlier in this chapter, women are disproportionately victims in intimate partner violence, with outcomes ranging from psychological injury to death. Many social scientists view these various exposures to violence as examples of women's power disadvantages in most cultures. While psychoanalytical observers might suggest that a masculine need to control women through violence derives from insecurity and fear, whatever the sources, oppression and victimization of women remain a problem worldwide.

In recent years, the United Nations has adopted as one of its major goals: the elimination of violence against women. Recognizing that attitudes fostering violence are deeply embedded in many traditional cultures, the UN has taken a stance that both respects culture and advocates for change (Jensen, 2006). This stance is based on a number of basic premises described in Box 26-6.

Clearly, the approaches implied in the premises are directed mostly to traditional cultures. For this reason the premises may seem at first glance to relate less to the problems women face in modern North American and European settings where the roots of gender violence may lie in the "cycle of violence" rather than in cultural values. Some reflection, however, will show that most of these premises have relevance to ending violence in countries like the United States. Perhaps some readers will have an awareness of the "Take Back the Night" campaigns (available at http://www.takebackthenight.org) to publicize and end sexual violence against women. The authors encourage all readers to look briefly at the "TBTN" Web site and reflect on which of the UN's premises seem to have been effective for this organization and its campaigns on behalf of women—and men.

Rape as a Form of Violence

While men are occasionally the victims of rape, the majority of rapes are perpetrated by men with women as victims. It is critical to understand that rape is violence and that in sexual negotiation there is no ambiguity: "no" means simply *no*. Even in the United States, some women believe that sexual gratification is a primary motivation for rape and that rape victims play a role in the causation of rape (Lee, Pomeroy, Yoo, & Rheinboldt, 2005). Even in our culture it has taken some time to get widespread acceptance that rape can occur between intimate partners or even married couples. Neither marriage nor cohabitation gives one member of a couple the right to touch without consent. Any touching of another individual without their consent is classified as assault (or depending on circumstances, **battery**, and if that touching has sexual content, it may legally constitute rape. There appears to be a continuum between bullying (called by some "sexual bullying") and sexual assault, and both occur with some frequency and probably at all ages during dating (Fredland, 2008). Even though many persons conceptualize rape as assault by a stranger (Lee et al., 2005) the majority of rapes are committed by persons known to the victim.

Nurses will frequently need to provide care to women who have been raped, and this requires special sensitivities. Box 26-7 lists the characteristics of responses of the nursing diagnosis Rape-Trauma Syndrome to illustrate the client needs. Emotional and physical needs must come first. Serious genital trauma occurs as a consequence of rape (especially when the victim is young, or virginal, or the rape involves anal intercourse). Non-genital trauma from blows, weapons, or strangling is more common and may need urgent attention. All rape victims need support and comfort. Once the immediate physical needs have been met, women will generally need a full physical and pelvic examination conducted by someone with excellent forensic skills. Preserving the chain of evidence can be critical for prosecution. Even if a woman says she does not want to press charges, it is important to collect specimens for evidence as she may change her mind days or even weeks later. Of course, here, too, "no" means *no*—examinations must be fully consensual. One of the purposes of an examination is to exclude sexually transmitted infections (including cervical cancer with a Pap smear if that has not been done within the recommended period). Some women will need and want post-coital contraception, and under some circumstances presumptive treatment for sexually transmitted infections (including HIV) may be given. Pregnancy testing is often needed to assure that any medications given are safe if there is a preexisting pregnancy. All women who have been victims of sexual violence should have the leisured opportunity to talk with a skilled sexual assault counselor and have carefully arranged physical and psychological follow-up. Substance use or abuse is sometimes associated with sexual violence, and any needs for counseling or other treatment around alcohol or other drugs should be ascertained. Depending on the policies of the facility in which the examination is done, it may be necessary to involve police personnel. Capable and sensitive police assistance—in most cases by a female officer—can help a woman decide whether to press charges. Special circumstances arise when the rape victim is very young or developmentally disabled.

BOX 26-6
UNITED NATIONS PREMISES FOR STRATEGIES TO ELIMINATE VIOLENCE AGAINST WOMEN

- Recognizing that culture is dynamic and often quite open to change. Change must be guided carefully with respect for underlying values.
- Understanding the local context. Violence toward women is typically embedded in cultural beliefs including myths and traditions. Understanding these will help bring about change.
- Gathering and reporting facts. When facts come from credible sources, people will more likely use them to make needed change.
- Adopting a rights-based approach. Women have the right to live free of violence; especially if abused, they have the right to enjoy accessible and sensitive health care and needed legal and social services.
- Allowing community involvement. Projects whose goal is to reduce women's exposure to violence must have the support and counsel of the communities in which they take place.
- Involving men in the process. Since men are the primary cause of violence toward women, their involvement is a necessary part of ending that violence. Many projects seek the participation of male community leaders, sports figures, and other celebrities.
- Taking a public health view. Violence is a severe threat to women's mental and physical health. Helping communities to see the public health benefits of ending violence toward women has proven effective in getting widespread acceptance of programs.
- Changing both laws and attitudes. In some countries laws permit or abet violence toward women. Not only must these laws be changed, but focused advocacy must help communities understand why new laws must be respected and obeyed.
- Involving local non-governmental organizations (NGOs). Local NGOs can be effective forces for cultural change because their involvement with communities helps them make connections with opinion leaders. Successful NGOs know how to maintain cultural respect and at the same time bring about needed change.
- Engaging local power structures including faith-based organizations. When not only men, but other power brokers in the community see the value and rightness of eliminating gender violence, they will help sway community opinion and action in needed directions.
- Involving people personally. Change comes about when the majority of people accept new norms of belief and behavior. This acceptance, in turn, derives from dialogue and the opportunity to weigh the personal costs and benefits of change. When people have well-led forums for public discussion they are more likely to accept the need for changing community behaviors.
- Separating the values underlying a harmful practice from the practice itself. Most practices, no matter how harmful they are to women (genital cutting, often called female circumcision, and honor killing are two important examples) serve a perceived purpose within the cultures that support them. While these practices are completely unacceptable from a rights point of view, people are less likely to resist change if wise cultural brokers can work to establish alternative rituals or practices that meet the same cultural needs but do not cause harm or injury to women. Communities are more likely to reject violent behaviors if in the process their culture is not eroded by necessary change.
- Expanding options for women. Without economic opportunities and self-sufficiency, women will not gain power.
- Seeking unity. Change potentially provokes dissension and social fragmentation. Effective change helps communities stay focused on remaining intact despite needed and inevitable progress.
- Reaching young people. True change takes place over generations and requires modifying the beliefs and values of the young without devaluing the culture to which they belong.
- Raising community awareness with creativity and the use of popular culture. As with men, sports figures, and community power brokers, a campaign using local musicians and artists can have important successes. Media are important as well.

From Jensen, L. (2006). *Ending violence against women.* New York, United Nations. Available at http://www.unfpa.org/upload/lib_pub_file/679_filename_endingvaw.pdf as accessed August 4, 2008.

BOX 26-7
NANDA'S CHARACTERISTICS OF RESPONSES TO RAPE-TRAUMA SYNDROME

EXAMPLES OF DEFINING CHARACTERISTICS

- Disorganization
- Change in relationships
- Confusion
- Physical trauma
- Suicide attempts
- Denial
- Guilt
- Humiliation
- Embarrassment
- Mood swings
- Powerlessness
- Nightmare and sleep disturbances
- Vulnerability
- Depression
- Inability to make decisions
- Anger
- Anxiety
- Shame
- Fear

COMPOUND REACTION

- Change in lifestyle
- Emotional reaction
- Multiple physical symptoms
- Reactivated symptoms of such previous conditions

SILENT REACTION

- Increased anxiety during interview, for example, blocking of associations, long periods of silence, minor stuttering, physical distress
- Sudden onset of phobic reactions
- No verbalization of the occurrence of rape
- Abrupt changes in relationships with men
- Increase in nightmares
- Pronounced changes in sexual behavior

From *Nursing Diagnoses: Definitions & Classification, 2009–2011*, by NANDA International, 2009, Philadelphia: Author.

RESEARCH Highlight 26–3

Mental Health after Sexual Violence: The Role of Behavioral and Demographic Risk Factors

STUDY PURPOSE

The researchers looked for associations between mental health sequelae and prior sociodemographic and behavioral factors for persons who had been exposed to sexual violence.

METHODS

Using an existing database, the South Carolina (2005) data from the Behavior Risk Factors Survey done by the CDC, researchers looked for associations/correlations between having reported being a victim of sexual violence and behavioral risk factors and poor mental health. Specifically, the researchers tried to identify demographic, social, and behavioral factors that may mediate mental health after exposure to sexual violence.

FINDINGS

Poor mental health among those who experienced sexual violence was associated with younger age, lower income, lower educational attainment, lack of emotional support, and lack of health insurance. Behavioral factors significantly associated with better mental health (after controlling for socioeconomic status) were healthy diet ($p = .05$), exercise ($p = .02$), and not smoking ($p = .0001$). Alcohol use was not associated with mental health.

IMPLICATIONS

Treatment after sexual violence should include attention to risk factors including low income, low educational attainment, and lack of emotional support, and to the protective influence of behavioral factors including a healthy diet, exercise, and not smoking. The authors comment that "Comprehensive integrated models of care addressing mental, physical, and social sequelae of sexual violence are needed"(p. 175).

Source: "Mental Health after Sexual Violence: The Role of Behavioral and Demographic Risk Factors," by Lisa Vandemark and Martina Mueller. (2008). *Nursing Research*, *57*(3), 175–181.

In both these circumstances it is crucial that highly experienced experts in rape participate in needed discussion and examinations. If there is a language barrier, interpreter services must be arranged. It is never appropriate for family members to act as interpreters in a case involving sexual violence.

NURSING PERSPECTIVES ON VIOLENCE

Nursing theories assist nurses in planning care for clients who are survivors of interpersonal violence and sexual assaults. The self-care deficit theory and crisis theory are especially helpful in planning nursing care for abused and neglected clients and rape survivors.

SELF-CARE DEFICIT THEORY

As explained in Chapter 3, "Theory as a Basis for Practice," and Chapter 14, "The Client Experiencing Depression," Orem's (1991) Self-Care Deficit Theory views nurses' work as doing for the client that which he cannot do for himself. Clients who experience interpersonal abuse and sexual assaults are often in a crisis and unable to care for all of their own needs. They may have severe physical injuries and psychological problems, such as depression and anxiety. They may need assistance in performing self-care activities that preserve and promote their health, life, and state of well-being. Orem calls the ability of clients to provide for their own self-care activities self-care agency. An abused or sexually assaulted client is likely to experience self-care deficit when the therapeutic self-care demand exceeds the client's self-care agency. Nursing interventions can be appropriate in addressing clients' self-care demands. For example, the nurse must first look after the client's need for safety and make sure that the client has a place to be that the client perceives to be safe and secure. Next, the nurse may attend to health demands, such as nutrition, sleep, and emotional support. The nursing goal is to support the client in making her own decisions while providing the structure for the client's needs to be met.

CRISIS INTERVENTION THEORY

Interpersonal violence and sexual assaults often create a crisis for clients. (See Chapter 11, "The Client Undergoing Crisis," for an in-depth explanation of the nature of crisis.) Crisis theory is a practical theory to use with clients experiencing a crisis. Aguilera (1998) has identified specific steps involved in the techniques of crisis intervention. Clients generally remain in treatment for one to six weeks.

The first phase is the assessment of the client and his problem. It includes an accurate assessment of the precipitating event and the resulting crisis that brought the client to seek professional help. If the client is a high suicidal risk, then a referral is made for consideration of hospitalization.

The second phase is the planning of therapeutic interventions. This phase is designed to restore the client to at least his precrisis level of equilibrium. The nurse needs to determine when the crisis occurred. Clients often do not seek help for one to two weeks after the crisis, but may do so within the first 24 hours. The nurse needs to assess the extent to which the crisis has disrupted the client's life. She should assess his strengths, coping skills used successfully in the past but not being used presently, alternative coping skills that are not presently being used, and his support system. The effect the crisis is having on the client's significant others also needs to be assessed.

The third phase involves the nursing interventions, which include helping the client gain an understanding of the crisis and get in touch with his feelings, examining alternative ways of coping, and helping him utilize his support system.

The last phase is resolution of the crisis and anticipatory planning. The nurse assists the client in making realistic plans for the future and discusses ways in which the present experience may help in coping with future crises (Aguilera, 1998, pp. 18–21).

Orem's self-care theory and Aguilera's crisis theory are complementary and ideal to use with clients who are survivors of interpersonal abuse and sexual assault. They promote self-reliance and advocate empowering clients to resolve their problems.

NURSING RESPONSIBILITIES

To begin to adequately provide care to survivors of violence, nurses first need to deal with their own feelings and beliefs about it. It can take nurses time to work through their own thoughts and beliefs about interpersonal violence, sexual assault, and political violence. Nurses need to identify any stereotypical beliefs that they may have about survivors and perpetrators. It is difficult for some nurses to be comfortable asking clients if they have been abused. Further, nurses need to avoid "rescuer fantasies" that may interfere with their ability to assess the real needs of survivors and their families.

Nurses need to be knowledgeable about the dynamics of intimate partner violence. They need to keep in mind that the client they are caring for, regardless of the setting, may be in an abusive relationship. In most settings, the nurses will be working as a member of an interdisciplinary team.

Nurses must know their state's legal requirements for reporting clients who are survivors of interpersonal violence and the specific requirements in their communities and agencies. Failure by a registered nurse to report actual or suspected abuse of clients of any age may constitute unprofessional conduct within the meaning of their state's Nursing Practice Act.

Nurses and other health professionals are mandated to report children who have experienced interpersonal violence and sexual assault to law enforcement or child protective services. If an adult client has been sexually assaulted, the report is made to law enforcement. In most states, if elderly clients are physically or sexually abused, a report is made to law enforcement or adult protective services.

All health care agencies need to educate nurses about the dynamics of interpersonal abuse. Survivors of abuse seek treatment not only for their immediate injuries, but also for the health problems that result from interpersonal violence, such as stress-related illnesses (anxiety, sleep disturbance) and chronic health care problems.

FUTURE DIRECTIONS

The U.S. Public Health Services identified violence as a critical public health problem. The United States ranks first among industrial nations in violent death rates. The federal government has a number of initiatives that are aimed at stopping interpersonal violence and sexual assault.

When Congress incorporated the Healthy People 2010 objectives into national legislation, it identified violent and abusive behavior as a national concern and a priority area. The CDC is the lead agency for this objective. The specific objectives for this initiative include reducing maltreatment and fatalities of children, the rate of physical assault by current or former intimate partners, the annual rate of rape or attempted rape, sexual assault other than rape, physical assaults, physical fighting among adolescents, and weapon carrying by adolescents on school property (U.S. Department of Health and Human Services, 2000).

The National Center for the Prevention and Treatment of Child Abuse and Neglect was established in 1972 at the University of Colorado as a resource for issues of child abuse and neglect. It provides professional training, consultation, program development and evaluation, and research in all forms of child abuse and neglect (http://www.kempecenter.org).

Victory over Violence (VOV) is a youth-sponsored initiative to help young people identify and counteract the root causes of violence in their lives and in their communities. It began its outreach programs in 1999 as a response to growing concerns over the rise in youth-related violence. It has sponsored over 3,000 grassroots discussions in the United States, with more than 110,000 people "taking the pledge" to lead nonviolent lives (http://www.vov.com/).

The Office on Violence against Women (OVW), a component of the U.S. Department of Justice, was created in 1995 to implement the Violence Against Women Act (VAWA) and subsequent legislation, and provide national leadership against domestic violence, sexual assault, and stalking (http://www.ovw.usdoj.gov/). One of OVW's initiatives is the President's Family Justice Center Initiative. This is a pilot program for planning and the developing comprehensive domestic violence victim service and support centers. The goal is to make the survivor's search for help and justice less burdensome by bringing professionals who provide an array of services to domestic violence survivors together in one location (U.S. Department of Justice: OVAW, 2007).

The National Center on Elder Abuse (NCEA), administered under the auspices of the National Association of State Units on Aging, is dedicated to educating the public about elder abuse, neglect, and exploitation, and its tragic consequences. It is a national resource for elder rights, law enforcement and legal professionals, public policy leaders, researchers, and the public (Teaster, Dugar, Mendiondo, et al, 2006).

All of these efforts indicate that U.S. society may finally be willing to do something besides give lip service to preventing interpersonal violence and sexual assault. Nurses need to be actively involved in community efforts to eliminate family violence from our society.

APPLICATION OF THE NURSING PROCESS 26-1

ASSESSMENT

There is no comprehensive assessment tool that offers conclusive evidence that violence has occurred. Nurses need to act like detectives when assessing clients, since clients or their abusers will rarely admit to abuse or violence. Nurses need to make direct observations of the client and family members. For example, does the child seem afraid of the caregiver? Does the caregiver hit the child? These observations are clues that more probing is necessary.

In order to properly assess survivors of abuse, nurses need to know the symptoms that are commonly seen in interpersonal violence and sexual assaults and the common characteristics of the abusers. Many of the symptoms are subjective, so the nurse and the health care team will need to piece together the evidence to determine if interpersonal violence has occurred or if clients are at risk for violence. Psychological abuse is a particularly difficult area to assess, as emotional relationships are very culture bound, and words and emotions that may be harmful in one family are not necessarily so in another family.

The interview provides an opportunity for nurses to question clients about interpersonal violence. The type of questions the nurse asks survivors of interpersonal violence or sexual assault will depend on the age of the survivor, the suspected type of abuse, and the situation.

NURSING DIAGNOSIS

Nurses will need to do a more extensive examination when the history or behavioral symptoms indicate interpersonal abuse. Clients will need to have physical examinations to assess the extent of their injuries and to collect forensic evidence to prove who assaulted them. A traumagram, or body

(*Continues*)

APPLICATION OF THE NURSING PROCESS 26-1 (Continued)

map (a drawing of the front and back of a nude human figure), is generally used by the nurse or physician to mark on the figure the location of all visible injuries. Each state has legally mandated procedures for collecting evidentiary material, and nurses need to be sure that the legal "chain of evidence" pertaining to collection of forensic samples is unbroken. The medical record should document the injuries and nursing and medical treatment that may serve as legal evidence of the client's condition. Nurses need to know their state's requirements and their agency's protocol for collecting and documenting evidence.

When clients are seen soon after experiencing interpersonal violence or sexual assault, their nursing and medical examinations can add to their trauma. They may be experiencing *Anxiety* (Herdman, 2009) and Acute Stress Disorder (DSM-IV-TR, 2000) that may interfere with ability to cooperate with the nursing and medical examinations. They can disrupt the client's cognitive perceptions, rendering memory of events incomplete or inaccurate. If they are examined several weeks to months after the assaults, they may be experiencing symptoms of *Post-trauma syndrome* (NANDA-I) and Post-Traumatic Stress Disorder (DSM-IV-TR). Other nursing diagnoses that may be applicable for clients who suffer from interpersonal violence or sexual assault will depend on their injuries.

OUTCOME IDENTIFICATION

Outcomes for clients suffering from abuse and violence must be carefully and thoughtfully considered and developed in conjunction with the client. Nurses must be careful to avoid projecting their personal opinions and desires onto the client's situation and should focus energies instead on effecting changes that are realistic and achievable for the client. This may be particularly difficult to do, since cases of abuse and violence are often emotionally charged for all parties involved, and it may be a challenge for the nurse to identify outcomes that are in the best interests of the client and in line with the client's wishes. The nurse needs to remain as impartial as possible while being a client advocate and work to outline intermediate steps that can be taken toward reaching an ultimate goal.

PLANNING/INTERVENTIONS

Planning care for survivors of abuse and their families will require input from the clients and a survey of their resources to ensure that the targeted care is in line with their expectations and commitments. Nursing interventions directed at primary prevention of interpersonal violence are those that reduce or control the causative factors associated with interpersonal violence and sexual assaults. Interventions directed toward potential abusers, survivors, and society in general are included. By identifying families at high risk for abuse, nurses can help the family plan efforts to modify those risk factors. This may include increasing the family's coping skills, thus improving self-esteem and sense of competence. It may involve treating existing psychopathology or substance abuse, discussing developmental issues, and providing emotional support and relief from stress. It can include identifying and referring cases of child abuse and children of battered women for counseling since a major risk factor of partner abuse is growing up in a violent home.

Primary prevention includes strengthening individuals and families by providing support and enrichment to at-risk individuals and families so they can cope more effectively with multiple life stressors and demands. It also includes changing the individuals' and families' perception that violence is an acceptable mode of conflict resolution. Prevention further includes empowering survivors of abuse by helping them learn to care for and protect themselves from the imposition by others. For example, children can be taught in health care settings or schools what to do if they are being abused. Primary prevention also includes nurses giving clients anticipatory guidance. For example, by anticipating the challenges of toddlerhood, nurses can acknowledge that this can be a difficult period for parents and can provide practical advice about constructive discipline. They can teach college freshmen about date rape and how to avoid vulnerable situations.

(Continues)

APPLICATION OF THE NURSING PROCESS 26-1 (Continued)

They can encourage families with dependent elderly members to use respite care services and day care programs. The support and anticipatory guidance can enhance the family and clients' competency and diminish the likelihood of using violence or being abused.

Primary prevention directed toward society involves measures of advocacy and political activity. Nurses can advocate for state and national policies and programs that benefit children and families, the elderly, and battered women.

Secondary prevention involves early detection and treatment for interpersonal violence. The two major goals of secondary prevention are to protect the survivor from further abuse and to break the cycle of violence. This may require medical and mental health treatment for survivors of interpersonal violence, reporting the abuse (or suspected abuse) to authorities, and removing the survivor from the abusive situation. Promoting safety of the survivor may mean placement of an abused child in foster care or arranging for an abused spouse or elderly person to go to a temporary shelter. It may involve encouraging family members to seek counseling and treatment for substance abuse problems. It involves potential abusers recognizing their tendency to be abusing and seeking help.

The goal of tertiary prevention is to provide appropriate supportive and rehabilitative services to violent families to prevent further abuse and neglect. High-risk families should receive follow-up care for ongoing supervision to prevent further abuse from occurring. Since many high-risk families are involved with multiple agencies, case management and agency collaboration are essential. When nurses care for abused clients, they need to coordinate their care with other community health and social service agencies. Their clients may be involved with their county department of social services, public health departments, battered women's shelters, legal assistance programs, and home health agencies.

EVALUATION

Evaluation of the effectiveness of the nursing interventions and the plan of care will include assessment of the client and any changes in behavior, attitude, or family circumstances. Progress toward goals that were identified with the client (and family, as appropriate) should be considered, and any that were not met should be carefully reviewed for achievability within the time frame, appropriateness to the client's developmental level, and realistic expectation given the circumstances. Coping mechanisms used by the client should be evaluated for their effectiveness, and the client should be redirected to strategies that may prove more effective.

Both nurses and clients need to keep in mind that progress toward achieving goals can be anywhere from very fast (removing a client from an immediate abusive situation) to painfully slow (changing attitudes toward abuse that have developed over a lifetime or changing responses and coping mechanisms used to deal with violent situations). As in identifying outcomes and planning care, the nurse must exercise caution in evaluating progress according to the client's needs, not the nurse's perception of what those needs may or should be.

NURSING CARE PLAN: NURSING PROCESS FORMAT 26-1

Elizabeth is experiencing Rape-Trauma Syndrome in an acute phase. She had been invited to a fraternity party, where she was raped by her date. After she was raped, she left the party alone. On the way back to her dorm she vomited in the street several times. The few people she saw on the way home did not approach her. She felt as if she looked like a coed who had had too much to drink. She said to herself, "I am simply disgusting." When she arrived at her dorm, she went into the bathroom before going to her room. She looked into the mirror and saw herself as ravaged, debased, her hair matted. She had vomit on her

(Continues)

NURSING CARE PLAN: NURSING PROCESS FORMAT 26-1 (Continued)

dress, legs, and shoes. The sight of herself made her sick again. She went into her room, where her roommate was sleeping. She put her clothes into a plastic bag and started crying. She douched and then showered for a half hour, but still did not feel clean. She returned to her room and tried to sleep. She wept off and on for hours, reliving every moment of the evening. She concluded that she was naive and an ignorant fool for having wanted her date to like her because he was a senior and so poised and good-looking. She had had too much beer and had been too trusting. She felt humiliated and degraded. Her roommate heard Elizabeth crying and asked if she was all right. She was too humiliated and ashamed to tell her. She felt that she was in a nightmare.

If Elizabeth had been seen the next morning at the student health center, the following care plan would be appropriate.

ASSESSMENT

Elizabeth is experiencing classic symptoms of Rape-Trauma Syndrome. Elizabeth has feelings of helplessness, anger, embarrassment, humiliation, and self-blame; gastrointestinal problems (nausea, vomiting, and anorexia); sleep disturbance; and skeletal muscle tension. She felt responsible for the rape because she had been flattered that Jimmy asked her out.

NURSING DIAGNOSIS 1 *Rape-Trauma Syndrome, acute phase*, related to forced intercourse, as evidenced by emotional reactions and physical symptoms.

OUTCOMES	NIC	NURSING ACTIONS	EVALUATION
• Elizabeth will acknowledge that she has been raped.	• Abuse protection support • Counseling • Coping enhancement	Assist Elizabeth in being able to accept that she has been raped by: • Reassuring Elizabeth that she is in a safe environment • Using active and empathetic listening skills • Communicating unconditional acceptance of Elizabeth and her situation	Elizabeth stated that she trusted the nurse and felt safe at the health center. Elizabeth confided in the nurse that she had been raped. She admitted that she was having difficulty talking about the rape.

NURSING DIAGNOSIS 2 *Ineffective coping*, related to situational crisis (rape), as evidenced by expression of anxiety and verbalization of inability to cope.

OUTCOMES	NIC	NURSING ACTIONS	EVALUATION
• Elizabeth will verbalize her feelings of anxiety, fear, and guilt. • Elizabeth will admit that she did not cause the rape. • Elizabeth will identify coping behaviors she used during the rape.	• Coping enhancement • Decision-making support • Counseling	• Encourage Elizabeth to discuss her reactions to the rape, including her feelings of anger, fear, guilt, rage, and helplessness. • Provide Elizabeth with anticipatory guidance and discuss the common emotional and social reactions to rape. • Encourage Elizabeth to make her own decisions.	Elizabeth acknowledged that how she was feeling and behaving was normal for someone who had been raped. Elizabeth admitted that she had begged Jimmy not to rape her and that she had tried to fight him off while he was raping her.

(Continues)

NURSING CARE PLAN: NURSING PROCESS FORMAT 26-1 (Continued)

OUTCOMES	NIC	NURSING ACTIONS	EVALUATION
• Elizabeth will seek support from family and friends to help her. • Elizabeth will verbalize an understanding of the Rape-Trauma Syndrome. • Elizabeth will be actively involved in resolving her crisis. • Elizabeth will identify family and friends who will support her during this crisis. • Elizabeth will return to and function at pre-rape level within a 6-week period.		• Assist her in identifying her immediate concerns. • Encourage her to confide in her parents and her roommate. • Obtain permission from her to talk with her parents and her roommate about the dynamics of the Rape-Trauma Syndrome. • Advise her of the benefit of obtaining counseling to help her deal with the traumatic event. • Provide her with a list of counselors who specialize in treating rape victims and strongly encourage her to seek therapy.	Elizabeth verbalized that she did not cause the rape but felt that she had put herself in a vulnerable situation. Elizabeth admitted that she had felt ashamed to call her family. Elizabeth consented to contacting her parents and telling them about being raped. Elizabeth, with the help of the nurse, confided in her roommate that she had been raped. Elizabeth's roommate helped her develop a plan so Elizabeth would feel safe attending her classes. Elizabeth verbalized the need for counseling to help her deal with her reactions to the rape. Elizabeth made an appointment with a rape crisis counselor before leaving the health center.

NURSING DIAGNOSIS 3 *Disturbed body image*, related to psychosocial perception, as evidenced by verbalization of negative feelings about body and feelings of helplessness and powerlessness.

OUTCOMES	NIC	NURSING ACTIONS	EVALUATION
• Elizabeth will acknowledge how the rape has affected how she feels about herself. • Her self-esteem will be restored within 6 weeks.	• Body image enhancement • Emotional support	• Help Elizabeth identify specific behaviors she used to prevent the rape. • Help Elizabeth feel less like a victim and more like a survivor of rape.	Elizabeth acknowledged that she felt better about herself after talking with the nurse. Elizabeth stated that she felt more in control of her emotions.

(Continues)

NURSING CARE PLAN: NURSING PROCESS FORMAT 26-1 (Continued)

REFLECTIVE QUESTIONS

1. **ASSESSMENT**
   What else should we take into account with Elizabeth?
2. **NURSING DIAGNOSIS**
   Are there other diagnoses that might better manage Elizabeth's issues?
3. **OUTCOMES**
   What do you think Elizabeth thought about these goals? Would they have to be mutual?
4. **NURSING ACTIONS**
   Could the same strategies that were used with Elizabeth work for other rape survivors? Where does the care need to be personalized?
5. **EVALUATION**
   What else should be considered with clients who have been raped? Do plans always work? How would we know if they worked for Elizabeth? What do you think will work with other clients?

NURSING CARE PLAN: NURSING PROCESS FORMAT 26-2

Vera is a survivor of domestic violence. She is married to Tom and they have two children. Since the birth of their second child, Tom becomes jealous of the attention that Vera gives the baby. About a month after the birth of the baby, Vera is seen in the emergency room for physical injuries. Tom is with her and will not let her out of his sight. The nurse, suspecting that Vera has been abused, tells Tom to remain in the waiting room. She provides Vera a quiet, private examination room so she can have a private interview with her.

ASSESSMENT

Vera was seen in the emergency room for physical injuries related to her husband's hitting her and throwing her against the wall. Vera told the nurse that the abuse was all her fault. She did not know what to do. She still had hope that Tom would change. She believed that their children needed him as a father. She stated that she felt blue. Vera stated that she was afraid that Tom would abuse her again. She stated that she was afraid that he would retaliate against her if the abuse were reported to law enforcement. Vera stated that she could not tell her family about the abuse. Her friends had told her that she should leave Tom, but they did not understand that he was not always bad. He loved her and the children. Vera stated that she was not familiar with the community resources.

NURSING DIAGNOSIS 1 *Risk for injury* as a result of physical abuse by her husband.

OUTCOMES	NIC	NURSING ACTIONS	EVALUATION
• Vera will develop a trusting relationship with the nurse. • Vera will admit her husband abused her. • Vera will be treated for her injuries.	• Presence • Abuse protection support: Domestic Partner	• Interview Vera in a private place. • Reassure Vera that she is in a safe place. • Interview Vera and be with her during the physical examination.	Vera stated that she felt safe the emergency room. Vera reported that she had been abused by her husband.

(Continues)

NURSING CARE PLAN: NURSING PROCESS FORMAT 26-2 (Continued)

OUTCOMES	NIC	NURSING ACTIONS	EVALUATION
		• Encourage Vera to discuss the battering incidents. • Obtain a history of her abusive relationship.	She was given a physical examination by the emergency room physician. She had no broken bones but did have old and new bruises on her face, abdomen, breasts, and upper extremities. She was given treatment for her injuries.

NURSING DIAGNOSIS 2 *Ineffective coping*, related to a situational crisis secondary to ongoing cycle of violence, as evidenced by inability to ask for help.

OUTCOMES	NIC	NURSING ACTIONS	EVALUATION
• Vera will verbalize her feelings, strengths, and needs. • Vera will state that she does not deserve to be battered.	• Counseling • Coping enhancement	• Provide crisis counseling. • Encourage Vera to express her feelings. • Accept and acknowledge Vera's state of confusion. • Help Vera identify her strengths and help her reestablish feelings of control.	Vera admitted that she did not deserve to be beaten by Tom. She admitted that she was ashamed to contact her family.

NURSING DIAGNOSIS 3 *Powerlessness*, related to lifestyle of helplessness, as evidenced by verbalization of fear for her safety and that of her children.

OUTCOMES	NIC	NURSING ACTIONS	EVALUATION
• Vera will verbalize alternatives she has available to her and her children. • Vera will have thought through a safety plan.	• Self-esteem enhancement • Decision-making support • Teaching	• Offer Vera support, but leave the final decision to stay or leave Tom to Vera. • Discuss with Vera her responsibility to report abuse. • Consult with the physician to determine whether the nature of the injuries warrants reporting the abuse to authorities.	Vera did not feel that her situation was bad enough to leave Tom. The nurse and physician made a report to law enforcement. They informed Tom and Vera of their legal responsibilities to report the abuse. They discussed a safety plan with Vera.

(*Continues*)

NURSING CARE PLAN: NURSING PROCESS FORMAT 26-2 (Continued)

NURSING DIAGNOSIS 4 *Deficient knowledge*, related to unfamiliarity with information resources, as evidenced by statements about lack of information about community resources.

OUTCOMES	NIC	NURSING ACTIONS	EVALUATION
• Vera will identify resources and services that are available to her.	• Anticipating guidance • Teaching	• Give Vera anticipatory guidance. • Discuss community resources available to Vera, such as shelters, social services, and job training programs.	Vera is more knowledgeable about available resources. She may consider contacting her family.

REFLECTIVE QUESTIONS

1. **ASSESSMENT**
   Should the assessment of Vera's situation include an interview with Tom? Do you think his involvement would help or hinder Vera's progress and recovery?
2. **NURSING DIAGNOSIS**
   What other psychosocial diagnoses might apply to Vera? Are additional diagnoses related to physical status appropriate?
3. **OUTCOMES**
   Would Tom be likely to support those outcomes for Vera? How important do you think his support would be to Vera's progress?
4. **NURSING ACTIONS**
   Do you think Vera will continue to respond as positively to the care plan once Tom is back in the picture?
5. **EVALUATION**
   How can you ensure Vera's continued commitment to protecting herself?

KEY CONCEPTS

- Violence is a major public health problem.
- Structural violence is a concept that provides understanding of the predictable impact of misuse of privilege and power on vulnerable segments of the population.
- Interpersonal violence includes child, partner, and elder abuse by family members; it involves clients being physically, psychologically, financially, or sexually abused.
- Intimate partner violence is usually abuse against women; it involves physical, emotional, financial, and frequently sexual abuse; it usually increases in severity and frequency and can escalate to homicide of either partner.
- Sexual assault is a crime of violence and power, not sexual passion.
- Nurses are in a position to assess and intervene in incidents of interpersonal violence and sexual assault; they need to understand the dynamics of violence to intervene effectively.
- Bullying and workplace incivility are forms of violence and can perpetrate considerable harm to victims.
- Political violence and war are global in impact and leave many people injured, desperate, and in great need of safety and compassion from those in more privileged situations.
- Interpersonal survivors of violence may exhibit both physical and psychological signs and symptoms of abuse; the nurse should assess clients for both.

- Nurses are mandated by law to report known or suspected cases of child abuse, and in some states elder abuse and sexual assault.
- Primary prevention is the single most important method of preventing interpersonal violence and sexual assaults.
- Secondary prevention of interpersonal violence is directed toward protecting the survivor and breaking the cycle of violence.
- Advocacy and political action are the most important methods of dealing with political results of war, human trafficking, and violence perpetrated against refugees.

REVIEW QUESTIONS

1. A nurse is treating a rape victim in the emergency room. The nurse's primary goal for this encounter would be which of the following?
   1. Have the victim talk with the police
   2. Convince the victim that not all men are like her attacker
   3. Encourage the victim to acknowledge and express feelings about the incident
   4. Encourage the victim to stop thinking about the trauma that she just experienced

2. A nurse is treating an eight-year-old boy for an injury. Which of the following observations about the child would indicate to the nurse that the child had possibly been abused?
   1. Scrapes on the knees and elbows
   2. Crying due to the pain of the injury
   3. Looks to the parents for care and comfort during the examination
   4. Withdrawn and displays no reaction to the pain of the injuries

3. A nurse is examining an elderly widow with clear signs of physical abuse. After inquiring about the abuse, the client states that she doesn't want the nurse to disclose her abuse to anyone. The nurse's next action should be which of the following?
   1. Continue to pressure the client to speak with the authorities regarding the abuse
   2. Promise not to tell anyone about the abuse and keep the client's secret due to nurse/client confidentiality
   3. Lie to the client, saying that she will not inform the authorities, then immediately inform adult protective services anyway
   4. Tell the client that the nurse is mandated by law to inform adult protective services about any cases of suspected elderly abuse, and do so

4. A child is seen in the emergency room for burns on her face and chest. The mother tells the nurse that the child knocked over a pot of water. Further assessment reveals that the child has several old bruises on her body. A review of the child's X-rays revealed that the child has had several broken bones that have now healed. The nurse should do which of the following?
   1. Tell the mother that she should supervise the child better
   2. Contact the authorities because the child may have been abused
   3. Ask the doctor to talk with the mother
   4. Call the police and have the mother arrested

5. A 45-year-old woman is being treated by the nurse in the ER for a dislocated shoulder. During the treatment, the woman confides in the nurse that her husband dislocated her shoulder during an argument. She goes on to explain that he has become much more violent with her since he lost his job six months ago. Which of the following would be the most therapeutic response by the nurse?
   1. Tell the client that the violence will stop once her husband finds employment again
   2. Ask the client what she said during the argument that caused her husband to become violent with her
   3. Recommend that the woman acquire a firearm or another weapon to protect herself from future altercations with her husband
   4. Explain to the woman that there are resources available to help her and her husband in this situation and provide her with information about those resources

6. The nurse is assigned to work with a community group on the prevention of violence. In a meeting with the community members, the nurse is most likely to indicate that which individual is at highest risk for being a victim of a violent crime?
   1. A 68-year-old Hispanic male who recently retired
   2. A 50-year-old Caucasian woman who works evenings
   3. A 36-year-old Asian male who owns the local grocery store
   4. A 16-year-old African American boy who attends the local high school

7. A woman is brought to the emergency room after being raped in an alley. The nurse caring for the woman would understand that the motivation to rape a person is based on the perpetrator's need for which of the following?
   1. Need to express love
   2. Need for control
   3. Need for attention
   4. Need for sexual release

LEARNING ACTIVITIES

1. Describe the difference between the WHO's definition of violence and the concept of structural violence.
2. Describe situations in our society where violence is most likely to occur.
3. What are your responsibilities in reporting child abuse, elder abuse, intimate partner violence, and sexual assaults?
4. What is a nurse's role in efforts to combat bullying and workplace incivility?
5. What is a nurse's role in global efforts to combat political violence, human trafficking, and the plight of refugees?
6. What theories would influence your interactions with clients who are victims of violence?
7. What nursing interventions would you think about using for an abused client?
8. What characteristics are seen in children, elders, and partners who are abused and their abusers?
9. What would you include in your assessment of an abused client?
10. Describe nursing interventions that can be used in primary, secondary, and tertiary prevention of interpersonal violence.

*Study*WARE™ CONNECTION

Using your *Study*WARE™ CD-ROM

1. Complete the Flashcard activity for this chapter.
2. Review the audio glossary for key terms in this chapter.
3. Explore the other games and activities that support this chapter.

REFERENCES

AACN. (2005). AACN standards for establishing and sustaining healthy work environments: A journey to excellence. *American Journal of Critical Care, 14,* 187–197.

Aguilera, D.C. (1998). *Crisis Intervention, theory and methodology* (8th ed). St Louis: Mosby.

American Psychiatric Association. (2000). *Diagnostic and statistical manual of mental disorders* (4th ed, Text Rrevised). Washington, DC: Author.

Anderson, M., Kaufman, J., Simon, T.R., Barrios, L., Paulozzi, L., Ryan, G., Hammond, R., Modzeleski, W., Feucht, T., Potter, L., & School-Associated Violent Deaths Study Group. (2002). School-associated violent deaths in the United States, 1994–1999. *Journal of the American Medical Association, 287*(8), 983.

Anonymous. (2005). *Fact sheet: Elder abuse prevalence and incidence.* Washington, DC. National Center on Elder Abuse. Retrieved August 1, 2008, from http://www.ncea.aoa.gov/NCEAroot/Main_Site/pdf/publication/FinalStatistics050331.pdf.

Anonymous. (2007). *Assessment of US government efforts to combat trafficking in persons in fiscal year 2006.* Available at http://www.usdoj.gov, as accessed August 5, 2008).

Banyard, V. L. (2008). Measurement and correlates of prosocial bystander behavior: The case of interpersonal violence. *Violence and Victims, 23,* 83–97.

Barrows, J., & Finger, R. (2008). Human trafficking and the healthcare professional. *Southern Medical Journal, 101,* 521–524.

Baschetti, R. (2008). Genetic evidence that Darwin was right about criminality: Nature, not nurture. *Medical Hypotheses, 70,* 1092–1102.

Basile, K. C., Arias, I., Desai, S., & Thompson, M. P. (2004). The differential association of intimate partner physical, sexual, psychological, and stalking violence and posttraumatic stress symptoms in a nationally representative sample of women. *Journal of Trauma and Stress, 17,* 413–421.

Bauer, N. S., Lozano, P., & Rivara, F. P. (2007). The effectiveness of the Olweus Bullying Prevention Program in public middle schools: A controlled trial. *Journal of Adolescent Health, 40,* 266–274.

Bitondo-Dyer, C., Connolly, M-T., & McFeely, P. (2000). The clinical and medical forensics of elder abuse and neglect. In R. J. Bonnie, & R. B. Wallace. (2002). *Elder mistreatment. Abuse, neglect, and exploitation in an aging America.* Washington, DC: National Academies Press.

Blass, T. (2004). *The man who shocked the world: The life and legacy of Stanley Milgram.* New York: Basic Books.

Blumstein, A., Rivara, F. P., & Rosenfeld, R. (2000). The rise and decline of homicide—and why. *Annual Review of Public Health, 21,* 505–541.

Bonnie R. J., & Wallace, R. B.(2002). *Elder mistreatment. Abuse, neglect, and exploitation in an aging America.* Washington, DC: National Academies Press.

Breiding, M. J., Black, M. C., & Ryan, G. W. (2008). Chronic disease and health risk behaviors associated with intimate partner violence–18 U.S. states/territories, 2005. *Annals of Epidemiology, 18,* 538–544.

Breitman, N., Shackelford, T. K., & Block, C. R. (2004). Couple age discrepancy and risk of intimate partner homicide. *Violence and Victims, 19,* 321–342.

Brodsky, B. S., & Stanley, B. (2008). Adverse childhood experiences and suicidal behavior. *Psychiatric Clinics of North America, 31,* 223–235.

Brymer, M. J., Steinberg, A. M., Sornborger, J., Layne, C. M., & Pynoos, R. S. (2008). Acute interventions for refugee children and families. *Child and Adolescent Psychiatric Clinics of North America, 17,* 625–640.

Butterfield, F. (1996). *All God's children.* New York: Harper Perennial.

Cartwright, R. (2004). Sleepwalking violence: A sleep disorder, a legal dilemma, and a psychological challenge. *American Journal of Psychiatry, 161,* 1149–1158.

Chambliss, L. R. (2008). Intimate partner violence and its implication for pregnancy. *Clinical Obstetrics and Gynecology, 51*, 385–397.

Child Welfare Information Gateway. (2007) *Mandatory reporters of child abuse and neglect: Summary of state laws.* Retrieved July 31, 2008, from http://www.childwelfare.gov/systemwide/laws_policies/statutes/mandaall.pdf.

Danis, F. S. (2003). The criminalization of domestic violence: What social workers need to know. *Social Work, 48*, 237–246.

Daro, Deborah. (2006). *World perspectives on child abuse.* West Chicago, Illinois: International Society for the Prevention of Child Abuse and Neglect.

Devinsky, O. (2008). Postictal psychosis: Common, dangerous, and treatable. *Epilepsy Currents, 8*, 31–34.

Dyer, C. B., Goodwin, J. S., Pickens-Pace, S., Burnett, J., & Kelly, P. A. (2007). Self-neglect among the elderly: A model based on more than 500 patients seen by a geriatric medicine team. *American Journal of Public Health, 97*, 1671–1676.

El-Bassel, N., Gilbert, L., Wu, E., Go, H., & Hill, J. (2005). Relationship between drug abuse and intimate partner violence: A longitudinal study among women receiving methadone. *American Journal of Public Health, 95*, 465–470.

Erez, E. (2002). Domestic violence and the criminal justice system: An overview. *Online Journal of Issues in Nursing, 7*, 4.

Erickson, P. G., Butters, J. E., Cousineau, M. M., Harrison, L., & Korf, D. (2006). Alcohol and Violence International Team, 2006. Girls and weapons: An international study of the perpetration of violence. *Journal of Urban Health, 83*, 788–801.

Ernst, A. A., Weiss, S. J., Enright-Smith, S., Hilton, E., & Byrd, E. C. (2008). Perpetrators of intimate partner violence use significantly more methamphetamine, cocaine, and alcohol than victims: A report by victims. *American Journal of Emergency Medicine, 26*, 592–596.

Farmer, P., & Sen, A. K. (2003). *Pathologies of power: Health, human rights, and the new war on the poor.* Berkeley: University of California.

Fernandes, C. M., Bouthillette, F., Raboud, J. M., Bullock, L., Moore, C. F., Christenson, J. M., et al. (1999). Violence in the emergency department: A survey of health care workers. *Canadian Medical Association Journal, 161*, 1245–1248.

Fiske, S. T., Harris, L. T., & Cuddy, A. J. (2004). Why ordinary people torture enemy prisoners. *Science, 306*(5701), 1482–1483.

Fredland, N. M. (2008). Sexual bullying: Addressing the gap between bullying and dating violence. *ANS Advances in Nursing Science, 31*, 95–105.

Gates, D. M., Ross, C. S., & McQueen, L. (2006). Violence against emergency department workers. *Journal of Emergency Medicine, 31*, 331–337.

Gilligan, J. (1997). *Violence: Reflections on a national epidemic.* New York: Vintage Books.

Gur, R. E., Loughead, J., Kohler, C. G., Elliott, M. A., Lesko, K., Ruparel, K., et al. (2007). Limbic activation associated with misidentification of fearful faces and flat affect in schizophrenia. *Archives of General Psychiatry, 64*, 1356–1366.

Gushulak, B. D., & MacPherson, D. W. (2000). Health issues associated with the smuggling and trafficking of migrants. *Journal of Immigrant Health, 2*, 67–78.

Hall, J., Whalley, H. C., McKirdy, J. W., Romaniuk, L., McGonigle, D., McIntosh, A. M., et al. (2008). Overactivation of fear systems to neutral faces in schizophrenia. *Biological Psychiatry, 64*, 70–73.

Henderson, A. D. (2003). Nurses and workplace violence: Nurses' experiences of verbal and physical abuse at work. *Nursing Leadership, 16*, 82–98.

Hendricks, S. A., Jenkins, E. L., & Anderson, K. R. (2007). Trends in workplace homicides in the U.S., 1993–2002: A decade of decline. *American Journal of Industrial Medicine, 50*, 316–325.

Herdman, H. (Ed). (2009). *Nursing diagnosis: Definitions and Classifications: 2009–2011.* Oxford: Wiley-Blackwell.

Hesketh, K. L., Duncan, S. M., Estabrooks, C. A., Reimer, M. A., Giovannetti, P., Hyndman, K., et al. (2003). Workplace violence in Alberta and British Columbia hospitals. *Health Policy, 63*, 311–321.

Hill, J., & Nathan, R. (2008). Childhood antecedents of serious violence in adult male offenders. *Aggressive Behavior, 34*, 329–338.

Hodgins, S. (2008). Review. Violent behaviour among people with schizophrenia: A framework for investigations of causes, and effective treatment, and prevention. *Philosophical Transactions of the Royal Society of London B: Biological Sciences, 363*, 2505–2518.

Houston, E., & McKirnan, D. J. (2007). Intimate partner abuse among gay and bisexual men: Risk correlates and health outcomes. *Journal of Urban Health, 84*, 681–690.

Huesmann, L. R., & Taylor, L. D. (2006). The role of media violence in violent behavior. *Annual Review of Public Health, 27*, 393–415.

Hughes, F. A., Thom, K., & Dixon, R. (2007). Nature & prevalence of stalking among New Zealand mental health clinicians. *Journal of Psychosocial Nursing and Mental Health Services, 45*, 32–39.

Human Rights Watch. (1995). *Rape for profit: Trafficking of Nepali girls and women to India's brothels.* Human Rights Watch.

Human Rights Watch. (2007). Available at http://www.hrw.org, as accessed August 5, 2008.)

Hutchinson, M., Vickers, M., Jackson, D., & Wilkes, L. (2006). Workplace bullying in nursing: Towards a more critical organisational perspective. *Nursing Inquiry, 13*, 118–126.

Hwang, L. (2007). Environmental stressors and violence: Lead and polychlorinated biphenyls. *Review of Environmental Health, 22*, 313–328.

Insel, B. J., & Gould, M. S. (2008). Impact of modeling on adolescent suicidal behavior. *Psychiatric Clinics of North America, 31*, 293–316.

Jensen L. (2006). *Ending violence against women.* New York: United Nations. Retrieved August 4, 2008, from http://www.unfpa.org/upload/lib_pub_file/679_filename_endingvaw.pdf.

Jones-Webb, R., & Wall, M. (2008). Neighborhood racial/ethnic concentration, social disadvantage, and homicide risk: An ecological analysis of 10 U.S. cities. *Journal of Urban Health, 85*(5), 662–676.

Karch, D. L., Lubell, K. M., Friday, J., Patel, N., Williams, D. D., Centers for Disease Control and Prevention (CDC) 2008. Surveillance for violent deaths—National Violent Death Reporting System, 16 states, 2005. *MMWR Surveillance Summary, 57*, 1–45.

Keller, A. S., Ford, D., Sachs, E., Rosenfeld, B., Trinh-Shevrin, C., Meserve, C., et al. (2003). The impact of detention on the health of asylum seekers. *Journal of Ambulatory Care Management, 26*, 383–385.

Kirk, D. S. (2008). The neighborhood context of racial and ethnic disparities in arrest. *Demography, 45*, 55–77.

Kohrt, B. A., Jordans, M. J., Tol, W. A., Speckman, R. A., Maharjan, S. M., Worthman, C. M., et al. (2008). Comparison of mental health between former child soldiers and children never conscripted by armed groups in Nepal. *Journal of the American Medical Association, 300*(6), 691–702.

Korman, L. M., Collins, J., Dutton, D., Dhayananthan, B., Littman-Sharp, N., & Skinner, W. (2008). Problem gambling and intimate partner violence. *Journal of Gambling Studies, 24*, 13–23.

Kramer, M., & Schmalenberg, C. (2008). Confirmation of a healthy work environment. *Critical Care Nurse, 28,* 56–63.

Krug E. G., Dahlberg L. L., Mercy J. A., Zwi, A. B., & Lozano, R. (2002). *World report on violence and health.* Geneva: World Health Organization.

Laajasalo, T., & Häkkänen, H. (2006). Excessive violence and psychotic symptomatology among homicide offenders with schizophrenia. *Criminal Behavior and Mental Health, 16,* 242–253.

Lee, J., Pomeroy, E. C., Yoo, S. K., & Rheinboldt, K. T. (2005). Attitudes toward rape: A comparison between Asian and Caucasian college students. *Violence against Women, 11,* 177–196.

Leyland, A. H. (2006). Homicides involving knives and other sharp objects in Scotland, 1981–2003. *(Oxford) Journal of Public Health 28,* 145–147.

Mack, A. (2007), *Human security brief 2007.* Burnaby, British Columbia: Simon Fraser University. Retrieved August 4, 2008, from http://www.humansecuritybrief.info.

McEwan, T. E., Mullen, P. E., & Mackenzie, R. (2008). A study of the predictors of persistence in stalking situations. *Law and Human Behavior, 33*(2), 149–158.

McKenna, B. G., Poole, S. J., Smith, N. A., Coverdale, J. H., & Gale, C. K. (2003). A survey of threats and violent behaviour by patients against registered nurses in their first year of practice. *International Journal of Mental Health Nursing, 12,* 56–63.

Mechanic, M. B., Weaver, T. L., & Resick, P. A. (2008). Mental health consequences of intimate partner abuse: A multidimensional assessment of four different forms of abuse. *Violence against Women, 14,* 634–654.

Melhem, N. M., Brent, D. A., Ziegler, M., Iyengar, S., Kolko, D., Oquendo, M., et al. (2007). Familial pathways to early-onset suicidal behavior: Familial and individual antecedents of suicidal behavior. *American Journal of Psychiatry, 164,* 1364–1370.

Muehlenhard, C. L., & Kimes, L. A. (1999). The social construction of violence: The case of sexual and domestic violence. *Personality and Social Psychology Review, 3,* 234–245.

Nansel, T. R., Craig, W., Overpeck, M. D., Saluja, G., Ruan, W. J., & Health Behaviour in School-aged Children Bullying Analyses Working Group. (2004). Cross-national consistency in the relationship between bullying behaviors and psychosocial adjustment. *Archives of Pediatric and Adolescent Medicine, 158*(8), 730–736.

National Center on Elder Abuse. (1998). *National elder abuse incidence study.* Washington, DC: National Center on Elder Abuse. Retrieved August 1, 2008, from http://www.aoa.gov/eldfam/elder_rights/elder_abuse/ABuseReport_Full.pdf.

National Institute for Occupational Safety and Health (NIOSH) (1995). "Preventing Homicide in the Workplace: Workers in Certain Industries and Occupations are at Increased Risk of Homicide." *NIOSH Alert,* Publication No. 93–109.

Newman, L. K., & Steel, Z. (2008). The child asylum seeker: Psychological and developmental impact of immigration detention. *Child and Adolescent Psychiatric Clinics of North America, 17,* 665–683.

North American Diagnosis Association (NANDA) (2009). NANDA-I Nursing diagnoses: Definitions & Classifications, 2009–2011. United Kingdom: John Wiley & Sons.

Olds, D. L. (2002). Prenatal and infancy home visiting by nurses: From randomized trials to community replication. *Prevention Science,* 3, 153–172.

Palmiotto, M. (2008). *Community policing* (2nd ed). Sudbury, MA: Jones and Bartlett.

Pulay, A. J., Dawson, D. A., Hasin, D. S., Goldstein, R. B., Ruan, W. J., Pickering, R. P., et al. (2008). Violent behavior and DSM-IV psychiatric disorders: Results from the national epidemiologic survey on alcohol and related conditions. *Journal of Clinical Psychiatry, 69,* 12–22.

Reid, R. J., Bonomi, A. E., Rivara, F. P., Anderson, M. L., Fishman, P. A., Carrell, D. S., et al. (2008). Intimate partner violence among men prevalence, chronicity, and health effects. *American Journal of Preventive Medicine, 34,* 478–485.

Richards, A. K., & Richards, A. D. (1997). Gambling, death, and violence: Hollywood looks at Las Vegas. *Psychoanalytical Reviews, 84,* 769–788.

Sarkar, N. N. (2008). The impact of intimate partner violence on women's reproductive health and pregnancy outcome. *Journal of Obstetrics and Gynaecology, 28,* 266–271.

Schmalenberg, C., & Kramer, M. (2008). Clinical units with the healthiest work environments. *Critical Care Nurse, 28,* 65–77.

Sedlak, A. J., & Broadhurst, D. D. (1996). *Third national incidence study of child abuse and neglect.* Washington, DC: U.S. Department of Health Education and Welfare.

Shaw, J., Amos, T., Hunt, I. M., Flynn, S., Turnbull, P., Kapur, N., et al. (2004). Mental illness in people who kill strangers: Longitudinal study and national clinical survey. *British Medical Journal, 328,* 734–737.

Shaw, J., Hunt, I. M., Flynn, S., Amos, T., Meehan, J., Robinson, J., et al. (2006). The role of alcohol and drugs in homicides in England and Wales. *Addiction, 101,* 1117–1124.

Shawyer, F., Mackinnon, A., Farhall, J., Sims, E., Blaney, S., Yardley, P., et al. (2008). Acting on harmful command hallucinations in psychotic disorders: An integrative approach. *Journal of Nervous and Mental Disorders, 196,* 390–398.

Silove, D., Steel, Z., & Mollica, R. (2001). Detention of asylum seekers: Assault on health, human rights, and social development. *Lancet, 357,* 1436–1437.

Simonoff, E., Elander, J., Holmshaw, J., Pickles, A., Murray, R., & Rutter, M. (2004). Predictors of antisocial personality. Continuities from childhood to adult life. *British Journal of Psychiatry, 184,* 118–127.

Simons, S. (2008). Workplace bullying experienced by Massachusetts registered nurses and the relationship to intention to leave the organization. *Advances in Nursing Science, 31*(2), 48–59.

Sivarajasingam, V., Shepherd, J. P., Matthews, K. (2003). Effect of urban closed circuit television on assault injury and violence detection. *Injury Prevention, 9,* 312–316.

Slater, M., Antley, A., Davison, A., Swapp, D., Guger, C., et al. (2006). A virtual reprise of the Stanley Milgram obedience experiments. *PLoS ONE, 1*(1), e39. doi:10.1371/journal.pone.0000039

Smith-Khuri, E., Iachan, R., Scheidt, P. C., Overpeck, M. D., Gabhainn, S. N., Pickett, W., et al. (2004). A cross-national study of violence-related behaviors in adolescents. *Archives of Pediatrics and Adolescent Medicine, 158,* 539–544.

Spunt, B., Brownstein, H., Goldstein, P., Fendrich, M., & Liberty, H. J. (1995). Drug use by homicide offenders. *Journal of Psychoactive Drugs, 27,* 125–134.

Stevens, V., De Bourdeaudhuij, I., & Van Oost, P. (2000). Bullying in Flemish schools: An evaluation of anti-bullying intervention in primary and secondary schools. *British Journal of Educational Psychology, 70*(Pt. 2), 195–210.

Stevens, V., Van Oost, P., & De Bourdeaudhuij, I. (2000). The effects of an anti-bullying intervention programme on peers' attitudes and behaviour. *Journal of Adolescence, 23,* 21–34.

Stewart, D. E., & Gajic-Veljanoski, O. (2005). Trafficking in women: The Canadian perspective. *Canadian Medical Association Journal, 173,* 25–26.

Stiegel, L. (2006). Recommendations for the elder abuse, health, and justice fields about medical forensic issues related to elder abuse and neglect. *Journal of Elder Abuse and Neglect, 14*, 41–81.

St-Pierre, I., & Holmes, D. (2008). Managing nurses through disciplinary power: A Foucauldian analysis of workplace violence. *Journal of Nursing Management, 16*, 352–359.

Stuart, G. L., Temple, J. R., Follansbee, K. W., Bucossi, M. M., Hellmuth, J. C., & Moore, T. M. (2008). The role of drug use in a conceptual model of intimate partner violence in men and women arrested for domestic violence. *Psychology of Addictive Behaviors, 22*, 12–24.

Teaster, P. B., Dugar, T. A., Mendiondo, M. S., Abner, E. L., Cecil, K. A., Otto, J. M. (2006). The 2004 Survey of Adult Protective Services: Abuse of Adults 60 Years of Age and Older. The National Center on Elder Abuse URL: http://www.ncea.aoa.gov/NCEAroot/Main_Site/pdf/2-14-06%20FINAL%2060+REPORT.pdf.

Thompson, R. S., Bonomi, A. E., Anderson, M., Reid, R. J., Dimer, J. A., Carrell, D., et al. (2006). Intimate partner violence: Prevalence, types, and chronicity in adult women. *American Journal of Preventive Medicine, 30*, 447–457.

Tyrer, P., Cooper, S., Herbert, E., Duggan, C., Crawford, M., Joyce, E., et al. (2007). The Quantification of Violence Scale: A simple method of recording significant violence. *International Journal of Social Psychiatry, 53*, 485–497.

U.S. Department of Health and Human Services (2000). *Healthy People 2010: Understanding and Improving Health*. Washington, DC: authors.

U.S. Department of Health and Human Services (DHHS), Administration for Children and Families, Office of Child Abuse and Neglect. (2003). Child Abuse and Prevention Treatment Act. Washington: US DHHS.

U.S. Office of Disease Prevention and Health Promotion. *Healthy People 2010*. Washington, DC: Author.

U.S. Department of Justice. (2007). The President's family justice center initiative best practices. http://www.justice.gov/archive/ovw/docs/family_justice_center_overview_12_07.pdf.

U.S. Department of Justice. (2008). *Attorney general's annual report to Congress and assessment of the U.S. government activities to combat trafficking in persons fiscal year 2007* (available at http://www.usdoj.gov, as accessed on August 5, 2008).

Volavka, J. (2004). *Neurobiology of violence*. (2nd ed). Washington, DC, American Psychiatric Press. Retrieved July 31, 2008, from http://books.google.ca/books?id=5eerwIWolXIC&pg=PA165&source=gbs_toc_r&cad=0_0&sig=ACfU3U3wbFDAHblY9o95T8En3eLk9PZNcg#PPA178,M1.

Waller, J. (2002). *Becoming evil: How ordinary people commit genocide and mass killing*. New York: Oxford University Press.

Walton-Moss, B.J., & Campbell, J. (2002). Intimate partner violence: implications for nursing. *Online Journal of Issues in Nursing, 7*(1), 6.

Williams, K.R., & Guerr, N.G.. (2007). Prevalence and predictors of Internet bullying. *Journal of Adolescent Health, 41*(6 Suppl), S14–21.

Wood, K., Lambert, H., & Jewkes, R. (2007). "Showing roughness in a beautiful way": Talk about love, coercion, and rape in South African youth sexual culture. *Medical Anthropology Quarterly, 21*, 277–300.

World Health Organizaion (WHO). (2002) *World Report on Violence and Health*, Geneva: WHO

Yaffe, M. J., Weiss, D., Wolfson, C., & Lithwick, M. (2007). Detection and prevalence of abuse of older males: Perspectives from family practice. *Journal of Elder Abuse and Neglect, 19*, 47–60.

Zeitler, M. S., Paine, A. D., Breitbart, V., Rickert, V. I., Olson, C., Stevens, L., et al. (2006). Attitudes about intimate partner violence screening among an ethnically diverse sample of young women. *Journal of Adolescent Health, 39*, 119. e1–8.

SUGGESTED READINGS

Anderson, L. A., & Whiston, S. C. (2005). Sexual assault education programs: A meta-analytic examination of their effectiveness. *Psychology of Women Quarterly, 29* (4, December).

Antecol, H., & Cobb-Clark, D. (2003). Does sexual harassment training change attitudes? A view from the federal level. *Social Science Quarterly, 84*(4), 826–842.

APHA. (2001). Preventing genocide. *American Journal of Public Health, 91*(3), 512–513.

Barlow, H. (2007). *Dead for good: Martyrdom and the rise of the suicide bomber*. Boulder: Paradigm Publishers.

Barmash, P. (2005). *Homicide in the biblical world*. New York: Cambridge University Press.

Baumeister, R. F. (1999). *Evil: Inside human violence and cruelty*. New York: W. H. Freeman.

Bloom, M. (2005). *Dying to kill: The allure of suicide terror*. New York: Columbia University Press.

Bograd, M. (1990). Why we need gender to understand human violence. *Journal of Interpersonal Violence, 5*, 132–135.

Bonner, M. (2006). *Jihad in Islamic history: Doctrines and practice*. Princeton: Princeton University Press.

Bowen, L. K., Gwiasda, V., & Brown, M. M. (2004). Engaging community residents to prevent violence. *Journal of Interpersonal Violence, 19*(3), 356–367.

Bromley D. G., & Gordon, M. J., (Eds.). (2002). *Cults, religion, and violence*. New York: Cambridge University Press.

Burstyn, J. N. (Ed.). (2001). *Preventing violence in schools: A challenge to American democracy*. Mahwah, NJ: Lawrence Erlbaum Associates.

Centers for Disease Control and Prevention. (2004). *Sexual violence prevention: Beginning the dialogue*. Atlanta, GA: Centers for Disease Control and Prevention.

Centers for Disease Control and Prevention. (2006). *Preventing violence against women: Program activities guide*. Atlanta, GA: Centers for Disease Control and Prevention.

Cook, D. (2005). *Understanding jihad*. Berkeley: University of California Press.

Cornelius, T. L., & Resseguie, N. (2006). Primary and secondary prevention programs for dating violence: A review of the literature. *Aggression and Violent Behavior, 12*, 364–375.

Ehrenreich, B. (1997). *Blood rites: Origins and history of the passions of war*. New York: Metropolitan Books.

Ellens, J. H., (Ed.). (2004). *The destructive power of religion: Violence in Judaism, Christianity, and Islam*. 4 vols. Westport, CT: Praeger.

Farrell, A. D., & Flannery, D. J. (2006). Youth violence prevention: Are we there yet? *Aggression and Violent Behavior, 11*(2), 138–150.

Finkelhor, D. (2007). Prevention of sexual abuse through educational programs directed toward children. *Pediatrics, 120*(3), 640–645.

Gibson, E. L., & Matthews, S. (Eds.). (2005). *Violence in the New Testament*. New York: T & T Clark.

Gourevitch, P. (1998). *We wish to inform you that tomorrow we will be killed with our families: Stories from Rwanda.* New York: Farrar Straus and Giroux.

Greene, J., & Pranis, K. (2007). Gang wars: The Failure of enforcement tactics and the need for effective public safety strategies. Retrieved July 30, 2008, from http://www.streetgangs.com/bibliography/2007/0707gangwars.pdf.

Hammond, W. R., Whitaker, D. J, Lutzker, J. R., Mercy, J., & Chin, P. M. (2006). Setting a violence prevention agenda at the Centers for Disease Control and Prevention. *Aggression and Violent Behavior, 11*(2), 112–119.

Hayden, T. (2005). *Street wars: Gangs and the future of violence.* New York: The New Press.

Ignatieff, M. (1998). *The warrior's honor: Ethnic war and the modern conscience.* New York: Metropolitan Books.

Kahn, A. S. (2004). What college women do and do not experience as rape. *Psychology of Women Quarterly, 28*(1, March).

Kidder, T. (2004). *Mountains beyond mountains: The quest of Dr. Paul Farmer, a man who would cure the world.* New York: Random House.

Kilmartin, C., Allison, J. (2007). *Men's violence against women: Theory, research, and activism.* Mahwah, NJ: Lawrence Erlbaum Associates.

Kilpatrick, D. G. (2004). What is violence against women? Defining and measuring the problem. *Journal of Interpersonal Violence, 19*(11), 1209–1234.

Krakauer, J. (2004). *Under the banner of heaven: A story of violent faith.* New York: Anchor Books.

Lutzker, J. R. (2006). Violence prevention: Expanding the applied science. *Aggression and Violent Behavior, 11*(2), 111.

Miller, E., Decker, M. R., Silverman, J. G., & Raj, A., (2007). Migration, sexual exploitation, and women's health: A case report from a community health center. *Violence against Women, 13,* 486–497.

Miller, T. W., Kraus, R. F., & Veltkamp, L. J. (2005). Character education as a prevention strategy in school-related violence. *Journal of Primary Prevention, 26*(5, September), 455–466.

MMWR. (2007). The effectiveness of universal school-based programs for the prevention of violent and aggressive behavior. A report on recommendations of the Task Force on Community Preventive Services. *Morbidity and Mortality Weekly Report, 56*(RR-7, August 10).

Molnar, B. E., Roberts, A. L., Browne, A., Gardener, H., & Buka, S. L. (2005). What girls need: Recommendations for preventing violence among urban girls in the U.S. *Social Science & Medicine, 60*(10), 2191–2204.

Naim, M. (2005). *Illicit: How smugglers, traffickers and copycats are hijacking the world economy.* New York: Doubleday.

Queen, W. (2005). *Under and alone: The true story of the undercover agent who Infiltrated America's most violent outlaw motorcycle gang.* New York: Random House.

Rinehart, J. F. (2006). *Apocalyptic faith and political violence: Prophets of terror.* New York: Palgrave Macmillan.

Ryan, C., Anastario, M., & DaCunha, A. (2006). Changing coverage of domestic violence murders: A longitudinal experiment in participatory communication. *Journal of Interpersonal Violence, 21*(2), 2009.

Simons S. (2008). Workplace bullying experienced by Massachusetts registered nurses and the relationship to intention to leave the organization. *Advances in Nursing Science* 31(2):E48–59.

Singer, P. W. (2006). *Children at war.* Berkeley: University of California Press.

United Nations Population Fund. (2006). *Programming to address violence against women: Ten case studies.* New York: United Nations Population Fund.

Vigil, J. D. (2003). *Rainbow of gangs: street cultures in the mega-city.* Austin: University of Texas Press.

Waller, J. (2002). *Becoming evil: How ordinary people commit genocide and mass killing.* New York: Oxford University Press, 2002.

Wrangham, R., & Wilson, M. (2004). Collective violence: Comparisons between youths and chimpanzees. *Annals of the New York Academy of Sciences, 1036*: 233–256.

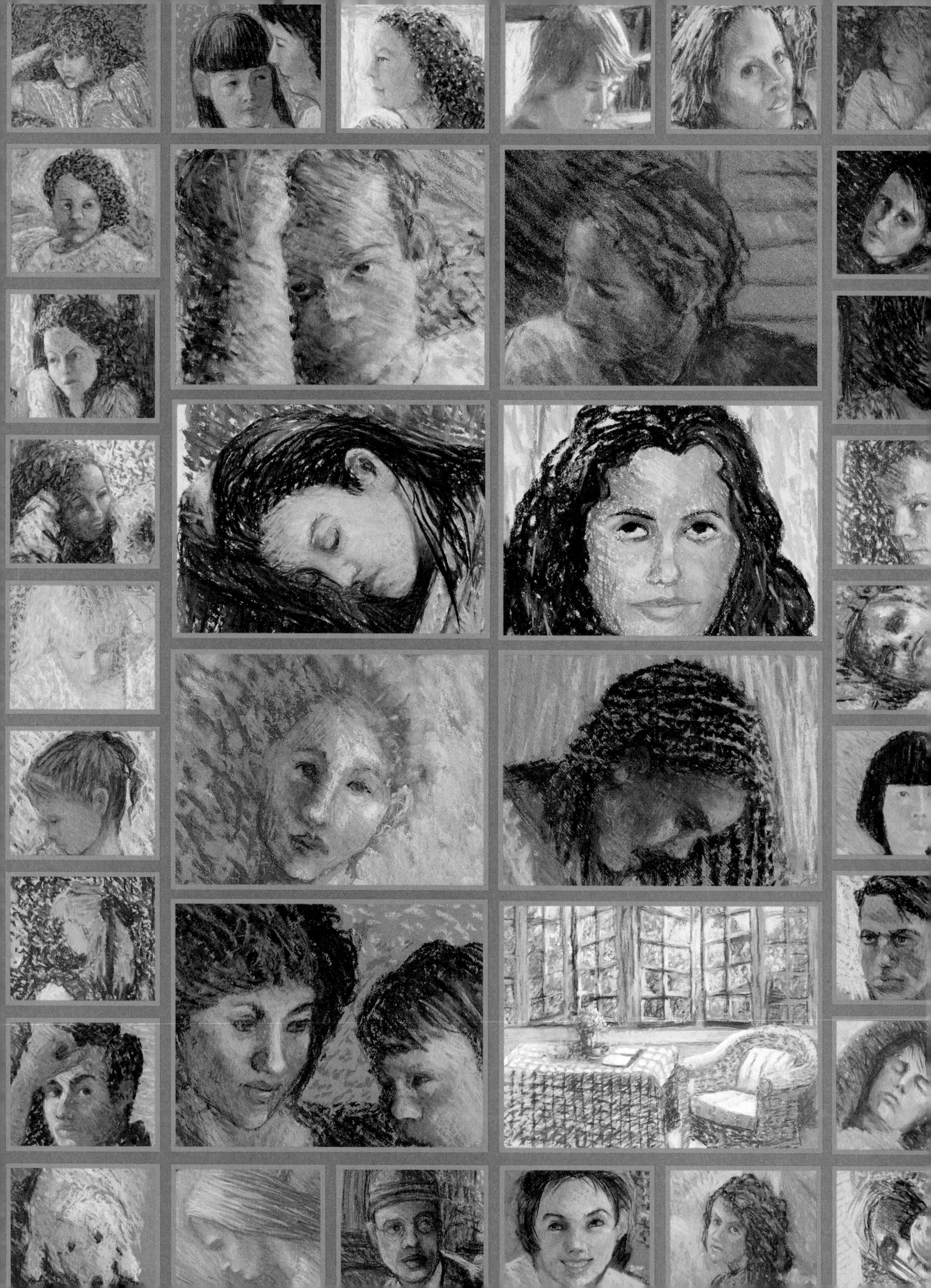

UNIT 4 Nursing Interventions and Treatment Modalities

What drugs are prescribed to treat individuals suffering from psychiatric disorders? What are the doses and side effects of these medications? How can nurses participate in the individual care of persons with mental illness? How do nurses provide mental health care to families? What is the nurse's role in group therapy? How can nurses influence the mental health of communities? What unique or special therapies are available to people with mental illness?

These questions are discussed in this unit entitled *Nursing Interventions and Treatment Modalities.*

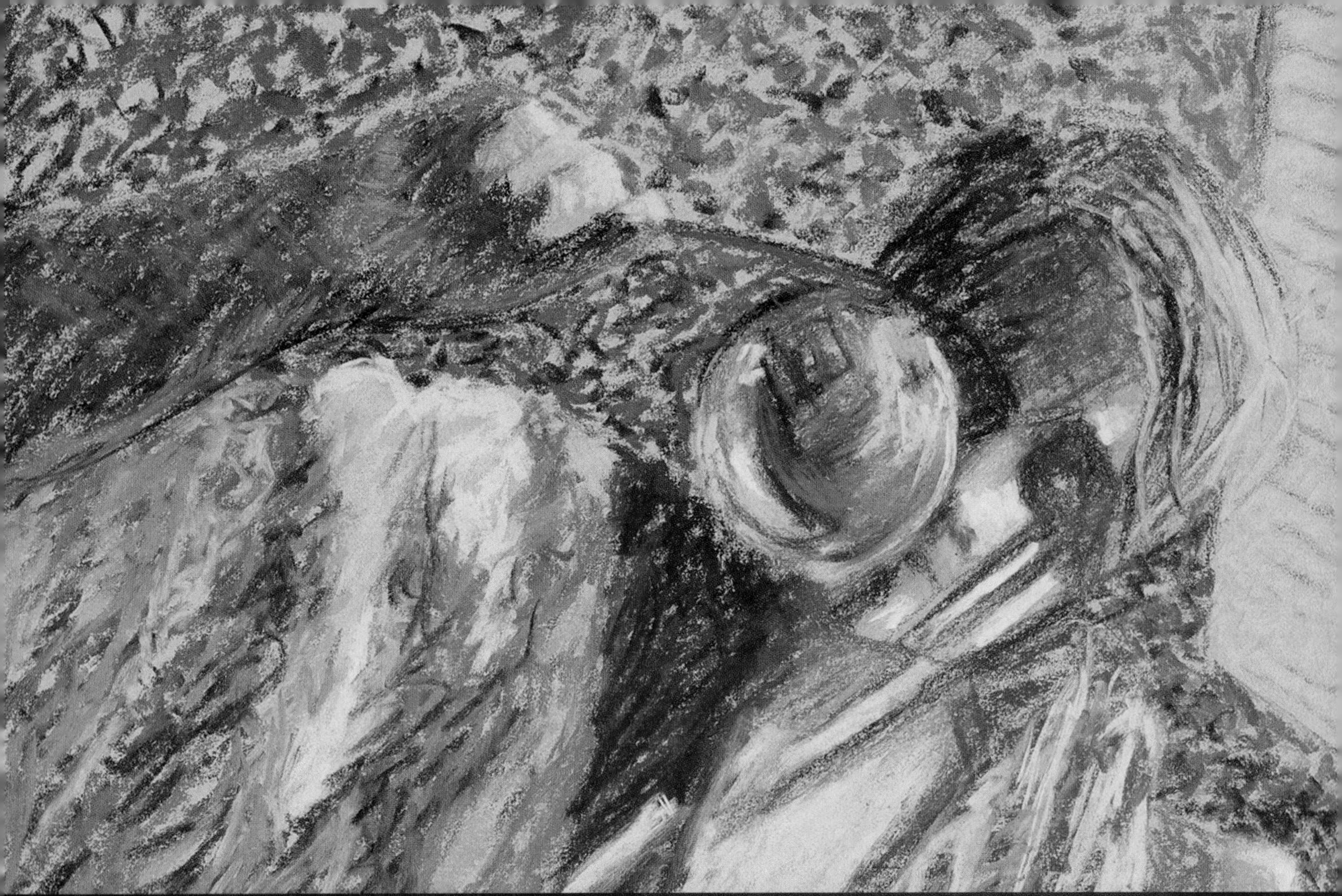

Genie in a Bottle

Use of Medications in Psychiatric Care

Nurses must have current and accurate information regarding medications ordered for their clients. This chapter provides information on major groups of psychotropic drugs; however, every nurse needs to know where to find information on all drugs. Consider the following:

- ***Do you know where to find drug information on the psychiatric unit where you are completing your student placement? Review the sources available there.***
- ***Does your outpatient clinic have drug resources available to both staff and clients?***
- ***Do you have a means of obtaining information through computer searching of a database?***
- ***Have you already purchased a pharmacology book? A drug handbook?***

Please review the sources of information available to you. Ensure that you have the means to obtain information when needed.

CHAPTER 27

Pharmacology in Psychiatric Care

CHRIS PAXOS
LAWRENCE E. FRISCH

CHAPTER OUTLINE

COMPETENCIES

Upon completion of this chapter, the reader will have general reference information on the major psychotropic drugs related to:

- Antipsychotics
- Mood disorders
- Anxiety and sleep disorders
- Stimulants
- Drugs used to treat chemical dependency

KEY TERMS

Akathisia
Antipsychotic Drugs
Blood-Brain Barrier
Dystonia
Half-Life
Neuroleptic Malignant Syndrome
Oculogyric Crisis
Serotonergic Syndrome
Tardive Dyskinesia
Therapeutic Window

This chapter provides reference information on the major psychotropic drugs. While each of the chapters dealing with psychopathology discusses drugs that may be used for specific conditions, detailed information is presented in this chapter to provide a source of information on major drugs used in psychiatric care. The nurse will find discussion on the history of psychotropic medications, medications used to treat psychosis, medications used to treat mood disorders, medications for anxiety and sleep disorders, stimulants, and drugs used to treat chemical dependency.

This chapter addresses only a few of the potentially most important drug interactions that the nurse must be prepared to anticipate. Many clients receive multiple psychiatric medications, and many individuals who are treated with these medications are also receiving therapies for nonpsychiatric conditions. Further, many persons take over-the-counter and herbal medications that may interact with prescribed treatments. The use of a computer- or "handheld"-based pharmacology program such as *ePocrates* can be invaluable in ensuring correct dosages and monitoring for potential interactions. Finally, this chapter uses the terms *drug* and *medication* interchangeably. While this synonymy is technically correct, the popular connotation of *drugging* may imply to some a kind of treatment that differs from that implied by the term *medicating*. Similarly, for some clients and caregivers, the word *drug* more likely refers to an abused substance than a helpful treatment. For these reasons, many nurses prefer to avoid the term *drug* when referring to psychiatric medications. Pharmacologists, on the other hand, think of drugs largely as chemical substances that act at specific receptor sites within the body. For these scientists, the word *drug* has a narrower and more precise meaning than does the word *medication*. Since this is a chapter on pharmacology, we believe that the use of the term *drug* is both defensible and at times preferable. Nonetheless, we recognize the importance of a distinction in clinical practice, and we encourage students to consult with instructors, mental health providers, and perhaps even clients to determine which usage is most appropriate in their own work settings.

HISTORY OF PSYCHIATRIC MEDICATION

The era of modern psychiatric drug treatment is less than 60 years old. Until very recently, only sedative/hypnotics (barbiturates, bromides, chloral hydrate) and stimulants (most commonly amphetamines) were used to affect individuals' moods, assist with sleep, and treat agitation or psychosis. Treatments were rarely effective, and unwanted side effects (including drug dependency) were common. Therapeutic options expanded rapidly beginning in the mid-twentieth century. While some kinds of drugs now in modern use were discovered or synthesized prior to the mid-twentieth century, virtually all the studies establishing modern drug effectiveness were carried out after 1950. The one exception to this description may be lithium. In 1886, John Aulde and Carl Lange recognized that lithium could be used to control symptoms of what was later called Bipolar Disorder (Schou, 1989). However, these early observations were forgotten, to be rediscovered by Cade and Schou in the mid-twentieth century (Schou, 1989).

The basic chemical structure underlying both tricyclic antidepressants and phenothiazine antipsychotics was initially synthesized in 1889. It was not until the early 1950s that pharmacological investigation led to modifications of this iminodibenzyl structure. These modifications produced both antidepressant and antipsychotic medications from remarkably similar underlying molecular structures. Benzodiazepine drugs for treatment of anxiety were first synthesized in the mid-1950s and released for clinical use in 1960. Carbamazepine (Tegretol) and divalproex (Depakote and others), used as alternatives to lithium in the management of Bipolar Disorder, were also brought into clinical practice as anticonvulsants at about this time. Much more recent pharmacological research has resulted in important therapeutic advances such as second-generation antipsychotics (clozapine) and selective serotonin reuptake inhibitors (fluoxetine [Prozac] and others). Current pharmacological treatments have serious deficiencies, of which the most important is that (as with

RESEARCH Highlight 27–1

Serendipity and SAR

For many years, lack of knowledge of neurochemistry, neurophysiology, and ethical concerns led to the very slow development of psychiatric medications. Serendipity refers to the fortuitous discovery of an effect of a drug that was not expected. For example, chlorpromazine was discovered in a search for new antihistamines and sedatives. Imipramine was discovered to be an antidepressant while being tested for antipsychotic properties. For many years, most psychiatric medications were developed "accidentally" while searching for another property.

Structure-activity relationship (SAR) is a complicated way of saying that if two drugs are chemically and structurally similar, they probably will produce similar effects, but perhaps one will have fewer side effects or be more effective. This process has led to many more psychotropic medications than random searching for neurologically effective substances.

The rapid discovery of the many chemical receptors in the brain, along with the development of sophisticated biotechnology, has allowed the cloning of drug receptors and the more rational development of drugs that act specifically at a given receptor, thus reducing side effects and increasing efficacy. However, the function of many brain receptors remains unknown despite extensive investigation. New discoveries may lead to further dramatic changes in psychiatric care.

many chronic diseases) they serve to control symptoms rather than to cure psychiatric disorders. Also, psychiatric drugs are not effective for, or tolerated by, a significant portion of affected individuals, often those with the most disabling symptoms. Despite these important limitations of current practice, the use of psychiatric medications offers great benefits to many clients. These benefits will continue to increase as ever more effective treatments are developed and brought into practice.

HOW AND WHY PSYCHIATRIC MEDICATIONS WORK

Understanding psychiatric medications requires a basic understanding of pharmacology and the concepts of administration, absorption, distribution, elimination, and metabolism. Many psychiatric medications are given orally (p.o.), and some are given parenterally, usually by the intramuscular (i.m.) route. Only rarely are psychiatric medications given intravenously (i.v.) or subcutaneously (subcut). Rectal administration (p.r.) of psychiatric medications is now quite uncommon. Most drugs are absorbed quite predictably when given by a parenteral route, but oral administration may be significantly affected by foods, stomach acidity (often modified by antacids), and the nature of the drug itself. Once absorbed, drugs distribute throughout the body depending on their solubility in water and fat and on their tendency to bind to proteins. Fat-soluble drugs tend to distribute widely in the body; protein-bound drugs may be very slow to diffuse out of the bloodstream. These characteristics affect drug actions. Once in the body, most drugs are eliminated by excretion (usually into the urine by the kidney or into the bile or feces by the liver). Prior to excretion, drugs are almost always metabolized, most often by the liver but occasionally by lungs or even skin. Some metabolic products are biologically inactive and are directly excreted; other metabolic products are even more active than are the original drugs. Many substances have pharmacological activity only after they have been metabolized into biologically active metabolites.

The potential effects of any drug are a complex balance of each of these factors: absorption, distribution, metabolism, and elimination. Another term for this balance is *pharmacokinetics*. In most cases, the goal of drug administration is the achievement of a "steady" pharmacokinetic state (often called steady state) in which the amount of drug absorbed is constantly balanced by the competing processes of distribution, elimination, and metabolism. It is often difficult to predict blood or tissue levels of a drug from the dose alone because pharmacokinetic relationships between absorption and steady state may not be linearly related to dose. Measurements of blood levels may be required to ensure appropriate dosing. Knowing something of a drug's half-life may help estimate pharmacokinetics, especially when combined with knowledge of absorption, distribution, metabolism, and elimination. The **half-life** is the time (typically in hours) that it takes for plasma concentrations of a drug to decrease to half of an initial value. After seven half-lives, less than 1% of a drug remains in the plasma. For a short-acting drug, such as triazolam, which has a half-life as short as 1.5 hours, seven half-lives may be very short (about 10 hours), whereas a long half-life drug such as fluoxetine (half-life of 3 days) and its metabolite, norfluoxetine, may not be fully eliminated for several weeks.

While these pharmacokinetic factors are important for understanding the drug's steady state, nurses often want to know how long it takes a drug to act after administration. Most drug handbooks offer information on onset of action. Onset clearly varies with the mode of administration and is typically shorter for drugs given parenterally (especially intravenously) than for drugs given orally. Some psychiatric drugs are intended to have a significant effect after the first dose. Antipsychotic drugs, hypnotics, and anxiolytics most commonly have rapid single-dose effects. Other psychiatric drugs only work after a steady state has been achieved, typically several weeks after administration begins. The nurse studying psychopharmacology will need to understand which drugs are given for their acute effect and which are expected to work only after some days or weeks.

The concept of **blood-brain barrier** is also very important for understanding drug effects in psychiatric mental health nursing. Most psychiatric drugs act on the central nervous system and must therefore leave the bloodstream to enter the interstitial fluid, the cerebrospinal fluid (CSF), and/or the cells of the brain. The capillary blood vessels of the brain are uniquely resistant to the passage of large molecules (such as drugs) from the bloodstream to the central nervous system. Many drugs circulate in the blood bound to protein, and these protein-drug complexes are almost completely excluded by the capillary barrier between blood and brain. Fat-soluble drugs can often pass through capillary membranes, and many molecules are actively transported across capillary cell walls into the brain. Some drugs cannot cross the blood-brain barrier in an active form, but will cross in an inactive form that is later changed into the active metabolite within the brain. For example, levodopa (L-dopa), used to treat parkinsonism, is converted to dopamine once it is transported across capillary walls.

Most drugs have their effect either because they bind to a specific brain receptor or because they have an effect on one or more brain neurotransmitter systems (see Figure 27-1). For example, virtually all antipsychotic medications bind strongly to brain receptors for dopamine. In contrast, monoamine oxidase inhibitors disrupt the breakdown/recycling of monoamine neurotransmitters that are released at neural synapses. This interference with the enzyme monoamine-oxidase effectively increases the concentration of a range of neurotransmitters throughout the brain (as well as in other parts of the neuroendocrine system). While few psychoactive drugs have completely "pure" actions, receptor binding and neurotransmitter modulation together explain much of the success of contemporary psychopharmacology. Considerable research is currently directed toward understanding basic mechanisms of drug action. New mechanisms of drug action may emerge from the evolving understanding of brain function and its relationship to psychiatric disorders.

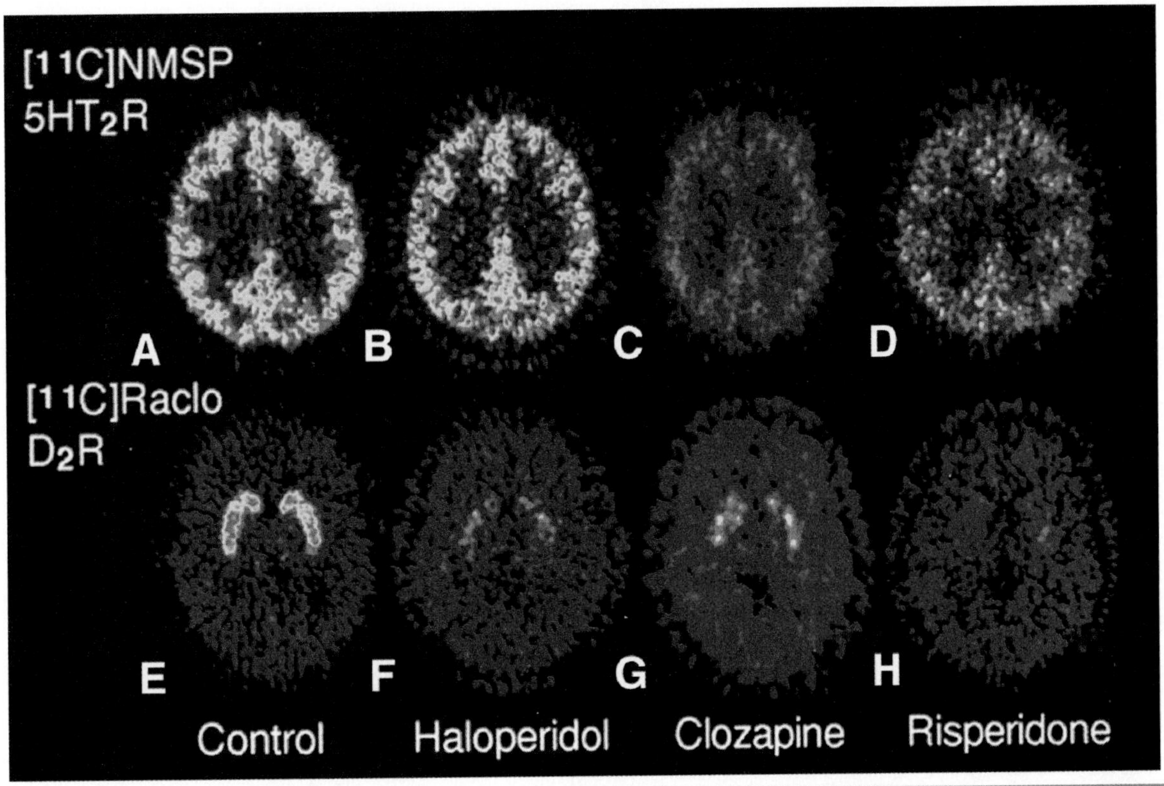

FIGURE 27-1 **PET images of antipsychotic drug binding sites. PET studies can show how drugs bind to brain tissue. In this study, haloperidol does not seem to bind to serotonin receptors (compare control A with the haloperidol-treated B). However, clozapine and risperidone do bind to serotonin receptors (compare control A with treated patients C and D). All three drugs bind to dopamine 2 receptors (bottom images: F, G, H). Yellow and red/orange are PET images of receptors available to bind with drugs. As drugs bind to receptors and they become unavailable, then the PET image changes to blue, green, or purple.** (FROM "CHEMICAL BRAIN ACTIVITY IN SCHIZOPHRENIA" BY G. SEDVALL AND L. FARDE. *LANCET*, 1995, *346* (8977), 746. REPRINTED WITH PERMISSION FROM ELSEVIER.)

ANTIPSYCHOTIC DRUGS

Antipsychotic drugs are administered to control the symptoms of psychosis such as hallucinations, and bizarre or paranoid behavior. These drugs calm without sedation or reduction in alertness. A number of antipsychotic medications are considered in this section, but at present these are best thought of as falling into two categories: first-generation drugs and second-generation drugs. First-generation drugs have been in use for several decades and share both effectiveness and the risk of certain important side effects. Among the most important first-generation drugs are haloperidol (Haldol), chlorpromazine (Thorazine), thioridazine (Mellaril), fluphenazine (Prolixin), and trifluoperazine (Stelazine). Haloperidol is classified as a butyrophenone antipsychotic, whereas the others listed belong to the drug family called phenothiazines. The chemical structures of some of these agents are shown in Figure 27-2, and aspects of their pharmacology are discussed later in this section. In recent years a variety of other antipsychotic medications have come into common use. In many settings, they have replaced the first-generation drugs nearly completely, though growing evidence of associated cardiovascular risk may change clinical practice somewhat. Collectively, these second-generation drugs are often referred to as "atypical" antipsychotics or atypical neuroleptics. Among the commonly prescribed atypical antipsychotics are aripiprazole (Abilify), risperidone (Risperdal), clozapine (Clozaril), olanzapine (Zyprexa), quetiapine (Seroquel), and ziprasidone (Geodon). Paliperidone (Invega), the primary active metabolite of risperidone, is the newest atypical antipsychotic currently available.

INDICATIONS AND EVIDENCE FOR EFFECTIVENESS

Antipsychotic medications are effective treatment for psychoses whether caused by psychiatric or medical conditions. However, since many medically induced psychotic states are transient, treatment may not be necessary for brief or mild psychosis. The major psychotic disorders—schizophrenia and manic-depressive psychosis—respond well to antipsychotics. Symptoms for which antipsychotic treatment is often used include hallucinations, delusions, and disorganized thought processes, including paranoia. In the course of schizophrenic illness, such antipsychotic-responsive symptoms are termed "positive" symptoms because they result in socially disruptive behaviors. As emphasized in Chapter 13, the *negative symptoms* of schizophrenia (withdrawal, lack of initiative, failure to maintain hygiene) do not respond to classical antipsychotics, and while they may briefly improve after treatment with the "atypical" antipsychotic clozapine (Clozaril; Kopelowicz, Zarate, Tripodis, Gonzalez, & Mintz, 2000;

Low Potency Phenothiazines

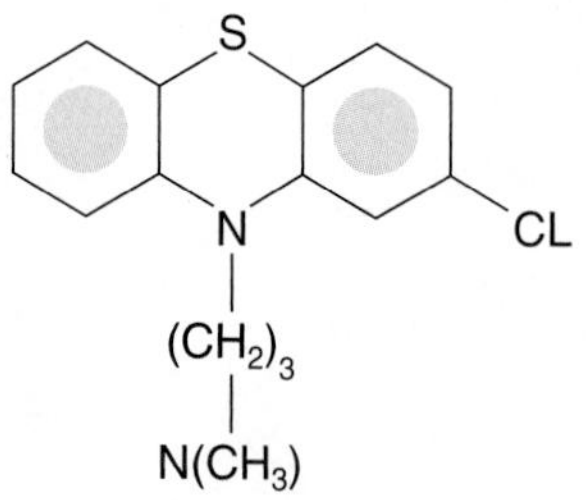

Chlorpromazine

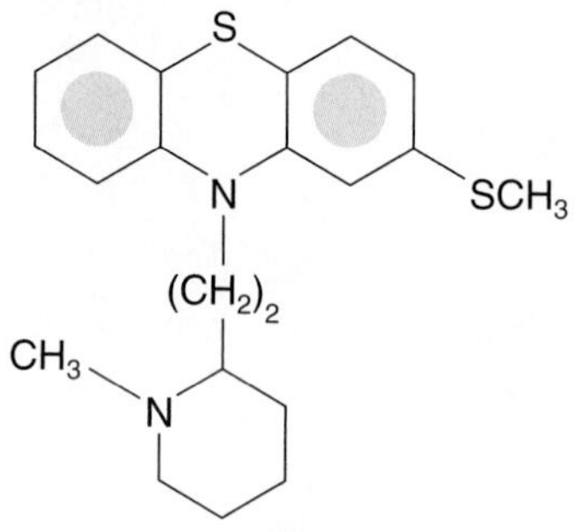

Thioridazine

High Potency Phenothiazines

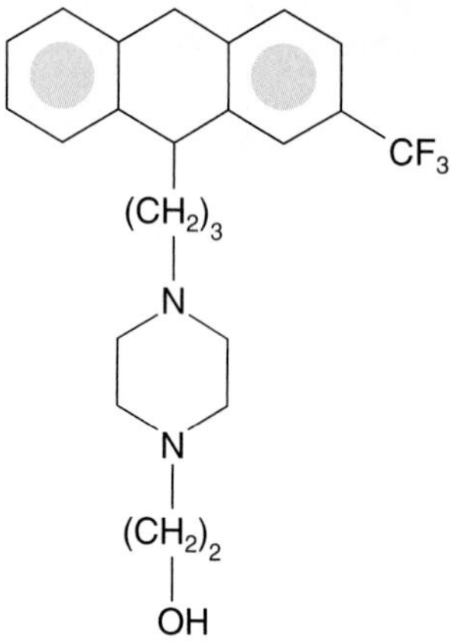

Fluphenazine

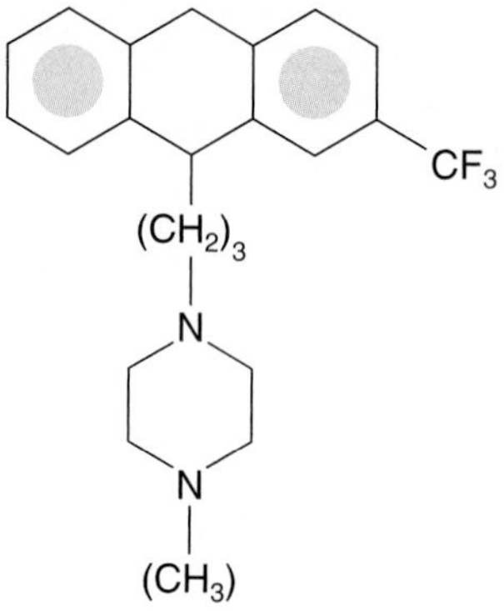

Trifluoprazine

Other Heterocyclic Antipsychotics

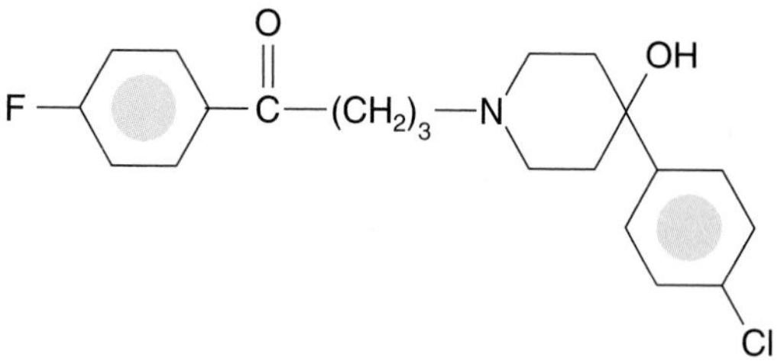

Haloperidol

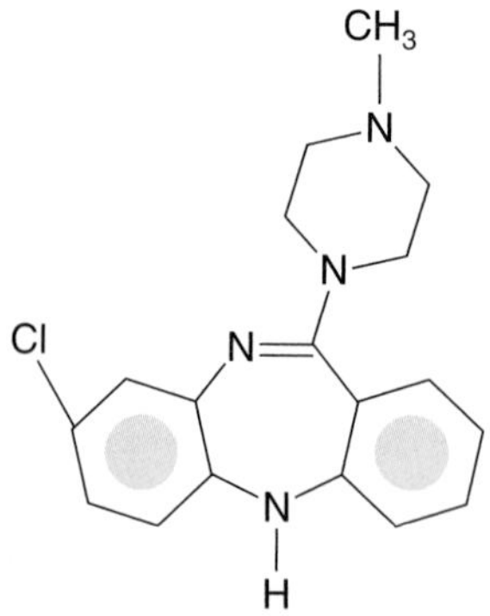

Clozapine

FIGURE 27-2 **Chemical Structure of Selected Antipsychotics** (DELMAR/CENGAGE LEARNING.)

NURSING ALERT 27-1

Drug Risks in Pregnancy

Drugs are placed into one of five categories describing the risk during pregnancy:

Category A
Clinical studies have not demonstrated risk to the fetus during the first trimester of pregnancy; no risk has been demonstrated in later trimesters.

Category B
Animal studies indicate no adverse effects on the fetus, but there are no studies in humans, OR animal studies have demonstrated an adverse effect, but studies in pregnant women have not demonstrated a risk to the fetus during the first trimester of pregnancy and there is no evidence of risk in later trimesters.

Category C
Animal studies have shown an adverse effect on the fetus, and there are no human studies. Risk during pregnancy cannot be ruled out; the potential benefits of the drug may outweigh the potential risks.

Category D
There is positive evidence of risk to the human fetus if the drug is used during pregnancy. Potential benefits of the drug may outweigh the potential risks.

Category X
Studies in animals or humans demonstrate fetal abnormalities or adverse reactions that indicate fetal risk. The use of the drug in pregnancy is contraindicated; there is no potential benefit that outweighs the known risks.

Rosenheck, Dunn, Peszke, Cramer, Xu, Thomas, et al. 1999), there is a broad consensus that new treatments are needed (Kirkpatrick & Galderisi, 2008). There are conflicting data on whether atypical antipsychotics differ among one another (Sprague, Loewen, & Raymond, 2004), but increasing evidence casts doubt on any superiority to first-generation agents (Manschreck & Boshes, 2007). Clozapine has been shown to be significantly more effective than other atypical antipsychotics and is used for treatment of refractory schizophrenia (McEvoy, Lieberman, Stroup, Davis, Meltzer, Rosenheck et al., 2006). These benefits come, however, along with side effects that may be life-threatening and that require frequent monitoring of blood counts. In most settings, atypical antipsychotics are now prescribed more frequently than are first-generation agents and, whether or not they are more effective, appear to be better tolerated when judged by the likelihood of continuing treatment without a change in medication (Jaffe & Levine, 2003; Manschreck & Boshes, 2007). Not only are antipsychotics effective in controlling symptoms

NURSING TIP 27-1

Neuroleptics and Antipsychotics

In the course of your professional duties, you may hear the term *neuroleptic* used in reference to a medication. This is an older term for *antipsychotics* that now is used less to refer to a medication than to the neurological side effects. The preferred term is *antipsychotic*—it is clearer as to its use and more hopeful in its meaning. However, many physicians continue to use the terms interchangeably, and you should always consider what is meant when the term *neuroleptic* is used.

of acute psychosis, they have been shown by a number of studies to be effective in preventing relapse in individuals with chronic disorders. Combining ongoing antipsychotic treatment with social support can reduce the likelihood of relapse and may even lead to remission of disease in some persons (Schooler, 2006).

PHARMACOLOGY

There are nearly 20 antipsychotic drugs in clinical use in the United States and many more worldwide. These drugs can be grouped in several ways:

Grouping by Chemical Class

While pharmacologists view the antipsychotic drugs as falling into a number of chemical categories, for most practicing mental health professionals the distinction between classical or "first-generation" antipsychotics and "second-generation" antipsychotics (sometimes still termed "atypicals") is the only useful distinction. This distinction emphasizes major differences in side effect profiles and costs. The second-generation medications have different and often fewer side effects than first-generation drugs, and they are often considerably more costly.

Antipsychotic drugs can be classed as phenothiazines, thioxanthenes, butyrophenones, dibenzoxazepines, dihydroindolones, dibenzodiazepines, and benzisoxazoles. The phenothiazines, together with the next four categories (thioxanthenes, butyrophenones, dibenzoxazepines, and dihydroindolones), comprise the "classical" antipsychotic drugs, most of which have been in clinical use for several decades.

Because chemical names are complex, nurses and mental health professionals find it practical to classify antipsychotic drugs into broad groups: (1) phenothiazines and the other classical agents, and (2) the newest drugs—clozapine (Clozaril), risperidone (Risperdal), olanzapine (Zyprexa), quetiapine (Seroquel), ziprasidone (Geodon), aripiprazole (Abilify), and paliperidone (Invega). Especially in combination with a variety of other medications, clozapine may effectively treat psychotic clients not helped by classical agents, but this benefit comes at the risk of occasional life-threatening bone marrow depression, a potential of some cardiac complications

(Rathore, Masani, & Callaghan, 2007), and dose-dependent lowering of the seizure threshold.

Grouping by Potency Class

Antipsychotic medications are commonly grouped by the amount of drug required to achieve an effect. Two phenothiazines—fluphenazine (Prolixin) and trifluoperazine (Stelazine)—and a butyrophenone—haloperidol (Haldol)—are classified as "high potency" because only a few milligrams have significant antipsychotic effects. The "low-potency" drugs—chlorpromazine (Thorazine), thioridazine (Mellaril)—typically achieve effects comparable to a few milligrams of high-potency drugs with doses of approximately 100 mg. Beyond this 50-fold difference in absolute dose needed to achieve similar effects, there are some additional differences between potency classes. For example, the low-potency drugs are more sedating, anticholinergic, and cause more orthostasis, whereas the high-potency drugs are more likely to produce certain troublesome complications (see following discussion of adverse reactions). The majority of drugs fall into an intermediate-potency range and also have intermediate sedative and adverse effects.

Non-Antipsychotic Drugs Commonly Used in the Treatment of Psychosis

Psychotic persons are often treated with benzodiazepines (discussed in the section on anxiety) and may be given antidepressants or mood stabilizers, or both, if they have psychosis due to or complicated by mood disorder. These latter drugs are occasionally useful in managing psychosis but are not antipsychotics. They are discussed in the section on mood disorders. Many psychotic persons are treated simultaneously with antipsychotic drugs and with antiparkinsonian or anticholinergic agents, or both. The antiparkinsonian and anticholinergic drugs are used to counteract antipsychotic medication side effects rather than for their specific effects on psychosis. These medications will be considered in a subsequent section describing adverse reactions to antipsychotic drugs.

As noted in Chapter 13, much current evidence suggests that schizophrenia (and perhaps other psychoses as well) involves excessive activation of brain D_2 dopamine receptors. (A more general discussion of the nature of receptors appears in Chapter 4.) Antipsychotic drugs are all strong blockers of dopamine D_2 receptors in the brain. Clozapine blocks D_2, but also has effects on other dopamine receptors (D_1 and D_4) as well as several other neurotransmitter systems. This wider range of action may explain the enhanced effectiveness of clozapine, in comparison with other "classical" antipsychotics. The atypical antipsychotic, aripiprazole (Abilify), is unique in that it functions as a partial agonist at D_2 (as well as D_3) receptors (Grunder, Fellows, Janouschek, Veselinovic, Boy, Brocheler, et al., 2008).

The phenothiazines, thioxanthenes, and dibenzoxazepines have a similar chemical structure, each with a central ring flanked on each side by two aromatic rings. The central ring is in turn linked to one of several longer chains, modifications of which may have a strong effect on drug potency. Because their chemical structure typically lacks highly polar regions, the antipsychotic drugs are not very water soluble, and as a result they have a high affinity for fatty tissues such as lung, brain, and adipose stores. Because of this fat affinity, lower doses may be required in very thin persons; however there are no standard recommendations to change dosage based on body weight or composition. This affinity affects how they are metabolized and excreted in the body. Figure 27-2 illustrates the chemical structure of selected antipsychotics.

Dose/Administration

All of the currently available antipsychotic drugs are well absorbed when given either orally or by intramuscular injection. Injection typically produces significant clinical effects within 15 to 30 minutes, whereas oral administration more commonly takes 1 to 4 hours. Many of the antipsychotics are formulated as both pills and a liquid concentrate. Absorption of the liquid preparations is often somewhat faster than the pills. Oral absorption can be decreased by foods, coffee, smoking, and some other drugs. Many antipsychotic drugs are rapidly metabolized by the liver before they actually reach the bloodstream. Parenteral administration avoids both variable absorption and such "first-pass" metabolism. Consequently, parenterally administered medication not only works faster, but also often has a greater clinical effect because of higher brain bioavailability.

The dosage of antipsychotics varies with the drug chosen and with the prescribing practice of the psychiatric clinician. On arrival in the bloodstream following either oral or parenteral administration, most antipsychotic drugs are tightly bound to serum proteins. Only unbound drug—typically less than 10% of that circulating in the plasma—is available to cross the blood-brain barrier and exert an antipsychotic effect on the brain. Once in the bloodstream, antipsychotic drugs are generally metabolized by the liver and excreted. Paliperidone (Invega) undergoes relatively little metabolism (Dolder, Nelson, & Deyo, 2008), so that as a result approximately 80% is renally excreted. Free drug (i.e., drug not bound to serum protein) may pass rapidly into fatty tissues, finding its way to the liver only after some delay. This means both that long dosing intervals (single daily doses) are practical and that drug may remain in the brain (and body fat stores) far longer than measured serum levels would suggest. The second-generation antipsychotics are metabolized in the liver through the P450 system, which both increases susceptibility to drug interactions and potentially poses a risk of toxicity in the presence of liver disease (Zhang, Ramzan, & Murray, 2007).

As noted previously, some first-generation antipsychotic drugs such as fluphenazine decanoate (Prolixin) and haloperidol decanoate (Haldol LA) have been specifically formulated to have a very long duration of action. These long-acting drugs are given by injection only and are manufactured as a preparation of drug dissolved in sesame oil. The sesame oil slows the diffusion of drug into adjacent muscle, and as a consequence, absorption is significantly delayed. Once the drug diffuses out of the oil and reaches muscle, the antipsychotic medication is rapidly absorbed and becomes biologically active. Absorption from oil is so slow that it takes up to three months of weekly injections for a pharmacological steady state to be reached. After achieving steady state, a balance is attained between drug that reaches the brain and drug that is excreted by the liver. As a result, serum levels and clinical effects stabilize. Other first-generation depot drugs include flupenthixol, clopenthixol, moloperidol, and zuclopenthixol, but none of these are available for use in the United States.

While for many years only first-generation antipsychotics were available in long-acting depot forms, risperidone is now marketed in an injectable form using "microspheres" rather than sesame oil. Injectable risperidone (Risperdal Consta) is approved for dosing every two weeks. Preliminary data suggest that this medication is well tolerated, with a low incidence of tardive dyskinesia (see following) and other side effects (Harrison & Goa, 2004). It is likely that other long-acting second-generation formulations such as iloperidone (a chemical relative of risperidone and ziprasidone) or paliperidone palmitate will be on the market soon and may need administration only every four weeks. Students should remember that several injectable medications—haloperidol is an example—are formulated in both short- and long-acting forms whose onset of action, dosages, and site of administration (long-acting drugs cannot currently be given in the biceps) differ significantly. It is always important to assess the reason for intramuscular administration and to be certain that a preparation appropriate to the desired indication has been chosen. Long-acting injections may be useful for patients with repeated nonadherence to oral treatment. Other special second-generation antipsychotic formulations include orally disintegrating tablets, such as olanzapine (Zyprexa Zydis), risperidone (Risperal M-Tab), aripiprazole (Abilify Discmelt), and clozapine (FazaClo). Such formulations can be useful when clients are reluctant or are unable to swallow oral medications. Olanzapine (Zyprexa), aripiprazole (Abilify), and ziprasidone (Geodon) are also available as injections.

Drug Actions

The pharmacological actions of antipsychotics are complex. In general, these medications have two major characteristics: (1) they all bind to brain dopamine receptors, and (2) probably as a result of that binding, they produce a degree of indifference to both external and internal stressful stimuli. This indifference is associated with relatively little sedation or inhibition of pain responses and leads to a calming effect without reducing alertness or sensitivity to pain. Other medications that induce a degree of indifference to stress (e.g., narcotics and sedatives) produce sedation or a direct blockade of pain perception. Dependency does not occur with antipsychotic medications, but clients should typically taper their use of these medications rather than stop abruptly. While second-generation antipsychotics also have an effect on dopamine receptors, they differ from the first-generation drugs in also acting at receptors for serotonin (Meltzer, Li, Kaneda, & Ichikawa, 2003).

Drug Interactions

Because antipsychotic drugs are most commonly metabolized by the liver, other medications that affect the rate of hepatic drug detoxification may have an effect on antipsychotic drug excretion. In recent years, psychiatrists have attempted to keep antipsychotic doses as low as possible so as to avoid common adverse effects. Interactions that raise drug levels—the drug cimetidine (Tagamet) is an example—may increase antipsychotic effects and lead to increased side effects. The interaction between antipsychotics and cimetidine is particularly troublesome since cimetidine is widely promoted for dyspepsia and is available without prescription.

> **NURSING ALERT 27-2**
>
> **Tagamet and Antipsychotics**
>
> **Tagamet (cimetidine), an over-the-counter drug for dyspepsia, may inhibit the metabolism of antipsychotics, resulting in increased levels and effects.**

Some antipsychotic medications may themselves affect the way in which other medications are metabolized. Anticonvulsant medications such as carbamazepine (Tegretol, Equetro), used either for seizure control or for mood stabilization, may lower plasma concentrations of antipsychotics. The commonly used mood stabilizer lithium also has a highly significant potential interaction with antipsychotics. This interaction occurs only rarely, but may result in profound and permanent neurological impairment. While antipsychotics and lithium are frequently used together without problems, this combination requires close monitoring for signs of neurological disorder (Jeffries, Remington, & Wilkins, 1984). Tricyclic antidepressants are also frequently combined with antipsychotics; this combination may cause additive side effects in terms of sedation and cardiovascular effects. Fluoxetine and other serotonin reuptake inhibitors may significantly increase antipsychotic drug levels and lead to serious adverse reactions; fortunately, this interaction is rare (Goff & Baldessarini, 1995). Some cardiac drugs (particularly quinidine, procainamide, and epinephrine) may interact with low-potency antipsychotics; the administration of epinephrine to persons taking medications such as chlorpromazine may result in severe hypotension. First-generation antipsychotics may interact with drugs such as erythromycin, ketaconazole, and a variety of other mostly psychiatric drugs to prolong the cardiac QT interval. QT prolongation is discussed following. Very high levels of caffeine intake may worsen psychosis despite antipsychotic administration (Lucas et al., 1990). Antacids, especially those formulated as gels (Amphogel, Gelusil), may decrease oral antipsychotic drug absorption and should not be administered within four hours of an antipsychotic dose.

Use During Pregnancy/Lactation

There are no specific known contraindications to the use of many antipsychotic medications in pregnancy, although most clinicians try to use the minimum possible dose and to avoid administration in early pregnancy and near the time of delivery (ACOG Practice Bulletin, 2008; McCauley-Elsom, & Kulkarni, 2007). Antipsychotic medications are excreted in breast milk, so that breast feeding is contraindicated when these medications must be used following delivery.

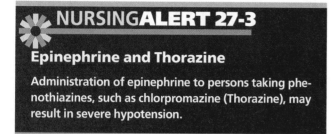

NURSINGALERT 27-3

Epinephrine and Thorazine

Administration of epinephrine to persons taking phenothiazines, such as chlorpromazine (Thorazine), may result in severe hypotension.

Side Effects

Potentially troublesome side effects of first-generation antipsychotic medications include constipation, dry mouth, blurred vision, postural hypotension, urinary hesitancy or retention, weight gain, and sedation. Most of these are anticholinergic effects that may be minimized by choosing drugs with relatively lower anticholinergic action—for example, haloperidol (Haldol), trifluoperazine (Stelazine), and fluphenazine (Prolixin).

Side effects from second-generation (atypical) antipsychotics vary among different agents, but weight gain has proven among the most troublesome complications. While the exact mechanism is unknown, the result is often significant weight gain. Effects on various receptors (e.g., histaminic) or other metabolic and endocrine factors may play a role as well. Weight gain has been associated with the development of type 2 diabetes (Ashim, Warrington, & Anderson, 2004) and with abnormal patterns of blood lipids (Melkersson & Dahl, 2004). Olanzapine and clozapine seem to be the worst offenders in terms of weight gain, lipids, and risk for diabetes. These metabolic effects, while not unknown, are less common with ziprasidone and aripiprazole (Baptista, Zarate, Joober, Colasante, Beauliew, Paez, et al., 2004). Recent data suggest that these metabolic changes are associated with an enhanced risk of heart disease (Davidson, 2002; Haddad, 2004). A consensus statement regarding monitoring parameters for metabolic effects of atypicals was issued by the American Diabetes Association, American Psychiatric Association, American Association of Clinical Endocrinologists, and the North American Association for the Study of Obesity (American Diabetes Association, 2004).

Adverse Effects

Antipsychotic medications have great potential for serious adverse affects. The classical agents such as thioridazine (Mellaril), haloperidol (Haldol), and chlorpromazine (Thorazine) frequently produce a variety of movement disorders. These include akathisia, dystonia, drug-induced parkinsonism, and tardive dyskinesia. Of these conditions, **akathisia** is the most common and consists of a subjective sense of restlessness with a perceived need to pace or otherwise move continuously. It is easy for the nurse to mistake akathisia for anxiety or agitation. (See the nursing tip on how to differentiate akathisia, anxiety, and agitation.) **Dystonia** consists of sustained, involuntary muscle spasms; these most commonly involve the head and neck, but may occasionally occur in other muscle groups. One of the most dramatic dystonic reactions is **oculogyric crisis**, in which extraocular muscle spasm forces the eyes into a fixed, usually upward gaze. Parkinsonism results in tremor and an unsteady shuffling gait; the features of drug-induced parkinsonism may closely resemble those of true idiopathic parkinsonism. The distinction between these two conditions may occasionally be difficult, but idiopathic parkinsonism most commonly occurs in older individuals who have no history of antipsychotic drug use. In contrast, drug-induced parkinsonism is common and occurs in up to 30% of individuals who take long-term antipsychotic medications. These three conditions—akathisia, dystonia, and parkinsonism—usually respond rapidly to antipsychotic dosage reduction, anticholinergic drugs, or diphenhydramine (Benadryl). Parenteral diphenhydramine is usually given for acute dystonia, but akathisia is often treated with the beta-blocker propranolol (Inderal), dosage reduction, or switching antipsychotics (Crismon, Argo, & Buckley, 2008).

The fourth movement disorder seen with antipsychotic drugs, tardive dyskinesia, is a more significant adverse effect because it may prove long-lasting despite withdrawal of antipsychotic medication. **Tardive dyskinesia** is a neurological disorder characterized by involuntary movements, most commonly of the tongue and lips. Grimacing, sucking movements, and lip smacking are among the most common tardive dyskinesias. When tardive dyskinesia affects the trunk and extremities, the result may be slow and irregular movements that diminish during relaxation and disappear during sleep. On occasion tardive dyskinesia may be so severe as to interfere with walking, eating, or even breathing. Tardive dyskinesia may improve or disappear when medications are stopped and may even improve with continued administration of classical antipsychotics (Marder & Van Putten, 1995, p. 257). While prevention is crucial, switching to clozapine may be a useful strategy for tardive dyskinesia (Crismon et al., 2008).

NURSINGTIP 27-2

Differentiating Akathisia, Anxiety, and Agitation

Akathisia

Assess for:

- Describing "feeling antsy"
- Inability to sit still
- Pacing floor
- Not being frightened

Anxiety

Assess for:

- Expressing thoughts of worry or concerns
- Having fears, even if unable to state the source of the worry
- Often having somatic symptoms

Agitation

Assess for:

- Exhibiting escalating anxiety and anger
- Vocalizing concerns/complaints
- Possibly demonstrating destructive behavior

Anticholinergic drugs are often used to treat medication-related movement disorders, but they are also frequently given along with antipsychotics in an effort to prevent the development of neurological symptoms. Common anticholinergic drugs include trihexyphenidyl (Artane) and benztropine (Cogentin). These drugs are usually given orally, but benztropine may be administered either orally or parenterally. The oral dosage of trihexyphenidyl ranges from 5 to 15 mg daily, usually in two or more doses. The side effects of anticholinergics are predictable from their inhibition of the cholinergic nervous system: dry mouth, nasal dryness, urinary hesitancy, blurred vision, orthostatic hypotension, decreased sweating, constipation, and sedation. The anti-parkinsonian drug amantadine (Symmetrel) is also frequently used in treating drug-induced movement disorders. Amantadine is given only orally, typically in a dose of 100 to 200 mg twice a day. Side effects are common, particularly in the elderly, and may include drowsiness, confusion, depression, and toxic psychosis. Seizures may occasionally be precipitated, and anticholinergic side effects are not uncommon.

Tardive dyskinesia occurs in at least 5% of persons who continue on antipsychotic medications for more than a year, and its incidence increases significantly with longer durations of treatment. In an effort to reduce the prevalence of tardive dyskinesia, the American Psychiatric Association Task Force on Tardive Dyskinesia (1992) has recommended a set of basic guidelines for management of persons needing antipsychotic treatment:

1. Continue medication use only when there is objective evidence that antipsychotic medications are effective treatment for a given individual.
2. Use the lowest effective dose of antipsychotic medications.
3. Be very cautious in prescribing antipsychotic medications to individuals at highest risk of developing tardive dyskinesia: children, the elderly, and individuals with affective disorders.
4. Conduct regular physical examinations to seek evidence of tardive dyskinesia.
5. On diagnosis (or especially worsening) of tardive dyskinesia, consider dosage reduction and substitution of other treatments. Utilize informed consent during antipsychotic administration.

Data suggests that atypical antipsychotics generally cause movement disorders less frequently than first generation antipsychotics. Risperidone (Risperdal) has been associated with the most, while clozapine (Clozaril) and quetiapine (Seroquel) with the least (Weiden, Preskorn, Fahnestock, Carpenter, Ross, Docherty, et al., 2007). Clozapine is only very rarely associated with movement disorders, including tardive dyskinesia. However, seizures do occur in some persons, and 1% to 2% of persons on clozapine develop bone marrow suppression, which may progress to fatal agranulocytosis. Safe use of clozapine requires weekly monitoring of white blood cell counts for the first six months of therapy, followed by every two weeks for the second six months. If white blood cell counts remain normal, monitoring may be extended to every four weeks. Therapy should be permanently discontinued if the white cell count falls below 2000. Pharmacologists are currently trying to develop antipsychotic medications with the effectiveness of clozapine but without its potentially fatal adverse effects. Olanzapine appears to share some of the benefits of clozapine without any significant risk of bone marrow suppression (Gómez, Sacristán, Hernández, Breier, Ruiz Carrasco, Antón Saiz, et al., 2000). It remains unclear whether olanzapine is as effective as clozapine in treating resistant psychosis, but preliminary data suggest comparable effectiveness (Tuunainen, Wahlbeck, & Gilbody, 2000).

Neuroleptic Malignant Syndrome

This syndrome is yet another serious complication of antipsychotic medications. All of the antipsychotic medications, including clozapine, may occasionally result in **Neuroleptic Malignant Syndrome**. This unusual disorder is associated with sudden fever, rigidity, tachycardia, hypertension, and decreased levels of consciousness. Fever can rise to exceedingly high levels, and death may occur. These individuals are usually thought incorrectly to have an infectious condition, and unnecessary investigations and antibiotic treatment may delay diagnosis. Rapid treatment is required for survival, but this requires a high index of suspicion. Treatment includes discontinuation of antipsychotics and the potential administration of a variety of medications, including amantadine, bromocriptine, dantrolene, and benzodiazepines (Strawn, Keck, & Caroff, 2007). Neuroleptic Malignant Syndrome, a diagnosis of exclusion, clinically resembles malignant hyperthermia, a condition seen during surgical anesthesia in genetically predisposed individuals.

Excess Deaths among Clients Treated with Antipsychotics

As noted in Chapter 13, there has been concern that antipsychotic medications may be associated with sudden death. The FDA has issued a "black box" warning on the use of antipsychotic medications in the elderly treated for dementia-related psychosis. Initially that warning involved only second-generation drugs, but it has subsequently been extended to all antipsychotics. The relative hazard of excess death has been most evident in the elderly, but it likely exists at younger ages as well, though the absolute risk is likely considerably lower (Sicouri & Antzelevitch, 2008). One proposed mechanism has been prolongation of the cardiac QT interval, an effect that has been attributed to other medications and can be associated with lethal arrhythmias. There is evidence that a variety of drugs used in psychiatric mental health can prolong the QT interval, and among these are first-generation antipsychotics—particularly thioridizine, pimozide, and haloperidol, especially when given intravenously (Zemrak & Kenna, 2008). The risk of prolonged QT interval increases with age and during co-administration of a variety of medications. Among these are anti-infective agents (notably some oral antifungals and erythromycin) and a variety of other psychiatric drugs including many antidepressants. The safe prescription of antipsychotic medications requires attention to other medications that may interact adversely.

A potentially more important risk involving second-generation antipsychotics is their association with weight gain, metabolic syndrome, diabetes, and enhanced cardiovascular risk. These complications are all linked together: increased abdominal fat increases the risk of diabetes and lipid abnormalities, each of which is a strong risk factor for cardiovascular disease including heart attack and stroke. While some experts believe that persons with schizophrenia have increased cardiovascular risk even in the absence of antipsychotic treatment, there is strong evidence for significant cardiac risk among persons, especially women, taking second-generation drugs (McEvoy et al., 2006; Arango, Bobes, Aranda, Carmena, Garcia-Garcia, Rejas, et al., 2008). Persons with schizophrenia have a life expectancy that is 15 years lower than the general population (Hennekens, Hennekens, Hollar, & Casey, 2005). While suicide accounts for some of this difference, the majority of risk derives from cardiovascular disease. Preventing the cardiovascular risk that is almost certainly increased by antipsychotic medications is among the major challenges of treating schizophrenia.

Summary of Antipsychotics

Antipsychotic medications are frequently used in psychiatric nursing and in general medical practice. Chlorpromazine, long-acting fluphenazine, and haloperidol are included in the World Health Organization list of essential drugs for primary care (Wig, 1993). The nurse should be familiar with the indications, side effects, and adverse effects of both orally administered and parenteral antipsychotics. Table 27-1 presents a summary of selected antipsychotic drugs. Although second-generation neuroleptics are more costly on a per-dose basis than are agents such as haloperidol, in many psychiatric settings the second-generation neuroleptics such as risperidone and olanzapine are preferentially used as initial treatments for clients with previously untreated psychosis. The CATIE trial's finding that second-generation antipsychotics (with the exception of clozapine) were not better at treating schizophrenia than were first-generation drugs makes it likely that first-generation drugs will become more widely used for initial treatment until research leads to new, and perhaps safer, antipsychotic drugs (Manschreck & Boshes, 2007). However, despite cardiovascular risk concerns, the second-generation antipsychotics remain first-line agents for the treatment of various psychiatric disorders.

DRUGS FOR TREATING MOOD DISORDERS

Drugs for treating mood disorders are used either to treat depressed mood (antidepressants) or to treat mania (mood stabilizers). While these drugs rarely act quickly and are not invariably effective, they can greatly enhance clients' well-being and useful functioning.

Indications and Evidence for Effectiveness

Pharmacological treatment for mood disorders is most commonly indicated when both client and provider agree that modification of mood would lead to enhanced well-being and functioning. On rare occasions persons may be given mood-modifying medication against their will, but such administration is invariably court ordered and given only to convicted criminals whose psychiatric hospitalization replaces a prison sentence.

Effectiveness data for antidepressants is well established for severe depression requiring hospitalization as well as for tricyclic medications. Selective serotonin reuptake inhibitors (SSRIs) have become widely used despite relatively limited evidence for their effectiveness, especially for mild to moderate depression (Kirsch, Deacon, Huedo-Medina, Scoboria, Moore, & Johnson, 2008). While tricyclic antidepressants have traditionally been less expensive than other antidepressants such as SSRIs, the generic availability of many SSRIs has made costs between antidepressant drug classes comparable. Trazodone is an agent with cost and side effects profile midway between tricyclics and SSRIs; this makes trazodone a popular choice for many prescribers. Nonetheless, many clinicians favor SSRI antidepressants because they are probably safer in intentional overdose, a significant risk in depressed individuals. Concerns about safety are discussed further under "adverse effects."

Drugs for treating mood disorders generally fall into four categories: tricyclic (and related) antidepressants, SSRIs, monoamine oxidase inhibitors (MAOIs), and mood stabilizers. There are an increasing number of agents, however, that fall outside these categories. Each one of these categories will be discussed separately in the sections that follow. The tricyclic medications include imipramine (Tofranil), desipramine (Norpramin or Pertofrane), amitriptyline (Elavil), nortriptyline (Pamelor), clomipramine (Anafranil), trimipramine (Surmontil), doxepin (Sinequan), and protriptyline (Vivactil). Amoxapine (Asendin), a tetracyclic, and maprotiline (Ludiomil), a heterocyclic, are closely related to these in their structure and effects. Several other compounds—trazodone (Desyrel), bupropion (Wellbutrin), venlafaxine (Effexor), and nefazodone (Serzone)—are not chemically related to the tricyclics but are quite similar in their antidepressant effects; these will be discussed in the section on tricyclics and related antidepressants. The SSRIs include fluoxetine (Prozac), sertraline (Zoloft), paroxetine (Paxil), escitalopram (Lexapro), citalopram (Celexa), and fluvoxamine (Luvox). Escitalopram (Lexapro) is the S-enantiomer of citalopram (Celexa). Two other drugs with both serotonin (SSRI) and norepinephrine receptor effects are venlafaxine (Effexor) and duloxetine (Cymbalta). Desvenlafaxine (Pristiq), a metabolite of venlafaxine (Effexor), is the newest antidepressant available. The MAOIs include phenelzine (Nardil), tranylcypromine (Parnate), and selegiline (Emsam in a formulation applied as a skin patch). Mood stabilizers include lithium and several anticonvulsants—primarily valaproic acid or divalproex (Depakote) and carbamazepine (Tegretol). Some clinicians use additional drugs in treating mood disorders; among these are the benzodiazepine alprazolam (Xanax), the antianxiety drug buspirone (BusPar), and stimulants such as amphetamines.

The neurobiology of depression is highly complex and is briefly reviewed in Chapter 14. A major current theory explaining depression states that depressed individuals have persistent abnormalities in the concentration and distribution of biogenic amines that serve as neurotransmitters within the brain. Most antidepressant medications in common use exert some measurable effect on levels of brain neurotransmitters, most commonly norepinephrine or serotonin, or both. The

TABLE 27-1 Antipsychotic Medications

GENERIC NAME	TRADE NAME	MODE OF ADMINISTRATION	SEDATION	EXTRA-PYRAMIDAL	ANTICHOLINERGIC	ORTHOSTATIC HYPOTENSION	MARROW SUPPRESSION	DOSE RANGE (MG)	PLASMA LEVELS (MG/ML)
Phenothiazines									
Chlorpromazine	Thorazine	p.o., p.r., i.m., i.v.	3+	2+	2+	2+	0	30–800	up to 2.0
Thioridizine	Mellaril	p.o.	3+	1+	3+	3+	1+*	150–800	—
Fluphenazine	Prolixin	p.o., i.m./subcut	1+	3+	1+	1+	0	5–40	0.13–2.8
Trifluoperazine	Stelazine	p.o., i.m.	1+	3+	1+	1+	0	2–20	—
Perphenazine	Trilafon	p.o.	2+	2+	1+	1+	0	10–64	—
Thioxanthene									
Thiothixene	Navane	p.o., i.m.	1+	3+	1+	1+	0	8–30	2–57
Butyrephenone									
Haloperidol	Haldol	p.o., i.m.	1+	3+	1+	1+	0	1–30	up to .05
Dibenzoxazepine									
Loxapine	Loxitane	p.o., i.m.	2+	3+	1+	2+	0	40–100	—
Dibenzodiazepines									
Clozapine	Clozaril	p.o.	3+	1+	3+	3+	4+	300–900	—
Olanzapine	Zyprexa	p.o., i.m.	2+	1+	2+	2+	0	5–20	—
Quetiapine	Seroquel	p.o.	2+	1+	2+	2+	0	150–800	—
Benzisoxazole									
Risperidone	Risperdal	p.o., i.m.	1+	3+	1+	1+	0	2–16	—
Ziprasidone	Geodon	p.o., i.m.	1+	0–1+	0–1+	1+	0	20–160	—
Aripiprazole	Abilify	p.o., i.m.	1+	0	0–1+	0	0	10–30	—

*Chlorpromazine and thioridazine have had associated agranulocytosis more frequently than other first generation agents.

SSRIs typically have negligible effects on norepinephrine systems, but are quite specific moderators of brain serotonin levels.

Plasma norepinephrine levels are also linked to mania (Swann, et.al. 1990), but theories about causes of mania are less well developed than are those pertaining to depression. Nonetheless, lithium and other mood-stabilizing medications used in the treatment of bipolar disorder act widely in the brain and seem to affect the release of norepinephrine, serotonin, and dopamine (another biogenic amine neurotransmitter; Lenox & Hahn, 2000).

Tricyclic and Related Antidepressants

Tricyclic and related drugs were the first antidepressants to come into clinical use, and these medications still have important roles in treating mood disorders. Although many tricyclic and related antidepressants are available, there are few significant differences among them. Imipramine was the first of the tricyclic drugs to be released, but no data demonstrate that any of the more recently introduced medications are more effective in treating depression. All of the cyclic antidepressants (tricyclic, tetracyclic, and heterocyclic) have a wide range of biochemical actions in the brain and elsewhere (Potter, Manji, & Rudorfer, 1995). These actions often result in side effects, and most choices among drugs are made in an effort to minimize such effects. These choices may be somewhat artificial since once in the body the liver modifies many of these drugs. For example, amitriptyline is converted by the liver to nortriptyline, and imipramine to desipramine. In general, imipramine or amitriptyline is used when sedation is a desired side effect, doxepin when both sedation and anxiety reduction are of primary importance, desipramine or nortriptyline when sedation is to be avoided, and protriptyline when some level of psychological stimulation is desired. Trazodone has a very different (and generally milder) spectrum of side effects when compared with tricyclic and heterocyclic antidepressants, but it may be less effective for the management of severe depression.

Dose/Administration

Antidepressants are only given orally, are typically well absorbed, and reach peak plasma concentrations in two to six hours. Sedation and side effects of antidepressants are seen within several hours of taking these medications—clients often report improved sleep patterns from the first night. Antidepressant effect, as with virtually all the antidepressants, is generally regarded as delayed, usually for two to six weeks from the beginning of treatment (though the existence of this delay is not universally accepted (Mitchell, 2006)). Doses are usually begun quite low and increased gradually (typically at intervals of one to four weeks) until clinical improvement occurs (Potter et al., 1995). Cyclic antidepressants generally have half-lives of approximately 24 hours and can usually be given once daily. The half-lives of trazodone, amoxapine, bupropion, and venlafaxine are shorter, and these drugs are generally given in divided doses. Total daily doses must be individualized based on response, side effects, and (occasionally) blood levels. Although assays for therapeutic (and toxic) blood levels are available for most of the tricyclic medications, they are of clear value only for nortriptyline, imipramine, and desipramine (Potter et al., 1995). Amitriptyline also has suggested therapeutic plasma concentrations. The use of nortriptyline often requires careful monitoring of blood levels because antidepressant effects are not seen below 50 ng/mL or above 150 ng/mL. Therapeutic dosage ranges for most other medications are approximately 100 to 200 mg daily. Except in the elderly, there is usually no need to measure levels until daily doses of 300 to 350 mg are exceeded. Clients with depression are commonly treated for at least six months. For many persons, maintenance treatment should be continued indefinitely. Those for whom long-term treatment should be considered include persons with profound depression, frequently recurring depression (two or more episodes of major depression probably justify long-term treatment), and suicidal ideation or attempts.

Drug Actions

Tricyclic and related antidepressants are usually, but not invariably, effective in relieving symptoms of depression. Individuals with relatively short duration of symptoms (less than a year) and with unipolar and/or melancholic depression are most likely to benefit from treatment. While some studies have suggested that trazodone is less effective than tricyclics in treating severe depression (usually defined as depression requiring hospitalization), its effectiveness for less severe forms of depression is generally accepted. Trazodone has a significant antianxiety effect in some individuals, and this effect is often seen well before depression improves. The nurse following a client receiving trazodone may observe less reported anxiety or may observe changes in the client's appearance or reaction to stressful situations. When antidepressant effects of trazodone and the cyclic antidepressants become evident after two to four weeks, the client will report improved mood, better and more restful sleep, and gradual loss of the primary depressive symptoms of anhedonia and dysphoria.

Tricyclic antidepressants have a number of indications beyond depression. Chief among these are the treatment of Panic Disorder (primarily with imipramine or nortriptyline), Obsessive-Compulsive Disorder (with clomipramine), and psychotic depression with delusions (primarily with amoxapine, an antidepressant chemically related to antipsychotic medications). Tricyclic antidepressants also have important uses in treating neuropathic pain such as that occurring after herpes zoster (shingles), as well as in prevention of migraine attacks. Imipramine is approved for treatment of nocturnal enuresis in children.

Drug Interactions

Cyclic antidepressants have a large number of potential interactions with other drugs, but many of these are of doubtful significance (Gillman, 2007). Students with an interest in the pharmacology of antidepressants including a comprehensive review of drug interactions are encouraged to read the article by Gillman that is available online at http://www.pubmedcentral.nih.gov (article title: "Tricyclic antidepressant pharmacology and therapeutic drug interactions updated"). Many of the cyclic drugs have significant anticholinergic side effects, and these may be enhanced to the point of toxicity by other anticholinergic drugs. This interaction is potentially most serious in the elderly and may be produced by antipsychotics, antihistamines, some general anesthetics and premedicating agents, and narcotic pain relievers, particularly meperidine. Norepinephrine may interact with some tricyclics, and even the small amount found in local anesthetics may potentially cause hypertension or arrhythmias if more than about 5 cc is injected (Yagiela, Duffin, & Hunt, 1985). Whereas the safety of oral sympathomimetics and inhaled bronchodilators is occasionally questioned, the combination of these medications with tricyclics seems to be safe (Ciraulo, Creelman, Shader, & O'Sullivan, 1994). Tricyclics may interact significantly with SSRIs and MAOIs; these interactions may produce significant elevations of tricyclic dosages and hypertensive crises, respectively. Serotonergic syndrome is also possible. Nortriptyline is probably less likely to interact adversely with other drugs than are other currently available tricyclics. Citalopram and escitalopram may have fewer interactions than other SSRIs, though SSRIs in general have a high likelihood of important interactions (Gillman, 2007). Cimetidine, available both by prescription and over the counter, may impair metabolism of tricyclic antidepressants and lead to elevated blood levels with resultant toxicity. Clients needing H2 blockade should preferentially take an alternative medicine such as ranitidine (Zantac). Alcohol adds to central nervous system (CNS) depression that is produced by many antidepressant drugs (most cyclics and trazodone), and alcohol-related impairment may occur after fewer drinks in persons taking these medications. All clients should be informed of this potentially significant interaction.

Use During Pregnancy/Lactation

Cyclic antidepressants should generally not be taken during pregnancy. With the exception of maprotiline (Ludiomil), all of the cyclic drugs are classified in either risk category D (positive evidence of risk) or C (risk cannot be ruled out). Maprotiline is classified in category B (no evidence of risk in humans). All SSRIs fall into pregnancy category C, with the exception of paroxetine (Paxil), which is category D. When the mother's well-being is judged to require antidepressant treatment, usually an SSRI should be used as there is enough experience with SSRIs in pregnancy to be reasonably certain that benefits outweigh risks in almost all persons (Addis & Koren, 2000).

NURSINGALERT 27-4

Alcohol and Antidepressants

Alcohol adds to the CNS depression produced by antidepressants, and clients must be made aware that alcohol-related impairment occurs after fewer drinks than in persons not taking these medications.

Side Effects

Cyclic antidepressants are sometimes called "dirty drugs" by psychiatrists and other mental health clinicians because they act on so many different receptor systems. Many of the actions of antidepressants on receptor systems probably have little or no direct relationship to antidepressant effects, but they are responsible for most drug side effects. While each of the cyclic medications has a different side effects profile, most have some effect on each of the following receptor systems: cholinergic (also called muscarinic), histaminergic, alpha-adrenergic, and dopaminergic. Anticholinergic effects include blurred vision, dry mouth, rapid heart rate, constipation, urinary retention, and perhaps impaired memory function. Antihistaminic effects include weight gain, sedation, and interaction with other drugs that cause CNS depression. Alpha-adrenergic effects include postural hypotension, dizziness, and potential interaction with some antihypertensive medications. Antidopaminergic effects include movement disorders and endocrine changes (see adverse effects). Cyclic medications all have side effects in each of these categories, although desipramine and nortriptyline probably have the best side effects profile of this group of drugs. Nortriptyline may have both greater efficacy and safety (both in overdose and drug interaction) than many other antidepressants (Gillman, 2007). Amitriptyline and maprotiline may be more likely than others to cause prolongation of the cardiac QT interval, a condition that can lead to arrhythmia or even sudden death. QT prolongation may be a particular risk when multiple medications are prescribed together; a particularly risky combination may be amitriptyline and the first generation antipsychotic thioridizine (Vieweg & Wood, 2004). Trazodone has no anticholinergic effect, moderate alpha-adrenergic effect (typically manifested by postural hypotension), and very little antidopaminergic effect.

Adverse Effects

The most significant adverse effects of cyclic antidepressants are seen in accidental or intentional overdose. These drugs typically have a very limited therapeutic margin, and fatal overdose may occur with ingestion of only a few days' supply. There appears to be considerable difference of safety in overdose even among the cyclic drugs. Nortriptyline has a level of risk in overdose that is significantly better than other tricyclics and comparable to that of SSRIs (Gillman, 2007). In contrast, deaths have occurred with only 1000 mg of amitriptyline, while it is not uncommon for clients to take 150 to 300 mg daily. It is usually recommended that clinicians not dispense more than 1000 mg of these drugs at a time unless suicidal risk is judged completely absent. Symptoms of overdose include CNS depression, widening of electrocardiogram (EKG) QRS complexes with associated heart block, shock, seizures, and dangerous temperature elevations. Some data suggest that antidepressants may increase the risk of suicide, especially in persons with a history of impulsive or aggressive behavior (Charney, Miller, Licinia, & Salomon, 1995). All classes of antidepressants now carry a black box warning regarding increased risk of suicidal thinking and behavior in children, adolescents, and young adults up to the age of 24. This issue is discussed further in Chapter 14. Overdose is not necessary for tricyclic-associated fatalities to occur; occasional unexplained, and presumably drug-related, deaths in children taking tricyclics continue to be reported and may be related to prolongation of the QT interval or other related cardiac effects (Sicouri & Antzelevitch, 2008).

Trazodone, along with most other noncyclic antidepressants, is relatively free of direct cardiac side effects and probably safer in overdose than are cyclic medications. Nonetheless, trazodone may produce severe postural hypotension that, especially in the elderly, can cause falls, fractures, or perhaps even cardiovascular events such as stroke or myocardial infarction. Trazodone should probably be avoided in geriatric individuals. Trazodone may rarely cause priapism (sustained and painful erection) in men, usually in the first weeks of treatment. This complication may require surgical treatment and may result in permanent impotence. For this reason, and despite the rarity of priapism, many clinicians avoid the use of trazodone in men. Nefazadone does not cause priapism or other sexual dysfunction, but otherwise is quite similar to trazadone. Through their inhibition of dopaminergic pathways, tricyclics and occasionally other antidepressants may increase levels of the hormone prolactin. This may result in galactorrhea (leakage of milk from one or both breasts) in women and in loss of libido in both men and women. All of the cyclic antidepressants have a small chance of inducing seizures, even in persons who have not previously had epilepsy. Although remarkably free from other adverse effects, bupropion, a noncyclic antidepressant, has been among the antidepressants most likely to produce seizures in ordinary clinical use—though these occur quite uncommonly and are likely rarer in persons receiving the sustained use formulation used for smoking cessation than in those treated for depression with short-acting preparations (Alper, Schwartz, Kolts, & Khan, 2007).

NURSINGTIP 27-3

Monitoring the Use of Cyclic Antidepressants

- Antidepressants such as amitriptyline have a limited therapeutic margin.
- The therapeutic dose (300 mg/day) is such that a 3–4 day supply is equivalent to a lethal dose.

Nursing actions:

- Assess suicidal risk.
- Assess how often prescription is being refilled.
- Assess if the drug is being taken daily.
- May conduct pill counts to determine if the drug is being taken or stored.
- Blood levels of the drugs are indicated if there is a concern about dose.

Selective Serotonin Reuptake Inhibitors

In recent years, a number of drugs have been developed whose actions primarily involve serotonin-related pathways. The tricyclic clomipramine was first among these, but in more recent years a series of selective serotonin reuptake inhibitors (SSRIs) has come into widespread clinical use. Fluoxetine (Prozac), sertraline (Zoloft), paroxetine (Paxil), citalopram (Celexa), and escitalopram (Lexapro) are among the most commonly prescribed prescription medications. As noted before, cyclic antidepressants and other closely related drugs show effects on a variety of brain neurotransmitters. These multiple actions are associated both with antidepressant effectiveness and with side and adverse effects. The SSRIs offer antidepressant effect with relatively few short- and long-term side effects. This benefit comes at two costs, however: accumulating evidence of suboptimal effectiveness in milder depression (Kirsch et al., 2008), and a significant risk of drug interactions, perhaps especially with fluoxetine and fluvoxamine (Gillman, 2007).

The SSRIs have most often been used as first-line medications for depressed individuals, particularly outpatients with moderate depression. While studies have clearly established the effectiveness of SSRIs compared with placebo in severe depression, no study has demonstrated any enhanced effectiveness of SSRIs over cyclic antidepressants. Their effectiveness in mild depression has also been questioned (Kirsch et al., 2008). With the exception of fluoxetine's long metabolic effect after discontinuation, there are few clinical differences between SSRIs and no apparent pharmacological reason to select one SSRI over another other than the possible lower risk of pharmacokinetic drug interactions with escitalopram and citalopram (Spina, Santoro, & D'Arrigo, 2008). Paroxetine may be slightly more anticholinergic and cause more weight gain than other SSRIs (Ables & Baughman, 2003).

Most SSRIs are now available with generic alternatives or on drug store prescription discount programs, significantly lowering their monthly cost. Since no data suggest SSRIs are more effective than tricyclics, they are often chosen because they are perceived to have fewer side effects and a greater margin of safety in overdose. There is evidence, however, that in comparison to SSRIs, nortriptyline (a tricyclic antidepressant) may have greater efficacy, fewer drug interactions, and comparable overdose safety (Gillman, 2007).

The SSRIs have been shown to be of value in a number of conditions other than depression. For example, SSRIs are clearly effective in treating Obsessive-Compulsive Disorder; fluoxetine and fluvoxamine are well documented to be of value in this condition. In addition, paroxetine and sertraline have also gained approval for this indication. Fluoxetine and several other SSRIs have been shown to improve symptoms in bulimia. Fluoxetine, paroxetine, and sertraline have been approved for use in Panic Disorder. Premenstrual syndrome ("late luteal phase dysphoric disorder") has been shown to respond well to SSRIs in a number of patients, with fluoxetine the only SSRI currently approved for the disorder. Escitalopram and paroxetine are useful for Generalized Anxiety

Disorder, while paroxetine and sertraline are approved for Social Anxiety Disorder. Other data suggest benefit in a variety of other conditions, including Post-Traumatic Stress Disorder, migraine, chronic pain, and alcohol dependency/abuse.

The SSRIs inhibit the reuptake of serotonin after it is released at the neuronal synapse. This means that serotonin is present for a longer time, and as a consequence its action is augmented. Because they augment or amplify the effect of serotonin released at synapses, SSRIs function as if they were directly stimulating brain serotonin pathways. In reality, that stimulation is brought about by naturally released serotonin because SSRIs increase the effect of an individual's own serotonin release. In most persons, such an increase in serotonergic effect is enough, after a period of time, to improve symptoms of depression.

Pharmacologically, the various SSRIs are strikingly different in the degree to which they inhibit reuptake of both serotonin and several other neurotransmitters. Paroxetine seems to be among the strongest inhibitors of serotonin reuptake, but it also inhibits uptake of norepinephrine and dopamine. Sertraline is a bit less potent in its inhibition of serotonin reuptake, but has even more inhibition of dopamine uptake than paroxetine. In contrast, fluvoxamine differs little from sertraline in its effects on serotonin reuptake, but it is strikingly ineffective in altering dopamine uptake (Boyer & Feighner, 1991). These differences among the various SSRIs are pharmacologically interesting, but there is as yet no evidence that they have any clinical importance. All of the SSRIs significantly alter serotonin effects at the synapse; the differences in their effects on other neurotransmitters so far seem relatively unimportant.

Dose/Administration

The SSRIs are all well absorbed after oral administration and are widely distributed throughout the body (including the brain). Dosage of SSRIs must be individualized and differs for each preparation. Compared with other antidepressants, most of the SSRIs have a fairly narrow therapeutic dose "window." Sertraline, for example, may be given in doses from 50 mg up to 200 mg, but effectiveness may decrease as dosage exceeds 200 mg (Tollefson, 1995). Blood levels of SSRIs have not been shown to be of clinical use in assessing nonresponse or toxicity. As with cyclic antidepressants, it is generally thought that SSRIs take some time to work, typically at least a month, though some effect on depression may be seen after 10 to 14 days. Based on this clinical belief, doses are rarely altered until after three to four weeks have elapsed, and it is often taught that there may be no benefit in raising the dose for up to eight weeks (Schweizer, Rickels, Amsterdam, Fox, Puzzuolu, & Weise 1990). In contrast, more recent but still somewhat preliminary data suggest that an SSRI antidepressant effect can be seen within three days and is quite significant within three weeks (Mitchell, 2006). While an antidepressant switch is still indicated if a medication does not produce the desired effect after an appropriate waiting period, there is no good evidence to guide clinicians how to select the next medication to try (Ruhe, Huyser, Swinkels, & Schene, 2006). Convenience may dictate some choices; for example, the SSRI drug fluoxetine is marketed in a long-acting form that allows once-weekly oral administration.

With the exception of fluoxetine, most SSRIs have elimination half-lives of about 24 hours. Fluoxetine's elimination half-life is somewhat longer, 24 to 72 hours, but unlike other SSRIs, fluoxetine has major metabolites that themselves have half-lives of up to 15 days. This means that in clinical use fluoxetine is uniquely long acting and has significant effects for many days after discontinuation. This characteristic is useful in preventing emergence of depressive symptoms if one or more doses are missed, but may be a problem either when side effects require discontinuation or when it is necessary to switch to another medication (such as a tricyclic or an MAOI) that may interact with fluoxetine. A full five-week "washout" period is recommended before starting a new medication. If the long-acting fluoxetine preparation is used, an even longer washout is required. This may greatly delay effective treatment for individuals who do not respond to fluoxetine. The washout period for other SSRIs is generally two weeks (American Psychiatric Association, 2000). This washout is very critical and hence longer when moving from SSRI treatment to administration of an MAOI because MAOIs may interact dangerously with residual SSRIs long after the last dose has been given.

Drug Actions

All of the SSRIs can probably relieve symptoms of depression after two to four weeks. Some patients benefit from even longer trials of six or more weeks. Clients report enhanced mood and decreased concern about thoughts or problems that previously would have upset or worried them. The SSRIs are often useful in management of Obsessive-Compulsive Disorder (though usually at higher dose than for the management of depression). As with depression, improvement of Obsessive-Compulsive Disorder is also delayed for some weeks. Many clients with depression also report significant anxiety, a symptom that generally decreases or disappears as medication brings depression under control. Symptoms of Panic Disorder also tend to resolve during treatment with SSRIs, although agoraphobia, commonly seen along with Panic Disorder, is less consistently improved.

Drug Interactions

As noted later, SSRI side and adverse effects are relatively mild; in contrast, the risk of drug interactions with these drugs may be of more concern than with many of the cyclic antidepressants (Gillman, 2007). Fluvoxamine and paroxetine interact with warfarin (Coumadin). Cimetidine (Tagamet; available over the counter as well as by prescription) may raise SSRI concentrations by impairing hepatic metabolism. Some clinicians combine SSRIs and tricyclics in an effort to utilize the latters' sedative qualities, but this practice may not always be safe because SSRIs may raise tricyclic blood levels and increase risk of toxicity. Monoamine oxidase inhibitors may interact significantly with SSRIs, and as noted previously, because of relatively long elimination half-lives, at least two weeks should be allowed for drug washout between stopping an SSRI and starting an MAOI (five weeks for "short acting" fluoxetine).

The SSRIs are less likely to increase the sedative or intoxicating potential of alcohol than are cyclic medications. Whereas sertraline absorption is affected when taken with or near meals, other SSRIs are uninfluenced by food.

A rare and potentially serious drug interaction (usually with an MAOI) is called the **serotonergic syndrome** and resembles somewhat symptoms seen in intentional SSRI overdose. Symptoms include agitation, sweating, increase in neuromuscular tone, fever, hyperreflexia, tachycardia, and hypertension (Dvir & Smallwood, 2008). On occasion coma and even death may occur. The serotonergic syndrome is most commonly seen following drug interaction between an SSRI and an MAOI. Many other agents such as meperidine (Demerol) and the antibiotic, linezolid (Zyvox), have been associated with drug interactions that have caused the serotonergic syndrome (Boyer & Shannon, 2006). As with overdose, treatment is largely supportive.

Use During Pregnancy/Lactation

Most SSRIs have been given a category C rating for pregnancy safety, with paroxetine having a D rating. An earlier study claimed that fluoxetine taken in late pregnancy increased the risk of premature birth and led to higher frequency of respiratory and other problems in the newborn period (Chambers, Johnson, Dick, Feley, & Jones, 1996). More recent studies on 17 newborns whose mothers were prescribed SSRI medications during pregnancy show differences in newborn arousal and behavior that seem to be attributable to the medications (Zeskind & Stephens, 2004). Whether these effects persist or have long-term consequences remains to be established. Animal studies do not suggest harm, and there are no human data contraindicating use of the drug in pregnancy. These drugs do appear in breast milk in approximately the same concentration as serum. While no data suggest harm to infants from absorbing SSRIs during breast feeding, many clinicians counsel caution in combining breast feeding and SSRI administration until long-term studies are available documenting safety for the infant (Misri, Kostaras, & Kostaras, 2000).

Side Effects

Overall, the SSRIs are among the best tolerated antidepressants. In short-term trials, 10% to 20% of patients have discontinued SSRIs because of side effects, compared with 30% to 35% taking tricyclic medications (Tollefson, 1995). Common side effects include anxiety, headache, and gastrointestinal disturbance (nausea, diarrhea). The SSRIs are particularly likely to interfere with sexual functioning (erection in men and orgasm in both men and women). Clients may not volunteer that they are experiencing these side effects, so it is important for the nurse to inquire explicitly about any sexual dysfunction. Since depression is itself associated with decreased libido and sexual functioning, it may occasionally be difficult to be certain whether reported sexual dysfunction is due to the drug or to depression itself. The SSRIs, particularly fluoxetine, can cause akathisia, a symptom of restlessness discussed in this chapter as a side effect of antipsychotic medications.

Although it was initially thought that SSRIs lead to weight *loss*, further experience with these agents has identified weight gain as a major side effect of several of these agents and of many of the newer non-SSRI antidepressants as well. If they are prescribed a medication known to be associated with weight gain, nurses should counsel clients about proper diet and exercise (Ferguson, 2001). For those with pre-existing obesity, diabetes, or other contributing risks for obesity or its complications, medications such as bupropion with a relatively low tendency to cause weight gain may be considered.

Adverse Effects

The SSRIs are generally free of serious adverse effects, even in intentional overdose. Deaths have occurred following SSRI overdoses, particularly when taken in combination with alcohol. However, death is a rare complication of SSRI overdose, and most patients recover uneventfully with supportive care. Venlafaxine, while not technically an SSRI, has been associated with overdose fatalities (Deshauer, 2007) as has citalopram (Flanagan, 2008). Serotonergic syndrome, discussed earlier under drug interactions, may occasionally occur without known administration of any drug other than SSRIs. As noted earlier, symptoms include agitation, sweating, rigidity, fever, hyperreflexia, tachycardia, and hypertension. Treatment is largely supportive but must be given with vigilance to avoid a potentially fatal outcome. An important concern has been the increased incidence of suicidal ideation and completed suicide in some persons taking SSRI medications (Dudley, Hadzi-Pavlovic, Andrews, & Perich, 2008). The concerns have primarily involved adolescents and young adults and have been largely focused on paroxetine. Nonetheless, available data suggest a potentially increased risk for nearly all of the SSRI drugs with the possible exception of fluoxetine. The Food and Drug Administration (FDA) has required antidepressant manufacturers to place black box package warnings. In Britain, psychiatrists are no longer allowed to prescribe SSRIs other than fluoxetine to young persons. This decision was taken in part because of the apparent enhanced risk of suicide and in part because of evidence that medications commonly prescribed to treat depression in children (notably paroxetine and venlafaxine) were seemingly ineffective for this indication (Garland, 2004). An important unresolved question is whether there is increased risk of suicidal ideation or attempt in *adults* treated with second-generation antidepressants (Seemuller, Riedel, Obermeier, Bauer, Adli, Mundt, et al., 2008). There is a fuller discussion of this controversy in Chapter 14.

Monoamine Oxidase Inhibitors

Monoamine oxidase inhibitors (MAOIs) are a group of drugs notable for their similar pharmacological actions, their good effectiveness in treatment of depression, and their potentially dangerous interactions with both drugs and foods. The MAOIs are useful "second-line" drugs for treating mood disorders, but can only be used safely with careful monitoring in highly motivated clients.

Indications and Evidence for Effectiveness

The MAOIs have demonstrated effectiveness in depression, Panic Disorder, some other anxiety disorders (social phobia, Obsessive-Compulsive Disorder, Post-Traumatic Stress Disorder), and bulimia. The "classical" nonselective agents isocarboxazid (Marplan), phenelzine (Nardil), and tranylcypromine (Parnate) have generally been regarded as second- or third-line antidepressant medications, to be tried when tricyclics or SSRIs fail. A double-blind crossover study found phenelzine effective in the majority of clients who failed a trial of imipramine (McGrath, et al., 1993). Many of these clients had atypical depression (see Chapter 14), a condition for which MAOIs and SSRIs are probably more effective than are tricyclic agents. Some data suggest that dysthymia (see Chapter 14) may respond more effectively to MAOIs than to tricyclics, but as with atypical depression, most clinicians are likely to utilize SSRIs for these individuals. Elderly clients may respond particularly well to MAOIs.

As more selective reversible MAOIs are released, these medications may become even more widely used. Recently developed MAOIs seem to interact less significantly with foods and medications, have fewer side effects, and are probably at least as effective as the older MAOI agents. The FDA's release of selegiline, particularly in a formulation administered by a skin patch requiring change every 24 hours, has offered an entirely new approach to MAOI usage that likely has fewer complications from food and drug interactions (Robinson & Amsterdam, 2008).

Pharmacology

The MAOIs act by blocking an enzyme (monoamine oxidase) whose primary purpose is to metabolize three important brain neurotransmitters (norepinephrine, serotonin, and dopamine) to biologically inactive forms. The inhibition of monoamine oxidase prevents the breakdown of the neurotransmitters and increases the concentration of these substances within neuronal cells. Over several weeks, this pharmacological effect results in changes in the number of cell-surface receptors for the involved neurotransmitters. Pharmacologists attribute the clinical usefulness of MAOIs both to this change in receptor levels and to increased amine levels. The MAOIs are commonly categorized by whether or not they fit into the following three groups: (1) those that belong to the chemical family of "hydrazines," (2) those that inhibit monoamine oxidase reversibly, and (3) those that are selective for one of the two forms of monoamine oxidase, MAO-A or MAO-B. The most frequently prescribed MAOI, phenelzine (Nardil) is a hydrazine that is a nonreversible inhibitor and is nonselective. Tranylcypromine (Parnate) is a similar nonhydrazine drug. Moclobemide remains unreleased in the United States, but it is both selective for MAO-A and reversible. Reversible inhibitors may be safer if food or drug interactions occur. MAO-A affects primarily dopamine and norepinephrine metabolism, whereas MAO-B is relatively selective for serotonin. It seems highly likely that reversible MAO-A inhibitors offer clinical advantages and will soon be available in the United States. Pure MAO-B inhibitors are not in common clinical use, and there is little evidence to suggest that selective inhibitors offer any benefit over nonselective drugs. While selegiline may have a greater affinity for MAO-B, it inhibits both MAO-A and MAO-B at transdermal doses. Selegiline (Emsam) is the only transdermal antidepressant available.

Dose/Administration

The MAOIs are all given orally, are well absorbed, and reach peak plasma levels within approximately one hour. The half-life is about 12 hours, but because most of these drugs have long-acting metabolites, at least two weeks should elapse between stopping an MAOI and starting a different antidepressant. The MAOIs should be stopped gradually to avoid significant side effects.

Phenelzine is given three times per day with a rapid increase of dose from 15 to 20 mg. Total daily doses up to 90 mg are often used initially, but as the desired effects are seen, the dosage is often reduced to as little as 15 mg daily or every other day. Tranylcypromine is given two times per day at 15 mg/dose. Increases are made fairly slowly over two to four weeks. When desired response is achieved, dosage is also dropped to low levels—typically 10 to 20 mg daily.

Transdermal selegiline (Emsam) is likely a safer medication than any of the previous drugs. Co-administration of a number of medications must still be avoided (a partial list includes most other antidepressants, and a variety of vasoconstrictors, anticonvulsants, and sympathomimetic drugs—as, for example, might be found in cold medications). Food limitations still apply to persons using the patch at doses of 9 mg/24 hours and 12 mg/24 hours. According to the manufacturer (Emsam [package insert]. Princeton, NJ: Bristol-Myers Squibb; 2008 February) the lower dose of 6 mg/24 hours does not require dietary restrictions.

Drug Actions

The MAOIs are used for depression of all degrees of severity. Tranylcypromine is somewhat more commonly employed in very severe depression and may have an effect sooner than other antidepressants, sometimes within 10 days. Tranylcypromine is chemically related to amphetamines (see the next general section on miscellaneous drugs for depression) and like amphetamines produces a stimulant effect that may contribute to drug effectiveness. Otherwise, like other categories of antidepressants, MAOIs take three to four weeks to improve symptoms of depression. As noted before, monoamine oxidase inhibition occurs quite rapidly, especially with irreversible inhibitors, but antidepressant effect typically takes some time to develop. This delay suggests that enzyme inhibition is only one of the effects that lead to improvement of depressive symptoms.

Drug Interactions

Significant drug interactions occur with MAOIs and may be quite serious (Rapaport, 2007). Since MAOIs inhibit the metabolism and detoxification of biogenic amines, ingestion of these substances or their analogues may result in prolonged and severe stimulation of nervous system pathways. The major drug interaction risks are other antidepressants (particularly SSRIs), narcotic analgesics (especially meperidine [Demerol] and dextromethorphan, a common ingredient in nonprescription cough medications such as Robitussin-DM), and various preparations containing sympathomimetic drugs. The latter include a variety of decongestants and cold medications. The SSRIs are sometimes purposefully used with MAOIs, and many experts feel the risks have been exaggerated. Surgery is particularly dangerous for persons on MAOIs because of the potential inadvertent administration of meperidine to control postoperative pain. The interaction between meperidine and MAOIs may result in coma, fever, and hypertension. Other drug-MAOI interactions may be dangerous and result in very high blood pressure, headache, sweating, and palpitations. Severe interactions may progress to decreased consciousness, extreme fever, intracranial hemorrhage, and death. Inadvertent medication interactions can be treated with a calcium channel blocker, typically nifedipine (Procardia). Usually a single oral dose will rapidly lower blood pressure and block the effects of drug interaction. When nifedipine is ineffective, phentolamine (Regitine) may be given intravenously. Sympathomimetic drugs pose somewhat uncertain and variable risks. In general, "direct" sympathomimetics such as epinephrine, norepinephrine, phenylephrine, isoproterenol, and methoxymine have the least serious interactions. "Indirect" sympathomimetics include amphetamine, methamphetamine, ephedrine, pseudoephedrine, phenylpropanolamine, and others. Many of these medications are available either as stimulant street drugs or as common ingredients in over-the-counter cough and cold treatments. Individuals on MAOIs must exercise great care to avoid these indirect sympathomimetics. Symptoms are similar to the meperidine interaction and include hypertension, agitation, fever, convulsions, and coma.

Food and Alcohol Interactions

One of the major deterrents to the use of MAOIs is that a number of foods react strongly with these medications to produce serious reactions identical to those that accompany the interaction between MAOIs and sympathomimetics or meperidine. Most offending foods contain significant amounts of the amino acid tyramine, which is an indirect sympathomimetic agent. Individuals taking MAOIs must avoid foods containing more than 6 mg of tyramine. Intake between 6 and 10 mg provokes a moderate reaction: elevated blood pressure, headache, restlessness. Ingestion of 25 mg or more may result in severe symptoms requiring emergency treatment. Death may occasionally occur from such dietary indiscretions. Few if any foods have more than 25 mg of tyramine in a single serving, though some "strong" cheeses may have as much as 15 to 17 mg. Aged cheddar cheese (often labeled "sharp") contains 7.5 mg per slice, whereas Swiss gruyere has 1.9 mg. Salami has 5.6 mg per serving, whereas liverwurst has only 0.1 mg. Sauerkraut has very high tyramine levels, and fairly high amounts are found in banana peels (though not in the fruit itself). Alcoholic beverages may interact with MAOIs, though not all experts agree on the potential seriousness of such interaction. Some imported beers have moderate tyramine concentrations; Guinness Extra Stout, for example, has slightly over a milligram per bottle. Red wines have small amounts of tyramine per 4-ounce serving, generally half a milligram or less. White wines, whiskey, gin, and vodka are probably safe in quantities up to 4 ounces. Even this restriction may be conservative since consuming a liter of Dubonnet would likely result in intake of less than 2 mg of tyramine (Ciraulo, et al. 1994). Clearly, individuals on MAOIs must be carefully instructed on avoiding risky foods and beverages. Selecting foods that can be safely consumed is not difficult but requires vigilance, especially when eating in restaurants. When MAOIs are prescribed, the nurse will need to assist the client in acquiring the necessary skills to avoid dangerous medication or food interactions.

NURSING ALERT 27-5

Demerol and MAOIs

- **Meperidine (Demerol) should not be given to persons taking MAOIs!**
- **There is a severe interaction between MAOIs and meperidine that produces fever, hypertension, and coma.**

NURSING ALERT 27-6

MAOIs and Dextromethorphan (Robitussin-DM, Delsym)

Persons taking MAOIs must be alerted to the fact that over-the-counter medications with dextromethorphan, a common ingredient of cough medication, interact with MAOIs, producing hypertension, fever, and possibly coma.

Use During Pregnancy/Lactation

The MAOIs are category C agents in pregnancy. Human data are sparse, and animal data suggest teratogenic potential for some agents. These drugs are usually avoided during pregnancy. Little data exist on use during lactation, and it is probably unwise to use these medications in lactating mothers.

BOX 27-1
FOODS TO BE AVOIDED BY PERSONS TAKING MAOIs

FOODS TO BE COMPLETELY AVOIDED:

- Sharp (old) cheddar cheese
- Salami
- Sauerkraut
- Beer containing yeast
- Yeast extracts
- Wine containing yeast
- Avocados (overripe)
- Caviar
- Fava beans

FOODS THAT CAN BE CONSUMED IF USED IN MODERATION:

- Chocolate
- Coffee

Side Effects

Common side effects of nonselective MAOIs are decreased heart rate, hypotension (which may lead to dizziness or syncope), and a variety of anticholinergic symptoms: dry mouth, blurred vision, and urinary hesitancy. Central nervous system symptoms occur on occasion and include agitation, anxiety, insomnia, and euphoria. Sexual dysfunction, weight gain, peripheral neuropathy, and impaired speech may sometimes occur as side effects. Newer MAOI agents such as moclobemide are remarkably generally free of these side effects, but may occasionally cause nausea.

Adverse Effects

The most serious adverse effects of nonselective, nonreversible agents include syncope from hypotension, potentially resulting in physical injury and either hepatic abnormality or bone marrow suppression. Routine monitoring of liver functions or blood counts are usually not necessary. On occasion MAOIs can produce hypomania or full-blown psychosis. Clients with a history of mania or hypomania should generally be placed on mood stabilizers rather than antidepressants. When selective MAO-A inhibitors are released, they will probably come into fairly widespread usage because they are generally free of serious adverse effects. Table 27-2 presents a summary of MAOIs as well as the antidepressants.

Miscellaneous Antidepressant Drug Categories and Drug Combinations

It has been convenient to think of antidepressants as divided neatly into three categories: tricyclics, SSRIs, and MAOIs. This classification has always omitted some medications that do not fit into one of those categories, so it is rapidly becoming outmoded. As more is understood of the basic neurophysiology of mood disorders, pharmaceutical companies are working to develop drugs with greater specificity (and therefore fewer unwanted side effects) and with more rapid onset of antidepressant action. The result has been a proliferation of new drugs that in turn create new categories: (1) serotonin noradrenergic reuptake inhibitors (SNaRIs), (2) selective noradrenaline reuptake inhibitor (NaRI), and (3) noradrenergic and specific serotonergic antidepressants (NaSSAs). Venlafaxine and duloxetine are SNaRIs; Mirtazapine is a NaSSA; and Reboxetine (not available in the United States) is a NaRI. There is some limited evidence that adding noradrenergic effect to serotonergic antidepressants may offer a small benefit (Papakostas, 2007), but in most mental health units the process of selecting an antidepressant is either arbitrary or governed by cost considerations.

Venlafaxine (Effexor, Effexor XR) and duloxetine (Cymbalta) are serotonin noradrenergic reuptake inhibitors. Venlafaxine inhibits serotonin at lower doses, while noradrenergic reuptake blockade occurs at higher doses in its dosing range. Conversely, duloxetine inhibits both serotonin and norepinephrine across its entire dosing range. Both antidepressants may cause elevations in blood pressure. Venlafaxine's metabolite, desvenlafaxine, is marketed as the antidepressant Pristiq. Duloxetine, which carries a risk of liver toxicity, is also formally approved for diabetic neuropathic pain and fibromyalgia (Teter, Kando, Wells, & Hayes, 2008).

Other available antidepressants include bupropion (Wellbutrin) and mirtazapine (Remeron). Bupropion inhibits the reuptake of dopamine and norepinephrine. Advantages include little weight gain and lack of sexual side effects. A significant adverse reaction is bupropion's ability to lower the seizure threshold. Mirtazapine acts as an antagonist at presynaptic alpha2 receptors and various serotonin receptors. Important side effects include sedation, weight gain, and possible increases in lipid levels. Interestingly, more sedation is noted at lower doses and less sedation at higher doses.

Finally, nefazodone (Serzone) is similar to trazodone in terms of its mechanism of action. Major differences include a black box warning for nefazodone regarding hepatoxicity as well as its potent inhibition of cytochrome P450 3A4.

Several medications have some utility in managing depression, although they are not usually considered to be first-line antidepressants. Among these are alprazolam (Xanax), amphetamines or other stimulant medications, and buspirone (BuSpar). Each of these drugs has other primary indications (anxiety and Panic Disorder for alprazolam, Attention-Deficit Disorder for amphetamines, and Generalized Anxiety Disorder for buspirone). While lacking Food and Drug Administration approval for depression, each of these three medications has some demonstrated effectiveness for depression. Buspirone has been shown effective in a number of trials, but quite large doses are required, often as high as 60 mg daily. Such high doses (two to four times the usual dose for treating anxiety) are very expensive, and although safe and relatively well tolerated, buspirone is unlikely to find

Table 27-2 Antidepressant Medications

GENERIC NAME	ANTITRADE NAME	ANTI-CHOLINERGIC	EPHRINE-SEDATION	ORTHOSTASIS	NOREPINEPHRINE BLOCKING ACTIVITY	SEROTONIN BLOCKING ACTIVITY	HALF-LIFE (HOURS)	DOSE RANGE (MG/DAY)
Tertiary tricyclics								
Amitriptyline	Elavil	4+	4+	2+	2+	2+	31–46	25–300
Doxepin	Sinequan, Adapin	2+	3+	2+	1+	2+	08–24	25–300
Imipramine	Tofranil	2+	2+	3+	2+	4+	11–25	25–300
Trimipramine	Surmontil	2+	3+	2+	1+	1+	07–30	50–300
Secondary amines								
Amoxapine	Asendin	3+	2+	1+	3+	2+	08–30	50–600
Desipramine	Norpramin	2+	1+	1+	4+	2+	12–24	25–300
Nortriptyline	Pamelor	2+	2+	1+	2+	3+	18–44	30–100
Protriptyline	Vivactil	3+	1+	1+	4+	2+	67–89	15–600
Phenethylamines	(SNaRIs)							
Venlafaxine	Effexor	0	0	0	3+	3+	05–11	75–375*
Tetracyclic amines								
Maprotiline	Ludiomil	2+	2+	1+	3+	1+	21–25	50–225
Mirtazapine	Remeron	1+	2+	0	0	0	20–40	15–45
Phenylpiperazines								
Nefazodone	Serzone	1+	3+	3+	3+	3+	2–4	200–600
Trazodone	Desyrel	1+	3+	2+	0	3+	4–9	150–600
Aminoketones								
Bupropion	Wellbutrin	1+	0	0	1+	1+	08–24	200–450
SSRIs								
Fluoxetine	Prozac	0	0	0	1+	4+	>72	10–80
Paroxetine	Paxil	0	0	0	1+	4+	10–24	10–60†
Sertraline	Zoloft	0	0	0	1+	4+	24	50–200
Citalopram	Celexa	0	0	0	1+	1+	16–24	40
Escitalopram	Lexapro	0	0	0	1+	1+	27–32	5–20
MAOIs								
Phenelzine	Nardil	0	0	1+	0	0	6–8	30–90
Tranylcypramine	Parnate	0	0	1+	0	0	6–8	10–40

*375 mg for immediate release. Recommended maximum of 225 mg for extended-release
†Paroxetine CR: dosage 12.5–62.5 mg

wide use. Habituation and abuse limit the usefulness of alprazolam and stimulants.

Several additional drugs have shown promise in treating refractory depressive symptoms when combined as "augmentation" with other more standard medication regimens (Nelson, 2007). Lithium may be given in combination with tricyclics, SSRIs, or MAOIs. These combinations may produce quite rapid antidepressant response (48–72 hours) in individuals who have failed other treatments, but it is more common for medications to take several weeks to improve symptoms. Evidence from several studies supports the effectiveness of lithium in reducing suicide risk among clients with Bipolar Disorder (Tondo & Baldessarini, 2000). Similar benefits have been claimed for lower-dose augmentation therapy of unipolar depression (Schule, Baghai, Eser, Nothdurfter, & Rupprecht, 2008). When combined with tricyclics for the treatment of unresponsive depression, thyroid hormone has been found as effective as lithium and significantly better than placebo (Joffe, Singer, Levitt, & MacDonald., 1993), but the role, if any, for this hormone in the management of depression remains elusive (Cooper-Kazaz & Lerer, 2008).

Like lithium, second-generation antipsychotics may reduce the risk of suicide, and they also seem to act as effective augmenting agents when combined with antidepressants (Papakostas, Peterse, Nierenberg, Murakami, Alpert, Rosenbaum, et al., 2004; Reeves, Batra, May, Zhang, Dahl, & Li, 2008). It seems likely that this combination of SSRI or similar medications with a second-generation antipsychotic will become more widely used even when managing suicidality is not the primary clinical focus (Keitner, Garlow, Ryan, Ninan, Solomon, Nemeroff, et al., 2008). Aripiprazole (Abilify) is currently the only second-generation antipsychotic currently approved as an adjunct treatment for Major Depressive Disorder.

Mood Stabilizers

Mood-stabilizing medications are typically used to control the symptoms of mania and, once controlled, to prevent its recurrence. The most commonly utilized antimanic drugs are lithium (Lithobid, Eskalith), carbamazepine (Tegretol), and two very closely related drugs: valproic acid (Depakene) and divalproex (Depakote).

Other anticonvulsant drugs—notably gabapentin (Neurontin)—have come into use both as mood stabilizers in their own right and as antidepressant augmenting agents. Since the evidence supporting effectiveness is somewhat uncertain, these drugs are generally used only when other treatments have proven ineffective.

Indications and Evidence for Effectiveness

Mood stabilizers are indicated for the management of mania. They can be used both to treat acute mania and to prevent the recurrence of mania in individuals who have a history of manic episodes. Antidepressants can provoke manic episodes in bipolar individuals (including those with Bipolar II Disorder where only hypomania has previously occurred). Prior treatment with mood stabilizers can prevent this occasional and undesirable outcome.

Numerous studies show that both divalproex and lithium are effective in the control and prevention of mania. About 80% of individuals respond to lithium, though response is typically delayed by at least one to two weeks. Lithium is generally effective in controlling depressive symptoms in individuals with Bipolar Disorder, so that most of these persons do not need other antidepressants. The data for other mood stabilizers are less well established, but antimanic effects have been most convincingly shown for carbamazepine. Since 1978, multiple studies have shown that carbamazepine is more effective than placebo in the control of mania. Most of these studies are small, but the effectiveness of carbamazepine has been adequately established (Stoner, Nelson, Lea, Marken, Sommi, & Dahmen, 2007). A longer-acting form of carbamazepine allows dosing intervals to be reduced to twice daily—improving ease of administration and probably enhancing client adherence (Weisler, Keck, Swann, Cutler, Ketter, Kalali, et al., 2005). Some data also suggest that certain types of mania, including rapid-cycling mania, may respond better to carbamazepine than to lithium (Delgado & Gelenberg, 1995). Lamotrigine, like divalproex and carbamazepine primarily an anti-epilepsy drug, is also effective in controlling symptoms of mania. In general, either lithium or divalproex is used as primary treatment, with the other mood stabilizers employed only if lithium fails or is not tolerated. Divalproex may, however, be particularly effective in managing adolescents with mania or hypomania. In this group of clients it may frequently be the first mood stabilizer utilized. The combination of mood stabilization and a second-generation antipsychotic such as olanzepine is commonly used for managing mania (Vieta, Panicali, Goetz, Reed, Comes, Tohen, et al. 2008), but at least one study suggests that carbamazepine alone is equally effective and associated with fewer adverse effects (Tohen et al., 2008).

Pharmacology

The neurobiology of mania is as yet incompletely understood, and as a result the precise mechanism of action of the mood stabilizers remains unknown. One of the extraordinary characteristics of lithium is that it has virtually no psychotropic effects in nonmanic individuals. Lithium is neither a sedative nor a depressant drug, and it appears not to affect mood in persons who do not have mania.

Lithium is well absorbed after an oral dose and is not metabolized in any way after absorption. Peak levels occur within two to four hours, longer with extended release preparations, after ingestion of a single dose. Lithium is not bound to protein and is excreted almost completely by the proximal tubules of the kidney. Once in the circulation, lithium has a mean half-life of 18 hours; there is considerable range in this half-life (10 to 30 hours) so that lithium levels are often required to establish the appropriate dose. Individuals whose clearance of lithium is more rapid will have lower serum levels at a given dose, whereas those with slower clearance will have higher levels. Since lithium has a narrow **therapeutic window** (blood levels only a little above the therapeutic range may lead to serious adverse effects), blood levels can allow both effective and safe administration.

Carbamazepine (Tegretol) is most commonly used as an anticonvulsant but has become more widely used in the management of mania as well. Like lithium, carbamazepine is absorbed after oral dosage, but unlike lithium, it is metabolized by the liver and circulates in the plasma almost completely bound to protein. The absorption of carbamazepine is also somewhat delayed and is quite variable from individual to individual. Peak levels may not be reached until 24 hours after a dose. The half-life of carbamazepine is also variable and ranges from 10 to 20 hours in individuals who have taken the drug for some weeks. Carbamazepine has the property of inducing increased levels of the enzymes that metabolize it in the liver. As a result, the half-life is much longer in the first few days that the drug is taken or after a single dose.

Divalproex more closely resembles lithium in its absorption. Peak concentrations are reached after one to four hours, and the half-life is about 15 hours. Like carbamazepine, divalproex is strongly bound to plasma proteins and is metabolized in the liver (though by a different enzymatic pathway than the one that acts on carbamazepine).

Dose/Administration

Lithium dosage is typically 1800 mg (two 300-mg capsules or tablets given three times daily) for acute mania and 900 to 1200 mg total daily dose (typically in three divided doses) for maintenance. All lithium administration needs to be accompanied by careful monitoring of serum levels, but this is particularly true when high doses are utilized. Lithium levels are most commonly maintained between 0.6 and 1.2 mEq/L, though levels up to 1.5 mEq/L are sometimes required for control of acute symptoms. Levels much above 1.5 mEq/L are often associated with unacceptable symptoms of toxicity such as lethargy and dizziness. Very high levels may produce EKG changes and potentially fatal cardiac toxicity.

Carbamazepine is administered in divided doses with a total of 400 to 1200 mg given daily. Levels are frequently measured, and as in seizure control, the desirable levels are between 4 and 12 mcg/mL. Divalproex is similarly given in doses of 500 to 1500 mg daily to achieve levels of 50 to 125 mcg/mL.

Drug Actions

The specific antimanic pharmacological actions of lithium remain unknown (Lenox & Hahn, 2000). Chemically, lithium is a metallic element closely related to sodium and is chemically recognized as sodium in brain pathways. This substitution may affect the way that neurotransmitters react, and it certainly influences many of the aspects of lithium side effects and toxicity to be discussed later. Lithium appears to affect cellular handling of sodium, and there is some evidence that intracellular sodium is elevated in Bipolar Disorder (Huang & El-Mallakh, 2007). Anticonvulsant drugs such as carbamazepine and divalproex (valproic acid) have effects on brain electrical functions. These effects reduce the brain's susceptibility to disorganized electrical activity, which produces seizure disorders, but their relationship to the control of mania remains incompletely understood.

Drug and Food Interactions

Since lithium interacts with body sodium metabolism, any drug that affects sodium levels may interact with lithium. Common antihypertensives such as ACE inhibitors (lisinopril, enalapril) may increase lithium levels. Diuretics (often used to combat the lithium side effect of peripheral edema) may influence lithium effectiveness and safety by lowering serum sodium through increased excretion, thereby increasing sodium reabsorption and hence elevating lithium levels. Similarly, since lithium and sodium share the same pathways for renal excretion, a low-salt diet may result in decreased lithium excretion and therefore high lithium levels. Many nonsteroidal anti-inflammatory drugs (NSAIDs), including a variety of nonprescription medications, can affect sodium excretion and increase lithium levels. This risk occurs with ibuprofen (Motrin, Advil), naproxen (Aleve), and probably ketoprofen (Orudis). A variety of prescription anti-inflammatory drugs can have similar effects: indomethacin (Indocin), piroxicam (Feldene), and phenylbutazone (Butazolodin). The NSAID sulindac (Clinoril) may be an exception to this drug interaction. Haloperidol (potentially used to treat psychosis in Bipolar Disorder) may interact to produce a dangerous encephalopathic syndrome potentially leading to permanent CNS damage. Aminophylline, less commonly used for asthma than in past years but still relatively frequently prescribed, can decrease lithium levels and precipitate manic relapse.

Carbamazepine is strongly affected by interactions with the large number of drugs that affect the liver cytochrome system. Erythromycin may specifically interact with carbamazepine and raise blood levels, leading to toxicity. Cimetidine (Tagamet), widely used and available without prescription, can have similar effects.

Since divalproex and valproic acid are also metabolized by the liver, they have a number of potential interactions that may be of clinical importance. Each prolongs anticoagulant effects in clients treated with warfarin (Coumadin) and increases the effects of MAOIs. Valproic acid may increase levels of lamotrigine. Lower doses of lamotrigine should be used.

Use During Pregnancy/Lactation

Lithium is potentially cardiotoxic and is usually not advised during pregnancy. Lithium teratogenicity is probably limited to the first trimester, and some psychiatrists will prescribe lithium for women in more advanced stages of pregnancy. Nonetheless, manic individuals may exhibit poor sexual decision-making as part of their manic condition and as a consequence may not infrequently become pregnant while on lithium. They may also fail to seek prenatal care early in the first trimester and as a consequence may remain on lithium during the first 8 to 12 weeks in which important organ systems (particularly the vulnerable circulatory system) are undergoing morphogenesis. Fortunately, the teratogenic risk of lithium seems relatively low, and fetal malformation occurs only rarely. Carbamazepine and divalproex *may* have less risk during early pregnancy and are sometimes substituted for lithium. However, depakote is classified as pregnancy category D, with a black box warning concerning teratogenic effects during pregnancy including neural tube defects. The management of mania during pregnancy is a difficult problem that should be undertaken with expert consultation.

Side Effects

Lithium has a spectrum of side effects that are often troubling to clients. Almost everyone who takes this medication develops thirst and polyuria because of the effect of lithium on the kidney. Another very common side effect is tremor, most noticeable in fine motor activities such as writing, buttoning clothes, and sewing. This tremor can be particularly troublesome to artistic individuals who need good fine motor coordination for their work. Weight gain is less common, but does occur in up to 30% of individuals. A smaller percentage of persons experience chronic diarrhea, which can also be an early sign of toxicity and, when of recent onset, requires that blood levels be measured immediately. The nurse can assist clients to distinguish between nuisance side effects and those that, like diarrhea, can be warning signs for more serious adverse effects. Thyroid enlargement and even frank hypothyroidism may occur in persons taking lithium. Thyroid abnormality is less common than other side effects, but does occasionally occur and may require treatment. Most individuals on lithium should have periodic measurements of their thyroid function (usually thyroid-stimulating hormone [TSH]). Other side effects include a host of dermatological effects, including acne, psoriasis, and folliculitis.

Carbamazepine is generally better tolerated than is lithium, although occasional individuals may have dizziness, and drowsiness often occurs, at least initially. Unfortunately, carbamazepine may seriously affect bone marrow function and, occasionally, liver enzymes. Fatal agranulocytosis (loss of all functioning polymorphonuclear white blood cells) may result if blood counts are not carefully monitored. Agranulocytosis leads to serious infections and may not infrequently prove fatal. Persons beginning carbamazepine treatment generally require frequent (usually weekly) testing of blood counts and often of liver enzymes as well. The frequency of testing may decrease if results remain normal over time.

Divalproex is generally very well tolerated, but has occasionally been associated with fatal liver damage, especially in children with epilepsy. Individuals on divalproex may benefit from careful monitoring of liver functions to help avoid this catastrophic outcome. The nurse can assist clients to remember to get any needed blood testing and to be alert for symptoms (loss of appetite, darkened urine, lightened stool, yellow color to skin, profound fatigue) that may indicate impending liver failure. Divalproex has also been associated with cases of life-threatening pancreatitis (Gerstner, Busing, Bell, Longin, Kasper, Klostermann, et al., 2007). Symptoms may include nausea, vomiting, and abdominal pain. Lamotrigine has relatively few common side effects, but it is occasionally associated with Stevens-Johnson syndrome, a potentially fatal allergic skin condition or severe liver failure (Overstreet, Costanza, Behling, Hassanin, & Masliah, 2002). Persons taking this medication should be instructed to stop it if they have the symptoms of liver disease noted before, any unusual skin rash, or develop sores in their mouth. Combining valproate or lamotrigine with other drugs may increase the risk of liver

NURSING TIP 27-4

Assessing for Lithium Toxicity

Symptoms: Depend on Serum Levels

Levels of 2 to 3 mEq/L:

- Agitation
- Ataxia
- Blurred vision
- Confusion
- Choreoathetoid movements
- Dysarthria
- Hyperreflexia
- Hypertonia
- Maniclike behavior
- Myoclonic twitching
- Slurred speech
- Tinnitus
- Incontinence
- Vertigo

Levels over 3 mEq/L:

- Arrhythmias
- Coma
- Hypotension
- Peripheral vascular collapse
- Seizures
- Spasticity
- Stupor
- Twitching of muscle groups

Treatment

- Early symptoms are treated by decreasing the dose or stopping treatment for 24 to 48 hours.
- Late symptoms are treated with gastric lavage, restoration of fluid and electrolyte balance, and increasing lithium excretion by giving aminophylline, mannitol, or urea.

Nursing Actions

- Observe carefully for symptoms of lithium toxicity.
- Report symptoms of toxicity whenever observed.
- Educate client to make own observations.
- Any situation where the client may lose excess sodium (as in heavy sweating during exercise) may produce lithium toxicity.

toxicity, and as in the case described previously (Overstreet et al., 2002), stopping medications may not prevent disease progression.

Adverse Effects

Divalproex and carbamazepine are relatively safer in overdose and with inadvertent high blood levels than is lithium. Lithium toxicity may be fatal as a result of cardiac arrhythmias. Individuals on lithium need to be alert for situations in which they may lose excess sodium, as in heavy sweating (such as occurs with vigorous physical exercise). Under such conditions, lithium toxicity may occur without any change in lithium intake. As noted before, drug interactions (including interactions with drugs commonly available without prescription) may also result in dangerously high lithium levels.

Second-Generation Antipsychotics

A recent development in the treatment of Bipolar Disorder has been the recognition that second-generation antipsychotics are effective for the management of mania—both acutely and in long-term follow-up (Vieta & Sanchez-Morena, 2008). These agents have been used alone and in combination with conventional mood stabilizers lithium and divalproex. They appear to improve depressive symptoms (McIntyre & Katzman, 2003) and may also decrease the risk of suicide. The first-generation antipsychotics, while of some value in acute treatment of mania, have not been shown to be effective in long-term management of this condition. The pharmacology, side effects, and adverse effects of these agents are discussed earlier in this chapter.

Summary of Drugs for Treating Mood Disorders

Mood disorders may reflect either depressed or expansive (manic) abnormalities or a combination of both. Whereas lithium is generally used to treat both depression and mania, the majority of drugs for mood disorders are targeted to either mood depression or mania. Drugs for depression fall into three categories: classical agents (most often tricyclics such as amitriptyline, imipramine, or related drugs such as trazodone), SSRIs (fluoxetine, sertraline, and paroxetine are among the most commonly used), and MAOIs (currently available nonselective MAOIs include phenylzine and tranylcypromine). Lithium, carbamazepine, and divalproex are commonly used to stabilize mood in persons with Mania or Bipolar Disorder. Second-generation antipsychotics are increasingly used in the management of acute mania. While mood stabilizers are most commonly prescribed by psychiatric specialists, antidepressants are widely used in general medical practice and frequently prescribed or furnished by nurse practitioners. Many of these drugs (in particular, amitriptyline, imipramine, lithium, carbamazepine, and divalproex) are included in the World Health Organization list of essential drugs for primary care (Wig, 1993). The nurse should be familiar with the indications, side effects, and adverse effects of the major classes of medications for mood disorders. The nurse who cares for persons taking lithium or MAOIs will need to combine expert knowledge of drug and food interactions with highly proficient client teaching skills; only through this combination can these valuable medications be administered without serious risk.

DRUGS FOR TREATING ANXIETY AND SLEEP DISORDERS

Acute symptoms of anxiety and insomnia are most commonly treated with benzodiazepines. Other medications useful on occasion include buspirone for generalized anxiety, antidepressants for Panic Disorder and Social Phobia, beta blockers for performance anxiety, and a variety of agents for insomnia. Antihistamines, antidepressants, barbiturates, and antipsychotics are sometimes prescribed for anxiety. Current best practice for the treatment of most anxiety disorders involves the use of antidepressants—typically SSRIs or related drugs. Dosages and side effects are as given in the section on depression in this chapter, though initial doses of SSRIs may be lower when treating some anxiety disorders. Persons commonly self-medicate anxiety with a range of drugs, including ethanol and illegally acquired tranquilizers of many sorts. It is probable that self-medication occurs for other psychiatric disorders as well, but anxiety disorders cause such acute symptoms and respond so quickly to sedatives that self-medication is common.

Indications and Evidence for Effectiveness

While they have many clinical uses, benzodiazepines have been most distinctly shown to be effective for generalized anxiety and Panic Disorder. Although all benzodiazepines may be equally effective for Panic Disorder, alprazolam (Xanax) was the first benzodiazepine approved for this treatment. There is no evidence that any other similar medication is more effective, but fairly high alprazolam doses are required: often 3 to 6 mg daily. Clinicians may use long half-life drugs (diazepam [Valium]) when daily administration is required, but may prefer relatively shorter half-lives (i.e., lorazepam [Ativan]) when clients are more likely to benefit from intermittent symptom-driven treatment. The selection of hypnotic medications was discussed previously and requires balancing onset of action, morning drowsiness, and rebound insomnia. Triazolam (Halcion) is particularly likely to produce rebound insomnia and may result in anterograde amnesia.

Pharmacology

As previously noted, the clinical effectiveness of benzodiazepines was first discovered in the mid-1950s. These medications have been in wide use since and remain among the most commonly prescribed of all drugs. Benzodiazepines are

BOX 27-2
HISTORY AND DEVELOPMENT OF SOME PSYCHOTROPIC MEDICATIONS

Since the earliest times alcohol was known as an effective sedative and mood-altering agent. Laudanum, a mixture extracted from opium poppies, has been around since the 1700s, and herbals such as valerian have been used as sedatives for centuries. These three medications were probably the only truly effective sedative/psychotropic agents used medically until the nineteenth century. In the middle nineteenth century, a number of sedatives were discovered, including bromide salts, chloral hydrate (also known as a Mickey Finn, when placed in an alcoholic drink to produce unconsciousness for illicit purposes), paraldehyde, urethane, and sulfonal. Although these agents did sedate people, most had severe side effects and are now banned, with the exception of chloral hydrate, which is sometimes used as a sleep aid, and paraldehyde, which is still occasionally used for treating alcoholic withdrawal.

In 1903, barbital was discovered and found to be an effective, useful sedative without severe side effects. Phenobarbital came along in 1912 in a search for anticonvulsant agents and was discovered to be both effective for certain types of epilepsy and a useful sedative. Phenytoin, an anticonvulsant still used today, was discovered at about the same time in the continuing search for antipsychotic sedatives. The 1950s and early 1960s were called the "age of the barbiturates." These drugs were widely and casually prescribed before their addiction potential and dangerous interaction with alcohol were known. Marilyn Monroe died of an overdose combination of alcohol and a barbiturate. Amphetamines were also widely prescribed during the mid-twentieth century, and many people took a barbiturate to sleep and an amphetamine to wake up. With the recognition of the dangers of these drugs, the FDA regulated their prescribing, and physicians began to modify their attitudes toward these drugs as well.

In 1950, the first true anxiolytic agent was developed, meprobamate (Miltown). Sales of meprobamate skyrocketed, surprisingly enough, because the television comedian Milton Berle was taking it and made frequent jokes and references about it on his TV show, the most watched program at the time.

In 1957, a major advance occurred with the discovery of chlordiazepoxide (Librium), an anxiolytic with less sedative properties than the barbiturates, with fewer serious side effects, and which in appropriate doses allowed quite normal functioning. Beginning in 1961, the benzodiazepine era virtually erupted like a volcano, with over 3,000 forms synthesized, 120 tested, and currently 35 in use worldwide. Perhaps one of the most interesting developments in anxiolytic drugs is buspirone (BuSpar). It appears to be nonaddictive, does not impair normal functioning, and is effective after two to three weeks. Many of these drugs serve a valid medical purpose in the short-term treatment of anxiety and as sleep aids, and can also be used to calm agitated psychotic clients. They are, of course, also drugs of abuse for some individuals, with the notable exception of buspirone (BuSpar).

frequently diverted to street sales and are readily available for illicit purchase. Benzodiazepines may produce dependence and are often abused along with other agents (especially alcohol). Subsequent research has shown that there is a benzodiazepine receptor in the mammalian brain and that this receptor is closely tied to the inhibitory neurotransmitter gamma aminobutyric acid (GABA; see Figure 27-3). Benzodiazepines may increase the effectiveness of GABA, but may also act separately by affecting brain metabolism of serotonin and norepinephrine (Ballenger, 1995). Zolpidem is a nonbenzodiazepine drug that nonetheless binds to benzodiazepine receptors and produces sleep induction with little effect on anxiety.

Barbiturates, now primarily used for anesthesia induction and seizure control, also augment brain GABA inhibitory effects but through a somewhat different molecular mechanism than that of benzodiazepines. Alcohol probably also exerts its anxiolytic and sedative effects, at least in part through enhancement of GABA transmission (Nishinto, Mignot, & Dement, 1995).

All the benzodiazepines are readily absorbed after oral administration and often reach peak levels within an hour or less. Diazepam (Valium, Diastat AcuDial) acts particularly quickly after oral administration. Lorazepam and midazolam (Versed) can be given intramuscularly, and diazepam is frequently given intravenously (most commonly for seizures, but occasionally for anxiety) or applied as a rectal gel. Nearly a dozen benzodiazepines are available for clinical use, and these vary most significantly in their half-lives. Triazolam, for example, has a half-life of only six hours and no clinically significant metabolites. As a result, triazolam is classified as a short-acting benzodiazepine. In contrast, diazepam has both a long half-life (nearly 24 hours) and active metabolites with similar long half-lives. The effect of metabolites can be quite important: flurazepam (Dalmane) itself has quite a short half-life (two to three hours), but its major metabolite has a half-life of more than two days. As a result, this commonly used sedative may prolong daytime drowsiness when used for treating insomnia.

Dose/Administration

Benzodiazepine doses are quite specific for the individual drugs chosen and vary over a rather wide range. Alprazolam (short to intermediate half-life) and clonazepam (long half-life) are perhaps the two most commonly used

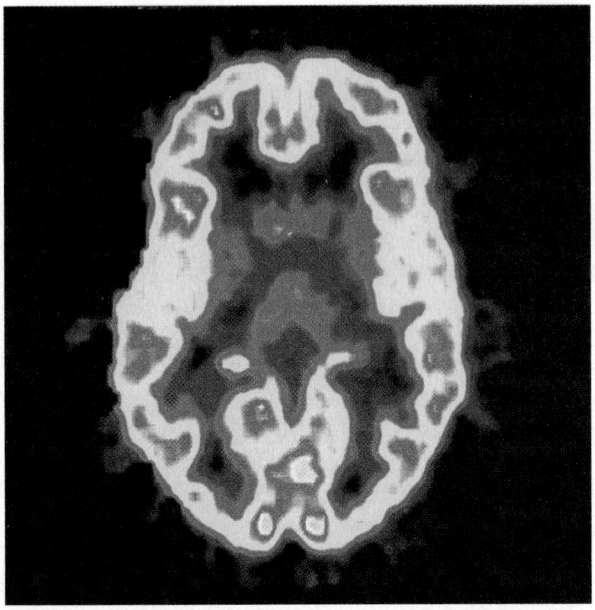

FIGURE 27-3 **PET image of benzodiazepine receptors. Areas of high binding to benzodiazepines are represented as white, orange/red, and yellow. Note that almost all binding occurs in the cortex. Compare the degree of binding in the frontal lobes (lower part of the image) with the PET scan of opioid receptors (Chapter 17). These latter two images show very few frontal lobe binding sites.** (FROM "ADDICTION: BRAIN MECHANISMS AND THEIR RELATED IMPLICATIONS," BY J. D. NUTT. *LANCET*, 1985, 347(8993), 33–35. REPRINTED WITH PERMISSION FROM ELSEVIER.)

benzodiazepine medications for treating anxiety. Alprazolam (Xanax) daily doses range from 0.75 to 8 mg daily, with a common range of 1.5 to 3 mg. Clonazepam (Klonopin) is generally given in a dosage range of 1.5 to 10 mg daily.

Drug Actions

Benzodiazepines exert a significant effect on GABA-ergic CNS pathways and produce both sedation and a marked decrease in subjective anxiety. These drugs induce sleep, decrease frequency of awakenings, slightly decrease rapid eye movement (REM) sleep, and moderately decrease slow-wave or deep Stage 3 to 4 sleep. Individuals who take benzodiazepines for sleep generally report an increased subjective sense of sleep quality. Sleep latency (the time to fall asleep) is significantly decreased by short half-life benzodiazepines such as triazolam, but these medications frequently produce rebound insomnia on subsequent nights. Longer half-life benzodiazepines take somewhat longer to produce sleep and cause some hangover the next day. Temazepam (Restoril) is a commonly prescribed hypnotic medication with an intermediate half-life and an onset of action within two to three hours. Many other medications such as eszopiclone, zaleplon, and ramelteon are used for management of insomnia. The interested reader might wish to consult one of several discussions of this topic (Passarella and Duong, 2008; Ramakrishnan & Scheid, 2007; Budur, Rodriguez, & Foldvary-Schaefer, 2007).

Drug and Food Interactions

There are few benzodiazepine drug interactions of clinical significance. Alcohol is additive with the sedative effects of benzodiazepines and will produce increased drowsiness if taken along with these medications. The combination of alcohol and large amounts of benzodiazepines can produce fatal respiratory depression and coma. This is a particular problem since some clients find that combining alcohol with benzodiazepines, perhaps especially clonazepam, produces a desirable "high."

Use During Pregnancy/Lactation

Benzodiazepines are commonly prescribed to and self-administered by women of child-bearing age. There is little firm data on which to base recommendations for benzodiazepine use during pregnancy. Alcohol and barbiturates clearly cause fetal damage, but a "fetal benzodiazepine syndrome" has not been unequivocally defined. Most benzodiazepines, including clonazepam (Klonopin), are pregnancy category D and are contraindicated during pregnancy. Risks during breast feeding are likely smaller, and in contrast to most other psychiatric medications, lower drug concentrations are found in milk than in plasma. Risks and benefits should be weighed whether to discontinue nursing or the benzodiazepine. Estazolam (ProSom), flurazepam (Dalmane), quazepam (Doral), temazepam (Restoril), and triazolam (Halcion) are category X drugs and, according to the manufacturers' package inserts of each, contraindicated in women who are or may become pregnant.

Side Effects

Benzodiazepine side effects are largely limited to sedation, interference with safe driving, and occasional amnesia. Paradoxical reactions of increased agitation or anger may occur.

Adverse Effects

Severe adverse effects are rare, even in intentional overdose. Deaths have occurred in combination with alcohol and other substances, but are unusual. The major adverse effects of benzodiazepines involve physical dependence. When given these medications over prolonged periods, many individuals have symptoms of increased anxiety and, rarely, seizures on abrupt withdrawal. Withdrawal should be accomplished slowly over several weeks and is most commonly a problem with alprazolam, a drug with a relatively short half-life. When withdrawal from alprazolam is required, many clinicians first switch their clients from alprazolam to a longer-acting drug such as diazepam or clonazepam, and then proceed with a slow withdrawal.

Nonbenzodiazepine Drugs for Anxiety and Sleep Disorders

While the benzodiazepines are widely used for management of anxiety and insomnia, they are not the only medications of value for treating these conditions and their tendency to produce dependency makes them unsatisfactory for many clients requiring long-term therapy. Some anxiety disorders, most notably post-traumatic stress, do not respond well to benzodiazepines, and evidence suggests that SSRIs are more effective in Generalized Anxiety Disorder (Davidson, 2004). Buspirone (BuSpar) is a unique antianxiety agent that has no effects on the benzodiazepine-GABA receptor. As a consequence, it produces relief of anxiety with virtually no sedation. Zolpidem (Ambien) does act on the benzodiazepine receptor, but it does not have the chemical structure of a benzodiazepine. As a consequence, zolpidem produces only sedation; it does not provide any relief from anxiety. Propranolol (Inderal), a beta blocker, has little demonstrated effect on anxiety, but it has proved useful when performance anxiety produces physical symptoms such as tremor or difficulty speaking. Administration of propranolol prior to activities such as public speaking or playing a musical instrument can sometimes improve performance by reducing tremor or other manifestations of nervousness. There is some limited role for beta blockers in other anxiety disorders. Antidepressants (and very rarely antipsychotics) can sometimes be helpful for control of anxiety or insomnia. As noted previously, trazodone seems particularly anxiolytic and is often used to combat onset insomnia in anxious and depressed individuals.

Buspirone

Buspirone was released in 1986 as an anxiolytic drug. Pharmacologically, buspirone bears some resemblance to antipsychotic medications, but even in high doses it both lacks antipsychotic effects and fails to produce tardive dyskinesia or other movement disorders. There is no evidence for habituation to or dependency on buspirone. Buspirone is well absorbed orally and has a short half-life. Unlike benzodiazepines, which affect anxiety within minutes to hours, the effect of buspirone is delayed, often to as much as seven weeks, and it may prove less effective (Chessick, et al., 2006)—especially in those who have already taken benzodiazepines. While not all individuals respond to buspirone (some data suggest that those who have previously been treated with benzodiazepines may be more likely to be poor responders), when response does occur, buspirone is as effective as benzodiazepines in the management of Generalized Anxiety Disorder. Buspirone has few side effects and almost no drug interactions. As a substrate of cytochrome P450 3A4, inhibitors and inducers of this enzyme may increase or decrease the effects of buspirone, respectively. Dizziness, headache, and nausea occur occasionally, but frequently improve with continued administration. Because of the relatively short half-life, doses need to be given three times daily. This need for a multiple dosage regimen, slow onset of action, and buspirone's relatively high cost are its primary disadvantages. Buspirone in high doses is an effective antidepressant and is often used along with other antidepressant drugs as an augmentation agent when monotherapy has failed (Doggrell, 2006). It is not effective in Panic Disorder but may have some benefit in Social Phobia. Results in Obsessive-Compulsive Disorder remain ambiguous. Buspirone is safe in overdose, has no effect on alertness or other job-related functions, and is free of abuse potential. Despite this nearly ideal profile, buspirone is not used widely in psychiatric practice, probably because of its slow onset and its very high cost. With generic formulations available, the cost of buspirone has decreased.

Beta Blockers

Beta blockers act peripherally to inhibit the beta-adrenergic receptor. They also have generalized CNS effects of sedation, fatigue, and occasionally depression. This sedative effect may produce some mild antianxiety effect, but beta blockers have at best only a minimal effect on generalized anxiety and probably no significant benefit in Panic Disorder. In contrast, there is some evidence to support the use of beta blockers in Social Phobia, especially, as noted earlier, when symptoms of autonomic arousal are debilitating. These symptoms include tremulousness, blushing, tachycardia, and subjective fear. Such symptoms are often mediated through peripheral beta-adrenergic stimulation and may be blocked with propranolol. Fear responds least well, and some studies have suggested no benefit of beta blockers on Social Phobia. Obsessive-Compulsive Disorder does not respond to propranolol, but Post-Traumatic Stress Disorder may respond somewhat, particularly when symptoms of autonomic arousal are prominent.

Zolpidem and Zaleplon

Zolpidem (Ambien) is a nonbenzodiazepine that nonetheless acts through the benzodiazepine receptor. Zolpidem has been marketed as a drug for treating insomnia, and in this use it may have some theoretical advantages over benzodiazepine hypnotics. Among these advantages are zolpidem's short half-life without rebound drowsiness. Long-acting benzodiazepines tend to produce early morning drowsiness, whereas short-acting benzodiazepines may "wear off" in the middle of the night, leading to nocturnal wakefulness and daytime sleepiness. Zolpidem, in contrast, seems to produce restful sleep that lasts through the night. Unlike benzodiazepines, zolpidem appears also not to reduce the amount of REM sleep. It is thought to have little or no abuse or dependency potential, and it does not seem to affect next morning alertness or job performance. Long-term usage of hypnotic drugs is generally discouraged, but where necessary, zolpidem would seem to be an appropriate medication for pharmacological management of chronic insomnia. Ramelteon (Rozerem; Reynoldson, Elliott, & Nelson, 2008) and eszopiclone (Lunesta; Hair, McCormack, & Curran, 2008) are among several newer agents that have differing pharmacology but are apparently safe for both short- and relatively long-term treatment. Ramelteon acts as an agonist at melatonin receptors and is not a controlled medication, a possible benefit over zopidem (Ambien), zaleplon (Sonata), and eszopiclone (Lunesta).

Zaleplon, like zolpidem, acts on the GABA receptor, but in a different way than do the benzodiazepines. These two drugs are fairly similar in their actions and clinical use; however, zaleplon is eliminated more quickly so that it may be more effective in inducing sleep onset than in maintaining uninterrupted sleep. On the other hand, the quicker elimination may result in fewer symptoms on awakening (Drover, 2004) and perhaps in lessened risk of driving impairment in the four to six hours after the medication is taken (Verster, Volkerts, Schreuder, Eijken, van Heuckelum, Veldhuijzen, et al., 2002). Zaleplon, zolpidem, and eszopiclone have been associated with hypersensitivity reactions, and various troublesome behaviors, such as driving while asleep, have been reported.

Antidepressants and Antipsychotics

Some clinicians use antidepressants to treat insomnia. Amitriptyline, doxepin, and trazodone are highly sedating and may help clients fall asleep. These medications are particularly useful when patients have coexisting insomnia and depression. It is generally regarded as atypical clinical practice to use antidepressants to treat insomnia in patients who do not meet DSM-IV-TR criteria for depression. Some clinicians use highly sedating antipsychotics such as thioridazine or quetiapine for sleep disorders, especially in the elderly (Salzman, Satlin, & Burrows, 1995). In some cases the benefits of such treatment may outweigh the risks, but it is unlikely that antipsychotic drugs should be widely employed for this purpose.

Antihistamines

The sedating antihistamine diphenhydramine (Benadryl) has been approved for over-the-counter sales as a hypnotic. Diphenhydramine does produce drowsiness and probably decreases the time to sleep onset. Studies do not show improved sleep quality in persons taking diphenhydramine (Cole & Yonkers, 1995). The anticholinergic side effects of this drug may be significant, especially in the elderly, and tolerance to its sedative effects develops rapidly (Passarella & Duong, 2008). Such side effects include blurred vision, urinary hesitancy or obstruction, and impaired sweating and temperature regulation. Diphenhydramine appears on the revised list of "potentially inappropriate" medications in the elderly (Fick, Mion, Beers, & Waller, 2008) and should generally be avoided in older persons.

Summary of Antianxiety Drugs

As the reader of this book's chapter on anxiety disorders (Chapter 12) will recognize, anxiety causes profound human distress. Currently available medications can provide dramatic relief for clients suffering from symptoms of anxiety. Benzodiazepines are widely used and are generally effective treatments for anxiety, but they are rarely satisfactory for long-term treatment and may be inferior in effectiveness to SSRIs for some common anxiety disorders (Davidson, 2004). Benzodiazepines are widely used for insomnia, though their effectiveness for anything other than acute use is uncertain. Zolpidem and the similar drug zaleplon are probably more effective and better tolerated than are benzodiazepines. Newer drugs such as ramelteon and eszopiclone offer additional treatment options for chronic insomnia given that long-term use of benzodiazepines may result in dependence and withdrawal symptoms. Buspirone is a sometimes-effective but expensive and slow-acting antianxiety medication that does not carry any risk of habituation or dependence. Some anxiety disorders (Obsessive-Compulsive Disorder, Panic Disorder) are primarily treated with antidepressant medications (most commonly SSRIs), and some antidepressants, notably trazodone, are particularly effective anxiolytics. Anxiolytics are frequently used in psychiatric nursing and in general medical practice. Diazepam is included in the World Health Organization list of essential drugs for primary care (Wig, 1993). Table 27-3 provides a summary of antianxiety and hypnotic medications.

DRUGS FOR TREATING SUBSTANCE ABUSE AND DEPENDENCY

Substance abuse is discussed in some detail in Chapter 17. Medications have a useful role in bringing about abstinence from some substances that cause physical dependency. They may also be used to treat symptoms of physical withdrawal. Drugs may help maintain abstinence—either by directly substituting for the substance of abuse (methadone for heroin, nicotine by patch or gum for smoking) or through the unique aversive conditioning of disulfiram (Antabuse), which produces a highly unpleasant set of physical symptoms when alcohol is ingested. Many drugs used in managing substance-related conditions have other roles as antidepressants, antipsychotics, or antianxiety medications and have been discussed previously in this chapter. However, there are some agents used primarily or exclusively in managing substance abuse, dependency, and withdrawal.

Substances with Little Role Outside Substance Abuse or Withdrawal

This somewhat arbitrary classification of medications includes methadone, buprenorphine, disulfiram, nicotine (for replacement in persons quitting smoking), varenicline and opioid receptor antagonists.

Methadone

Methadone is a relatively long-acting narcotic that is useful in both acute detoxification and in long-term maintenance of previously opioid-dependent individuals. A longer-acting derivative of methadone, LAAM (l-α-acetyl-methadol), was discontinued by its manufacturer.

Short-term use of methadone may reduce the intensity of withdrawal symptoms and allows detoxification using an easily administered oral regimen. Methadone doses for

TABLE 27-3 Selected Antianxiety and Hypnotic Medications

GENERIC NAME	TRADE NAME	MEDICATION TYPE	CLINICAL USE	DOSAGE (MG/DAY)	HALF-LIFE (HOURS)	SPEED OF ONSET (P.O.)
Alprazolam	Xanax	Benzodiazepine	Antianxiety	0.75–4	12–15	Intermediate
Chlordiazepoxide	Librium	Benzodiazepine		15–100	5–30	Intermediate
Clonazepam	Klonopin	Benzodiazepine	Antianxiety, anticonvulsant	1.5–20	18–50	Intermediate
Diazepam	Valium	Benzodiazepine	Antianxiety anticonvulsant	5–40	20–80	Rapid
Lorazepam	Ativan	Benzodiazepine	Antianxiety	2–4	10–20	Intermediate
Flurazepam	Dalmane	Benzodiazepine	Hypnotic	15–30	2–3	Very rapid
Midazolam	Versed	Benzodiazepine	Sedative	i.m. or i.v., dosage usually based on weight	1–12	Very rapid
Temazepam	Restoril	Benzodiazepine	Hypnotic	15–30	8–15	Intermediate
Triazolam	Halcion	Benzodiazepine	Hypnotic	0.125–0.5	1.5–6	Rapid
Buspirone	BuSpar	Serotonin and dopamine agonist	Antianxiety	10–60	2–3	Slow (weeks)
Zolpidem	Ambien	Nonbenzodiazepine but binds to benzodiazepine receptors	Hypnotic	5–10	1.5–5	Very rapid
Zaleplon	Sonata	Nonbenzodiazepine but binds to benzodiazepine receptors	Hypnotic	5–10	1	Very rapid

withdrawal are typically 40 mg or less given initially and then reduced by 10% to 20% daily until the individual is drug free after one to two weeks. Such a regimen may make withdrawal easier than suddenly stopping the intake of opioids. Such sudden stopping often leads to unpleasant symptoms (tearing, runny nose, nausea, agitation, and piloerection) and is frequently termed "cold turkey" withdrawal. Unlike alcohol withdrawal, which may occasionally be dangerous, cold turkey withdrawal from opioids, while distinctly uncomfortable, is not dangerous.

Long-term methadone maintenance is far more controversial since it substitutes oral methadone for injection drugs without any goal of eventually achieving a drug-free status. Advocates of methadone maintenance claim that it reduces criminality and (unless other injection substances are involved) should eliminate needle use—of immense importance in controlling spread of injection-associated infectious agents, notably HIV, hepatitis B, and hepatitis C. Methadone maintenance currently must be given through clinics specifically licensed for this purpose. Clients who "earn" the privilege of self-administration are typically given a week's supply of methadone and are subject to periodic urine testing to evaluate use of substances other than methadone. Other clients go to the clinic daily to receive their methadone. Relatively high doses of 60 to 80 mg are often given daily, and additional services of counseling and medical and psychiatric care are often provided. Regulations require that current physiological dependence be documented and that the individual have been opioid dependent for at least a year. Special rules apply to clients under 18 years of age. Long-term methadone treatment remains a controversial but well-established approach to the management of opioid dependence.

Buprenorphine (Sporer, 2004) has been approved for outpatient management of addiction to opioids after having been used with apparent success in Europe. In 2002, the FDA announced the classification of buprenorphine as a Schedule III narcotic. This means that it can be prescribed by physicians in ordinary office practice—unlike methadone, which (at least until recently) could only be given out in a clinic approved for the treatment of opioid addiction. Prescribers must become certified to prescribe Suboxone for office-based treatment of opioid dependence. Buprenorphine is used both for detoxification/withdrawal and for ongoing maintenance. When used for maintenance, it is combined with the narcotic antagonist naloxone to counter psychoactive symptoms and respiratory depression in the event that it is injected as a drug of abuse. Evidence is insufficient to judge whether buprenorphine offers any advantage over methadone (Amato, Davoli,

Ferri, Gowing, & Perucci, 2004), but it may be indicated in situations where methadone is unavailable or not effective.

Disulfiram

Disulfiram is an inhibitor of the enzyme aldehyde dehydrogenase, which catalyzes a major step in the breakdown of alcohol. When the enzyme is inhibited and an individual drinks alcohol, blood concentrations of the toxic metabolite acetaldehyde increase significantly. Acetaldehyde produces unpleasant symptoms of flushing, tachycardia, nausea, vomiting, and hypotension. Especially in medically fragile individuals, these symptoms may prove life threatening. Because of associated risks, disulfiram is used only with highly selected individuals who have good physical health and a high chance of remaining abstinent. However, even in such carefully selected individuals, disulfiram may occasionally produce serious illness, including fatal hepatitis. This risk must be balanced against the severe morbidity, and even mortality, caused by alcoholism itself (Chick, 1999). Studies show that disulfiram maintenance can significantly reduce drinking (Fuller et al., 1986). The dose is typically 250 mg daily, though larger doses may be given, especially when dosing intervals exceed one day. The relatively long half-life of disulfiram ensures that several days must elapse between stopping medication and safely drinking alcohol; this long half-life probably decreases the likelihood of impulsive relapse. However, perhaps not surprisingly, the major difficulty with disulfiram as primary treatment for alcohol dependency is the difficulty in assuring long-term compliance with the medication. Such compliance may be enhanced by frequent clinic visits (including giving medication under observation every three to four days) and by enlisting others (visiting nurse, significant other) in ensuring compliance. Disulfiram may also reduce craving for cocaine even in persons who do not also use alcohol (George, Chawarski, Pakes, Carroll, Kosten, & Schottenfeld, 2000).

Acamprosate

Acamprosate (Campral) has been approved for the maintenance of alcohol abstinence. It appears to balance GABA and glutamate activity. The recommended dose of acamprosate is two 333 mg tablets (each dose should total 666 mg) taken three times daily. Acamprosate is not metabolized, an advantage for patients with varying degrees of liver impairment according to the drug's package insert.

Nicotine Replacement

Smoking is an issue of particular concern to mental health nursing because of the high incidence of smoking among psychiatric clients. Alcohol abusers and schizophrenic individuals have especially high tobacco consumption. Depression and abuse of a variety of non-nicotine substances are also associated with tobacco abuse (Cornish, McNicholas, & O'Brien, 1995). Many individuals have nicotine dependency without any other diagnosable DSM-IV-TR condition. Chemical replacement of nicotine may allow some highly dependent persons to quit more easily. Adhesive patches (Habitrol, Nicoderm, and others) supply a steady quantity of nicotine. Chewing gum (Nicorette) and patches have both shown enhanced one-year abstinence rates compared with placebo (Anonymous, 1995b; Benowitz, 1993). These products may be purchased without prescription. Nicotine nasal spray (Nicotrol NS) is also available and may prove useful for some individuals. The nurse can assist clients in assessing their readiness to quit, in setting a "quit date," in assessing potential risks to successful quitting, and in finding a support group to enhance quitting success. In some settings, the nurse can serve as a resource when a client is having difficulties with nicotine abstinence. The antidepressant bupropion (Zyban), in a long-acting formulation, is effective in promoting nicotine abstinence. Whether other antidepressants have similar benefits remains unproven. Varenicline (Chantix), a partial activator (agonist) of brain nicotine receptors (more technically, the nicotinic acetylcholine receptor) has proven relatively effective in the management of nicotine dependence. Short-term quit rates may be higher with varenicline than with other treatments, however there is some evidence of associated depression and suicidal ideation in users (Cahill, Stead, & Lancaster, 2008). The FDA is in the process of weighing the evidence and has so far issued two warnings about the potential risk of depression during or after varenicline administration (Hughes, 2008).

Opioid Receptor Antagonists

Opioid receptor antagonists have been available for many years (naloxone, nalmefene, naltrexone, and others). These medications may be life saving when clients present with respiratory depression and coma due to narcotic agonists. Giving 0.4 to 0.8 mg of naloxone intravenously will dramatically reverse symptoms of narcotic overdose, but will often precipitate symptoms of withdrawal as clients awaken. The precipitation of withdrawal by injection of naloxone is sometimes used as a criterion for physical dependency (the establishment of which is required for entry into a methadone program). The long-acting receptor antagonist naltrexone is sometimes used for relapse prevention in a manner analogous to disulfiram. A single oral dose will block the subjective effects of administered opioids for up to several days. In contrast to disulfiram, no adverse reaction occurs if a person on naltrexone uses an opioid, but because of naltrexone receptor antagonism, there is no opioid "high" to rekindle a desire for continuing use. (Such long-acting receptor blockade could theoretically pose difficulties if an acute injury or unexpected surgery required narcotic pain relief.) Naltrexone relapse prevention requires a higher level of motivation for abstention than is seen in most opioid-dependent individuals. This medication may work best for dependent professionals who have undergone detoxification and whose continuing licensure and maintenance of a (usually) prosperous livelihood require documented freedom from opioid use. Intriguingly, naltrexone has also been shown to be of some value in promoting abstinence and is approved for the treatment of alcohol dependence. Whether it will have long-term benefit for alcohol dependence is currently uncertain, though studies using long-acting injectable forms of naltrexone are promising (Ciraulo, Dong, Silverman, Gastfriend, & Pettinati, 2008). Vivitrol, a once-monthly injection of naltrexone, is currently available.

Other Medications of Use in Managing Substance Dependence

Many of the drugs used in managing individuals dependent on a variety of substances have been discussed previously in this chapter in their roles as antidepressants, anxiolytics, and antipsychotics. Antidepressants, particularly imipramine, may be of value in reducing alcohol consumption in depressed individuals with alcohol dependency. Haloperidol and benzodiazepines are often used to manage excitement and toxic psychosis seen in acute phencyclidine (PCP) and stimulant drug intoxication. The vitamin thiamine is frequently given intravenously to alcoholics for prevention of Wernicke's encephalopathy, a serious complication that is most likely to occur when adequate nutrition is reestablished. Wernicke's encephalopathy (often called "Wernicke's syndrome") is characterized by confusion, memory loss, and abnormalities of cranial nerve function. Untreated, it can lead to death, permanent memory loss, or other neurological impairment. Early intravenous administration of glucose plus thiamine results in rapid, often complete, improvement in neurological functioning. Intravenous glucose (along with thiamine) is the treatment of choice for alcohol-induced hypoglycemia, and long-acting benzodiazepines (commonly diazepam and chlordiazepoxide [Librium]) are used in management and prevention of alcohol withdrawal. Clonidine (Catapres), an alpha-adrenergic agonist primarily employed to treat hypertension, has come to play a significant role in reducing symptoms of withdrawal from opioids and perhaps from nicotine as well. As noted earlier, the antidepressant bupropion has demonstrated effectiveness in reducing symptoms of nicotine withdrawal.

> **NURSINGALERT 27-7**
>
> **Thiamine and Alcohol-Induced Hypoglycemia**
>
> When hydrating alcoholics, thiamine must also be given. The alcoholic person is hypoglycemic. When hydration increases glucose metabolism, the client uses up thiamine stores and there is an increased body requirement for thiamine. Failure to give thiamine prior to fluids and glucose may result in permanent neurological damage.

STIMULANT DRUGS

Clinically useful stimulant drugs include dextroamphetamine, methylphenidate (Ritalin), dexmethylphenidate (Focalin), and lisdexamfetamine (Vyvanse). Dexmethylphenidate is an enantiomer of methylphenidate, while lisdexamfetamine is a prodrug that is converted to dextroamphetamine. Stimulant drugs (including these substances, but also cocaine, methamphetamine, and others) are major substances of abuse, but they also have significant benefits when used under clinical supervision. The use of stimulants as antidepressants was discussed previously in this chapter but remains controversial. These medications may work best in combination with other antidepressants and may be particularly useful in severely depressed, medically ill older individuals in whom rapid relief of symptoms is important to avoid suicide or physical deterioration. Stimulants may also be freer of significant side effects than other antidepressants but have significant cardiovascular warnings. Furthermore, stimulants carry warnings detailing possible psychiatric events such as new onset psychosis. Atomoxetine (Strattera) is a non-stimulant that inhibits the reuptake of norepinephrine.

Stimulant medications have their best-documented uses in the management of Narcolepsy and Attention-Deficit Hyperactivity Disorder. There is little controversy surrounding stimulant use in Narcolepsy, a condition in which daytime sleepiness can make many common activities (notably driving) hazardous. Stimulant drugs reduce daytime sleepiness but must be given on a chronic basis, presumably for the individual's lifetime. Stimulants seem to be particularly effective for adult Attention-Deficit Disorder (Wender, Reimherr, Wood, & Ward, 1985), although other medications such as the antidepressants bupropion or desipramine and the newer agent atomoxetine may be effective with less potential for abuse in susceptible individuals (Wilens, 2004). Stimulants are now much less commonly recommended for narcolepsy than in the recent past. The atypical stimulant modafinil (Provigil) has proven effective in combating daytime sleepiness from narcolepsy (and other sleep-related conditions), and sodium oxybate (Xyrem) may also play a useful role. Treatment of children with Attention-Deficit Disorder is somewhat more controversial. Many parents and clinicians are concerned about use of highly psychoactive controlled substances in young children, particularly since the demonstrated benefits, while consistent, are only modest and last only as long as the medication is given. Short-term benefits in behavior and learning have been clearly demonstrated, but prolonged administration of these drugs to children raises a number of serious issues involving safety, efficacy, and clinical wisdom (Schachar & Tannock, 1993). Among these are a small risk of sudden death (less than one per million prescriptions) and elevation in blood pressure that has prompted significant FDA concern about cardiac risk from long-term administration (Nissen, 2006). Stimulants also carry warnings pertaining to growth suppression concerns in children. Atomoxetine (Strattera) has become popular for treating children with ADHD because it is not a

REFLECTIVE THINKING 27-1

The Drug-Receptor Hypothesis

For many years, the philosophy behind the use of a medication was "if it works, use it." Paul Ehrlich was the first scientist to see the possibility of targeting medicines at a specific cause or organism, sometimes referred to as the "magic bullet" hypothesis. As knowledge of drug actions increased, the mechanism of drug action, or exactly how they worked, began to be studied. It was primarily the work of Ehrlich that led to the concept that the effect of drugs is due to their interaction with specific receptors. Today, we have discovered receptors for benzodiazepines, morphine, serotonin, nicotine, and marijuana. This implies that the body produces substances naturally that act at these receptors. In the early 1970s, endorphins were discovered, naturally occurring peptides in the body that act at the morphine receptor. Acetylcholine acts at the nicotinic receptors, and amandamide and 2-arachidonylglycerol (2-AG) act at the so-called marijuana receptors. Scientists still do not know the biological functions of amandamide and 2-AG. Once a receptor is discovered, it can be cloned, receptor blockers synthesized, and function examined.

This drug receptor hypothesis can change the way one thinks about medications. What do you think the implications are of the statement that the body may produce substances that act at the receptors identified? How have plants "learned" to produce substances that act so strongly on our brain receptors?

NURSINGTIP 27-5

Nursing Implications in Pharmacotherapeutics

The nurse's role is to understand the reason that each medication is prescribed, to administer the medications safely, and to assess for untoward effects. Further, the nurse has an important role in client (and family) education, so that the client understands the drug, how to take it, and how to observe for side effects. For cross-reference, medications listed in this chapter are also described in chapters focusing on psychopathology, where the medication would be indicated in treatment of the condition.

controlled substance as compared to stimulants. However, the FDA has also issued warnings about atomoxetine—both for apparent increased risk of suicidal ideation and for rare, but potentially fatal, liver disease. These concerns make prescribing decision difficult for individuals with ADHD needing pharmacological treatment. There is increasing data that modafinil (Provigil) may have a role in the management of ADHD in children and adolescents (Biederman & Pliszka, 2008) and also perhaps in adults under some circumstances (Mann & Bitsios, 2008), however, recent warnings of hypersensitivity reactions may limit its use.

One of the earliest lessons nurses learn from working with psychiatric clients is that responses to medications are sometimes unpredictable. Even when studies show that a medication works for a given disorder, there is no certainty that any given individual will respond satisfactorily to that drug. A switch to a second drug in the same class may be effective for some, whereas for others an entirely different class of medications may be needed. As with effectiveness, side effects may be highly variable from person to person. For example, even with the use of classic neuroleptic agents such as haloperidol, tardive dyskinesia develops in only some treated individuals. At present this variability is beneficial and harmful responses to drug treatment seem random. However, increasing evidence suggests that much of the observed difference in drug response is due to measurable host factors. In other words, the person receiving medication has a series of metabolic responses to the specific drug given that determine both the drug's effectiveness and its side-effects profile. Much data further suggest that the different ways people react to drugs are not random, but instead are genetically programmed. We likely inherit a range of enzyme systems that respond to and metabolize drugs; in this view, the effect (and side effects) of a drug are a balance between the drug's inherent pharmacological properties and our own body's response to and metabolism of the drug. Many scientists feel strongly that as we develop the ability to analyze the human genome one of the most important benefits will be an increasing ability to predict how an individual is likely to respond to a given drug. This knowledge would allow us to begin therapy confident of a response and of relative freedom from serious side effects. One of the current puzzles and challenges of psychopharmacology is that some treatments, particularly for mood disorders, do not work rapidly; even effective medications may take three weeks or more to have the desired effect. With genetic-derived understanding of an individual's predicted response to drugs we might also be able to select medication that would work faster. These issues have been discussed in some detail for pharmacogenomics in general (Belle & Singh, 2008; Campbell & Levitt, 2008) as well as for psychiatric care of children and adolescents (Anderson & Cook, 2000).

KEY CONCEPTS

- Psychotropic medications are an important and often an essential mode of treatment.
- Since the advent of modern pharmaceuticals, there have been many drugs developed as antipsychotic, antidepressant, and antianxiety medications.
- Each category of medication has helped us learn something about the etiology of mental disease.
- While medications help to alleviate symptoms, they do not cure the underlying problem or condition that causes the symptom.

REVIEW QUESTIONS

1. After taking Thorazine for two days, a client complains of dry mouth (anticholinergic effect). Which medication will be most effective in addressing the client's complaint?
   1. Valium
   2. Mellaril (thioridizine)
   3. Cogentin
   4. Trilafon (perphenazine)

2. The client is admitted to the emergency department for an opiate overdose. The physician orders Catapres to be given stat. Which assessment should the nurse do prior to giving the medication?
   1. Check the client's vital signs including blood pressure
   2. Observe the client's pupillary reaction
   3. Verify that a chest X-ray was been completed
   4. Observe the client for hyperreflexia

3. A client is seen in the clinic with symptoms of moderate depression. At the completion of the visit, the client is given an appointment with the nurse and a prescription for an antidepressant. The nurse would understand that which of the following medications would be most appropriate for this client?
   1. Tricyclic
   2. SSRI
   3. MAOI
   4. Lithium

4. Prior to administering Antabuse the nurse should do which of the following?
   1. Check the client's chart to determine that a chest X-ray has been ordered
   2. Determine that the client has not had alcohol in the last two weeks
   3. Check the client's temperature, pulse, and respiration
   4. Provide the client with written literature regarding Antabuse

5. The physician has ordered that a client with severe depression be placed on an MAO inhibitor. The nurse's teaching plan should include the fact that which of the following could occur if the client eats foods high in tyramine?
   1. Hypertensive crisis
   2. Constipation and dry mouth
   3. Orthostatic hypotension
   4. Urinary frequency

LEARNING ACTIVITIES

1. Review the medications ordered for each client you care for during your psychiatric mental health nursing course.

2. Explain the following for each medication:
   a. Reason for drug to be ordered
   b. How you know if your client is on a therapeutic dose
   c. Side effects and adverse effects

3. For each of your clients, evaluate the level of compliance in taking drugs.

4. Describe specific activities you can do to increase compliance with the therapeutic regimen.

StudyWARE™ CONNECTION

Using your StudyWARE™ CD-ROM

1. Complete the Flashcard activity for this chapter.
2. View the Multimedia Animations that accompany this chapter.
   a. Acetylcholine
   b. Depressants
   c. Dopamine
   d. Dopaminergic
   e. Drugs and Anxiety
   f. Seratonergic
   g. Seratonin
   h. Stimulants
   i. Stress Response
3. Review the audio glossary for key terms in this chapter.
4. Explore the other games and activities that support this chapter.

REFERENCES

Ables, A. Z., & Baughman, O. L., 3rd. (2003). Antidepressants: Update on new agents and indications. *American Family Physician, 67*(3), 547–554.

ACOG. (2008). Practice Bulletin: Clinical management guidelines for obstetrician-gynecologists number 92, April 2008 (replaces Practice Bulletin number 87, November 2007). Use of psychiatric medications during pregnancy and lactation. (2008). *Obstetrics & Gynecology, 111*(4), 1001–1020 CN - ACOG Committee.

Addis, A., & Koren, G. (2000). Safety of fluoxetine during the first trimester of pregnancy: A meta-analytical review of epidemiological studies. *Psychological Medicine, (1)*, 89–94.

Alper, K., Schwartz, K. A., Kolts, R. L., & Khan, A. (2007). Seizure incidence in psychopharmacological clinical trials: An analysis of Food and Drug Administration (FDA) summary basis of approval reports. *Biological Psychiatry, 62*(4), 345–354.

Amato, L., Davoli, M., Ferri, M., Gowing, L., & Perucci, C. A. (2004). Effectiveness of interventions on opiate withdrawal treatment: An overview of systematic reviews. *Drug and Alcohol Dependency, 73*(3), 219–226.

American Diabetes Association. (2004). Consensus development conference on antipsychotic drugs and obesity and diabetes. *Diabetes Care, 27*, 596–601.

American Psychiatric Association Task Force on Tardive Dyskinesia. (1992). *Tardive dyskinesia: A task force report of the American Psychiatric Association.* Washington, DC: American Psychiatric Press.

American Psychiatric Association,. (2002). *Diagnostic and statistical manual of mental disorders* (4th ed -Text Revised). Washington, DC: Author.

Amsterdam, J. D. (2003). A double-blind, placebo-controlled trial of the safety and efficacy of selegiline transdermal system without dietary restrictions in patients with major depressive disorder. *Journal of Clinical Psychiatry, 64*(2), 208–214.

Anderson, G. M., & Cook, E. H. (2000). Pharmacogenetics. Promise and potential in child and adolescent psychiatry. *Child and Adolescent Psychiatry Clinics of North America, 9*(1), 23–42.

Anonymous. (1995a). Nefazodone for depression. *The Medical Letter, 37*, 33–34.

Anonymous. (1995b). Use of nicotine to stop smoking. *The Medical Letter, 37*, 6–8.

Arango, C., Bobes, J., Aranda, P., Carmena, R., Garcia-Garcia, M., Rejas, J., et al. (2008). A comparison of schizophrenia outpatients treated with antipsychotics with and without metabolic syndrome: Findings from the CLAMORS study. *Schizophrenia Research, 104*(1–3), 1–12.

Ashim, S., Warrington, S., & Anderson, I. M. (2004). Management of diabetes mellitus occurring during treatment with olanzapine: A report of six cases and clinical implications. *Journal of Psychopharmacology, 18*(1), 128–132.

Association, A. P. (2000). Practice guideline for the treatment of patients with major depressive disorder (revision). American Psychiatric Association. *American Journal of Psychiatry, 157*(Suppl. 4), 1–45.

Ballenger, J. C. (1995). Benzodiazepines. In A. F. Schatzberg & C. B. Nereroff (Eds.), *The American Psychiatric Press textbook of psychopharmacology* (pp. 215–230). Washington, DC: American Psychiatric Press.

Baptista, T., Zarate, J., Joober, R., Colasante, C., Beauliew, S., Paez, X., et al. (2004). Drug induced weight gain, an impediment to successful pharmacotherapy: Focus on antipsychotics. *Current Drug Targets, 5*(3), 279–299.

Belle, D. J., & Singh, H. (2008). Genetic factors in drug metabolism. *American Family Physician, 77*(11), 1553–1560.

Benowitz, N. L. (1993). Nicotine replacement therapy: What has been accomplished—can we do better? *Drugs, 45*, 157–170.

Biederman, J., & Pliszka, S. R. (2008). Modafinil improves symptoms of attention deficit/hyperactivity disorder across subtypes in children and adolescents. *Child and Adolescent Psychiatiry Clinics of North America, 17*(2), 439–458.

Boyer, E. W., & Shannon, M. (2005). The serotonin syndrome. *New England Journal of Medicine, 352*(11), 1112–1120.

Boyer, W. F., & Feighner, J. P. (1991). The efficacy of selective serotonin uptake inhibitors in depression. In J. P. Feighner & W. F. Boyer (Eds.), *Selective serotonin reuptake inhibitors* (pp. 89–108). Chichester, England: Wiley.

Budur, K., Rodriguez, C., & Foldvary-Schaefer, N. (2007). Advances in treating insomnia. *Cleveland Clinic Journal of Medicine, 74*(4), 251–252, 255–258, 261–262.

Cahill, K., Stead, L. F., & Lancaster, T. (2008). Nicotine receptor partial agonists for smoking cessation. *Cochrane Database of Systematic Reviews* (3).

Campbell, D. B., & Levitt, P. (2008). Future of individualized psychiatric treatment. *Pharmacogenomics, 9*(5), 493–495.

Chambers, C. D., Johnson, B. A., Dick, L., Feley, R., & Jones, K. L. (1996). Birth outcomes in pregnant women taking fluoxetine. *New England Journal of Medicine, 335*(14), 1010–1015.

Charney, D. S., Miller, H., Licinia, J., & Salomon, R. (1995). Treatment of depression. In A. F. Schatzberg & C. B. Nemeroff (Eds.), *The American Psychiatric Press textbook of psychopharmacology* (pp. 587–588). Washington, DC: American Psychiatric Press.

Chessick, C. A., Allen, M. H., Thase, M., Batista Miralha da Cunha, A.B., Kapczinski, F. F., de Lima, M. S., & dos Santos Sousa, J. J., (2006). Azapirones for generalized anxiety disorder. *Cochrane Database of Systematic Reviews* (3).

Chick, J. (1999). Safety issues concerning the use of disulfiram in treating alcohol dependence. *Drug Safety, 20*(5), 427–435.

Ciraulo, D. A., Creelman, W. L., Shader, R. I., & O'Sullivan, R. L. (1994). Antidepressants. In D. A. Ciraulo, R. I. Shader, D. J. Greenblatt, & W. L. Creelman (Eds.), *Drug interactions in psychiatry* (2nd ed.). Baltimore: Williams & Wilkins.

Ciraulo, D. A., Dong, Q., Silverman, B. L., Gastfriend, D. R., & Pettinati, H. M. (2008). Early treatment response in alcohol dependence with extended-release naltrexone. *Journal of Clinical Psychiatry, 69*(2), 190–195.

Cole, J. O., & Yonkers, K. A. (1995). Nonbenzodiazepine anxiolytics. In A. F. Schatzberg & C. B. Nereroff (Eds.), *The American Psychiatric Press textbook of psychopharmacology* (p. 231). Washington, DC: American Psychiatric Press.

Cooper-Kazaz, R., & Lerer, B. (2008). Efficacy and safety of triiodothyronine supplementation in patients with major depressive disorder treated with specific serotonin reuptake inhibitors. *International Journal of Neuropsychopharmacology, 11*(5), 685–699.

Cornish, J. W., McNicholas, L. F., & O'Brien, C. P. (1995). Treatment of substance-related disorders. In A. F. Schatzberg & C. B. Nereroff (Eds.), *The American Psychiatric Press textbook of psychopharmacology* (p. 719). Washington, DC: American Psychiatric Press.

Crismon, M. L., Argo, T. R., & Buckley, P. F. (2008). Schizophrenia. In J. T. Dipiro, R. L. Talbert, G. C. Yee, G. R. Matzke, B. G. Wells, & L. M. Posey (Eds.), *Pharmacotherapy: A pathophysiologic approach* (pp. 1099–1122). New York: McGraw-Hill.

Davidson, J. R. (2004). Use of benzodiazepines in social anxiety disorder, generalized anxiety disorder, and posttraumatic stress disorder. *Journal of Clinical Psychiatry, 65*(Suppl. 5), 29–33.

Davidson, M. (2002). Risk of cardiovascular disease and sudden death in schizophrenia. *Journal of Clinical Psychiatry, 63*(Suppl. 9), 5–11.

Delgado, P. L., & Gelenberg, A. J. (1995). Antidepressant and antimanic medications. In G. O. Gabbard (Ed.), *Treatments of psychiatric disorders* (pp. 1131–1168). Washington, DC: American Psychiatric Press.

Deshauer, D. (2007). Venlafaxine (Effexor): Concerns about increased risk of fatal outcomes in overdose. *Canadian Medical Association Journal, 176*(1), 39–40.

Doggrell, S. A. (2006). After the failure of citalopram for depression, what next? *Expert Opinion on Pharmacotherapy, 7*(11), 1515–1518.

Dolder, C., Nelson, M., & Deyo, Z. (2008). Paliperidone for schizophrenia. *American Journal of Health-System Pharmacy, 65*(5), 403–413.

Drover, D. R. (2004). Comparative pharmacokinetics and pharmacodynamics of short acting hypnosedatives: Zaleplon, Zolpidem, and zopiclone. *Clinical Pharmacokinetics, 43*(4), 227–238.

Dudley, M., Hadzi-Pavlovic, D., Andrews, D., & Perich, T. (2008). New-generation antidepressants, suicide and depressed adolescents: How should clinicians respond to changing evidence? *Australian and New Zealand Journal of Psychiatry, 42*(6), 456–466.

Dvir, Y., & Smallwood, P. (2008). Serotonin syndrome: A complex but easily avoidable condition. *General Hospital Psychiatry, 30*(3), 284–287.

Ferguson, J. M. (2001). SSRI antidepressant medications: Adverse effects and tolerability. *Primary Care Companion to Journal of Clinical Psychiatry, 3*(1), 22–27.

Fick, D. M., Mion, L. C., Beers, M. H., & Waller, J. (2008). Health outcomes associated with potentially inappropriate medication use in older adults. *Research in Nursing & Health, 31*(1), 42–51.

Flanagan, R. J. (2008). Fatal toxicity of drugs used in psychiatry. *Human Psychopharmacology, 23*(Suppl. 1), 43–51.

Fuller, R. K., Branchey, L., Brightwell, D. R., Derman, R. M., Emrick, C. D., Iber, F. L., James, K. E., Lacoursiere, R. B., Lee, K. K., Lowenstam, I., Maany, I., Neiderhiser, D., Nocks. J. J. & Shaw, S. (1986). Disulfiram treatment of alcoholism: A Veterans Administration cooperative study. *Journal of the American Medical Association, 256*, 1449–1455.

Garland, E. J. (2004). Commentary: Facing the evidence: Antidepressant treatment in children and adolescents. *Canadian Medical Association Journal, 170*(4) 1.

George, T. P., Chawarski, M. C., Pakes, J., Carroll, K. M., Kosten, T. R., & Schottenfeld, R. S. (2000). Disulfiram versus placebo for cocaine dependence in buprenorphine-maintained subjects: A preliminary trial. *Biological Psychiatry, 47*(12), 1080–1086.

Gerstner, T., Busing, D., Bell, N., Longin, E., Kasper, J. M., Klostermann, W., et al. (2007). Valproic acid-induced pancreatitis: 16 new cases and a review of the literature. *Journal of Gastroenterology, 42*(1), 39–48.

Gillman, P. K. (2007). Tricyclic antidepressant pharmacology and therapeutic drug interactions updated. *British Journal of Pharmacology, 151*(6), 737–748.

Goff, B., & Baldessarini, R. J. (1995). Antipsychotics. In D. A. Ciraulo, R. I. Shader, D. J. Greenblatt, & W. L. Creelman (Eds.), *Drug interactions in psychiatry* (2nd ed., pp. 147–173). Baltimore: Williams & Wilkins.

Gómez, J. C., Sacristán, J. A., Hernández, J., Breier, A., Ruiz Carrasco, P., Antón Saiz, C., et al. (2000). The safety of olanzapine compared with other antipsychotic drugs: Results of an observational prospective study in patients with schizophrenia (EFESO Study). Pharmacoepidemiologic Study of Olanzapine in Schizophrenia. *Journal of Clinical Psychiatry, 61*(5), 335–343.

Grunder, G., Fellows, C., Janouschek, H., Veselinovic, T., Boy, C., Brocheler, A., et al. (2008). Brain and plasma pharmacokinetics of aripiprazole in patients with schizophrenia: An [18F]fallypride PET study. *American Journal of Psychiatry, 165*(8), 988–995.

Haddad, P. M. (2004). Antipsychotics and diabetes: A review of non-prospective data. *British Journal Psychiatry Supplement, 47*, S80–86.

Hair, P. I., McCormack, P. L., & Curran, M. P. (2008). Spotlight on eszopiclone in insomnia. *CNS Drugs, 22*(11), 975–978.

Harrison, T. S., & Goa, K. L. (2004). Long-acting risperidone: A review of its use in schizophrenia. *CNS Drugs, 18*(2), 113–132.

Hennekens, C. H., Hennekens, A. R., Hollar, D., & Casey, D. E. (2005). Schizophrenia and increased risks of cardiovascular disease. *American Heart Journal, 150*(6), 1115–1121.

Huang, X., Lei, Z., & El-Mallakh, R. S. (2007). Lithium normalizes elevated intracellular sodium. *Bipolar Disorders, 9*(3), 298–300.

Hughes, J. R. (2008). Smoking and suicide: A brief overview. *Drug and Alcohol Dependence, 98*(3), 169–178.

Jaffe, A. B., & Levine, J. (2003). Efficacy and effectiveness of first-and second-generation antipsychotics in schizophrenia. *Journal of Clinical Psychiatry, 64*(Suppl. 17), 3–6.

Jeffries, J., Remington, G., & Wilkins, J. (1984). The question of lithium/neuroleptic toxicity. *Canadian Journal of Psychiatry, 29*, 601–605.

Joffe, R. T., Singer, W., Levitt, A. J., & MacDonald, C. (1993). A placebo controlled comparison of lithium and triiodothyronine augmentation of tricyclic antidepressants in unipolar refractory depression. *Archives of General Psychiatry, 50*, 387–393.

Keitner, G. I., Garlow, S. J., Ryan, C. E., Ninan, P. T., Solomon, D. A., Nemeroff, C. B., & Keller, M.B. (2008). A randomized, placebo-controlled trial of risperidone augmentation for patients with difficult-to-treat unipolar, non-psychotic major depression. *Journal of Psychiatric Research, 43*(3), 205–214.

Kirkpatrick, B., & Galderisi, S. (2008). Deficit schizophrenia: An update. *World Psychiatry, 7*(3), 143–147.

Kirsch, I., Deacon, B. J., Huedo-Medina, T. B., Scoboria, A., Moore, T. J., & Johnson, B. T. (2008). Initial severity and antidepressant benefits: A meta-analysis of data submitted to the Food and Drug Administration. *PLoS Med, 5*(2).

Kopelowicz, A., Zarate, R., Tripodis, K., Gonzalez, V., & Mintz, J. (2000). Differential efficacy of olanzapine for deficit and nondeficit negative symptoms in schizophrenia. *American Journal of Psychiatry, 157*(6), 987–993.

Lenox, R. H., & Hahn, C. G. (2000). Overview of the mechanism of action of lithium in the brain: Fifty-year update. *Journal of Clinical Psychiatry, 61*(Suppl. 9), 5–15.

Lucas, P. B., Pickar, D., Kelsoe, J., Rapaport, M., Pato, C. & Hommer, D. (1990). Effects of the acute administration of caffeine to patients with schizophrenia. *Biological Psychiatry, 28,* 35.

Mann, N., & Bitsios, P. (2008). Modafinil treatment of amphetamine abuse in adult ADHD. *Journal of Psychopharmacology, 23*(4), 468–471.

Manschreck, T. C., & Boshes, R. A. (2007). The CATIE schizophrenia trial: Results, impact, controversy. *Harvard Review of Psychiatry, 15*(5), 245–258.

Marder, S. R., & Van Putten, T. (1995). Antipsychotic medications. In A. F. Schatzberg & C. B. Nemeroff (Eds.), *The American Psychiatric Press textbook of psychopharmacology.* Washington, DC: American Psychiatric Press.

McCauley-Elsom, K., & Kulkarni, J. (2007). Managing psychosis in pregnancy. *Australian and New Zealand Journal of Psychiatry, 41*(3), 289–292.

McEvoy, J. P., Lieberman, J. A., Stroup, T. S., Davis, S. M., Meltzer, H. Y., Rosenheck, R. A. et al. (2006). Effectiveness of clozapine versus olanzapine, quetiapine, and risperidone in patients with chronic schizophrenia who did not respond to prior atypical antipsychotic treatment. *American Journal of Psychiatry, 163,* 600–610.

McGrath, P. J., Stewart, J. W., Nunes, E. V., Ocepek-Welikson, K., Rabkin, J. G., Quitkin, F. M., & Klein, D. F. (1993). A double-blind crossover trial of imipramine and phenelzine for outpatients with treatment-refractory depression. *American Journal of Psychiatry, 150,* 118–123.

McIntyre, R., & Katzman, M. (2003). The role of atypical antipsychotics in bipolar depression and anxiety disorders. *Bipolar Disorders, 5*(Suppl. 2), 20–25.

Melkersson, K., & Dahl, M. L. (2004). Adverse metabolic effects associated with atypical antipsychotics: Literature review and clinical implications. *Drugs, 64*(7), 701–723.

Meltzer, H. Y., Li, Z., Kaneda, Y., & Ichikawa, J. (2003). Serotonin receptors: Their key role in drugs to treat schizophrenia. *Progress in Neuro-psychopharmacology and Biological Psychiatry, 27*(7), 1159–1172.

Misri, S., Kostaras, D., & Kostaras, X. (2000). The use of selective serotonin reuptake inhibitors during pregnancy and lactation: Current knowledge. *Canadian Journal of Psychiatry, 45*(3), 285–287.

Mitchell, A. J. (2006). Two-week delay in onset of action of antidepressants: New evidence. *British Journal of Psychiatry, 188,* 105–106.

Nelson, J. C. (2007). Augmentation strategies in the treatment of major depressive disorder. Recent findings and current status of augmentation strategies. *CNS Spectrums, 12*(12, Suppl. 22), 6–9.

Nemeroff, C. B. (2007). Prevalence and management of treatment-resistant depression. *Journal of Clinical Psychiatry, 68*(Suppl. 8), 17–25.

Nishinto, S., Mignot, E., & Dement, W. C. (1995). Sedative-hypnotics. In A. F. Schatzberg & C. B. Nemeroff (Eds.), *The American Psychiatric Press textbook of psychopharmacology* (p. 410). Washington, DC: American Psychiatric Press.

Nissen, S. E. (2006). ADHD drugs and cardiovascular risk. *New England Journal of Medicine, 354*(14), 1445–1448.

Nutt, D. J. (1995). Addition: Brain mechanisms and their related implications. *Lancet, 347*(8993), 33–35.

Overstreet, K., Costanza, C., Behling, C., Hassanin, T., & Masliah, E. (2002). Fatal progressive hepatic necrosis associated with lamotrigine treatment: A case report and literature review. *Digestive Diseases and Science, 47*(9), 1921–1925.

Papakostas, G.I. (2007). Limitations of contemporary antidepressants: tolerability. *Journal of Clinical Psychiatry, 68(Suppl 10),* 11–17.

Papakostas, G. I., Peterse, T. J., Nierenberg, A. A., Murakami, J. L., Alpert, J. E., Rosenbaum, J. F., et al. (2004). Ziprasodone augmentation of selective serotonin reuptake inhibitors (SSRIs) for SSRI-resistant major depressive disorder. *Journal of Clinical Psychiatry, 65*(2), 217–221.

Passarella, S., & Duong, M. T. (2008). Diagnosis and treatment of insomnia. *American Journal of Health-System Pharmacy, 65*(10), 927–934.

Potter, W. Z., Manji, H., & Rudorfer, M. (1995). Tricyclics and tetracyclics. In A. F. Schatzberg & C. B. Nemeroff (Eds.), *The American Psychiatric Press textbook of psychopharmacology* (p. 145). Washington, DC: American Psychiatric Press.

Ramakrishnan, K., & Scheid, D. C. (2007). Treatment options for insomnia. *American Family Physician, 76*(4), 517–526.

Rapaport, M. H. (2007). Dietary restrictions and drug interactions with monoamine oxidase inhibitors: The state of the art. *Journal of Clinical Psychiatry, 68*(Suppl. 8), 42–46.

Rathore, S., Masani, N. D., & Callaghan, P. O. (2007). Clozapine-induced effuso-constrictive pericarditis. Case report and review of the literature. *Cardiology, 108*(3), 183–185.

Reeves, H., Batra, S., May, R. S., Zhang, R., Dahl, D. C., & Li, X. (2008). Efficacy of risperidone augmentation to antidepressants in the management of suicidality in major depressive disorder: A randomized, double-blind, placebo-controlled pilot study. *Journal of Clinical Psychiatry, 69*(8), 1228–1336.

Reynoldson, J. N., Elliott, E., Sr. & Nelson, L. A. (2008). Ramelteon: A novel approach in the treatment of insomnia. *Annals of Pharmacotherapy, 42*(9), 1262–1271.

Robinson, D. S., & Amsterdam, J. D. (2008). The selegiline transdermal system in major depressive disorder: A systematic review of safety and tolerability. *Journal of Affective Disorders, 105*(1–3), 15–23.

Rosenheck, R., Dunn, L., Peszke, M., Cramer, J., Xu, W., Thomas, J., et al. (1999). Impact of clozapine on negative symptoms and on the deficit syndrome in refractory schizophrenia. Department of Veterans Affairs Cooperative Study Group on Clozapine in Refractory Schizophrenia. *American Journal of Psychiatry, 156*(1), 88–93.

Ruhe, H. G., Huyser, J., Swinkels, J. A., & Schene, A. H. (2006). Switching antidepressants after a first selective serotonin reuptake inhibitor in major depressive disorder: A systematic review. *Journal of Clinical Psychiatry, 67*(12), 1836–1855.

Salzman, C., Satlin, A., & Burrows, A. B. (1995). Geriatric psychopharmacology. In A. F. Schatzberg & C. B. Nemeroff (Eds.), *The American Psychiatric Press textbook of psychopharmacology* (p. 812). Washington, DC: American Psychiatric Press.

Schachar, R., & Tannock, R. (1993). Childhood hyperactivity and psychostimulants: A review of extended treatment studies. *Journal of Child and Adolescent Psychopharmacology, 3,* 81–97.

Schooler, N. R. (2006). Relapse prevention and recovery in the treatment of schizophrenia. *Journal of Clinical Psychiatry, 67*(Suppl. 5), 19–23.

Schou, M. (1989). *Lithium treatment of manic-depressive illness* (4th ed., rev.). Basel, Switzerland: Karger.

Schule, C., Baghai, T. C., Eser, D., Nothdurfter, C., & Rupprecht, R. (2008). Lithium but not carbamazepine augments antidepressant efficacy of mirtazapine in unipolar depression: An open-label study.

World Journal of Biological Psychiatry, Jan 25, 1–10 Epub ahead of print.

Schweizer, E., Rickels, K., Amsterdam, J. D., Fox, I, Puzzuoli, G, & Weise, C. (1990). What constitutes an adequate antidepressant trial for fluoxetine? *Journal of Clinical Psychiatry, 51*, 8–11.

Sedvall, G., & Farde, L. (1995). Chemical brain activity in schizophrenia. *Lancet, 346*(8977) 746.

Seemuller, F., Riedel, M., Obermeier, M., Bauer, M., Adli, M., Mundt, C., et al. (2008). The controversial link between antidepressants and suicidality risks in adults: Data from a naturalistic study on a large sample of in-patients with a major depressive episode. *International Journal of Neuropsychopharmacology*, 1–9.

Sicouri, S., & Antzelevitch, C. (2008). Sudden cardiac death secondary to antidepressant and antipsychotic drugs. *Expert Opinion on Drug Safety, 7*(2), 181–194.

Spina, E., Santoro, V., & D'Arrigo, C. (2008). Clinically relevant pharmacokinetic drug interactions with second-generation antidepressants: An update. *Clinical Therapeutics, 30*(7), 1206–1227.

Sporer, K. A. (2004). Buprenorphine: A primer for emergency physicians. *Annals of Emergency Medicine, 43*(5), 580–584.

Sprague, D. A., Loewen, P. S., & Raymond, C. B. (2004). Selection of atypical antipsychotics for the management of schizophrenia. *Annals of Pharmacotherapy, 38*(2), 313–319.

Stoner, S. C., Nelson, L. A., Lea, J. W., Marken, P. A., Sommi, R. W., & Dahmen, M. M. (2007). Historical review of carbamazepine for the treatment of bipolar disorder. *Pharmacotherapy, 27*(1), 68–88.

Strawn, J. R., Keck, P. E., Jr., & Caroff, S. N. (2007). Neuroleptic malignant syndrome. *American Journal of Psychiatry, 164*(6), 870–876.

Swann, A. C., Secunda, S. K., Stokes, P. E., Davis, J.M., Koslow, J.M., & Maas, J.W. (1990). Stress, depression and mania; Relationship between perceived role of stressful events and clinical and biochemical characteristics. *Acta Psychiatrica Scandinavica, 81*, 389–397.

Teter, C. J., Kando, J. C., Wells, B. G., & Hayes, P. E. (2008). Depressive disorders. In J. T. Dipiro, R. L. Talbert, G. C. Yee, G. R. Matzke, B. G. Wells, & L. M. Posey, (Eds.), *Pharmacotherapy: A pathophysiologic approach* (pp.1123–1139). New York: McGraw-Hill.

Tohen, M., Bowden, C. L., Smulevich, A. B., Bergstrom, R., Quinlan, T., Osuntokun, O., Wang, W. V., Oliff, H. S., Martenyl, F., Kryzhanovskaya, L. A., & Griel, W. (2008). Olanzaprine plus carbamazeprine v. carbamazeprine alone in treating manic episodes. *British Journal of Psychiatry, 192*(2), 135–143.

Tollefson, G. D. (1995). Selective serotonin reuptake inhibitors. In A. F. Schatzberg & C. B. Nemeroff (Eds.), *The American Psychiatric Press textbook of psychopharmacology* (p. 167). Washington, DC: American Psychiatric Press.

Tondo, L., & Baldessarini, R. J. (2000). Reduced suicide risk during lithium maintenance treatment. *Journal of Clinical Psychiatry, 61*(Suppl. 9), 97–104.

Tuunainen, A., Wahlbeck, K., & Gilbody, S. M. (2000). Newer atypical antipsychotic medication versus clozapine for schizophrenia. *Cochrane Database System Review* (2), CD000966.

Verster, J. C., Volkerts, E. R., Schreuder, A. H., Eijken, E. J., van Heuckelum, J., Veldhuijzen, D. S., et al. (2002). Residual effects of the middle-of-the-night administration of zaleplon and zolpidem on driving ability, memory functions and psychomotor performance. *Journal of Clinical Psychopharmacology, 22*(6), 576–583.

Vieta, E., Panicali, F., Goetz, I., Reed, C., Comes, M., Tohen, M., et al. (2008). Olanzapine monotherapy and olanzapine combination therapy in the treatment of mania: 12-week results from the European Mania in Bipolar Longitudinal Evaluation of Medication (EMBLEM) observational study. *Journal of Affective Disorders, 106*(1–2), 63–72.

Vieta, E., & Sanchez-Moreno, J. (2008). Acute and long-term treatment of mania. *Dialogues in Clinical Neuroscience, 10*(2), 165–179.

Vieweg, W. V., & Wood, M. A. (2004). Tricyclic antidepressants, QT interval prolongation, and torsade de pointes. *Psychosomatics, 45*(5), 371–377.

Weiden, P. J., Preskorn, S. H., Fahnestock, P. A., Carpenter, D., Ross, R., Docherty, J. P., et al. (2007). Translating the psychopharmacology of antipsychotics to individualized treatment for severe mental illness: A Roadmap. *Journal of Clinical Psychiatry, 68*(Suppl. 7), 1–48.

Weisler, R. H., Keck, P. E., Jr, Swann, A. C., Cutler, A. J., Ketter, T. A., Kalali, A. H., et al. (2005). Extended-release carbamazepine capsules as monotherapy for acute mania in bipolar disorder: A multicenter, randomized, double-blind, placebo-controlled trial. *Journal of Clinical Psychiatry, 66*(3), 323–330.

Wender, P. H., Reimherr, J., Wood, D., & Ward, M. (1985). A controlled study of methylphenidate in the treatment of attention deficit disorder, residual type, in adults. *American Journal of Psychiatry, 142*, 547–552.

Wig, N. N. (1993). Rational treatment in psychiatry, perspectives on psychiatric treatment by level of care. In N. Sartorius, G. de Girolamo, G. Andrews, G. A. German, & L. Eisenberg (Eds.), *Treatment of mental disorders* (pp. 423–441). Washington, DC: American Psychiatric Press.

Wilens, T. E. (2004). Impact of ADHD and its treatment on substance abuse in adults. *Journal of Clinical Psychiatry, 65*(Suppl. 3), 38–45.

Yagiela, J. A., Duffin, S. R., & Hunt L. M. (1985). Drug interactions and vasoconstrictors used in local anesthetic solutions. *Oral Surgery Oral Medicine Oral Pathology. 59*, 565–571.

Zemrak, W. R., & Kenna, G. A. (2008). Association of antipsychotic and antidepressant drugs with Q-T interval prolongation. *American Journal of Health-System Pharmaists, 65*(11), 1029–1038.

Zeskind, P. S., & Stephens, L. E. (2004). Maternal selective serotonin reuptake inhibitor use during pregnancy and newborn neurobehavior. *Pediatrics, 113*(2), 368–375.

Zhang, W. V., Ramzan, I., & Murray, M. (2007). Impaired microsomal oxidation of the atypical antipsychotic agent clozapine in hepatic steatosis. *Journal of Pharmacology and Experimental Therapeutics, 322*(2), 770–777.

SUGGESTED READINGS

Enger, C., Weatherby, L., Reynold, R. F., Glasser, D. B., & Walker, A. M. (2004). Serious cardiovascular events and mortality among patients with schizophrenia. *Journal of Nervous and Mental Disease, 192*(1), 19–27.

Fuller, M. A. (2004). *Drug information handbook for psychiatry.* Hudson, OH: Lexi-Comp, Inc.

Rankin, E. (2000). *Quick reference to psychopharmacology.* Clifton Park, NY: Thomson Delmar Learning.

Schatzberg, A. F., & Schatzberg, C. B. (2004). *The American Psychiatric Publishing textbook of psychopharmacology* (3rd ed.). Washington, DC: American Psychiatric Publishing.

Spratto, G., & Woods, A. (2006). *2006 PDR Nurse's drug handbook.* Clifton Park, NY: Thomson Delmar Learning.

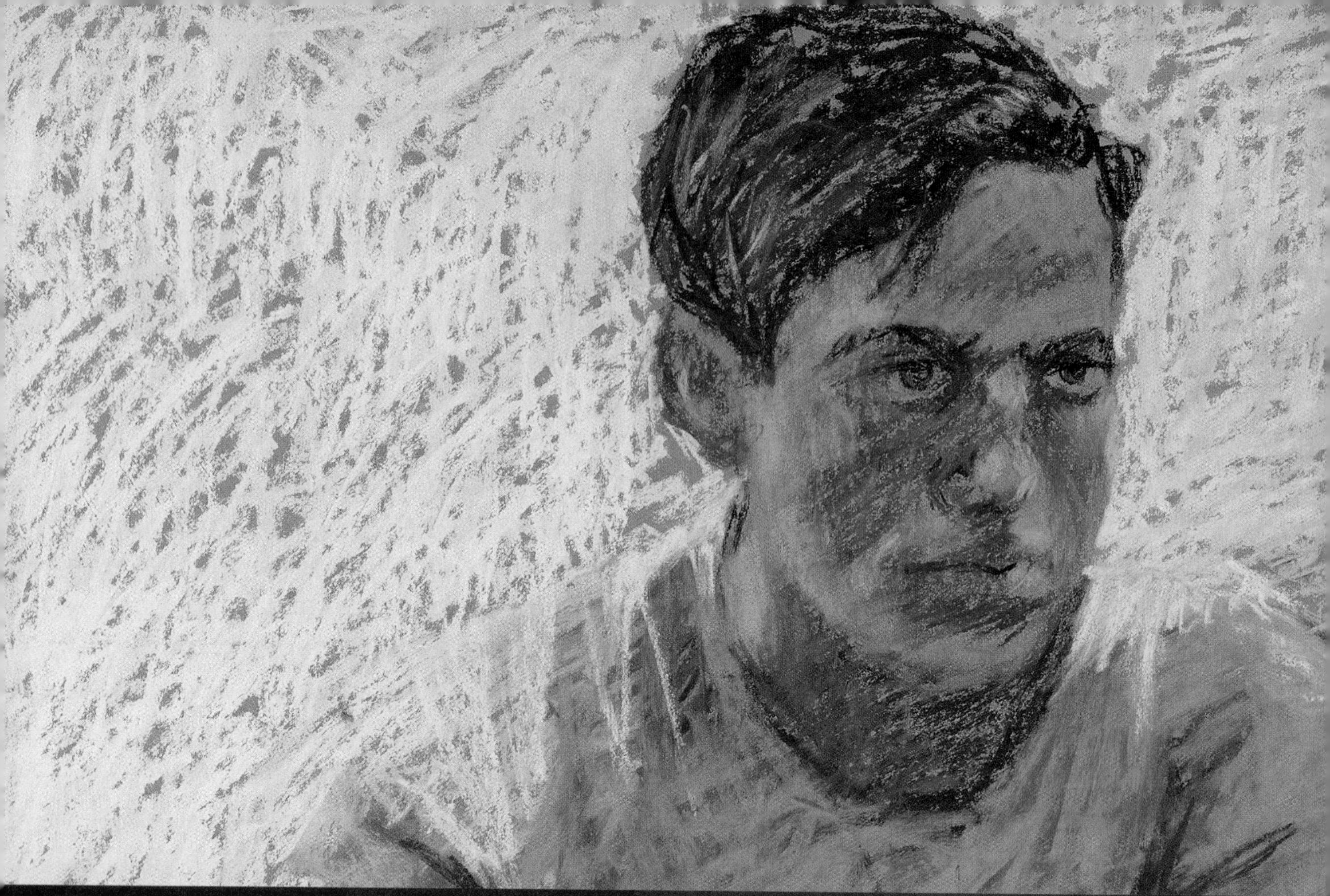

Psychotherapy

Consider the reasons clients might seek individual therapy:

- ***Many persons seek a therapist during a time of crisis and change.***
- ***Others seek therapy to deal with a specific issue (for example, the breakup of a relationship) and then find there are other concerns that underlie the current issue.***
- ***Still others seek therapy because their feelings and behaviors have impaired their ability to function effectively.***

As you work with clients, consider the reasons that each is seeking care at this time and begin to evaluate how the motivation for treatment affects the type of therapy that will best meet the client's immediate needs.

CHAPTER 28

Individual Psychotherapy

Noreen Cavan Frisch
Lawrence E. Frisch

CHAPTER OUTLINE

COMPETENCIES

Upon completion of this chapter, the reader should be able to:

1. Define *psychotherapy.*
2. Describe various approaches to therapy, including:
   - Psychoanalysis
   - Psychodynamic therapy
   - Interpersonal therapy
   - Cognitive-behavioral therapy
   - Client-centered therapy
3. Suggest ways that psychotherapeutic approaches are used in nursing practice.
4. Relate major psychotherapeutic approaches to nursing theory.
5. Describe the research base of psychotherapeutic interventions.

KEY TERMS

Behaviorally Oriented Therapy	Confrontation	Psychoanalysis
Catharsis	Experience-Oriented Therapy	Psychodynamic Therapy
Clarification	Insight-Oriented Therapies	Psychotherapy
Client-Centered Therapy	Interpersonal Therapy	Repression
Cognitive-Behavioral Therapy	Interpretation	Suggestion

Psychotherapy is the treatment of mental or emotional disorders through psychological rather than physical methods (although it is often done in conjunction with somatic therapy, especially medications). Often, psychotherapy is referred to as "talk therapy." Psychotherapy can be done with individuals or with groups (see Chapter 30). Individual psychotherapy is the use of psychological techniques applied in a one-on-one setting. The techniques are designed to help persons overcome mental distress and illness for the purpose of assisting those individuals to reach their optimum level of health. Psychotherapy has several characteristics that make it an important study for psychiatric nurses:

1. Data clearly establish the effectiveness of individual psychotherapy for a number of specific therapies targeted to specific disorders.
2. Many of the techniques of psychotherapy are of value to nurses in their daily work, both with psychiatric clients and with others.
3. Psychotherapy has potential relevance to all settings in which psychiatric nursing is carried out: inpatient, outpatient, and home care.
4. Developments in the not so distant past have placed a strong emphasis on brief treatment techniques in psychotherapy.
5. More recent developments in psychotherapy have validated the longer-term use of psychotherapies for many individuals with chronic mental disorders.

It is important for nurses to understand how psychotherapies differ so that they can help clients choose appropriate treatment.

Only a few decades ago, individuals seeking counseling or therapy would have had few options: primarily lengthy, intensive psychoanalysis. Today, there are multiple approaches to therapy. Some of these approaches derive from psychoanalysis and rely on helping individuals gain insight into feelings and behaviors; these are known as **insight-oriented therapies**. Other therapies are **behaviorally oriented**. They help individuals to gain tools that allow them to change behavior (and often feelings). Yet a third group of therapies is **experience-oriented**. These attempt to create an experience that will facilitate growth and personal development. The purpose of this chapter is to acquaint the nurse with major approaches to psychotherapy. However, because many different types of professionals offer psychotherapy, it is important to begin with a brief discussion of the identity and credentials of individuals who commonly offer psychotherapeutic services.

PROVIDERS OF THERAPY

Clients seeking therapy may be seen by a psychiatrist (MD), a psychologist (PhD), a nurse (RN, MSN, DNP, or PhD), a social worker (MSW), or a therapist/counselor. Although the distinction between psychotherapy and counseling may be vague, psychotherapy is typically more intense and frequently more likely to be directed to persons with serious psychopathology. Counseling is more commonly sought by individuals experiencing acute situational crisis (see Chapter 10). Counselors are more often educated at the master's level and are less likely to have experience with seriously ill individuals.

Registered nurses may provide counseling and client education related to crisis, stress, and mental health and may also provide referral to community sources for both therapy and counseling. In addition, experienced psychiatric nurses may provide client support and carry out interventions that are based on any of the psychotherapeutic approaches. In some settings, nurses in advanced practice roles (MSN, DNP, CNS, or PhD) provide both counseling and psychotherapy; in some states, these practitioners may also perform physical examinations and prescribe medications.

An important concept in psychotherapy is the role of the therapist and the role of the client. A major medical textbook presents the view that, for psychiatry, the therapist must take on the role of "helper" and the client must take on the role of "help seeker." The therapist, as the helper, is seen as the expert who sets the roles, rules, and boundaries of the verbal interchange in the therapy session (Ursano & Silberman, 2003). In contrast, a nursing role is, by definition, a more collaborative one. Thus, as readers become acquainted with the various approaches to psychotherapy described in the following section, they are encouraged to consider these roles of helper and help seeker from within a nursing perspective as the similarities and contrasts will be addressed in the later sections of this chapter.

MAJOR APPROACHES TO PSYCHOTHERAPY

Virtually all of the many varieties and schools of psychotherapy can be grouped into one of three categories: insight-oriented therapy, behaviorally oriented therapy, and experience-oriented therapy. There are many specific types of therapy within each category, but if the nurse understands the principles underlying each major category, then he will be able to understand the principles of new or unfamiliar psychotherapeutic techniques.

INSIGHT-ORIENTED THERAPY

Psychoanalysis

Psychoanalysis is the oldest and best known of the insight-oriented therapies. It is derived from the Freudian view of psychosexual development (see Chapter 3). Psychoanalysis is a form of psychotherapy focusing on the uncovering of unconscious memories and processes: "Psychoanalysis is based on the observation that individuals are often unaware of many of the factors that determine their emotions and behavior. These unconscious factors may create unhappiness, sometimes in the form of recognizable symptoms and at other times as troubling personality traits, difficulties in work or in love relationships, or disturbances in mood and self-esteem" (American Psychoanalytic Association, 2008).

The goal of the psychoanalytic treatment is to demonstrate to the client how unconscious factors affect current relationship and behavior patterns. The treatment traces the patterns of behavior and relationships back to their origin in infancy or childhood. Through the process of reexperiencing life circumstances and interactions with the analyst, the client becomes both intellectually and emotionally aware of the underlying sources of difficulties. The client provides the analyst with clues to the unconscious sources of current difficulties—through identification of certain patterns of behavior, in the subjects that he finds hard to talk about, or in the ways he relates to the analyst. During the psychoanalytic process, the client grapples with insights, going over them again and again with the analyst, as well as repeatedly addressing these insights in daily life, in dreams, and in fantasies.

The process of psychoanalysis is highly individualized, and its course is dictated both by the nature of the presenting problem and by the personalities and backgrounds of both

The Persistence of Memory

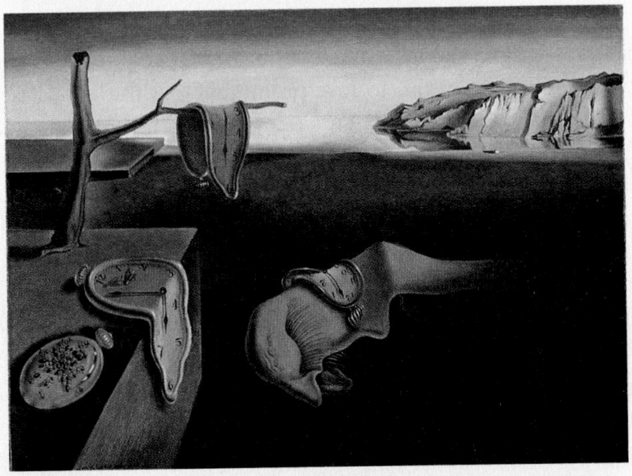

The landscape and subject evoke a dream or nightmare. Perhaps a pun on the distortion of time often experienced in dreams, the deformed watches may also be symbols from a frightening past—hence the title. This picture seems to demand a formal interpretation, but it is hard to believe that any would succeed short of detailed psychoanalysis of the painter himself. Painted during Freud's lifetime, this work strongly suggests the mysteries, and perhaps even the potential dangers, of deeply probing the unconscious self through psychoanalytic therapy.

analyst and client. For this reason it is often hard to describe a "typical" psychoanalysis. Most psychoanalysts believe in the process of **repression**, in which painful memories, thoughts, or experiences are actively kept out of conscious awareness. These memories may have highly emotional content; for example, such memories may involve violence or sexual experiences. The analyst's goal is to uncover unconscious experiences and to interpret them to a client who finds them painful and frightening.

Psychoanalytic theory assumes that clients actively resist coming to an understanding of repressed, unconscious thoughts or feelings. Because of this resistance, the analyst must use specific therapeutic techniques that help the client grow in his willingness to accept uncomfortable conscious or unconscious thoughts and change dysfunctional behaviors. Some of these techniques are summarized in Table 28-1. This table provides an example of a typical client-analyst interaction in a therapy session. In this session, the therapist is using the techniques of **confrontation** and **clarification** to assist the client to see that she is dealing with irritation and anger in a passive and indirect way. The purpose of the session would be to identify if the client has a long-standing pattern of dealing with anger this way, to explore the origins of the pattern, and ultimately to gain insights that will permit the client to adopt more active and direct methods of dealing with anger: "Eventually the [client's] life—his or her behavior, relationships, sense of self—changes in deep and abiding ways" (American Psychoanalytic Association, 2008).

Although psychoanalysis was the predominant therapeutic approach to mental illness throughout much of the twentieth century, it began to lose prominence in the 1980s and 1990s, only to regain a new resurgence in recent years. In 2004, one psychoanalytically oriented editorialist commented that psychoanalysis's "present position in psychiatry is at best precarious" (Bateman, 2004). However, in 2008, one finds increasing attention being paid to psychoanalysis not only as a therapy, but as a method of learning about the mind and a theory from which to understand the workings of the mind (American Psychoanalytic Association, 2008). Psychoanalysis focuses primarily on reporting case studies and on refining an elaborate theoretical basis whose origins go back to the nineteenth-century writings of Sigmund Freud. As a therapy, psychoanalysis requires frequent (several times per week) sessions between the client and analyst where the client is encouraged to explore and uncover the meaning of past experiences and to use insights gained to understand and interpret current life events. Psychoanalysis has been contrasted with nonpsychoanalytic approaches to mental illness that have undertaken well-designed empirical trials of effectiveness and have attempted to develop an understanding of psychiatric disorders at the molecular level and through complex imaging procedures. In recent years there have been substantive efforts to empirically document the evidence base supporting the effectiveness of this treatment. For example, the Stockholm Outcome of Psychoanalysis and Psychotherapy Project assessed the outcomes of psychoanalysis and psychodynamic psychotherapy in clients followed for up to three years after the completion of therapy (Sandell, Bloberg, Lazar, Carlsson, Broberg, & Schubert, 2000). While satisfactory outcome measures are difficult to define for studies of this sort (Vaughan, Marshall, Mackinnon, Vaughan, Mellman, & Roose, 2000), the Stockholm project provided some evidence that clients treated with psychoanalysis improved steadily even after therapy had concluded. It is difficult to predict to what degree the discipline of psychoanalysis will continue to play a major role among psychiatric treatment. Several additional studies have been conducted, with recent reports in the literature of the benefits of psychoanalysis in the treatment of clients with complex and severe mental disorders (Leichsenring & Rabung, 2008). These researchers report that

TABLE 28-1 Techniques Used in Psychoanalysis

TECHNIQUE	EXAMPLE
Suggestion: a technique in which the analyst tentatively interprets the client's thoughts, actions, or dreams.	Analyst states, "Your recurrent dreams about taking tests may be an indication of your worry about success."
Catharsis: the experience of release that occurs by bringing unconscious thoughts through to consciousness in efforts to cure psychological symptoms.	Client states, "I feel relieved, I can now see that the fearful figure in my dream is my father."
Confrontation: the analyst directly challenges the client's behavior or thought, usually intended to provoke a reaction from the client. Such reactions are intended to overcome emotional barriers to change.	Analyst states, "You are relating to your boss the same way you relate to your father."
Clarification: the analyst describes the client's behavior, pointing out a pattern that is not recognized by the client.	Analyst states, "You have a pattern of dealing with anger by laughing. That is an indirect means of expressing anger."
Interpretation: the analyst brings her understanding of the client's unconscious processes to explain behavior.	Analyst states, "You are angry with me because I'm telling you the same things your mother told you."

BOX 28-1
SAMPLE CLIENT-ANALYST INTERACTION IN THERAPY

Therapist: How do you feel when I indicate to you that you are passive?

Client: I don't like it. (The client is laughing, but it is quite evident that she is irritated.)

Therapist: But you are smiling.

Client: I know, Well . . . maybe that is my way of expressing my irritation.

Therapist: Then you are irritated?

Client: A little bit . . . yeah . . .

Therapist: A little bit?

Client: Actually, quite a bit. (The client is laughing.)

Therapist: Let's look at what happened here. I brought to your attention your passivity, your noninvolvement. You got irritated and angry with me and the way you dealt with your irritation was by smiling.

From *Short-term Dynamic Psychotherapy* by H. Delano, 1980, New York: Jason Aronson.

long-term therapy yields stable positive outcomes for patients with personality disorders, multiple mental disorders, and chronic mental disorders. They go on to state that some clients with chronic conditions do not benefit from short-term psychotherapy. It seems that clients do benefit from the steady, frequent, and close attention that psychoanalysts provide. Such an idea is supported by the writings of a University of Southern California law professor who has lived most of her life with schizophrenia; Professor Elyn R. Saks remains an enthusiast for psychoanalytic "talk therapies" that made a difference in her life and the management of her illness (Saks, 2007).

Psychoanalysis is inherently lengthy and, for this reason, quite costly. Clients have traditionally paid their analyst directly for psychotherapeutic services, although in recent years some insurance plans have included coverage for psychological treatment, including psychoanalysis. As the realities of managed care have become increasingly evident, there has been a growth of interest in therapeutic techniques that can provide needed psychological insights in a shorter and thus more cost-effective time. Prominent among these techniques is a psychotherapeutic technique called psychodynamic therapy.

Psychodynamic Therapy

Psychodynamic therapy is based on psychoanalytic principles and interpretations. Psychodynamic therapy attempts to replace full psychoanalysis with a process that focuses on selected therapeutic issues so as to get more rapidly to what the therapist perceives to be the core of the individual's psychological distress. The goal of psychodynamic therapy is improved functioning rather than complete personality reconstruction. Psychodynamic therapy may take place over a few months or weeks, rather than the years occupied by traditional psychoanalysis. In at least one study comparing brief psychodynamic interventions with "usual care," suicidal outpatients who received four therapy sessions had significant improvements in level of depression and in subsequent episodes of self-harm (Guthrie et al., 2001).

Both psychoanalysis and psychodynamic therapy begin with two assumptions: First, it is assumed that the client is seeking therapy and is trying as hard as possible to work with the therapist; second, it is assumed that the client has basic abilities of cognition and insight. These approaches to therapy may be difficult to carry out with individuals who have significant psychological problems, including psychosis, substance abuse, and personality disorders. Even less disabling problems such as phobia or obsessional symptoms may make a psychodynamic approach untenable (Worchel, 1990). A meta-analysis summarizing evidence for psychodynamic psychotherapy in schizophrenia and other severe mental illness found few studies on which to base any conclusion (Malmberg & Fenton, 2001). Additional work is ongoing to document and validate evidence on which to base recommendations for this treatment.

REFLECTIVE THINKING 28-1

Psychoanalysis Techniques

Consider your own behavior and coping mechanisms. Do you find that you, intentionally or not, employ some of the techniques of psychoanalysis in your own behavioral strategies? What patterns can you recognize in your thoughts and behaviors?

Interpersonal Therapy

Not all insight-based therapy is derived from the psychoanalytic perspective. **Interpersonal therapy**, also insight-based, is based on the recognition that psychological distress frequently occurs in conjunction with disturbed human relationships. Interpersonal therapy is based on the interpersonal theories of Sullivan and the related nursing theory of Peplau (see Chapter 3).

During interpersonal therapy, the client enters into a relationship with the therapist and is helped to examine patterns of relationships and interactions with others. It is assumed that the client can use the experience of a positive therapeutic relationship, coupled with insights about past relationships, to establish meaningful, positive relationships with others outside the therapy sessions. Whereas psychoanalysis and its less intense cousin, psychodynamic therapy, search for their insights deep within the individual's unconscious mind, interpersonal therapy seeks to provide its clients with insight into the processes of daily life and human interaction. As for all of the numerous insight-based therapies, the goal is enhanced self-understanding leading to enhanced personal and interpersonal success. Nursing research studies evaluating the effects of interpersonal therapy have suggested that the approach is useful for clients with mood disorders and eating disorders (Crowe & Lutz, 2005a). These same authors state that a benefit of interpersonal therapy is that it emphasizes action rather than reflection and helps people to make meaningful connections with others (Crowe & Lutz, 2005b).

NURSINGTIP 28-1

Sample Homework Assignments in Cognitive-Behavioral Therapy

- Reading: may include books, workbook material, or relevant articles
- Written assignments: keeping a journal or log of day-to-day events
- Experiential activities: planned activities that involve risk taking or trying out new behaviors in a safe setting

Behaviorally Oriented Therapy

In recent years, the predominance of psychoanalytic methods has been giving way to a newer approach to the mind: cognitive-behavioral psychology. **Cognitive-behavioral therapy** is not about gaining insight into the presumed childhood origins of problems. It is not just about venting feelings or talking about problems. Rather, cognitive-behavioral therapy focuses on practical results. The main issue is not how an individual got to be the way he is; it is helping that individual make practical changes. Cognitive-behavioral therapy has several distinct characteristics:

1. It is result oriented. The therapy begins with assisting the client to define goals and then proceeds to monitor progress toward those goals.
2. It is short term. For most clients, the goals of the therapy can be accomplished quickly, often within 5 to 20 sessions.
3. It is self-help oriented. The therapist is a coach or teacher who helps the client learn how to manage his own life better. The client learns new tools for living his life and dealing with life's challenges.

The major goals of cognitive-behavioral therapy are to provide cost-effective care for a wide range of problems; to alter clients' interpretations of themselves by changing their behavior, environment, or cognition directly; to increase clients' coping skills; and to increase the likelihood that gains made during therapy will be maintained once therapy is terminated.

Cognitive therapies are concerned with how the client thinks about himself. Behavioral therapies focus on precisely what the client does. Together, the cognitive-behavioral approach attempts to change both a client's beliefs and his behavior. The therapy rarely addresses why a client feels or acts in a certain way; it is sufficient to ascertain only that this feeling or action is undesirable. Often, the therapist will work with her client to determine specifically in what settings the undesired thoughts or behaviors occur. The therapist then helps the client focus on alternatives to the specific thoughts or actions and works to help the client feel that he can truly use these alternatives.

The therapy becomes behaviorally oriented because the therapist gives the client "homework assignments" to complete in between therapy sessions. For example, a client dealing with problems of anger and risk for violence may be asked to keep a journal detailing feelings of anger, situations bringing on angry feelings, and immediate behaviors following angry feelings. The therapist and the client will review the journal during the following therapy session to identify thoughts and behaviors that can be used to replace the patterns that are causing trouble for the client.

Cognitive-behavioral therapy is frequently used in the treatment of depression. From this standpoint, the therapy may be based on three principles:

1. Moods, feelings, and depression are created and maintained by one's thoughts and feelings. In this view, beliefs come first, feelings follow.
2. In depression, the majority of one's thoughts are negative; the individual has difficulty focusing on any positive aspects of a life situation.
3. In depression, one's negative thoughts and negativity are often irrational or distorted or bear little relationship to reality.

First, the client learns to recognize the presence of negative and disturbing thoughts. For example, a depressed person may think that his feelings of guilt derive from having done something bad, even if he has no idea what the bad deed may have been. Most depressed persons have such negative thoughts. One of the initial goals of therapy is to help such persons identify negative thoughts and to see these thoughts as harmful, abnormal, and the root cause of feelings of depression. The therapist may ask the client to write down all of the negative thoughts he experiences. Then, the client may be asked to analyze each thought and explain why it is irrational or exaggerated. Finally, the client is asked to substitute a nondepressed, positive thought in place of the negative one. Clients are coached in doing this until the substitution of the positive for negative thoughts becomes natural and automatic. Therapy actually teaches the client to recognize a series of specific thought distortions common in depression. Box 28-2 summarizes some of these common thought distortions. Any of these thought distortions can be harmful and lead to continued depression. For example, a client who engages in "all-or-nothing" thinking will interpret life

REFLECTIVE THINKING 28-2

Sadness in Your Past

Remember a time when you felt sad or depressed. What thoughts or behaviors did you exhibit? At the time, did you view these thoughts as rational or irrational? Do you hold the same opinion now, after some time has passed? Do you feel that there were any interventions that might have changed these negative thoughts and behaviors?

experiences to be either good or bad and see nothing in between. Thus, if the client finds fault with any part of a task he has performed, he will interpret the whole endeavor as bad. If, on the other hand, a client engages in "reasoning from feeling," he may think, for example, that if he has not slept well one night, he cannot either feel well or be well.

While cognitive-behavioral therapists most often treat depression, other problems that have been successfully addressed by cognitive-behavioral therapy include anxiety, anger, sexual dysfunction, chronic pain, substance abuse, and eating disorders. By its nature, cognitive-behavioral therapy requires that the client be intellectually intact. It is inappropriate to conduct cognitive-behavioral therapy with one who is psychotic or demented or unable or unwilling to cooperate actively with the therapist.

While much of the previous discussion has focused on depression, behaviorally oriented therapies have also proven effective in treating anxiety (Deacon & Abramowitz, 2004). "Exposure" therapies have been widely used, particularly for phobias. Exposure involves reproducing a feared experience either in reality or through realistic simulation. Phobias involving fear of heights, spiders, and flying have been successfully treated through these means. More controversial applications of exposure therapies include the techniques of "flooding," "implosive therapy," and "imaginal desensitization," which have been used in therapy of Post-Traumatic Stress Disorder. These three techniques, respectively, may employ elements of the original traumatic experience, recalled memories of the trauma, or visual cues, which are intended to evoke the traumatic experience. In each case the goal is to re-create something of the original experience in a controlled therapeutic setting. There is some evidence that these uses of exposure may be effective, but it remains uncertain whether this form of therapy is more effective than other forms of psychological treatment.

BOX 28-2
COMMON THOUGHT DISTORTIONS ADDRESSED IN COGNITIVE-BEHAVIORAL THERAPY

- All-or-nothing thinking: seeing things only in absolutes
- Overgeneralization: interpreting every small setback as a never-ending pattern of defeat
- Dwelling on negatives: ignoring multiple positive experiences
- Jumping to conclusions: assuming that others are reacting negatively without definite evidence
- Pessimism: automatically predicting that things will turn out badly
- Reasoning from feeling: thinking that if one feels bad, one must be bad
- Obligations: living life around a succession of too many "shoulds," "shouldn'ts," "musts," "oughts," and "have-tos"

EXPERIENCE-ORIENTED THERAPY

Experience-oriented therapy focuses on the client's experiences as an agent for producing change. The client's experience is facilitated by a therapist who has assessed the client and who directs experiences to produce a calculated change in behavior and feeling. Unlike insight-oriented therapy, experience-oriented processes do not emphasize the individual's discovery of unconscious knowledge, and unlike behaviorally oriented therapy, the experience-oriented techniques do not require any "homework" or other efforts to consciously change thoughts and behaviors. Experience-oriented therapy engages the client in new interactions and in new ways-of-being within the therapy session.

Client-centered therapy (founded by Carl Rogers) is an example of experience-oriented therapy. Client-centered therapy is based on the idea that every individual has a store of internal resources and self-understanding, and that these inner resources can be brought out when the therapist is open, nonjudgmental, and empathic (Figure 28-1). The therapist seeks to be uniformly supportive and kind. The therapist does not interpret client behaviors; rather, the therapist attempts only to understand the client's inner feelings. The therapist offers respect and protection of the client's autonomy. The client is viewed as the expert about himself—the therapist is a supportive facilitator rather than an authority figure. The therapist will answer questions, give explanations, and shape experiments for the client to try. For example, the client may be asked to role-play with the therapist in a session. The therapist may play the client's boss, in an effort to bring an experience into the present, so that the client may interpret his emotions and actions.

In contrast to psychoanalysis, in which the analyst attempts to overcome the client's repression of painful thoughts, this shaping of experiences is done gently, with the client's full cooperation. The client experiences therapy as a safe, empowering encounter with a kind and caring therapist. This encounter provides the grounding experience from which the client can try out new behaviors and grow

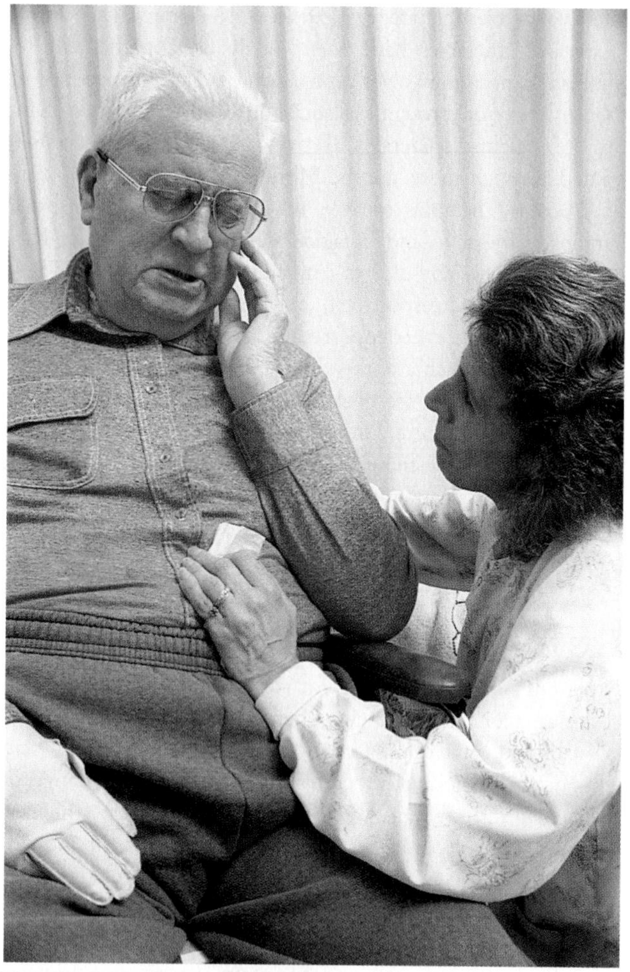

FIGURE 28-1 **Clients undergoing individual therapy may become emotional as they recall significant personal life events. The nurse who embodies empathy, support, and caring will best be able to assist clients in dealing with the myriad emotions that surface during therapy sessions.** (DELMAR/CENGAGE LEARNING.)

interpersonally and emotionally. The therapy ideally results in the client's ability to see self differently and to promote self-growth and maturation.

RESEARCH BASE FOR PSYCHOTHERAPEUTIC INTERVENTIONS

Studies of insight-oriented therapies apply only to those individuals who are motivated enough to qualify for psychodynamic treatments. One psychodynamic therapist writes: "The therapy is not considered successful unless the patient is not only symptom free, but also the patient's maladaptive character defenses are replaced with adaptive character defenses. At the termination, the patient must have both cognitive and emotional insight into the structure of his pathology" (Worchel, 1990, p. 214) There is a mounting body of evidence supporting the use of psychoanalysis and psychodynamic therapies, as researchers and practitioners document the outcomes of current practices (Leichsenring & Leibling, 2003); Leichsenring & Rabung, 2008).

Interpersonal therapy that addresses the specific interpersonal content surrounding episodes of psychological distress has been shown to be effective. Studies validate that short-term interpersonal therapy is highly effective in the management of major depression, particularly in young and middle-aged adults with unipolar symptoms. The combination of medication and interpersonal therapy has been shown to be more effective than either treatment alone in the management of major depression. Recent investigations indicate that interpersonal therapy is useful in treating depression in adolescents (Mufson, Dorta, Wickramaratine, Nomura, Olfson, & Weissman, 2005), dysthymia, and other forms of depression (Markowitz, 2008; Markowitz, Kocsis, Christos, Bleiberg, & Carlin, 2008).

Many studies have established that task-oriented therapies, including cognitive and cognitive-behavioral therapies, are effective treatment for many psychological conditions. Cognitive therapy has been shown to be effective treatment for depression, substance abuse, anxiety disorders, eating disorders, and personality disorders (Wright, Beck, & Thase, 2003).

Experience-oriented and client-centered therapies are difficult to assess, and there are few, if any, studies on treatment outcome, perhaps largely because the therapist does

NURSING TIP 28-2

Psychotherapy and Cultural Sensitivity

To be an effective therapist, you must understand the experiences, the worldview, and the values of your clients. In an increasingly diverse society, you must be continually aware of potential areas of bias or misunderstanding.

A classic 1980 study provides the best example of such biases. Li-Repac (1980) had white and Chinese American therapists rate both white and Chinese American clients. White clinicians rated the Chinese American clients as *anxious*, *awkward*, *confused*, *nervous*, and *reserved*, whereas the Chinese American clinicians used words such as *alert*, *dependable*, *friendly*, and *practical* for the same clients. The Chinese American clinicians rated the white clients as *active*, *aggressive*, and *rebellious*, whereas the white clinicians rated the same clients as *affectionate*, *adventurous*, and *capable*. These findings point out how easily the ethnic or cultural background of the therapist can influence therapy. Since much has been done since 1980 to increase awareness of and sensitivity to one ethnic and cultural group to the experiences and behaviors of other groups, it is possible that findings would be different if one replicated this study today (see also Chapter 7).

not define the expected outcome prior to the start (or even conclusion) of therapy.

PSYCHOTHERAPY AND CULTURAL SENSITIVITY

Several studies have been done on the effectiveness of psychotherapy in persons from varied cultural and ethnic backgrounds. Because effectiveness of psychotherapy is related to multiple variables, such studies are difficult to conduct and findings may be inconclusive. However, the available research does seem to indicate that psychotherapy is effective in individuals, regardless of background. Most investigations further indicate that an ethnic match between client and therapist does not affect outcomes. However, there is some evidence of assessment bias that is related to the background of the therapist.

PSYCHOTHERAPY IN NURSING PRACTICE

In an era in which public and professional discussions often focus on the role of medication to treat mental distress and there is ever-increasing emphasis on the biological basis of mental disease, it is important to recognize that individual psychotherapy remains an important and well-validated therapeutic tool. Many clients are helped through processes that allow them to gain insight, to examine their thoughts and behaviors, and to try out new ways of relating to others.

Nurses in virtually any area of practice will encounter professional therapists who offer many different approaches to treatment. A 2009 Internet search resulted in a list of more than 40 distinct approaches to therapy. Some of these therapies are relatively conventional (brief psychotherapy, psychoanalysis, client-centered therapy), while others may be viewed as unconventional (videotherapy, ritual therapy, or persuasion therapy). Each therapy has its strong proponents and clearly unique benefits. Clients may often seek the nurse's opinions regarding the value of specific therapeutic approaches.

Some nurses in advanced practice roles function as therapists, offering direct service to clients. These nurses have additional education in individual therapy, and many have experienced therapy themselves as a means to gain insight into their own professional and personal behaviors. Other nurses, however, may employ specific psychotherapeutic techniques to assist clients in all clinical settings. For example, a nurse may use the psychodynamic technique of **interpretation** to offer a **suggestion** of how she perceives the client is handling a crisis. The statement, "While you are in the hospital, it seems difficult for you to take on the dependent role of client," offers an interpretation of the client's behavior, expresses empathy, and opens up areas for discussion between nurse and client. Techniques of cognitive-behavioral therapy that help the client look at his thought patterns may be used as well. For example, asking a client to identify something positive about his work performance, rather than dwelling on negatives, may be the first step for the client to reframe his thinking about himself. Principles of experiential therapies, with emphasis on a caring, humanistic

BOX 28-3
DIFFERENT KINDS OF THERAPIES

- Adventure therapy
- Analytical psychotherapy
- Art therapy
- Autogenic training
- Bibliotherapy
- Brief psychotherapy
- Client-centered therapy
- Cognitive-affective behavior therapy
- Cognitive-behavioral therapy
- Dance therapy
- Directed reverie therapy
- Dream therapy
- Ego state therapy
- Encounter group therapy
- Ethnocultural therapy
- Existential psychotherapy
- Experiential psychotherapy
- Expressive psychotherapy
- Family therapy
- Gestalt therapy
- Hypnotherapy
- Individual psychotherapy
- Insight therapy
- Logotherapy
- Marathon therapy
- Multimodal therapy
- Persuasion therapy
- Play therapy
- Primal therapy
- Process experiential psychotherapy
- Psychoanalysis
- Psychodrama
- Rational-emotive therapy
- Reality therapy
- Recreation therapy
- Relationship therapy
- Ritual therapy
- Self-psychology
- Short-term dynamic therapy
- Therapeutic writing
- Transactional analysis
- Video therapy

relationship, fit well in practice directed by nursing theory in which the goal is to provide a safe psychological environment for the client to explore the meaning of his life, his work, his illness, or his current circumstance.

Two other principles of psychotherapy derived from the psychoanalytic literature are the concepts of transference and countertransference. While these are technical terms, their meaning is fairly straightforward and is readily applicable to nursing activities both with psychiatric clients and with persons suffering from a variety of nonpsychiatric conditions. *Transference* refers to the tendency of clients to relate to their therapist in ways reflecting their own past experiences with specific important other persons in their early lives. In transference, client emotions can be either positive or negative. Some clients develop intense romantic feelings toward their therapist, while others find themselves angry and hostile. Nurses who work closely with clients will frequently find themselves to be the recipients of transference emotions. It is important to recognize these emotions and to recognize that, at least according to traditional psychoanalytic theory, they are really directed not to the nurse but to a person in the client's early life (parent, sibling, loved one) whose memory the nurse somehow evokes. This evocation is almost always unconscious: the client rarely recognizes the underlying reasons for his or her emotions until they are explained by a psychotherapist. A psychoanalytic therapist typically uses his or her understanding of a client's transference to help the client gain insights that can bring about emotional growth. In contrast, most nurses do not have the training and skills to use transference in this way. Instead, for the majority of nurses it is sufficient to recognize when clients are experiencing strong emotions toward them. In most cases transference should be discussed with clients, but the majority of nurses will find that this can be done professionally only under the guidance of experienced supervisors or mental health professionals. Above all, nurses need, of course, to avoid entering into personal relationships with clients—especially relationships that have romantic content. Such relationships threaten the nurse's ability to provide care and may represent an unethical crossing of important professional boundaries.

Countertransference occurs when the nurse experiences strong emotional feelings *toward the client.* While such feelings may be hostile, countertransference seems to cause the most difficulty when the feelings are positive or romantic. It is not unusual or inherently wrong for nurses to experience warm or even romantic feelings for their clients. What *is* wrong is for nurses to fail to recognize the psychological origins of these feelings in the phenomenon of countertransference. It is rarely appropriate for the nurse to express his or her feelings to the client, and it is never appropriate to allow a therapeutic relationship to cross therapeutic boundaries into social interaction or romance. If countertransference feelings are strong or difficult for the nurse to deal with, he or she needs to discuss the situation with an experienced supervisor or liaison psychiatric provider. In most cases, acknowledging that feelings exist and that they have their origin in the psychoanalytic phenomenon of countertransference will allow the nurse to remain detached while still being supportive and helpful. Therapists learn in their training that their role is to be a supportive guide for the client's recovery rather than the client's personal friend. This sense of detachment is equally important for nurses, who need to realize that detachment is not the same as indifference. Caring and support are therapeutic, but intense emotional attachment is a form of countertransference that almost always works against the nurse's ability to facilitate growth and healing.

Nursing Theory

Professional practice increasingly requires that nurses understand their care from a theory base. Thus, it is reasonable to ask how psychotherapeutic approaches fit with the philosophy of nursing theory.

Psychoanalysis and psychodynamic therapy are most consistent with nursing theories that emphasize human development and the influence of past experiences on present behaviors. Peplau's nursing theory is particularly compatible with a psychoanalytic and interpersonal therapy, and its development was directly influenced by the interpersonal theory and by concepts of psychoanalysis. Peplau identifies needs, frustrations, conflict, and anxiety as important factors that a nurse should explicitly evaluate in the context of a client's past history and present circumstances (Belcher & Fish, 1995).

Cognitive-behavioral therapy is consistent with nursing theories emphasizing adaptation, for example, Callista Roy's theory (see Chapter 3). Roy's theory assumes that behavior is adaptive and that changes in the environment (internal or external) can affect the client's feelings and behavior.

There is a very strong philosophical similarity between the nursing concept of human care and the client-centered approach of experience-oriented psychotherapy. In nursing, caring is a unique philosophy that emphasizes the nurse-client relationship and places value on positive regard, acceptance, human care, and nurturance. These qualities are an implicit part of the client-centered psychotherapeutic approach. Nurse theorists from Leininger to Watson to Erickson have repeatedly emphasized the caring aspects of nursing as the priority of focus. Nursing theories based on caring and client-centered psychotherapy seem to share a series of assumptions:

1. In contrast to therapeutic objectivity, caring within a nurse-client relationship maintains a therapeutic perspective, where feelings are acknowledged and integrated into a framework of understanding.
2. Caregivers can experience an existential or spiritual significance to their involvement with the client.
3. Nurses who are experienced in caring can respond to their own experiences and intuition to guide practice.
4. Self-disclosure of the therapist is acceptable when directed toward the goal of shared human experiences.
5. The therapist accepts the client's view of his world, and the client determines desired outcomes.
6. Instilling hope is an important aspect of caring.

These assumptions describe a therapeutic process that emphasizes humanistic caring with a focus on experiences shared between the client and nurse.

Collaborative Interventions

Like any area of nursing practice, psychiatric care is a discipline in which the nurse must work as a member of a treatment team composed of representatives of several professions. The team approach may dictate the nurse's style of intervention with his clients. For example, if the treatment team elects to use a psychodynamic approach, the nurse's interventions must be grounded in the principles of psychodynamic therapy. In contrast, if the treatment approach is cognitive-behavioral, the nurse must plan interventions consistent with identifying thoughts and changing behavioral outcomes. In such a collaborative setting, nurses must understand the treatment approaches selected for each client and then must ensure that nursing interventions are consistent with those of other team professionals.

REFLECTIVE THINKING 28-3

Characteristics Clients Wish for in Their Therapists

Based on a study of clients,* researchers found that clients want their therapists to:

- **be warm, calm and responsive**
- **listen attentively**
- **be understanding, and**
- **balance specific questions and comments with listening.**
- **What do you think you can do to make yourself the kind of therapist-nurse clients wish for?**
- **How do you listen, understand, respond, and maintain the needed balance between talking and listening?**

*From Littauer, H, Sextun, H., & Wynn, R., (2005). Qualities clients wish for in their therapists. *Scandinavian Journal of Caring Science, 19,* 28–31.

NURSING PROCESS

When a nurse provides individual psychotherapy, the nurse is functioning as a therapist such that all professional actions are grounded in the theory or approach of the therapy. However, the nurse will choose and apply a therapy that is consistent with her nursing role and beliefs. The statement at the beginning of this chapter about psychotherapy from a medical model suggests that the therapist is the "expert" and the client is the "seeker of help." While a nursing expert will interact as an expert with a client seeking help, the balance of power and the sense of "expertness" may change in both subtle and profound ways as nurses enter into the field of psychotherapy. In nursing, it is not unusual to consider the client an "expert" on himself (Lamprecht, et al., 2007), thus rendering the client a more collaborative role than traditional psychotherapy. Also, it is important to note that while therapists make assessments of their clients and plan the therapy according to assessment data, therapists do not apply the nursing process. The nursing process requires assessment and analysis of data that results in a nursing diagnosis. Psychotherapy does not require a nursing diagnosis, and in some cases (for example, client-centered therapy), the therapist would not make a diagnosis of any kind. Analysis of data in psychotherapy is done according to the theory. For example, assessment of depressed emotions could be interpreted as anger toward self (psychodynamic therapy), as a manifestation of negative thinking (cognitive-behavioral therapy), or as the client's experience of his world (client-centered therapy). It is irrelevant to the therapy whether or not the client behaviors could be labeled according to a standard nursing diagnosis. The nursing process requires outcome identification as well, and in psychoanalytic, psychodynamic, and client-centered therapy, the therapist does not identify outcomes. It is a challenge, then, for nurses entering the role of psychotherapist to bring a nursing perspective to that role and to find the balance between being a therapist and being a professional nurse.

The nurse's role in individual psychotherapy reminds one that professional nurses do more than apply the nursing process, and that the nursing process was never intended to document every activity a professional nurse provides. In some areas of advanced practice—psychotherapy as a prime example—the nurse is engaged in professional activities outside the nursing process.

KEY CONCEPTS

- Individual psychotherapy is the treatment of mental or emotional disorders through one-to-one encounters with a therapist/counselor.
- Therapies can be organized into three basic approaches: insight-oriented, behaviorally oriented, and experience-oriented.
- Psychoanalysis and psychodynamic therapy are insight-oriented therapies grounded in Freudian theory.
- Interpersonal therapy is insight-oriented and based on the belief that psychological distress occurs in conjunction with disturbed human relationships.

- Behaviorally oriented therapies focus on outcomes and give clients specific tasks or activities to assist them in achieving outcomes.
- Cognitive-behavioral therapy sets out to change a client's attitudes and behaviors.
- Experience-oriented therapy directs the client through specific experiences in a caring, therapeutic encounter.
- Nursing interventions may be grounded in any of the psychotherapeutic approaches.
- Psychotherapeutic approaches can be used within the framework of nursing theory.
- To date, no research has shown that one therapy is better than the others; all have benefit to clients.
- In a managed-care environment, the nursing challenge is to provide care that is affordable, accessible, and accountable.

REVIEW QUESTIONS

1. The goal of psychoanalytic theory is which of the following?
   1. Assist the client to make changes in their thinking process
   2. Understand the client's inner feelings and offer support
   3. Help the client identify patterns of relationships and interactions with others
   4. Uncover and interpret the client's experiences that have been unconsciously repressed

2. A client is being seen for short-term therapy with an Advance Practice Registered Nurse (APRN). The major approach taken by the nurse would be which of the following?
   1. Set goals for the client
   2. Focus on the central issue
   3. Use a confrontational approach
   4. Set limits on client's behavior

3. The therapist is working with a client who demonstrates a very pessimistic attitude. The client constantly complains that nothing has gone right in his life. He is constantly getting fired from jobs, his children hate him, and his wife wants a divorce. The therapist requests that the client keep a journal and record each time something has gone wrong in his life over a two-week period. The therapist is most likely using an approach grounded in which of the following types of therapy?
   1. Cognitive therapy
   2. Psychoanalytic therapy
   3. Behavioral therapy
   4. Gestalt therapy

4. A therapist is conducting a session with a client admitted for treatment of alcoholism. The therapist is experiencing difficulty expressing empathy for the client because her own father had been an alcoholic. As the therapist interacts with the client, she remembers the pain that her father's addiction had caused the family. The therapist is most likely experiencing which of the following?
   1. Regression
   2. Transference
   3. Depersonalization
   4. Countertransference

5. A client tells her therapist, "I enjoy meeting with you. You give me great advice just like my mother and you are usually right." The client's comments indicate that which of the following processes is occurring?
   1. Regression
   2. Transference
   3. Depersonalization
   4. Countertransference

6. Therapists who base their therapy on the theories of caring recognize that an important aspect of caring is which of the following?
   1. The instillation of hope
   2. Effective use of transference
   3. The importance of reminiscing
   4. The therapist maintaining all control

7. The Advance Practice Registered Nurse (APRN) is using the FRAME model as a tool when conducting brief intervention with a client who has recently been discharged from the alcohol treatment facility. The nurse would plan to meet with the client for how many sessions?
   1. 1–4
   2. 5–8
   3. 8–12
   4. 12–16

LEARNING ACTIVITIES

1. How do you distinguish between psychodynamic and interpersonal therapy?
2. Have you observed a client who has had cognitive-behavioral therapy? Describe the client's condition and how the approach was used.
3. Explain how experience-oriented therapy fits with Watson's nursing theory.
4. Do you think that the mandates of managed care will lead to an increased use of cognitive-behavioral therapy? Explain your answer.
5. What research is needed to expand our knowledge of psychotherapeutic approaches?

*Study*WARE™ CONNECTION

Using your *Study*WARE™ CD-ROM

1. Complete the Flashcard activity for this chapter.
2. Review the audio glossary for key terms in this chapter.
3. Explore the other games and activities that support this chapter.

REFERENCES

American Psychoanalytic Association. (2008). Homepage, at http://www.apsa.org/

Bateman, A. W. (2004). Psychoanalysis and psychiatry—is there a future? *Acta Psychiatrica Scandinavica* (Editorial), *109*, 161–162.

Belcher, J. R., & Fish, L. J. B. (1995). Hildegard E. Peplau. In J. George (Ed.), *Nursing theories: The base for professional nursing practice* (4th ed., pp. 49–66). Norwalk, CT: Appleton & Lange.

Crowe, M., & Lutz, S. (2005a). Interpersonal psychotherapy: An effective psychotherapeutic intervention for mental health nursing practice. *International Journal of Mental Health Nursing, 14*, 24–31.

Crowe, M., & Lutz, S. (2005b). Recovering from depression: A discourse analysis of interpersonal psychotherapy. *Nursing Inquiry, 12*(1), 43–50.

Deacon, B. J., & Abramowitz, J. S. (2004). Cognitive and behavioral treatments for anxiety disorders: A review of meta-analytic findings. *Journal of Clinical Psychology, 60*, 429–441.

Elkin, I. (1994). The NIMH treatment of the depression collaborative research program: Where we began and where we are. In A. Bergin & S. Garfield (Eds.), *Handbook of psychotherapy and behavior change* (pp. 114–139). New York: Wiley.

Evans, M., Hollon, S., DeRubeis, R., Plasecki, J., Grove, W., Garvey, M., et al. (1992). Differential relapse following cognitive therapy and pharmacotherapy for depression. *Archives of General Psychiatry, 49*, 802–808.

Fava, G. A., Rafanelli, C., Grandi, S., Conti, S., & Bellaurdo, P. (1998). Prevention of recurrent depression with cognitive behavioral therapy: Preliminary findings. *Archives of General Psychiatry, 55*(9), 816–820.

Guthrie, E., Kapur, N., Mackway-Jones, K., Chew-Graham, C., Moorey, J., Mendel, E., Marino-Francis, F., Sanderson, S., Turpin, C., Boddy, G., & Tomenson, B. (2001). Randomised controlled trial of brief psychological intervention after deliberate self-poisoning. *British Medical Journal, 323(7305)*, 135–138.

Lamprecht, H., Laydon, C., McQuillan, C., Wiseman, S. Williams, I. Gash, A. Reilly, J. & Winship, G. (2007). Single-session solution-focused brief therapy and self-harm: A pilot study. *Journal of Psychiatric & Mental Health Nursing, 14*(6), 601–602.

Leichsenring, F., & Leibing, F. (2003). The effectiveness of psychodynamic theory and cognitive behavior therapy in treatment of personality disorders: A meta-analysis. *American Journal of Psychiatry, 160*(7), 1223–1232.

Leichsenring, F., & Rabung, S. (2008). Effectiveness of long-term psychodynamic psychotherapy. *Journal of the American Medical Association, 300*(13), 1551–1565.

Lewinsohn, P. M., & Clarke, G. N. (1999). Psychosocial treatments for adolescent depression. *Clinical Psychology Review, 19*(3), 329–342.

Li-Repac, D. (1980). Cultural influences on clinical perception: A comparison between Caucasian and Chinese-American therapists. *Journal of Cross-Cultural Psychology, 11*, 327–342.

Malmberg, L., & Fenton, M. (2001). Individual psychodynamic psychotherapy and psychoanalysis for schizophrenia and severe mental illness. *Cochrane Database Systematic Review* (2), CD001360.

Markowitz, J. C. (2008). Evidenced-based therapies for depression. *Journal of Occupational Environmental Medicine, 50*(4), 437–440.

Markowitz, J. C., Kocsis, J. H., Christos, P., Bleiberg, K., & Carlin, A. (2008). Pilot study of interpersonal psychotherapy versus supportive psychotherapy for dysthymic patients with secondary alcohol abuse of dependence. *Journal of Nervous and Mental Disorders, 196*(6), 468–274.

Miklowitz, D. J. (2008). Adjunctive psychotherapy for bipolar disorder: State of the evidence. *American Journal of Psychiatry (Epub ahead of print).*

Mojtabai, R., Nicholson, R. A., & Carpenter, B. N. (1998). Role of psychosocial treatments in management of schizophrenia: A meta-analytic review of controlled outcome studies. *Schizophrenia Bulletin, 24*(4), 569–587.

Mufson, L., Dorta, K. P., Wickramaratine, P., Nomura, Y., Olfson, M., & Weissman, M. M. (2005). A randomized effectiveness trial of interpersonal psychotherapy for depressed adolescents. *Evidenced Based Mental Health, 8*(1), 11.

Rogers, C. (1951). *Client-centered therapy.* Boston: Houghton Mifflin.

Saks, E. E. (2007). *The center cannot hold: My journey through madness.* New York: Hyperion.

Sandell, R., Bloberg, J., Lazar, A. Carlsson, J., Broberg, J., & Schubert, J. (2000). Varieties of long-term outcome among patients in psychoanalysis and long-term psychotherapy. A review of findings in the Stockholm Outcome of Psychoanalysis and Psychotherapy Project (STOPP). *International Journal of Psychoanalysis, 81*(Pt. 5), 921–942.

Sherman, J. J. (1998). Effects of psychotherapeutic treatment of PTSD: A meta-analysis of controlled clinical trials. *Journal of Trauma Stress, 11*(3), 413–435.

Ursano, R. J., & Silberman, E. K. (2003). Psychoanalysis, psychoanalytic psychotherapy, and supportive psychotherapy. In R. E. Hales and S. C. Yudofsky (Eds.), *The American textbook of clinical psychiatry* (4th ed., pp. 1177–1206). Washington, DC: American Psychiatric Publishing, Inc.

Vaughan, S. C., Marshall, R. D., Mackinnon, R. A., Vaughan, R., Mellman, L., & Roose, S. P. (2000). Can we do psychoanalytic outcome research? A feasibility study. *International Journal of Psychoanalysis, 81*(Pt. 3), 513–527.

Worchel, J. (1990). Short-term dynamic psychotherapy. In R. Wells & V. Giannetti (Eds.), *Handbook of the brief psychotherapies* (pp. 193–216). New York: Plenum.

Wright, J. H., Beck, A., & Thase, M. (2003). Cognitive therapy. In R. E. Hales and S. C. Yudofsky (Eds.), *The American textbook of clinical psychiatry* (4th ed., pp. 1245–1284). Washington, DC: American Psychiatric Publishing, Inc.

SUGGESTED READINGS

Freud, S. (1953–1974). In J. Strachey (Ed.), *The standard edition of the complete psychological works of Sigmund Freud.* London: Hogarth Press and Institute for Psychoanalysis.

Peplau, H. (1952). *Interpersonal relations in nursing.* New York: Putnam.

Saks, E. E. (2007). *The center cannot hold: My journey through madness.* New York: Hyperion.

Sullivan, H. S. (1953). *The interpersonal theory of psychiatry.* New York: Norton.

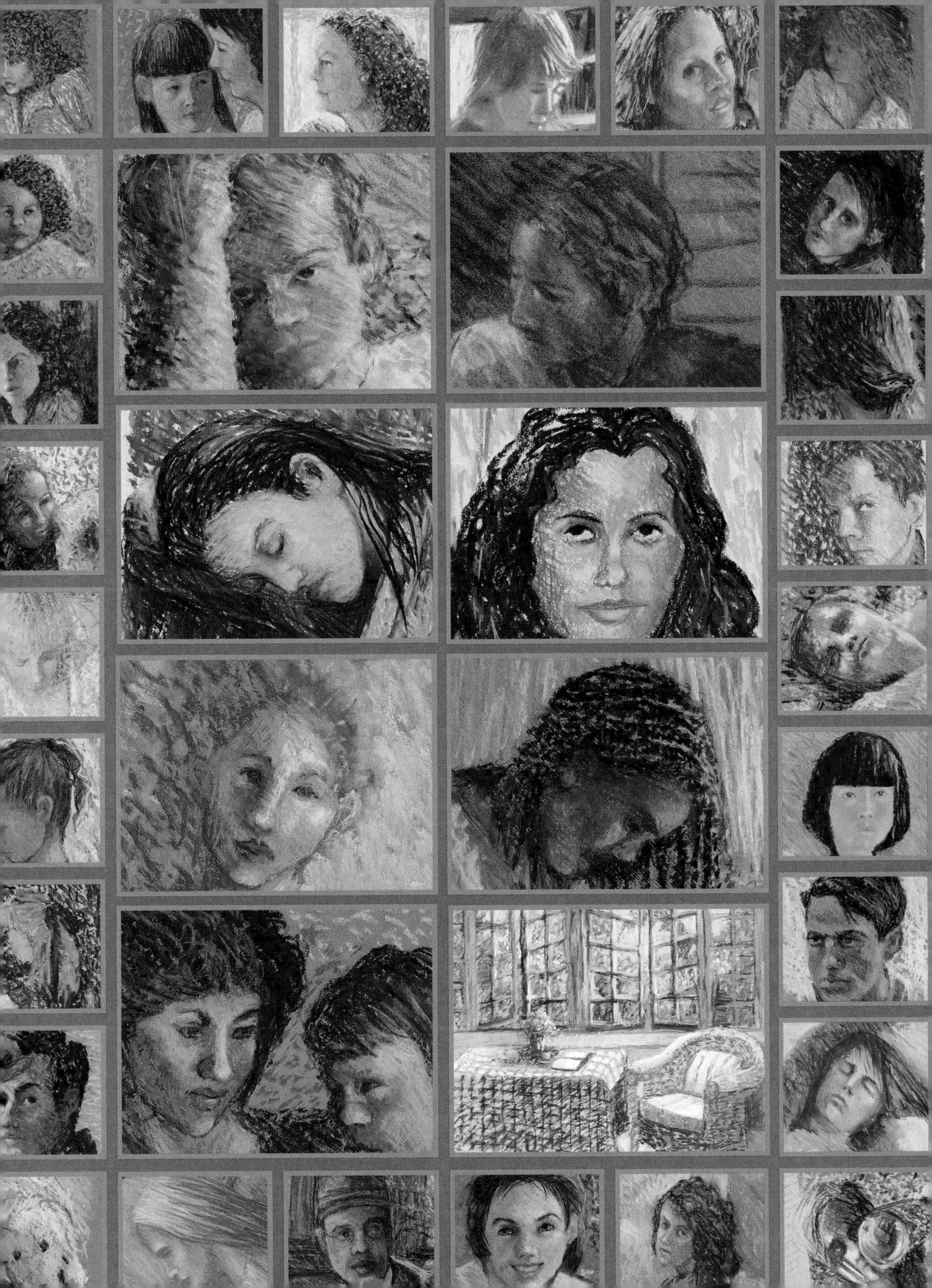

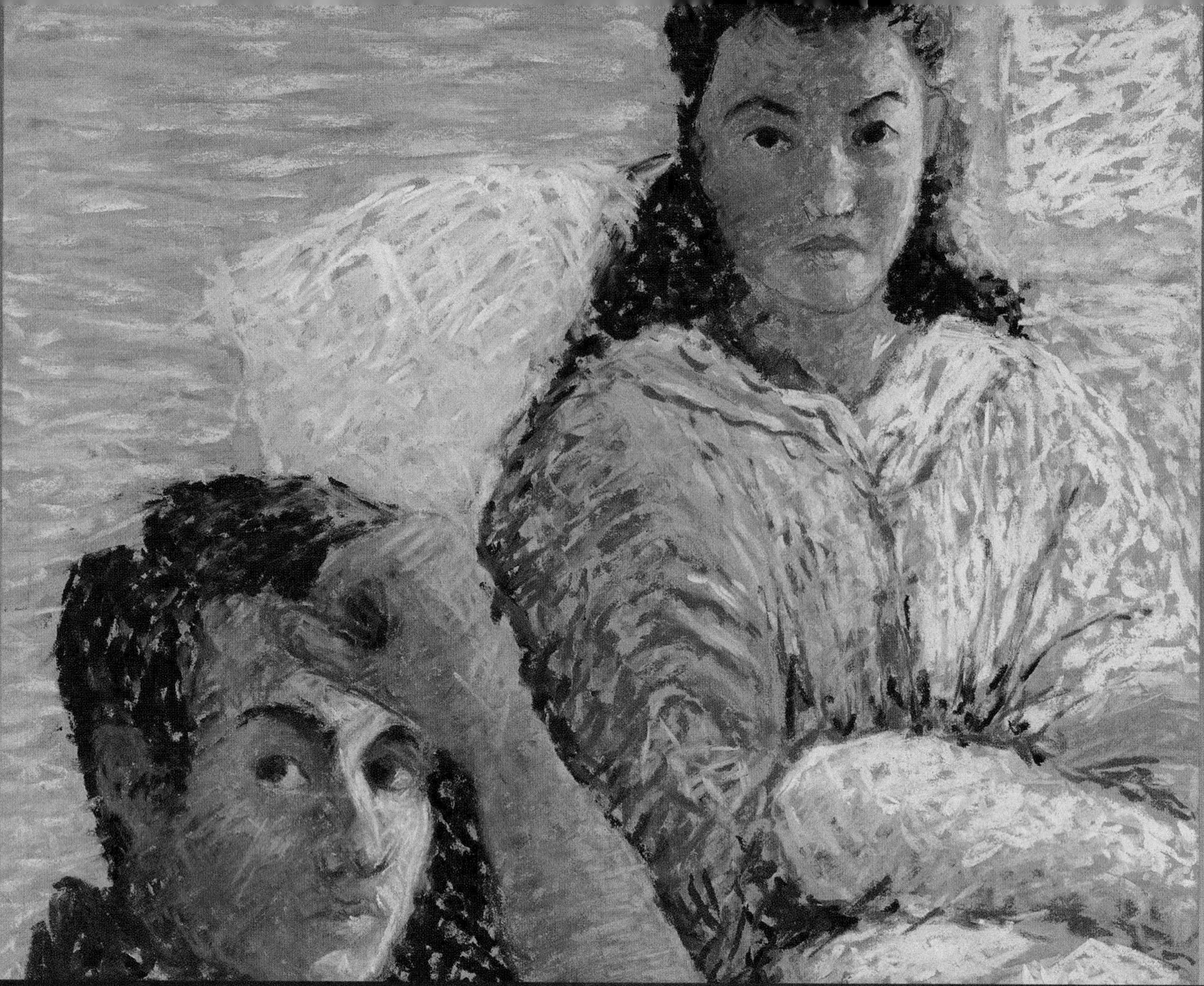

So Now What?

Your Family

You have been a member of a family all of your life. This is an area where you have much experience and expertise! Think about your family in two ways: First, think about your family as the context (background) of your growing up.

- *Consider ways in which your family taught you how to understand others and society.*
- *Describe ways that your family offered you support or encouragement to do something, or ways that your family did not.*
- *Examine how your adult means of coping may have been learned from early experiences within your family household.*
- *If you have siblings, consider your similarities and differences, given that you were raised in the same environment.*

Second, think about your family as a whole.

- *Consider your own family as a group. Do you react or respond as one unit to others outside of the family?*
- *What stages of family development has your family gone through?*
- *What are the patterns of family behavior characteristic of your family as a whole?*

As you begin this chapter, consider two views of the family: as the context for care and as the focus of care. Use your experience within your own family to examine those situations in which one or the other approach is most appropriate.

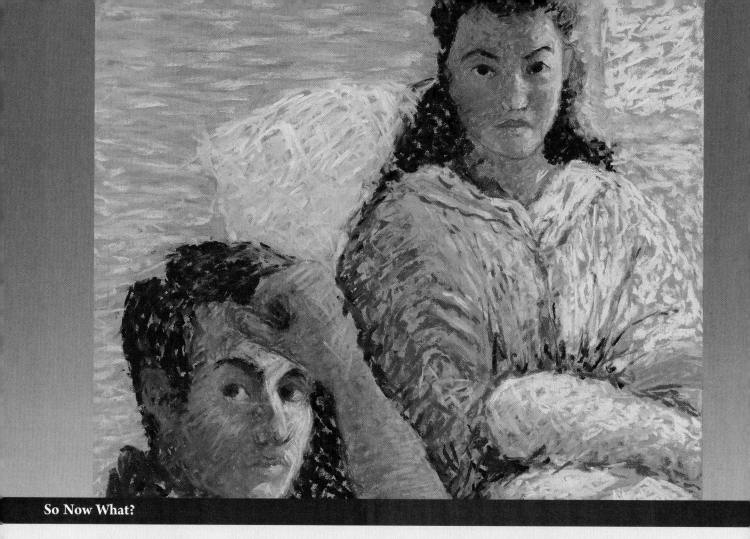

CHAPTER 29

Family Therapy

JANE KELLEY
NOREEN CAVAN FRISCH

CHAPTER OUTLINE

COMPETENCIES

Upon completion of this chapter, the reader should be able to:

1. Define differing nursing approaches to working with families.
2. Apply the concepts of family development and family life cycle to assessments of families.
3. Describe Bowen's family theory, and make an assessment of family level of differentiation.
4. Explain structural family theory, and describe the nurse-therapist's role of entering into the family interactions and structure.
5. Use communication theory and the techniques of therapeutic communication to assist families in improving interfamilial communication.
6. Use the NANDA-I taxonomy to document family nursing diagnoses.
7. Complete family assessments using nursing assessment tools.
8. Use the nursing process to establish a plan of care for families in the psychiatric mental health setting.

KEY TERMS

Circular Communication
Differentiation
Ecomap
Emotional Cutoff
Family
Family Attachment Diagram
Family Projection Process
Genogram
Interventive Questions
Multigenerational Transmission Process
Nuclear Family Emotional System
Power
Relativistic Thinking
Sibling Position
Societal Regression
Triangulation

Nurses recognize that psychiatric and physical illnesses have great impact on families. The family can be the individual's first source of support and stability or it can be part of the problem that leads to ineffective coping. This chapter explores the nature of nursing interventions with families, how nurses care for families, the various theories that guide nursing actions, and the interventions used by nurses with families in psychiatric mental health settings. The goals are to provide the reader with the background to give client care within the context of family and home life, and to provide care to the family as a unit, when appropriate.

WHAT IS A FAMILY?

To assess a family, the nurse must determine what constitutes a family. First, there is the family of origin, or the family of one's birth and the family of procreation. Some people think of a mother, father, and their children when they think of family. But in today's world, many different groups might be considered family. One way to decide which individuals make up a family is to limit family to those who live in the same household under the same roof. Another way to determine family is to include the nuclear family of mother, father, and their children, wherever they reside. But what about extended family members, such as grandparents, who may or may not reside in the same household? And what about blended families of couples with children of former marriages? Or unmarried couples, gay and lesbian couples, persons living in communes, and other groupings of individuals that may consider themselves to be families?

Traditionally, *family* was defined as relationships of blood, marriage, or adoption. But by the mid-1980s, family nursing moved to incorporate a broader definition believed to be more relevant to the times. As early as 1985, one could find reference to family as being characterized by commitment, mutual decision making, and shared goals. For instance, the definition of **family** is a social system composed of two or more persons who coexist within the context of some expectations of reciprocal affection, mutual responsibility, and temporal duration (Department of Family Nursing, Oregon Health Sciences Center, 1985, quoted in Hanson & Boyd, 1996, p. 6).

Another definition is offered by the National Institute of Mental Health (1995): The family is a "network of mutual commitment." And a definition by family oriented primary care physicians is: "The family is a social system composed of two or more persons who coexist within the context of some expectations of reciprocal affection, mutual responsibility, and temporal duration." This definition is broad enough to incorporate newer forms of family. But a simple definition that is used in this text to define family is: The family is composed of all those persons the client says it includes.

Given the complexity of families, there is one relatively simple way to decide if a group of persons should be considered a family: Ask family members which individuals make up

NURSING TIP 29-1

Defining Families

Remember that it is the family members, not the nurse, who determines which individuals constitute their family unit. The family is who they say they are!

BOX 29-1
SAMPLE OF DEFINITIONS OF FAMILIES THROUGHOUT THE YEARS, AS REPORTED BY BOMAR (2004)

- *Legal.* A family is a group of two or more persons residing in the same household who are related by blood, marriage, or adoption (U. S. Census Bureau, 2002).
- *Family Science.* A family is two or more persons who are committed to each other and who share intimacy, resources, decisions, and values (Olson & DeFrain, 1994, p. 9).
- *Sociology.* Family is an intimate association of persons who are related to one another by blood, a marriage, formal or informal adoption, or appropriation; often sharing a common residence (Billingsley, 1992).
- *Family Therapy.* Family is a "natural social system" with rules, ascribed roles, power structures, intricate communication, and a reciprocal emotional attachment that varies across the family life course (Goldberg & Goldberg, 2002).
- *Family Nursing.* A family is two or more persons who are joined together by bonds or sharing and emotional closeness and who identify themselves as being a part of the family (Friedman, Bowden, & Jones, 2003).
- *Family Systems Nursing.* Family is a group of individuals who are bound by emotional ties, a sense of belonging, and a passion for being involved in one another's lives (Wright, Watson, & Bell, 1996, p. 45).
- *Family Health Care Nursing.* Family refers to two or more individuals who depend on one another for emotional, physical, and economical support. The members are self-defined (Hanson, Gedaly-Duff, & Kaakinen, 2005, p. 7).

their family. When the family members agree on this point, the family is designated. In a case of disagreement, the nurse can note the disagreement and include as the designated family the persons who interact most often as the family unit.

VIEWS OF THE FAMILY

Nurses have long recognized the importance of the family as a context for a client's illness and care, but an interest in incorporating the family as a unit into care has emerged more recently. The literature suggests that the client of the family nurse may be (Bomar & McNeely, 1996):

- The individual as client with the family as context
- The entire family unit as client
- The family interactional systems of dyads, triads, or other groupings as client
- Family aggregates (families sharing similar issues) as client

Figure 29-1 illustrates these four approaches.

Family as Context

In the family-as-context approach, the individual is the focus of care, and the family is part of the environment, serving as a base of support or stress for the client. This approach to family nursing has had its roots in pediatric and maternal-child nursing (Hanson & Boyd, 1996). The impact and consequences of illness and treatment are considered in light of the family members' needs to adjust or adapt to changes. For example, changes in one person's diet will affect cooking and eating behaviors within the family. Further, from this perspective, changes in family structure (an obvious one being the birth of a baby) clearly have an impact on the family life. The nurse will assess the meaning and significance of each event, illness, stressor, or change to the family as a whole and assist in whatever way possible to help the family make positive adjustments that promote health for each member. For nursing services provided under this framework, the nurse focuses on one family member as the "client" and views the family within the context of affecting the health, treatment, and management of the therapeutic regimen for the client.

Family as Client

In the family-as-client approach, the family itself is considered the focus of care. Here the "family is considered the sum of its individual members, and the focus is on every individual member" (Hanson & Boyd, 1996, p. 25). This approach to families is used often in primary care settings, where each person within the family is assessed for health needs and each client is known and understood in relation to the family group. Family nurse practitioners and family practice physicians commonly use this approach, making a clear distinction between care provided in primary care offices and care provided by physician specialists who see only individuals without knowing or assessing the family unit.

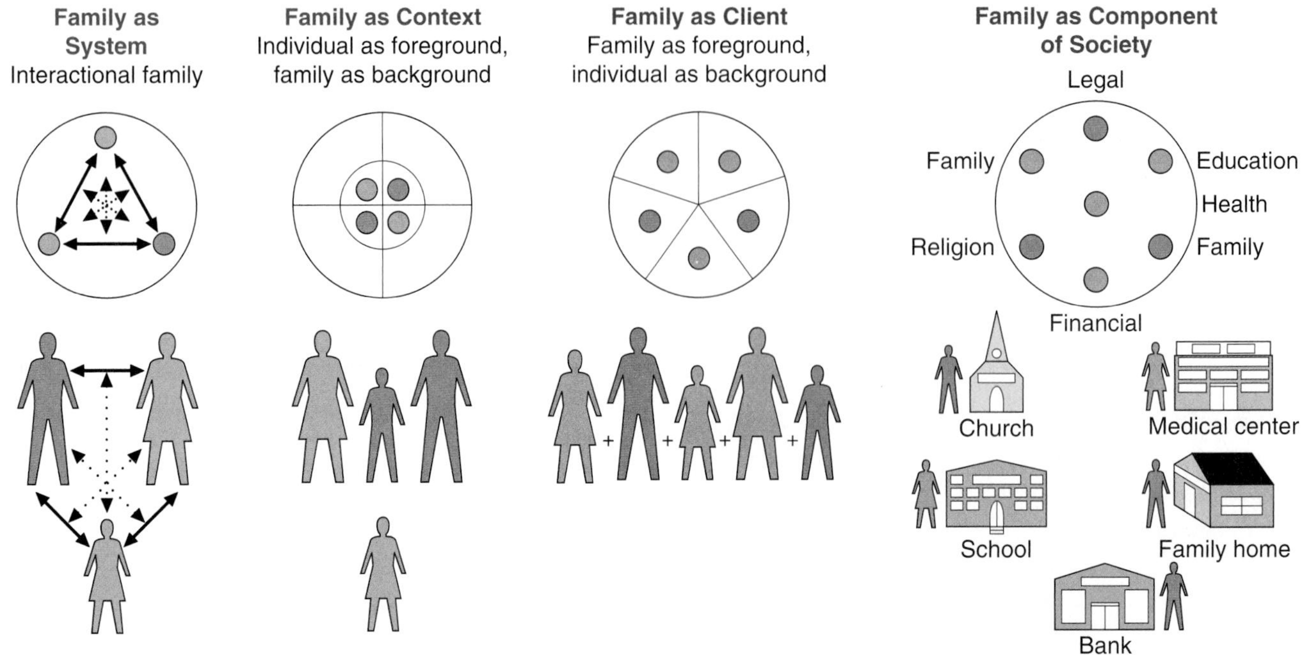

FIGURE 29-1 **Approaches to family nursing** (FROM *FAMILY HEALTH CARE NURSING: THEORY, PRACTICE AND RESEARCH*, BY S. HANSON & S. BOYD, 1996, PHILADELPHIA: F.A. DAVIS.)

FAMILY AS SYSTEM

In the family-as-system approach, the family is viewed as more than the sum of its individual parts. If a significant event affects one family member, there is an impact on others. The nurse assesses both the individual members *and* the family group simultaneously. Systems theory suggests that the individuals within a family are emotionally connected such that any important event that affects one family member will have an effect on others as well. According to systems theory, when people are connected to each other in some meaningful way, events will necessitate a change or adjustment in all other parts of the system. It is helpful to think of the family as in balance. A family works to achieve a state of equilibrium. Then, if something happens to one member, the equilibrium is upset and the relationships, supports, and tasks of everyday living need to be readjusted (Frisch & Kelley, 1996). This family systems approach is used in mental health nursing, and the nurse focuses on the significant event, its impact on the individual, and its impact on the family unit. This family systems approach is also frequently used in family therapy.

FAMILY AS COMPONENT OF SOCIETY

An emerging view of the family in nursing is to understand the family as a component of society (Hanson & Boyd, 1996). The family is one of many of society's institutions, understood by some to be the basic or primary unit. The family interacts with other social institutions (schools, churches, legal bodies, economic institutions) and either receives or provides communication or services. Social scientists have developed this interpretation of families, and the approach is being used by nurses in the community (Hanson & Boyd, 1996).

APPROACHES TO FAMILY NURSING

Although discussions of family nursing suggest that nurses in one setting or specialty use one of the four approaches to family nursing, in mental health practice, psychiatric nurses use all of these perspectives. For example, when providing follow-up care to a client with Bipolar Disorder recently discharged to home, the nurse assesses the impact on the family as a whole of the client's illness, hospitalization, and need to be medicated on lithium. The family is viewed as the context in which continued treatment and management of the condition take place. In another setting or situation, the psychiatric nurse therapist will see a family in therapy as a group, viewing the family as an interactional system. In such a case, the nurse may focus on family interactions and how the family members can support one another to assist each member to meet the needs of the others. When dealing with major societal problems, such as those observed with youth drug addiction and violence, the psychiatric nurse must understand the family as a component of the larger society. Lastly, the family may be understood as the client by the community mental health nurse providing care to one member, understanding that care to each individual family member must be provided for each individual member to maintain health. Table 29-1 provides examples of each of the four approaches used in the psychiatric mental health setting. It is clearly not a situation in which one approach is "better" than another or one approach is more suitable to psychiatric nursing than the other. The nurse must have an understanding of each approach to appropriately choose the strategy that will provide the best outcome for each individual situation. Further, the level of nursing education will dictate when the nurse will provide the care and when referral should be made to one with more specialized skill and expertise.

Nurses intervene after assessing. Nurses have to determine methods for assessing families before they can determine interventions. Theories about how to look at families abound, and each determines a different way to assess what is operating within the family. Also, these assessment approaches are applied to many family and family member disorders or illnesses. Psychiatric disorders are the focus of this text, but illnesses often affect the mental health of the family or its members. For instance, Rogerson (2006) describes family intervention with people suffering from dementia, and Lewandowski, Morris, Drauker, and Risko (2007) describe how chronic pain affects the family system and how the family in turn can affect maintaining and perpetuating the chronic pain.

FAMILY THEORIES

As there are several distinct approaches to nursing of families, there are also several theories of families that influence and guide nursing practice. The following discussion provides background on the major theoretical approaches used in psychiatric nursing care. As will be seen, each theoretical approach provides a framework from which to understand families, and each provides guidance as to the nursing approach that will be most useful for the family unit.

Family Developmental Theory

Nurses are familiar with developmental theory to describe individual growth and development. Duvall's (1979) Family Development Theory is a similar model applied to families and incorporates eight chronological stages that include predictable tasks that families need to master before proceeding to the next stage. The stages are beginning family, child-bearing family, family with preschool children, family with teenagers, family launching young adults, families with middle-aged parents, and family in retirement. Family tasks include such challenges for the beginning family as adjusting to married life to make space for children and for the family with adolescents as shifting parent-child relationships to permit adolescents to move into or out of the family system (see Table 29-2). It is clear that Duvall's stages of family development are based on a traditional family structure and are defined by the ages of children. For use with modern families, other authors have suggested a Family Life Cycle Model that emphasizes typical transitions of most families that are connected to comings and goings of family members and require reorganization of roles and rules within the family (Wright & Leahey, 2000). In the Life Cycle Model, emphasis is placed on family resources rather than deficits, on transitions rather than stages, and on the family's ability to integrate both stability and change. Assessment of family development evaluates "patterns of continuity, identity, and stability that can be maintained while new behavioral patterns are changing" (p. 67). Table 29-2 presents work that extends Duvall's theory to include family development for other than traditional families, life-cycle stages for three differing North American family types: (1) the traditional married couple with children; (2) the divorced or post-divorced family; and (3) the remarried couple with children.

Nursing Interpretations Based on Family Development

Assessing a family's stage in the family life cycle process aids the nurse in both identifying the level of anxiety the family might be experiencing and understanding the tasks the family is trying to accomplish (Figure 29-2). Many times family members are not fully aware of the complexities of the developmental or transitional tasks they face. For example, a new mother who expresses anxiety by wondering why it is so difficult to incorporate her infant into the family, return to work in six weeks, keep the house in order, and feel good about

Table 29-1 Four Approaches to Family Nursing in Psychiatric Mental Health Care

APPROACH	USE IN PSYCHIATRIC MENTAL HEALTH	NURSE PREPARATION
Family as context	Individual is client. Management of individual care requires family support. Family needs education or explanation, or both.	Undergraduate
Family as client	Each family member is known to the nurse. Care to individuals is part of care to the family unit. Family practice setting	Nurse in primary care Nurse practitioner
Family as system	Use of therapeutic communication to enhance family communication. Family in therapy	Undergraduate Graduate
Family as component of society	Family problems viewed from a public health and societal perspective.	Undergraduate and graduate

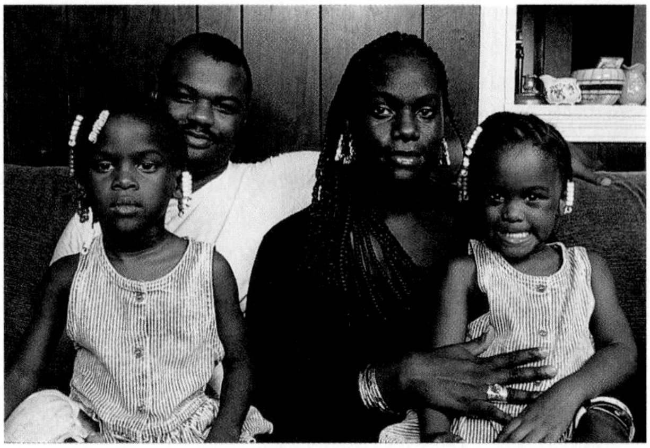

FIGURE 29-2 **Families go through predictable growth stages as members are challenged to adapt to developmental transitions of the family unit combined with changing needs of individual members.** (DELMAR/CENGAGE LEARNING.)

her physical appearance may need support that she and her family are facing one of the most difficult transitions for today's young families—that of joining child rearing, new roles of parenting, and meeting financial and household tasks. The nurse may give tremendous support to such a new mother by explaining some of the tasks typically associated with families with infants. Likewise, a couple going through divorce may seek out support from a nurse by asking what to expect of children, and how to allay some of their anxiety. The nurse may explain that finding ways to continue effective parenting is difficult for all parents going through divorce and will offer continued support for the custodial parent and child. Nurses have established support groups for children of divorce that aim to increase the child's ability to communicate more openly with parents and other caregivers (Rich, Molloy, Hart, Ginsberg, & Mulvey, 2007). Thus, similar to using individual developmental theory to understand a person's anxiety going though life challenges, using family developmental theory helps a nurse by giving new dimension and depth to understanding families.

Bowen's Family Theory

Bowen's theory views each family as being within a multigenerational context and suggests that patterns of family interactions tend to repeat themselves over generations (Kaakinen & Hanson, 2004). Eight interwoven concepts capture the familial and emotional interaction patterns: differentiation, triangulation, family projection process, multigenerational transmission process, nuclear family emotional system, sibling position, emotional cutoff, and societal regression (Bowen, 1978). Because of the centrality of the differentiation concept, key elements related to differentiation are described. A brief explanation of the other concepts follows. This explanation presents Bowen's theory as used by nurses.

Differentiation is the process of unfolding, growth, and maturation, leading to a balance between emotional and intellectual components. Differentiation is the basis of Bowen's theory, and the goal of therapy is to increase the level of differentiation. A summary of key elements of the concept (Frisch & Kelley, 1996) notes that Bowen views persons as having both an emotional and an intellectual level of functioning. The emotional level is associated with lower brain centers and relates to feelings. The intellectual level is associated with the cerebral cortex or higher brain centers and relates to cognition. Bowen suggests that the emotional and intellectual systems of an individual are connected neurologically and the degree of connectedness varies among persons.

This degree of connectedness between emotional and intellectual systems of a person dramatically affects the person's functioning, especially in social circumstances such as family. The greater the balance between the intellectual process of thinking and the subjective process of feeling (a high differentiation of self), the better the individual (or family) is at managing anxiety, acting in a thoughtful, nonreactive manner, and having intimate relationships while maintaining a separate sense of self. The family whose adult members have a high level of differentiation is flexible in its interactions, seeks to support all members, understands each member as unique, and encourages members to develop differently from one another. Family roles are assigned on the basis of knowledge, skill, and interest.

Low Level of Differentiation

When there is a low level of differentiation, the person (or family) is governed by emotions, acts impulsively, has difficulty delaying gratification, cannot step back and analyze a situation before reacting, and cannot maintain intimate interpersonal relationships. Much like a two-year-old child (developmentally at a low level of differentiation), the individual cannot give empathy, understanding, or love to another.

A two-year-old child readily exhibits behaviors and actions consistent with a low level of differentiation. The child lives in the present, knows what he wants, and cannot understand the concept of delayed gratification. The child wants what he wants now! Emotions dominate actions. The child laughs or cries and experiences fear and anger, love and hate, all within a few moments. Intimate interpersonal relationships are not possible because the child cannot give empathy, understanding, or love to another. The child at this age is only able to accept and enjoy the attentions of another.

Young children are not the only individuals who exhibit low levels of differentiation. Many adults have not developed the connections between their emotional and intellectual components. These adults may be functioning well in other aspects of their lives; for example, they may be fully employed and successful in work roles. However, their emotions dominate relationships with others such that they are unable to form intimate relationships. They make decisions impulsively, on the basis of emotions. The adult functioning at this level is not able to step back from a situation and analyze what is happening and instead reacts emotionally to situations. Intense, short-term, often serial relationships are common.

Table 29-2 Family Life-Cycle Stages and Tasks for Three Types of Family Life Cycles

STAGE	TASK
Middle-Class North American Family Life Cycle	
1. Leaving home: single young adult	a. Differentiating self in relation to family of origin b. Developing intimate peer relationships c. Establishing self in relation to work and financial independence
2. Marriage: the joining of families	a. Forming marital system b. Realigning relationships with extended families and friends to include spouse c. Making decisions about parenthood
3. Families with young children	a. Adjusting marital system to make space for children b. Joining in child-rearing, financial, and household tasks c. Realigning relationships with extended family to include parenting and grandparenting roles
4. Families with adolescents	a. Shifting parent-child relationships to permit adolescents to move into or out of system b. Refocusing on midlife marital and career issues c. Beginning shift toward joint caring for older generation
5. Launching children and moving on	a. Renegotiating marital system as a dyad b. Developing adult-to-adult relationships between grown children and their parents c. Realigning relationships to include in-laws and grandchildren d. Dealing with disabilities and death of parents (grandparents)
6. Families in later life	a. Maintaining own and/or couple functioning and interest in the face of physiological decline: exploring new familial and social role options b. Making room in the system for the wisdom and experience of elderly people, supporting the older generation without overfunctioning for them c. Dealing with loss of spouse, siblings, and other peers and preparation for death; life review and integration
Divorce and Postdivorce Family Life Cycle	
1. Deciding to divorce	a. Accepting one's own part in the failure of the marriage
2. Planning the breakup of the system	a. Working cooperatively on problems of custody, visitation, and finances b. Dealing with extended family about the divorce
3. Separation	a. Mourning loss of nuclear family b. Restructuring marital and parent-child relationships and finances; adapting to living apart c. Realigning relationships with extended family; staying connected with spouse's extended family
4. Divorce Postdivorce: single-parent (custodial)	a. Retrieving hopes, dreams, and expectations from the marriage b. Making flexible visitation arrangements with ex-spouse and his or her family c. Rebuilding own financial resources d. Rebuilding own social network
Postdivorce: single-parent (noncustodial)	a. Finding ways to continue effective parenting relationship with children b. Maintaining financial responsibilities to ex-spouse and children c. Rebuilding own social network
Remarried Family Life Cycle	
1. Entering the new relationship; conceptualizing and planning the new marriage and family	a. Recommitting to marriage and to forming a family b. Developing openness and avoiding pseudomutuality in the new relationship c. Planning financial and coparental relationships with ex-spouse d. Planning to help children deal with fears, loyalty conflicts, and membership in two systems e. Realigning relationships with extended family to include new spouse and children f. Planning maintenance of connections for children with extended family of ex-spouse(s)

(Continues)

TABLE 29-2 (Continued)

2.	Remarriage and reconstitution of family	a. Restructuring family boundaries to allow for inclusion of new spouse-stepparent b. Realigning relationships and financial arrangements throughout subsystems to permit interweaving of several systems c. Making room for relationships of all children with custodial and noncustodial parents and grandparents d. Sharing memories and histories to enhance stepfamily integration

Source: Nurses and Families: A Guide to Family Assessment and Intervention (4th ed.), by L. Wright and M. Leahey, 2005, Philadelphia: F. A. Davis. Adapted with permission.

Moderate Level of Differentiation

A person at this stage of development is less dominated by the emotional system. However, emotions dominate much of the person's relationships. Intellectually, the person tends to engage in dualistic thinking. The person views the world in terms of black and white. Things are either good or bad; people are either smart or stupid, loved or rejected. The person may have a closeness to another, but finds that in a positive relationship he will "fuse" or enmesh with the other person. The goal of a relationship is to please the other person, and the individual loses himself.

People at this level form relationships, some of which last over periods of years. However, these people find that life becomes rule bound. They do "what is right" and stick to rules, commitments, and decisions. They expect others to do the same, and they are judgmental. Such an individual is unable to see the context of a situation or comprehend that an understanding of the context of a situation could lead to a different understanding of the event. A person at a moderate level of differentiation is unable to "step into another person's shoes" and cannot see the world from another's perspective.

High Level of Differentiation

People at a high level of differentiation have a balance between emotions and intellect. These people express emotions and understand them at the same time. They are able to feel anger and step back from that anger to understand what caused it. These people are able to temper anger by using intellectual functioning. They exhibit **relativistic thinking** and are able to understand the contextual nature of the world. This thinking enables them to understand events from multiple perspectives and to evaluate the circumstances and contexts of events. For individuals at this level of differentiation, the world is not a black-and-white place where decisions are grounded in rules. Decisions are not a matter of rules or a matter of doing what is right or doing what is expected; rather, decisions are made on the basis of the context, the impact, and the outcome. A person at this level of differentiation can form intimate relationships and appreciate the uniqueness of self and of others.

Family Dynamics and Level of Differentiation

Families take on a character that reflects the level of differentiation of the adult family members. Families whose adult members operate at a low level of differentiation exhibit impulsive patterns of interactions. They make decisions without thinking through the effects and consequences. They relate on an emotional level. They often will exhibit spousal abuse and other forms of violence, as they are unable to use intellectual powers to check an emotion as strong as anger. A family whose adult members have developed to a moderate level of differentiation exhibits rigid patterns of interactions. The family is bound by rules and order. Each family member is expected to have defined roles, and the family does not tolerate any variations in expected roles or behaviors.

In contrast, a family whose adult members have developed to a high level of differentiation is flexible in its interactions. The family actively seeks to support all of its members. Because the adults are able to see the world from another person's perspective, the family understands each member as unique and encourages family members to develop differently from one another. Family roles are assigned on the basis of knowledge, skill, and interest. Table 29-3 presents a summary of family patterns according to level of differentiation.

In addition to the concept of differentiation, there are seven major concepts from Bowen's theory. **Triangulation** is a relational pattern among persons. It is an emotional configuration involving three family members. One way of thinking about a triangle is "two people avoiding an issue by pulling in an outside person" (Shealy, 1988, p. 547). While triangles exist in all families, a pattern can be established where two persons avoid dealing with issues and closeness by using the third person to evade stress. For instance, a couple experiencing a stressful relationship may pull in the wife's mother or a child as a third person in the relationship, and the husband may react by withdrawing from his wife and involving himself in his work. Thus, the anxiety is diluted as it shifts to be borne by three instead of two. Because a triangle has much higher tolerance for anxiety than a relationship of two persons, most family relationships operate with triangles. The amount of interaction is

TABLE 29-3 Level of Differentiation and Family Patterns

PARAMETER	LOW DIFFERENTIATION	MODERATE DIFFERENTIATION	HIGH DIFFERENTIATION
Mode of operation	Emotions dominate relationships	Emotions dominate relationships; intellect plays a role	Emotions and intellect in balance
Anxiety level	High	Moderate	Low
Thought patterns	Live in present; will not think ahead	Dualistic thinking	Relativistic thinking
Family dynamics	Impulsive	Rigid	Flexible

Source: Healing Life's Crises: A Guide for Nurses, by N. Frisch and J. Kelley, 1996, Clifton Park, NY: Delmar Cengage Learning.

usually relatively balanced, and shifts occur to maintain this balance. If one member withdraws, the other two move closer.

The **family projection process** describes the situation where adult family members deal with their own anxiety in relationships by projecting the anxiety onto a child. When this family projection process goes through successive generations, it is called the **multigenerational transmission process**. When the family projection process targets one child, that child is believed to have limited chances of reaching a high level of differentiation. Therefore, this child will likely choose a spouse or partner with a similarly low level of differentiation, and the family patterns will continue across generations.

The **nuclear family emotional system** describes how a family manages anxiety. Besides projecting the anxiety onto a child, the family may manage the anxiety through marital conflict or distance or through dysfunction of a spouse. **Sibling position**, or birth order of children, plays a role in analysis of expected behavioral characteristics based on birth order. When a child did not exhibit predicted behaviors, Bowen would examine if parental anxiety focused on this child. He noted a tendency for siblings in certain positions to assume certain roles and behaviors, such as an older child being responsible and taking on the role of caretaker of the other children, and sometimes taking on the role of adult family members as well.

Emotional cutoff is Bowen's term for a family member's efforts to distance self from family to reduce anxiety. For some families the process of children's distancing themselves from their parents in order to become independent results in emotional cut off. In particular, children caught in families with low to moderate levels of differentiation need to cut themselves off in order to achieve any autonomy. Finally, Bowen's concept of **societal regression** is used to describe the process of how intense anxiety leads to emotionally based decisions. In response to increasing or chronic anxiety, families' decisions become emotional rather than intellectual. Situations of extreme anxiety, such as during war or severe economic crises, produce such emotionally laden responses in virtually all families.

Nursing Interpretations Based on Bowen's Theory

Assessment of the family level of differentiation is the single most important aspect of understanding family dynamics. If a nurse knows the family's level of differentiation, the nurse also knows how the family thinks, what is important to the family, and how to communicate with the family on an appropriate level.

For example, knowing that a family is at a low level of differentiation, a nurse seeks to develop trust with the family and provide experiences that will help the adults develop cognitive skills to understand their emotions. The literature provides examples of how nurses and therapists help impulsive, violent persons deal with anger, and these are excellent examples of effective ways of dealing with persons with low differentiation. For example, one technique includes having a person keep an "anger journal," wherein the client keeps track of when the anger occurred and what brought it on. The person is taught to identify the anger and accept it as part of living. Further, the person is asked to remove himself from the situation so that escalation of the emotion cannot occur. Both drinking alcohol and driving must be avoided. The person learns to take time out by going for a walk or engaging in some other nonhurtful activity until the anger

REFLECTIVE THINKING 29-1

The Multigenerational Projection Process

It is very difficult for people to believe the simple fact that every persecutor was once a victim. Yet it should be very obvious that someone who was allowed to feel free and strong from childhood does not have the need to humiliate another person (Miller, 1983).

cools down. Thus, the person learns, in the instance of anger, how intellectual skills (that is, identifying the anger and using a contract to perform some nonhurtful activity) can be used to avoid negative expressions of the emotion. In this process, the person learns one method of using intellectual functioning to balance an emotion. For many clients, this is the first step in moving toward a higher level of differentiation. Here the nurse is working with an individual client using assessment of the family from Bowen's family theory and using the family as the context in which to provide care. Understanding that changes in one family member will affect the rest of the family, the nurse can predict changes in family health and dynamics by working with one family member.

In contrast, a family at a high level of differentiation needs nursing care that facilitates members' own abilities to feel emotions and understand events. The family members have many skills in dealing with their own situations, but will often seek nursing care at a time of crisis or when facing a new and difficult task. The family will need help from the nurse, and the nurse recognizes that the adult family members are able to view their situation from one another's perspectives. The nurse may choose to see the family as a unit and focus on facilitating communication and problem solving.

Structural Family Theory

Structural family theory, developed by Minuchin (1974), posits that a family operates as a system such that a family with a dysfunction has some underlying structure that serves to maintain equilibrium in an unhealthy or dysfunctional way. Minuchin (1974) suggests that family structure creates an organization or foundation for the ways in which families interact. Therapy within this framework seeks to change the underlying family organization and structure, thus bringing about change in each family member's position within the group.

From this perspective, a person is seen as a social being, and each person's experience is based on his relationship with others in his environment. Family structures include two systems of constraints: a generic system, involving rules governing family organization, position, and power, and an idiosyncratic system, involving mutual expectations of family members (Minuchin, 1974).

Power has to do with the influences each family member has on the family processes and functioning. Some distribution of power is essential to maintain order. It is assumed that there is a power hierarchy such that parents have different levels of authority than do children. Optimally, parents have a sense of shared power, and children are given power on the basis of their level of maturity and responsibility.

Within a family, each member belongs to a number of subsystems. These subsystems can be formed by generation (parents and children and grandchildren), by sex (male and female family members), by interest (those who play music together), or by function (those who have jobs outside the home and those who do not). These subsystems are related to each other according to rules and patterns. Often, these rules develop in a family over time and are never articulated to family members. These rules can be taken for granted and may be unconscious. Often, it is only when a person outside the family sphere points out that the rules exist and dictate behavior that family members begin to see their own organization and learn that other families may not behave in a similar manner. Part of the nurse's role is to help the family understand its own structure and how its rules can positively or negatively affect its functioning.

Families that are dysfunctional will frequently have a "target" family member—the person with the problem that is causing the family to seek professional help. There may be a young child who cannot behave kindly toward others at preschool, or there may be a depressed teenager. When structural family theory is used as a basis for therapy, the goal of the therapy is to uncover the family structure, that is, its rules and organization that allows the problem behavior to persist. For example, the preschooler may have learned he has more power within the family if he acts up at school and has to be taken home. The depressed teenager may be reacting to controls that will not allow him to become independent and competent. Only when the family members understand their rules and patterns are they able to make changes. Thus, structural family therapy deals with feedback between circumstances and the person(s) involved.

Different from other forms of therapy, structural family therapy is a therapy of action. The nurse using this approach joins the family in interactions with the goal of changing the family structure. The nurse's work is in the present, in interactions with the family as a whole. When the nurse joins the family system and participates in interactions, the interactions between and among all other family members are altered. Thus, the family members have a chance to experience new circumstances of interactions with each other and to see both themselves and one another in a new light.

Nursing Interpretations Based on Structural Family Theory

To use structural family theory as a therapist, the nurse must be trained as a therapist and will see the family members in sessions together. Advanced practice nurses may use this approach in both inpatient and outpatient psychiatric settings.

However, the theory may help a nurse who is not in an advanced practice role to understand a broader perspective on client problems than what is commonly discussed in many inpatient units. Minuchin (1992) provides an important description of a 10-year-old boy with a diagnosis of Attention-Deficit Disorder. The child had been hospitalized in a child psychiatric unit for one year of his life and had been placed on numerous medications. When Minuchin was called in to consult on the case, he received a detailed case history, on which he reflected: "The precision with which the ten people talking with me cover up the narrowness of their point of view impresses me" (p. 4). These professionals were looking at the child as a neurological system, completely devoid of life experiences. Minuchin's beginning approach with the family was to view the child in interaction with his family. Minuchin was the only professional to point out that the child would remain in the hospital as long as his mother could not control him. The problem is the fit between the mother and child, not simply the child. Expanding one's own views of family and "problem family members" will permit nurses to serve as client advocates and may open doors for referrals and services for those receiving nursing care and screening.

By way of example, consider another client situation. A mental health nurse working for the public schools is called because a 10-year-old girl, Gail, is acting out in class. She is not paying attention to her teacher, she is calling out to attract attention to herself, and she is making fun of some of the other children in the class. The nurse making an assessment from a structural family theory approach would first find out what is going on with the child's family and what reasons might explain the current change in the girl's behavior. Talking to the mother, the nurse learns that Gail's younger brother, Tommy, has been diagnosed with leukemia and that the family is experiencing a crisis situation in efforts to come to terms with his illness and to obtain appropriate care for him. Gail's behavior takes on a very different interpretation as the nurse assesses that Gail feels powerless and isolated as the family structure changes to meet the needs of her brother. Using structural family theory, the nurse can help the parents to understand Gail's anxiety and coping. Through a better understanding of the family structure and changes, the nurse, parents, and teacher can help to plan methods of returning power to Gail. The theory provides a means of helping the parents look further to the impact of Tommy's illness on each of them and the family as a whole. These understandings provide insights that assist in coping.

Communication Theory

Many theorists and therapists have focused on communication as the area within families needing attention and correction. Communication theorists have presented the view that verbal and nonverbal communication influence the behaviors of all family members. Internationally known family therapist Virginia Satir intentionally focuses her work on communication. The goal of Satir's family therapy is to improve communication to the point of making all family communication clear, accurate, and meaningful (Satir, 1967).

Watzlawick, a communication theorist, presented four axioms, or rules, of communication that nurses have found useful in assisting communication within families. These axioms are (Watzlawick, Beavin, & Jackson, 1967):

1. All behavior, whether nonverbal or verbal, is communication and conveys a message.
2. All communication defines a relationship.
3. Persons communicate both verbally and nonverbally; the former presents more content, whereas the latter informs more about the relationship.
4. All communication is either symmetrical (equality exists and either person is free to take the lead) or complementary (one leads and the other follows).

Satir (1967) emphasized nonverbal communication patterns. She identified roles that family members take on, for example, the placater (the one who fixes every problem), the blamer (the one who accuses others), and the computer (the nonemotional thinking person). She used these roles to help persons see themselves in relationship to others in their family. She identified an important goal for the family therapist as helping family members to see each other, not as bad or mean, but as people whose communications are not always clear.

Nursing Interpretations Based on Communication Theory

Nurses involved with families can use all of the skills of communication theory to help family members learn how to communicate their messages effectively. (For techniques of therapeutic communication, see Chapter 5.) These techniques can be used by the nurse in sessions with all family members present to clarify communication, to affirm that messages are being heard and understood, and to provide a role model for effective listening and participation in the communication process. Nurses use these techniques in formal therapy sessions in an office and also in less formal situations such as during a home visit. In each of these cases, the nurse can view the family unit as the client.

Wright and Leahey (2005) provide an adaptation of communication theory to nursing through their work on the Calgary Family Assessment Model and the Calgary Family Intervention Model. They note that there is a pattern of **circular communication** in most relationships. Circular communication is a predictable pattern of communication and response between two people. Because the patterns are repeated again and again, the family members are often unaware of them. The nurse can point them out, resulting in surprise, awareness, and then ability to change. A common negative circular communication is described in the following example: An angry wife is criticizing her husband; the husband's response is to feel anger and to withdraw; the wife becomes angrier and criticizes more; the husband becomes angrier and withdraws further. Each sees the other person as the problem. A nurse pointing out the communication as circular, unending, and negative is able to help the couple see themselves differently and thus make a decision to change.

Family Spirituality

An area often omitted in assessing and intervening with families, especially in family nursing, is family spirituality. When spirituality is addressed, it is usually approached from the point of view of each individual family member rather than as family spirituality, or family spiritual health. An approach to spiritual assessment and interventions for families has been proposed by Tanyi (2006). Tanyi uses the common differentiation of religion from spirituality, describing spirituality as "the search for meaning and purpose in life, meaningful relationships, individual family member spirituality, family values, beliefs, and practices, which may or may not be religiously based, and the ability to be transcendent" (p. 1).

Tanyi notes findings of the positive impact of spirituality in facilitating marital and family functioning; in maintaining family cohesion and resilience; in positive adjuctment to loss

Table 29-4 Guidelines for Spiritual Assessment of Families

Meaning and purpose
- Who or what does the family consider the most meaningful?
- What gives the family meaning in their daily routines?
- What gives the family peace, joy, and satisfaction?

Strengths
- What gives the family strength?
- What helps the family to deal with crises?
- What does the family do in order to rebuild their strength?

Relationships
- What do family members like about their family?
- Does the family have a relationship with God/Higher Power, universe, Other? If yes, how do they describe it?
- Is the family involved in community-based spiritual activities? If yes, which ones?

Beliefs
- What are the family's beliefs? And what do these beliefs mean to their health?
- Does the family practice rituals such as prayer, worship, or medication?

Individual family member spirituality
- How do family members express/describe their spirituality? And what does this mean to their health?
- Are there conflicts between family members because of their spiritual views?
- If yes, what is the impact, if any, on the individuals' and family's health?

Family's preference for spiritual care
- How does the family describe/express their spiritual views?
- Can the family give examples of how nurses can integrate their spiritual views when working with them?
- Does the family consider any one their spiritual leader? And if necessary, can the spiritual leader be contacted to assist with providing care to the family?

Source: R. Tanyi, 2006, Spirituality and family nursing: Spiritual assessment and interventions for families, *Journal of Advanced Nursing*, *53*(3), 287–294 [online version, p. 3].

Table 29-5 Guidelines to Spiritual Interventions for Families

Spiritual support
- Be present and available to the family in a non-hurried manner
- Respect the family's spiritual orientation and support their practices
- Encourage and support comments that reflect the family's need for spiritual growth

Spiritual well-being
- Support and encourage the family's use of spiritual resources as desired
- Assist the family in locating spiritual groups and resources in their community
- Support, acknowledge, and applaud verbalized comments of peace, harmony, and satisfaction with family circumstances and relationships
- Encourage continual spiritual growth

Spiritual distress
- Attempt to determine the reason(s) for the distress, and support the family's efforts to examine their beliefs and values
- Acknowledge the family's position, but if necessary, obtain their consent to consult with a spiritual leader of their preference
- Provide research-based evidence to the family about the positive impacts of spirituality on family health and functioning
- Continue to display empathy, acceptance, and kindness in a non-judgmental manner

Source: R. Tanyi, 2006, Spirituality and family nursing: Spiritual assessment and interventions for families, *Journal of Advanced Nursing*, *53*(3), 287–294 (online version, p. 4).

of a family member; in coping with disabilities; in coping with caregivers' burdens, and other family challenges.

The goals of family spiritual assessment, according to Tanyi, are "(1) to support and enhance families' spiritual well-being and development; (2) to discern spiritual distress and its effects on overall family health; and (3) to ascertain ways to incorporate family spirituality when providing care" (p. 3).

Tanyi proposes example guidelines for spiritual assessment and intervention. These guidelines are presented in Tables 29-4 and 29-5.

APPLICATION OF THE NURSING PROCESS 29-1

ASSESSMENT

Family assessment involves interviewing, observing, and creating diagrams of information for pattern analysis. The nurse must begin with assessment designed to obtain information about the family as well as its individual members. While several assessment tools exist and may be helpful, the Family Assessment Tool is suggested as a means of obtaining detailed information about a family and its members' views of their own strengths and problems. The tool was modified on the basis of the work of several family nursing experts. A brief version of the Family Assessment Tool is presented in Table 29-6 (the complete version appears at the end of this chapter in the Resource section) and is modified only slightly from the Calgary Family Assessment Model developed by Wright and colleagues.

TABLE 29-6 Family Assessment Tool: Brief Version

I. Identifying data
II. Graphic family diagrams
  A. Genogram
  B. Family attachment diagram
  C. Ecomap
III. Family structure
  A. Internal structure
    1. Family composition
    2. Gender
    3. Sexual orientation
    4. Rank order
    5. Subsystems
    6. Boundaries
    7. Power structure
  B. External structure
    1. Extended family
    2. External systems
  C. Context
    1. Race/ethnicity
    2. Social class
    3. Religion and spirituality
    4. Environment
IV. Family development/life cycle
  A. Stages
  B. Tasks
  C. Attachments
V. Family function
  A. Instrumental functioning
    1. Activities of daily living
  B. Affective and socialization functioning
    1. Affective
    2. Socialization
  C. Expressive functioning
    1. Emotional communication
    2. Verbal communication
    3. Nonverbal (and paraverbal) communication
    4. Circular communication
    5. Problem solving
    6. Roles
    7. Alliances/coalitions
    8. Influence and power
      a. Instrumental
      b. Psychological
      c. Corporal
  D. Health care functioning
    1. Beliefs (about health care)
    2. Health practices

Source: Calgary Family Assessment Model, in *Nurses and Families: A Guide to Family Assessment and Interventions* (4th ed.), by L. Wright and M. Leahey, 2005, Philadelphia: F. A. Davis. With modifications based on information from M. M. Friedman, V. R. Bowden, & E. G. Jones, (2003). *Family Nursing: Theory and Practice* (3rd ed.), Englewood Cliffs, NJ: Prentice Hall. (Integrated adaption with permission of Wright Leahey/FA Davis).

(Continues)

APPLICATION OF THE NURSING PROCESS 29-1 (Continued)

In addition to recording basic assessment information in narrative form, there are three diagrams that can be used to depict large amounts of information about the families in a graphic form. The three diagrams are the genogram, the attachment or interaction diagram, and the ecomap.

> **NURSINGTIP 29-2**
>
> **Family Assessment**
>
> Keep in mind that family assessment is also in a sense family intervention, as the assessment process requires communication and information gathering from different family members.

The **genogram** is a graphic depiction of a family tree that records information about family members and their relationships for at least three generations (McGoldrick & Gerson, 1985). There are various ways to construct genograms, and each will provide a tangible illustration of family information. A genogram helps the nurse to keep the whole family in mind as a unit, even if the nurse is caring for one family member at a time. A genogram can be constructed during the first encounter with a family and can be kept as part of the clinical record.

Inasmuch as families repeat behaviors and patterns across generations, a genogram presents a representation of family patterns. A genogram depicts the family tree, with information on pertinent health history (most notably, major illnesses and cause of death) and social history (births, deaths, marriages, separations, divorces). The information is obtained from the family members themselves, and the genogram can be shared with the family members. Often, patterns emerge that were unnoticed by the family members. For example, in a family where parents and grandparents had a history of multiple separations and divorces, a family may see that there is a tendency toward ending marriage.

Other families may have a history of persistent and chronic health problems that create stress and difficulty across generations. Many nurses find that a genogram can be used as a basis for discussion with families and that the information opens up areas for prevention and risk management. Figure 29-3 provides a basic form for a three-generation genogram. The case study at the end of this chapter provides an example of a completed genogram.

A **family attachment diagram** is a representation of the reciprocal nature and quality of the affectional ties between the family members. Some authors suggest that the family interaction pattern symbols be inserted into the genogram (McGoldrick & Gerson, 1985); however, because of confusion that can occur when too many symbols are used in a genogram, the attachment diagram is presented separately in this text. Figure 29-4 illustrates the

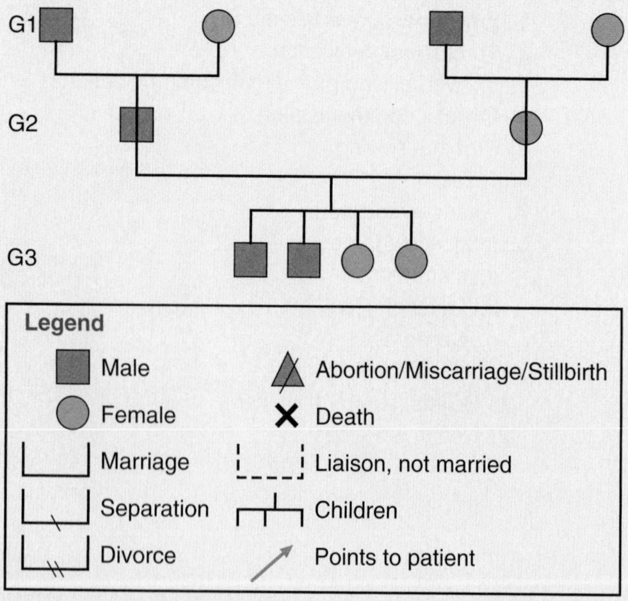

FIGURE 29-3 **Basic genogram form** (DELMAR/CENGAGE LEARNING)

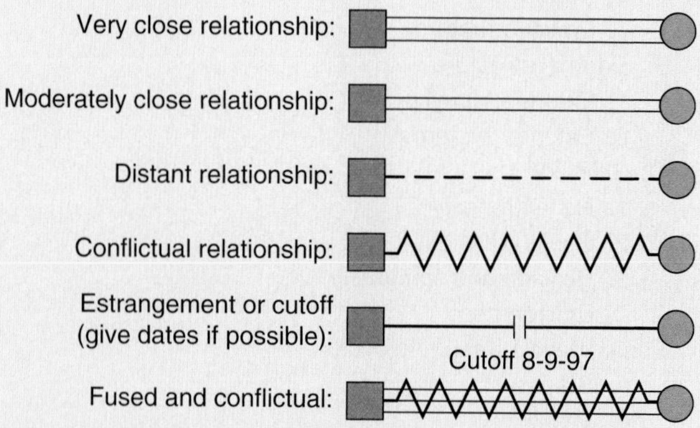

FIGURE 29-4 **Symbols used in an attachment diagram** (FROM *GENOGRAMS IN FAMILY ASSESSMENT*, BY MONICA MCGOLDRICK AND RANDY GERSON. COPYRIGHT © 1985. REPRINTED WITH PERMISSION OF W. W. NORTON COMPANY, INC.)

(*Continues*)

APPLICATION OF THE NURSING PROCESS 29-1 (Continued)

symbols used in such a diagram. The case study at the end of this chapter illustrates the application of a family attachment diagram.

Lastly, the **ecomap** depicts the family members' interactions with systems outside the family. The diagram is similar to the attachment diagram in that it depicts the nature of the family members' relationships with institutions, agencies, and significant people outside the group designated as immediate family. The strength and positive or conflictual nature of relationships with such groups as the extended family, neighbors, friends, work, school, and the health care system are diagrammed.

In construction of an ecomap, the immediate family is put in a center circle. The significant individuals, organizations, or agencies with which the family members interact are put in circles surrounding the center circle. The nature of the relationship between the family member and the outer circle is represented by straight lines (strong communication), number of lines (more lines indicate a stronger relationship), dotted lines (tenuous connection), and zig-zag lines (stressful connection). Further, arrows may be placed on the lines to indicate flow of energy and resources. Figure 29-5 depicts the symbols and form used in an ecomap. See the case study at the end of the chapter for an illustration of the application of an ecomap in family assessment.

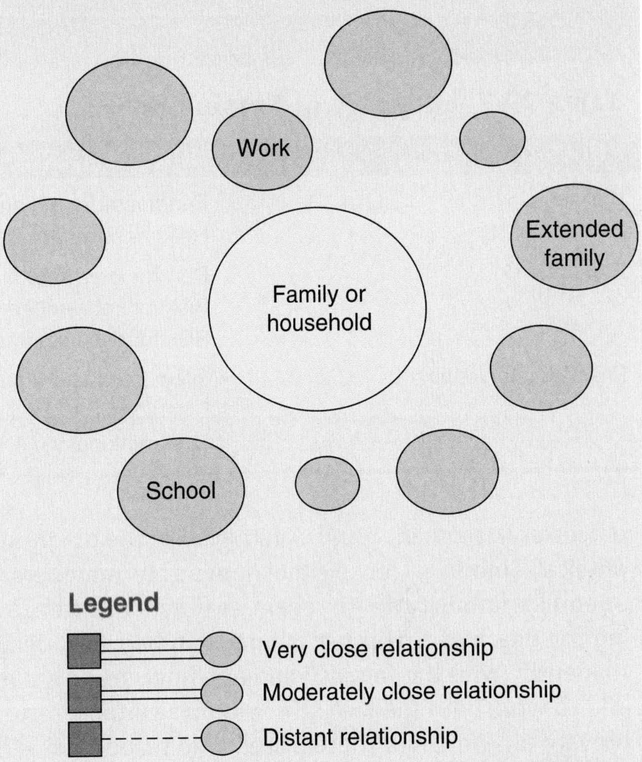

FIGURE 29-5 **Symbols and form used in a family ecomap** (FROM A. HARTMAN. *FINDING FAMILIES: AN ECOLOGICAL APPROACH TO FAMILY ASSESSMENT AND ADOPTION.* COPYRIGHT © 1979. REPRINTED BY PERMISSION OF SAGE PUBLICATIONS.)

In addition to their value in family assessment, the construction of the diagrams serves as an intervention with the family. When the nurse shares the diagrams with the family members, new insights are drawn as patterns are noted.

NURSING DIAGNOSIS

In work with families, the NANDA-I taxonomy of nursing diagnoses provides a language to identify nursing concerns regarding the family unit. There are diagnoses specifically dealing with the family unit, and through the development of axes to the existing diagnoses, there is opportunity to identify any diagnosis as pertaining to the family as a whole. (See Chapter 4 for a detailed description of the NANDA-I diagnoses.)

There are diagnoses specifically pertaining to families; these are related to family processes, family coping, and home maintenance management (NANDA-I, 2009). Each of these diagnoses may be used to describe the various nursing roles in problem intervention, preventive care, and promotion of wellness. These are used extensively by nurses in psychiatric and community settings who document care under a nursing model. Each will be discussed below and reflect nursing diagnoses that require wellness, prevention, and problem interventions.

FAMILY PROCESSES

Family processes is a phrase that refers to family functioning. A family that normally functions well and experiences a crisis or change leading to a disruption of family processes is considered to have *Interrupted family*

(Continues)

APPLICATION OF THE NURSING PROCESS 29-1 (Continued)

TABLE 29-7 Language of Nursing Roles

ROLES	NURSING LANGUAGE
Wellness	Readiness for enhanced family processes Readiness for enhanced family coping
Prevention	Risk for interrupted family processes Risk for imbalanced family coping Risk for dysfunctional family processes
Problem intervention	Interrupted family processes Disabled family coping Dysfunctional family processes

processes (Herdman, 2009). A family with the diagnosis *Interrupted family processes* is unable to meet the physical, emotional, or spiritual needs of its members. This family requires support to find a new adjustment or equilibrium in order to regain its function. Often, a family undergoing a maturational change or experiencing the death of a member or birth of a baby will demonstrate *Interrupted family processes.* A nursing role is to identify with the family when and how the new event or situation affected their typical family functioning and to work with the family in finding a suitable resolution. This diagnosis, however, may be used either to prevent a problem (if there is reason to suspect risk—risk for interrupted family processes) or (if the family wants) to examine and make changes in how they function (readiness for enhanced family functioning).

Typical uses of this diagnosis to illustrate the three nursing roles are given in the following examples:

1. A nurse in a community geriatric day care center is called on to make home visits to a family. One of the center's clients, Mr. Lawrence, a 68-year-old man with dementia, has just moved in with his daughter and her family. The client has reached a point where he is unable to safely care for himself, and the family believes that the best care could be provided by having him move into their home. The family unit consists of the client's daughter and her husband, their 25-year-old son who lives with his own family five miles away, and an 18-year-old daughter living at home and going to school. The wife does not work outside the home and is ready to accept the role of caregiver to her father. The nurse obtains a family history that indicates the family has functioned well in the past and that the family members all view themselves as close and supportive. With this information, the nurse may use the diagnosis of *Interrupted family processes* related to family adjustments dictated by changed living arrangements and the need for Mr. Lawrence to receive care from his daughter. In using this diagnostic statement, the nurse is identifying that the family is facing changes, these changes will put them in a state of imbalance, and they will have to change many of their family patterns.
2. While talking with a woman who has brought her child in for a school athletic physical, a nurse in a primary care clinic discovers that the family is about to move to another city, about 200 miles away. The family will face changes in jobs (both parents are professionals who have already secured employment in the new location), and all three school-aged children will be in a new elementary school. This nurse may use the diagnosis of *Risk for interrupted family processes* related to the upcoming change and inevitable adjustment to a new living situation.
3. A school nurse is talking with the mother of a 10-year-old with asthma about the child's medications and activity level when the mother states that she is expecting her second child. The mother begins to ask the nurse questions regarding how a new baby in the home may affect her 10-year-old child, and also relates that both parents have begun to give some thought to the changes that will occur in their

(*Continues*)

APPLICATION OF THE NURSING PROCESS 29-1 (Continued)

home once the new baby arrives. This nurse uses the diagnosis of *Readiness for enhanced family processes* to indicate that there is an opening for her to initiate work with the family to promote wellness and a positive adjustment.

FAMILY COPING

Family coping refers to the family's patterns of interactions that have to do with its ability to provide sufficient and effective support, encouragement, or assistance to its members facing illness or threats to well-being.

Disabled family coping refers to the situations where the family has insufficient coping patterns to deal with a new challenge. The nurse is usually called in to assist the family because there is a target event (for example, an incidence of spousal abuse) that draws attention to the ineffective family patterns. In situations where the family as a whole, or one of its members, expresses willingness to change their means of interactions, the nurse may use the wellness diagnosis label of *Readiness for enhanced family coping*. For example, a situation where one family member states he will seek therapy to assist himself and the family to support one another in a more positive way exhibits an admission that the current coping patterns are not adequate and expresses, both by actions and words, a desire to make changes.

HOME MAINTENANCE

Home maintenance refers to the family's ability to independently maintain a safe and growth-promoting immediate environment for its members. Defining characteristics include the subjective expression from the family for help in the area of home maintenance and objective data of a disorderly home environment, accumulation of dirt and waste, and overtaxed family members who do not have the resources (emotional, physical, or financial) to provide for a safe and supportive home environment.

Community nurses may make this diagnosis when it is clear that a family requires services or supports to maintain a desirable environment. For example, consider a nurse visiting the home of a new mother with a five-day-old baby who assesses that the mother is undergoing significant postpartum depression. The nurse will first take appropriate steps to see that the mother is evaluated and treated for her condition. Second, the nurse will also assess the home environment and may well observe that the young mother and her family have been unable to meet the basic needs of providing and keeping food in the home, caring for the baby, and maintaining a clean, safe environment. The nurse could make a diagnosis of *Impaired home maintenance* and work with the family to find community resources to assist until the mother and other family members have sufficient resources to maintain the household. In another situation, the same community nurse may visit a young, single mother who is doing well with her new baby—both physically and emotionally—but finds that the new mother is asking the nurse for assistance in organizing and maintaining her apartment now that the baby has arrived. The nurse could make a diagnosis of *Readiness for enhanced home maintenance* while providing care to this mother.

OTHER NURSING DIAGNOSES

It is increasingly important for nurses to direct their attention to the ongoing needs of families who become the caregivers of members who, by the nature of their psychiatric illness, are unable to safely care for themselves. *Caregiver role strain* is an identified nursing diagnosis (NANDA-I, 2009) and is one that may be underutilized in community mental health. One nurse author has documented that families of persons with severe mental illness often live in anguish because of stressors of the caregiving role (Parker, 1993). Nurses should assess for emotional distress, including signs of grief, guilt, anger, powerlessness, and fear. The family providing care needs to be included as part of the team that is caring for the client. Parker warns that "many families have been deeply wounded by being given the role of caregiver to persons with severe mental illness, without any preparation or support. Mental health providers

(*Continues*)

APPLICATION OF THE NURSING PROCESS 29-1 (Continued)

must redress this wrong" (p. 21). Parker goes on to recommend that families be provided with education regarding the illness of their family member and suggests that family self-help groups are a viable source of support in many communities.

In addition to identifying specific diagnoses addressing families, nurses using nursing diagnoses have suggested that any nursing diagnosis can be used, with the unit of analysis being an individual, family, or community group (Hoskins, 1991; Warren, 1991). The thinking behind this idea is that there could be an introduction of axes into the taxonomy such that the nurse could identify the appropriate unit receiving nursing care (see Chapter 4). Thus, potentially any diagnosis on the NANDA-I-approved list can be applied to family nursing. For example, diagnoses such as *Powerlessness*, *Imbalanced nutrition*, or *Decisional conflict* could be made to underscore that the problem the nurse is seeing has to do with underlying familial patterns or structures. The nursing role could be to treat individual members of the family with these nursing concerns; however, it is often most appropriate to see the family as a whole and to provide care at the level of the family. Thus, the axis indicating that the diagnosis pertains to the family group along with interventions such as family therapy or communication counseling is an important way to indicate the family nursing role. Family therapy covers many approaches, including short- or long-term time frames. Short-term approaches, such as that of the Calgary Family Systems Unit (Wright & Leahey, 2005; Wright, Watson, & Bell, 1996) and a very short-term single-session approach described for adolescents in Australia (Goodman & Happell, 2006) are among those useful to psychiatric nurses.

OUTCOME IDENTIFICATION

When a nurse diagnoses a family problem, the nurse and family together must define outcomes. Often the family members will simply say, "We don't want to feel so frustrated," or "Things have got to change . . . this family is no fun anymore." Only as the nurse works with the family over time will the nurse and family begin to identify real, achievable outcomes. In the beginning it is enough to state that the family wishes to work with the nurse to effect a change.

Outcomes will be dictated by the theoretical approach. For example, if a nurse were using communication theory to effect change, the outcome would be that the family members would state a change in communication and a new understanding of each other's communications. In another example, if a nurse used Bowen's concept of differentiation, a goal of interventions for a family at a low level of differentiation would be that the family members would learn to step back from problem situations and think or talk about them before reacting emotionally.

PLANNING/INTERVENTIONS

Once assessments have been completed and outcomes identified, the nurse will plan needed care and interventions. Nursing interventions may be directed toward an individual within the context of the family or toward the family as a unit. Current nursing interventions include family therapy on a structural or systems model and family therapy directed at improving communication. Such therapy will be based on the theoretical perspectives previously described.

Nurses who are not functioning as nurse-therapists typically provide interventions in the areas of:

1. Educating and informing families of their illnesses, resources, and treatment regimens, and working with family members to provide effective management of illness
2. Providing support for caregivers of psychiatric mental health family members (see Sin, Moore, & Newell, 2007, for an example of psycho-educational support for caregivers of young adults with early onset psychosis)
3. Using techniques of therapeutic communication to assist families to improve their interfamily communication

(*Continues*)

APPLICATION OF THE NURSING PROCESS 29-1 (Continued)

RESEARCH Highlight 29-1

Family Intervention Sessions

STUDY PROBLEM/PURPOSE

To examine the effectiveness of therapeutic conversations with families (through family sessions) in alleviating health complaints among adolescent girls in a school setting.

METHODS

Four girls with recurrent subjective health complaints and their families were included in the study. Three sessions were held with each family, using genograms, ecomaps, interventive questions, and other family nursing interventions. Practicing school nurses were also present. A therapeutic letter was sent to each family at the end of the sessions. The Strengths and Difficulties Questionnaire was used as a pre-and post-test measure. Evaluative interviews were carried out with the families and with the school nurses.

FINDINGS

The families reported feeling relief and described positive affective, behavioral, and cognitive changes as a consequence of the interventions. The school nurses experienced the family sessions as time-saving and easy-to-use tools in their work involving the family.

IMPLICATIONS

When schoolchildren's recurrent mental health problems are addressed, this may reduce future suffering.

Source: "Family Intervention Sessions," by Eva Clausson and Agneta Berg, 2008, *Journal of Family Nursing*, *14*(2), 289–313.

4. Assisting families to modify their home environment to provide a supportive environment for safety, interaction, and health
5. Serving as case manager or resource person, or both, to help families obtain services and referrals.

These interventions may be considered supportive in that they assist the family members to make the best adjustments possible to the situations in which they find themselves. These interventions focus on the human response to health problems, the nursing role becoming one of supporting the family's adjustment (Hanson & Boyd, 1996).

A differing approach to family nursing interventions is presented by the Calgary Family Intervention Model (CFIM). This model is based on several theoretical foundations, concepts, and components (Wright & Leahey, 2005) and is a "strengths-based, resiliency-oriented model that focuses on promoting, improving, and/or sustaining effective family functioning in three domains: cognitive, affective and behavioral" (p. 153–154). Using this model, the nurse begins interventions by determining the predominant domain of family functioning (cognitive, affective, or behavioral) that needs changing. Recommended interventions are selected from two categories: interventive questions (which are a specific form of therapeutic communication) and other interventions.

Interventive questions are circular questions used to uncover the explanations of the problem to understand and discover relationships and connections between individuals, events, ideas, and beliefs (Wright & Leahey, 2005). Four types of circular questions are described: difference questions (exploring differences between people, relationships, time, ideas, and beliefs); behavioral effect questions (exploring the effect of one person's actions on another); hypothetical or future-oriented questions (questions that explore outcomes, the what-if questions); and triadic questions (questions posed to a third person about the relationship between two others). These four types of circular questions can be used to trigger exploration and change in any of the family functional domains. Table 29-8 illustrates examples of circular questions in the domain of family functioning.

(*Continues*)

APPLICATION OF THE NURSING PROCESS 29-1 (Continued)

Table 29-8 Examples of Circular Questions to Invite Change in Family Functioning

DOMAIN OF FAMILY FUNCTIONS	DIFFERENCE	BEHAVIORAL EFFECT	HYPOTHETICAL/ FUTURE-ORIENTED	TRIADIC
	Explores differences between people, relationships, time, ideas, beliefs	Explores connections between the effect of one family member's behavior on another	Explores family options and alternative actions or meanings in the future	Question posed to a third person about the relationship between two other people
COGNITIVE Offer new ideas, opinions, information, education	*To mother*—What is the best advice you have been given about managing your daughter's eating disorder? *To mother*—Who would benefit most from more information?	*To mother*—How do you make sense of your husband's refusal to discuss your daughter's condition?	*To daughter*—What do you think will happen if you begin to believe the prescribed diet will not make you fat?	*To mother*—If your daughter begins to regain her weight, what will your husband think about it?
AFFECTIVE Reduce or increase intense emotions	*To daughter*—Who in the family is most worried about your eating disorder?	*To daughter*—How does your mother show her concern for your health?	*To mother*—If your daughter begins to eat the prescribed diet, what do you think her mood will be? Sad? Mad? Resigned?	*To daughter*—When your dad gets angry with you, how does your mother feel?
BEHAVIORAL Assist to behave differently toward one another	*To mother*—Who in the family is best at getting your daughter to take her medicine?	*To daughter*—What could your father do that would indicate to your mother that he understands her fears?	*To mother*—How long do you think it will take before your husband opens himself to your daughter's need for treatment?	*To daughter*—If your father were willing to share his feelings with your mother, what do you think he would say?

Source: Nurses and Families: A Guide to Family Assessment and Interventions (3rd ed.), by L. Wright and M. Leathey, 2000, Philadelphia: F. A. Davis. Adapted with permission.

Other interventions cited by Wright and Leahey are similar to those described by others; they are interventions aimed at offering support, education, encouragement, and hope. Table 29-9 provides examples of other interventions.

EVALUATION

Evaluation of a nurse's work with any family depends, of course, on the stated outcomes. Families often want to feel better about themselves, about their shared lives. The nurse will not be able to change the family's life circumstances, but may significantly change the family's reactions to it.

(Continues)

APPLICATION OF THE NURSING PROCESS 29-1 (Continued)

TABLE 29-9 Nursing Interventions with Families

DOMAIN	INTERVENTIONS
Cognitive	Commending family and individual strengths Offering information/opinions Reframing Encouraging Externalizing the problem
Affective	Validating/normalizing emotional responses Encouraging the telling of illness narratives Drawing forth family support
Behavioral	Encouraging family members to be caregivers and offering caregiver support Encouraging respite Devising rituals

Note: Interventions do not pertain to only one domain, but dividing by domains may start the process of thinking through how they can be used.

Source: Nurses and Families: A Guide to Family Assessment and Interventions (3rd and 4th eds.). by L. Wright and M. Leahey, 2000/2005, Philadelphia: F. A. Davis. Adapted with permission.

When terminating with a family because the work of the nurse is accomplished, one means of assisting the family to maintain a new level of functioning is to ask a question about what each family member will do to maintain the change. Thus, in terminating, the nurse helps the family members to continue their positive work.

NURSING CARE PLAN: NURSING PROCESS FORMAT 29-1

Caroline Milton is a 20-year-old college student from an affluent family. She attends a small, private college. She has distinguished herself in her academic courses and in tennis, as well as in her role as a campus leader. She is noted for her peacemaking skills and her desire to please. She is soft spoken and quite beautiful, except that she is somewhat thin even for the fashion norm of her age. Caroline and her family are referred to the family nurse by her physician when her mother and the physician determine that there is a strong likelihood that Caroline is developing an eating disorder. At the initial interview, the nurse discovers that the parents believe that Caroline has always been the "perfect child," never causing any trouble, always following the rules, and making the family proud. They cannot understand her desire to lose so much weight, and they worry about her health.

The father, William, is head of a successful business that he inherited from his father, John. The mother, Marie, is very active in various volunteer organizations. The family places high value on serving the community and strictly following the rules of their Protestant religion.

Caroline has become very thin and is still losing weight, and her mother is very concerned about the possibility that Caroline has an eating disorder. The father is less concerned and believes that Caroline is

(*Continues*)

NURSING CARE PLAN: NURSING PROCESS FORMAT 29-1 (Continued)

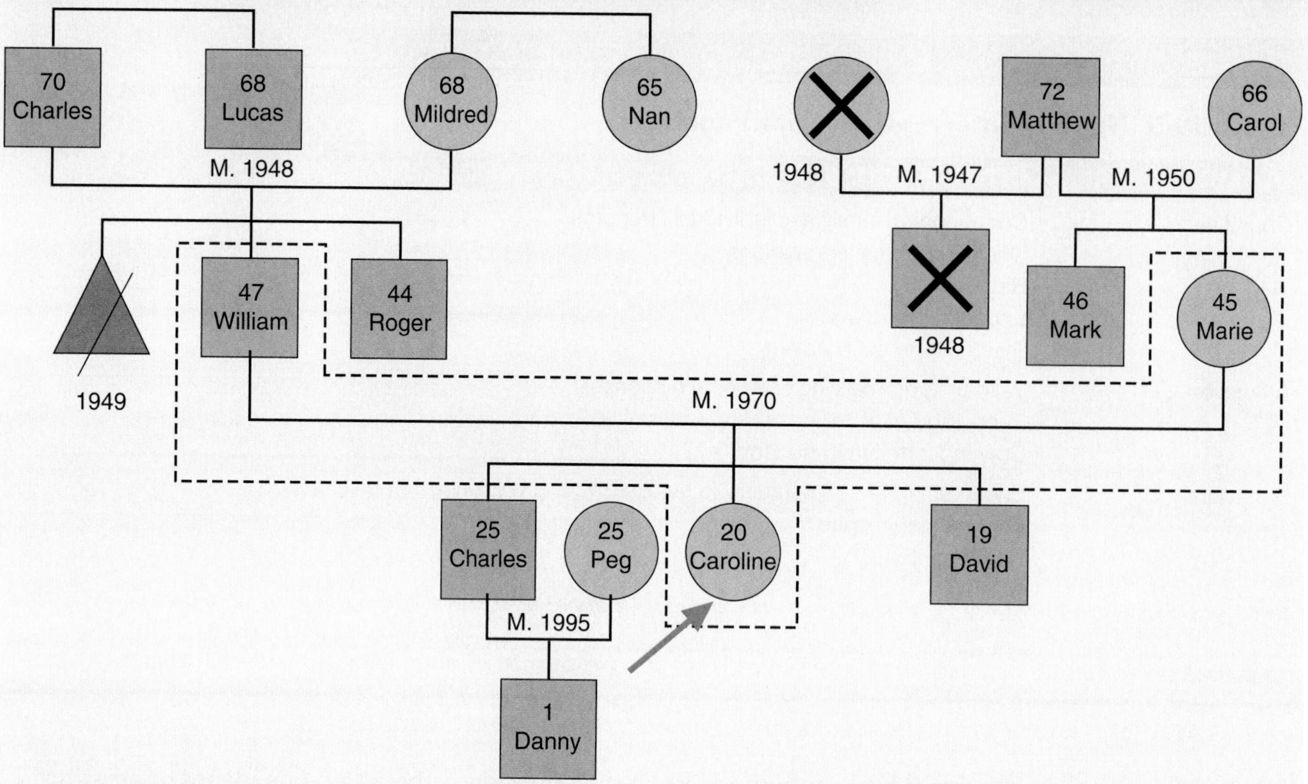

FIGURE 29-6 **Milton family genogram** (DELMAR/CENGAGE LEARNING)

beautiful, even if a bit thin, and that if she would just start eating more of the "right things" she would be fine again. He states that he does not have time to attend family sessions with the nurse at this time of the business year, but may attend later.

ASSESSMENT

The Milton family identifies Caroline's eating pattern as the presenting problem.

GENOGRAM

The nuclear family consists of 47-year-old William, his wife, Marie (45 years old), a son, Charles (25 years old), Caroline (20 years old), and another son, David (19 years old). William is the first-born son to survive, following a miscarriage, and has one younger brother. William's father was also an oldest son with one younger brother. Marie is the younger sister of an older brother. Marie's father's first wife died giving birth to a stillborn baby (see Figure 29-6).

FAMILY ATTACHMENTS

The parents describe their home life as "normal" and harmonious. Caroline has two brothers, Charles, who graduated from college with honors and now works with his father, and David, who became rebellious in high school, dropped out of college, and now lives in a commune out West. The parents say that they cannot understand David and guess that he will "come to his senses" someday—soon, they hope. While describing the family interactions when David was at home, the family reveals that Caroline would try to make peace between the parents and her brother. The mother would spend much time talking with Caroline about the situation, but the father would become angry with the mother and Caroline, withdraw, and spend more and more time at work and with the older son. Since Caroline has been at college, her father

(Continues)

NURSING CARE PLAN: NURSING PROCESS FORMAT 29-1 (Continued)

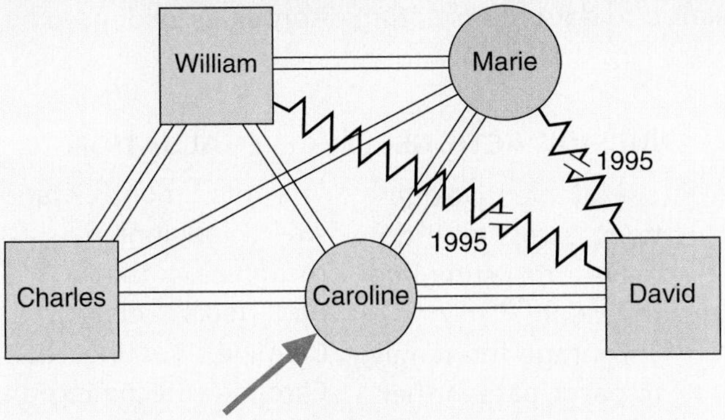

FIGURE 29-7 **Milton family attachment diagram** (DELMAR/CENGAGE LEARNING.)

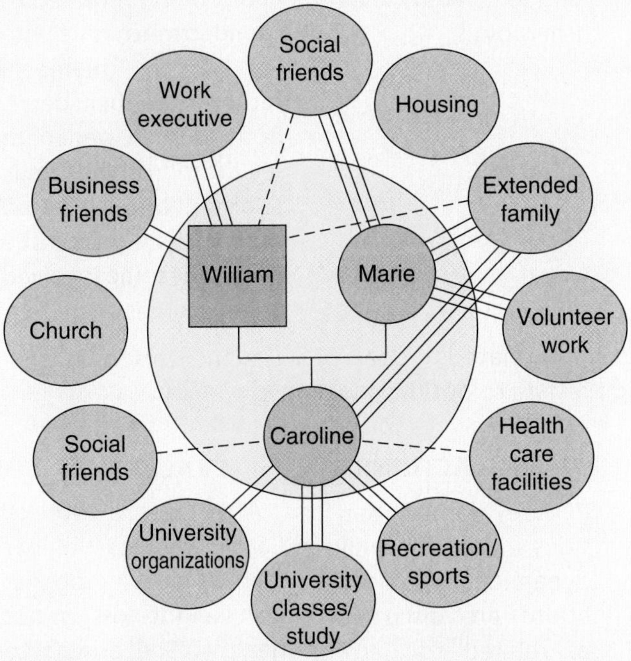

FIGURE 29-8 **Milton family ecomap** (DELMAR/CENGAGE LEARNING.)

has expressed high expectations for her success, attends many ceremonies, and on occasion takes her to dinner to celebrate (see Figure 29-7).

ECOMAP

The ecomap reveals that William is enmeshed with his work, spends time with Marie mostly at business and community social gatherings, and spends time with Charles at work or discussing work-related matters. Marie spends much of her time with her community volunteer efforts, as well as with friends shopping, planning events, and visiting her parents and inviting them to dinner regularly. She and Caroline have lunch out, or Caroline comes home for dinner and to do her laundry twice a week. Caroline studies many hours and is very involved in a sorority and in her campus leadership activities. She practices tennis daily for one-and-a-half hours, except Sundays. She visits one set of grandparents every two weeks, making sure that she distributes her time equally between the couples. She communicates with David through letters and occasional telephone calls, and sees Charles and his wife and baby at her parent's home for occasional dinners (see Figure 29-8).

INTERPRETATION OF FAMILY ASSESSMENT DATA

The Milton family perceives itself to be both a nuclear family and a multigenerational family whose members all reside in the same city, except for David, who has been essentially cut off from the family for over a year. Gender roles have been traditional, with the men working outside the home and bearing the financial responsibility for the family and the women, although educated, investing their time in volunteer and social activities.

FAMILY DEVELOPMENT/LIFE CYCLE

The Milton family is in the "launching of young adults" stage. Marie and William have invested little time in the tasks of the parental life-cycle stage of launching children and moving on as a couple.

LEVEL OF DIFFERENTIATION

The family is at a moderate level of differentiation. There seems to be a suppression of emotion. Emotions, or the suppression thereof, tend to dominate personal relationships. There is evidence of dualistic thinking, and there are rigid patterns of interactions that are bound by rules and order. Neither Charles nor Caroline has differentiated self from the family; David has physically removed himself from the family, and it is not known if he has resolved his emotions and allowed himself to be autonomous emotionally.

(Continues)

NURSING CARE PLAN: NURSING PROCESS FORMAT 29-1 (Continued)

NURSING DIAGNOSIS 1 *Interrupted family processes*, related to daughter's eating disorder, as evidenced by inability or unwillingness to express feelings.

OUTCOMES	NIC	NURSING ACTIONS	EVALUATION
• Within 1 month of weekly sessions with the nurse, family members will begin to identify that change in communication patterns would help them to understand one another and deal with Caroline's eating disorder.	• Family process maintenance • Family integrity promotion	• Use interventive questions, across each domain, to stimulate reflection. • Encourage the family to participate in therapy as a unit, especially the father, who previously was unwilling to commit time to therapy.	Within 1 month, Marie was beginning to recognize that she had fears related to Caroline's eating and Caroline's becoming an adult that she had not expressed. Caroline expressed ambivalence about being required to spend so much time with her family members rather than her peers. Both women began to see the men in the family as distant and requested that William make the time to become involved in the sessions.

NURSING DIAGNOSIS 2 *Readiness for enhanced family coping*, related to goals of self-actualization, as evidenced by Caroline's moving toward a health-promoting lifestyle to optimize wellness.

OUTCOMES	NIC	NURSING ACTIONS	EVALUATION
• Within 1 month, Caroline will state, with the support of her family, that her eating patterns need attention in order to maximize her health.	• Family coping enhancement	• Initiate family sessions in which family dynamics and expectations are discussed as related to Caroline's eating habits (e.g., desire to please, desire to succeed, expectations of perfection).	After several weeks, Caroline agrees with her family's assessment that her weight loss is not healthy. She admits to feeling pressure from her family, especially her father, to succeed effortlessly at all she does, including looking good and healthy. She agrees, with her family's help, to begin monitoring her eating patterns in an effort to identify problem areas and behaviors.

(Continues)

NURSING CARE PLAN: NURSING PROCESS FORMAT 29-1 (Continued)

REFLECTIVE QUESTIONS

1. **ASSESSMENT**
   What other family issues should be considered as possibly having an impact on Caroline's health and family position? Do you think sibling position is relevant in this case? What about the fact that Caroline is the first female born into her father's family in over three generations? Do you think this fact brings with it certain expectations, given the nature of this family?
2. **NURSING DIAGNOSIS**
   Why did the nurse choose communication as the priority diagnosis? What would happen if another diagnosis were selected?
3. **OUTCOMES**
   How do you know if outcomes selected were appropriate? What would you tell the family if you believed family members could enhance their communication with one another? Are there other ways you could draw attention away from Caroline's eating and on to other issues?
4. **NURSING ACTIONS**
   Examine the questions presented in Table 29-8. Provide examples of other interventive questions you might use.
5. **EVALUATION**
   Once the family members have begun to see their own patterns of communication, what do you think the nurse can do to clarify and support each member? Do you think reflective questions are appropriate? Does this approach include collaboration with the family members?

KEY CONCEPTS

- Nurses provide care to families using four approaches: (1) viewing the family as the context for care of an individual, (2) viewing the family as a unit, (3) viewing the family as a system, and (4) viewing the family as a component of society.
- Family theories give a framework for understanding and interpreting family patterns.
- Bowen's theory is founded on the concept of differentiation.
- Structural theory emphasizes family rules and organization.
- Communication theory stresses family communication patterns and focuses on assisting family members with clear, honest, and open communication.
- Family assessment includes evaluation of family patterns and identification of stressors and strengths.
- The NANDA nursing diagnoses give the nurse a means of documenting the need for family care under a nursing model.
- Nursing interventions with families include providing information/education, serving as facilitator of effective communication, working as a family therapist, providing assessment and referrals to social agencies, and evaluating and treating actual and potential family health problems, enhancing the family functioning when a window of opportunity exists.
- Evaluation of outcomes depends on goals set by the nurse and family members. Initially, specific outcomes may not be identified, but over time, the nurse and family should identify specific, measurable goals.

REVIEW QUESTIONS

1. A nurse is assigned to conduct family sessions with a family that consists of a mother, father, and three adolescents. To provide effective care, the nurse must realize that the average family in this stage of development would need to perform which of the following tasks?
   1. Establishing couple identity
   2. Shifting parent-child relationships to permit adolescents to move into or out of the family system
   3. Realigning relationships with extended family to include parenting and grand-parenting roles
   4. Dealing with loss of spouse, siblings, and other peers and preparation for death

2. According to Bowen's theory of family, when a couple experiencing a stressful relationship involves a mother-in-law in the problem, which of the following is occurring?
   1. Triangulation
   2. Scapegoating
   3. Social regression
   4. Multigenerational transmission

3. According to communication theory related to working with families, which of the following is correct?
   1. Communication should be random and not situation specific
   2. All behavior, whether nonverbal or verbal, is communication and conveys a message
   3. Communication in a family should always be verbal and between equal partners
   4. Nonverbal communication between family members represents content

4. An advanced practice nurse is conducting family therapy with a multigenerational family. Her assessment reveals blurring of family roles, inconsistency in providing discipline for the children, and knowledge deficit related to parenting. The father was recently fired from his job and spends the day watching television and drinking. The children are often truant from school, and the grandparents are in need of medical attention. An appropriate nursing diagnosis for this family would include which of the following?
   1. Interrupted family process
   2. Dysfunctional family process
   3. Risk for family dysfunction
   4. Inappropriate family communication

5. Several members of a family were recently killed in a car accident. The remaining members have experienced difficulty resuming previous levels of functioning. An appropriate diagnosis for this family would be which of the following?
   1. Disabled family coping
   2. Inappropriate family communication
   3. Family depression
   4. Readiness or enhanced home maintenance

LEARNING ACTIVITIES

1. Provide case examples of nurses' work in the following:
   a. The family as context
   b. The family as a unit
   c. The family as a system
   d. The family as a unit of society

2. Which care settings lend themselves to each of the above (a–d)?

3. Examine a family you know well from the perspective of each of the family theories discussed (Bowen, structural, and communication).

4. Describe a nursing focus with a family having to do with each nursing role: wellness, prevention, and problem identification.

5. Familiarize yourself with family nursing assessment tools by completing one on a family.

6. Complete a genogram, a family attachment diagram, and an ecomap on your own family. Identify patterns.

*Study*WARE™ CONNECTION

Using your *Study*WARE™ CD-ROM

1. Complete the Crossword Puzzle activity for this chapter.
2. Review the audio glossary for key terms in this chapter.
3. Explore the other games and activities that support this chapter.

REFERENCES

American Heritage Dictionary (2nd ed.). (1982). Boston: Houghton Mifflin.

Billingsley, A. (1992). *Climbing Jacob's ladder.* New York: Simon & Schuster.

Bomar, P. J. (2004). *Promoting health in families* (3rd ed.). Philadelphia: Saunders.

Bomar, P., & McNeely, G. (1996). Family health nursing role: Past, present and future. In P. Bomar (Ed.), *Nursing and family health promotion* (2nd ed., pp. 3–21). Philadelphia: Saunders.

Bowen, M. (1978). *Family therapy in clinical practice.* New York: Jason Aronson.

Duvall, E. (1979). *Marriage and family development* (5th ed.). Philadelphia: J. B. Lippincott.

Friedman, M. (1992). *Family nursing: Theory and practice* (3rd ed.). Norwalk, CT: Appleton & Lange.

Friedman, M., Bowden, V. R., & Jones, E. (2003). *Family nursing: Research, theory and practice.* Upper Saddle River, NJ: Prentice Hall.

Frisch, N., & Kelley, J. (1996). *Healing life's crises, a guide for nurses.* Clifton Park, NY: Thomson Delmar Learning.

Goldberg, I., & Goldberg, J. (2002). *Counseling today's families.* (4th ed.). Pacific Grove, CA: Brooks/Cole.

Goodman, D., & Happell, B. (2006). The efficacy of family intervention in adolescent mental health. *International Journal of Psychiatric Nursing Research, 12*(1), 1364–1377.

Hanson, S. M. H. (2001). *Family health care nursing* (2nd ed.). Philadelphia: F. A. Davis.

Hanson, S. M. H., & Boyd, S. T. (1996). Family nursing: An overview. In S. M. H. Hanson & S. T. Boyd (Eds.), *Family health care nursing: Theory, practice and research* (pp. 4–37). Philadelphia: F. A. Davis.

Hanson, S. M. H., Gedaly-Duff, V., & Kaakinen, J. (2005). *Family health care nursing: Theory, practice & research* (3rd ed.). Philadelphia: F.A. Davis.

Hartman, A. (1979). *Finding families: An ecological approach to family assessment and adoption.* Thousand Oaks, CA: Sage Publications.

Haneon, S., Gedaly-Duff, V., & Kaakinen, J. (2005). *Family health care nursing* (3rd ed.). Philadelphia: F.A. Davis.

Herdman, H. (Ed). (2009). *Nursing diagnosis: Definitions and Classifications: 2009–2011.* Oxford: Wiley-Blackwell.

Hoskins, L. M. (1991). What is the focus of Taxonomy II? Nursing diagnosis axes. In R. M. Carroll-Johnson (Ed.), *Classification of nursing diagnoses: Proceedings of the ninth conference* (pp. 35–37). Philadelphia: J. B. Lippincott.

Kaakinen, J., & Hanson, S. M. H. (2004). Theoretical foundations for family health nursing practice. In P. J. Bomar, *Promoting health in families* (3rd ed., pp. 93–113). Philadelphia: Saunders.

Leff, J., Berkowitz, R. N., Shavit, N., Strachan, A., Glass, I., & Vaughn, C. (1990). A trial of family therapy versus a relatives' group for schizophrenia: Two-year follow-up. *British Journal of Psychiatry, 157,* 571–577.

Lewandowski, W., Morris, R., Drauker, C., & Risko, J. (2007). Chronic pain and the family: Theory-driven treatment approaches. *Issues in Mental Health Nursing, 28,* 1019–1044.

McDaniel, S. H., Cambell, T. L., Hepworth, J., & Lorenz, A. (2005). *Family-oriented primary care* (2nd ed.). New York, NY: Springer.

McGoldrick, M., & Gerson, R. (1985). *Genograms in family assessment.* New York: Norton.

Miller, A. (1983). *Unintentional cruelty hurts, too. For your own good: Hidden cruelty in child-rearing and the roots of violence* (pp. 247–253). New York: Farrar, Straus, Giroux.

Minuchin, S. (1974). *Families and family therapy.* Cambridge, MA: Harvard University Press.

Minuchin, S. (1992). *Family healing.* New York: Free Press.

NANDA International. (2009). *Nursing diagnoses: Definitions and classification, 2009–2011.* Philadelphia: Author.

National Institute of Mental Health (1995). *Family Interventions and HIV/AIDS.* Retrieved September 7, 2009, from http://grants.-nih.gov/grants/guide/rfa-files/RFA-MH-95-002.html

Olson, D. G., & DeFrain, J. (1994). *Marriage and the family.* Mountain View, CA: Mayfield.

Parker, B. A. (1993). Living with mental illness: The family as caregiver. *Journal of Psychosocial Nursing and Mental Health Services, 31,* 10–21.

Rich, B. W., Molloy, P., Hart, B., Ginsberg, S., & Mulvey, T. (2007). Conducting a children's divorce group: One approach. *Journal of Child & Adolescent Psychiatric Nursing, 20*(3), 163–175.

Rogerson, H., (2006). Family work with people with dementia. *Nursing Older People, 18*(7), 1–31.

Satir, V. (1967). *Conjoint family therapy.* Palo Alto, CA: Science and Behavior Books.

Shealy, A. H. (1988). Family therapy. In C. Beck, R. Rawlins, & S. Williams (Eds.), *Mental health-psychiatric nursing, a holistic life-cycle approach* (pp. 543–557). St. Louis: Mosby.

Sin, J., Moone, N., & Newell, J. (2007). Developing services for the carers of young adults with early-onset psychosis: Implementing evidence based practice on psycho-educational family interventions. *Journal of Psychiatric Mental Health Nursing, 14,* 282–290.

Tanyi, R. (2006). Spirituality and family nursing: Spiritual assessment and interventions for families. *Journal of Advanced Nursing, 53*(3), 287–294 [Online version, pp. 1–9].

U.S. Census Bureau. (2002). *Current population survey (CPS)—Definitions and explanations.* Retrieved April 20, 2003, from http://www.census.gov/population/www/cps/spsdef.html.

Warren, J. (1991). Implications of introducing axes into a classification system. In R. M. Carroll-Johnson (Ed.), *Classification of nursing diagnoses: Proceedings of the ninth conference* (pp. 38–44). Philadelphia: J. B. Lippincott.

Watzlawick, P., Beavin, J., & Jackson, D. (1967). *The pragmatics of human communication.* New York: W. W. Norton.

Wright, L., & Leahey, M. (1994). *Nurses and families: A guide to family assessment and interventions* (2nd ed.). Philadelphia: F. A. Davis.

Wright, L., & Leahey, M. (2000). *Nurses and families: A guide to family assessment and interventions* (3rd ed.). Philadelphia: F. A. Davis.

Wright, L., & Leahey, M. (2005). *Nurses and families: A guide to family assessment and interventions* (4th ed.). Philadelphia: F. A. Davis.

Wright, L. M., Watson, W., & Bell, J. (1996). *Beliefs: The heart of healing in families and illness.* New York: Basic Books.

RESOURCE: FAMILY ASSESSMENT TOOL (COMPLETE VERSION)

I. **Identifying Data**
  A. Family name
  B. Address, telephone
  C. Identified individual client (if any) and client's presenting problem
  D. Family's presenting problem

II. **Graphic Family Diagrams**
  A. Genogram
  B. Family attachment diagram
  C. Ecomap

III. **Family Structure**
  A. Internal structure
    1. Family composition (see genogram)
      a. Family type (nuclear, single parent, three generational, etc.)
      b. Who does the family consider to be family?
      c. Changes in family composition. Has anyone recently moved out or in?
    2. Gender (questions to ask the family members)
      a. What are expected behaviors for men? For women?
      b. How should a man behave toward a woman?
      c. How should a woman behave toward a man?
      d. Should men express emotion?
      e. Should women be competitive?
      f. What effect has your parents' ideas had on your views about masculinity and femininity?
      g. Would you like your child to believe differently about masculinity and femininity?
    3. Sexual orientation
      a. At what age did you first engage in sexual activity?
      b. When your younger brother told your mother that he was homosexual, how did your mother respond? Was there a change in her caretaking role with your brother?
      c. How did your parents respond when your sister said that she and her lesbian partner were adopting a child?
    4. Rank order (position of the individual within the family in terms of age and gender; refer to genogram)
      a. How many siblings do you have? Are you the oldest? Youngest? Middle?
      b. Are you an older/younger sister/brother?
      c. Is your spouse an older/younger sister/brother?
      d. Are the spouses' birth rank orders likely to be complementary (e.g., older brother, younger sister) or competitive (e.g., older brother, older sister)?
      e. How many children do you have?
      f. Do any patterns appear when the genogram and family attachment diagram are examined for rank order?
    5. Subsystems (refer to family attachment diagram)
      a. Are there any family subgroups with close emotional ties? Subgroups who do activities together?
      b. What do the women do as a group without the men? The men without the women?
      c. How do you feel when a subgroup does things together without you?
    6. Boundaries
      a. Does the family boundary tend to be diffuse, rigid, or permeable?
      b. Are family members enmeshed? Disengaged? Is this true for all members? Only in special situations?
      c. Is there someone outside/inside the family you would talk to if you felt sad or stressed? Happy? Would anyone in the family not like your talking to that person?
    7. Power structure
      a. Who makes decisions within the family?
      b. Who handles family finances?
      c. Who disciplines the children?
      d. Who decides family activities?
      e. In a disagreement, who has the last say?
      f. Are family members satisfied with the present power structure?
      g. On a family power continuum, does the family seem more chaotic (no leader), egalitarian, or dominated by an individual? If dominated, by whom?
  B. External structure
    1. Extended family (see genogram, family attachment diagram, and ecomap)
      a. Is the extended family significant to the family's functioning?
      b. Are extended family members available when needed to support the family?
    2. External systems (e.g., work, social agencies, health facilities; see ecomap)
      a. What relationship is there between the family and external systems?
      b. How regularly do they interact?
      c. Are external systems overinvolved or underinvolved with the family?
      d. If the family is seeking help from an agency, do the family and agency agree on the problem definition and proposed solution?
  C. Context
    1. Race/ethnicity

a. If immigrants, what is the country of origin? Length of time in the United States?
b. Language spoken in the home? In the neighborhood? Level of facility with English?
c. What is the family's ethnicity (self-identified)?
d. Does the family live in a neighborhood of the same ethnicity?
e. Is the family's social network of the same ethnicity? Exclusively, or are persons of other ethnicities included, too?
f. How traditional are the family's practices regarding dress, diet, home life? Regarding family roles and power structure? Regarding illness and health care?
g. Does the family have more than one ethnic or racial makeup?
h. What difference can you notice between practices of relatives of different ethnic/racial origins and your own?

2. Social class
a. Into what social class would the family be classified (based on cultural, social, and economic factors)?
b. How does the family classify themselves with respect to social class?
c. Does the family consider their income to be adequate?
d. Does the family receive financial assistance? From what source(s)?

3. Religion and spirituality
a. Are there obvious signs of religious influence (in the home, on persons)?
b. Do family members identify an affiliation with religious organization(s)?
c. Are religious controversies a source of problems within the family?
d. Who most actively participates in religious activities?
e. Who is considered to be the most spiritual among the family members?
f. Do family members find their spiritual beliefs to be a resource for them?

4. Environment
a. Characteristics of the residence (if assessed)
(1) Is the residence adequate and safe for the family's needs?
(2) How satisfied is the family with their housing arrangements?
b. Characteristics of the neighborhood
(1) Neighborhood type (rural, farm, urban, suburban, inner city, industrial, residential)
(2) Neighborhood condition (cleanliness, age, how well maintained, how safe)
(3) Neighborhood and community demographics
(4) How available and accessible are community agencies and resources?
c. Family/neighborhood interactions
(1) Family's geographic mobility. How long in this neighborhood? This residence?
(2) Does the family have a social support system within the community?
(3) Which family members use what community services or agencies? How frequently? (refer to ecomap)
(4) How satisfied is the family with the community and its resources?
(5) Is the family aware of most community resources?

IV. **Family Development/Life Cycle**
A. Stages
What is (are) the present family life cycle stage(s)? Designate present family life cycle stage(s):
1. Middle-class North American
2. Divorce and postdivorce
3. Remarried
4. Professional
5. Low income
6. Adoptive

B. Tasks
1. How well is the family fulfilling developmental tasks appropriate to the present family life cycle stage?
2. Does the family describe a balance between satisfaction and stress drawn from the developmental tasks?

C. Attachments
1. Does the pattern of attachments (see family attachment diagram) reflect the tasks of the present life cycle stage?

V. **Family Function**
A. Instrumental functioning
1. How well is the family able to carry out routine activities of daily living, such as eating, sleeping, preparing meals?
2. Does a family member's illness affect any of the family's daily activities?
3. Is the family able to meet caregiving needs of an ill family member?

B. Affective and socialization functioning
1. Affective
a. Do family members perceive and respond to the needs of other members?
b. Are family members' needs being met by the family?
c. Do family members provide mutual support and nurturance to each other?
d. Is there a sense of closeness and intimacy among family members?
e. How does the family deal with separateness and connectedness of its members?

2. Socialization
   a. Are the family's child-rearing practices appropriate for healthy socialization of the children?

C. Expressive functioning
1. Emotional communication
   a. Do all family members express a broad range of emotion (e.g., happiness, sadness, anger, affection)?
   b. Does one group (e.g., parents) express an emotion (e.g., anger) while another group (e.g., children) does not?
   c. Are family members' verbal messages congruent with nonverbal messages?
   d. Do family members firmly and clearly express their feelings and needs?
   e. Do family members seek or discourage feedback to their ideas and behaviors?
   f. Do family members listen attentively to one another?
   g. Do members react negatively to messages from other members?
   h. Do members respond on the basis of unclarified assumptions and make judgmental statements?
   i. How are emotional messages communicated within the family?
   j. Are there areas that are closed off for discussion within the family?
2. Verbal communication
   a. Is there a pattern of direct communication, or are messages displaced onto others?
   b. Are verbal messages clearly stated, or is meaning distorted and masked?
3. Nonverbal (and paraverbal) communication
   a. Do nonverbal communications match verbal content of messages?
   b. What can be inferred from other family members' nonverbal behaviors when one member is talking?
   c. What effect does the nonverbal behavior of one family member have on another (e.g., sadness expressed nonverbally by daughter to mother's discussion of nearing death)?
4. Circular communication
   a. Is a pattern of circular communication evident (negative or adaptive)?
5. Problem solving
   a. Is the family generally able to solve its own problems effectively?
   b. Are problems usually identified by someone within the family or by someone from outside? If within, by whom?
   c. What are the family's solution patterns? From whom is help sought?
6. Roles
   a. What formal roles are fulfilled by individual family members? By subgroups?
   b. Are these roles acceptable to the family and consistent with family expectations?
   c. How competently do family members fulfill these roles?
   d. Is there flexibility in role performance when needed?
   e. What informal or covert roles exist in the family?
   f. What purpose do these covert roles serve?
   g. Is there a transgenerational pattern of dysfunctional covert roles?
   h. Who were the role models for family members?
7. Alliances/coalitions
   a. Are two-person relationships within the family complementary and symmetrical?
   b. Is there evidence of triangles in the three-person relationships within the family?
   c. Are there cross-generational patterns of coalitions?
8. Influence and power (instrumental, psychological, corporal)
   a. What objects or privileges, if any, are used to reinforce behaviors (e.g., money, television watching, candy, vacation)?
   b. What psychological methods are used to reinforce behaviors (e.g., praise, approval, criticism, guilt induction)?
   c. Is corporal control used (e.g., hugging, spanking, other forms of physical contact)?
   d. Is the influence method most used by the family consistent? Based on encouragement or punishment?
   e. Which parent is best at getting the child to take medicine?
   f. When one parent dominates the conversation, what does the other parent do?

D. Health care function
1. Beliefs (about a health problem)
   a. What do the family members believe about the etiology, treatment, and prognosis of a health problem, the role of health care professionals, the role of the family, and the level of control the family has relative to the health problem?
   b. Are the family members' beliefs congruent, or do they disagree?
   c. What does the family believe about the availability and usefulness of resources, medication, and treatment?
   d. What influence does the family believe the health problem has on the family?
   e. What strengths does the family believe it has at present for coping with the health problem?
   f. What concerns does the family have related to its ability to handle the health problem?
2. Health practices
   a. Are the family's dietary practices healthy for the family members?
   b. Do factors such as finances, knowledge of nutrition and food safety, or cultural practices

serve as a source of risk to family dietary practices?

c. What function do mealtimes serve for the family?
d. Are family sleep and rest habits meeting family needs?
e. Are family exercise and recreation patterns adequate and healthy to meet family members' needs?
f. What is the pattern of drug and substance use in the family?
g. Does the family encounter unsafe levels of environmental hazards?
h. Are the family's cleanliness and hygiene practices within the limits of safety?
i. Do family members practice dental hygiene and preventive care?
j. What is the three-generational pattern of family health? Are illness or behavior patterns evident?

From *Nurses and Families: A Guide to Family Assessment and Interventions* (4th ed.), by L. Wright and M. Leahey, 2005, F. A. Davis Philadelphia:. With modifications based on the Friedman Family Assessment Model (Short Form) from M. M. Friedman, V. R. Bowden, & E. G. Jones. (2003). *Family nursing: Research, theory & practice* (5th ed.). Prentice Hall Englewood Cliffs, NJ:. (Integrated adaptation created with permission Wright and Leahey/FA Davis)

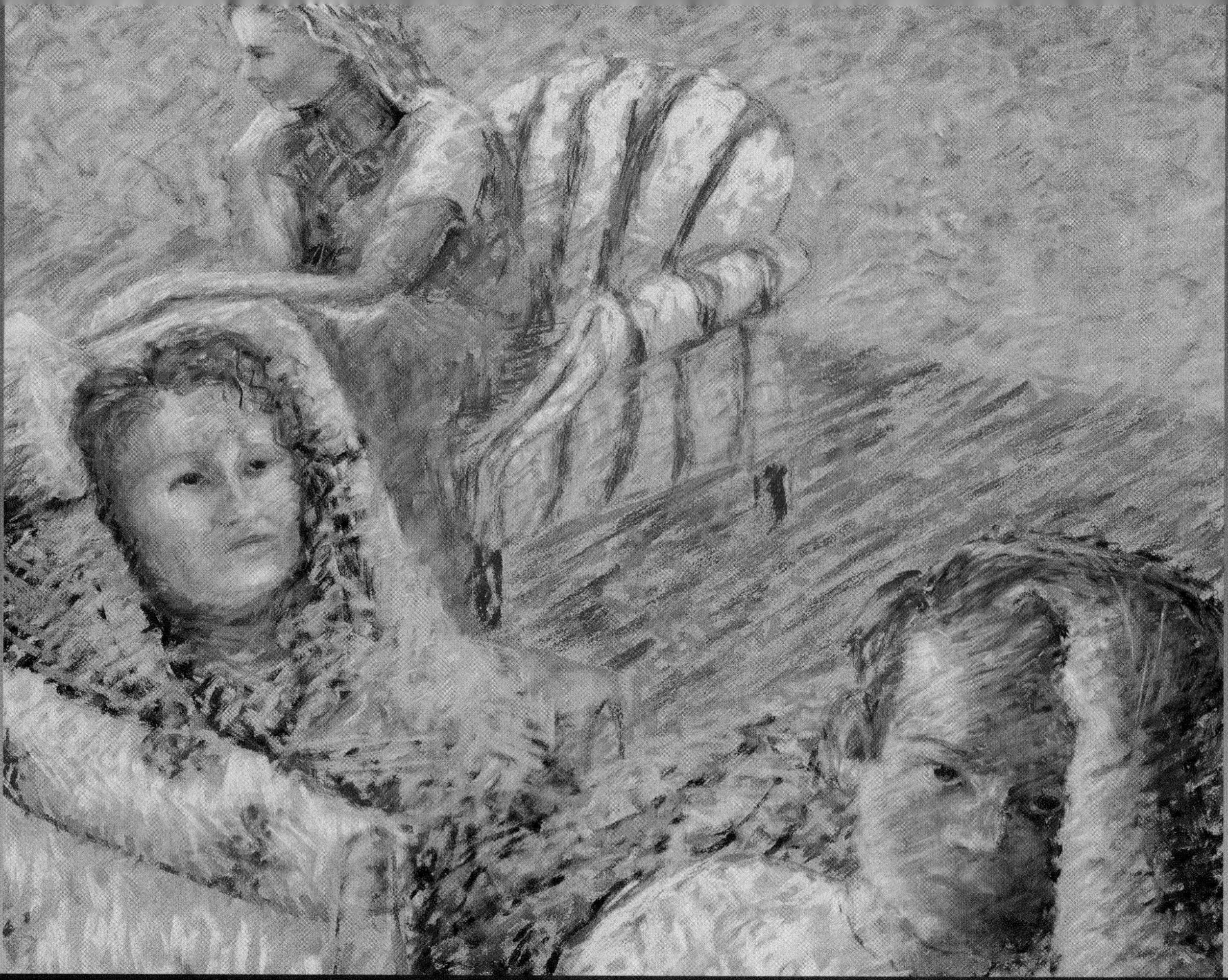

Group Work

Reflections on Groups

Try to remember situations in which:

- ***Other students in a class asked the very question you were thinking about asking.***
- ***Someone with whom you were socializing expressed a feeling that was the same as yours, for example, "That movie scared me!"***
- ***Another person reached out to you and demonstrated empathy, such as another nurse at work, saying, "You must be tired today because your baby is sick at home. Can I help you with your work?"***

How did your feelings about the situation change when you realized that someone else shared the same thoughts as you or empathized with your position?

Consider how you have been helped by persons whose relation to you is that you and they are part of a group—a class, a social group, or a work group. Purposeful use of groups allows a nurse to offer help to clients in a similar way.

CHAPTER 30

Group Therapy

NOREEN CAVAN FRISCH

CHAPTER OUTLINE

COMPETENCIES

Upon completion of this chapter, the reader should be able to:

1. Outline the three phases of group work: orientation phase, working phase, and termination phase.
2. Explain the terms *group dynamics*, *group content*, and *group process*.
3. Analyze the dynamics of a group session.
4. Define nursing roles with groups in the psychiatric mental health nursing setting.
5. Explain major theoretical approaches used in group therapy.
6. Explain the nursing role in supportive groups.
7. Compare and contrast different types of groups (socialization, recreation, educational, reality orientation, reminiscence, and self-help) in terms of purpose, nursing interventions, and evaluation.

KEY TERMS

Closed Group
Group
Group Content
Group Dynamics
Group Leader/Facilitator
Group Process
Open Group
Self-Help Groups
Supportive Groups
Therapy Groups

In an increasing number of situations, nurses are called on to work with groups of clients, and in psychiatric mental health care, the nurse has many different roles in the group setting. For example, a nurse may see a group of clients in therapy sessions; facilitate a support group for persons who share a particular problem; plan and carry out recreational activities for a client group that has a need to socialize; or provide client education information to a client group. The purpose of this chapter is to give the reader descriptive background information on the nature of group work in mental health nursing and to provide knowledge about different types of groups and different approaches to working with a client group. A nurse with knowledge of group process and group dynamics can increase her effectiveness in work with many kinds of clients.

GROUPS

A **group** is a collection of persons who comes together in some way that makes them interdependent. A group, therefore, may be a client group who comes together for mutual support and therapy once a week or a group of persons admitted to a chemical dependency unit who are a group by nature of being on the unit at the same time. For purposes of this chapter, two types of groups are discussed: **therapy groups**—groups of persons that come together to receive psychotherapy in a group setting—and **supportive groups**—groups of persons that come together for the primary purpose of offering support, education, and/or socialization/recreation.

The members of a group are usually strangers coming together for some purpose. There is a **group leader** or **facilitator**, the person who invites or selects group members according to what the group can accomplish and who helps to identify the purpose and goals of the group. A group is referred to as open or closed. An **open group** is one where participants may come and go, depending on their individual needs. In an open group, participants may come for as many sessions as they perceive they need; open groups are common on inpatient units and as self-help groups. In contrast, a **closed group** begins with a certain number of participants and is not open to new members. Closed groups are often found in outpatient settings and often have a focus on psychotherapy. Some groups are ongoing, that is, they meet indefinitely, whereas others meet only for a certain period of time. Box 30-1 lists some of the benefits of group (rather than individual) interventions.

PHASES OF GROUP WORK

Whatever the kind of group, virtually all groups go through phases of work identical to those described in Chapter 5 relating to the nurse-client relationship: the orientation phase, the working phase, and the termination phase (Table 30-1).

ORIENTATION PHASE

In a group, the orientation phase is the time during the initial meetings of the group when the leader/facilitator introduces the reason for bringing the individuals into the group. In the orientation phase, the participants begin to get to know one

BOX 30-1
BENEFITS OF GROUP INTERVENTIONS

BENEFITS FOR CLIENT:
- Able to learn from others' experiences
- Able to observe others in social interaction; others are role models
- Able to try out new ways of interaction in a supportive environment
- Have a place to belong; a group identity

BENEFITS FOR THE GROUP LEADER:
- Able to serve several clients at once; cost and time effective
- Able to provide additional social and supportive interactions to clients
- Can draw on strengths and ideas of group to arrive at creative solutions

another, and the group members set the stage for the group work that will come later. It is essential in every group that the participants establish a level of trust with one another. Therefore, there are rules of group behavior that must be made explicit at the outset. For example, participants are asked to agree to treat one another in a respectful manner and to try to understand and value each member. Further, participants agree that information shared in the group sessions is confidential, so that no one member need fear that personal disclosure would or could result in gossip or discussion with others outside of the session. Other group rules or expectations may include regular attendance (indicating a commitment to the group), encouragement of verbal expression, and participation of all group members.

The group leader/facilitator has the responsibility to ensure that all members of the group know and agree to the rules of behavior, and this is an essential step in establishing trust. Further, the group leader/facilitator has the responsibility to ensure that all members know and agree to any requirements for payment of fees and such matters as shared responsibility for setting up rooms, putting chairs away, and the like. Sometimes group rules are formalized with a written contract; sometimes a verbal agreement is all that is needed.

The orientation phase is a time of give and take, often a time of testing to see if the group is really accepting, or nonjudgmental, or to see if the group notices and cares about such matters as one participant's absence. Particularly during the orientation phase, participants feel anxiety, and there are frequently long pauses of silence. The group leader/facilitator must permit the silences to occur, allowing the group participants to deal with their own feelings. The leader/facilitator will use techniques of therapeutic communication to draw out members who are silent and withdrawn, and to ensure that one or two persons do not take over the entire discussion. The goal for this phase is that the participants develop a sense of belonging to the group. This sense of belonging occurs over time and only when the participants get to know and trust one another. Group members feel a sense of cohesion and a sense of belonging once the orientation phase is complete.

NURSINGTIP 30-1

Guidelines for Behavior of Group Members

- Ensure that all statements made in group are confidential.
- Allow other group members time to speak.
- Consider the needs of each group member.
- Provide other group members with your respect and attention.
- Contribute to the group by sharing your opinions, experiences, and feelings whenever you are comfortable doing so.

TABLE 30-1 Three Phases of Group Work

PHASES	GROUP TASKS	ROLE OF GROUP LEADER
Orientation	Get to know one another Set out rules and expectations Build cohesion	Help to make members comfortable and feel welcome Ensure expectations are clear Set atmosphere of respect and trust
Working	Actively accomplish purposes of the group	Keep group on task Support individual members accomplishing goals Describe how purposes have (or have not) been accomplished
Termination	Prepare for separation Help one another plan for the future	Acknowledge contributions of each member Acknowledge the group experience

Working Phase

The working phase refers to the time when the participants are actively accomplishing the purposes of the group: They may share their feelings and fears with one another; they may try out new behaviors; they may confront similar problems; and they may point out behavior patterns to one another. The group participants learn to rely on one another for honest feedback, for support, and to be there to listen and care. The leader/facilitator serves to guide the group to achieve its goals by keeping discussions related to group goals, by ensuring that each participant is having his or her needs met, and by serving as a role model for behaviors such as showing respect, listening, responding honestly, and providing nonjudgmental support.

If and when counterproductive behaviors such as ignoring or monopolizing occur, the group leader/facilitator will point out the behavior, explain why it is counterproductive, and let the group participants develop their own skills in working together. For example, if one group member spends all of his time talking and does not permit others to join in or respond, the leader might say, "I notice that you, Howard, have a lot to say tonight, but maybe someone else also has something to say; let's give time for others to speak." In another situation, if one group member has expressed an idea and there is no response, the other group members might go on to a different topic. The leader might say, "Vera expressed a thought a few minutes ago, and I didn't hear a response to her. Let's go back and consider what Vera said." Thus, the working phase of the group provides the participants with a safe place to learn about their behaviors and to achieve their own goals related to the group, which often include trying out new behaviors in a supportive and kind environment.

Termination Phase

Termination of a group occurs when it is a time-limited, closed group and the number of sessions comes to an end, or when an open group no longer needs to meet because the purposes have been met. Termination brings about inevitable feelings of change, often including loss or sadness of parting. The group members may want to provide support to one another during parting, and the leader/facilitator can serve as a resource. For many groups, a ritual celebration is an important way to mark the event. This celebration may be as simple as bringing food to share with one another during the last meeting or as elaborate as providing each member with a written remembrance of his or her contribution or something that resembles a "graduation" ceremony. Each type of ritual provides a way for members to meet the transition of stepping into a new role. The leader/facilitator may be in a position to help the participants consider alternatives in marking the last group meeting as a significant event in their life and work. The leader/facilitator also helps each participant to see that participation in the group has benefited him or her in some way, by stating how each member has taken a step toward achieving some individual goal in the process of helping one another.

GROUP DYNAMICS, GROUP CONTENT, AND GROUP PROCESS

Group dynamics refers to the underlying forces that work to produce behavior patterns within groups. The group dynamics include both the group content and the group processes. **Group content**, as implied by its name, refers to the specific problems, topics, or conditions addressed by the group as a whole. **Group process** refers to the interaction (verbal and nonverbal) between the group members. Process also refers to all of the factors that contribute to the group purposes. The role taken by each individual and the resultant behaviors in the group are part of the group process. For example, the group leader/facilitator is the person "in charge" of the group. One person may take on the role of

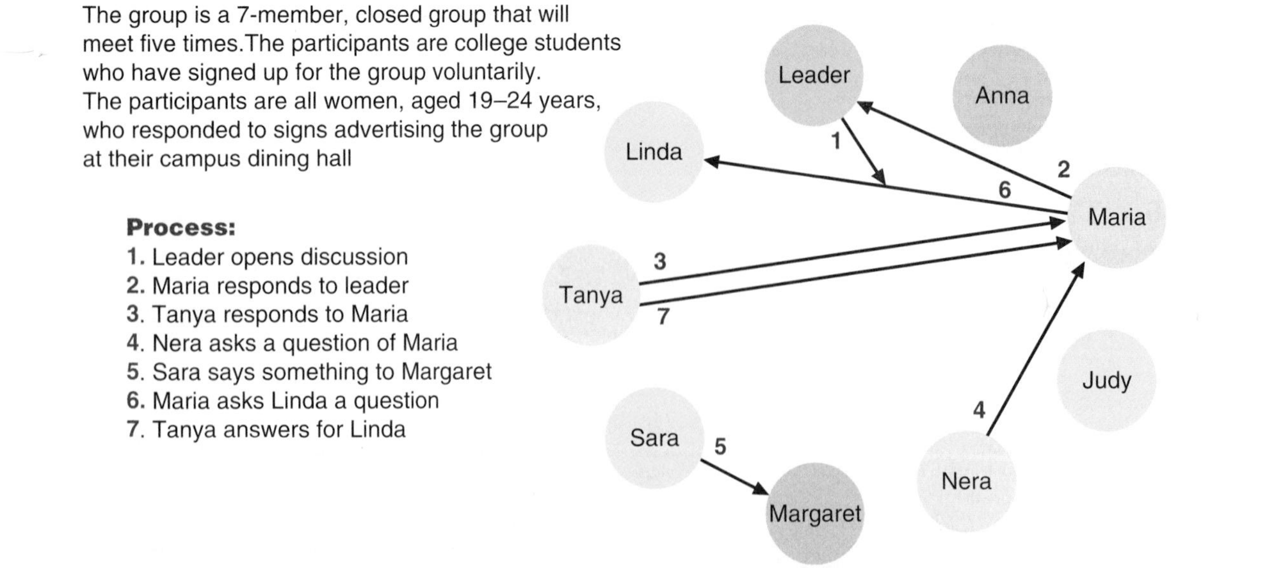

The group is a 7-member, closed group that will meet five times.The participants are college students who have signed up for the group voluntarily. The participants are all women, aged 19–24 years, who responded to signs advertising the group at their campus dining hall
Process:
1. Leader opens discussion
2. Maria responds to leader
3. Tanya responds to Maria
4. Nera asks a question of Maria
5. Sara says something to Margaret
6. Maria asks Linda a question
7. Tanya answers for Linda
Leader
Anna
Linda
Maria
Tanya
Judy
Sara
Nera
Margaret
1
2
3
4
5
6
7

FIGURE 30-1 **Sample group dynamics: assertiveness training group** (DELMAR/CENGAGE LEARNING.)

being friendly and agreeable within the group; another person may seem unfriendly and may frequently disagree with the group. Or, in a different situation, one person may take on the role of being timid and unable to answer questions; another person may "come to her rescue" and answer questions for her. When a scenario such as the one involving a timid participant is played out in the group, it is the responsibility of the group leader to notice the process and comment on it. For example, the group leader might say, "I notice that Maria seems to answer the questions for Joe. Joe, do you want to answer for yourself?" In doing so, the leader makes explicit the interactions between the two individuals and may challenge the timid person to take on a more active or direct role. The group leader also may comment and respond to the group content; however, it is the group process that brings forward many unconscious and unnoticed means of interaction. Attention to process is the factor most likely to stimulate growth in group participants. Refer to Figure 30-1 for a sample sequence of group dynamics for the first few minutes of a voluntary assertiveness training group session. In the figure, there are arrows that indicate the direction of the communications. For example, in communication 1, the leader speaks to the group (the arrow goes to the center). In communication 2, group participant Maria responds to the leader. In communication 3, Tanya responds to Maria, and so on. Looking at the diagram, it becomes clear that Maria is the central focus for communications during the first few interactions of this group session. Identification of the central focus is part of the group leader's role—to observe for the dynamics of group interaction. There will always be one person who is the focus for a conversation, and the leader will expect that this role shifts when the conversation moves on. If it did not, the leader might well make a process comment, such as, "I note that Maria has commented on this issue and some have agreed with her, does anyone else see this issue from a different perspective?"

Understanding group dynamics is also enhanced by determining the roles that individual group member may take. For example, one person may be the "helper" in the group and someone else may be the "controller." Box 30-2 provides definitions of the most common roles that group members assume.

Preparation of Group Leaders/Facilitators

The educational and experiential background for group leaders will be dictated by the purpose of a group. If the group is a therapy group, using a distinct psychological/psychiatric theoretical approach, the nurse functioning as group therapist will need graduate-level education and experience in group therapy. On the other hand, if the group is primarily an educational group, providing clients with information about medication and assisting them in establishing methods of compliance with medication and food regimens, the nurse will be appropriately prepared at the undergraduate level. If the group is dealing with issues related to recovery from chemical addiction, the nurse will need preparation at the undergraduate level along with extensive continuing education in the areas of drug and alcohol abuse. Current recommendations of professional organizations such as the American Nurses Association (ANA) and the American Group Psychotherapy Association (AGPA requires at least a master's level preparation for individuals carrying out group therapy). Table 30-2 provides examples of commonly

BOX 30-2
ROLES GROUP MEMBERS MAY TAKE

- Problem solver: one who tries to work through situations and reach a resolution of issues
- Controller: one who tries to direct group conversation and activities
- Talker: one who talks more than others, frequently dominating discussions
- Silent one: one who is shy and retiring, who does not participate (or rarely participates) in discussions
- Nay sayer: one who predicts negative outcomes
- Supporter: one who attempts to be kind and helpful to all
- Intimidator: one who takes over, who scares off others
- Devil's advocate: one who finds fault with seemingly everyone and everything

TABLE 30-2 Nursing Roles in Groups, with Associated Educational Preparation

ROLE	EDUCATIONAL PREPARATION
Nurse therapist	Graduate
Cotherapist	Graduate
Facilitator, socialization or recreation group	Undergraduate
Leader, support group for clients with specific illness, such as breast cancer	Undergraduate, with continuing preparation in group dynamics and the content of the group
Leader, educational	Undergraduate, with preparation group in the content area
Facilitator/resource person to self-help groups	Undergraduate

occurring nursing roles in group settings and suggests the appropriate educational level for the nurse assuming those roles.

A group leader or facilitator takes responsibility to manage the group. The Nursing Interventions Classification lists many of the activities of a group leader, which include: determining (or interpreting) the group's purpose, beginning and ending the group on time, addressing the issues of group rules, giving the group a sense of direction, providing social reinforcement, planning structured activities (when appropriate), moving the group toward the working phase as soon as possible, and dealing with individual and whole group termination (Bulecheck, Butcher, & Dochterman, 2008). Nursing Tip 30-2 provides some examples of how a leader may take control or manage a group situation.

Typical personal characteristics of group leaders include being sociable, friendly, and comfortable in small-group situations. Styles of group leaders do vary—some may be more reflective and others may be more spontaneous and talkative. However, all successful group leaders will have well-developed techniques of therapeutic communication, observation, and listening. Further, successful group leaders will be comfortable with silences.

Number of Group Leaders

In establishing a group, the nurse will consider whether the groups will be led or facilitated by one or two persons. Traditionally, there has been one group leader. However, group therapists noted real benefits of having two leaders and began recommending two co-leaders. Two leaders provide a perspective on group process and dynamics from two points of view, and this always adds to the analysis of group activities. Further, there could be fewer interruptions in the actual group session, for if one person is needed away from the session or to provide individual counseling or support, one of the leaders may go and the other can stay with the group. Group participants have the opportunity to observe a collaborative and positive relationship between the two group leaders, and this interaction may serve as the only role model some clients have for adult-to-adult collaboration. At times, when one of the leaders is male and the other female, the ability to relate equally well to group members of both genders becomes easier. A nurse setting up a group, then, will consider the possible benefits of co-leaders and may decide to invite another to collaborate.

> **NURSING TIP 30-2**
>
> **Group Management**
>
> In situations where a group seems unproductive, the group leader can redirect the group most readily by making a comment on the group process, for example:
>
> - "We're talking about what was on TV last night, as a group we are not focusing on what brought us here. Let's get back to the topic at hand."
>
> OR
>
> - "I noticed that Tanya has become the spokesperson for the group. She presents opinions and feelings for all our members. Does everyone agree with this direction?"

APPROACHES TO THERAPY GROUPS

There are several theoretical approaches to group therapy currently used in practice. Major approaches will be discussed following.

Psychoanalytic Approach

Psychoanalysis was developed as a therapy for individual clients (see Chapter 27). Only after the development of a kind of systems approach in which any small group could be viewed as a whole could psychoanalytic techniques be applied in a small-group setting. Typically, a therapist using this approach in group work is providing individual therapy to all of the group members and brings the persons together for the group to achieve additional benefits that only a group can provide.

Psychoanalysis is described in Chapter 27 of this text and emphasizes the client's growth through the uncovering of the client's unconscious self and awareness of past experiences. These discoveries provide insight into current patterns and difficulties. Concepts such as *resistance, transference,* and *working through* are central to the theory of psychoanalysis. It is expected that the client will exhibit resistance, or opposition, to attempts to draw out unconscious and unrecognized patterns. Transference is the result of the client's either distorting or misperceiving the behaviors of another (typically the therapist), due to unconsciously viewing the therapist as someone from his past. Understanding one's own resistance and transference is central to growth. Working through is the process of taking new insights and using them for change.

Some goals of psychoanalytic therapy are very well achieved in group settings. Some examples were provided by Shaffer and Galinsky in their descriptions of models of group therapy (1989):

1. The client may learn that other people can disclose their problems openly and that they gain some relief in doing so.
2. The client learns that he is not alone in having problems and others have similar difficulties.
3. The client may reexperience early family relationships in a setting that is emotionally safe.

4. The client may be able to see and understand his own transferential relationships with both the therapist and other group members.
5. The client may gain more direct and immediate feedback as to the ways in which others perceive his style and defenses than is possible in normal social life or in individual therapy.

Further, the use of group therapy from a psychoanalytic perspective permits the client to wean himself from a prolonged, excessively soul-searching, and sometimes dependent relationship on the therapist that often may occur in individual psychoanalysis (Shaffer & Galinsky, 1989) and allows the client to get on with the business of making life changes and moving effectively back into the world. Thus, the psychoanalytic approach is an effective approach for client groups, particularly when the clients are at a point in their therapy where they can benefit from interactions with others rather than remain only in individual therapy.

Interpersonal Groups

The interpersonal theory of Sullivan (1953) and the interpersonal psychiatrist forms the basis for working with groups (see Chapter 27). According to this approach, group members examine their interactions. The therapist's goal is to help the client identify interpersonal difficulties and to encourage more successful styles of relating to others. Specifically, the group leader helps the members to make connections between their "here and now" responses and their past behaviors and experiences outside the group (Montgomery, 2002). Although interpersonal theory can be used in individual therapy, the group setting offers a good context in which to assist the client to develop differing interpersonal styles.

Peplau, the nursing theorist whose work is grounded in interpersonal theory, believed that the closeness of a therapeutic relationship can build trust, empathy, and growth toward healthy behaviors (George, 2002). Gerrick and Ewashen (2001) write that group therapy from an interpersonal perspective can be used with inpatient adolescents because it proves a safe and therapeutic forum to promote healthy exploration, change, and empowerment. Group therapy can provide this kind of therapeutic relationship with others in the group. A positive group experience will put the client in a situation where he is accepted by others and begins to experience satisfying relationships with others. The focus of the group and the therapist is to provide a place where all group members are accepted, where they can interact with one another openly and honestly, where they can identify with others as "belonging," and where they receive honest and constructive feedback regarding relationship styles.

Existential Groups

Based on the work of existential philosophers, an existential approach to therapy emerged in the 1950s and 1960s that shifted attitudes away from a "scientific" approach to human experience (as exemplified in Freudian psychology and causality) toward an approach that emphasized human subjective experience. Existential psychology includes beliefs in the ideas that each person has a need to give meaning to his life, and in so doing there is an inevitable fear of death; each person's unconscious contains forces for courage and creativity as well as for violence and cruelty; and in a therapeutic relationship the therapist and client are more equal than unequal because each has to reconcile the same problems of existence (Shaffer & Galinsky, 1989). The existential approach also requires the therapist to accept all aspects of the client, including the client's freedom to resist treatment.

In nursing, theories of human becoming and human care (Parse, 1996, 1998; Watson, 1988, 2005) have been clearly influenced by existential thought. These theories emphasize the relationship between nurse and client, strive for mutuality and spontaneity, are grounded in the notions of human care, and attend to the importance of the client's subjective experience of his life.

From an existential perspective, in group therapy the group leader may be seen as the person in the group most experienced in the search to understand the meaning of existence and striving to live a life of authenticity and honesty. The group becomes a place where individuals can experience one another, seek to establish relationships based on equality and mutuality, and explore and ultimately give up self-confirmations based on others' notions of what they should be. The group members provide strong support for all participants who strive to relate to one another from an "authentic" base.

Cognitive-Behavioral Groups

Like a cognitive-behavioral approach to individual therapy (see Chapter 28), a cognitive-behavioral approach to group work is concerned with the thought processes and the behavioral patterns of the clients. Unlike other approaches that focus on the "why" of behavior, this approach focuses on the attitudes. The cognitive-behavioral therapists assume that negative attitudes or negative thinking will result in an interpretation that the world is "bad," and this thinking will result in maladaptive behavior patterns. Lonergan is one of the therapists that initially developed this approach (1994) and has become a leader in the field. Her work suggests that believing that if one part of a system changes the other parts of the system will change allows therapists to reason that changing the negative attitudes and thoughts into positive ones will result in changed behavior and better adjustment.

An example of this approach is as follows: If a person is depressed, he may spend his whole day thinking that the world is a destructive place and that he should just "give up" and not try to achieve anything. A cognitive approach to therapy would have this man acknowledge his negative thinking, and the therapist would try to help him see how his views are destructive. The therapist might suggest that he consciously stop the negative thinking and put a more positive idea in its

RESEARCH Highlight 30-1

The Evaluation of Cognitive Behavioral Therapy on Patient Depression and Self Esteem

STUDY PROBLEM/PURPOSE

To evaluate the results of a 12-week cognitive-behavioral therapy group for patients diagnosed with depression.

METHODS

The study used an experimental design with patients being randomly assigned to an experimental or control group. Experimental group patients received the group therapy treatments, and the control group patients were offered the same treatment only after completion of the data collection. Pre- and post-therapy group assessments were done using standard measures of self-esteem and depression. The therapy group was conducted by a nurse experienced in the therapeutic approach.

FINDINGS

When compared to the control group, the experimental group patients demonstrated improvements in areas of depression relief and enhancement self-esteem, and these improvements remained after one month following treatment.

IMPLICATIONS

Such groups are potentially very useful for clients in outpatient settings who experience depression. Given the prevalence of depression in society, group therapy is an important and efficient adjunct to care.

Source: "The Evaluation of Cognitive Behavioral Therapy on Patient Depression and Self-Esteem," by T. W. Chen, R. B. Lu, A. J. Chang, D. M. Chu, & K. R. Chou, 2006, *Archives of Psychiatric Nursing*, *20*(1), 3–11.

place. This would be rather like seeing a glass as half full instead of seeing it as half empty. Positive affirmations and making positive statements about self ("I am able to take this test today") represent one technique often used to assist persons to develop a more positive way of thinking. Also, a technique of reframing is used to assist a client to reframe an event into its most positive light. For example, "I lost this job, but the next one may be even better" would be a means of reframing a bad situation into a more positive and hopeful one.

Cognitive-behavioral groups work with clients to assist all to monitor negative thoughts, recognize the connections between their thoughts and actions, and substitute reality-based interpretations of life events. Group members gain support from one another as they examine their own attitudes and behaviors and observe others doing the same.

Psychodrama

Psychodrama is a group therapy approach that encourages expression of feelings that underlie personal problems through use of spontaneous, dramatic role-play (Shaffer & Galinsky, 1989). The dramatic acting out of situations and scenes significant to the client is important in allowing the client to "relive" events, to feel the emotions as if the event was happening once again, but in the psychodrama, the client has the ability to reformulate the problems. The psychodrama functionally puts the client back into the situation, rather than simply encouraging one to talk about the situation. The client uses other members of the group to play roles of persons in the drama. This technique forces the client to "show" other group members how persons in the drama/life situation would respond by taking on various roles to demonstrate. Thus, the client must be able to take on roles of significant persons (boss, mother, father, siblings, etc.) and, for at least a short while, to speak from their perspective and take on their worldview.

The technique of psychodrama originated with the work of Moreno in 1970, and the concept has now been in existence for well over 30 years. Some psychodrama groups are held in "theaters" expressly designed for this purpose; others are held in more typical group therapy rooms, where the center of the group becomes the "stage."

The emphasis in psychodrama is on the "here and now." If a group member is disturbed about something that happened yesterday or 10 years ago, that situation is brought into the present in a drama, and its impact on the client's here-and-now behavior is explored. The psychodrama is a powerful technique, in that there are no means of hiding behind feelings or leaving emotions unfinished or without closure. The drama puts the client into the situation such that a resolution must be found. The psychodrama occurs within a very supportive environment in which the client may explore past events, relive uncomfortable emotions in a safe, secure, and helpful environment, and try out new means of handling similar situations in the present life.

APPROACHES TO SUPPORTIVE GROUPS

A nurse does not have to be in an advanced practice role to provide care to a client group, for there are many situations where nurses apply the nursing process and give care to a group. Some of them are discussed next: socialization groups, recreation groups, education groups, reality orientation groups, reminiscence groups, and self-help groups. The reader is encouraged to identify additional situations where a nurse might intervene with a group in practice settings. The following discussion serves as a guide to the kind of group activities common in psychiatric mental health nursing.

RESEARCH Highlight 30-2

Changes in Eating Behavior Following Group Therapy for Women Who Binge-eat

STUDY PROBLEM/PURPOSE

To assess the outcome of a pilot intervention of weekly group therapy sessions over 6 months for women with eating disorders.

METHODS

The researchers used pre/post-test design without a control group to evaluate the effectiveness of a group therapy approach that integrated several group therapy models. There were nine participants in the study. The group therapy methods included educational approaches, cognitive-behavioral approaches, as well as exploration of issues such as family influences, self-image, and self-agency. The outcome measures included standardized tests of binge eating behaviors and results of interview data addressing the participants' experience of the group sessions and their awareness of self-image, body image, and relationship with food.

FINDINGS

The study results show positive effects on the measure of eating behavior that reached statistical significance. Qualitative interview data indicated a positive impact on eating behavior, thoughts about eating, changes in dichotomous thinking, and changes in dietary behavior.

IMPLICATIONS

This study demonstrates the possible effectiveness of an integrated group therapy approach for clients with eating disorders. Clearly, the integrated group method may be helpful to other clients as well.

Source: D. Seamoore, J. Buckroyd, & D. Stott. 2006. Changes in eating behavior following group therapy for women who binge eat: A pilot study. *Journal of Psychiatric and Mental Health Nursing*, *13*, 337–345.

RESEARCH Highlight 30-3

Long-Term Effects of Teaching Behavioral Strategies for Managing Persistent Auditory Hallucinations in Schizophrenia

STUDY PROBLEM/PURPOSE

To document the effects of a class designed to teach behavioral management strategies to people with schizophrenia with a goal of reducing the negative characteristics of the disease.

METHODS

Participants attended sessions for 10 weeks and were evaluated for 12 months after the conclusion of the session.

FINDINGS

Participants were characterized as feeling more in control, less distractible, and less anxious. They reported that their experiences of hearing voices were less frequent.

IMPLICATIONS

The clients who participated in the study recommended that others do so as well. The psychoeducational approach was effective in this case and should be further evaluated for outpatients living with schizophrenia.

Source: "Long-Term Effects of Teaching Behavioral Strategies for Managing Persistent Auditory Hallucinations in Schizophrenia," by R. Buccheri, L. Trygstad, G. Dowling, R. Hopkins, K. White, J. Griffin, et al., (2004). *Journal of Psychosocial Nursing and Mental Health Services*, *18*(9), 20–27, 48–49.

Socialization Groups

For many mental health clients, there is a need for increased socialization and social contacts. Some persons have never developed basic skills of conversation with others; other persons specifically express the need and desire to have friends; some persons are affected by the negative symptoms of schizophrenia and have need for support in social activities. Socialization groups are group activities aimed at providing clients with experiences in social situations and assisting them to learn methods of interaction with others.

Typically, such groups are common on inpatient psychiatric units and in outpatient clinics. A group of persons comes together with a facilitator to interact with one another. The atmosphere in such a group is informal. Often, participants will sit in a lounge (with couches and comfortable chairs) rather than in a room designed for "group therapy." Clients are encouraged to talk about events that happened to them that day, plans for weekend activities, and the like, so that interaction between any given client and others is increased. There is no goal to provide in-depth therapy or analysis—the purpose is to increase interactions and develop social skills. Socialization groups can be helpful for those situations where the client needs assistance in establishing social relationships, as in situations of those experiencing the negative symptoms of schizophrenia, those with early dementia, and with others who are facing stress and adjustment/developmental difficulties.

Recreation Groups

The recreation group is an extension of the socialization group. The purpose is to plan and experience activities for enjoyment, camaraderie, and socialization. Participants come together with a facilitator to plan activities such as picnics, fishing trips, trips to the movies, and the like, so that a group of otherwise isolated clients who might stay in their rooms is able to participate in a structured activity. Over time, persons who participate in recreation groups develop a repertoire of activities, some of which they find enjoyable. The overall purpose is to introduce clients to activities that they might choose to continue outside of the group and also to encourage movement, interaction, and travel to places within the community.

Educational Groups

Nurses are quite familiar with the need for client education. Whenever a nurse brings a group of clients together who have similar needs for health education, that nurse is engaged with the group as his client. There are two main purposes for providing education in group settings: (1) It is more cost effective to teach a group of people together than it is to provide education on a one-to-one basis, and (2) bringing the group together provides the benefits of universality (each client learns he is not alone and that other people have the same or similar needs and difficulties). Clients may benefit by listening to the questions and concerns raised by other group members. Further, bringing a group of clients together provides them with some socialization with one another, although this may not be the express purpose of the education group.

Reality Orientation Groups

In situations where mental health clients, nursing home residents, or residents of board-and-care facilities are out of touch with reality, the reality orientation group serves to reorient the client to time, place, and season, and to provide information of current events of note. These groups are often conducted in inpatient settings in rooms where groups of clients may be gathered for another purpose, such as a day room or dining room. The facilitator of the group will state the place, date, and time to provide basic orientation. Frequently, the facilitator or one of the participants will read from a daily newspaper to orient the group to current events. Participants in the group may be asked to comment on news events. Often, important personal events may be announced, for example, birthdays, anniversaries, visits by family members, and the like. The purpose of such groups is orientation as well as promoting social interaction and involvement in daily activities and current events.

Reminiscence Groups

Groups for the elderly that are specifically aimed at permitting reminiscence or life review are considered helpful when a person is at a developmental stage in which he is feeling he has completed his life and has a need to look back over significant events. These groups are particularly effective at encouraging socialization and self-esteem. Strategies used in reminiscence groups include sharing photos of important life events, storytelling around a theme (e.g., "what school was like when I was in eighth grade" or "when I played football"), or describing family gatherings at holiday times. (See Chapter 24 for a discussion of these groups.)

Self-Help Groups

The 1990s may well have been the age of the self-help group. **Self-help groups** are groups of persons coming together who are facing a common difficulty. They purposefully seek out others so that they may give and receive support with others whose experience is very similar to theirs. Often, persons attending self-help groups explain that others in their lives who do not face their problems cannot really understand what they are going through. Alcoholics Anonymous (AA) is probably the best known and largest self-help group (see Chapter 16). Other self-help groups include groups for persons who are facing a life-threatening illness, groups for persons with a specific medical diagnosis (e.g., breast cancer), women's support groups, men's support groups, groups for parents of children with particular problems, groups for caregivers of family members requiring physical care in the home, and mothers' groups for women with infants and preschoolers. These groups may be organized and facilitated by group members; however, in many situations, nurses or other professionals serve as facilitators. In such cases, the nurse may have identified the need for such a supportive group in her community and taken steps to set up the group (i.e., securing a meeting room, helping with publicity, and providing support to those persons who wish to meet in a group). Often, as in the case of a group for women with breast cancer, the nurse will attend the group and serve as a facilitator and resource person to the women coming together for mutual support.

The self-help group is empowering to those who attend because participants learn they are not alone, and they can provide help to one another. Further, they develop a sense of camaraderie and support, often supplying each other with personal telephone numbers and support outside of the group.

In the age of computer technology, there are several self-help groups emerging "online" where persons from around the country can join a discussion group over the Internet. This is a new means of persons reaching out to learn of others' experiences and provides an increased means of support, particularly to persons who are facing a relatively rare physical health problem or individuals who are homebound. Over time, the number of self-help discussion groups over the Internet will continue to increase. Persons can find such self-help groups through a search engine of the Internet, for example, a Netscape search under the name of a particular illness will usually provide a link to a self-help group, if one exists.

APPLICATION OF THE NURSING PROCESS 30-1

As in individual psychotherapy (see Chapter 28), a nurse therapist conducting a therapy group does not apply the nursing process per se. The nursing process requires the steps of assessment, analysis and diagnosis, outcome identification, planning/interventions, and evaluation. Although a therapist will assess group members and apply strategies to assist clients toward healthful outcomes, a therapist is guided by the psychotherapeutic theory. A therapist's assessment will be in terms of that specific theory and will not lead to a nursing diagnosis. Further, in some approaches to group therapy (the existential group, for example), the therapist will not identify outcomes, but rather will focus the experience in the present. Thus, the nurse functioning as group therapist is in a different role than the nurse applying the nursing process to clients in supportive groups.

In working with supportive groups, the nurse will apply the nursing process, much as in any other area of nursing. The nurse will complete an assessment of needs, and these assessment data of individuals may indicate that a group of persons, known to the nurse, could benefit from group interactions. Areas of need are identified (nursing diagnoses), and target outcomes are established and outlined. Then, planning the group itself is a nursing intervention aimed at meeting a group of clients' individual needs. Assessments and evaluation of individual client outcomes are also important in documenting the nursing role in client care.

The following case examples are presented to illustrate the nursing role in establishing, implementing, and evaluating group interventions, highlighting the emphasis on the supportive group roles that undergraduate-prepared nurses are expected to carry out.

REFLECTIVE THINKING 30-1

Group Therapy

The nurse has the skills and the license to assess and provide care for clients as a group in many settings. Psychiatric mental health nursing is a specialty where the nurse frequently may combine personal expertise in group process and dynamics, experience in client education, and personal creativity to establish and manage supportive groups. Consider the client population currently under your care. How would you approach assessing the need for group interventions? What benefits can you envision to a group approach to providing care to your client population? How could you initiate group activities? What checkpoints would you outline to monitor the group's progress toward the goals you have established?

CASE EXAMPLE 30-1

The Socialization Group on an Inpatient Unit

Nurse Bob is working on an inpatient psychiatric unit for persons who require hospitalization over a period of 1 month or longer. Most of the clients on the unit carry a *Diagnostic and Statistical Manual of Mental Disorders,* Fourth Edition-Text Revision (DSM-IV-TR) diagnosis of schizophrenia, although others on the unit may be hospitalized for Bipolar Disorder, Major Depression, or other diagnoses.

Assessment

Bob notices that there are five persons on the unit who rarely leave their rooms unless specifically asked to go somewhere or when told it is time for meals. These clients have a program of activities that

(*Continues*)

CASE EXAMPLE 30-1 (Continued)

includes recreational and occupational activities and individual therapy. Bob believes that each of these persons could benefit from a socialization group.

Bob begins with an assessment of each of the five individuals. May, a 60-year-old woman who has had repeated psychiatric hospitalizations, was admitted to the unit five days ago from a board-and-care home because she was hallucinating. May is having her medication evaluated and has been encouraged to participate in unit activities. May, however, spends her time alone. She interacts with Bob on a one-to-one basis and says she has "no one to talk to." Joe is a 25-year-old man who has had a history of paranoid ideations. He has been on the unit for two weeks. He is not actively hallucinating now, keeps to himself, but interacts with others who approach him. Sharon is a 30-year-old housewife who was finding herself unable to carry out daily activities at home. She expresses feeling "depressed" and "tired." She was hospitalized for evaluation of major depression/psychosis. She appears in touch with reality, is withdrawn, and keeps herself isolated from others. Ed is a long time client in Bob's unit. He is hospitalized frequently for schizophrenia due to noncompliance with medications. Ed was found by neighbors last week wandering in the streets, out of touch with reality, and unable to give his name to his neighbor. He is hospitalized for his own protection and to evaluate his need for medication and supervision on hospital discharge. Susan is a 40-year-old woman with much the same history as Ed. She is on Bob's unit awaiting placement in a board-and-care home where she will receive supervision.

Nursing Diagnosis

The nursing diagnoses that Bob has identified are *social isolation; impaired social interaction;* **and** *risk for loneliness.*

Outcome Identification

The expected outcome for the group is to increase social contact among the five persons on the unit. Bob will serve as facilitator, bringing the clients together and helping to initiate conversation and discussion.

Planning/Interventions

Bob concludes that a structured socialization group would be indicated for all of these five persons. The purpose of the group would be to provide an activity each morning wherein the group participants would be encouraged to interact with one another. Bob has developed a rapport with each client as an individual and believes they would attend a morning session after breakfast at his urging. He explains his assessment and treatment plan at a unit team meeting, and others agree that Bob should set up a one-half-hour socialization group to meet each morning. Bob discusses the group with each individual client and plans to have the first meeting tomorrow.

Evaluation

Bob will evaluate the degree to which each person in the group increases social contact. He will first observe and evaluate if each person contributes to the group meetings by talking and listening to others. Further, he will observe the clients on the unit outside of the group sessions and evaluate if the number of social contacts increases.

CASE EXAMPLE 30-2

The Reality Orientation Group in a Geriatric Day Care Facility

Two student nurses, Mario and John, are assigned to work each Wednesday morning at a geriatric day care center where frail elderly come for meals, activities, physical therapy, and nursing care. Mario and John have noticed that there are several clients who have trouble remembering the day of the week, and a few have sometimes been confused about where they are. Comments such as "What is the name of this place?" and "Am I at home?" and "Will my daughter be here?" have indicated to Mario and John that at least some of the clients could benefit from daily reality orientation.

Assessment

Further assessment of the clients indicates to Mario and John that, of 25 clients, at least 15 have had some difficulty with orientation in the past. The average age of the clients at the facility is 78 years, with the range being 64 to 96 years. Mario and John discuss their plans with their nursing instructor and with the day care staff. All agree some form of orientation group is indicated. Mario and John plan for such a daily group and conduct the group themselves on Wednesdays; center staff agree to conduct the group when Mario and John are not there.

Nursing Diagnosis

The nursing diagnosis that Mario and John have identified is *Impaired environmental interpretation syndrome.*

Outcome Identification

Mario and John expect that with initiation of the orientation sessions, each client at the center will show signs of progress in being oriented to person, place, and time every morning; use of the calendar is designed to serve as a reminder to clients throughout the day. Further, their use of a local newspaper should serve to keep participants informed regarding local and national issues.

Planning/Interventions

The group will meet for a 15-minute session every morning at 10 A.M. when the clients at the facility have a morning snack. The facilitator of the group introduces himself and gives the month, day, and year and places an X on a large calendar on the wall of the meeting room. Then, the facilitator discusses activities to be done at the center that day. Next, the facilitator reads selected items from a local newspaper, emphasizing current local and national events. The participants are asked to comment on the news items. Discussion may last for up to 10 minutes.

Evaluation

Mario and John will evaluate the degree to which the clients demonstrate improvement in reality orientation. They will observe how well clients are oriented to person, place, and time. They will listen for client discussion of current events. Further, Mario and John will observe if the clients refer to the calendar on the wall at any time later in the day.

CASE EXAMPLE 30-3

An Educational Group for Parents/Support Persons of Young Adults Diagnosed with Schizophrenia

Tara is a community mental health care nurse who is making follow-up home visits to clients served by a community outpatient mental health clinic. She identifies six young adults (aged 17 to 25 years) on her caseload that have been diagnosed with schizophrenia within the past six months. She understands that management of their illness requires support from family members. Each of these young adults is living with relatives, four with their parents, one with an aunt, and one with his older brother. During a home visit, she identified the person who is serving as the primary support person to each of the clients and plans an educational group to meet once a week for two months to provide information to the caregivers/support persons.

Assessment

Tara assessed that each identified family member requires further information on the disease of schizophrenia, its management, its genetic base, and the meaning of their loved one's living with the illness. Further, each family member requires information on medications used to treat the condition and the role of therapy. All require information on community services and what to do if their family member becomes sick, threatening, or potentially violent. Families have each disclosed to Tara that they live in fear that their family member will go "out of control" and they will not know what to do.

Nursing Diagnosis

The nursing diagnoses Tara is addressing are *Deficient knowledge* related to the therapeutic management and support of a family member with schizophrenia, and *Risk for caregiver role strain* related to being in a setting of caring and supporting a family member with a chronic psychiatric illness.

Outcome Identification

Tara believes that the educational group will not only provide these family members with needed information, it will also serve to let each know he is not alone, will provide a support network for families facing similar difficulties, and will engage the families as an active part of the treatment team who will be caring for these clients in years to come.

Planning/Interventions

Tara has planned educational sessions to meet once a week for two months, covering the topics of the disease of schizophrenia, including what is known about the genetic base of the disease, its pharmacological management, and the meaning of negative symptoms. Further, Tara has planned 15 to 20 minutes at the end of her teaching session for discussion of topics relevant to each family member. Tara also will provide a box where any participant may write down a question and leave it for her to cover in one of the following sessions. She uses this technique to encourage questions one might feel too shy to ask but that are important enough for group discussion.

Evaluation

Tara will evaluate the success of the group in two ways. First, she will determine through individual contacts with the families if the information provided was understood and is being applied in the home setting. Second, she will observe the level of interaction and support the participants give one another during and after the sessions. She will observe for informal communication and spontaneous discussion of common issues.

KEY CONCEPTS

- There are two types of groups with which nurses are involved: therapeutic and supportive.
- All groups go through the three phases of relationship: orientation, working, and termination.
- Therapy groups are conducted on the basis of identified theoretical frameworks.
- Supportive groups are designed to meet specific client needs.
- Supportive groups are conducted within the framework of the nursing process.

REVIEW QUESTIONS

1. An advanced practice nurse is asked to develop a group that can help the clients with their thought processes and behavioral patterns. The nurse would most likely develop which of the following types of groups?
   1. Psychoanalytic group
   2. Interpersonal group
   3. Cognitive-behavioral group
   4. Existential group

2. A client with a dual diagnosis Bipolar Disorder and Alcoholism is ready for discharge. The nurse would include referring the client to which of the following groups that can provide support so that he remains alcohol free?
   1. A self-help group such as AA
   2. A socialization group for single people
   3. An educational group
   4. A psychoanalytic group

3. A nurse is conducting group sessions with a group of elderly clients. The nurse plans to have each of the group members share their experiences of the good times they have had on family vacations. The nurse is most likely conducting which of the following types of group therapy found to be useful with the elderly?
   1. Self-help groups
   2. Reminiscence groups
   3. Socialization groups
   4. Reality orientation groups

4. A client enters the community group meeting dressed inappropriately. The best approach by the nurse is to do which of the following?
   1. Tell the client that she is dressed like a street person
   2. Ask the other group members to comment on the client's attire
   3. Escort the client to her room and assist her to find more appropriate attire
   4. Ignore the client's inappropriate attire

5. At what phase of group work is the goal of having members develop a sense of belonging to the group usually addressed?
   1. Pre-orientation phase
   2. Orientation phase
   3. Working phase
   4. Termination phase

6. One afternoon, two advanced practice nurses conducted a group for the women on the psychiatric unit. Throughout the group meeting, one of the group members found fault with everyone and every aspect of the group. When the group ended, the two nurses had a debriefing session to discuss the process and content of the group meeting. Their evaluation revealed that the member, who always found fault with everything, had been functioning in which group role?
   1. Controller
   2. Problem solver
   3. Nay sayer
   4. Devil's advocate

LEARNING ACTIVITIES

1. Describe the difference between a therapy group and a supportive group.
2. Observe a group therapy session (if at all possible) and document the group dynamics.
3. Identify which of the major approaches to group therapy might be most useful for a specific group of clients you know.
4. Describe how you could set up a supportive group to meet client needs that you have identified.

StudyWARE™ CONNECTION

Using your StudyWARE™ CD-ROM

1. Complete the Concentration activity for this chapter.
2. Review the audio glossary for key terms in this chapter.
3. Explore the other games and activities that support this chapter.

REFERENCES

Buccheri, R., Trystad, L, Dowling, G., Hopkins, R., White, K., Griffin, J., et al., (2004). Long-term effects of teaching behavioral strategies for managing persistent auditory hallucinations in schizophrenia. *Journal of Psychosocial Nursing and Mental Health Services, 18*(9), 20–27, 48–49.

Bulecheck, G., Butcher, H., & Dochterman, J. (2008). *Nursing interventions classification* (5th ed.). St. Louis: Mosby.

Chen, T. W., Lu, R. B., Chang, A. J., Chu, D. M., & Chou, K. R. (2006). The evaluation of cognitive behavioral therapy on patient depression and self-esteem. *Archives of Psychiatric Nursing, 20*(1), 3–11.

Gerrick, D., & Ewashen, C. (2001). An integrated model for adolescent inpatient group therapy. *Journal of Psychiatric and Mental Health Nursing, 8*(2), 165–171.

George, J. (2002). *Nursing theories: The basis for professional nursing practice* (5th ed). Norwalk CT: Appleton & Lange.

Keen, E. (1970). *Three faces of being: Toward an existential clinical psychology*. Englewood Cliffs, NJ: Prentice-Hall.

Lonergan, E. C. (1994). Using theories of group therapy. In H. S. Barnard & K. R. MacKenzie (Eds.), *Basics of group psychotherapy* (pp. 189–216). New York: Guillford.

Montgomery, C. (2002). The role of dynamic group therapy in psychiatry. *Advances in Psychiatric Treatment, 8*, 34–41.

Moreno, J. L. (1970). *Psychodrama* (3rd ed.). New York: Beacon House.

Parse, R. (1996). *Theory of human becoming*. New York: National League for Nursing.

Parse, R. R. (1998). *The human becoming school of thought*. Thousand Oaks, CA: Sage.

Seamoore, D., Buckroyd, J., & Stott, D. (2006). Changes in eating behavior following group therapy for women who binge eat: A pilot study. *Journal of Psychiatric and Mental Health Nursing, 13*, 337–345.

Shaffer, J., & Galinsky, M. D. (1989). *Models of group therapy*. Englewood Cliffs, NJ: Prentice-Hall.

Sullivan, H. S. (1953). *Interpersonal theory of psychiatry*. New York: Norton.

Watson, J. (2005). *Caring science as sacred science*. Philadelphia: Davis.

Watson, J. (1988). *Nursing science of human care*. New York: National League for Nursing.

SUGGESTED READINGS

Beiling, P. J., McCabe, R. E., & Antony, M. M. (2006). *Cognitive-behavioral therapy in groups*. New York: Guilford Press.

Yalom, I. D., & Leszcz, M. (2005). *Theory and practice of group psychotherapy* (5th ed.). New York: Basic Books.

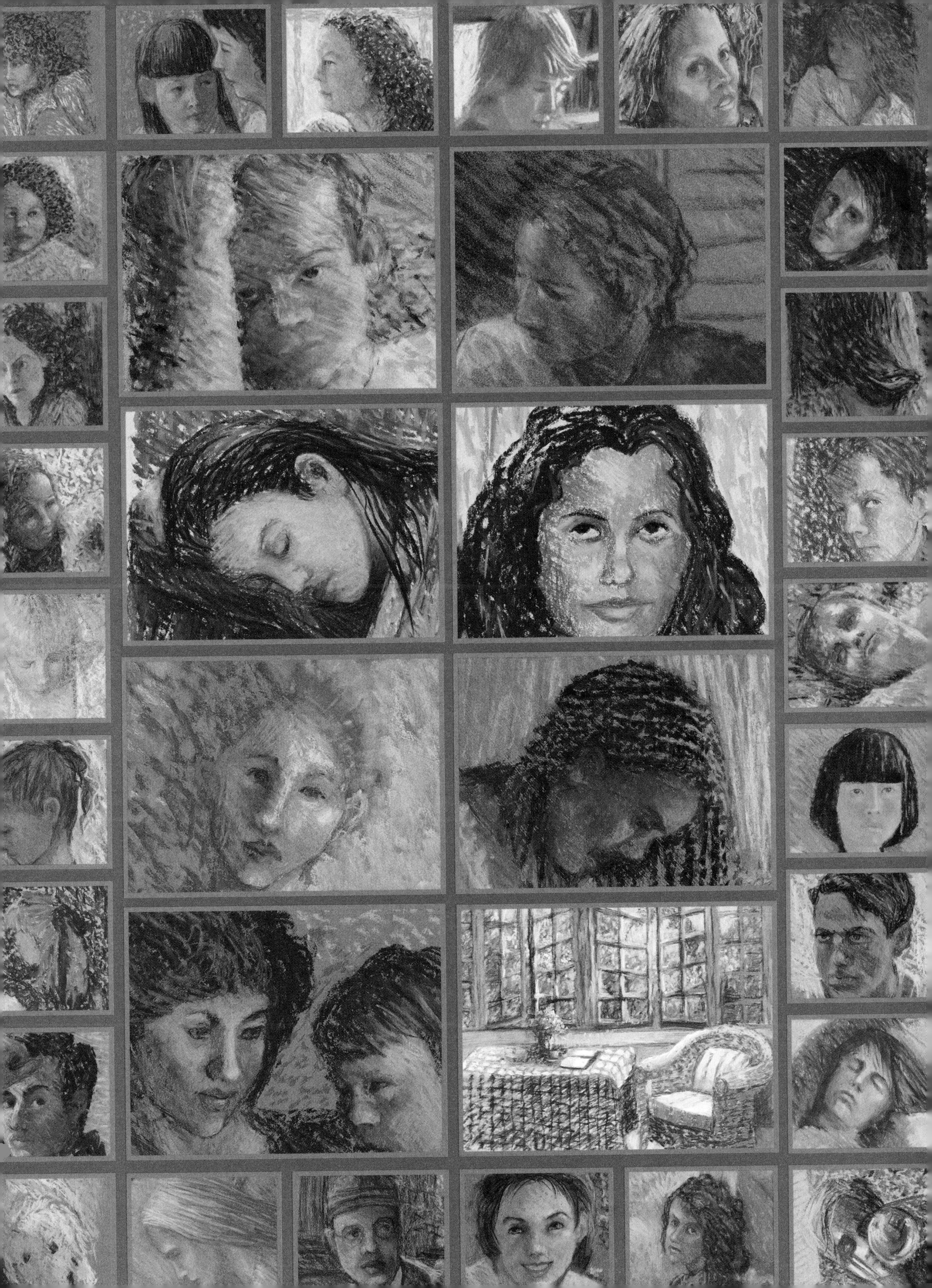

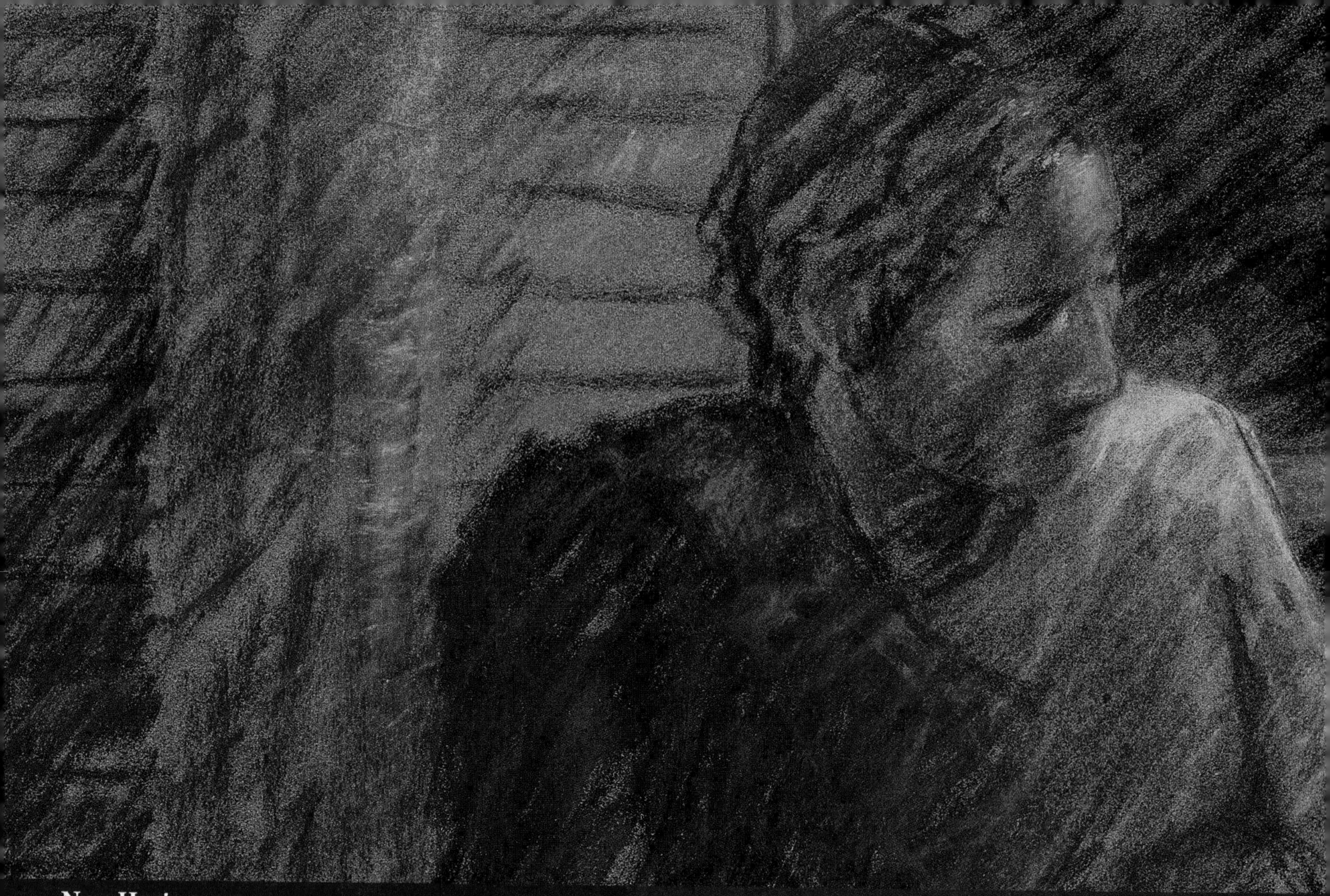

New Horizons

Considering Community Health Nursing

- *What is the relationship between community health nursing, public health nursing, and home health nursing?*
- *How is the focus of mental health care changing?*
- *What is meant by a community-based, population-focused approach to planning, delivering, and evaluating nursing care?*
- *What are the goals of community-based mental health care?*
- *What is the nurse's role in designing, managing, monitoring, and evaluating systems of care that address mental health problems experienced by aggregates (population groups)?*

Consider these questions as you read this chapter.

CHAPTER 31

Community Mental Health Nursing

GENEVIEVE M. BARTOL

CHAPTER OUTLINE

COMPETENCIES

Upon completion of this chapter, the reader should be able to:

1. Describe the changing focus of care in the field of mental health.
2. Explain a conceptual framework for nursing practice with aggregates (population groups).
3. Explain selected strategies that can be used to improve the health status of aggregates (population groups).
4. Describe nursing practice with aggregates (population groups).

KEY TERMS

Aggregate
Assertive Community Treatment (ACT)
Capitation
Case Management
Community Health Nursing
Community Mental Health
Community Support System (CSS)
Deinstitutionalization
Home Health Nursing
Managed-Care
Population
Primary Prevention
Programs for Assertive Community Treatment (PACT)
Prospective Payment Systems
Public Health Nursing
Secondary Prevention
Tertiary Prevention

The terms *public health nursing* and *community health nursing* are sometimes used interchangeably. Public health nursing was first used by Lillian Wald in 1893 (Figure 31-1). Wald realized that individual nursing care was not sufficient for the people she served. Clients who lived in squalid conditions and could not buy nourishing food would not get well without proper housing and food. According to Wald, nurses working in the community who addressed social, economic, and environmental conditions that influenced health engaged in **public health nursing** (Dieckmann, 2008).

By the 1960s, many nurses were practicing in the community, but not necessarily practicing public health. The term *community health nursing* was coined to describe nurses who practice in community settings. Over time, community health nursing was viewed by some nurses as a broad term that applies to all nurses working in community settings. Some nurses insist that public health nursing does not fit under the umbrella of community health nursing. **Community health nursing** is defined in this chapter as the synthesis of nursing and public health practice to promote, maintain, and conserve the health of population aggregates in the community. **Population** refers to an aggregate of persons in the community who share a common characteristic, such as age or a diagnostic category. **Aggregate** refers to a population or defined group.

Still, the debate about the proper use of these terms continues today and is further confounded by the advent of home health nursing. **Home health nursing** refers to the delivery of health services in the home under the direction of a health care agency. Home health services are an outgrowth of shortened hospital stays in an era of cost containment. Sometimes hospitals establish home health programs to quickly move clients from hospitals to the community. Some psychiatric nurses engaged in private practice provide home health services. Private home care agencies are also beginning to serve psychiatric clients. Psychiatric home care, which may include help with housework and companionship, is considered a major factor in maintaining clients in the home (Sebastian & Martin, 2008). The use of these terms is not simply a semantic question, but may well shape the role of nurses in health care (Kearney-Nunnery, 2008). In this chapter, **community mental health** is viewed as a synthesis of community health nursing and public health with particular emphasis on mental health (though not to the exclusion of physical health).

THE CHANGING FOCUS OF CARE

Before 1840, people who were mentally ill were generally placed in prisons, asylums, and county homes. Only the wealthy could afford the luxury of a private hospital. The purpose for placement in any of these settings was to protect the ill person from harming others or being harmed, neither of which was ensured by the arrangement.

In 1841, Dorothea Dix, a former school teacher who was distressed by the poor care given to the mentally ill, personally crusaded for enlightened treatment. Dix insisted that each state assume responsibility for its own mentally ill residents. Her efforts led to the establishment of 32 state mental hospitals throughout the United States. Most of the hospitals were built in rural areas, where the environment was considered healthful and clients could be removed from the communities who feared them. Consequently, the people who entered the state psychiatric hospitals left their communities at the door and were often forgotten by those they left behind (Thompson-Heisterman, 2008).

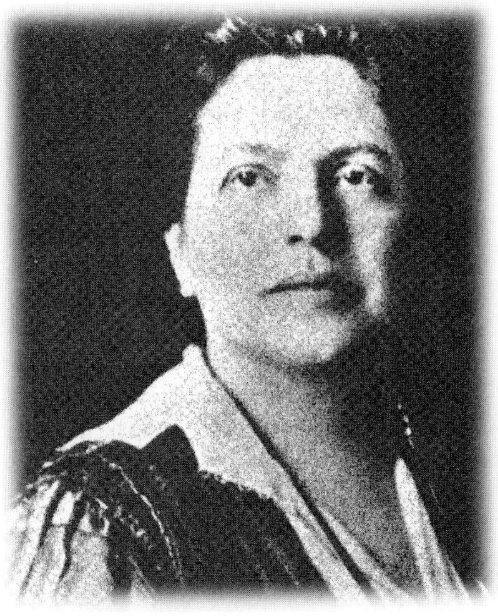

FIGURE 31-1 **Lillian D. Wald** (COURTESY: AMERICAN NURSES ASSOCIATION.)

By 1900, the state hospitals were overcrowded and understaffed. The construction of new hospitals had not kept pace with the growing population. Once again concern arose as the conditions in state psychiatric hospitals deteriorated. Demands for community-based mental health services prompted federal legislation that shaped the development of the community mental health concept (Thompson-Heisterman, 2008).

The move to the community received a major impetus in 1908 with the publication of Clifford Beers's book *A Mind That Found Itself* (Beers, 1921). In this book, Beers graphically describes his experiences as a client in a psychiatric hospital and advocates for better treatment for the mentally ill. He is credited with the establishment of the Connecticut Society for Mental Hygiene, whose purpose was to educate the public about mental illness. In 1909, the National Committee for Mental Hygiene was founded. Within the next 10 years, 19 state mental hygiene societies were formed (Stanhope & Lancaster, 2003). Consumer interest in mental health steadily increased thereafter. The National Alliance for the Mentally Ill (NAMI) was the first consumer group to advocate for better services. Today there are at least seven consumer advocacy and self-help organizations. "The community health principles that are the underpinnings of practice include the right to mental health services delivered in the least restrictive environment, consumer involvement in treatment, advocacy and rehabilitation services" (Thompson-Heisterman, 2008, p. 791).

FEDERAL GOVERNMENT IN MENTAL HEALTH CARE

The shift in responsibility for mental illness from states to the federal government began with the passage of the Social Security Act in 1935. This change was in response to the economic and social problems of the era, and was based on the concept that if local communities could not effectively care for their ill members, the federal government should take responsibility (Thompson-Heisterman, 2008).

World War II brought additional attention to the problem of mental illness. Almost 6% of draftees were barred from service because of existing mental illness (Stanhope & Lancaster, 2003). As a nation, we had to acknowledge that mental illness was a major problem.

A significant increase in the government's involvement in mental health followed the war. The National Mental Health Act of 1946 was passed in an attempt to improve care for the growing number of psychiatric patients. The U.S. government awarded grants to the states to develop mental health programs outside state hospitals. Psychiatric units and outpatient psychiatric services were set up in general hospitals. In 1946, the National Institute of Mental Health (NIMH) was established and charged with the responsibility for mental health in the United States. Legislation was designed to apply a community health approach to promoting mental health and preventing mental illness. In actuality, the medical model, with its emphasis on individual psychotherapy, remained dominant because adequate funding for community services was not provided with the legislation (Thompson-Heisterman, 2008).

In 1955, the Joint Commission on Mental Health and Illness was established by Congress to survey the nation's mental health needs and to recommend new approaches to improve mental health care (Thompson-Heisterman, 2008). This commission, made up of representatives of 36 organizations and agencies selected by NIMH, published their report in 1961. Their historic document, *Action for Mental Health*, emphasized the need for better training for caregivers, early and intensive treatment for the acutely ill, and improvements in education and research of mental illness. President John F. Kennedy appointed a cabinet-level committee to review the report and to make recommendations for federal action. In 1963, Kennedy called for a new approach that would return mentally ill clients to their local communities. The concept of the comprehensive community mental health center was born. Community mental health centers were constructed through the joint efforts of federal and state governments (Thompson-Heisterman, 2008).

In 1963, Public Law 88-164, the Mental Retardation Facilities and Community Mental Health Centers Construction Act, was passed. This act was designed to provide comprehensive mental health services to all residents in a specific area. The designated service area usually included about 75,000 to 200,000 people and was referred to as a catchment area. Each center was required to provide five essential services to qualify for funding. The five services included inpatient care for clients requiring short-term hospitalization, partial hospitalization incorporating day and night care, outpatient treatment, 24-hour emergency help, and consultation/education for the community. Additional supplementary services, such as diagnostic services, vocational counseling, research, and evaluation were encouraged. Money, based on a declining formula of federal support over a 51-month period, was allocated to the states to launch the centers. The plan did not work where state or local funds did not increase sufficiently

BOX 31-1
SERVICES INCLUDED IN COMPREHENSIVE MENTAL HEALTH CENTERS

ESSENTIAL SERVICES

- Inpatient care for patients requiring short-term hospitalization
- Partial hospitalization incorporating day and night care
- Outpatient treatment
- Twenty-four–hour emergency help
- Consultation/education for the community

SUGGESTED ADDITIONAL SUPPLEMENTARY SERVICES

- Diagnostic services
- Vocational counseling
- Research
- Evaluation

to compensate for the declining federal support, and the services provided were uneven. Unfortunately, adequate community services were not always available, and clients once again suffered neglect (Thompson-Heisterman, 2008).

President George W. Bush established the New Freedom Commission on Mental Health by executive order in 2002 to recommend ways in which the federal government can help states increase accesses to mental health care and improve the quality of public programs. The commission identified five major barriers to mental health care within the current system: (1) fragmentation and gaps in care for children; (2) fragmentation and gaps in care for adults with serious mental illness; (3) high unemployment and disability for people with serious mental illness; (4) older adults not receiving care; and (5) mental health and suicide prevention not yet a national priority. The commission made recommendations in regard to how care is delivered; focusing on symptom management and accepting long-term disability are not acceptable. Rather, mental health services and support should promote recovery and build resilience so that people with mental illness are able to meet life's challenges (Miller, 2003).

Deinstitutionalization

Beginning in the late 1960s, the increased availability of psychotropic medications and the promise of saving money heightened the movement of clients toward community care. Many psychiatric hospital beds were eliminated, and clients were returned to families or placed in supervised nursing homes, rest homes, and apartments. This shift of clients and mental health services from state mental hospitals to community settings is referred to as **deinstitutionalization.** It was believed that the mentally ill would be better cared for in their home communities surrounded by those who were not mentally ill. Unfortunately, adequate support services were not in place in many communities, and a decreased quality of life for the mentally ill resulted. Clients were often returned to hospitals, stabilized, and discharged again in a cycling pattern (sometimes described as the "revolving door"). Some discharged clients did not return to the hospital and became homeless or were imprisoned (Satel, 2003; Report of the Federal Task Force on Homelessness and Severe Mental Illness, 1992; Thompson-Heisterman, 2008).

In 1974, NIMH began to study the problems resulting from deinstitutionalization. Consumers, family members, and mental health professionals were asked for input about the services needed. The concept of an organized network of people committed to helping persons with severe mental illness meet their needs and move toward independence, known as the **community support system (CSS)**, resulted. Returning the mentally ill to large, isolated hospitals was no longer considered a viable option. The CSS concept comprises an entire array of treatment, life-support, and rehabilitation services.

It is the community mental health centers that have the primary responsibility for developing and implementing CSS for their catchment areas. The essential components of CSS include client identification and outreach, mental health treatment, health and dental care, crisis response services, protection and advocacy, rehabilitation, family and community support, peer support, income support, and entitlement and housing (NIMH, 1987; see Figure 31-2).

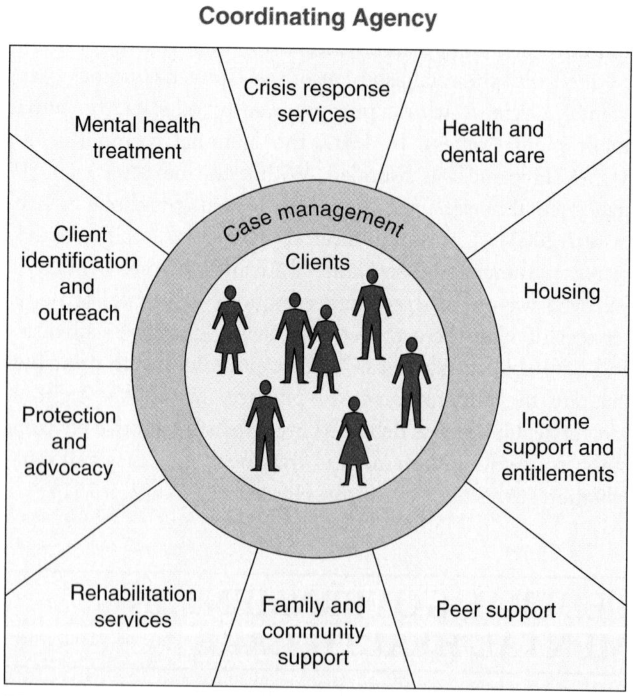

FIGURE 31-2 Components of a Community Support System (CSS) (COURTESY: NATIONAL INSTITUTE OF MENTAL HEALTH, ROCKVILLE, MD.)

BOX 31-2
RECOMMENDATIONS OF THE COMMISSION'S FINAL REPORT, JULY 2003

ACHIEVING THE PROMISE: TRANSFORMING MENTAL HEALTH CARE IN AMERICA

- Advance and implement a national campaign to reduce the stigma of seeking care and a national strategy for suicide prevention.
- Address mental health with the same urgency as physical health.
- Develop an individualized plan for every adult with a serious mental illness and every child with a serious emotional disturbance.
- Involve consumers and families fully in orienting the mental system toward recovery.
- Align relevant federal programs to improve access and accountability for mental health services.
- Create a Comprehensive State Mental Health Plan.
- Protect and enhance the rights of people with mental illness.
- Improve access to quality care that is culturally competent.
- Improve access to quality care in rural and geographically remote areas.
- Promote the mental health of young children.
- Improve and expand school mental health programs.
- Screen for co-occurring mental and substance abuse disorders and link with integrated treatment strategies.
- Screen for mental disorders in primary health care, across the life span, and connect to treatments and supports.
- Accelerate research to promote recovery and resilience, and ultimately to care for and prevent mental illness.
- Advance evidence-based practices using dissemination and demonstration projects, and create a public-private partnership to guide their implementation.
- Improve and expand the workforce, providing evidence-based mental health services and supports.
- Develop the knowledge base in four understudied areas: mental health disparities, long-term effects of medications, trauma, and acute care.
- Use health technology and telehealth to improve access and coordination of mental health care, especially for Americans in remote areas or in underserved populations.
- Develop and implement integrated electronic health record and personal health information systems.

From "Reform and Revolution: President Bush's New Freedom Commission," by J. E. Miller, 2003, *NAMI Advocate*, *25*(1), pp. 12–13.

Legislation known as the Amendments of 1975 (Public Law 94-63) provided a more stable funding for community mental health centers to develop CSSs. Monies were provided for specialty areas, including child care, aging, court screening, care for discharged clients, transitional services, and substance abuse counseling. Funding was extended in 1977. Legislative mandates and incentives facilitated the movement toward a community-based system of care (Lauterbach, 2001; Thompson-Heisterman, 2008).

The efforts to improve services for the mentally ill continued despite financial difficulties because of the strong advocacy movements (Donley, 2008; Lauterbach, 2001). Research, moreover, demonstrated that community-based care was cost effective. The CSS, which includes components of other human services, such as housing support and coordination across the fragmented human service system, was promoted. In 1985, for example, the Robert Wood Johnson Foundation, in collaboration with the U.S. Department of Housing and Urban Development, sponsored a $100 million program for communitywide projects that would consolidate and expand services for the long-term mentally ill. The Social Security Administration (SSA) sent SSA workers into mental health settings to improve the process of determining disability. Health services, social services, and housing and income needs for the mentally ill require coordination and cooperation to provide successful community-based care. The CSS model was viewed as the most appropriate model for caring for the mentally ill in the community (NIMH, 1987). Philosophically, the community is believed to have an abundant source of resources for mental health consumers and their families (Drake, Green, Mueser, & Goldman 2003). The CSS model is designed to help clients assess those resources.

Of course, there are also forces resisting the movement to community-based care (Lauterbach, 2001). The concern of state hospital employees for their jobs, families' anxiety about long-term care requirements, public fear and discrimination, state and federal battles over authority, and inadequate support services for clients in the community exert

TABLE 31-1 Examples of Case Management Activities

ACTIVITY	EXAMPLE
Identification	Identifying a client who is missing his or her outreach appointments for medication checks and providing additional services to ensure proper treatment
Assessment	Calling the client who missed an appointment to determine why the appointment was missed
Service planning	Holding a care conference for a client who is having difficulty adjusting to a job situation
Linkage with services	Making an appointment for a client with a vocational rehabilitation counselor
Monitoring service	Making a follow-up call to find out if the client kept the appointment with the vocational counselor and received help
Advocacy	Speaking to a client's landlord to arrange for necessary repairs

significant pressure for a return to inpatient care. Moreover, insurance companies often will provide reimbursement for inpatient services but not for outpatient services.

NAMI continues to advocate for quality care and plays a leading role in the development and coordination of nine peer-directed education and support programs. For example, NAMI offers a free 12-week educational program for families, partners, and friends of individuals with serious mental illness. Scientific evaluation shows that participants gain a greater understanding of mental illness, cope better with the strains of illness, worry less, and feel greatly empowered to navigate the health care and political systems to obtain improved treatment and services. In another sponsored program, the NAMI Connection Recovery Support Group, people living with mental illness attend a weekly 90-minute session in which participants learn from one another's experiences and offer one another encouragement and understanding (NAMI, 2009).

CASE MANAGEMENT

Case management is a constellation of services that includes screening, assessment, care planning, arranging for service delivery, monitoring, reassessment, evaluation, and discharge for the purpose of ensuring continuity of care. As Figure 31-2 shows, case management is integral to the CSS. Case managers, a position often held by nurses, help seriously mentally ill persons build skills and access supports so they can function as independently as possible. Six activities form the core of case management: identification and outreach, assessment, service planning, linkage with needed services, monitoring service delivery, and advocacy. See Table 31-1 for examples of case management activities.

The major goal of case management is to help the mentally ill person remain in the community. Case management services for the seriously mentally ill is the key component of CSS that coordinates all the other services and ensures that needed services are received. Assertive community treatment (ACT) programs, psychological rehabilitation (clubhouses), and intensive case management are central to preventing relapse (Thompson-Heisterman, 2008).

High-quality, general case management programs are effective. The case manager plans and brokers services and advocates on behalf of clients in a community support system as described earlier. Case managers are mobile and provide crisis services. A single case manager, however, is typically responsible for about 25 to 30 clients. Case managers, therefore, cannot always provide enough individualized help. Some seriously mentally ill clients need the help of a more intensive program, known as **Assertive Community Treatment (ACT)** (Thompson-Heisterman, 2008). This model provides a full range of medical, psychosocial, and rehabilitation services by a community-based, multidisciplinary team that operates 7 days a week, 24 hours a day, and is responsible for only about 10 to 12 clients. The model presumes that bringing care to the client will more effectively develop needed skills and eliminate problems associated with missed appointments. For example, medications could be administered to the client in a timely manner, which would prevent exacerbation of symptoms. These intensive case management models are sometimes referred to as "hospitals without walls" (p. 792). Box 31-3 shows the services offered by **Programs for Assertive Community Treatment (PACT)**.

CONSUMER INVOLVEMENT

Advocacy for the mentally ill is still needed. In 1980, a federal law was passed because mentally ill persons were still found to be subject to abuse and neglect. For example, clients were being unnecessarily secluded or restrained. The Mental Health System Act (MHSA, 1980) adopted into law a Bill of Rights for persons receiving mental health treatment services. The Americans with Disabilities Act, which prohibited discrimination and promoted opportunities for persons with mental disorders, was passed in 1990. And in 1996, the Mental Health Parity Act addressed the discrepancy between

RESEARCH Highlight 31-1

Social Functioning in Schizophrenia

STUDY PROBLEM/PURPOSE

To examine the relationship of clinical factors and environmental opportunities to social functioning in young adults with schizophrenia.

METHODS

Used data from the long-term experimental evaluation of a PACT for 87 young adults with schizophrenia spectrum disorders. Data from two time points, 6 months apart, were used to test models predicting five social outcomes (network size, network reciprocity, sociosexual contact, satisfaction with social relationships, and loneliness) from positive symptoms, work involvement, living situation and residential mobility.

FINDINGS

Results revealed that (1) work involvement was associated with larger network sizes over a 6-month period; (2) experiencing an increase in positive symptoms over a 6-month period was associated with the loss of reciprocal network ties, a lessening of satisfaction with social relationships, and an increase in loneliness; and (3) neither living situation nor moving frequently was associated with later social outcomes.

IMPLICATIONS

The findings of this study suggest strong support for the role of short-term changes in positive symptoms and modest support for the role of work involvement in social outcome.

Source: "The Relationship of Clinical Factors and Environmental Opportunities to Social Functioning in Young Adults with Schizophrenia," by B. Angell and M. A. Test, 2002, *Schizophrenia Bulletin*, *28*(2), 259–271.

REFLECTIVE THINKING 31-1

PACT Services

- Which psychiatric clients would most likely benefit from a PACT?
- What are the expected benefits for the clients who are enrolled in a PACT?
- How can PACT teams be cost effective when they provide such intensive services?

mental health and medical-surgical benefits in employer-sponsored health plans (Thompson-Heisterman, 2008).

Consumer groups are a primary force in changing mental health care from a provider-driven to a consumer-driven delivery system (Francell, Conn, & Gray, 1988). NAMI educates, advocates, and lobbies on behalf of primary (current or former clients) and secondary (family members and significant others) consumers. Local chapters of NAMI serve as a forum for members to tell their stories and gain support and advice. As a result, consumers who once felt frustrated and helpless about their particular situations are beginning to recognize their right to information about mental illness and the options for treatment. Consumers are increasingly claiming their right to collaborate with health care providers in planning their care.

Also, NAMI is a major force for legislative changes on a state and national level and for programmatic changes on the local level. Members of NAMI channel their energies into positive, constructive efforts to improve the lot for the mentally ill. For example, NAMI struggles to eliminate stigmatization of the mentally ill by fighting the use of disempowering labels. Through their efforts, the terms we use changed from *chronically mentally ill* to *long-term mentally ill* and eventually to *seriously mentally ill.* These changes in wording spawn hope that mental illness, though serious, can be cured, and emphasize the view that mental illness is a brain disease for which a definitive cure may be found (Stanhope & Lancaster, 2003). At the same time, there is increasing documentation of the psychophysiology of body-mind relationships that clearly demonstrates mental illness does not reside solely in the brain and multiple interventions are appropriate (Bartol & Courts, 2008).

Consumer empowerment is also a goal of the CSS concept. Therefore, NIMH funds consumer organizing activities. The National Ex-Patient Teleconference and the National Mental Health Consumer Self-Help Clearing house and Alternatives, an annual consumer conference, are examples of collaborative projects funded by NIMH and consumer groups. In the past, families were often blamed for their members' illness. Now it is recognized that successful community-based care requires united efforts of clients, their families, caregivers, and society (Stanhope & Lancaster, 2003).

Families play a major role in the client's health status. Members of the family movement (e.g., NAMI, and others) advocate for protection, clinical services, and basic research. The health consumer movement emphasizes autonomy for the client. Nevertheless, both groups see optimal autonomy as a therapeutic goal. Evidence suggests that the feelings of emotional burden experienced by family members are directly related to the severity of stressors generated by the ill member. Moreover, it appears that emphasis on autonomy for the client may be the most effective way of relieving the family burden (Lefley, 1999). Research on families of clients with severe mental illness indicates that the caregiving burden can be significant. Nurses often need to intervene to prevent mental illness in family caregivers (Thompson-Heisterman, 2008).

The movement toward promoting self-determination for individuals with psychiatric disabilities through self-directed services is increasingly emphasized by consumer groups.

BOX 31-3
DESCRIPTION OF PACT SERVICES

1. Medication support
   - Order medications from pharmacy.
   - Deliver medications to clients.
   - Educate about medication.
   - Monitor medication compliance and side effects.
2. Rehabilitative approach to daily living skills
   - Do grocery shopping and cooking.
   - Purchase and maintain clothing.
   - Facilitate access to transportation.
   - Foster social and family relationships.
   - Educate about legal rights.
3. Family involvement
   - Provide crisis management.
   - Do counseling and psycho-education with family and extended family.
   - Coordinate with family service agencies.
4. Work opportunities
   - Give support in finding volunteer and vocational opportunities.
   - Serve as liaison with and educator for employers.
   - Serve as job coach for clients.
5. Entitlement
   - Assist with documentation.
   - Accompany clients to entitlement offices.
   - Manage food stamps.
   - Assist with redetermination of benefits.
6. Health promotion
   - Provide preventive health education.
   - Conduct medical screening.
   - Schedule maintenance visits.
   - Act as liaison for acute medical care.
   - Provide reproductive counseling and sex education.
7. Housing assistance
   - Find suitable shelter.
   - Secure leases and pay rent.
   - Purchase and repair household items.
   - Develop relationships with landlords.
   - Improve housekeeping skills.
8. Financial management
   - Plan budget.
   - Troubleshoot financial problems, for example, disability payments.
   - Assist with bills.
   - Increase independence in money management.
9. Counseling
   - Encourage problem-solving approach.
   - Facilitate integration into continuous work.
   - Orchestrate goals addressed by all team members.
   - Develop communication skills.
   - Coordinate a comprehensive rehabilitative approach.

Adapted from *Hospital without Walls*, by Duke University Medical Center: Division of Social and Community Psychiatry, Department of Psychiatry, 1993 (Study guide accompanying video *Hospital without Walls*).

Some suggest that funds ordinarily paid to service provider agencies should be transferred directly to people with psychiatric disabilities, using various formulas to account for direct, administrative, and other costs.

In 1991, NIMH and the National Advisory Mental Health Council (NAMHC) published a national plan of research to improve services for persons with severe mental disorders. The plan represents a systematic review of knowledge about the best ways to provide care for the severely and persistently mentally ill. Gaps in knowledge were identified and important questions formulated. The goal of finding ways to improve the quality of care provided to the mentally ill remains. The task is further complicated by the growing diversity of the population and the need to design culturally sensitive approaches. What works in some instances may not be appropriate in others.

The health promotion and disease prevention goals outlined in *Healthy People 2010* (USDHHS, 2000) address settings where people receive care (e.g., primary care, jail), populations at risk (such as children and adults with substance abuse disorders), and issues of cultural competence. The overall goals are to improve mental health and ensure access to quality and appropriate services (USDHHS, 2000).

Still, progress is slow and uneven. Deregulation legislation during the Reagan and Bush presidencies reduced federal authority and funding and shifted responsibility for health care back to the states. Fewer community-based public health programs and clinics served the poor as a result of the decrease in federal regulation and spending. Price control and competition were encouraged, and diagnostic-related grouping (DRG) was devised through amendments to the Social Security Act and the Medicare program (Donley, 2008).

The DRG is a construct that groups diagnoses into categories that require similar levels of resources. Payment for services is linked to a flat rate for each category. If the costs of treatment exceed the DRG payment allotted in that category, the provider is required to absorb the extra costs. While mental health did not initially come under the threat of

BOX 31-4
MENTAL HEALTH STATUS IMPROVEMENT

18.1 Reduce 6.0 suicide deaths per 100,000 population
18.2 Reduce suicide attempts by adolescents to 12-month average of 1%
18.3 Reduce homeless adults who have serious mental illness (SMI) from 25% to 19%
18.4 Increase employment of persons with SMI from 43% to 51%
18.5 Reduce eating disorder relapse rates

TREATMENT EXPANSION

18.6 Increase the number of persons who receive mental health screening and assessment in primary care
18.7 Increase the number of children with mental health problems who receive treatment
18.8 Increase the number of juvenile justice facilities that screen new admissions for mental health problems.
18.9 Increase the number of adults with SMI who receive treatment
18.10 Increase the proportion of persons with co-occurring substance abuse and mental disorders who receive treatment for both conditions.
18.11 Increase the number of community-based jail diversion programs for adults with SMI

STATE ACTIVITIES

18.12 Increase the number of states tracking consumers' satisfaction with the mental health services they receive
18.13 Increase the number of operational mental health plans that address cultural competence
18.14 Increase the number of operational mental health plans that address mental health crisis interventions, ongoing screening, and treatment services for elderly persons

From U.S. Department of Health and Human Services. *Healthy People 2010: National health and disease prevention objectives*, Volume II, Washington, DC, U.S. Government Printing).

DRGs, "the writing was on the wall," and concerns about cost increasingly guided treatment decisions. More attention was also directed to demonstrating the cost effectiveness of specific treatments.

In 1992, a report of the Federal Task Force on Homelessness and Severe Mental Illness noted that one out of every three homeless persons in the United States suffers from a severe mental illness. The task force stated that any successful effort to end homelessness among the seriously mentally ill must be pluralistic. Federal, state, and local governments, as well as providers, family members, voluntary organizations, and mental health consumers must take part in the effort. The recommendations of the task force emphasize the need for integration in care delivery systems that serve the mentally ill. Nevertheless, community-based mental health care has been clearly pronounced as a national goal (Lauterbach, 2001). Even the growth of home health nursing underscores the shift in the locus of care from hospitals to the community.

BOX 31-5
BILL OF RIGHTS FOR CLIENTS

1. The right to appropriate treatment in settings and under conditions most supportive and least restrictive to personal liberty
2. The right to an individualized written treatment plan, periodic review of treatment, and revision of plan
3. The right to ongoing participation in the planning of services and the right to a reasonable explanation of general mental condition, treatment objective, adverse effects of treatment, reasons for treatment, and available alternatives
4. The right to refuse treatment except in an emergency or as permitted by law
5. The right not to participate in experimentation
6. The right to freedom from restraint or seclusion
7. The right to a humane treatment environment
8. The right to confidentiality of records
9. The right to access to records except data provided by third parties or unless access would be detrimental to health
10. The right of access to telephone use, mail, and visitors
11. The right to know these rights
12. The right to initiate grievances when rights are infringed
13. The right to referral when discharged

From Mental Health System Act, 1980, 96th Congress, Public Law 96-398, Section 9501, Amendment to Senate Bill 1177, September 23, 1980.

MODELS FOR COMMUNITY MENTAL HEALTH NURSING

CLIENT-CENTERED MODEL

As noted earlier, community mental health nursing incorporates community nursing and public health nursing. Community nursing refers to nursing practice in the community

RESEARCH Highlight 31-2

Caregiver Stresses

STUDY PROBLEM/PURPOSE

To examine caregivers' stresses when living together or apart from clients with chronic schizophrenia.

METHODS

Ratings of stress and burden and mental symptoms, which were screened by the General Health Questionnaire (GHQ), were collected from two types of primary caregivers either living with (N = 37) or separately from (N = 38) a client with a chronic schizophrenic disorder.

FINDINGS

The stress levels and burden of caregivers were similar to those who were living together with clients, and around 25% of both groups met GHQ criterion for having a mental disorder. Multiple regression analyses of all subjects identified stress with the client's disorder and strain in their own marital relationships as most predictive of their subjective global stress ratings.

IMPLICATIONS

The findings of this study suggest that mental health services should aim to assist key caregivers of people with chronic schizophrenic disorders to manage stress whether or not the client lives in the same household as the caregiver.

Source: "The Caregiver's Stresses When Living Together or Apart from Patients with Chronic Schizophrenia," by T. M. Laidlaw, J. H. Coverdale, I. R. Falloon, and R. R. Kydd, 2002, *Community Mental Health Journal*, *38*(4), pp. 302–310.

(the emphasis is on the locus of the practice). Community nursing, as presently practiced, is client centered and eclectic in its approach. Case management and ACT described herein are interventions that would fit into the category of client-centered care.

Case Management Model

As noted earlier, some clients do not fit into one service system but require multiple systems simultaneously. For example, clients who have a dual diagnosis, such as a substance abuse problem and a psychiatric disorder, would require services from multiple providers. Some clients suffering from depression who attempt to self-treat their depression with alcohol, for example, may become addicted. Such clients will probably need the services of a psychiatrist, psychiatric nurse, social worker, substance abuse counselor, and perhaps even a vocational rehabilitation counselor. A case manager orchestrates the necessary services. Clients with mental illness who also have acquired immunodeficiency syndrome/human immunodeficiency virus (AIDS/HIV) need services from the general health sector as well as psychiatric services. Again, a case manager could take responsibility for coordinating all those services. Different models of case management, including those that involve paraprofessionals and peer assistance, are being tried (Bedell, Cohen, & Sullivan, 2000). Nurses, because of their unique preparation in a medical framework with a holistic orientation, are often best prepared to serve as a case manager for clients with complex problems.

Clients who are seriously mentally ill or homeless mentally ill may require the more intense services offered by ACT. These services would be directed toward maintaining such clients at their highest level of functioning in a community setting. Nurses are valuable members of such teams.

Capitation and Managed-Care Models

Reimbursement mechanisms that favor cost containment are influencing the patterns of service delivery in community mental health. Capitation and managed care, which are increasingly evident in the general health sector, are examples of **prospective payment systems**. Prospective payment systems provide a predetermined payment for a specific period of time or diagnosis for an individual client. Both these models have as their goal providing effective care at the lowest possible cost and include prospective payment systems.

Capitation is a funding mechanism in which all defined services for a specified period of time are provided for an agreed-on single payment. The payment is tied to the care of a particular client or group of clients. The provider contracts in advance to accept the risk for costs exceeding the agreed-on amount (Donley, 2008).

Managed care is not the same as case management even though the terms are often used interchangeably and they share a similar historical development (Buchda, 2008). **Managed-care** programs are prepaid health plans in which an identified intermediary is given authority to manage how and from whom the client (patient) may obtain services. When managed-care programs include mental health services in their benefit package, the services provided are under the constraints of whatever group provides payment (Donley, 2008). As efforts are made to contain the rising costs of health care, capitation and managed-care programs will have increasing influence in health care delivery.

Public Health Model

Caplan (1964) developed the guiding principles for community mental health nursing in the early years of the community mental health movement. In this model the client is the community rather than the individual, and the focus of practice is the factor that promotes or inhibits mental health. Caplan (1964) focused on preventive psychiatry and introduced three important terms: primary prevention, secondary prevention, and tertiary prevention. This terminology remains relevant to this day (Caplan & Caplan, 2000).

REFLECTIVE THINKING 31-2

Prevention Levels

There has been a rash of "copycat" suicides among 15- to 18-year-old persons in your catchment area in the past year. You notice that many of the suicides occurred during the spring term in two high schools. You are meeting with a group of concerned health professionals to define the problem, identify the major factors, and appraise the strategies that may reduce the incidence of suicide in the target aggregate. Which of the following interventions are representative of (a) primary prevention activities, (b) secondary prevention activities, and (c) tertiary prevention activities?

- Ongoing assessment of students who are receiving failing grades in school
- Teaching concepts of stress management at Parent-Teacher Association (PTA) meetings
- Sending crisis teams into the schools when a suicide has occurred
- Monitoring effectiveness of follow-up appointments in community mental health centers
- Operating a suicide hotline
- Writing an article on teenage suicide for the local newspaper
- Making referrals to support services (e.g., Big Brothers or Big Sisters) as indicated for teens who are seen at the community mental health center for depression
- Establishing a support group for teens dealing with the divorce of their parents
- Teaching the school nurse to identify signs of physical, sexual, and emotional abuse in students
- Supporting legislation for a recreational center for teens in a poor neighborhood
- Teaching parenting skills to prospective parents
- Conducting stress-reduction classes for high school students

Primary prevention refers to activities directed at reducing the incidence of mental disorder within a population.

Primary prevention is a community concept. Aggregates (population groups) at risk of developing the identified mental disorder and environmental factors that may contribute to that risk are targeted. *Population-focused practice* refers to the target population to which the intervention is directed. Primary prevention does not seek to prevent a specific person from developing a mental disorder. Rather, it reduces the risk for aggregates within a population through health promotion. Examples of primary prevention activities engaged in by nurses are (a) teaching classes on stress management to factory workers, (b) conducting support groups for children moving from a small local elementary school to a large consolidated high school, and (c) teaching parenting skills to single, teenage mothers.

Secondary prevention refers to activities directed at reducing the prevalence of mental disorders by shortening the duration of a sufficient number of established cases. This reduction is achieved by encouraging early referrals, decreasing barriers to early diagnosis, and providing effective treatment. Examples of secondary prevention activities engaged in by nurses are (a) staffing rape crisis centers, (b) operating shelters for abused women and their children, and (c) screening clients with debilitating chronic disease who are at high risk for developing depression.

Tertiary prevention activities are aimed at reducing the residual defects that are associated with mental disorders. Examples of tertiary prevention activities engaged in by nurses are (a) teaching social skills to clients enrolled in partial hospitalization programs, (b) monitoring the effectiveness of after-care services with follow-up appointments in community mental health centers, and (c) conducting medication groups for clients in group homes or other transition housing programs.

The services provided in the public health model are based on a community needs assessment. Descriptive statistics found in public records and reports provide social indicators that are highly correlated with mental health problems. Income level, marital status, population density, and crime statistics are examples of social indicators that may be used.

Epidemiological studies that examine the incidence and prevalence of mental disorders in a specific catchment area are also used. Chapter 8 in this text describes several major epidemiological studies that were conducted to assess the needs of large groups. Data from such studies often serve as the basis of the work done by task forces composed of experts from several disciplines who come together to explore the information and make recommendations for addressing the problems noted. An example of such a task force is given in the Report of the Federal Task Force on Homelessness and Severe Mental Illness (1992). *Healthy People 2010* (U.S. Department of Health and Human Services, 2000) is another example.

In addition, local community mental health centers regularly collect data on the people they serve. Aggregate data are used for the purposes of evaluation of local programs, for reports to funding sources, and to compile the statistics for government agencies. These data are available to legitimate researchers.

In the public health model, the role of the nurse is largely collaborative. The nurse, functioning as part of a team of health professionals (a) assesses the needs of the community; (b) identifies and determines priorities for high-risk aggregates (population groups); and (c) designs, implements, and evaluates appropriate interventions. Few nurses function primarily in this model partly because basic nursing education seldom prepares nurses adequately for this role. Instead, social workers and psychologists dominate administrative and

RESEARCH Highlight 31-3

Supported Employment

STUDY PROBLEM/PURPOSE

To examine the outcomes of supported employment 10 years after an initial demonstration project.

METHODS

Thirty-six clients, who had participated in a supported employment program at one of two mental health centers in 1990 or 1992, were interviewed 10 years after program completion about their employment history, facilitators to their employment, and their perceptions of how working affected areas of their lives.

FINDINGS

Seventy-five percent of the participants worked beyond the initial study period, with 33% who worked at least 5 years during the 10-year period. Current and recent jobs tended to be competitive and long term; the average job tenure was 32 months. Few clients, however, made the transition to full-time employment with health benefits. Clients reported improvements in self-esteem, hope, relationships, and control of substance abuse.

IMPLICATIONS

On the basis of this small sample, supported employment seems to be more effective over the long term, with benefits lasting beyond the first 1 to 2 years.

Source: "A Ten-Year Follow-Up of a Supported Employment Program," by M. P. Salyers, D. R. Becker, R. E. Drake, W. C. Torrey, and P. F. Wyzik, 2004, *Psychiatric Services*, *55*(3), 302–308.

managerial positions in the public health model. As nurses become better educated in community interventions, it can be surmised that nurses will return to exercise their original role in the community, and not be limited to tasks such as administering medications to the chronically mentally ill.

Nurses will increasingly function in a collaborative manner with many disciplines. For example, mounting evidence suggests that mental health problems relate to the built environment such as homes, schools, workplaces, parks, industrial areas, farms, and roadways. Preliminary research suggests that sustainable communities offer mental health benefits. Considering the complexity of our lived environment, understanding its influence on mental health demands a community-based, multilevel, and interdisciplinary research approach. Nurses need to appreciate the multiple aspects of what constitutes a healthful environment and be prepared to consult with persons responsible for the design and building of our environment (Srinivasan, O'Fallon, & Dearry, 2003).

FUTURE DIRECTIONS

Nurses are often valued in community mental health because of their traditional nursing skills, which are well known and readily accepted by psychiatrists. In the client-centered model, nurses already take responsibility for medication management and participate in outreach programs, such as family support groups. Nurses can be expected to serve as case managers and play an increasingly important role in the rehabilitation of long-term mentally ill clients. The added skills of nurse practitioners will make nurses even more valuable in the management of the seriously mentally ill. The variable educational preparation of nurses, however, complicates the situation. When salary scales are based on the number of years of basic preparation, nurses with associate degrees or diplomas compare unfavorably with psychologists and social workers with baccalaureate or master's degrees. At the same time, the salary scale for nurses working in hospitals is generally higher in contrast to that of nurses working in community mental health centers. Psychiatric nurses working in inpatient settings are developing an awareness of the need for rehabilitation services for clients who experience long-term mental illness. With the advent of managed care, more nurses will move to rehabilitation-oriented community-based settings, some of which may be under the auspices of the psychiatric inpatient unit (Lauterbach, 2001; Thompson-Heisterman, 2008). Community health nurses in a managed-care system will need to be prepared to serve clients who have mental health problems as well as other health problems (McElmurry, Park, & Busch, 2003). Nurses in all settings will need to expand beyond their traditional roles and take their place as members of interdisciplinary teams. Collaboration among all agencies is essential to providing quality care to the mentally ill.

Nurses for the twenty-first century will need to provide mental health care to an increasingly diverse society. An understanding of culture as a group of persons with common race or ethnicity and shared values, norms, and behaviors is not sufficient. There is increasing diversity within such groupings. A cultural assessment, one's own as well as that of one's client, is needed to provide culturally congruent mental health care. Efforts to reconcile the differences between the two cultural perspectives are required to design effective interventions. The acknowledgment of an emerging global perspective is essential to being a culturally competent nurse (Andrews & Boyle, 2008).

KEY CONCEPTS

- There are commonalities and differences among community health nursing, public health nursing, and home health nursing.
- Despite unevenness, the focus of mental health care is moving steadily toward community-based care.
- Community mental health centers strive to meet their goals of providing accessible, comprehensive mental health services, but fluctuation in funding is a continuing challenge.
- Deinstitutionalization of seriously mentally ill clients has dramatically altered the services provided by nurses working in community mental health centers.
- Consumers and their families are important collaborative partners in planning mental health care.
- Case management requires an understanding of the special needs of the target population, the individual, and community resources.
- Capitation and managed care are increasingly affecting services provided by community mental health centers.
- Nurses have skills that uniquely prepare them to work with the high-risk populations served by community mental health centers.

REVIEW QUESTIONS

1. The community health nurse plans to visit the area high schools to discuss the "Say No to Drugs" program to provide students with knowledge and techniques for avoiding alcohol use. The nurse's plan focuses on which level of prevention?
   1. Primary prevention
   2. Secondary prevention
   3. Tertiary prevention
   4. It is not a level of prevention

2. The nurse's discharge teaching for a client hospitalized for withdrawal from alcohol would include encouraging the client to attend Alcoholics Anonymous Association meetings several times per week after discharge. Attending these meetings would be considered which level of prevention?
   1. Primary prevention
   2. Secondary prevention
   3. Tertiary prevention
   4. It is not a level of prevention

3. The nurse works in a community health facility that utilizes a case management approach. The nurse knows that which of the following is characteristic of this form of distributing health care?
   1. Case management is a system that can be applied to any population in need without significant modification
   2. Case management requires an understanding of the special needs of the target population, the individual, and the community
   3. Case management works well in urban environments but has been largely ineffective in rural areas
   4. The case management method is only appropriate when dealing with clients with relatively minor bouts of mental illness

4. A comprehensive mental health center provides which of the following supplementary services?
   1. Diagnostic services, vocational counseling, research, and evaluation
   2. Counseling, 24-hour emergency help, diagnostic services, and evaluation
   3. Research, short and long-term hospitalization, and outpatient treatment
   4. Short-term hospitalization, partial hospitalization, outpatient treatment, and vocational counseling.

5. A pregnant client has come to the clinic for her regularly scheduled appointment. You notice that the client's gait is unsteady, her words are slurred, and she smells of alcohol. Important health teaching for the client regarding her drinking while pregnant would include which of the following?
   1. She is acting like an unfit mother
   2. The baby might have congenital anomalies
   3. The baby is not affected by her drinking
   4. The child could be born with fetal alcohol syndrome

LEARNING ACTIVITIES

1. Describe the changing focus of mental health care, and explain the major factors that influenced the change in focus.

2. What is meant by a community-based, population-focused approach to planning, delivering, and evaluating nursing care?

3. What are the goals of community-based mental health care?
4. Explain two models for practice for community mental health nursing.
5. What is the nurse's role in designing, managing, monitoring, and evaluating systems of care that address mental health problems experienced by aggregates?
6. Relate the process of community mental health planning for a specific aggregate.
7. Explain three selected strategies that can be used to improve the health status of a target aggregate (population group) in your community.
8. Name an intervention activity for each of the following categories: primary prevention, secondary prevention, and tertiary prevention.

*Study*WARE™ CONNECTION

Using your *Study*WARE™ CD-ROM

1. Complete the Flashcard activity for this chapter.
2. Review the audio glossary for key terms in this chapter.
3. Explore the other games and activities that support this chapter.

REFERENCES

Andrews, M. M., & Boyle, J. S. (2008). *Transcultural concepts in nursing care* (5th ed.). Philadelphia: Wolters Kluwer/Lippincott Williams & Wilkins.

Angell, B., & Test, M. A. (2002). The relationship of clinical factors and environmental opportunities to social functioning in young adults with schizophrenia. *Schizophrenia Bulletin, 28*(2), 259–271.

Bartol, G. M., & Courts, N. F. (2008). The psychophysiology of body-mind healing. In B. M. Dossey &, L. Keegan, (Eds.), *Holistic nursing* (pp. 601–615). Boston: Jones & Bartlett.

Bedell, J. R., Cohen, N. L., & Sullivan, A. (2000). Case management: The current best practices and the next generation of innovation. *Journal of Community Mental Health, 36*(2), 179–194.

Beers, C. W. (1921). *A mind that found itself.* Garden City, NY: Doubleday.

Buchda, V. L. (2008). Managing and providing care. In R. K. Kearney-Nunnery (Ed.), *Advancing your career: Concepts of professional nursing* (pp. 244–258). Philadelphia: F. A. Davis.

Caplan, G. (1964). *Principles of preventive psychiatry.* New York: Basic Books.

Caplan, G., & Caplan, R. (2000). Principles of community psychiatry. *Journal of Community Mental Health, 36*(1), 7–24.

Dieckmann, J. (2008). History of public health and community health nursing. In M. Stanhope & J. Lancaster. (2008). *Public health nursing: Population centered health care in the community* (7th ed., pp. 27–28). Philadelphia: Elsevier.

Donley, R. (2008). Health care agenda and reform. In R. K. Kearney-Nunnery (Ed.), *Advancing your career: Concepts of professional nursing* (pp. 403–416). Philadelphia: F. A. Davis.

Drake, R. E., Green, A. I., Mueser, K. T., & Goldman, H. H. (2003). The history of community mental health treatment and rehabilitation for persons with severe mental illness. *Community Mental Health Journal, 39*(5), 427–450.

Duke University Medical Center, Division of Social and Community Psychiatry, Department of Psychiatry. (1993). *Hospital without walls.* Study Guide for distribution with videotape. Francell, C. G., Conn, V. S., & Gray, D. P. (1988). Family perspectives of burden of care for chronically mentally ill. *Hospital and Community Psychiatry, 39,* 1296–1300.

Francell, C.G., Conn, V.S., & Gray, D.P. (1988). Family perspectives of burdon of care for the chronically mentally ill. *Hospital and Community Psychiatry,* 39, 1296–1300.

Kearney-Nunnery, R. K. (2008). *Advancing your career: Concepts of professional nursing.* Philadelphia: F. A. Davis.

Laidlaw, T. M., Coverdale, J. H., Falloon, I. R., & Kydd, R. R. (2002). Caregivers' stresses when living together or apart from patients with chromic schizophrenia. *Community Mental Health Journal, 38*(4), 303–310.

Lauterbach, S. S. (2001). Mental health in the community. In K. S. Lundy & S. Janes, *Community health nursing. Caring for the public's health* (pp. 836–861). Sudbury, MA: Jones & Bartlett.

Lefley, H. P. (1999). What does "community" mean for persons with mental illness? *New Directions in Mental Health Services, 83* (Fall), 3–12.

McElmurry, B. J., Park C. G., & Busch, A. G. (2003). The nurse-community health advocate team for urban immigrant primary health care. *Journal of Nursing Scholarship, 35*(3), 275–281.

Mental Health System Act. (1980). 96th Congress. Public Law 96-398, Sec. 9501, Amendment to Senate Bill 1177, September 23.

Miller, J. E. (2003, Summer/Fall). Reform and revolution: President Bush's New Freedom Commission. *NAMI Advocate, 25*(1), 11–12.

NAMI. (2009). *NAMI education training and peer support center programs.* Retrieved from: http://www.nami.org/namiland09/FullEducationProgramBook.pdf

National Institute of Mental Health (NIMH). (1987). *Toward a model plan for a comprehensive, community-based mental health system.* Rockville, MD: U.S. Public Health Service, Alcohol, Drug Abuse, and Mental Health Administration, Division of Education and Service System Liaison.

Report of the Federal Task Force on Homelessness and Severe Mental Illness. (1992). *Outcasts on main street* (ADM 92-1904). Washington, DC: Author.

Salyers, M. P., Becker, D. R., Drake, R. E., Torrey, W. C., & Wyzik, P. F. (2004). A ten-year follow-up of a supported employment program. *Psychiatric Services, 55*(3), 302–308.

Satel, S. (2003, November 1). Out if the asylum, into the cell. *New York Times,* Opinion.

Sebastian, J. G., & Martin, K. S. (2008). The nurse in home health and hospice. In M. Stanhope & J. Lancaster. (2008). *Public health nursing: Population-centered health care in the community* (7th ed.; pp. 960–961). Philadelphia Elsevier.

Srinivasan, S., O'Fallon, L. R., & Dearry, A. (2003). Creating healthy communities, healthy homes, healthy people: Initiating a research agenda on the built environment and public health. *American Journal of Public Health, 93*(9) 1446–1450.

Stanhope, M., & Lancaster, J. (2003). *Community and public health nursing* (6th ed.). St. Louis: Elsevier Science.

Thompson-Heisterman, A. (2008). Mental health issues. In M. Stanhope & J. Lancaster, *Public health nursing: Population-centered health care in the community* (7th ed.; pp. 784–805). Philadelphia Elsevier.

U.S. Department of Health and Human Services. (2000). *Healthy People 2010.* Washington, DC: U.S. Government Printing Office.

SUGGESTED READINGS

Babiss, F. (2004). *Ethnographic study of mental health treatment and outcomes: Doing what works.* Binghamton, NY: Haworth Press.

Bellack, A. S. (2006). Scientific and consumer models of recovery in schizophrenia: Concordance, contrasts, and implications. *Schizophrenia Bulletin, 33*(3), 432–442.

Engstrom, T. H. & Robison, W. L. (2006). *Health care reform: Ethics and politics.* Rochester, NY: University of Rochester Press.

Glasser, W. (2004). *Warning: Psychiatry can be hazardous to your mental health.* New York: Harper Collins.

Kovner, A. R., & Knickman, J. R. (2008). *Jonas and Kovner's health care delivery in the United States.* (Eds). New York: Springer.

Stanhope, M., & Lancaster, J. (2006). *Foundations of nursing in the community* (2nd. ed.). St. Louis: Mosby Elsevier.

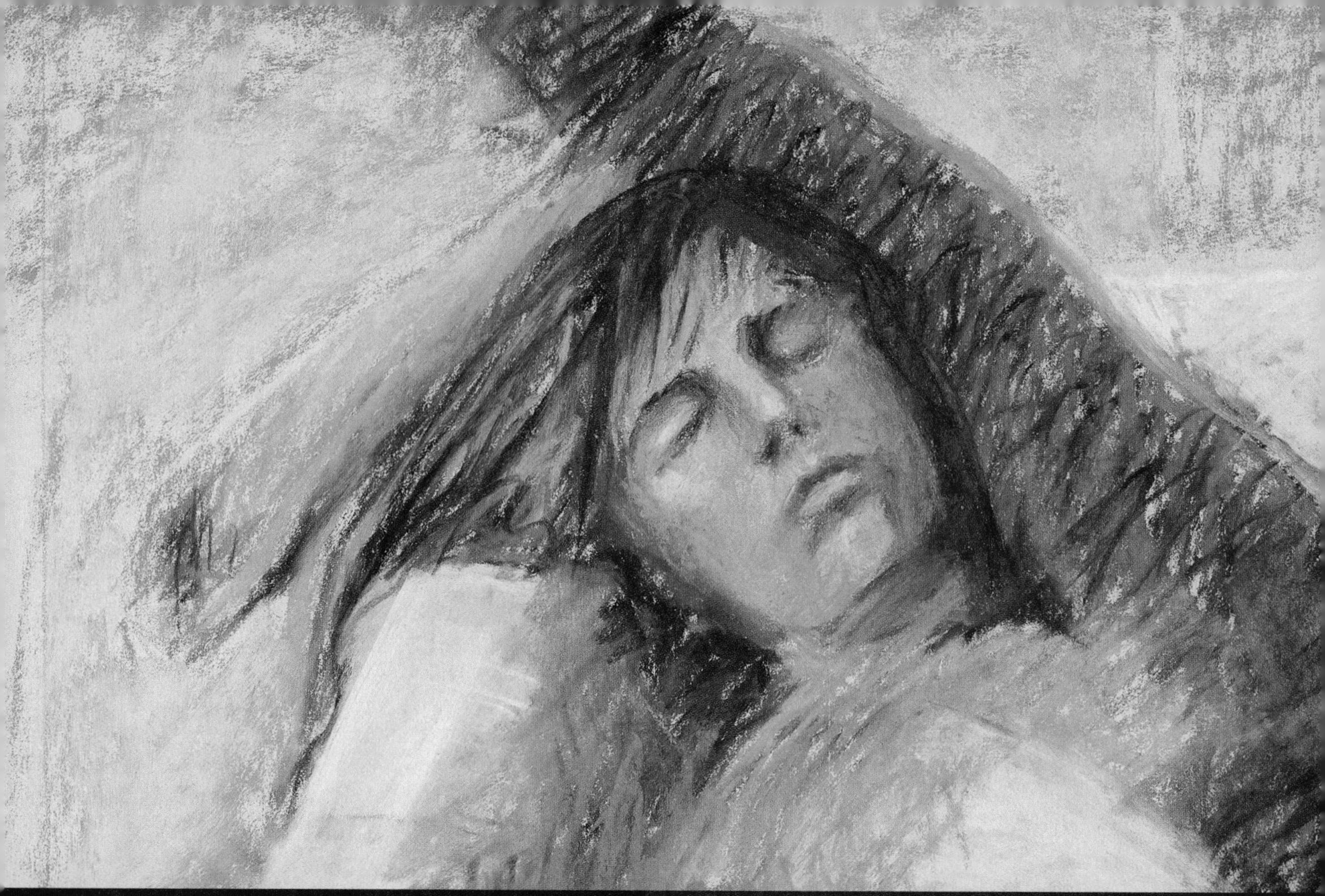

Relax, Close Your Eyes

Using Complementary Therapies in Daily Life

Different people deal with stress and tension in various ways. What do you do to relax? Do you take a warm bath or soak your feet? Sit under a tree? Fantasize? Play a sport or do some physical exercise?

- *Try practicing guided imagery informally to help you manage stressful situations. Close your eyes and imagine that you are in your favorite place. Involve as many of your senses as you can (sight, smell, touch, hearing, etc.). Do you experience any changes in your level of relaxation as a result of completing this exercise?*
- *Have you ever used music as a form of emotional outlet, perhaps to relieve stress or to help deal with painful emotions such as sadness or loneliness? What type(s) of music do you find to be uplifting in such situations?*
- *Think about the role of physical touch in your own life. Do you come from a family background where expression of comfort and support through physical touch is encouraged or discouraged? As a nursing professional, how comfortable would you be with using appropriate physical touch with a client?*

CHAPTER 32

Complementary and Somatic Therapies

NOREEN CAVAN FRISCH
LAWRENCE E. FRISCH

CHAPTER OUTLINE

COMPETENCIES

Upon completion of this chapter, the reader should be able to:

1. Describe the use of six complementary modalities as nursing interventions in psychiatric mental health care: relaxation and guided imagery, hypnosis, massage, energy-based modalities (therapeutic touch [TT] and healing touch), music therapy, and animal-assisted therapy.
2. Intervene to control escalating anger in a client.
3. Describe the use of physical restraints and seclusion in control of violent behavior.
4. Describe the use of light therapy for treatment of seasonal affective disorder (SAD).
5. Describe the current indications for electroconvulsive therapy (ECT), and provide nursing care to a client undergoing the procedure.

KEY TERMS

Anger Control Assistance
Animal-Assisted Therapy
Complementary Modalities
Electroconvulsive Therapy (ECT)
Energy-Based Modalities
Guided Imagery
Healing Touch
Hypnosis
Light Therapy (Phototherapy)
Massage
Music Therapy
Relaxation
Seclusion
Somatic Therapies
Therapeutic Imagery
Therapeutic Massage
Therapeutic Touch (TT)

The goal of the chapter is to broaden the reader's knowledge of the scope of nursing practice relevant to psychiatric mental health care by providing the reader with information on a wide range of interventions commonly used in psychiatric mental health nursing. The chapter is divided into three sections: one on complementary modalities, one on somatic interventions within the domain of nursing practice, and the third section on collaborative interventions. **Complementary modalities** are those modalities used as an adjunct to medical care and psychiatric treatment that are thought to have effects on stress, sleep disturbance, anxiety, or other emotions. Other interventions, known as **somatic therapies**, comprise a miscellaneous set of therapies that have long been used in the management of psychiatric symptoms, for example, use of seclusion or physical restraints to control anger. Both complementary and somatic modalities have a useful role in modern-day nursing care, and each of the interventions discussed in the chapter is listed in the fifth edition of the Nursing Interventions Classification (NIC; discussed in Chapter 4). Each of these interventions is presented along with specific practice examples to illustrate recommended and appropriate use. In addition, the section on nursing collaborative interventions for specific psychiatric somatic therapies outlines the nursing care required for the client undergoing specific procedures that must be ordered and carried out with physician/psychiatrist orders.

COMPLEMENTARY MODALITIES

Table 32-1 provides a summary of the complementary modalities discussed in this section and indicates when the modality is most useful in psychiatric mental health care. The discussion on individual modalities will serve as an introduction, but is not comprehensive. Since there is no standard listing of complementary modalities, we have almost certainly omitted some that readers (or their clients) would find of interest. Each of the modalities and techniques described requires further study and, in many cases, certification as a practitioner to incorporate into practice. Refer to the resource list at the end of the chapter for contact information regarding further study. Because these therapies are quite different and often greatly influenced by skills, techniques, and setting, good empirical assessments of their effectiveness have been difficult to perform. Several authors have reviewed the available evidence on treatment effectiveness (Mamtani & Cimino, 2002; Mantle, 2002). Readers must not forget that many clients seek out these modalities in addition to, or sometimes in lieu of, conventional psychiatric therapies (Elkins, Rajab, & Marcus, 2005). As a result, the nurse needs to ask about clients' interest in and involvement with complementary therapies, even if she does not personally provide them.

RELAXATION

Relaxation is defined as a psychophysiological state characterized by parasympathetic dominance involving multiple visceral and somatic symptoms, including the absence of physical, mental, and emotional tension (Kolkmeier, 1988). Relaxation permits a person to quiet himself, retreat mentally from his surroundings, and decrease tension, anxiety, or pain.

The term *relaxation response* was first used by Herbert Benson when referring to the psychophysiological state where muscles are relaxed; tension is released; blood pressure, heart rate, and respiratory rate are decreased; the brain

TABLE 32-1 Complementary Modalities in Psychiatric Mental Health Care

MODALITY	DEFINITION	USE IN PSYCHIATRIC MENTAL HEALTH CARE
Relaxation	Use of techniques to elicit a relaxation response	Antidote to stress/anxiety
Guided imagery	Use of sensory images to enhance relaxation and healing	Helpful in reducing depression and overcoming addictions
Hypnosis, hypnotherapy	Assisting the client to an altered state of consciousness	Adjunct to psychotherapy; helpful in overcoming addictions
Massage	Stimulation of the skin and underlying tissues	Produces relaxation; helpful to induce sleep; meets client's need for "safe" touch
Energy-based modalities	Nursing interventions based on the concept of the human energy field	Helpful in reducing anxiety/stress, working through grief, and assisting in addictions recovery
Music therapy	Use of music to alter behavior, emotions, and/or physiology	Reduces anxiety; promotes sleep
Pet-assisted therapy	Use of animals to provide affection, attention, diversion, and relaxation	Decreases feelings of loneliness; increases socialization; provides diversional activities

is in the alpha state; and the parasympathetic nervous system is activated. When the parasympathetic system is activated, the person feels calm (as opposed to the sympathetic system associated with the fight-or-flight response); the alpha brain wave state is a deepened state of relaxation. Assisting a client to achieve a relaxation state is an "antidote to stress" and helps the client to access inner resources that may have been obscured by the anxious state (Shames, 1996). The nurse understands that many times people are told to "just relax" and find they cannot. Relaxation is a skill that requires learning and practice. It is an art and also an expression or process (Anselmo, 2009). Nurses also find that relaxation is a practice that helps nurses themselves in areas of self-care and readiness to be fully present in their work with clients.

Several techniques are used by nurses to activate the relaxation response. All begin by starting in a quiet, relaxed area, breathing deeply, and concentrating on quiet and calm. Progressive muscle relaxation (PMR) is a technique of alternately tensing and relaxing muscle groups throughout the body to become aware of tensions and the contrast between muscle tension and relaxation. Persons undergoing PMR are led through sessions by the nurse, who coaches them to assume a comfortable position and suggests the process of tensing and releasing major muscle groups (working from the feet to the head):

> *The client is first encouraged to take several deep breaths and relax. He is then advised to feel his feet on the floor. Next he is told to squeeze the muscles in his feet and perhaps scrunch his toes and tighten his feet until his feet feel small, perhaps round. Then, the client is told to relax those muscles. This technique serves to focus attention on body parts, one by one, and to make the client very aware of what it feels like when that part is tense, and how it feels to relax that same part. (Shames, 1996, p. 74)*

Persons receiving PMR as a treatment are able to get in touch with tensions and become aware of how these tensions are affecting their physical body. For clients completing this technique, there is frequently a sense of relief and a subjective sense of letting go of the tensions. PMR is particularly helpful for clients who feel tense, anxious, or agitated, and may be preferable to passive exercises (Anselmo, 2009).

Other relaxation techniques include "countdown" and eye muscle tightening and relaxing. Countdown is a technique in which the client is advised to count down slowly from 10 to 0 and to feel both refreshed and relaxed when he reaches 0. Eye muscle tightening and relaxing is done while the client is in a comfortable position with his eyes open. He is instructed to focus intently on an object, which results in a certain amount of eye muscle tightening and fatigue. He is then instructed to relieve the fatigue by closing his eyes. Shames (1996) states: "The juxtaposition of the tightening followed by the relaxation encourages the onset of a relaxed state" (p. 75).

Many clients will learn that they can induce their own relaxation response at home after practicing the techniques and sometimes with the addition of an audiotape that leads them through the process of PMR. The purpose of using relaxation techniques in nursing practice is to help the client first acknowledge the degree to which he feels tension and anxiety, to provide a contrast to the daily experience of tension by teaching relaxation, and to give the client the ability to use relaxation therapy as a self-help intervention. A comprehensive review and meta-analysis based on 11 clinical trials has shown that relaxation therapies clearly benefit clients with depression, though the degree of benefit was likely not

Dhârâna
by Frederick Horgman Varley

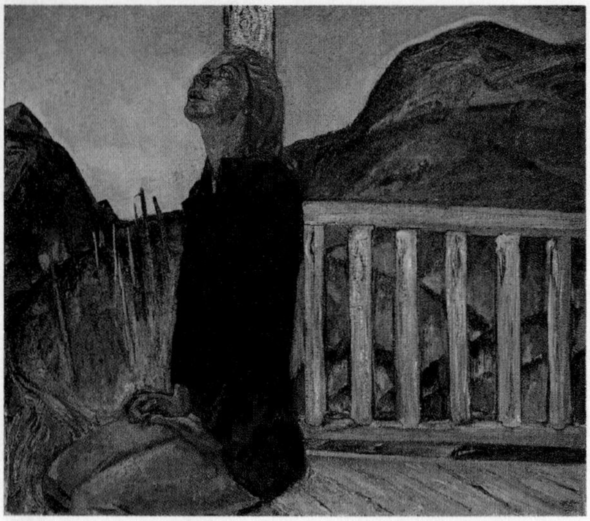

Courtesy: Fredrick Horgman Varley, Canadian 1881–1969, Copyright © 1932. Canadian 1881–1969 Oil on canvas 86.4 × 101.6 cm. Art Gallery of Ontario, Toronto. Gift from the Albert H. Robson Memorial Subscription Fund, 1942.

While never abandoning his strong Christian beliefs, Varley was deeply attracted to Eastern thought and to the mysteries of nature revealed in the remote Canadian wilderness. (See his painting of Arctic icebergs in Chapter 7.) *Dhârâna* combines his appreciation of nature and of the spirit in one powerful vision of deep meditation.

as great as with more conventional psychotherapy (Jorm, Morgan, & Hetrick, 2008). Further studies will be required to determine whether the combination of conventional treatment and relaxation offers added benefit. A similar review was unable to show comparable benefit for meditation in anxiety and concluded as well that further studies are needed (Krisanaprakornkit, Krisanaprakornkit, Piyavhatkul, & Laopaiboon, 2006). A study involving more than 100 healthy adults did show that brief training in meditation-based relaxation was able to significantly reduce feelings of anxiety and depression as measured on a variety of standardized psychological instruments (Lane, Seskevich, & Pieper, 2007). However, the absence of a control group in this study and the inclusion only of persons "interested in learning meditation for stress reduction," along with limited follow-up, make the validity of the authors' conclusions uncertain.

Guided Imagery

A technique that goes hand in hand with relaxation, guided imagery builds on the relaxation response and adds visual or other sensory images to enhance the relaxation and to present an image for the client that is one of healing (Reed, 2007). **Therapeutic imagery** is defined as the ability to take one's natural thought processes and to direct these thoughts in a creative way, potentiating a positive outcome. Shames (1996) defined **guided imagery** as an "unconditional process in which the practitioner leads the subject with specific words, suggestions, symbols, or images to elicit a positive response" (p. 71).

One example of a simple guided imagery technique is a "pleasant memory technique" in which a client who is comfortable and relaxed is told to close his eyes and is given the suggestion to think back to an enjoyable event. Thinking of a pleasant event can bring many positive sensations to the client, as he will remember sights, sounds, and smells of a joyful time. For example, one client might remember being in his grandmother's kitchen, smelling and eating homemade bread; another might remember walking in an attractive park, with sounds and smells of being in the woods. This technique can be extended to ask the client to think of a "special place" or a "safe place" where he has positive memories. A client can use his imagination to remember a place and experience being there. This technique has been useful when nurses are working with clients who will be undergoing medical procedures that are uncomfortable, or scary, or both. The nurse can suggest that the client return to the pleasant place brought up in his memory and think about being there rather than in the medical office, dentist's chair, or other similarly negative situation. The nurse will assist the client in developing the scene by asking questions such as: "How does it look?" "What does it smell like?" "What does it feel like?" The nurse chooses words or phrases that convey positive images and may suggest sensations like floating, releasing, washing away the pain/discomfort, and so on. To end a guided imagery session, the nurse will encourage the patient to express thoughts and feelings about the experience to whatever degree the client is comfortable disclosing his personal experiences.

Relaxation and guided imagery techniques have great use in nursing practice. As mentioned earlier, there is use in preparing clients to go through procedures, but there are other documented uses as well. Relaxation and imagery have long been used in maternity care for preparation for and management of labor and childbirth. One nurse researcher has documented the use of guided imagery in hospitalized, depressed children and found it is an effective technique in reducing measured depression (Bufe, 1994). Guided imagery is beneficial for clients undergoing chemotherapy and cancer treatments (Troesch, Rodehaver, Delaney, & Yanes, 1993; Sloman, 1995; Roffe, Schmidt, & Ernst, 2005). Others have documented a positive role of imagery in assisting clients to overcome addictions (Wynd, 1992; Zimmerman, 1989). These techniques, however, have not been as helpful for clients with severe anxiety disorders; for example, a client experiencing panic attacks will not be able to concentrate on the relaxation exercises and may in fact become more anxious when asked to do so. However, in situations where the client is undergoing stress, relaxation and imagery are two nursing interventions that give nurses tools to use in a highly stressful world (Reed, 2007). They are noninvasive techniques that can assist the client to regain control, both for the moment as in using imagery while undergoing a procedure or in the long term as in using imagery to give up an addiction such as cigarette smoking.

The nurse is cautioned, however, that imagery is never recommended for use with clients who are psychotic or who have a background of schizophrenia: "It is generally considered that these people are often bombarded with too many images already, and are unable to differentiate between those they choose to envision and those that plague their mental processes involuntarily" (Shames, 1996, p. 95). The therapeutic use of imagery demands an ability to sustain one's focus and concentration, and clients who are psychotic or schizophrenic are usually unable to maintain these components.

The processes of relaxation and guided imagery are discussed here for nursing practice at the elementary level. These interventions are both listed and described in the NIC (Bulechek, Butcher, & Dochterman, 2008). Both of these techniques, however, can be practiced at intermediate and advanced levels for those who seek additional education. The technique called interactive guided imagery was developed by the faculty at the Academy for Guided Imagery in Mill Valley, California. Interactive guided imagery is described as "a powerful modality for helping a patient/client connect with the deeper wellsprings of what is true for them at cognitive, affective, and somatic levels" (Shames, 1996, p. 32). More quantitative evaluations of the effect of guided imagery have been less optimistic, showing a small benefit that may diminish over a few months. The use of imagery requires education, and the reader is referred to the list of resources at the end of the chapter for further information.

Current research in guided imagery seeks to determine characteristics of people who are able to generate a vivid mental image and to experience those images as real. It is believed that some people are more able to image (or have greater "imagery ability") than others. Thus, a means to evaluate imagery ability will provide the nurse with a sense of which clients are most likely to benefit from imagery interventions. Kwekkeboom has developed two tools for this purpose: the Imagery Ability Questionnaire (IAQ) and the Kids Imagery Ability Questionnaire (KIAQ) and reports an acceptable measure of validity and reliability for the tools (Kwekkeboom, 2000; Kwekkeboom, Maddox, & West, 2000). Some of the characteristic of those who can image include responsiveness to stimuli, synesthesia, enhanced cognition, vivid reminiscence, and enhanced awareness. Persons who can image respond positively to statements such as "I can picture a country scene that is so real I can feel that I'm there."

Nursing research on imagery, stress reduction, and touch therapy have shown significant benefit when used to reduce anxiety in clients undergoing invasive cardiac procedures (Seskevich, Crater, Lane, & Krucof, 2004). In contrast, a study utilizing similar modalities with clients who had cancer accompanied by symptoms of anxiety and depression found improvements in depression (but not anxiety) with progressive muscle relaxation and guided imagery (Sloman, 2002).

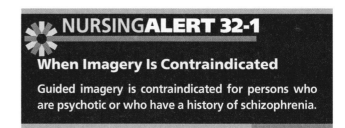

NURSINGALERT 32-1

When Imagery Is Contraindicated

Guided imagery is contraindicated for persons who are psychotic or who have a history of schizophrenia.

RESEARCH Highlight 32-1

Imagery in the Clinical Setting: A Tool for Healing

STUDY PROBLEMS/PURPOSE

To evaluate the use of individualized perioperative imagery sessions on patients' need for pain control in the postoperative period.

METHODS

An experimental group of 30 patients who were to have elective knee or hip replacement surgery were provided individualized imagery sessions. These sessions included relaxation and a "rehearsal" based on their desired outcomes of surgery, followed by a tape-recorded session that the patients could use at will, and a visit by the imagery nurse in the immediate post-surgery recovery period. Data on opioid use for pain post-surgery and an assessment of pain intensity were obtained from this group compared to control group data of 29 patients who received standard care.

FINDINGS

The experimental group demonstrated a significant decrease in perception of pain and a decrease in daily use of opioid pain medication postsurgery, compared to the controls.

IMPLICATIONS

Imagery techniques are noninvasive actions that the nurse and client may choose to use with potential to reduce use of pain medication and to reduce the subjective experience of postsurgical pain. Further research is indicated.

Source: "Imagery in the Clinical Setting: A Tool for Healing," by T. Reed, 2007, *Nursing Clinics of North America*, *42*, 261–277.

HYPNOTHERAPY

Hypnosis is defined as "assisting the client to an altered state of consciousness to create an awareness and a directed focus experience" (McCloskey & Bulechek, 2000, p. 384). The word *hypnosis* actually refers to the induction of sleep. In practice, hypnosis is a technique in which the practitioner is quite active in directing the client and the client is suggestible and in a very relaxed state. Hypnosis has been used in health care to varying degrees of success for centuries. Many anthropologists believe that some form of hypnosis, or trance state, has been used among all known primitive cultures. Its use in modern health care began in the late 1950s, when the technique was used to treat soldiers suffering from postwar traumas of World Wars I and II. The British Medical Society endorsed the practice of hypnosis in medical school education in 1955, and the American Medical Association (AMA) followed (Shames, 1996). Since then, the technique has been used in many areas of medical, dental, and nursing practice. Frequently, hypnosis is used to assist a client to gain relief from pain, which can be either acute (as in childbirth) or chronic (as in arthritis). Recent reports in nursing literature indicate that hypnosis can be successfully used in several areas of reproductive health, including sexual dysfunction, urinary incontinence, chronic pelvic pain, hyperemesis gravidarum, and pain relief during labor and delivery (Baram, 1995; Letts, Baker, Ruderman, & Kennedy, 1993). Other studies indicate a positive effect in pain management (Spira & Speigel, 1992) and in management of migraine (Matthew & Flatt, 1999). Research Highlight 32-2 provides data from a study on sleeping problems in child psychiatric liaison service (Hawkins & Polemikos, 2002). Hypnosis has also been used to alter physiological processes and to assist in changing behaviors such as smoking. For advanced practitioners, hypnotherapy—the use of hypnosis to achieve resolution of psychic trauma and distress—is used along with other forms of psychotherapy. It is important for nurses to understand, however, that memories invoked by hypnosis—vivid as they may be—may or may not accurately reflect true events. This uncertainty about validity of recalled experience may not be important in therapy, but it is vitally important in criminal cases where the use of hypnosis has had a controversial history (Newman & Thompson, 2001).

In nursing practice, the use of hypnosis is governed by licensure laws in each state. Nurses are advised to consult with their state board of nursing or their licensing body regarding regulation governing their locality. In all cases, nurses who practice hypnotherapy must have formal training in the use of the modality. Most often this training is accompanied by a graduate degree and always by a period of supervised work with a faculty member who is an advanced practitioner.

RESEARCH Highlight 32-2

Effectiveness of Hypnosis in Reducing Mild Essential Hypertension: A One-year Follow-up Study

STUDY PROBLEM/PURPOSE

The researchers sought to investigate whether a controlled hypnosis treatment is effective in reducing mild essential hypertension.

METHODS

Adults with hypertension volunteered for the study. The researchers divided the volunteers into two groups: an experimental group that received standard eight-session hypnosis treatments and a control group that was "wait-listed" for the hypnosis sessions. The hypnosis sessions were initiated with techniques to induce relaxation. The subjects were given self-hypnosis practice suggestions at the end of each session.

FINDINGS

For the experimental subjects, both systolic and diastolic blood pressure measures were reduced after the hypnosis treatments. These subjects also had significant reductions in anxiety scores. While many of these individuals practice self-hypnosis, this practice did not influence the findings.

IMPLICATIONS

Hypnosis can be effective in managing essential hypertension.

Source: "Effectiveness of Hypnosis in Reducing Mild Essential Hypertension: A One-year Follow-up Study," by M. C. Kay, 2007, *International Journal of Clinical and Experimental Hypnosis*, *55*(1), 67–83.

Massage and Touch

Massage is the stimulation of the skin and underlying tissues for the purposes of increasing circulation and inducing a relaxation response. Massage and the use of touch have long been a part of nursing practice. Massage techniques include the back rub, a very traditional part of care, frequently given to clients on bedrest, confined to wheelchairs, and before the hours of sleep. Also, techniques of stimulating the skin to increase circulation during bathing are massage techniques. These basic massage techniques are taught to student nurses and are included in texts of fundamentals of nursing skill. Many nurses are skilled in the basic massage movements of *effleurage* (long, soothing strokes) to increase circulation, *tapotement* (stimulating rapid percussive movements), and *petrissage* (kneading motions) for stimulation.

Therapeutic massage is an extension of massage techniques involving deep tissue and advanced massage techniques. Nurses providing therapeutic massage have received advanced education in massage, and many have become certified as massage therapists. The National Association of Nurse Massage Therapists (NANMT) is a resource for nurses wishing to obtain information on advanced education in therapeutic massage. Massage has obvious benefits in inducing relaxation, in assisting with sleep disturbances, and in offering the client contact involving touch. Case reports attest to the perceived benefit of massage therapy in mental health care (Garner, Phillips, Schmidt, Markulev, O'Connor, Wood, et al., 2008), though more formal evaluation remains elusive. Readers may be pleased to learn, however, that when nurses were the recipient of brief daily massages their measured levels of psychological stress decreased—even in the absence of changes in more objective physiologic measures (Bost and Wallis, 2006). For those in advanced massage practice, massage techniques can also assist in healing/repair of muscle trauma.

Simple touch—reaching out to physically contact another—is a therapy too often neglected in busy nursing practice.

Simpler than massage, touch is accessible to all nurses. Jackson and Keegan (2009) write that touch "is perhaps one of our most frequently used, yet least acknowledged of the five recognized senses" (p. 350). Touch is one mechanism of communicating caring, support, and nurturing to clients who may feel isolated and fearful. For example, reaching out to take a client's hand is a way to communicate caring and support. Often, touching a client on the shoulder is a means of letting the person know that the nurse is present and cares about the client.

Early studies documented that the elderly in particular have a need to be touched (Rozema, 1986). One study on the utilization of touch by health care personnel found that clients in the age range of 66 to 100 years received the least amount of touch, when compared with younger patients (Barnett, 1972). Clients in geriatric institutions may well place great importance and value on the smallest gesture of touch as touch leads to a feeling affinity and of belonging to community (Salzmann-Erikson & Erikkson, 2005; Jackson & Keegan, 2009). Particularly related to the elderly are research findings that have documented potential benefits of massage (especially the technique of effleurage) in reducing the risk of pressure ulcer (Duimel-Peeters, Halfens, Berger, & Snoecky, 2005). In mental health practice, massage is thought to be helpful in decreasing agitation in persons with dementia, decreasing stress for seriously ill inpatients that have unfulfilled needs for safe touch and producing calming effects.

Touch, of course, has many personal connotations to both nurses and their clients. The interpretation of touch is both culturally and familially derived. The nurse should never assume that any individual client wants to be touched, must assess the client's individual needs and desires before implementing any form of massage, and should never offer touch in situations where the client is uncomfortable with it. The best means of determining how the client feels is, for example, to state, "Here, you can hold my hand if you like while the procedure is being done," or "I'll put my hand on your shoulder, if you like, while you talk about yesterday's experiences in the group."

RESEARCH Highlight 32-3

Pilot Study Evaluating the Effect of Massage Therapy on Stress, Anxiety, and Aggression in a Young Adult Psychiatric Inpatient Unit

STUDY PROBLEM/PURPOSE

The study purpose was to examine the effectiveness of a relaxation massage therapy program in reducing stress, anxiety, and aggression on a young adult psychiatric inpatient unit.

METHODS

The researchers used a prospective, nonrandomized intervention study design. Participants were patients aged 15–25 years who were invited to participate in the study 24 hours post admission to the psychiatric unit. The massage therapy treatment was a daily, 20-minute session given to the patient who was fully clothed and sitting in a massage chair. Participants were assessed at baseline and prior to discharge from the unit.

FINDINGS

The average number of massage treatments provided to the participating patients was 4.3. Massage therapy had immediate beneficial effects on anxiety-related measures (anxiety, resting heart rate and saliva corisol levels), and may be a useful de-escalating tool for reducing stress and anxiety in hospitalized psychiatric patients.

IMPLICATIONS

This study shows that massage therapy treatments can be incorporated into the daily routine of such units. The authors suggest that massage could be offered to clients for a calming effect and to reduce agitation in lieu of reliance on PRN medications. Further studies in this area, particularly randomized studies, are indicated.

Source: "Pilot study evaluating the effect of massage therapy on stress, anxiety and aggression in a young adult psychiatric inpatient unit," by B. Garner, L. Phillips, H. Schmidt, C. Markulev, J. O'Connor, S. Wood, et al., 2008, *Australian and New Zealand Journal of Psychiatry*, *42*(5), 414–422.

Energy-Based Modalities

For purposes of this chapter, **energy-based modalities** refer to techniques for healing grounded in the notion of the human energy field. The reader will remember that Martha Rogers, the nurse theorist who developed the theory of nursing called the Science of Unitary Human Beings, defined the person as a unified whole possessing individual integrity that is more than and different from the sum of the parts (see Chapter 3). From this perspective, the human being is an energy field that is in constant interactions with the environmental fields.

With the perspective of a human energy field, the nurse can be viewed as an integral part of the client's environmental field. Thus, healing interventions can be performed where the "nurse uses his or her hands as a mediating focus in the continuing patternings of the mutual patient-environmental energy field process" (Meeham, 1990, p. 74). The best-known nursing intervention using the human energy field perspective is therapeutic touch. However, there are several other techniques and approaches based on the same or similar ideas of working within the client's energy field to balance the energy through interaction with the nurse. Figure 32-1 is an illustration of human interaction seen as an energy exchange of two energy fields. In energy-based work, the nurse develops skills to assess the balance of the client's field and effect changes through the nurse's own energy patterning.

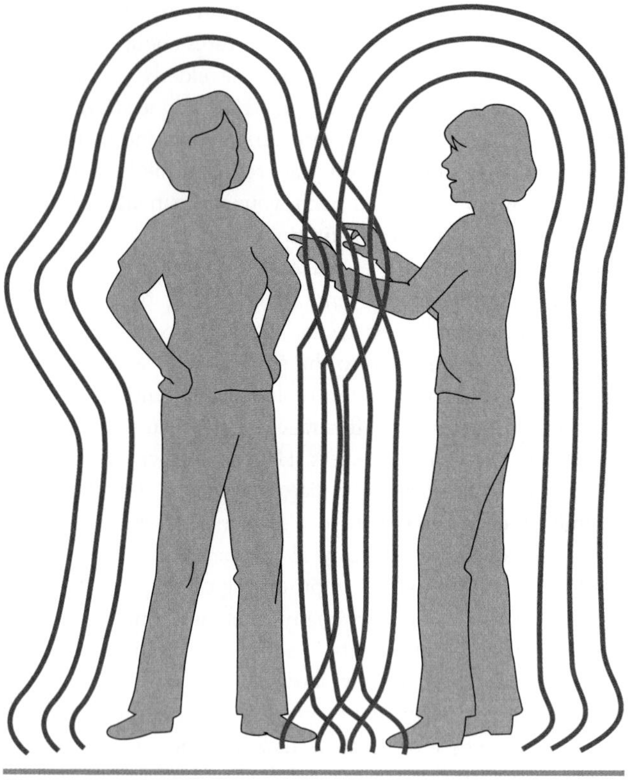

FIGURE 32-1 **Human interaction as an exchange of energy between two fields** (DELMAR/CENGAGE LEARNING.)

Therapeutic Touch

Therapeutic touch (TT) is a specific technique developed in the 1970s by Dolores Krieger (1979) at New York University. TT is a five-step process of centering; assessing the client's energy field; smoothing, or "unruffling," the field; modulating or transferring energy; and knowing when to stop. Krieger describes TT as "a contemporary interpretation of several ancient healing practices. These practices consist of learned skills for consciously directing or sensitively modulating human energies" (Krieger, 1993, p. 11). This five-step procedure is often referred to as the Krieger-Kunz Method of Therapeutic Touch, in acknowledgment of Krieger's work and that of her colleague, Dora Kunz.

The technique of TT has been widely investigated by nurses, beginning with Krieger herself. In 1988, Quinn published a review article of the state of TT research from the time period 1974 to 1986, and Scandrett-Hibdon did so in 1996. Work continues on the modality, and findings have shown TT to have a positive and consistent effect in producing a relaxation response. In some situations, TT has been effective in controlling headache pain, relieving pain in cancer treatments, reducing anxiety, promoting wound healing, and impacting the treatment of alcohol and drug abuse and the behavioral symptoms of dementia (Jackson, Kelley, McNeil, Meyor, Schlegel, & Eaton, 2008; Woods, Craven, & Whitney, 2005; Hagemaster, 2000; Keller & Bzdek, 1986; Gange & Toye, 1994; Olson & Sneed, 1995; Quinn, 1981, 1983; Wirth, Richardson, Eidelman, & O'Malley, 1993). While an extensive review of the research literature on TT is beyond the scope of this chapter, the reader is referred to the review articles cited and to the organization Nurse Healer's Professional Associates (see end of chapter) for detailed information on the topic. TT is currently listed in the NIC as a nursing intervention that involves "Attuning to the universal healing field, seeking to act as an instrument for healing influence, and using the natural sensitivity of the hands to gently focus and direct the intervention process" (Bulechek, et al., 2008, p. 751).

Healing Touch

Healing touch is a program of study that involves a "systematic approach to healing using several energy interventions that incorporate a variety of therapeutic maneuvers" (Scandrett-Hibdon, 1996, p. 27). Some of these interventions include full-body techniques, in which the maneuvers are used over the entire body to complete balancing of the entire energy field. Other techniques are localized to affect a specific clinical outcome, for example, a "mind-clearing" technique used for relaxation and to focus the mind (Mentgen, 1996). These healing touch techniques all involve work with the energy field

RESEARCH Highlight 32-4

Effects of Healing Touch on Stress Perception and Biological Correlates

STUDY PURPOSE/PROBLEM

The researchers investigated the effects of specific healing touch techniques on physiological and psychological relaxation.

METHODS

A quantitative study using repeated measures, quasiexperimental design was used with 30 healthy volunteer subjects. The subjects received two healing touch interventions: "hands moving" and "chakra connection." They were assessed through use of standardized measures of anxiety (State-Trait Anxiety Inventory), heart rate, blood pressure, muscle tension, skin conductance, and skin temperature.

FINDINGS

Physiological measures indicated that healing touch is associated with relaxation. Further, 63% of the participants described their experiences as relaxing.

IMPLICATIONS

Further study is needed, but study indicates that healing touch may promote relaxation in both the physiological and psychological domains.

Source: "Effects of Healing Touch on Stress Perception and Biological Correlates," by J. A. Maville and G. Bowen, 2008, *Holistic Nursing Practice*, *22*(2), 103–110.

and are based on the assumptions described previously. All of the healing touch techniques have been published and are available for the student wishing further information on the subject (Hover-Kramer & Mentgen, 2002).

Energy-Based Modalities in Psychiatric Mental Health Care

Hover-Kramer (1996; 2002) describes several uses of energy-based techniques in mental health care. She indicates that emotional distress, such as that seen during grief, depression, anxiety, and stress, causes imbalances in the energy field. When a psychotherapist is able to work with the energy field at the same time that he is working with the subjective and verbal expression of the distress, he is able to offer the client an additional powerful technique to help the client to restore harmony and balance. Hover-Kramer (1996; Hover-Kramer & Mentgen, 2002) suggests the usefulness of these techniques in working through the grief process, treating anxiety and stress, working with hyperactivity in children, and assisting in addictions recovery.

Music Therapy

The arts provide the nurse with an opportunity to work with clients in avenues that do not require verbal expression or the rational, cognitive processes. There are many times when the client is unable or unwilling to express emotion (particularly negative emotion) through words. Visual and expressive arts are a means of communication that circumvent the need for talk and permit the client and nurse to interact on emotional and intuitive levels. There is ample evidence that use of the arts can be highly therapeutic and of significant benefit in mental health practice.

Music therapy is concerned with the use of specific kinds of music and its ability to effect changes in behavior, emotions, and physiology (Grocke, Bloch, & Castle, 2008). The form of music therapy used primarily by nurses is providing music for the client that will help to achieve a specific change in behavior or feeling (McCloskey & Bulechek, 2000).

Guzzetta (1988) warned that the nurse is not to confuse music as therapy with music as entertainment or diversion. One hears music for enjoyment at a concert, and one hears music as diversion while being placed "on hold" on a telephone answering system. To be therapy, the goal is the reduction of psychophysiological stress, pain, anxiety, or isolation. According to Guzzetta (1988), music therapy has been shown to help clients relax, develop a sense of self-awareness, improve learning, and cope with a variety of psychophysiological dysfunctions.

Music can be used as a catalyst to facilitate mental suggestion and to enhance the client's self-healing. Music has been used in birthing rooms, in operating rooms, during massage therapy sessions, during counseling sessions, on psychiatric inpatient units, and during addictions treatment. It is believed that music therapy offers a response because music produces alterations in physiology. Music therapy is thought to reduce psychophysiological stress, pain, anxiety, and isolation (Morris, 2009).

RESEARCH Highlight 32-5

Complementary Therapy for Addiction: "Drumming Out Drugs"

STUDY PROBLEM/PURPOSE

The researcher examined drumming activities as a complementary modality being used in addiction treatments.

METHODS

The researcher observed drumming circles for substances abuse and interviewed counselors and Internet mailing list participants. A drumming circle pilot program was initiated.

FINDINGS

Research reviews indicated that drumming enhances recovery through inducing relaxation and enhancing theta-wave production of brain-wave synchronization. Drumming was experienced as pleasurable and as a technique that enhanced awareness of preconscious dynamics. Drumming also created a sense of connectedness, alleviating self-centeredness and isolation.

IMPLICATIONS

Drumming as a form of music therapy may have positive effects on treatment of addictions.

Source: "Complementary Therapy for Addiction: 'Drumming Out Drugs,' " by M. Winkelman, 2003, *American Journal of Public Health*, *93*(4), 647–651.

There is a skill in selecting music to be played for therapy. Certain types of music have been shown to produce physiological benefits consistently, regardless of the clients' ages, cultural backgrounds, and musical preferences—these are baroque, classical, and new age music. These forms of music usually have a beat that is slower than the human heart rate. Music for therapy is not necessarily the music a client would choose to hear for entertainment; however, there is always a matter of personal preference that must be assessed.

Pet-Assisted Therapy

The idea that pets can provide companionship, affection, and comfort is not new. In health care settings, however, the notion of bringing animals into agencies for the express purpose of providing therapy is still somewhat new. **Animal-assisted therapy** is the purposeful use of animals to provide affection, attention, diversion, or relaxation (Bulechek, et al., 2008). The concept is based on a growing knowledge of benefits that animals can provide to the sick, the elderly, and the isolated (Barba, 1995). Pets, particularly dogs, puppies, and cats, have been shown to decrease feelings of loneliness. One investigation suggests that visiting volunteers and pets to a nursing home recreate "an aura of domesticity for residents who had been cut off from home and families by age and illness" (Savishinsky, 1992, p. 1325). In one hospice program, the introduction of a resident miniature poodle appeared to have facilitated staff-client interactions, eased client-visitor relations, and improved staff and client morale on a situational basis (Chinner & Dalziel, 1991) or to meet the clients' need for socialization (Churchhill, Safaoui, McKabe, & Baun, 1999). In another setting, the presence of a dog facilitated socialization among nursing home residents attending a socialization group (Fick, 1993) or to meet the clients' need for socialization (Churchill et al., 1999). In addition, animals may be brought into a facility to meet the clients' need for diversional activity (Rantz, 1991). In these situations, the clients are encouraged to play with the animals, feed them, and groom them. The effects of animals on clients with psychiatric illnesses (and their caretakers) may occur in unexpected ways, perhaps best captured through anecdotal reports (Niksa, 2007). The use of animals for therapy is still being investigated, but there seems to be evidence that, at least for some clients, introduction of pets into the care facility has positive effects on emotions, socialization, and adjustment.

RESEARCH Highlight 32-6

Animal-Assisted Therapy in Patients Hospitalized with Heart Failure

STUDY PROBLEM/PURPOSE

The researchers sought to determine effects of a 12-minute hospital visit with a therapy dog for patients with advanced heart failure. Specifically, they wanted to determine whether visits with a therapy dog improved hemodynamic measures, lowered neurohormone levels, and decreased anxiety.

METHODS

A three-group, repeated measures design was used. One group received visits from a volunteer and a therapy dog, another group received visits from a volunteer, and the third group served as controls. Data were collected on a number of dependent variables, including blood pressure, heart rate, pulmonary arterial pressure, pulmonary capillary wedge pressure, right atrial pressure, cardiac index, systemic vascular resistance, epinephrine level, norepinephrine level, and state anxiety.

FINDINGS

Patients who received a visit from a volunteer and dog had lower cardiopulmonary pressures, neurohormone levels, and anxiety levels than did patients visited by a volunteer only, while heart rate, blood pressure, cardiac index, and SVR were not significantly affected by the intervention.

IMPLICATIONS

Further research is needed to assess the use of animal assisted therapy in the acute management of symptoms (e.g., dyspnea), in improving satisfaction of patients, and in potentially decreasing length of stay in the hospital. Other investigations are needed to determine whether this adjunctive therapy may positively contribute to the long-term treatment of patients with heart failure.

Source: "Animal-Assisted Therapy in Patients Hospitalized with Heart Failure," by K. M. Cole, A. Gawlinski, N. Steers, and J. Koterman, 2007, *American Journal of Critical Care*, *16*(6), 575–586.

NURSING ROLE IN SOMATIC INTERVENTIONS

ANGER CONTROL ASSISTANCE

Control of anger and escalating violence are an important part of psychiatric care. In inpatient units, one expects to be in contact with clients who are hospitalized because they are unable to control their own behaviors and are assessed to be a risk either to themselves or to others. Similarly, nurses in emergency departments should be prepared to interact with both clients and family members who are experiencing anger and at risk for losing control.

Anger control assistance is defined as a nursing intervention aimed at facilitation of the expression of anger in an adaptive and nonviolent manner (Bulechek et al., 2008). Being angry is associated with higher levels of serum cortisol—a stress hormone—which can affect mood and physical well-being. Intriguingly, wound healing may be slowed among persons whose levels of anger are higher (Gouin, Kiecolt-Glaser, Malarkey, & Glaser, 2008). While helping clients to decrease feelings of anger has not yet been shown to have physiological benefit (such as shortening wound healing or reducing risk of infection), it is very possible that further studies may demonstrate such benefits. Neither holding anger inside nor letting anger be expressed openly are thought to be psychologically healthy (Anonymous, 2008). In contrast, controlling anger may well lead to better physical and psychological health. For the psychiatric nurse, anger control includes establishing a basic level of trust and rapport with the client and using a calm and reassuring manner. The nurse should use every means possible to learn from the client (or his family/friends) what situations are likely to bring on anger. Further, the nurse should encourage the client to let the nursing staff know when he is feeling tension. Although the nurse has a responsibility to help the client learn to deal with his anger, she also has a clear duty to assess for inappropriate aggression and intervene before it is expressed.

Some of the techniques used in anger control include limiting access to frustrating situations, providing physical outlets for expression of anger or tension (such as punching

> **NURSING TIP 32-1**
>
> **Assessing for Risk of Violence**
>
> - Be aware of those clients with past history of violence and poor impulse control.
> - Observe the client's body language: Notice changes in behavior, words, or dress.
> - Assess for aggressive behaviors, increasing tensions, clenched fists, loud or angry tone of voice, narrowed eyes, and pacing.
>
> Remember that hostility tends to be contagious. Do not reciprocate with anger and hostility!

bags, large motor activities [sports], and use of anger journals), and ensuring that a client for whom anger is a problem is given enough personal space that he does not have to feel encroached on by others when he is unable to tolerate environmental stimuli. However, even when all of the techniques available are used to assist the client to remain in control, there are times when the client must be physically stopped from harming himself or others.

There are two commonly used interventions for situations where the client is out of control: use of physical restraints and use of seclusion. These external controls may be used only when there is no other option for protecting the client and others.

Physical Restraints

Physical restraints, usually leather straps, are used to immobilize a person who is clearly dangerous to self or others and there is sufficient risk of harm AND no other alternative is likely to prevent harm to the client or others (Bower, McCullough, & Timmons, 2003). Physical restraints may be applied only under the direction and supervision of a registered nurse and must comply with state laws regarding their use. In almost all cases, there must be a physician's order to apply the restraints, and there must be clearly documented evidence that the restraints were needed. Some of the observable behaviors indicating that restraints are necessary include increased motor activity, verbal and physical threats, overresponsiveness to stimuli, and actual physical assault.

To be effective, application of physical restraints must be done quickly, as soon as the decision is made that they are needed. Sufficient numbers of staff persons must be present to restrain the client, to maintain privacy from other patients during the process, and to maintain the client's dignity. The staff members should carry out the restraining procedure in a matter-of-fact, nonemotional manner and never give the indication that the restraints are being used as punishment. The reason for the restraints must be given to the client, for example, "We are going to restrain you now, because you are not in control of yourself. You will be restrained so that you can regain your control."

While in restraints, the client must be observed, and he cannot be left alone. The restraints are padded to avoid circulation problems and skin breakdown; however, these potential problems must be assessed. The nurse should ensure that the client is restrained in a position of anatomical alignment, that his vital signs are checked, that he is observed for any sign of circulatory impairment, and that a staff person is available to talk to the client. Basic needs for food, fluid, and elimination must be met. The client should not be restrained any longer than is absolutely necessary. In general, if the client requires restraints for longer than 2 hours, the restraints must be removed for at least 5 minutes every 2 hours, so that the extremity can be assessed. Clients must be observed at least every 15 minutes. The nurse should always check the institutional guidelines and policies for specific expectations because most inpatient facilities—especially those receiving accreditation by the Joint Commission for Accreditation of Healthcare Organizations (JCAHO)—have stringent restrictions on restraint application that include frequent documentation and (where clearly indicated) reordering. A survey of more than 50 emergency psychiatric services found that restraints were used in less than 10% of clients presenting with acute psychosis, and that when applied these were used only for a mean of 3.3 hours (Allen & Currier, 2004). These data suggest that many centers are appropriately conservative in their use of restraints, applying them rarely and only for limited periods of time. An interesting qualitative study in a long-term care facility for adults with learning difficulties found that staff reported that they used restraints only as a means of "last resort," whereas clients often perceived this not to be the case (Fish & Culshaw, 2005). Both staff and clients reported that the use of "time-outs" could be effective alternatives, and that thoughtful discussions after any use of restraints could be helpful. Whether these findings can be extrapolated to more conventional mental health settings is unclear. On the other hand, others have found that by using a specially trained consultant team it was possible to abolish restraint usage on a psychiatric unit (Sclafani, Humphrey, Repko, Ko, Wallen, & Digiacomo, 2008). In the more complex and fast-paced setting of a general emergency room it appears to be more difficult to provide effective alternatives to the use of restraints, though many such alternatives are often tried (Downey, Zun, & Gonzales, 2007). It is important to recognize that restraints are usually applied to persons who are psychotic or who are suffering from delirium (see Chapter 25). Delirium has many causes, including adverse response to medications—especially, but by no means uniquely, among the elderly. Nurses must make every effort to find treatable causes of delirium (Maldonado, 2008) before—or at least concurrent with—employing restraints to protect clients or others they might harm.

Seclusion

Seclusion is the process of confining a client to a single room. The room may be locked or unlocked, and it may have furnishings or it may not. The purpose of seclusion is to provide security, to remove the client from a situation of escalating anger and violence, and to remove the client who is hypersensitive to environmental stimuli from the stimulation of a hospital unit. Seclusion, like the use of physical restraints, can be used only when all other avenues for control have been exhausted. The client must be told what is happening and why. He must not be left alone; a staff member should be assigned to observe the client, usually from the doorway. Seclusion is an enforced "time-out" where the client is removed from the situation only long enough that he can calm down, regain a sense of control, and then reenter the unit. It should be noted that a general policy in many institutions is that suicidal clients should not be secluded; they may harm themselves, even if the staff have removed potentially dangerous objects and clothing. As in the case of physical restraints, there must be a physician's order to use seclusion, there must be clear documentation of the indications for seclusion, and there must be a record of staff observations and nursing care provided during the seclusion period. The JCAHO standards regard both restraints and seclusion as procedures that should be employed only as last resorts when all other interventions have failed. Since seclusion may also be applied to persons with delirium, the comments about identifying treatable causes of delirium made in the section about restraints also apply here.

Reentry of the Client to the Unit

When the client is ready to come out of restraints or seclusion, the nurse must reassure the client that the staff will assist him in learning how to deal with anger in a nonviolent way and take steps to help him. The nurse should establish the clear expectation that the client can and will learn to control his behavior. Some interventions that are useful are: to help the client identify what makes him angry, assist him to plan strategies to prevent the escalation of the anger, help the client to learn of calming measures (such as taking a "time-out"), and provide role models of persons who can appropriately deal with anger. In all situations where anger has been handled appropriately, the nurse should provide positive reinforcement (Bulechek et al. 2008).

Light Therapy

Light therapy (or **phototherapy**) is a treatment for individuals with Seasonal Affective Disorder (SAD; see Chapter 13), a nonpsychotic depression experienced during winter months. SAD is a cyclical illness, and in most cases, episodes begin in fall or winter and remit in spring. The prevalence of winter-type SAD appears to vary with latitude, age, and sex. Prevalence increases with higher latitudes, younger persons are at higher risk than older adults, and women comprise 60% to 90% of persons with the illness (American Psychiatric Association, 2000).

Light therapy is an intervention that provides artificial lighting, brighter than indoor lighting, to the environment of an individual experiencing SAD. It relieves symptoms in about 75% of persons with SAD and is as effective as conventional antidepressants in properly selected clients (Westrin & Lam, 2007). Light therapy needs to be administered by a knowledgeable professional and consists of exposing clients to artificial therapeutic lighting, which is about 5 to 20 times brighter than indoor lighting. Lights with a set of broad-spectrum fluorescent bulbs have been designed to produce the intensity and color of outdoor daylight. Persons with SAD sit in their homes with such lights and engage in their usual activities—eating, reading, and so on. A newer device, a "light visor" or "light goggle," has been developed so that a person can wear the device about the head. The advantage of such devices is that the person may walk around while receiving treatment. There is also evidence that small diode devices available without medical prescription can lead to benefit if used for 30 minutes daily on awakening and prior to 8 A.M. (Desan, Weinstein, Michalak, Tam, Meesters, Ruiter, et al., 2007). The amount of light required to achieve remission of symptoms seems to vary with individuals and with the intensity of the light. In general, the brighter the light, the more effective the treatment, though other options to bright light therapy are being explored for SAD including low-level, gradually increasing early morning illumination ("dawn therapy") and the use of high-density electrically negative ions (Terman & Terman, 2006).

Light therapy seems to have positive effects on depressive symptoms within one week of initiating treatment. While the mechanism of action is unknown, it is clear that light therapy is based on biological rhythms and provides the equivalent of bright outdoor light to persons living in dark winter climates. The nurses' role is to explain the treatment, assist the person to obtain and set up light sources in the home, and support their use. Light therapy is an important alternative to drug treatment for the nearly 15 million Americans who experience SAD.

COLLABORATIVE INTERVENTIONS IN PSYCHIATRIC SOMATIC TREATMENTS

Electroconvulsive Therapy

Electroconvulsive Therapy is a somatic treatment that, while rarely used in current psychiatric settings, has a role in the management and control of symptoms otherwise unresponsive to therapy and medication. **Electroconvulsive therapy (ECT)** is the passage of an electrical stimulus to the brain to produce a seizure. It has been used for more than a century, and, as a therapy, it has had its critics and its supporters. ECT emerged as a treatment in the 1930s at a time when psychiatrists believed that schizophrenia and epilepsy were incompatible (Keltner & Folks, 1993). Early advocates of ECT thought this treatment would result in dramatic cures for many disorders. And while there was a clearly documented effect for some conditions, the treatment did not prove to be the cure early advocates had hoped for. Although ECT was used for a wide range of disorders, it became increasingly clear that it was most effective in treatment of depressive illness and mania (Runck, 1985). See Table 32-2 for a summary of available evidence on its use.

TABLE 32-2 Indications for ECT Treatments

A systematic review of the literature on ECT revealed that there is a great need for continuing studies on its use and effectiveness. Based on available data, the authors report that:

- ECT is probably more effective than pharmacology in the short term.
- ECT is probably more effective that repetitive transcranial magnetic stimulation.
- Gains in effectiveness of ECT are achieved only at the expense of higher risk of cognitive side effects.
- ECT, either in combination with antipsychotics or without antipsychotics, is not more effective than antipsychotics alone in people with schizophrenia.
- More research is needed to examine the long-term efficacy and the cognitive side effects of ECT and its effectiveness/use in potential suicide cases.

Source: Greenhalgh, J., Knight, C., Hind, D., Beverly, C., & Walters, S. (2005). Clinical and cost-effectiveness of electroconvulsive therapy for depressive illness, schizophrenia, catatonia, and mania: Systematic reviews and economic modeling studies. *Health Technology Assessment*, *9*(9), 1–170.

During the 1960s and 1970s, ECT came under harsh criticism, and its use declined dramatically. In the ensuing years, the actual procedure for administering the treatment was changed, such that ECT is currently modified by brief anesthesia, relaxation with succinylcholine, and ventilation with oxygen. In the 1980s, the use of ECT increased once again, but only in highly selected cases. Currently, the indications for ECT include cases of major depression that have not responded to other treatments, severe suicidal tendencies, acute mania, and catatonia.

In current use of the technique, the client does not experience a full grand mal seizure, as in years past; a seizure may last for as little as 20 seconds. Those who read past accounts of ECT must remember that there is a clear distinction between the "old" ECT and its current use (Merton, 2008) and that the disturbing descriptions found in some novels are examples of the old procedure. A recent study evaluated the knowledge of and attitudes about ECT held by elderly (over 65 years), depressed clients (Bustin, Rapoport, Krishna, Matusevich, Finkelstein, Strejrevich, et al., 2008). The study enrolled participants from three countries: England, Canada, and Argentina. Results, across the three countries, showed that patient attitudes are negative to neutral, with 75% of the patients stating that they either thought that ECT was unsafe or they did not know if it was safe. Similarly, 73% of the patients said they would not accept ECT if offered or recommended as part of their treatment. Interestingly, the media served as the major source on information on ECT in Argentina, where in England and Canada the major source of information was talking to people who experienced ECT. The level of knowledge that these patients had about ECT was poor. While no similar studies exist in the American population, one might be concerned that the public attitude about ECT is probably not informed by actual knowledge of the treatment as to its benefits and risks.

In recent years, ECT has been safely and effectively applied to treatment of the elderly (Kamat, Lefevre, & Grossberg, 2003) and has been given successfully to outpatients (Dew & McCall, 2004). While the use of ECT in adolescents may be controversial, clinical guidelines have been written stressing the importance of informed consent and proper client selection (Ghaziuddin, Kutcher, & Knapp, 2004). ECT appears to be effective in adolescents who have mood disorders that have proven unresponsive to other forms of therapy.

Pharmacological Aspects of ECT

Modern ECT is administered under highly controlled settings and is quite safe, even for medically ill individuals (Knos, Sung, Cooper, & Stoundenine, 1990). In some settings an anesthesiologist always participates in ECT, whereas in others the psychiatrist serves to monitor anesthesia as well as to supervise shock administration. The ECT anesthesia typically involves a short-acting barbiturate (methohexital [Brevital]) followed by succinylcholine to produce muscle paralysis. As for many surgical procedures, premedication with atropine (usually 0.4 to 0.6 mg intramuscular or subcutaneous) is given an hour before ECT. Mechanical ventilation with 100% oxygen is provided prior to inducing electrical seizure activity and until the effects of succinylcholine paralysis wear off and the client is able to breathe on his or her own, typically about five minutes (Keltner & Folks, 1993).

Nursing Care

As for any procedure, a consent form must be signed. The client will receive nothing by mouth from midnight the night before the treatment, and preprocedure medications such as atropine must be given as ordered. The client should be asked to urinate before the treatment; hairpins, dentures, and so on should be removed. Vital signs should be taken and recorded. During the procedure, the nurse will assist in monitoring the vital signs and electroencephalography. Postprocedure, the nurse will monitor for respiratory difficulties and will continue to assess vital signs. ECT causes confusion, so the nurse will need to reorient the client and observe for level of confusion/orientation after each treatment and during a series of treatments.

Magnet Therapy

One of the most interesting developments among somatic therapies has been the use of transcutaneous magnetic therapy to treat depression and several other psychiatric disorders. In this treatment, a powerful magnet is placed on the skull, and specific brain regions are stimulated with pulsating fields. There is good evidence that this treatment leads to reversible changes in underlying brain activity (Speer, Willis, Herscovitch, Dauble-Witherspoon, Shelton, Benson, et al., 2003) although the effectiveness and potential role of magnetic therapy remains to be completely defined (Lisanby, Kinnunen, Crupain, 2002; Chang, 2004). Students still show conflicting results with some supporting benefit (Kauffmann, Cheema, Miller, 2004) while others seem to show no effect (Hausmann, Kemmler, Walpoth, Mechtcheriakov, Krammer-Reinstadler, Lechner, et al., 2004). There are even some reports that clients with affective disorders experience improved mood after certain kinds of magnetic imaging procedures (magnetic resonance imaging [MRI] spectroscopy). These findings have led to preliminary investigations of a variety of externally applied magnetic fields that may prove useful in the management of clients with psychiatric disorders (Rohan, Parwo, Stoll, Demolulos, Friedman, Dager, et al., 2004; Kayser, Bewernick, Axmacher, & Schlaepfer, 2009).

KEY CONCEPTS

- Complementary modalities, such as guided imagery, hypnosis, relaxation, massage, therapeutic touch, music therapy, and pet-assisted therapy, are nursing interventions that are being used as an adjunct to medical care and psychiatric treatments that are thought to have effects on stress, sleep disturbance, anxiety, and other emotions.
- Each of the complementary modalities addressed in this chapter is included in the Nursing Interventions Classification (NIC) and is being researched by nurses.
- Anger control assistance requires that the nurse develop a sense of trust with the client and carefully observe any signs of escalating anger.
- Use of physical restraints or seclusion, or both, is appropriate when there are no other means to ensure safety.
- Light therapy is a useful treatment for Seasonal Affective Disorder (SAD) and involves bringing high-intensity lighting into the homes and environments of affected individuals.
- Electroconvulsive therapy (ECT) is a treatment involving an electrical shock to the brain and is indicated in highly specific situations.

REVIEW QUESTIONS

1. What is the major role of the nurse during electroconvulsive therapy (ECT)?
   1. Administer the anesthesia
   2. Hold the client during the convulsion
   3. Monitor vital signs and electroencephalography
   4. Supervise the administration of electrical shocks

2. A nurse developing a care plan for an angry client would include exercise therapy as a part of the client's daily activity. Exercise therapy is included for which of the following purposes?
   1. It helps the client lose excess weight
   2. It provides an outlet for the client's anger
   3. It helps the client to feel more powerful
   4. It provides for this client a level of exercise required by all patients on the unit

3. When a nurse is interacting with a client who is hostile or angry, which of the following would be most important?
   1. Immediately have the client placed in restraints
   2. Approach the client in a calm and reassuring manner
   3. Tell the client that he will be sedated if he does not calm down
   4. Speak to the client in an equally hostile tone to demonstrate that the nurse is not intimidated

4. Which of the following individuals would be a good candidate for guided imagery therapy?
   1. A client having a psychotic episode
   2. A client with a history of schizophrenia
   3. A client suffering from pain after a surgery
   4. A client currently experiencing a severe panic attack

5. A nurse is utilizing hypnosis in treating a client. The nurse should be aware of what aspect of hypnotherapy?
   1. That memories recalled during the hypnotic trance may or MAY NOT be accurate.
   2. That any hypnotic suggestion the nurse gives the client while in a trance will be obeyed by the client, regardless of whether the client wants to or not.
   3. That hypnosis is most effective with people of limited intelligence, and least effective on people with higher IQs.
   4. That hypnosis has NOT been shown to be effective when dealing with physical ailments such as pain management or urinary incontinence.

LEARNING ACTIVITIES

1. For each of the complementary modalities listed, describe a client population for whom the intervention would be appropriate:
   a. Relaxation and guided imagery
   b. Hypnosis
   c. Massage
   d. Energy-based modalities
   e. Music therapy
   f. Pet-assisted therapy
2. Describe a situation where you observed escalating anger in a client.
3. Identify four things you can do to assist a client to gain control of his anger.
4. Describe the indications for physical restraints and seclusion. Examine the policy at your own facility.
5. Suggest ways you could support a client undergoing light therapy for SAD in his home.
6. Review the indications for ECT and the nursing responsibilities.

*Study*WARE™ CONNECTION

Using your *Study*WARE™ CD-ROM

1. Complete the Concentration activity for this chapter.
2. Review the audio glossary for key terms in this chapter.
3. Explore the other games and activities that support this chapter.

REFERENCES

Allen, M. H., & Currier, G. W. (2004). Use of restraints and pharmacotherapy in academic psychiatric emergency services. *General Hospital Psychiatry, 26*(1), 42–49.

American Psychiatric Association. (2000). *Diagnostic and statistical manual of mental disorders* (Fourth Edition-Text Revision). Washington, DC: Author.

Anonymous. (2008). Anger control: Harness its healing power. *Consumer Reports, 73*(7), 46.

Anselmo J. (2009). Relaxation. In B. Dossey and L. Keegan, *Holistic nursing: A handbook for practice* (5th ed., pp. 259–285). Boston: Jones and Bartlett.

Baram, D. A. (1995). Hypnosis in reproductive health care: A review and case reports. *Birth, 22,* 37–42.

Barba, B. E. (1995). The positive influence of animals: Animal-assisted therapy in acute care. *Clinical Nurse Specialist, 9,* 199–202.

Barnett, K. (1972). A survey of the current utilization of touch by health team personnel with hospitalized patients. *International Journal of Nursing Studies, 9,* 195–209.

Bost, N., & Wallis, M. (2006). The effectiveness of a 15 minute weekly massage in reducing physical and psychological stress in nurses. *Australian Journal of Advanced Nursing, 23*(4), 28–33.

Bower, F. L., McCullough, C. S., & Timmons, M. E. (2003). A synthesis of what we know about the use of physical restraints and seclusion with patients in psychiatric and acute care settings: 2003 update. *Online Journal of Knowledge Synthesis for Nursing, 10,* 1.

Bufe, G. (1994). Guided imagery with depressed children. In R. M. Carroll-Johnson (Ed.), *Classification of nursing diagnoses: Proceedings of the tenth conference* (p. 371). Philadelphia: J. B. Lippincott.

Bulechek, G. M., Butcher, H., & Dochterman, J. (2008). *Nursing interventions classification* (NIC; 5th ed.). St. Louis: Mosby.

Bustin, J., Rapoport, M. J., Krishna, M., Matusevich, C., Finkelstein, S., Strejrevich, S., & Anderson, D. (2008). Are patients' attitudes towards and knowledge of electroconvulsive therapy transcultural? A multi-national pilot study. *International Journal of Geriatric Psychiatry, 23,* 492–503.

Chang, J. Y. (2004). Brain stimulation for neurological and psychiatric disorders, current status and future directions. *Journal of Pharmacological and Experimental Therapies, 309*(1), 1–7.

Chinner, T. L., & Dalziel, F. R. (1991). An exploratory study on the viability and efficacy of a pet-facilitated therapy project within a hospice. *Journal of Palliative Care, 7,* 13–20.

Churchill, M., Safaoui, J., McKabe, B. V. V., & Baun, M. M. (1999). Using a therapy dog to alleviate the agitation and desocialization of people with Alzheimer's disease. *Journal of Psychosocial Nursing and Mental Health Services, 37*(4), 16–22, 42–43.

Cole, K. M., Gawlinski, A., Steers, N., & Koterman, J. (2007). Animal-assisted therapy in patients hospitalized with heart failure. *American Journal of Critical Care, 16*(6), 575–586.

Desan, P. H., Weinstein, A. J., Michalak, E. E., Tam, E. M., Meesters, Y., Ruiter, M. J., et al. (2007). A controlled trial of the Litebook light-emitting diode (LED) light therapy device for treatment of Seasonal Affective Disorder (SAD). *BMC Psychiatry, 7,* 38.

Dew, R., & McCall, W. V. (2004). Efficiency of outpatient ECT. *Journal of ECT, 20*(1), 24–25.

Doherty, D., Wright, S., Aveyard, B., & Sykes, M. (2006). Therapeutic touch and dementia care: An ongoing journey. *Nursing Older People, 18*(11), 27–30.

Downey, L. V., Zun, L. S., & Gonzales, S. J. (2007). Frequency of alternative to restraints and seclusion and uses of agitation reduction techniques in the emergency department. *General Hospital Psychiatry, 29*(6), 470–474.

Duimel-Peeters, I., Halfens, R., Berger, M., & Snoecky, L. (2005). Effects of massage as a method to prevent pressure ulcers: A review of the literature. *Ostomy and Wound Management, 51*(4), 70–80.

Elkins, G., Rajab, M. H., & Marcus, J. (2005). Complementary and alternative medicine use by psychiatric inpatients. *Psychological Reports, 96*(1), 163–166.

Fick, K. M. (1993). The influence of an animal on social interactions of nursing home residents in a group setting. *American Journal of Occupational Therapy, 47,* 529–534.

Fish, R., & Culshaw, E. (2005). The last resort? Staff and client perspectives on physical intervention. *Journal of Intellectual Disabilities,* 9(2), 93–107.

Gange, D., & Toye, R. C. (1994). The effects of therapeutic touch and relaxation therapy in reducing anxiety. *Archives of Psychiatric Nursing, 8,* 184–189.

Garner, B., Phillips, L. J., Schmidt, H. M., Markulev, C., O'Connor, J., Wood, S. J., et al. (2008). Pilot study evaluating the effect of massage therapy on stress, anxiety and aggression in a young adult psychiatric inpatient unit. *Australian and New Zealand Journal of Psychiatry, 42*(5), 414–422.

Ghaziuddin, N., Kutcher, S. P., & Knapp, P. (2004). Summary of the practice parameters for the use of eletroconvulsive therapy with adolescents. *Journal of the American Academy of Child and Adolescent Psychiatry, 43*(1), 119–122.

Gouin, J. P., Kiecolt-Glaser, J. K., Malarkey, W. B., & Glaser, R. (2008). The influence of anger expression on wound healing. *Brain, Behavior, and Immunity, 22*(5), 699–708.

Greenhalgh, J., Knight, C., Hind, D., Beverley, C., & Walters, S. (2005). Clinical and cost-effectiveness of electroconvulsive therapy for depressive illness, schizophrenia, catatonia, and mania: Systematic reviews and economic modeling. *Health Technology Assessment,* 9(9), 1–170.

Grocke, D., Bloch, S., & Castle, D. (2008). Is there a role for music therapy in the care of the severely mentally ill? *Australasian Psychiatry, 16*(6), 442–445.

Guzzetta, C. (1988). Music therapy: Healing the melody of the soul. In L. Keegan, B. Dossey, C. Guzzetta, & L. Kolkmeier (Eds.), *Holistic nursing practice* (p. 288). Rockville, MD: Aspen.

Hagemaster, J. (2000). Use of therapeutic touch in treatment of drug addictions. *Holistic Nursing Practice, 14*(3), 14–20.

Hamel, P. M. (1979). *Through music to the self.* Boulder, CO: Shambala Press.

Harvey, A. (1987, December 17). Music and health. *USA Today,* pp. 9–12.

Hausmann, A., Kemmler, G., Walpoth, M., Mechtcheriakov, S., Krammer-Reinstadler, K., Lechner, T., et al. (2004). No benefit derived from repetitive transcranial magnetic stimulation in depression: A prospective, single center, randomized, double blind, sham controlled "add on" trial. *Journal of Neurological and Neurosurgical Psychiatry, 75*(2), 320–322.

Hawkins, P., & Polemikos, N. (2002). Hypnosis treatment of sleeping problems in children experiencing loss. *Contemporary Hypnosis, 19*(1), 18–24.

Hilliard, D. (1995). Massage for the seriously mentally ill. *Journal of Psychosocial Nursing and Mental Health Services, 33,* 29–30.

Hover-Kramer, D. (1996). Interrelationships with psychotherapy. In D. Hover-Kramer (Ed.), *Healing touch: A resource for health care professionals* (pp. 189–199). Clifton Park, NY: Thomson Delmar Learning.

Hover-Kramer, D. & Mentgen, J. (2002). *Healing touch: A guidebook for practitioners,* Clifton Park, NY: Thomson Delmar Learning.

Jackson, C., & Keegan, L. (2009). Touch. In B. Dossey and L. Keegan, *Holistic nursing: A handbook for practice,* (5th ed., pp. 347–359). Boston: Jones and Bartlett.

Jackson, E., Kelley, M., McNeil, P, Meyor, E., Schlegel, L., & Eaton, M. (2008). Does therapeutic touch help reduce pain and anxiety in patients with cancer? *Clinical Journal of Oncology Nursing, 12*(1), 113–120.

Jorm, A. F., Morgan, A. J., & Hetrick, S. E. (2008). Relaxation for depression. *Cochrane Database of Systematic Reviews* (4).

Kamat, S. M., Lefevre, P. J., & Grossberg, G. T. (2003). Electroconvulsive therapy in the elderly. *Clinical Geriatric Medicine, 19*(4), 825–839.

Kauffmann, C. D., Cheema, M. A., & Miller, B. E., (2004). Slow right prefrontal transcranial magnetic stimulation as a treatment for medication-resistant depression: A double-blind placebo controlled study. *Depression and Anxiety, 19*(1), 59–92.

Kay, M.C. (2007). Effectiveness of hypnosis in reducing mild essential hypertension: A one-year follow-up study. *International Journal of Clinical and Experimental Hypnosis, 55*(1), 67–83.

Kayser, S., Bewernick, B., Axmacher, N., & Schlaepfer, T. E. (2009). Magnetic seizure therapy of treatment-resistant depression in a patient with bipolar disorder. The *Journal of ECT.* 25, 137–140.

Keller, E., & Bzdek, V. M. (1986). Effects of therapeutic touch on tension headaches. *Nursing Research, 35,* 101–105.

Keltner, N., & Folks, D. (1993). *Psychotropic drugs.* St. Louis: Mosby.

Knos, G. B., Sung, Y. F., Cooper, R. C., & Stoundenine, A. (1990). Electroconvulsive therapy-induced hemodynamic changes unmask unsuspected coronary artery disease. *Journal of Clinical Anesthesia, 2,* 37–41.

Kolkmeier, L. (1988). Relaxation: Opening the door to change. In L. Keegan, B. Dossey, C. Guzzetta, & L. Kolkmeier (Eds.), *Holistic nursing practice* (pp. 195–222). Rockville, MD: Aspen.

Krieger, D. (1979). *Living the therapeutic touch: Healing as a lifestyle.* New York: Dodd, Mead.

Krieger, D. (1993). *Accepting your power to heal the personal practice of therapeutic touch.* Santa Fe, NM: Bear & Co.

Krisanaprakornkit, T., Krisanaprakornkit, W., Piyavhatkul, N., & Laopaiboon, M. (2006). Meditation therapy for anxiety disorders. *Cochrane Database of Systematic Reviews* (1).

Kwekkeboom, K. L. (2000). Measuring imagery ability: Psychometric testing of the Imagery Ability Questionnaire. *Research in Nursing and Health, 23*(4), 301–309.

Kwekkeboom, K. L., Maddox, M. A., & West, T. (2000). Measuring imagery ability. *Journal of Pediatric Health Care, 14*(6), 297–303.

Lane, J. D., Seskevich, J. E., & Pieper, C. F. (2007). Brief meditation training can improve perceived stress and negative mood. *Alternative Therapies in Health and Medicine, 13*(1), 38–44.

Letts, P. J., Baker, P. R. A., Ruderman, J., & Kennedy, K. (1993). The use of hypnosis in labor and delivery: A preliminary study. *Journal of Women's Health, 2,* 335–341.

Lisanby, S. H., Kinnunen, L. H., & Crupain, M. J. (2002). Applications of TMS to therapy in psychiatry. *Journal of Clinical Neurophysiology, 19*(4), 344–360.

MacIntyre, B., Hamilton, J., Fricke, T., Ma, W., Mehle, S. & Michel, M. (2008). The efficacy of healing touch in coronary artery bypass surgery recovery: A randomized, clinical trial. *Alternative Therapies, 14*(4), 24–37.

Maldonado, J. R. (2008). Delirium in the acute care setting: Characteristics, diagnosis and treatment. *Critical Care Clinics, 24*(4), 657–722, vii.

Mamtani, R., & Cimino, A. (2002). A primer of complementary and alternative medicine and its relevance in the treatment of mental health problems. *Psychiatric Quarterly, 73*(4), 367–381.

Mantle, F. (2002). The role of alternative medicine in treating postnatal depression. *Complementary Therapies and Nurse Midwifery, 8*(4), 197–203.

Matthew, M., & Flatt, S. (1999). The efficacy of hypnotherapy in treatment of migraine. *Nursing Standard, 14*(7), 33–36.

Maville, J. A., & Bowan, G. (2008). Effect of healing touch on stress perception and biological correlates. *Holistic Nursing Practice, 22*(2), 103–110.

McClelland, D. C. (1979). Music in the operating room. *AORN Journal, 29*, 252–260.

McCloskey J. C., Bulechek G. M., (Eds.). (2000). *Nursing interventions classification (NIC)*, (3rd ed.). St Louis: Mosby.

Meeham, T. C. (1990). The science of unitary human beings and theory-based practice: Therapeutic touch. In M. Barrett (Ed.), *Visions of Rogers' science-based nursing*. New York: National League for Nursing.

Meek, S. S. (1993). Effect of slow stroke back massage on relaxation in hospice clients. *Image, 25*, 17–21.

Mentgen, J. (1996). Specific interventions for identified problems. In D. Hover-Kramer (Ed.), *Healing touch: A resource for health care professionals* (pp. 141–153). Clifton Park, NY: Thomson Delmar Learning.

Merton, A. (2008). The third way: ECT isn't what it used to be. *American Journal of Nursing, 108*(10), 88.

Mornhinweg, G. C., & Voignier, R. R. (1995). Music for sleep disturbance in the elderly. *Journal of Holistic Nursing, 13*, 248–254.

Morris, D. (2009). Music therapy. In B. Dossey and L. Keegan, *Holistic nursing: A handbook for practice* (5th ed., pp. 327–336). Boston: Jones and Bartlett.

Moss, V. A. (1988). Music and the surgical patient. *AORN Journal, 40*, 64–69.

Newman, A. W., & Thompson, J. W., Jr. (2001). The rise and fall of forensic hypnosis in criminal investigation. *Journal of the American Academy of Psychiatry and the Law, 29*(1), 75–84.

Niksa, E. (2007). The use of animal-assisted therapy in psychiatric nursing: The story of Timmy and Buddy. *Journal of Psychosocial Nursing & Mental Health Services, 45*(6), 56–58.

Olson, M., & Sneed, N. (1995). Anxiety and therapeutic touch. *Issues in Mental Health Nursing, 16*, 97–108.

Quinn, C., Chandler, C., & Moraska, A. (2002). Massage therapy and frequency of chronic tension headaches. *American Journal of Public Health, 92*(10), 1657–1661.

Quinn, J. (1981). *An investigation of the effect of therapeutic touch done without physical contact on the state of anxiety of hospitalized cardiovascular patients*. Unpublished doctoral dissertation, New York University .

Quinn, J. (1983). Therapeutic touch as energy exchange: Testing the theory. *Advances in Nursing Science, 6*, 42–49.

Quinn, J. (1988). Building a body of knowledge: Research on therapeutic touch. *Journal of Holistic Nursing, 6*(1), 37–45.

Rantz, M. (1991). Diversional activity deficit. In M. Maas, K. Buckwalter, & M. Hardy (Eds.), *Nursing diagnosis and interventions for the elderly* (pp. 299–312). Redwood City, CA: Addison-Wesley.

Reed, T. (2007). Imagery in the clinical setting: A tool for healing. *Nursing Clinics of North America, 42*(2), 261–277, vii.

Roffe, L., Schmidt, K., & Ernst, E. (2005). A systematic review of guided imagery as an adjuvant cancer therapy. *Psychooncology, 14*(8), 607–617.

Rohan, M., Parwo, A., Stoll, A. L., Demolulos, C., Friedman, S., Dager, S., et al. (2004). Low-field magnetic stimulation in bipolar depression using an MRI-based stimulator. *American Journal of Psychiatry, 161*(1), 93–98.

Rowe, M., & Alfred, D. (1999). The effectiveness of slow-stroke massage in diffusing agitated behaviors in individuals with Alzheimer's disease. *Journal of Gerontological Nursing, 25*(6), 22–34.

Rozema, H. (1986, September/October). Touch needs of the elderly. *Nursing Homes*, 42–43.

Runck, B. (1985). NIMH report: Consensus panel backs cautious use of ECT for severe disorders. *Hospital and Community Psychiatry*. 36(9), 943–946.

Salzmann-Erikson, M., & Eriksson, H. (2005). Encountering touch: A path to affinity in psychiatric care. *Mental Health Nursing Journal, 26*(8), 843–852.

Savishinsky, J. S. (1992). Intimacy, domesticity and pet therapy with the elderly: Expectation and experience among nursing home volunteers. *Social Science and Medicine, 34*, 1325–1334.

Scandrett-Hibdon, S. (1996). Research foundations. In D. Hover-Kramer (Ed.), *Healing touch: A resource for health care professionals* (pp. 27–42). Clifton Park, NY: Thomson Delmar Learning.

Sclafani, M. J., Humphrey, F. J., 2nd, Repko, S., Ko, H. S., Wallen, M. C., & Digiacomo, A. (2008). Reducing patient restraints: A pilot approach using clinical case review. *Perspectives in Psychiatric Care, 44*(1), 32–39.

Seskevich, J. E., Crater, S. W., Lane, J. D., & Krucof, M. W. (2004). Beneficial effects of noetic therapies on mood before percutaneous intervention for unstable coronary syndromes. *Nursing Research, 53*(2), 116–121.

Shames, K. (1996). *Creative imagery in nursing*. Clifton Park, NY: Thomson Delmar Learning.

Sloman, R. (1995). Relaxation and the relief of cancer pain. *Nursing Clinics of North America, 30*, 697–709.

Sloman, R. (2002). Relaxation and imagery for anxiety and depression control in community patients with advanced cancer. *Cancer Nursing, 25*(6), 432–435.

Speer, A. M., Willis, M. W., Herscovitch, P., Dauble-Witherspoon, M., Shelton, J., Benson, B. E., et al. (2003). Intensity-dependent regional cerebral blood flow during 1 Hz repetitive transcranial stimulation (rTMS) in health volunteers with H2150 positron emission tomography: Effects of primary motor cortex rTMS. *Biological Psychiatry, 54*(8), 818–825.

Spira, J. L., & Speigel, D. (1992). Hypnosis and related techniques in pain management. *Hospice Journal, 8*, 89–119.

Synder, M., Egan, E. C., & Burns, K. R. (1995). Efficacy of hand massage in decreasing agitation behaviors associated with care activities in persons with dementia. *Geriatric Nursing, 16*, 60–63.

Terman, M., & Terman, J. S. (2006). Controlled trial of naturalistic dawn simulation and negative air ionization for seasonal affective disorder. *American Journal of Psychiatry, 163*(12), 2126–2133.

Troesch, L. M., Rodehaver, C. B., Delaney, E. A., & Yanes, B. (1993). The influence of guided imagery on chemotherapy-related nausea and vomiting. *Oncology Nurses Forum, 20*, 1179–1185.

Van Kuiken, D. (2004). A meta-analysis of the effect of guided imagery practice on outcomes. *Journal of Holistic Nursing, 22*(2), 164–179.

Westrin, A., & Lam, R. W. (2007). Seasonal affective disorder: A clinical update. *Annals of Clinical Psychiatry, 19*(4), 239–246.

Winkleman, M. (2003). Complementary therapy for addiction: "Drumming out drugs." *Journal of Public Health, 93*(4), 647–651.

Wirth, D., Richardson, J. T., Eidelman, W. S., & O'Malley, A. C. (1993). Full-thickness dermal wounds treated with non-contact therapeutic touch: A replication and extension. *Complementary Therapies in Medicine, 1*, 127–132.

Woods, D. L., Craven, R., & Whitney, J. (2005). The effects of therapeutic touch on behavioral symptoms of persons with dementia. *Alternative Therapies, 11*(1), 66–74.

Wynd, C. A. (1992). Personal power imagery and relaxation techniques used in smoking cessation programs. *American Journal of Health Promotion, 6*, 184–189, 196.

Zimmerman, M. L. (1989). Using principles of relaxation, visualization, and guided imagery in the care of persons recovering from addictions. *Addictions Nursing Network, 1*, 9–11.

SUGGESTED READINGS

Dossey, B. (1997). *Core curriculum for holistic nursing*. Gaithersburg, MD: Aspen.

Dossey, B., Keegan, L., & Guzzetta, C. (2004). *Holistic nursing: Handbook for practice*. Gaithersburg, MD: Aspen.

Frisch, N., Dossey, B., Guzzetta, C., & Quinn, J. (2000). *Standards of holistic nursing practice*. Gaithersburg, MD: Aspen.

RESOURCES

Academy for Guided Imagery
30765 Pacific Coast Highway
Malibu, California 90265
http://www.academyforguidedimagery.com

American Holistic Nurses Association
P.O. Box 2130
Flagstaff, Arizona 86004-2130
http://www.ahna.org

Healing Touch International
445 Union Blvd., Suite 105
Lakewood, Colorado, 80228
http://www.healingtouch.net

Nurse Healers Professional Associates International
3760 South Highland Drive
Salt Lake City, Utah, 84104
http://www.therapeutictouch.org

UNIT 5 Additional Resources

What are some movies to watch that illustrate the experience of mental illness?

This question is answered in the content of this unique unit, *Additional Resources*.

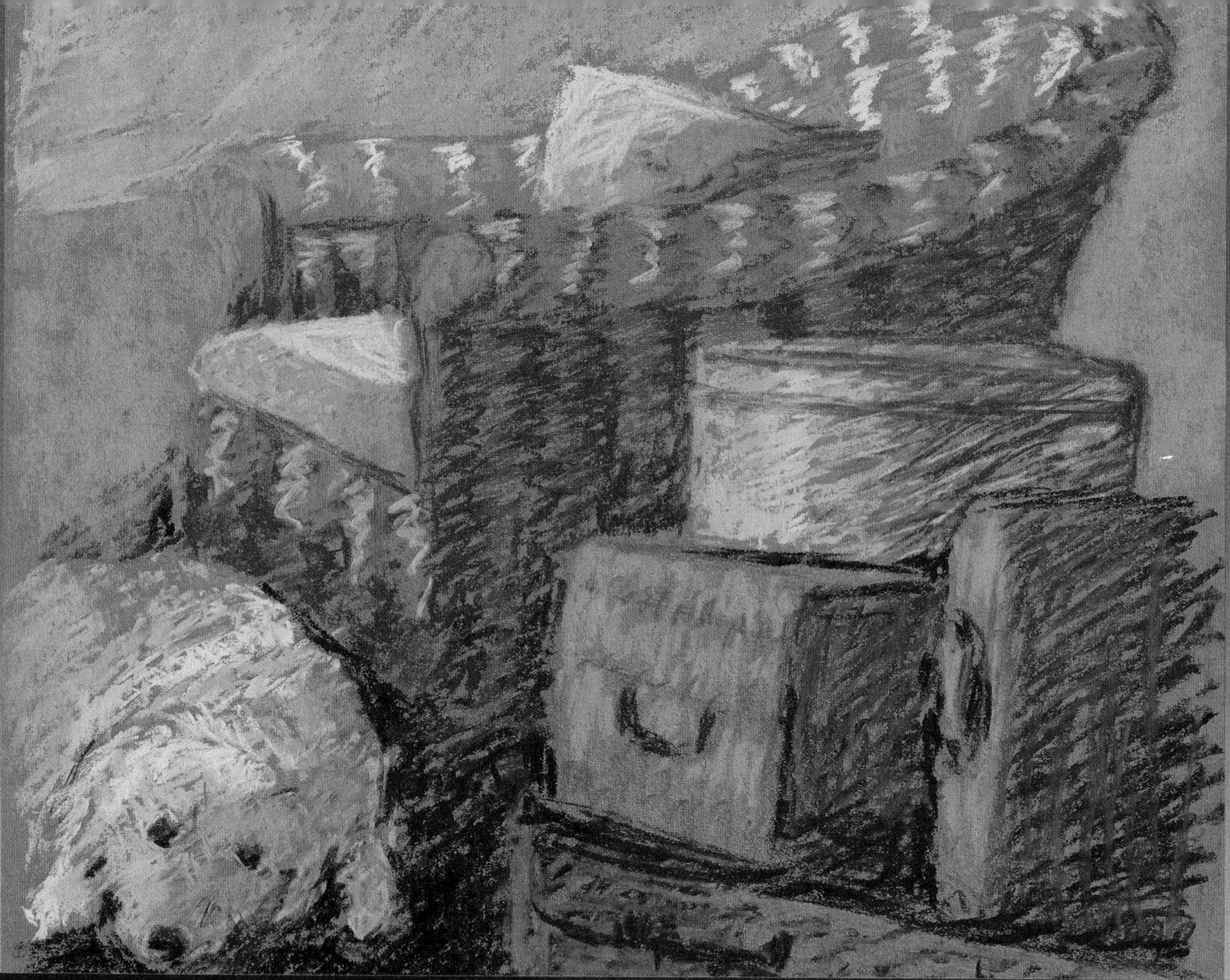

View Into...

Psychiatric Disorders: A Cinematic View

Many of the films in this chapter vividly capture the human experience of emotional distress. As you view each film, consider the following questions:

- ***Do the characters in the movies you are watching exhibit any traits of a specific psychiatric disorder?***
- ***What societal or cultural attitudes are reflected in the depiction of mental illness, its treatment, and the role of the nurse?***
- ***What ethical questions have arisen in the movies you are watching?***
- ***How do you react to the characters in each film? Does your knowledge of the field of psychiatric nursing change your response to the film or to its characters?***
- ***How would you use the film to help clients, families, populations, or health care staff to better understand mental illness or its treatment?***

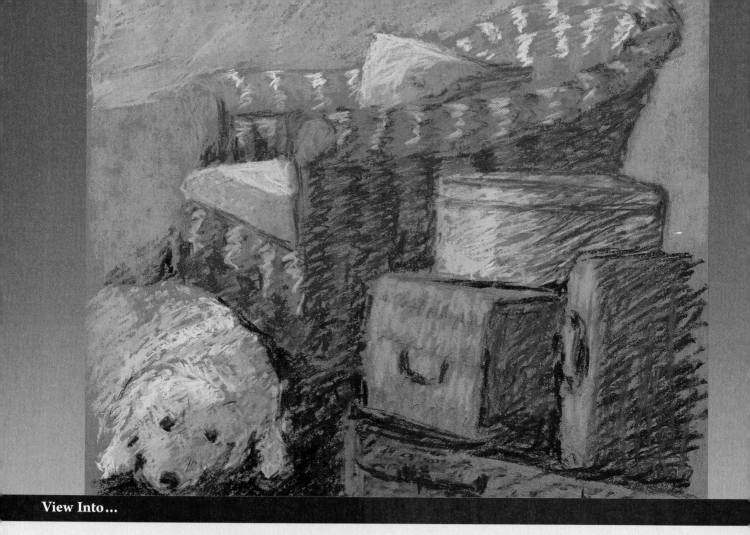

CHAPTER 33

Friday Night at the Movies

LAWRENCE E. FRISCH

CHAPTER OUTLINE

Shine (1996)
A Beautiful Mind (2001)
Spider (2003)
Tarnation (2004)
Canvas (2007)

Chapter 14: The Client Experiencing Depression

The Fire Within (1963)
Patch Adams (1998)
The Wrong Man (1956)
Ordinary People (1980)
Vincent and Theo (1990)
Off the Map (2005)

Chapter 15: The Client Experiencing Mania

A Fine Madness (1966)
Animal House (1978)
Mosquito Coast (1986)
The Butcher Boy (1998)
Mr. Jones (1993)
The Devil and Daniel Johnston (2006)

Chapter 16: The Client Who Is Suicidal

It's a Wonderful Life (1946)
The Slender Thread (1965)
Harold and Maude (1971)
The Virgin Suicides (2000)
Whose Life Is It Anyway? (1981)
The Big Chill (1983)
Sylvia (2003) also The Bell Jar (1979)
Wilby Wonderful (2005)

Chapter 17: The Client Who Abuses Chemical Substances

The Lost Weekend (1945)
I'll Cry Tomorrow (1955)
The Man with the Golden Arm (1955)
Panic in Needle Park (1971)
The Seven Percent Solution (1976)
Clean and Sober (1988)
Drugstore Cowboy (1989)
Postcards from the Edge (1990)
Affliction (1999)
Requiem for a Dream (1998)
Traffic (2000)
Blow (2001)
Candy (2006)

Chapter 18: The Client with a Personality Disorder

Gone with the Wind (1939)
Gypsy (1962)
Play Misty for Me (1971)
Pee Wee's Big Adventure (1985)
The House of Games (1987)
Bad Influence (1990)
Henry: Portrait of a Serial Killer (1990)
What about Bob? (1991)
Heavy (1995)
The Station Agent (2003)
The Assassination of Richard Nixon (2004)
Tell Them Who You Are (2004)
Head-On (2005)

Chapter 19: The Client Experiencing a Somatoform, Factitious, or Dissociative Disorder

The Barretts of Wimpole Street (1934)
Send Me No Flowers (1964)
Safe (1995)
Hannah and Her Sisters (1986)
Dr. Jekyll and Mr. Hyde (1932)
The Three Faces of Eve (1957)
Sybil (1976)
Dancer in the Dark (2000)

Chapter 20: The Client with Disorders of Self-Regulation: Sleep Disorders, Eating Disorders, and Sexual Disorders

The Mark (1961)
The Best Little Girl in the World (1981)
Dreamchild (1985)
Superstar: The Karen Carpenter Story (1987)
Life Is Sweet (1990)
The Haridresser's Husband (1990)
Le Cri de la Soie (1996)
My Own Private Idaho (1991)
The Piano Teacher (2002)

UNIT 3: SPECIAL POPULATIONS

Chapter 21: The Physically Ill Client Experiencing Emotional Distress

The Pride of the Yankees (1942)
The Elephant Man (1980)
The Shadow Box (1980)
Parting Glances (1986)
Beaches (1988)
Awakenings (1990)
Passion Fish (1992)
Iris (2001)
Talk to Her (2002)

Chapter 22: Forgotten Populations: The Homeless and the Incarcerated

Short Eyes (1977)
Dead Man Out (1989)

The Fisher King (1991)
The Lovers on the Bridge (1991)
The Saint of Fort Washington (1993)

Chapter 23: The Child

The 400 Blows (1959)
The Effect of Cosmic Rays on Man-in-the-Moon Marigolds (1988)
Small Change (1976)
Rain Man (1988)
Lorenzo's Oil (1992)
The Danish Poet (2006)

Chapter 24: The Adolescent

Mouchette (1967)
Gaby: A True Story (1987)
My Left Foot (1989)
Wildflower (1991)
Good Will Hunting (1997)
Bluebird (2004)

Chapter 25: The Elderly

The Last Laugh (1922)
Kotch (1971)
Harry and Tonto (1974)
Gin Game (1984)
Driving Miss Daisy (1989)
Age Old Friends (1989)
Children of Nature (1991)
A Woman's Tale (1991)
The Straight Story (1999)
Young@Heart (2007)

Chapter 26: Survivors of Violence or Abuse

Murmur of the Heart (1971)
Judgment (1990)
Sleeping with the Enemy (1991)
Mystic River (2003)
Mysterious Skin (2005)

UNIT 4: NURSING INTERVENTIONS AND TREATMENT MODALITIES

Secrets of the Soul (1926)
Freud (1962)
Pressure Point (1962)
Lilith (1964)
Frances (1982)
The Dream Team (1989)
Prince of Tides (1991)
Shall We Dance? (1996)
Prime (2005)

COMPETENCIES

This chapter is provided for the student to experience learning while enjoying a movie! Remember, learning is possible in many situations. Invite your friends to watch with you, keep up your skills in observation, and don't forget the popcorn!

ACKNOWLEDGMENT

We are grateful to Mary Sherman of Wichita State University for sharing the filmography developed for her class "Critical Studies in Film: Psychology, Psychiatry, and the Cinema." Some of these films have been selected for review in this chapter.

While only some nurses will practice exclusively in psychiatric settings, all will work closely with clients to help each achieve his or her optimum physical, emotional, and spiritual well-being. The subject of mental health nursing is human psychological makeup and variation—the normal varieties and the abnormal extremes of the human response to life events. Grief, loss, depression, anxiety, disordered thought, and substance use and abuse—these are among the essential human experiences, experiences not just of the psychiatrically disturbed, but also of many individuals at some time in their lives. The nurse who learns to listen to, understand, empathize with, and provide help for the emotional aspects of a client's life and illness will have at his or her disposal some of the most powerful tools of a skilled healer. The core of psychiatric mental health nursing involves the understanding of human experience, an understanding also sought by writers and, in recent decades, by film makers. The editors and authors of this book feel strongly that there is no better way to understand nursing clients and their varied psychiatric conditions and diagnoses than by entering into their lives through reading literature *or* by turning down the lights and experiencing the magic world of film. The purpose of this chapter is to offer summary descriptions of more than 100 films, each available on VHS video and/or DVD, that complement the various sections of the text. Some of these films were made for television and may be difficult to find in video rental stores, while others are among the most famous classic films. Some were made decades ago, and others are as recent as this textbook itself. No attempt has been made to censor this list, and many viewers may find the violence or sexuality in a few of the films to be disturbing. The authors have tried to indicate which films should be viewed selectively, and it should be possible to choose films from the given list that are consistently appropriate for adult viewers. Your "Friday Night at the Movies" need not be a Friday, nor does it have to be every week. We think, however, that the more of these films you are able to watch, the more we will achieve our goal of communicating to you something of the *experience* of human transitions and human distress. And, if you really get hooked on psychiatry-related movies, you will surely want a copy of psychiatrist Dr. David Robinson's *Reel Psychiatry—Movie Portrayals of Psychiatric Conditions* (Rapid Psychler Press, Port Huron, Michigan, 2003). We have found Dr. Robinson's book immensely helpful in selecting our "Playbill" for this chapter, and we have greatly enjoyed his insightful comments and reviews. Another great source for information and highly intelligent film reviews on psychological subjects is psychiatrist Dr. Roland Atkinson, whose "Psychflix" Web site is http://www.psychflix.com/.

Now the moment you have been waiting for—*Psychiatric Mental Health Nursing*'s Edition 4 nominations for the Celluloid Psychiatry Top 10. These are the movies that we think you will definitely want to see while you are learning about psychiatric nursing. We find these films to have a winning combination of entertainment value and real insights into the experience of mental illness. The films are listed in chapter order:

One Flew Over the Cuckoo's Nest
Matchstick Men (shared with *The Aviator)*
Spider (shared with: *Clean, Shaven*)
The Wrong Man
Ordinary People
Mr. Jones
Sylvia
Drugstore Cowboy
Shine
Dreamchild

UNIT 1: FOUNDATIONS FOR PRACTICE

Chapters 1, 2, and 7: Psychiatric Institutions, Psychiatric Care, and Cultural Considerations

The films in this section provide an introduction to psychiatric care and its special challenges both in the contemporary United States and at other times and places.

Down to Earth

(1917) Douglas Fairbanks Pictures

A remarkable silent-era film starring the great Douglas Fairbanks as the "liberator" of a mental institution in which his girlfriend has been placed. The film offers a marvelous view of a now-distant institutional world through the camera skills of a (then) young Victor Fleming, who went on to direct two immortal films: *Gone with the Wind* and *The Wizard of Oz*.

Day at the Races

(1937) MGM

In this Marx Brothers farce, Groucho plays a veterinarian who, through a series of not entirely accidental misunderstandings, becomes chief psychiatrist at an institution for the mentally ill. While neither a lifelike portrayal of an earlier era's mental institutions nor one of the Marx Brothers' greatest, this film is still an amusing spoof on psychiatry and the definition of sanity in a bureaucratic society.

Titticut Follies

(1964) Bridgewater Film Productions

This film is now almost impossible to obtain, though some libraries may have copies. *Titticut Follies* is a true-life documentary about the squalor and degradation experienced by patients at a large public mental institution near Boston. The public outcry that director Frederick Wiseman's film generated on its release gave great impetus to deinstitutionalization. The film is highly disturbing in its shocking depiction of dehumanization, but is a "must see" if it can be located.

King of Hearts

(1966) Compania Cinamatografica Montoro

A notable film about a war-torn French town repopulated by inhabitants of the local institution for the mentally ill. While decidedly odd in some ways, the society created by these "sick" individuals seems abundantly more sane than that of the world around them. This is a memorable film of great warmth, charm, and humanity.

Marat Sade

(1966) United Artists

An imagining of the eighteenth-century insane asylum where the infamous Marquis de Sade was housed for many years as a (probably thoroughly sane) threat to French public morals. In this film—as he did in real life—the Marquis produces a play with his fellow clients as actors. The film is intriguing, and it provides a somewhat fanciful view of the care of the mentally ill in another country and another era.

One Flew Over the Cuckoo's Nest

(1975) United Artists

A very fine film produced at the height of the deinstitutionalization movement. A sane, but personality-disordered, patient meets his match in the person of Big Nurse. This film defined a whole generation's view of mental health facilities and personnel. Its negative view of the abuse of medical and nursing authority contributed to public and legislative enthusiasm for the downsizing of mental health institutions. *One Flew Over the Cuckoo's Nest* is regarded by many as among the greatest films of the last 35 years.

Network

(1976) MGM/United Artists

This film tells the story of a television newscaster who develops a debilitating mental illness that severely interferes with his work. In the noncelebrity world, he might be expected to receive treatment and then return to this (or another) job. In this four-time Oscar-winning dramatic version of life lived in the limelight, the television network attempts to benefit financially from Peter Finch's illness, turning him into a celebrity in the process. The story is familiar at least to politicians: People in the public eye often must give up all hope of maintaining private lives, even in the face of serious health concerns.

The Ninth Configuration

(1979) Warner Brothers

See this strange movie along with *Twelve Monkeys,* or if you want to have a really bizarre movie evening, add *Being John Malkovich* as well. *The Ninth Configuration* is a story about a military hospital for the mentally ill where the uniformed inmates plot a rebellion under the watchful eye of the hospital commander (who may be as unbalanced as they are).

A Man Facing Southeast

(1986) Cinaquanon

A film from Argentina about an unexpected visitor to an institution for the mentally ill. The movie describes a psychologist's attempt to determine if the visitor is truly insane or if, as he claims, he is really an alien from another world. The movie offers insights into mental health care in another culture and raises intriguing questions about the nature of sanity.

The Madness of King George

(1994) Samuel Goldwyn Company

Another view of madness in a distant country and time, but this time it is the madness of King George III, the ruler of England at the time of the American Revolution. It is currently believed that George suffered from hereditary porphyria, a metabolic disorder that produces episodic abdominal pain and psychosis. In the movie George is odd, if not psychotic, and his caretakers give some insight into competing eighteenth-century views of psychiatric management.

Kids in the Hall: Brain Candy

(1996) Paramount Pictures

Most of the films reviewed in this chapter are serious attempts to depict and understand the human experience of mental illness. *Brain Candy* is the exception: a (more or less) comic story about the invention of a new antidepressant medication. While highly successful in reversing depression, the new drug, "Gleemonox," turns out to eventually cause irreversible coma in its users. The film turns improbable, but with a disturbing hint of truth, when the drug's promoters attempt to market the comatose state as a desirable outcome. *Brain Candy* is far from an accurate portrayal of depression, antidepressants, or even the ethical problems of postmarketing drug side effects. It *is* sometimes funny and would make a good Friday night break from studies.

The Madness of King George

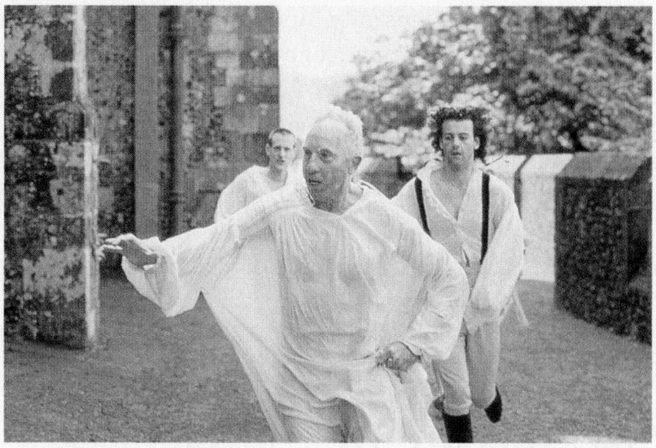

Courtesy: Sam Goldwyn/Channel Four/Close Call/The Kobal Collection

Twelve Monkeys

(1995) Universal Pictures

A combination of *Back to the Future, Outbreak,* and *On the Beach, Twelve Monkeys* stars Bruce Willis as a time-traveling envoy from a future haunted by a deadly virus. His romantic interest is a psychiatrist, so there's plenty of lunacy (including, some believe, the movie itself). It is a strange plot (what there is of it), a curious but compelling movie, and only peripherally about recognizable mental illness.

Being John Malkovich

(1999) Gramercy Pictures

One of the most valuable abilities a nurse can have is the skill of entering into the mind of another individual. The result is a better understanding of how the world looks "from the inside." Unless, that is, you are director Spike Jonze and you are making this movie. Somehow the seventh floor of a New York office building contains a tunnel that allows direct entry into the mind of the actor John Malkovich. Anyone crawling into the tunnel soon finds himself or herself inside this poor fellow's head and looking at the world through Malkovich's eyes. This "insight" lasts 15 minutes before the inhabitant is summarily ejected onto the soft shoulder of the New Jersey Turnpike. Jonze's idea of entering the client's mind is decidedly different from what most psychiatric nurses mean by this concept, but the results of taking the idea this literally are intriguingly whacky—and at times even thought provoking.

House of Fools

2003 (Paramount)

This Russian film about war and a Chechen asylum was filmed on location and "stars" mostly the residents of a real institution for the mentally ill, though with several "real" actors mixed in. This alone gives the movie a unique status—risking perhaps being a Russian *Titticut Follies.* But instead, it is closer to *King of Hearts* in its portrayal of the not-unrelated madnesses of war and insanity. And in this movie, as in *King of Hearts,* there's a strong connection between the two. Admirers of *The Station Master* (all three of these films are reviewed in this chapter) will not be surprised to see a dwarfed individual feature prominently. Critics almost uniformly disliked *House of Fools,* but we found it every bit as engrossing as our favorite, *King of Hearts,* and somehow even more real despite its fantastical mix of fact and fiction, actors and inmates.

UNIT 2: CLIENTS WITH PSYCHIATRIC DISORDERS

Chapter 11: The Client Undergoing Crisis

The films in this section depict real or (in the case of *On the Beach*) imagined physical or psychological crises and the human reactions that follow them.

Seventh Veil

(1945) Universal Pictures

The heroine is a pianist whose hands are severely burned in an accident. This crisis precipitates deep depression, suicidal thoughts, and seems to bring an end to the heroine's artistic career, but all is restored through hypnosis and psychotherapy. James Mason and Ann Todd make a memorable movie out of a melodramatic script.

On the Beach

(1959) United Artists

An antiwar movie about life after a nuclear holocaust. A remarkable cast—Gregory Peck, Anthony Perkins, Ava Gardner, and Fred Astaire—portrays one extreme of possible human crises.

Cleo from 5 to 7

(1962) Rome-Paris Films

This French film follows Cleo's wanderings through Paris while she waits to learn whether or not she has cancer. A well-respected film from the 1960s, *Cleo* realistically portrays the stress that comes from uncertainty about illness.

Grbavica

(2006) Coop 99

No crisis has affected more Europeans in recent years than the war in former Yugoslavia. Set in a suburb of Sarajevo, this is a deep, affecting, and perhaps cautiously optimistic film about the personal and emotional ravages of war seen as a crisis involving the whole of society. Unlike many war films, this one is not primarily about PTSD, but instead focuses on how the experience of war affects an entire generation—as seen here through the relationship of a mother and her coming-of-age daughter. The theme is hardly new, but the setting, and the two leading actresses, are memorable. This excellent movie is among the latest in a fine string of Bosnian film productions.

Chapter 12: The Client Experiencing Anxiety

Anxiety is one of the most common and most distressing human experiences. Many films powerfully depict anxiety in its various forms.

As Good as It Gets

(1997) Columbia/TriStar

A Jack Nicholson movie showcasing Obsessive-Compulsive Disorder (OCD), although in a character a bit too aggressive and unpleasant to not have some other Axis II diagnosis lurking in the background as well. Unpleasant he may be, but Nicholson's Melvin Udall—by trade the author of pulp novels—somehow manages to be immensely likeable as well. Believe it or not, despite the counting rituals and cleaning obsessions, this is a funny movie that easily makes our list of the best all-time psychiatric celluloid.

High Anxiety

(1977) 20th Century Fox

In this film, comic director Mel Brooks (*Blazing Saddles*) spoofs both fear of heights and some of Alfred Hitchcock's most famous thriller films. The leading character is a psychiatrist who is afraid of heights and gets caught up in solving a murder mystery that requires him to visit a number of very scary high places. Since such "exposure therapy" has been shown to be of value for persons with phobias, this otherwise whacky film contains a core of serious psychological truth.

Johnny Stecchino

(1991) MGM

OCD is only one of the subplots in this delightful Italian film about mistaken identity. Dante (Roberto Benigni), a charming

As Good As It Gets

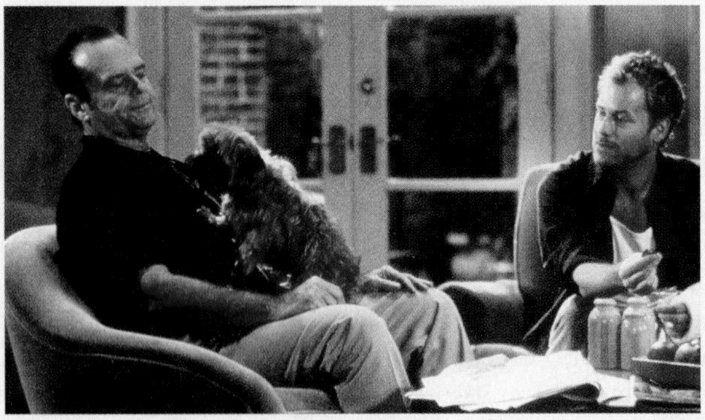

Courtesy: Tristar/Gracie Films/The Kobal Collection

but decidedly odd school bus driver with a best friend with Down syndrome, looks surprisingly like a notorious Mafioso who is also played, not surprisingly, by Benigni. Ever naive, Dante enjoys a free trip to Sicily—never suspecting that the beautiful woman who invites him there plans to have him bumped off by his Mafia look-alike's enemies. A series of improbable events puts Dante back in Rome and his look-alike underground. You may have seen Benigni in the better-known film *Life Is Beautiful*. *Johnny Stecchino* (Johnny Toothpick) lacks the later film's serious message, but not its comic charm and intensity.

The Fear Inside

(1992) Viacom

Agoraphobia makes the heroine of this film deathly afraid of the world outside her home. The strength of this movie is the realistic sense of ungrounded fear that it conveys. Not one of the all-time greats, but a good portrayal of a common anxiety disorder.

Copycat

(1995) Warner Brothers

In this film, Sigourney Weaver plays a criminologist whose near murder leads to a profound post-traumatic Agoraphobia. From the seclusion of her apartment she is able to help a trusting detective (Holly Hunter) find a vicious serial killer. Serial killers generally have Antisocial Personality Disorder, but the movie is not an extraordinary example of this psychiatric diagnosis. It does convey fairly accurately the terror that keeps persons with Agoraphobia out of situations in which they feel exposed and threatened. Few persons become agoraphobic because they, like Sigourney Weaver, have been assaulted and consequently suffer from PTSD. However, if you can tolerate gratuitously violent movies, you will come away from *Copycat* with a better understanding of the experience of Agoraphobia.

Vertigo

(1958, 1997) Paramount Pictures

A classic Alfred Hitchcock film (spoofed in Mel Brooks's *High Anxiety* discussed previously) in which the hero's fear of heights leads to the death of a friend and (perhaps) to the death of a mysterious woman who returns to haunt his days and nights. A great dramatic portrayal of two anxiety diagnoses: fear of heights and PTSD. *Vertigo,* rereleased in a much improved 1997 version, is widely acknowledged as one of the greatest of all motion pictures.

Little Voice

(1998) Miramax

A shy girl makes good. Little Voice (L.V.) is a young British woman with social phobia who—when the lights go out—can belt out 1940s hits with a voice that is anything but little. This wonderful film sets her social phobia in a small English town complete with overbearing mother and sleazy talent scout. Another must-see selection on our all-time psychiatric celluloid list.

Little Voice

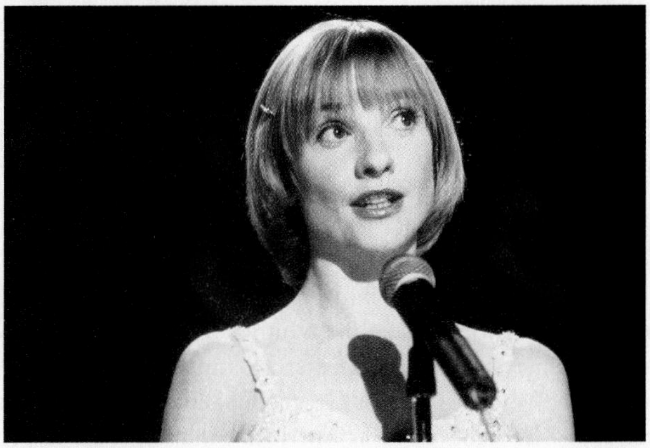

Miramax (Courtesy: The Kobal Collection)

The Aviator

(2004) Miramax Films

The famously reclusive Howard Hughes suffered from OCD, substance abuse, and perhaps also psychosis during his complex and tortured life. Some of his story is recounted in Chapter 12. A good deal more is found in this Martin Scorcese film about the middle years of Hughes' life, with Howard Hughes played by Leonardo DiCaprio. This film addresses many of the psychological issues in Hughes' life, but also chronicles a very compelling story involving one of mid-twentieth century America's wealthiest—and strangest—entrepreneurs.

Matchstick Men

(2005) Warner Brothers

Nicolas Cage plays a character who has nearly every anxiety disorder in the DSM as well as a good dose of Antisocial Personality Disorder—though, perhaps through ineptitude, he generally manages to cheat his victims only out of relatively small amounts of money. Providing further, if fictional, evidence that antisocial personality may be inherited, Cage's character's daughter from a long-past relationship emerges on the scene and becomes involved with her father in bigger scams that lead to trouble for all. Cage's portrayal makes the movie worth seeing, and Alison Lohman is particularly good as the wayward daughter.

Chapter 13: The Client Experiencing Schizophrenia

Filmmakers have been powerfully attracted to stories involving schizophrenia and other psychotic states. The results have been a number of fairly accurate portrayals of both the experience of schizophrenia and other psychotic states. Several of the films recommended here deal with delusions rather than full-blown schizophrenia.

David and Lisa

(1962) Continental Distributing

This is a classic film about psychotic mental illness. David and Lisa are institutionalized adolescents who fall in love and, as a consequence, pose immense problems for their paternalistic caretakers. A beautiful and touching movie.

They Might Be Giants

(1971) Universal Pictures

This film can be hard to find but makes a good antidote to the extreme seriousness of many other films on serious psychiatric subjects. The movie stars Joanne Woodward as a psychiatrist who treats actor George C. Scott for delusions of grandeur—he believes he is Sherlock Holmes. If he is pronounced insane and committed, Scott's money goes to another character in the film, so Woodward is under a lot of pressure to make the "correct" clinical decision. Parts of this film are very funny, and it serves as a good, if light-hearted, introduction to grandiose delusions.

The Story of Adele H.

(1975) Les Productions Artistes Associés

A young French woman becomes psychotic after her betrayal and rejection by an English soldier. She lives out her last years in an institution, writing letters in an indecipherable code. This movie captures the experience of psychosis as well as any film that has been made, and while sad, it is perhaps not as depressing as most other films about mood and thought disorders. It is beautifully photographed and directed by François Truffaut—a "must see." (French, with English subtitles.)

I Never Promised You a Rose Garden

(1977) New World

A film version of the popular 1960s book of the same name that portrays the development and treatment of schizophrenia in an adolescent woman. It is a realistic and touching film, but very hard to find in most video stores. The book is just as good and much easier to come by; be sure to see this one if you can locate it.

The Story of Adele H.

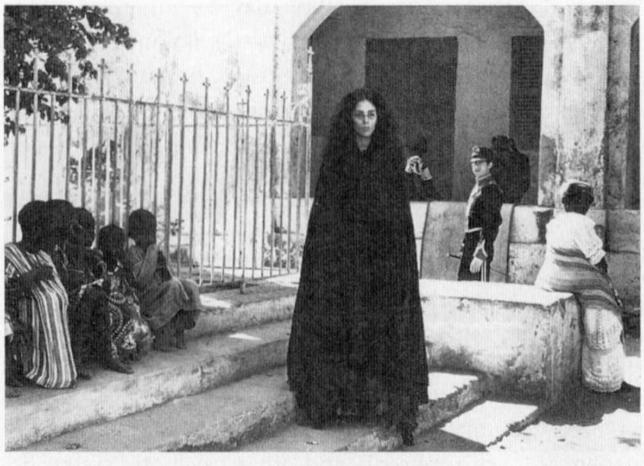

Films du Carosse/Artistes Associés (Courtesy: The Kobal Collection)

Clean, Shaven

(1993) Good Machine

It is hard to imagine a better, and more disturbing, movie about the experience of schizophrenia. This is a film starring Peter Greene (also in *Pulp Fiction*) as a young man with schizophrenia trying to survive in a confusing and sometimes terrifying world. While the film's soundtrack reflects seemingly random noise and disconnected speech, the camera brilliantly details Peter's obsessions and his fearful encounters with daily reality. The plot is loosely about Peter's search for a daughter from his pre-illness life and about the way schizophrenia robs him, but not completely, of the ability to love and be loved. Shocking, touching, and unnerving, *Clean, Shaven* is *the* movie about psychosis. It is not easy to watch, but it should not be missed.

Shine

(1996) Warner Brothers

See what you think about pianist David Helfgott's diagnosis in this film based on a true story of a pianist who recovers his career after years of mental illness. David almost certainly has schizophrenia, but he is a very isolated and unusual child well before the symptoms of this disorder surface. Does he have an underlying schizoid or even Schizotypal Personality Disorder? Or does he have Asperger's syndrome? What seems more clear is that David's father, Peter, suffers from Paranoid Personality Disorder. David is sometimes a bit too open and cheerful in adult life to be a convincing schizophrenic (or schizoid, or schizotypal personality), but this is a minor complaint about a wonderful story of triumph over severe mental illness. It is another top-ranking "psychiatric celluloid" feature.

A Beautiful Mind

(2001) Universal Pictures

Not your typical schizophrenic, real-life John Nash is a world-class mathematician who also suffers from delusions and hallucinations. The film is based on a true story, so it is hard not to believe that Nash was able to somehow gain control over his illness and to achieve success against odds. This work portrays both the positive and negative symptoms of schizophrenia, though, not surprisingly (in a film), visual hallucinations play a greater role than auditory. In real-life schizophrenia, the opposite is more commonly true. This is an engaging film, but not the most accurate evocation of the experience of schizophrenia. Try *Clean, Shaven* or *Spider* for more accuracy, but perhaps a bit less Hollywood. By the way, if you'd prefer an impressive *Bollywood* view of schizophrenia, try *Devrai (The Sacred Grove)*. While not strictly Bollywood (it's a Marathi language film—Bollywood films are in the Hindi language), *Devrai* is an Indian film about schizophrenia starring psychiatrist and well-known actor

A Beautiful Mind

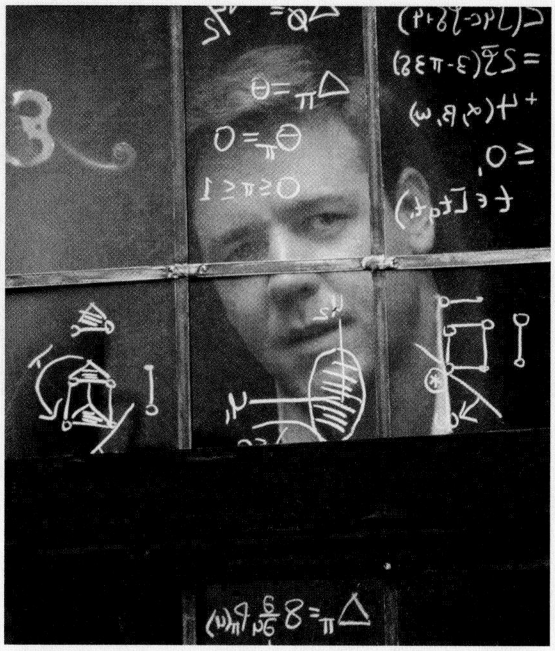

Courtesy: Dreamworks/Universal/The Kobal Collection

Dr. Mohan Agashe. Like *Canvas,* (reviewed below) the film's major focus is on the effect of schizophrenia on family members. With good sleuthing, you can probably see this film free on the Internet (we did, but unfortunately in a version lacking English subtitles for the dialogue). Fortunately, there's a nice plot summary to be found as well http://www.chowk.com/articles/9835, as accessed January 1, 2009.

Spider

(2003) Sony

As was discussed in Chapter 13, most persons with schizophrenia are not violent, however this film does describe a plausible occurrence—while arguably reinforcing a stereotype view of this disorder. Despite this caveat, Ralph Fiennes' performance as "Spider" is one of the best portrayals of schizophrenia ever done in film. Another "don't miss" film, if like most filmgoers you are not averse to movie violence. In this case, at least, the violence is not gratuitous.

Tarnation

(2004) Wellspring

This film is perhaps most famous for being shot on a budget of around $200 using home-edited video and computer shareware. Like *Canvas* (see following) it chronicles the experience of growing up in a family with a schizophrenic mother. This film portrays its director's mother as suffering from both schizophrenia and depression—a not rare combination often termed "schizoaffective disorder." This too is a "must see" film. You may have trouble finding it locally, but it is available through several mail-order rental services.

Canvas

(2007) Screen Media

Directed by Joseph Greco, whose own mother suffered from schizophrenia, this film is an affecting dramatization of the experience of growing up in a family like Greco's. This is his first film, and some critics thought its content leaned a little too much toward "made for TV" emotionality. However, the acting by Joe Pantoliano as husband of the mentally ill woman played by Marcia Gay Harden (who also acts exceptionally well) is reason enough to see this film.

Chapter 14: The Client Experiencing Depression

Loss and depression are nearly universal human experiences that a number of excellent films have explored sensitively.

The Fire Within

(1963) Nouvelles Editions de Films

As depressing as movies come, *The Fire Within*'s hero, despondent and alcoholic, becomes increasingly depressed after his psychiatric hospitalization. He gives up hope and calmly makes plans to kill himself. Based on the true story of the life of a well-known French writer, it is a realistic evocation of the very depths of despair.

Patch Adams

(1998) Universal Pictures

This film is a depiction of severe depression overcome through vision, commitment, and work. This is not the way things really turn out, and anyone who has heard the real-life charismatic Patch talk about either his depression or his vision will see how little of the man Robin Williams has captured on screen. Still, it is a mostly feel-good movie that hints at the power of health care idealism in a world dominated by medicine for money.

The Wrong Man

(1956) Warner Home Video

Yes it is old, but portrayals of profound—ultimately psychotic—depression do not get any better than this. In this film, starring Henry Fonda and Vera Miles, life circumstances lead to the development of depression in Vera's character, Rose. Of course, in real life it does not take your husband's false accusation of having committed a crime to precipitate depression, but what Alfred Hitchcock movie lets reality call the shots?

Ordinary People

(1980) Paramount Pictures

In this film, depression, suicide attempt, hospitalization, and electroconvulsive therapy all follow the accidental death of the hero Conrad's brother in a boating accident. Psychoanalysis comes to the rescue, with some fairly good scenes of therapist/client interaction. Conrad's mother—the source of many of his problems—could benefit from therapy as well.

Vincent and Theo

(1990) Arena Films

This textbook includes reproductions of a number of paintings by the great nineteenth-century artist Vincent van Gogh, who is the subject of this exquisite film about art, mental illness, and the love of friends and brothers. This is a beautiful and touching film that, despite Vincent's tormented life and eventual suicide, is probably more about art and love than mental illness.

Off the Map

(2005) Holedigger Studios

A largely accurate portrayal of severe depression in an unusual family living a remote "back to nature" lifestyle. If you like to see the extraordinary beauty of New Mexico on film, combined with a fetching story about odd but interesting people, then this is the film for you. Taking someone else's antidepressant medication, as depicted in this film, is neither wise nor recommended, even if the eventual outcome is positive.

Chapter 15: The Client Experiencing Mania

Movies are particularly useful for understanding mania because, unlike depression, which we all feel at some time, mania is an unusual experience of extraordinary intensity. Several films do a remarkable job of portraying this seriously disruptive mood disorder.

A Fine Madness

(1966) Warner Brothers

A probably manic poet cavorts through the fairly pleasant New York of the 1960s and survives the malignant efforts of his psychiatrists. (See this film along with *The Fisher King*, which shows an equally manic Robin Williams in a far more threatening modern New York.)

Animal House

(1978) Universal Pictures

A movie with an abundantly manic tone—so, it might seem, was John Belushi, who stars in *Animal House* and went on to a number of equally zany acting roles before his untimely death. The film's subject is fraternity life (or some fictional view of what fraternity life could be at its very worst); it includes moviedom's grossest foodfight. Primarily a cult film, but it does give a good sense of the energy that gives rise to manic behavior.

Don Juan de Marco

(1995) New Line Cinema

Yet another film about grandiosity. This hero is convinced he is truly Don Juan, the famous seducer of women immortalized in Mozart's opera *Don Giovanni*. It is an enjoyable recent treatment of delusions of grandeur and the energy that drives manic behavior.

Don Juan de Marco

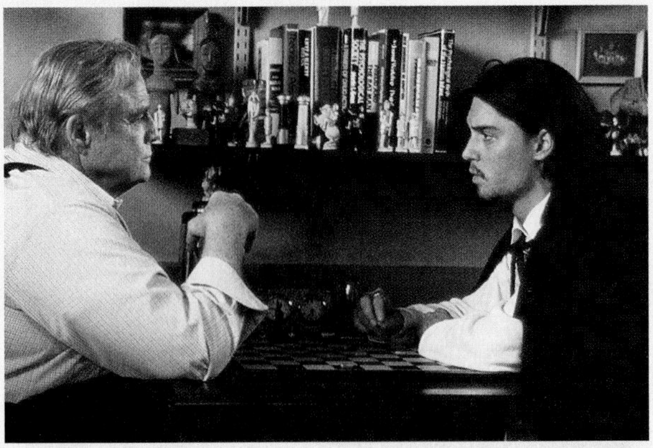

Courtesy: New Line/Zoetrope/The Kobal Collection

The Butcher Boy

(1988) Warner Brothers

Take your pick: either this film is about the development of personality disorder (probably antisocial) in a 12-year-old Irish boy or about the evolution of bipolar depression in his mother, Annie. Strictly speaking, it has to be the former, but we have put the movie in this section because of its accurate portrayal of serious mental illness, depression, and suicide. This is one of the very fine films from director Neil Jordan, who also directed the better known films *Crying Game* and *Mona Lisa*.

Mr. Jones

(1993) Columbia Tri-Star

There is much to dislike about this movie, perhaps its ending and especially its love affair between the manic-depressive patient (Mr. Jones) and his psychiatrist. While psychiatrists do continue to become emotionally involved with their clients, outside a Hollywood movie any romantic involvement is considered unethical and can lead to loss of licensure. Although actor Richard Gere is thoroughly convincing at both poles of his Bipolar Disorder, no other film we know of gives such a great portrayal of mania. Seeing this film, you may wish the psychiatrist would give Mr. Jones a little less attention and a little more lithium, but you will have a great understanding of what it means to be manic.

The Devil and Daniel Johnston

(2006) Sony Pictures

As you may know, Daniel Johnston is a singer/songwriter and cartoon artist from Texas who has suffered severely from mental illness during his life. Mania has had a huge impact on him

Mr. Jones

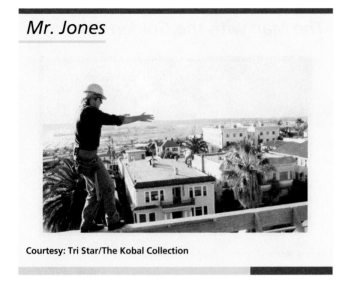

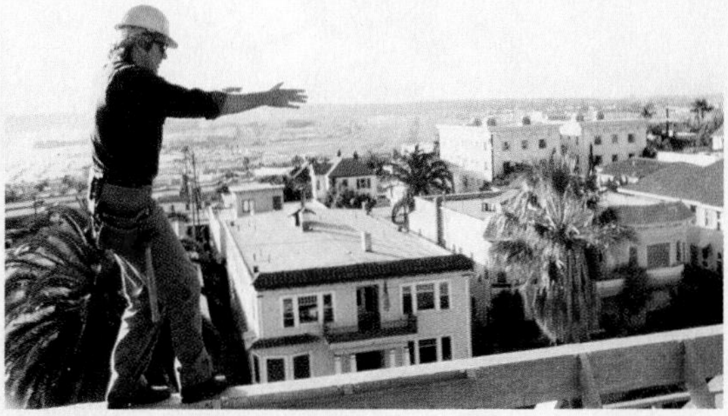

Courtesy: Tri Star/The Kobal Collection

as portrayed in this biopic chronicling his difficult years as well as his recent post-treatment successes in both music and art. Take a look at this film, whose title borrows from the famous 1941 film starring Walter Huston, *The Devil and Daniel Webster,* or at least look at Johnston's Web site, www.hihowareyou.com. Johnston is far from the only artist with bipolar disorder, but this film offers a valuable window into how powerful and widespread an effect this condition can have.

Chapter 16: The Client Who Is Suicidal

It's a Wonderful Life

(1946) RKO Pictures

This is a 1940s "feel good" film that evokes a postwar Hollywood view of optimism and hope. The hero, played by James Stewart, is saved from suicidal depression by an unlikely visit from a (heavenly) angel who shows him the love and warmth that truly surrounds his life. This film is sugary and far from an accurate depiction of the suicidal depths of depression. Few nonpsychotic individuals are saved from suicide by a celestial visitor, but this is otherwise vintage Hollywood at its best. *It's a Wonderful Life* would probably have walked away with all of the Oscars for 1946, but it was released the same year as the even greater *The Best Years of Our Lives.* See them together to understand how deeply the stresses of war affected American life in the 1940s.

The Slender Thread

(1965) Paramount Pictures

A film produced at a time when community mental health centers and suicide hotlines were first making their appearance. Adapted from a supposedly true story published in *Time Magazine,* the movie portrays a college student who answers a suicide hotline and has to keep the heroine talking long enough for police to trace the call before she dies of the sleeping pill overdose she has taken. In real life, and on the screen, the student saves the day and the young woman. It is probably not Hollywood's greatest film, but stars two of its best: Anne Bancroft and Sidney Poitier.

Harold and Maude

(1971) Paramount Pictures

A 1970s cult classic that looks wryly at youth, old age, and love. A suicidally depressed 20-something-year-old and an 80-year-old improbably fall in love; the result is at times very funny and often very touching. Harold and Maude is perhaps a bit dated, and its view of depression may be more theatrical than realistic, but this is an often remarkable "must see" film.

The Virgin Suicides

(1998) Universal Pictures

This film is not so much a psychological exploration of why teenage women kill themselves, "copycat" suicide, depression, or even family dysfunction, as it is something of all of these. A stunning first feature film by Sofia Coppola (director of *Lost in Translation*), this movie traces the permanent scars that suicide leaves on survivors as it evokes the world of a quiet 1970s Midwest suburb.

Whose Life Is It Anyway?

(1981) MGM

A funny movie that raised important questions about assisted suicide of the severely ill long before such questions reached wide public attention. Richard Dreyfuss plays a sculptor who becomes paraplegic and wants to die. The acting is excellent, and the issues remain contemporary many years after the film's release.

The Big Chill

(1983) Columbia Pictures

A friend's suicide leads to the reunion of a group of college friends who recall his life and its intermingling with their own. It is a beautiful and touching film about friendship, death, and changing eras and values.

The Bell Jar

(1979) AVCO Embassy Pictures

and

Sylvia

(2003) Focus Features

The Bell Jar is not a particularly great film and not particularly easy to find (probably for that reason). The book of the same name (see Chapter 15) is much better, but if you can find this film, it is worth seeing.

You will likely want to see this one along with the 2003 biopic of its author, Sylvia Plath, *Sylvia. Sylvia* conveys Plath's obsession with death and suggests a bipolar temperament unable to find a life-affirming way in marriage, in work, or on two continents.

Wilby Wonderful

(2005) Palpable Productions

This film describes "a day in the life" of one small Canadian town (Wilby) with enough present and past intrigue to last a lifetime. Suicidal ideation is only one of the many themes that run through the movie, but the film does give some insight, albeit often comical, into recurring suicidal despair. The world's real small-town Wilbys are usually far from wonderful, but this sleeper of a movie about suicide, and much else, is worth seeing—though outside of Canada it probably has to be rented by mail since it was never widely released.

Chapter 17: The Client Who Abuses Chemical Substances

It sometimes seems hard to find a film that *does not* depict excessive drinking or other substance misuse. Some films, such as those described below, do an extraordinary job of portraying the experience of substance dependence and addiction.

The Lost Weekend

(1945) Paramount Pictures

One of Hollywood's all-time great films and a stunning depiction of alcoholic denial, this film won four Oscars in 1945, including best picture. It remains eminently worth seeing despite a less-than-realistic ending.

I'll Cry Tomorrow

(1955) MGM

One of Susan Hayward's great 1950s films about an actress's struggle with alcoholism, this movie features a variety of notable period songs.

The Man with the Golden Arm

(1955) United Artists

This is a classic Frank Sinatra movie about heroin addiction. While 1955 audiences found the film shocking, it may seem somewhat melodramatic today. Realistically portraying many aspects of addict life, this is a film in the same spirit as William Burroughs' heroin memoirs (see Chapter 16). It was made just as the U.S. Congress was establishing penalties for drug possession and caught—or played on—the antidrug spirit of the day.

Panic in Needle Park

(1971) 20th Century Fox

Al Pacino's first major film, *Panic in Needle Park* is a realistic portrayal of substance abuse, crime, and prostitution. While crack cocaine has significantly changed the culture of addiction, this film still gives an accurate picture of the desperate lives of many substance abusers. Far less violent than Pacino's later films (*The Godfather*, *Scarface*), *Panic* is not for the easily depressed.

The Man with the Golden Arm

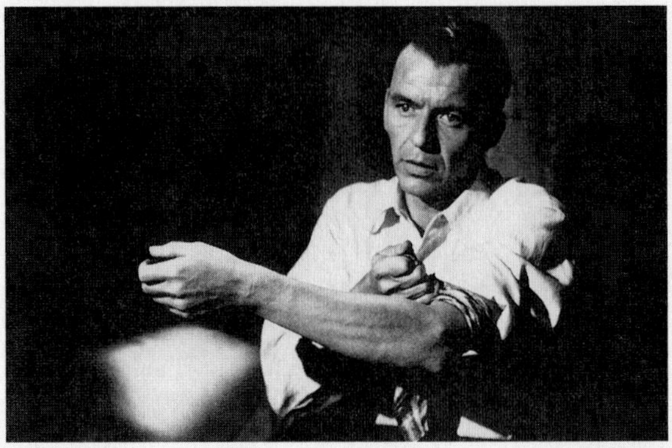

United Artists (Courtesy: The Kobal Collection)

The Seven Percent Solution

(1976) Universal Pictures

Dr. Watson meets Dr. Freud. Or rather, Sherlock Holmes is referred to Dr. Freud by his friend, Dr. Watson. The reason? Holmes's cocaine habit. Readers of this textbook will know that Freud was no stranger to cocaine himself, and while Conan Doyle never actually brought Dr. Freud into a Sherlock Holmes story, Freud and Holmes were more or less contemporaries. Here the founder of psychoanalysis is right at home solving a mystery. Lots of fun, for a Sherlock Holmes flick.

Clean and Sober

(1988) Warner Brothers

Morgan Freeman turns in a fine supporting performance while Michael Keaton plays a substance-abusing real estate salesman who struggles to kick his habit. It is a tough film that effectively captures some of the desperation behind addiction and substance abuse. Highly recommended.

Drugstore Cowboy

(1989) Avenue Pictures

This cops and robbers film is about abuse of prescription drugs and dramatically links pharmacy hold-ups with injection drug use. Today we think of drugs as primarily bought and sold on the street—largely because effective distribution networks likely keep prices lower than they would be if theft from "legitimate" sources was the primary route. But whatever the economic realities, this film is a great portrayal of the allegiances, superstitions, and cravings that link substance abusers to one another and to their abused substances. This is one of the truly great mental health-related films, and it is one of the films that helped to create successful non-Hollywood alternate film making in the United States.

Postcards from the Edge

(1990) Columbia Pictures

An amazing cast that includes Meryl Streep, Shirley MacLaine, Gene Hackman, and Richard Dreyfuss. Drug dependence (Meryl Streep's character) is only part of this story about an aspiring actress. Perhaps not one of Streep's all-time great performances, but a fast-paced and captivating movie worth seeing on a Friday night.

Affliction

(1999) Lions Gate Films

This is a story of alcohol abuse and its effect on two generations. Nick Nolte plays a small-town sheriff whose life has been dominated by his violent, alcoholic father. Part crime thriller, part character study, this is a compelling piece about the ways that substance abuse and family violence cast a very long shadow on troubled lives.

Requiem for a Dream

(1998) Artisan

This film is neither an antidrug movie nor a glorification of drug use. But it immerses the viewer in a drug-dominated world in which the four major characters—all with a claim on our emotions—live lives totally dominated by drug use. The rhythms of the film itself reflect drug use: the action speeds up and slows down dramatically depending on who has taken what drug. But this is no trick; the cinematography works, and the movie is dramatically compelling.

Traffic

(2000) USA Films

This film is not about substance abuse itself, but about the U.S. antidrug war that began in the late 1930s with the Food, Drug, and Cosmetic Act and gathered momentum through the 1960s. This Steven Soderbergh movie offers no solution to what is indeed a worldwide drug problem. But it does show how ineffective and misguided much of our antidrug legislation and enforcement has been over the past 70 years or more.

Requiem for a Dream

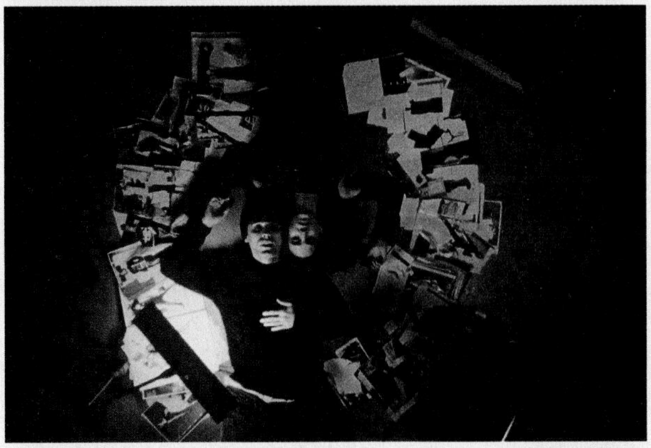

Artisan (Courtesy: The Kobal Collection)

Blow

(2001) New Line Cinema

Blow is another cocaine movie and another Johnny Depp film. Not every critic liked this movie, but it is a grim, exciting, and a pretty good depiction of the hold that cocaine can have on the body, mind, and pocketbook. The real-life subject of this film is probably still in jail on drug charges, but his story is a compelling view into the world of drug use and drug smuggling.

Candy

(2006) ThinkFilm

Another film starring Heath Ledger (*Brokeback Mountain*), but this time as a handsome and poetic heroin addict paired with fetching painter Abbie Cornish who's addicted to heroin and in love with him. This film, as many critics point out, doesn't stray far from the tragic storyline set out in *Man with a Golden Arm* or *Requiem for a Dream* (both reviewed previously). But its antiheroes are terrific and act convincingly even as their lives, finances, and physical appearances unravel in the throes of substance dependency.

Chapter 18: The Client with a Personality Disorder

With the exception of the antisocial personalities who flourish in *film noir* and inhabit most of Hollywood's most violent movies, few directors set out to depict any specific *Diagnostic and Statistical Manual of Mental Disorders,* Fourth Edition-Text Revision (DSM-IV-TR) personality disorder. However, elements of both the dramatic and the eccentric personality categories are frequently and effectively depicted in numerous films.

Gone with the Wind

(1939) Selznick International Films

On nearly anyone's list of all-time great movies, *Gone with the Wind* is far more than a study of Ashley Wilkes's Avoidant Personality Disorder. This immortal Hollywood epic runs for nearly four hours, and Ashley's avoidant personality is central to the story.

Gypsy

(1962) Warner Brothers

Gypsy is a musical adaptation of the Broadway play about (among other matters) Histrionic Personality Disorder. See the 1962 version starring Rosalind Russell and Natalie Wood, although there is a 1993 remake with Bette Midler in the title role.

Play Misty for Me

(1971) Universal Pictures

This was Clint Eastwood's first film as a director, and it is a powerful drama about a young woman who almost certainly has Borderline Personality Disorder (BPD). Not only does she cut her own wrists (not unusual for BPD), but her possessive emotional attachments turn decidedly homicidal (probably more characteristic of Hollywood movies than of BPD). But this is an exciting film that captures much of the roller-coaster experience of a relationship with someone who has a borderline personality.

Pee Wee's Big Adventure

(1985) Warner Brothers

Pee Wee is too charming to be schizoid, too socially committed to be avoidant, and probably too unique to have a clearly diagnosable personality disorder. Still, it would be hard to find a movie that gives a more sympathetic view of the problematic interaction between ordinary society and a distinctly "odd" personality. A great introduction to the topic of personality disorders and a delightful not-to-be-missed movie experience.

The House of Games

(1987) Filmhaus

Two personality disorders clash in this labyrinth of a crime thriller where nothing is ever what it seems to be. Uptight female psychiatrist (perhaps with OCD?) meets (no doubt about it: Antisocial Personality Disorder) gambler and con man. She's ready for a little change in her uptight style, but perhaps not for all that follows. Written and directed by David Mamet. If you have seen his *The Spanish Prisoner*, you'll want to see this film too; if you haven't, see both together. *The Spanish Prisoner* may be better, but they're both full of more mind-boggling twists than the road up Pike's Peak.

Play Misty for Me

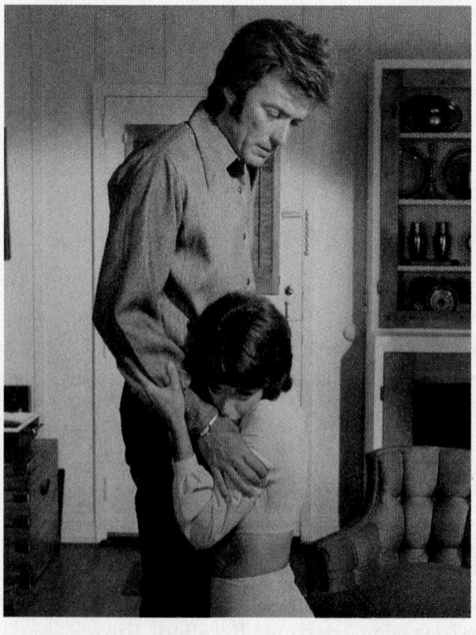

Universal (Courtesy: The Kobal Collection)

Pee Wee's Big Adventure

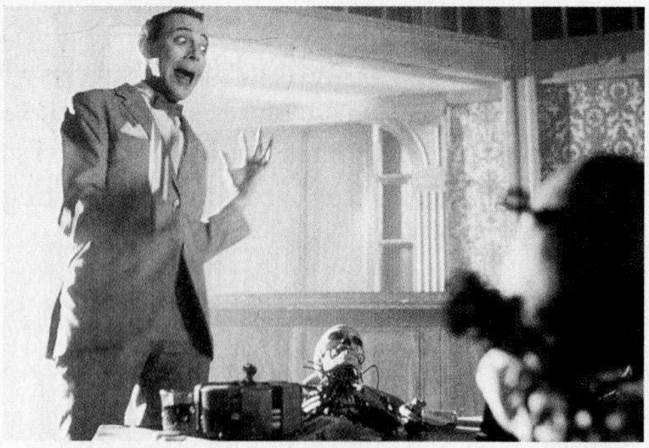

Warner Brothers (Courtesy: The Kobal Collection)

Bad Influence

(1990) MGM

This is a great portrayal of the conning type of Antisocial Personality Disorder, although it does have a murder or two thrown in. Alex, the antihero, manages to con his way into the life of Michael Boll, a young stockbroker, and, for a while at least, Michael's life takes a turn for the better. The film is at its best depicting the power that Alex's plotting and conniving has over the people with whom he comes in contact.

Henry: Portrait of a Serial Killer

(1990) Maljack

X-rated because of extreme violence, this film is definitely not for the faint hearted. However, for those who can stomach its real-life blood and gore, *Portrait* offers a minimally fictionalized view of Antisocial Personality Disorder. The film is based on the real life and violent deeds of a convicted serial killer.

What about Bob?

(1991) Buena Vista

Well, it is about Bill Murray as the client (Dependent Personality Disorder, it would appear) and Richard Dreyfus as the psychiatrist, and it is a great personality disorder flick.

Heavy

(1995) Columbia Tri-Star Home Video

Victor is an obese young man with a severe personality disorder that keeps him from all but the most limited forms of social relationships. His transformation through falling in love with a younger woman is touching but unbelievable.

What about Bob?

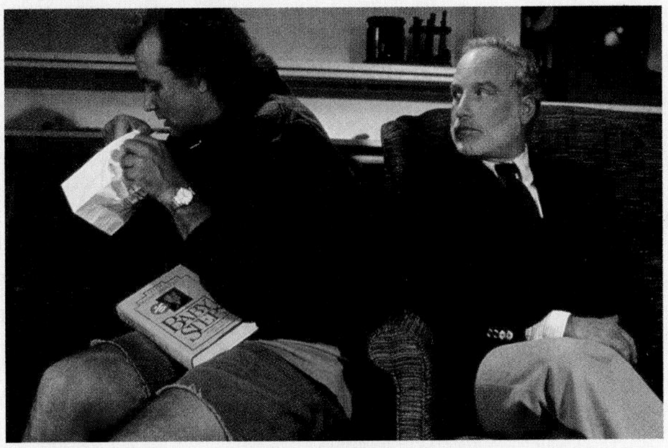

Touchstone (Courtesy: The Kobal Collection)

Nonetheless, *Heavy* is a good introduction to odd and eccentric characters.

The Station Agent

(2003) Miramax

Another avoidant personality film—maybe not better than *Gone with the Wind*, given that film is on most everyone's short list of all-time greats—but certainly more modern, and just as avoidant. In this film, boy does get girl (or rather boy who doesn't want girl gets girl who doesn't want boy—because she's in mourning for a dead son). Whether it matters that the avoidant boy is Peter Dinklage (who is a dwarf) we'll leave to you. Dinklage is a remarkable actor, and this film is surely worth seeing for his performance alone.

The Assassination of Richard Nixon

(2004)

Like many films in this chapter, this one tells what was a true story: secret service agents did foil an attempt on Richard Nixon's life. The would-be assassin (in real life Samuel Byck) is played—under a slightly modified name—by the great actor Sean Penn. Penn captures with great effectiveness the Paranoid Personality Disorder underlying the assassination plot. Penn's character moves from a frustrated sense of failure in nearly every aspect of his life to a fixation on Nixon's role in the Vietnam War. This fixation becomes delusional, and the Byck character creates a plot that ends in the death of two persons in addition to himself. This is an effective movie that shows how paranoid thinking can sometimes transform into dangerous delusion.

Tell Them Who You Are

(2004)

Another "fathers and sons" film, this movie describes growing up with a famous, highly narcissistic father, Haskell Wexler, who was one of Hollywood's most famous cinematographers, among whose many achievements (garnering five Oscars along the way) was filming *One Flew Over the Cuckoo's Nest* (reviewed previously). Both his sons have had respectable careers in film despite their father's domineering hypercritical character. This film features interviews with a multitude of famous Hollywood figures who know and comment on Haskell's personality. And the man himself, 83 at the time of filming, is on camera, at times taking charge of the film while he explains how he could have made many others' films much better than they were had he been given the chance. It is hard not to feel sorry for son Mark, as well as grateful to him for offering such a compelling portrait of a narcissistic personality in action.

Head-On

(2005) Strand Releasing

It's not that films about impulsive, suicide-attempting, women are rare. Depictions of Borderline Personality Disorder or its variants abound in the movies: *A Woman Under the Influence* (not reviewed here) and the slightly earlier *Play Misty for Me* are two fine examples (starring Gena Rowlands and Jessica Walter, respectively). But here we have the borderline world—heavily colored by cultural complexities—transposed to Turkish immigrants in Germany, and then back again to Turkey. This is a movie about which critics have been nearly uniformly enthusiastic, and it received a "Best European Film" award after its 2004 German release. A love story—not quite—a psych flick—well maybe not quite—and a "boy meets girl, boy loses girl"—well sort of; *Head-On* is a compelling, sometimes violent, movie that has much to say about life in our complex multicultural world.

Chapter 19: The Client Experiencing a Somatoform, Factitious, or Dissociative Disorder

The concept of multiple personalities has captured the popular imagination for many years. How real or common this abnormality is remains controversial among experts, but this controversy has not stopped film makers from producing at least three well-known films.

The Barretts of Wimpole Street

(1934) MGM

Few films feature somatization disorders, but this 1934 movie takes on the real-life story of nineteenth-century poets Robert Browning and Elizabeth Barrett. Until she met and married Browning, Elizabeth was confined to bed with a succession of ill-defined sicknesses. Somatization disorder may today present somewhat differently, but this film emphasizes what a profound effect somatization may have on an individual's life. While Freud attributed many of the symptoms of hysteria to repressed sexuality, falling in love is rarely the cure that it was for Elizabeth Barrett Browning.

Send Me No Flowerss

(1964) MCA Home Video

At last—a comedy! Here, Rock Hudson (with Somatization Disorder and the bad luck to overhear doctors talking about someone else's fatal disease) plans for his own imminent death by preparing to marry his wife off to his best friend. His wife (Doris Day) isn't quite sure what's going on, but suspects the worst (or rather what she thinks would be the worst), and the results—for the 1960s, anyway—are moderately funny.

Safe

(1995) Sony Pictures Classics

Safe is the story of a Los Angeles woman who becomes profoundly ill, perhaps as a result of exposure to chemical fumes and odors in her home environment. The illness progresses dramatically, and she receives little help from traditional medical or psychiatric care. Her search for healing in a highly unconventional and probably exploitive "therapeutic environment" highlights the complex interaction between physical and emotional factors in illness. The film portrays its heroine's illness as primarily somatic, but because "environmental sensitivity" is a highly controversial medical diagnosis, many psychiatrists would probably give Conversion Disorder as an alternative. This is a good introduction to the complexities of the somatoform disorders as well as some of their unusual medical mimics.

Hannah and Her Sisters

(1986) MGM

This is one of Woody Allen's best films starring (of course) Allen as—what else—Mickey, a client with a psychosomatic illness—or rather, as is often the case, a great deal of psychosomatic illnesses. If there is any doubt about Mickey's diagnosis, we are told explicitly by a screen title shot that he is a hypochondriac. And what a hypochondriac he is: X-rays, hearing tests, and other medical interventions follow one another with dizzying speed. A three-Oscar film that is more than worth watching.

Safe

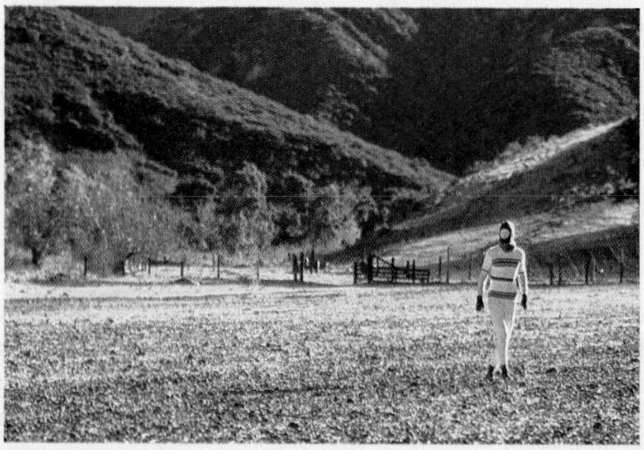

Courtesy: American Playhouse/Channel 4/The Kobal Collection

Dr. Jekyll and Mr. Hyde

(1911, 1920, 1932, 1941, 1968, 1973) 1932 Paramount Pictures

The Robert Louis Stevenson classic of split personality has been filmed at least six times. The 1932 version is arguably the best.

The Three Faces of Eve

(1957) 20th Century Fox

A 1957 drama starring Joanne Woodward (see *They Might Be Giants*, Chapter 12) as a psychologically distressed woman who turns out to have three distinct personalities. Not as many faces as *Sybil* (see below), but it is a far better film.

Sybil

(1976) NBC/Lorimar Television

A television production about a woman who seems to have had 16 separate personalities. While Dissociative Disorder is not a major topic of this book, the film makes for excellent drama and a good introduction to the somewhat controversial diagnosis.

Dancer in the Dark

2000 (Zentropa)

The film for Bjork fans: here she plays a young immigrant single mother trying to cope with her young son's troubling behavior and his—and her own—impending blindness. But wait, there's more: her character seeks escape from these and other troubles by retreating with almost fugue-like intensity to a fantasy world of music and dance à la Broadway musicals. This world eventually becomes more real for her than the bleak reality she faces in her daily life. Bjork wrote and sings the music—enough reason for many to see this movie that comes across powerfully because of beautiful cinematography blended with Bjork's compelling mix of singing, dancing, and acting.

Chapter 20: The Client with Disorders of Self-Regulation: Sleep Disorders, Eating Disorders, and Sexual Disorders

Film makers have frequently portrayed individuals who live "at the edge" of society and social norms. The disorders of regulation are not infrequently depicted in films and documentaries.

The Mark

(1961) 20th Century Fox

A study of pedophilia, this film effectively presents scenes from the life of a convicted child molester on his release from prison. From the early 1960s, but still a convincing portrayal and a moving film.

The Best Little Girl in the World

(1981) ABC Television

A fine 1980s TV movie about Anorexia Nervosa, this film can often be found in video rental stores and, if available, should not be missed.

Dreamchild

(1985) Universal Pictures

Lewis Carroll (his real name was Charles Dodgson) wrote *Alice in Wonderland*, but he also photographed naked young girls (amazingly, with their mothers' permission) and likely today would have been diagnosed as having pedophilia. This is a fictional movie about the "real" Alice, who, more than 70 years after her encounter with Carroll, remains haunted by his memory and the fictional creations of his imagination. *Dreamchild* is a beautiful movie about childhood reflected in old age; it features dream sequences filled with stunning Muppet characters. Only partly about pedophilia, it suggests how disturbing but "forgotten" childhood experiences can remain as subconscious images through an entire lifetime.

Superstar: The Karen Carpenter Story

(1987) Iced Tea Productions

In real life, Karen Carpenter was a highly successful 1960s popular singer who died at age 32 from complications of Anorexia Nervosa. This extraordinary 43-minute film features no human actors after the opening that depicts Karen's death, but only "barbie dolls" playing the roles of Karen and the often uncaring people around her. This film can be hard to locate, but is so unusual that it should definitely be seen as an introduction to eating disorders and the way in which society's expectations about behavior and appearance influence the way women live and die.

Life Is Sweet

(1990) Film Four International

An English movie about obsessive eating, *Life Is Sweet* is more accurately a movie about middle-class English life in which eating plays a disproportionately important role. Although not a clinical study of bulimia, this movie offers realistic portrayals of binging and purging behaviors and how they are hidden from friends and family.

The Hairdresser's Husband

(1990) TF1 Film Productions

A film about paraphilia: The hero has a hair fetish and finds happiness married to a woman who cuts others' hair. An unusual film about an unconventional subject, but overall pleasant entertainment despite a sad ending.

Le Cri de la Soie

(1996) Mimosa Productions

This is an odd but touching movie about a woman who is hospitalized because she has a fetish for silk and cannot resist stealing swatches of it from fabric stores. She is treated by a sympathetic doctor who, it turns out, is also a silk fetishist. Silk fetish is rare enough that the probability of such an encounter between therapist and client is highly unlikely. "The Scream of the Silk" is an attractive evocation of World War I France, but it also makes a particularly useful introduction to understanding paraphilia.

My Own Private Idaho

(1991) New Line Cinema

This film is about two drifters who earn their way through prostitution but are somehow looking for love and relatedness. It has become something of a gay cult movie, but it has strong appeal well beyond this audience. For this chapter, the most interesting feature is the recurrent sleep attacks due to narcolepsy experienced by the character Mike Waters (played by River Phoenix, opposite Keanu Reeves).

The Piano Teacher

(2002) Arte

This chapter is about sometimes disturbing psychiatric realities, and *The Piano Teacher* is a fitting accompaniment. There are many films about sexual sadomasochism, (most of which we confess we haven't watched), and it is likely that the majority of these come closer to soft—or even hard—porn than to movie art. *The Piano Teacher* is an important exception in that it is a riveting story brilliantly portrayed by Isabelle Huppert who won multiple prestigious awards (Cannes, Seattle Film Festival, San Francisco Film Critics, European Film Awards) for her performance. In January 2009 she was also named head of that year's Cannes Film Festival Jury—only the fourth woman ever to hold that position, which goes to show that critics like disturbing films about the margins of human sanity. Huppert's character is a notable pianist whose dark sexual fantasies come into actuality when she is pursued by a handsome young student who was—well—expecting something else. The audience, too, should expect some tough visual and emotional going. Avoid this one if you're queasy; no matter how brilliant the acting and filming, the subject matter could prove distasteful.

UNIT 3: SPECIAL POPULATIONS

Chapter 21: The Physically Ill Client Experiencing Emotional Distress

A few films have explored the human response to illness with great sensitivity.

The Pride of the Yankees

(1942) RKO Pictures

The great New York Yankees baseball player Lou Gehrig died young of the devastating neuromuscular disease amyotrophic lateral sclerosis. This 1942 Gary Cooper film tells his story vividly and movingly. For a more modern view of another extraordinary man's battle with this same neurological disorder, see *A Brief History of Time*, a biographical study of a great modern physicist confronting the same neurological handicap that felled Gehrig more than 50 years before.

The Elephant Man

(1980) Paramount Pictures

A somewhat fictionalized account of a man afflicted with a grotesquely deforming hereditary skin disease, probably neurofibromatosis. Based on a real story, this film boldly illustrates the rejection that deformed persons face in conventional society. Recent popular films have tended to offer generous and colorful portrayals of Victorian and turn-of-the-century British life; this film uses stark black-and-white images to detail Victorian upper class intolerance.

The Shadow Box

(1980) ABC/The Shadowbox Film Company

This film may be difficult to find, but it is a fine movie version of the prize-winning theater production excerpted in Chapter 9. A film that takes place in a hospice and explores the impending cancer death of three residents. Another powerful film starring Joanne Woodward (*The Three Faces of Eve*) and directed by Paul Newman (*The Verdict*).

Parting Glances

(1986) Rondo Pictures

An early account of two gay men coming to personal understanding of the tragedy of acquired immunodeficiency syndrome (AIDS). Less flamboyant than the Oscar-winning 1993 film *Philadelphia*, but, for many, *Parting Glances* may be a more moving film experience.

Beaches

(1988) Touchstone Pictures

Bette Midler stars in this film about friendship and dying. A touching story about the healing role of relatedness in life's crises.

Awakenings

(1990) Columbia Pictures

Awakenings is a dramatization of Oliver Sacks's book about the (temporary) effectiveness of the drug L-Dopa in restoring responsiveness to persons "frozen" by postencephalitic parkinsonism. Sacks's book reminds us that persons who seem unaware and even unconscious can sometimes be remarkably in touch with their environment. A decent movie with several Oscar nominations, *Awakenings* is worth seeing, especially if you cannot read the book. Robin Williams stars as a character based on Oliver Sacks himself, and the movie features Robert De Niro as one of the patients who "awaken" after L-Dopa treatment. More about neurology than psychiatry, it is an attractive film about the potential for modern pharmacology to change the lives of physically and mentally ill individuals.

Passion Fish

(1992) Atchafalaya

This film may not always avoid sentimentality, but it offers a touching and realistic portrayal of the difficulties posed by catastrophic spinal cord injury. A vigorous New York actress becomes paralyzed and returns to her home in the rural South. The film portrays her efforts to find personal fulfillment in her newly dependent role.

Iris

(2001) BBC

Iris Murdoch was famously a novelist and one-time philosophy professor at Oxford University whose books echoed many of the moral themes that a philosophy course might revolve around. Her personal life was a complex mix of domestic affection (marriage to fellow novelist and academic John Bayley) and—though biographical accounts vary somewhat—considerable personal cruelty, masochism, and, almost certainly, sexual promiscuity. *Iris* follows the memoirs of her decline into Alzheimer's written by husband John Bayley, but the film elects to bypass much of the emotional complexity of her pre-Alzheimer years (such as her long and perhaps at least somewhat secret affair with novelist Elias Canetti) or the content of her actual writing that Canetti described (writing in his eighties) as "Oxford tittle-tattle," but which millions of other readers have found thoughtful and engrossing. This is a movie about the dissolution of personality in the face of Alzheimer's. It also reflects the touching 40+ year marriage between two most unlikely partners, a partnership that brought creativity, fulfillment, and apparently a large measure of happiness to both. A very good film, with excellent acting by the two women who play Murdoch in youth and age (Kate Winslet and Dame Judi Dench), but a film—like the cottage that Iris and Bayley shared—with many unseen and very dusty corners.

Talk to Her

(2002) Sony

For nurses this is a cautionary tale. While we don't ever know for sure that Benigno is—not so benignly as his name implies—responsible for his comatose patient's pregnancy, his punishment is a reminder of how important it is for nurses to keep boundaries firmly in mind. But that's really the core of this film, which is about hope and caring, even when the latter become obsessions. While a few critics have found the story (two comatose women; two very different lovers) predictable and melodramatic, its screenplay won an Oscar in 2002. The film is a reminder that it does matter ever so much how we talk to and touch our clients—how and *that* we care about and for them—even as there are lines of professional comportment that must not be crossed.

Chapter 22: Forgotten Populations: The Homeless and the Incarcerated

Prison inmates are frequently depicted in modern films, but neither prisoners nor the homeless are given sympathetic hearings. A few films have approached these special populations with sensitivity.

Short Eyes

(1977) Short Eyes Entertainment

More a film about the harshness of prison life than pedophilia, this film describes the prison persecution of a convicted child molester. A highly realistic view of New York penal life, with excellent acting.

Dead Man Out

(1989) HBO Films

A convicted murderer becomes insane while waiting on Death Row. Can he be cured so that his execution can take place? Does society—and his psychiatrist—have a moral responsibility to return him to sanity for the purpose of facing his death sentence? An intriguing, thought-provoking, and exciting film. It is also an excellent film to see while reading about the ethics of mental health care.

The Fisher King

(1991) Columbia Pictures

A somewhat surrealistic film that is mostly perhaps about bipolar (manic-depressive) psychosis. Some will find the psychedelic portrayals of psychosis unconvincing, but this remarkable Robin Williams (*Dead Poets' Society, Mrs. Doubtfire*) film excels above all in capturing the desperation and squalor in which America's homeless live.

The Fisher King

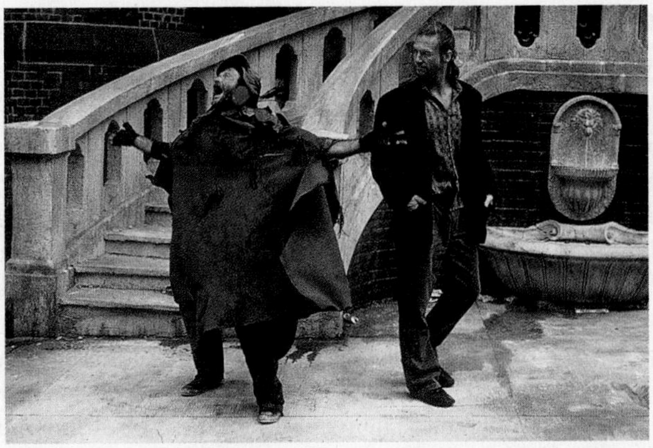

Courtesy: Columbia/Tri Star/The Kobal Collection

The Lovers on the Bridge

(1991) Films A2

Two young lovers (one of whom is played by the fabulous Juliette Binoche) are down and out street people in Paris. In the end, Binoche's character returns to her well-off middle-class world, a world her partner can never enter. Another star-crossed lovers movie, but with great cinematic passion. Grittier and probably more realistic than *The Fisher King* or *The Saint of Fort Washington,* this film provides an extraordinary vision of squalor and vibrancy in the life of the homeless on Paris streets (and bridges).

The Saint of Fort Washington

(1993) Carrie Productions, Inc.

This film about homelessness also gives a fairly convincing portrait of schizophrenia and of PTSD. Most of us look the other way when confronted by the reality of homelessness and the mental illness that often accompanies it. This film allows us to hide behind the camera and look fairly accurately at a world we might not otherwise see. At times the film focuses too much on the "drama" of physical violence and exploitation; it is probable that the day-to-day experience of homelessness involves far more "quiet desperation" than violence, but desperation does not sell movies.

Chapter 23: The Child

Children frequently appear in films, but movies about mentally ill children are relatively rare. The French director François Truffaut had a particular fondness for children and a remarkable vision of the bittersweet nature of childhood.

The 400 Blows

(1959) Les Films du Carosse

One of the great movies of the twentieth century, *The 400 Blows* attempts to capture the complexities of early adolescence as seen through the eyes of a 12-year-old boy. There is little explicitly about mental health in this film of growing up in France, but few artists have managed to convey the joys and trials of childhood with as little sentimentality as does François Truffaut in this semiautobiographical movie.

The Effect of Cosmic Rays on Man-in-the-Moon Marigolds

(1988) 20th Century Fox

This is possibly the longest movie title of the 1980s (though shorter than *Oh Dad, Poor Dad Mamma's Hung You in the Closet and I'm Feeling So Sad,* which preceded it as an off-Broadway play and then became a forgettable movie in 1967). *Cosmic Rays* is a story of growing up more or less successfully in a dysfunctional family. An oddly upbeat story directed by Paul Newman and starring both his wife, Joanne Woodward, and their daughter, Eleanor (Nell Potts), as Matilda, the family's survivor. Perhaps heartened by the fictional Matilda's fortitude in facing psychological adversity, Newman and Woodward have in real life funded many programs for children battling cancer and other childhood disabilities.

Small Change

(1976) Les Films du Carosse

Another Truffaut movie made almost 20 years after *The 400 Blows, Small Change* celebrates childhood—despite deprivation and parental neglect—as a golden time. More sentimental than its famous predecessor, *Small Change* is still a heartwarming film about the everyday lives of children.

Rain Man

(1988) United Artists

One of the classics of the 1980s, *Rain Man* stars Dustin Hoffman and Tom Cruise and won four Oscars. This is a story of two brothers, one autistic, and how as adults they come to find a relationship despite the serious emotional limitations of each of them. This relationship begins on fairly sordid terms as Cruise seeks out his abandoned brother only so he (Cruise) can inherit a fortune. The motives change as Cruise begins to develop genuine affection for a brother who can't express or perhaps even feel emotion. Hoffman is in one of his best roles as the autistic idiot savant brother who emerges from years of neglect and institutionalization to help deepen the emotional world of those around him.

Lorenzo's Oil

(1992) Universal Pictures

This film describes one family's real-life struggles to find a cure for their child's rare neurological disorder. This is a good film for health professionals to watch because it portrays hospitals, doctors, and nurses as they too often appear to anxious families in need: unhelpful, impersonal, and uncaring.

The Danish Poet

(2006) Microfilm

This movie wins the prize for the shortest film on our list (15 minutes), but in won the 2006 Oscar for best short animated film. It also won the prestigious Chicago Children's Film Festival's award that year. With wonderful narration by actress Liv Ullmann, it tells a story every child wants to hear: how their mother and father came to meet and fall in love. If you find it on the DVD featuring other 2006 Oscar-nominated shorts, you can see *Binta and the Great Idea* and *The West Bank Story* as well. Otherwise, you may be able see it (as we did, along with *Binta*) on the YouTube screening room.

Chapter 24: The Adolescent

Adolescents suffer from most of the same psychiatric disorders that affect adults, but their responses to these disorders are powerfully influenced by their developmental status. Some remarkable films have captured some of the poignancy of adolescent experience with mental illness and psychological distress.

Mouchette

(1967) Parc Films

Mouchette can be difficult to find and for some is difficult to watch. The story of a lonely, depressed adolescent, this film ends in her suicide. This film has a very Catholic viewpoint and, despite its somber story, can serve as an important reminder of the importance of spiritual values in a healthy life.

Gaby: A True Story

(1987) Columbia Tri-Star

A similar story to *My Left Foot,* this film is not as successful (no Oscars) or as emotionally powerful. With the aid of her supportive family, a young woman battles cerebral palsy to become a successful author.

My Left Foot

(1989) Palace/Ferndale Films

This movie won two Oscars (plus three additional nominations) for its portrayal of Christy Brown's triumph over devastating neurological impairment from cerebral palsy. The acting is superb, and the film, based on a true story, is a testimony to a mother's faith in her child's potential—a "must-see."

Wildflower

(1991) The Polone Company

A highly emotional film about physical illness (epilepsy, hearing loss) and child abuse, *Wildflower* suggests that friendship and goodwill can occasionally overcome the severest of human handicaps. This film raises important questions about families and social responsibility. It also serves as a reminder of the potential for adolescence as a time for growth and caring.

Good Will Hunting

(1997) Miramax

This is a film about psychotherapy—sort of—and Asperger's syndrome—again sort of—although Will seems to have more social skills (in his own way) than might be likely, given that diagnosis. The movie is pretty good, even if for the most part, the fictional Will isn't. He (Will Hunting) is something of a genius in the rough: more at home in the bars and tough streets of South Boston than at MIT (where he solves unsolvable math problems while working as a janitor). Sentenced to psychiatry instead of jail, Will enters therapy with Robin Williams. Williams's character has his own problems, which Will quickly recognizes, though ultimately the two of them form a kind of alliance to the benefit of both. Captures something of the challenge of Asperger's syndrome and perhaps also something of the intense honesty required for effective psychotherapy.

Good Will Hunting

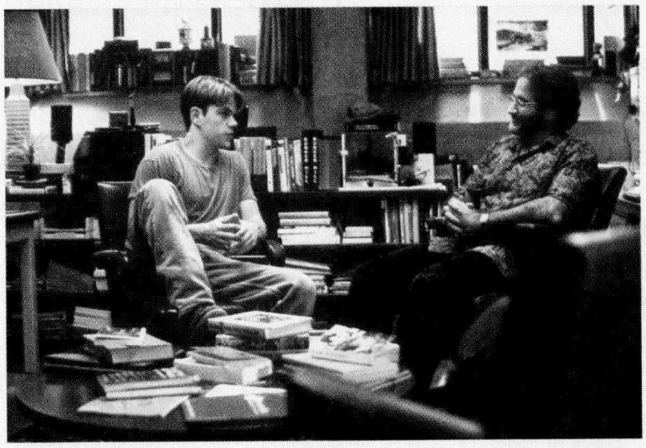

Miramax (Courtesy: The Kobal Collection)

Bluebird

(2004)

Don't confuse this film with several *Blue Bird* movies of an earlier era, and don't expect to find it at your local video shop. You'll have to get this Dutch made-for-TV movie by mail, but the trouble is worth it. The wonderful 13-year-old heroine is too bright, too energetic, and too grown up (in her own way) to fit in with her peers. This leads to a collision of idealism with a reality of derision and bullying that sets the stage for the movie's denouement. This film was written for children, so you can imagine that things do work out in the end. A wonderful short film for and about young adolescents.

Chapter 25: The Elderly

Old age is inevitably a time of loss, of either friends or personal capabilities or of both. It is also a time for growth, wisdom, and sometimes great joy. All of these attributes of elder life have been depicted in a number of fine films.

The Last Laugh

(1922) Fox Film Corporation

This silent film is about how in upper-class European society aging leads inevitably to loss of position and status. An influential film because of its technical innovations, but also a moving portrayal of the triumph of human dignity in the face of prejudice.

Kotch

(1971) Kotch Company Productions

A fine film, starring Walter Matthau and directed by Jack Lemmon, about the relationship between aging parents and their children.

Harry and Tonto

(1974) 20th Century Fox

This is a wonderful film about the travels of 70-something Harry and his cat Tonto. Art Carney stars in this film, which serves as a forceful reminder that aging need not lead to a loss of vitality or the ability to care deeply for others—human and animal alike. This film also reminds viewers that the quality of life can sometimes be greatly improved by slowing down its pace.

Gin Game

(1984) RKO Pictures

This is a celebrated film about love in a nursing home, starring Jessica Tandy (*Driving Miss Daisy*) and Hume Cronyn (*Age Old Friends*)—two wonderful actors in a warm and touching story.

Driving Miss Daisy

(1989) Warner Brothers

One of the most celebrated recent movie portrayals of aging, *Driving Miss Daisy* won a best picture Oscar in 1989. This film perhaps treats issues of race prejudice more directly than those of aging, but Jessica Tandy's portrayal of Daisy is particularly memorable.

Age Old Friends

(1989) Central Independent Television Plc.

This is a touching film about the effects of dementia on friendship and family ties. This movie features marvelous acting and highly realistic subject matter. A wonderful introduction to the special concerns and needs of the elderly and their children.

Children of Nature

(1991) Northern Arts Entertainment

A warm movie from a very cold country, this film in Icelandic (with English subtitles) is a charming tale of romance involving two nursing home residents.

A Woman's Tale

(1991) Illumination Films

This is a film about the last days of a vital 78-year-old. There is wonderful acting by Sheila Florence, who herself died of cancer soon after the film was completed. It is a very special movie about the richness of a fully lived life.

The Straight Story

(1999) Asymmetrical Productions

Directed by David Lynch, this is a poignant story about an elderly Iowan who decides it is time to visit his ill brother from whom he has long been estranged. Describing the trip as a "hard swallow of my pride," Alvin Straight sets out down the road, driving his lawnmower, and perhaps not surprisingly, encountering a range of other humans along the way. The film is based on a true story, but director David Lynch (who has rarely been known for telling straight stories) surely told the story of Straight's trip as a metaphor of human mortality: a Pilgrim's Progress, as John Bunyan put it 325 years before, "from this world to that which is to come"—the Celestial City located on the peak of Mt. Zion. And so it proved for the actor who played Alvin Straight. Richard Farnsworth killed himself at age 80, a year after the film was made. During the filming he had apparently suffered painfully from metastatic prostate cancer, but continued with filming in homage to Alvin Straight—who had in turn died two years previously after completing his long trip to his brother's home in ... Mt. Zion, Wisconsin.

Young@Heart

2007 Fox Searchlight

Young@Heart is a New England choir that doesn't let anyone in until they reach 70 and has been known to keep them in until age 100. Founded in 1982, the group has toured widely in Europe where they caught the attention of British film makers. At least two other films have been made about community choirs—one in the UK and the other in Norway (*Cool and Crazy*). But while *Cool and Crazy's* choir had only one 90-year-old, *Young@Heart* seemingly specializes in them. You'll love their rock music renditions: if James Brown can feel good when he sings, consider the meaning of his "I feel good" when belted out by an octogenarian. If we didn't already clue you in, *Young@Heart* was filmed during the two weeks before the group's annual home-town performance in Northampton, Massachusetts.

Chapter 26: Survivors of Violence or Abuse

It seems hard for many parents and moviegoers to find a film that is *not* about violence. The film world has been relatively slow to address intrafamilial violence and sexual abuse, but some excellent movies have treated these and related topics.

Murmur of the Heart

(1971) NEF Filmproduktion

There are few films about incest. *Murmur of the Heart* portrays an adolescent coming of age in France and depicts an episode of mother-son incest that apparently occurs without much consequence for either. It is not a terribly realistic view of a typical incestuous parental relationship—more commonly involving both a father/daughter pairing as well as some element of physical coercion or intimidation.

Judgment

(1990) HBO Films

This made-for-cable-television film dramatizes a true case of child sexual abuse perpetrated by a parish priest. An important truth in this story is that many parents know of their children's molestation but remain silent. Such "conspiracy of silence" is not an infrequent finding when children have been sexually abused, especially when the perpetrator is a parent.

Sleeping with the Enemy

(1991) 20th Century Fox

One of the better recent films about intrafamilial violence, this movie emphasizes the real danger and abject fear that affect many abused women's lives.

Mystic River

(2003) Warner Brothers

This is a film about the aftermath of child molestation, and perhaps also about the origins of Antisocial Personality Disorder in childhood. Most sexual assault of children is less grotesquely violent than the episode portrayed (most off-screen) in this film, and many children are abused by someone they know and trust rather than by a sadistic stranger, as in *Mystic River*. Still, for many children the scars of sexual abuse persist for a lifetime. A brilliant film with Sean Penn as a neighborhood sociopath and Tim Robbins as the adult victim of child molestation. There is more drama than psychiatric content in this film, but just for gripping entertainment it is another "must-see" if you did not catch it the first time around.

Mysterious Skin

(2005) Desperate Pictures

The seemingly unending media coverage of sexual abuse of young boys, and perhaps the success of *Mystic River* (see previous review) surely helped lead to the creation of this film—the outline of whose plot has a good deal in common with that of *Mystic River*. Two teenagers, abused in childhood by a baseball coach, eventually reunite to share their stories and to attempt healing. Like Penn's film, *Mysterious Skin* has wonderful acting, but the film appears to acknowledge that these boys suffered harm as much from what their parents didn't give them (love and attention) as from what their coach physically did to them. That's often the way it works with child abuse.

UNIT 4: NURSING INTERVENTIONS AND TREATMENT MODALITIES

Few directors set out to write films about psychiatric treatment modalities, but some films seem to help us understand better what treatments can "work" and occasionally why. Others have looked with interest at popular or controversial psychiatric treatments such as psychotherapy or electroshock therapy.

Secrets of a Soul

(1926) Neumann-Filmproduktion

A silent film about psychoanalysis and the interpretation of dreams. Beautiful film work, especially in the dream sequences, and a relatively painless introduction to the theory and practice of psychoanalytic therapy. Produced when Freud's influence and reputation were particularly strong.

Freud

(1962) U-1 Films

In this film, Freud has fallen a bit from intellectual favor in some circles. The film may be difficult to find, however, it is worth seeing if it can be located.

Pressure Point

(1962) United Artists

This is another intense film on the troubled relationship between therapist and client. The great actor Sidney Poitier plays a psychiatrist who must treat an imprisoned Nazi and racist. Based on a true story, this film dramatically addresses the difficulties that arise in therapy when personal values and beliefs separate therapist and patient.

Lilith

(1964) Columbia Pictures

Warren Beatty, playing a young psychotherapist, experiences countertransference as he falls in love with his patient and nearly loses his own sanity. This film raises more than just ethical questions and is worth seeing for its often realistic exploration of the difficult relational issues that can arise during intense therapy.

Frances

(1982) Brooks Films

This is a moving and tragic account of the mental illness of actress Frances Farmer, whose depression, substance abuse, and seemingly atrocious mental health care led to disaster. Frances ultimately had a prefrontal lobotomy, and the movie offers a dramatic portrayal of the worst effects of surgery for psychiatric conditions. Excellent acting by Jessica Lange keeps this film from being a melodrama about inept psychiatric treatment.

The Dream Team

(1989) Universal Pictures

A sometimes charming comedy about therapy, murder, and insanity, *The Dream Team* depicts four mentally ill individuals who leave their psychiatric unit on a furlough and, while losing their psychiatrist escort to an act of random violence, find themselves wandering freely (and off medication) in New York City. This movie offers a nice depiction of Axis II OCD (probably combined with delusions of grandeur). Three of the "escapees" are also interesting and well-cast "odd personalities" who may or may not truly be candidates for inpatient psychiatric care. The plot (preventing their psychiatrist's murder by the mob) is a bit far-fetched, but the movie is a worthy exercise in understanding and sympathizing with four unusual men trying to accomplish good against physical and psychological odds.

The Dream Team

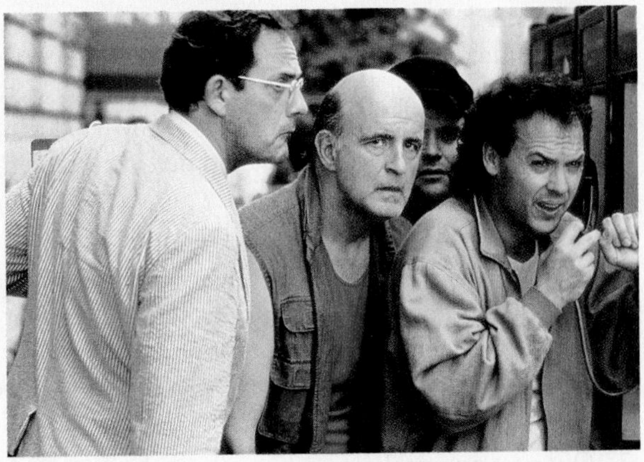

Universal (Courtesy: The Kobal Collection)

Prince of Tides

(1991) Columbia Pictures

A psychiatrist (played by Barbra Streisand) helps a pair of troubled twins sort out deeply troubled lives. This film is at times not a fully realistic portrait either of mental illness or psychiatry, but it is a fine story and a beautifully filmed movie. It received multiple Oscar nominations in 1991, including best picture and best actor.

Shall We Dance?

(1996) Miramax

This marvelous Japanese movie can be seen as a metaphor for the cognitive-behavioral therapy of depression. The hero is a middle-aged businessman who lives his life without pleasure from work, family, or social interaction. Walking down the street at night he is captivated by the image of a woman standing in a second-floor dance studio. Taken by her beauty, he conquers his shyness, physical ineptness, and the strong social disapproval of dancing in traditional Japanese culture. Practicing his steps as he works and walks, he begins to dance with the beautiful dance-studio instructor. Their relationship is limited to dancing, but it transforms his life into one of fullness and joy as dancing meets and overcomes dysthymia. (If you have missed *Strictly Ballroom*, see both of these films for a dancing treat!)

Prime

(2005) Prime Film Productions LLC

Meryl Streep stars in this film—yet another movie about (female) psychotherapists and the problems they encounter in keeping to boundaries. This one has a plot that is more unlikely than most and is also billed as a comedy. It may not have a lot to tell us about how psychotherapy is (or should be) done, but it's a good way to spend an entertaining Friday Night at the Psychiatric and Mental Health Nursing Movies. Bring your friends and enjoy!! Don't forget the popcorn.

REVIEW QUESTIONS AND ACTIVITIES

1. Consider how you might provide nursing care to one of the characters in the movies you saw. Write a nursing care plan for the character (include assessment questions, nursing diagnoses/DSM-IV-TR diagnoses, desired outcomes, and nursing interventions).
2. As a nursing professional, you may be caring for people with many of the psychiatric disorders you have seen depicted in these films. Consider what you can do to foster in yourself an attitude of understanding, empathy, and respect toward these people.
3. Our past personal experiences, family backgrounds, and relationships can affect our attitudes toward people with certain psychiatric disorders. Think about your reaction (either positive or negative) to one of the characters in the films you watched who remind you of someone you know. Did your past experience cause you to react more strongly to this character? If so, how might this affect your interaction with a client who has a similar disorder?
4. Think about the ethical questions that arose in one or more of the films you viewed. Were there nursing actions that you might handle differently? How would you treat a client experiencing that particular psychiatric disorder?
5. Some of these films portray mental health treatments and psychiatric personnel (nurses and psychiatrists) in a very negative way. Could clients watching these movies make decisions about their own treatment based on the films, rather than on reality?
6. Many of the films listed have scenes depicting romance between client and therapist. Some suggest that such romance is the basis for therapeutic success. What is "transference"? Is a therapist (or nurse) ever justified in having a romantic relationship with his or her clients?

APPENDIX A
DSM-IV-TR Classification

NOS = Not Otherwise Specified.

An *x* appearing in a diagnostic code indicates that a specific code number is required.

An ellipsis (...) is used in the names of certain disorders to indicate that the name of a specific mental disorder or general medical condition should be inserted when recording the name (e.g., 293.0 Delirium Due to Hypothyroidism).

If criteria are currently met, one of the following severity specifiers may be noted after the diagnosis:

Mild
Moderate
Severe

If criteria are no longer met, one of the following specifiers may be noted:

In Partial Remission
In Full Remission
Prior History

DISORDERS USUALLY FIRST DIAGNOSED IN INFANCY, CHILDHOOD, OR ADOLESCENCE

Mental Retardation

Note: *These are coded on Axis II.*

317	Mild Mental Retardation
318.0	Moderate Mental Retardation
318.1	Severe Mental Retardation
318.2	Profound Mental Retardation
319	Mental Retardation, Severity Unspecified

Learning Disorders

315.00	Reading Disorder
315.1	Mathematics Disorder
315.2	Disorder of Written Expression
315.9	Learning Disorder NOS

Motor Skills Disorder

315.4	Developmental Coordination Disorder

Communication Disorders

315.31	Expressive Language Disorder
315.31	Mixed Receptive-Expressive Language Disorder
315.39	Phonological Disorder
307.0	Stuttering
307.9	Communication Disorder NOS

Pervasive Developmental Disorders

299.00	Autistic Disorder
299.80	Rett's Disorder
299.10	Childhood Disintegrative Disorder
299.80	Asperger's Disorder
299.80	Pervasive Developmental Disorder NOS

Attention-Deficit and Disruptive Behavior Disorders

314.xx	Attention-Deficit/Hyperactivity Disorder
.01	Combined Type
.00	Predominantly Inattentive Type
.01	Predominantly Hyperactive-Impulsive Type
314.9	Attention-Deficit/Hyperactivity Disorder NOS
312.8	Conduct Disorder
	Specify type: Childhood-Onset Type/ Adolescent-Onset Type
313.81	Oppositional Defiant Disorder
312.9	Disruptive Behavior Disorder NOS

Feeding and Eating Disorders of Infancy or Early Childhood

307.52 Pica
307.53 Rumination Disorder
307.59 Feeding Disorder of Infancy or Early Childhood

Tic Disorders

307.23 Tourette's Disorder
307.22 Chronic Motor or Vocal Tic Disorder
307.21 Transient Tic Disorder
Specify if: Single Episode/Recurrent
307.20 Tic Disorder NOS

Elimination Disorders

___.__ Encopresis
787.6 With Constipation and Overflow Incontinence
307.7 Without Constipation and Overflow Incontinence
307.6 Enuresis (Not Due to a General Medical Condition)
Specify type: Nocturnal Only/Diurnal Only/Nocturnal and Diurnal

Other Disorders of Infancy, Childhood, or Adolescence

309.21 Separation Anxiety Disorder
Specify if: Early Onset
313.23 Selective Mutism
313.89 Reactive Attachment Disorder of Infancy or Early Childhood
Specify type: Inhibited Type/Disinhibited Type
307.3 Stereotypic Movement Disorder
Specify if: With Self-Injurious Behavior
313.9 Disorder of Infancy, Childhood, or Adolescence NOS

DELIRIUM, DEMENTIA, AND AMNESTIC AND OTHER COGNITIVE DISORDERS

Delirium

293.0 Delirium Due to ... *[Indicate the General Medical Condition]*
___.__ Substance Intoxication Delirium (refer to Substance-Related Disorders for substance-specific codes)
___.__ Substance Withdrawal Delirium (refer to Substance-Related Disorders for substance-specific codes)
___.__ Delirium Due to Multiple Etiologies (code each of the specific etiologies)
780.09 Delirium NOS

Dementia

290.xx Dementia of the Alzheimer's Type, With Early Onset *(also code 331.0 Alzheimer's disease on Axis III)*
.10 Uncomplicated
.11 With Delirium
.12 With Delusions
.13 With Depressed Mood
Specify if: With Behavioral Disturbance
290.xx Dementia of the Alzheimer's Type, With Late Onset *(also code 331.0 Alzheimer's disease on Axis III)*
.0 Uncomplicated
.3 With Delirium
.20 With Delusions
.21 With Depressed Mood
Specify if: With Behavioral Disturbance
290.xx Vascular Dementia
.40 Uncomplicated
.41 With Delirium
.42 With Delusions
.43 With Depressed Mood
Specify if: With Behavioral Disturbance
294.9 Dementia Due to HIV Disease *(also code 043.1 HIV infection affecting central nervous system on Axis III)*
294.1 Dementia Due to Head Trauma *(also code 854.00 head injury on Axis III)*
294.1 Dementia Due to Parkinson's Disease *(also code 332.0 Parkinson's disease on Axis III)*
294.1 Dementia Due to Huntington's Disease *(also code 333.4 Huntington's disease on Axis III)*
290.10 Dementia Due to Pick's Disease *(also code 331.1 Pick's disease on Axis III)*
290.10 Dementia Due to Creutzfeldt-Jakob Disease *(also code 046.1 Creutzfeldt-Jakob disease on Axis III)*
294.1 Dementia Due to ... *[Indicate the General Medical Condition not listed above] (also code the general medical condition on Axis III)*
___.__ Substance-Induced Persisting Dementia *(refer to Substance-Related Disorders for substance-specific codes)*
___.__ Dementia Due to Multiple Etiologies *(code each of the specific etiologies)*
294.8 Dementia NOS

Amnestic Disorders

294.0 Amnestic Disorder Due to ... *[Indicate the General Medical Condition]*
Specify if: Transient/Chronic
___.__ Substance-Induced Persisting Amnestic Disorder (refer to Substance-Related Disorders for substance-specific codes)
294.8 Amnestic Disorder NOS

Other Cognitive Disorders

294.9 Cognitive Disorder NOS

MENTAL DISORDERS DUE TO A GENERAL MEDICAL CONDITION NOT ELSEWHERE CLASSIFIED

293.89 Catatonic Disorder Due to ... *[Indicate the General Medical Condition]*
310.1 Personality Change Due to ... *[Indicate the General Medical Condition]*
Specify type: Labile Type/Disinhibited Type/Aggressive Type/Apathetic Type/Paranoid Type/Other Type/Combined Type/Unspecified Type
293.9 Mental Disorder NOS Due to ... *[Indicate the General Medical Condition]*

SUBSTANCE-RELATED DISORDERS

[a]*The following specifiers may be applied to Substance Dependence:*

With Physiological Dependence/Without Physiological Dependence

Early Full Remission/Early Partial Remission/Sustained Full Remission/Sustained Partial Remission

On Agonist Therapy/In a Controlled Environment

The following specifiers apply to Substance-Induced Disorders as noted:

[I]With Onset During Intoxication/[W]With Onset During Withdrawal

ALCOHOL-RELATED DISORDERS

Alcohol Use Disorders

303.90 Alcohol Dependence[a]
305.00 Alcohol Abuse

Alcohol-Induced Disorders

303.00 Alcohol Intoxication
291.8 Alcohol Withdrawal
Specify if: With Perceptual Disturbances
291.0 Alcohol Intoxication Delirium
291.0 Alcohol Withdrawal Delirium
291.2 Alcohol-Induced Persisting Dementia
291.1 Alcohol-Induced Persisting Amnestic Disorder
291.x Alcohol-Induced Psychotic Disorder
.5 With Delusions[I,W]
.3 With Hallucinations[I,W]
291.8 Alcohol-Induced Mood Disorder[I,W]
291.8 Alcohol-Induced Anxiety Disorder[I,W]
291.8 Alcohol-Induced Sexual Dysfunction[I]
291.8 Alcohol-Induced Sleep Disorder[I,W]
291.9 Alcohol-Related Disorder NOS

AMPHETAMINE (OR AMPHETAMINE-LIKE)–RELATED DISORDERS

Amphetamine Use Disorders

304.40 Amphetamine Dependence[a]
305.70 Amphetamine Abuse

Amphetamine-Induced Disorders

292.89 Amphetamine Intoxication
Specify if: With Perceptual Disturbances
292.0 Amphetamine Withdrawal
292.81 Amphetamine Intoxication Delirium
292.xx Amphetamine-Induced Psychotic Disorder
.11 With Delusions[I]
.12 With Hallucinations[I]
292.84 Amphetamine-Induced Mood Disorder[I,W]
292.89 Amphetamine-Induced Anxiety Disorder[I]
292.89 Amphetamine-Induced Sexual Dysfunction[I]
292.89 Amphetamine-Induced Sleep Disorder[I,W]
292.9 Amphetamine-Related Disorder NOS

CAFFEINE-RELATED DISORDERS

Caffeine-Induced Disorders

305.90 Caffeine Intoxication
292.89 Caffeine-Induced Anxiety Disorder[I]
292.89 Caffeine-Induced Sleep Disorder[I]
292.9 Caffeine-Related Disorder NOS

CANNABIS-RELATED DISORDERS

Cannabis Use Disorders

304.30 Cannabis Dependence[a]
305.20 Cannabis Abuse

Cannabis-Induced Disorders

292.89 Cannabis Intoxication
Specify if: With Perceptual Disturbances
292.81 Cannabis Intoxication Delirium
292.xx Cannabis-Induced Psychotic Disorder
.11 With Delusions[I]
.12 With Hallucinations[I]
292.89 Cannabis-Induced Anxiety Disorder[I]
292.9 Cannabis-Related Disorder NOS

COCAINE-RELATED DISORDERS

Cocaine Use Disorders

304.20 Cocaine Dependence[a]
305.60 Cocaine Abuse

Cocaine-Induced Disorders

292.89 Cocaine Intoxication
Specify if: With Perceptual Disturbances
292.0 Cocaine Withdrawal

292.81 Cocaine Intoxication Delirium
292.xx Cocaine-Induced Psychotic Disorder
.11 With Delusions[I]
.12 With Hallucinations[I]
292.84 Cocaine-Induced Mood Disorder[I,W]
292.89 Cocaine-Induced Anxiety Disorder[I,W]
292.89 Cocaine-Induced Sexual Dysfunction[I]
292.89 Cocaine-Induced Sleep Disorder[I,W]
292.9 Cocaine-Related Disorder NOS

Hallucinogen-Related Disorders

Hallucinogen Use Disorders

304.50 Hallucinogen Dependence[a]
305.30 Hallucinogen Abuse

Hallucinogen-Induced Disorders

292.89 Hallucinogen Intoxication
292.89 Hallucinogen Persisting Perception Disorder (Flashbacks)
292.81 Hallucinogen Intoxication Delirium
292.xx Hallucinogen-Induced Psychotic Disorder
.11 With Delusions[I]
.12 With Hallucinations[I]
292.84 Hallucinogen-Induced Mood Disorder[I]
292.89 Hallucinogen-Induced Anxiety Disorder[I]
292.9 Hallucinogen-Related Disorder NOS

Inhalant-Related Disorders

Inhalant Use Disorders

304.60 Inhalant Dependence[a]
305.90 Inhalant Abuse

Inhalant-Induced Disorders

292.89 Inhalant Intoxication
292.81 Inhalant Intoxication Delirium
292.82 Inhalant-Induced Persisting Dementia
292.xx Inhalant-Induced Psychotic Disorder
.11 With Delusions[I]
.12 With Hallucinations[I]
292.84 Inhalant-Induced Mood Disorder [I]
292.89 Inhalant-Induced Anxiety Disorder[I]
292.9 Inhalant-Related Disorder NOS

Nicotine-Related Disorders

Nicotine Use Disorder

305.10 Nicotine Dependence[a]

Nicotine-Induced Disorder

292.0 Nicotine Withdrawal
292.9 Nicotine-Related Disorder NOS

Opioid-Related Disorders

Opioid Use Disorders

304.00 Opioid Dependence[a]
305.50 Opioid Abuse

Opioid-Induced Disorders

292.89 Opioid Intoxication
Specify if: With Perceptual Disturbances
292.0 Opioid Withdrawal
292.81 Opioid Intoxication Delirium
292.xx Opioid-Induced Psychotic Disorder
.11 With Delusions[I]
.12 With Hallucinations[I]
292.84 Opioid-Induced Mood Disorder[I]
292.89 Opioid-Induced Sexual Dysfunction[I]
292.89 Opioid-Induced Sleep Disorder[I,W]
292.9 Opioid-Related Disorder NOS

Phencyclidine (or Phencyclidine-Like)–Related Disorders

Phencyclidine Use Disorders

304.90 Phencyclidine Dependence[a]
305.90 Phencyclidine Abuse

Phencyclidine-Induced Disorders

292.89 Phencyclidine Intoxication
Specify if: With Perceptual Disturbances
292.81 Phencyclidine Intoxication Delirium
292.xx Phencyclidine-Induced Psychotic Disorder
.11 With Delusions[I]
.12 With Hallucinations[I]
292.84 Phencyclidine-Induced Mood Disorder[I]
292.89 Phencyclidine-Induced Anxiety Disorder[I]
292.9 Phencyclidine-Related Disorder NOS

Sedative-, Hypnotic-, or Anxiolytic-Related Disorders

Sedative, Hypnotic, or Anxiolytic Use Disorders

304.10 Sedative, Hypnotic, or Anxiolytic Dependence[a]
305.40 Sedative, Hypnotic, or Anxiolytic Abuse

Sedative-, Hypnotic-, or Anxiolytic-Induced Disorders

292.89 Sedative, Hypnotic, or Anxiolytic Intoxication
292.0 Sedative, Hypnotic, or Anxiolytic Withdrawal
Specify if: With Perceptual Disturbances

292.81 Sedative, Hypnotic, or Anxiolytic Intoxication Delirium
292.81 Sedative, Hypnotic, or Anxiolytic Withdrawal Delirium
292.82 Sedative-, Hypnotic-, or Anxiolytic-Induced Persisting Dementia
292.83 Sedative-, Hypnotic-, or Anxiolytic-Induced Persisting Amnestic Disorder
292.xx Sedative-, Hypnotic-, or Anxiolytic-Induced Psychotic Disorder
.11 With Delusions[I,W]
.12 With Hallucinations[I,W]
292.84 Sedative-, Hypnotic-, or Anxiolytic-Induced Mood Disorder[I,W]
292.89 Sedative-, Hypnotic-, or Anxiolytic-Induced Anxiety Disorder[W]
292.89 Sedative-, Hypnotic-, or Anxiolytic-Induced Sexual Dysfunction[I]
292.89 Sedative-, Hypnotic-, or Anxiolytic-Induced Sleep Disorder[I,W]
292.9 Sedative-, Hypnotic-, or Anxiolytic-Related Disorder NOS

Polysubstance-Related Disorder

304.80 Polysubstance Dependence[a]

Other (or Unknown) Substance-Related Disorders

Other (or Unknown) Substance Use Disorders

304.90 Other (or Unknown) Substance Dependence[a]
305.90 Other (or Unknown) Substance Abuse

Other (or Unknown) Substance-Induced Disorders

292.89 Other (or Unknown) Substance Intoxication
Specify if: With Perceptual Disturbances
292.0 Other (or Unknown) Substance Withdrawal
Specify if: With Perceptual Disturbances
292.81 Other (or Unknown) Substance–Induced Delirium
292.82 Other (or Unknown) Substance–Induced Persisting Dementia
292.83 (or Unknown) Substance–Induced Persisting Amnestic Disorder
292.xx Other (or Unknown) Substance–Induced Psychotic Disorder
.11 With Delusions[I,W]
.12 With Hallucinations[I,W]
292.84 Other (or Unknown) Substance–Induced Mood Disorder[I,W]
292.89 Other (or Unknown) Substance–Induced Anxiety Disorder[I,W]
292.89 Other (or Unknown) Substance–Induced Sexual Dysfunction[I]
292.89 Other (or Unknown) Substance–Induced Sleep Disorder[I,W]
292.9 Other (or Unknown) Substance–Related Disorder NOS

SCHIZOPHRENIA AND OTHER PSYCHOTIC DISORDERS

295.xx Schizophrenia

The following Classification of Longitudinal Course applies to all subtypes of Schizophrenia:

Episodic With Interepisode Residual Symptoms (*specify if:* With Prominent Negative Symptoms)/Episodic With No Interepisode Residual Symptoms

Continuous (*specify if:* With Prominent Negative Symptoms)

Single Episode In Partial Remission (*specify if:* With Prominent Negative Symptoms)/Single Episode In Full Remission

Other or Unspecified Pattern

.30 Paranoid Type
.10 Disorganized Type
.20 Catatonic Type
.90 Undifferentiated Type
.60 Residual Type
295.40 Schizophreniform Disorder
Specify if: Without Good Prognostic Features/With Good Prognostic Features
295.70 Schizoaffective Disorder
Specify type: Bipolar Type/Depressive Type
297.1 Delusional Disorder
Specify type: Erotomanic Type/Grandiose Type/Jealous Type/Persecutory Type/Somatic Type/Mixed Type/Unspecified Type
298.8 Brief Psychotic Disorder
Specify if: With Marked Stressor(s)/Without Marked Stressor(s)/With Postpartum Onset
297.3 Shared Psychotic Disorder
293.xx Psychotic Disorder Due to ... *[Indicate the General Medical Condition]*
.81 With Delusions
.82 With Hallucinations
___._ Substance-Induced Psychotic Disorder (*refer to Substance-Related Disorders for substance-specific codes)*
Specify if: With Onset During Intoxication/With Onset During Withdrawal
298.9 Psychotic Disorder NOS

MOOD DISORDERS

Code current state of Major Depressive Disorder or Bipolar I Disorder in fifth digit:

1 = Mild
2 = Moderate
3 = Severe Without Psychotic Features
4 = Severe With Psychotic Features
Specify: Mood-Congruent Psychotic Features/Mood-Incongruent Psychotic Features
5 = In Partial Remission
6 = In Full Remission
0 = Unspecified

The following specifiers apply (for current or most recent episode) to Mood Disorders as noted:

[a]Severity/Psychotic/Remission Specifiers/[b]Chronic/[c]With Catatonic Features/[d]With Melancholic Features/[e]With Atypical Features/[f]With Postpartum Onset

The following specifiers apply to Mood Disorders as noted:

[g]With or Without Full Interepisode Recovery/[h]With Seasonal Pattern/[i]With Rapid Cycling

Depressive Disorders

296.xx	Major Depressive Disorder,
.2x	Single Episode[a,b,c,d,e,]
.3x	Recurrent[a,b,c,d,e,f,g,h]
300.4	Dysthymic Disorder
	Specify if: Early Onset/Late Onset
	Specify if: With Atypical Features
311	Depressive Disorder NOS

Bipolar Disorders

296.xx	Bipolar I Disorder,
.0x	Single Manic Episode[a,c,f]
	Specify if: Mixed
.40	Most Recent Episode Hypomanic[g,h,i]
.4x	Most Recent Episode Manic[a,c,f,g,h,i]
.6x	Most Recent Episode Mixed[a,c,f,g,h,i]
.5x	Most Recent Episode Depressed[a,b,c,d,e,f,g,h,i]
.7	Most Recent Episode Unspecified[g,h,i]
296.89	Bipolar II Disorder[a,b,c,d,e,f,g,h,i]
	Specify (current or most recent episode): Hypomanic/Depressed
301.13	Cyclothymic Disorder
296.80	Bipolar Disorder NOS
293.83	Mood Disorder Due to ... *[Indicate the General Medical Condition]*
	Specify type: With Depressive Features/With Major Depressive-Like Episode/With Manic Features/With Mixed Features
___.__	Substance-Induced Mood Disorder (refer to Substance-Related Disorders for substance-specific codes)
	Specify type: With Depressive Features/With Manic Features/With Mixed Features
	Specify if: With Onset During Intoxication/With Onset During Withdrawal
296.90	Mood Disorder NOS

ANXIETY DISORDERS

300.01	Panic Disorder Without Agoraphobia
300.21	Panic Disorder With Agoraphobia
300.22	Agoraphobia Without History of Panic Disorder
300.29	Specific Phobia
	Specify type: Animal Type/Natural Environment Type/Blood-Injection-Injury Type/Situational Type/Other Type
300.23	Social Phobia
	Specify if: Generalized
300.3	Obsessive-Compulsive Disorder
	Specify if: With Poor Insight
309.81	Posttraumatic Stress Disorder
	Specify if: Acute/Chronic
	Specify if: With Delayed Onset
308.3	Acute Stress Disorder
300.02	Generalized Anxiety Disorder
293.89	Anxiety Disorder Due to ... *[Indicate the General Medical Condition]*
	Specify if: With Generalized Anxiety/With Panic Attacks/With Obsessive-Compulsive Symptoms
___.__	Substance-Induced Anxiety Disorder *(refer to Substance-Related Disorders for substance-specific codes)*
	Specify if: With Generalized Anxiety/With Panic Attacks/With Obsessive-Compulsive Symptoms/With Phobic Symptoms
	Specify if: With Onset During Intoxication/With Onset During Withdrawal
300.00	Anxiety Disorder NOS

SOMATOFORM DISORDERS

300.81	Somatization Disorder
300.81	Undifferentiated Somatoform Disorder
300.11	Conversion Disorder
	Specify type: With Motor Symptom or Deficit/With Sensory Symptom or Deficit/With Seizures or Convulsions/With Mixed Presentation
307.xx	Pain Disorder
.80	Associated With Psychological Factors
.89	Associated With Both Psychological Factors and a General Medical Condition
	Specify if: Acute/Chronic
300.7	Hypochondriasis
	Specify if: With Poor Insight
300.7	Body Dysmorphic Disorder
300.81	Somatoform Disorder NOS

FACTITIOUS DISORDERS

300.xx Factitious Disorder
  .16 With Predominantly Psychological Signs and Symptoms
  .19 With Predominantly Physical Signs and Symptoms
  .19 With Combined Psychological and Physical Signs and Symptoms
300.19 Factitious Disorder NOS

DISSOCIATIVE DISORDERS

300.12 Dissociative Amnesia
300.13 Dissociative Fugue
300.14 Dissociative Identity Disorder
300.6 Depersonalization Disorder
300.15 Dissociative Disorder NOS

SEXUAL AND GENDER IDENTITY DISORDERS

Sexual Dysfunction

The following specifiers apply to all primary Sexual Dysfunctions:
Lifelong Type/Acquired Type
Generalized Type/Situational Type
Due to Psychological Factors/Due to Combined Factors

Sexual Desire Disorders

302.71 Hypoactive Sexual Desire Disorder
302.79 Sexual Aversion Disorder

Sexual Arousal Disorders

302.72 Female Sexual Arousal Disorder
302.72 Male Erectile Disorder

Orgasmic Disorders

302.73 Female Orgasmic Disorder
302.74 Male Orgasmic Disorder
302.75 Premature Ejaculation

Sexual Pain Disorders

302.76 Dyspareunia (Not Due to a General Medical Condition)
306.51 Vaginismus (Not Due to a General Medical Condition)

Sexual Dysfunction Due to a General Medical Condition

625.8 Female Hypoactive Sexual Desire Disorder Due to ... *[Indicate the General Medical Condition]*
608.89 Male Hypoactive Sexual Desire Disorder Due to ... *[Indicate the General Medical Condition]*
607.84 Male Erectile Disorder Due to ... *[Indicate the General Medical Condition]*
625.0 Female Dyspareunia Due to ... *[Indicate the General Medical Condition]*
608.89 Male Dyspareunia Due to ... *[Indicate the General Medical Condition]*
625.8 Other Female Sexual Dysfunction Due to ... *[Indicate the General Medical Condition]*
608.89 Other Male Sexual Dysfunction Due to ... *[Indicate the General Medical Condition]*
___.__ Substance-Induced Sexual Dysfunction *(refer to Substance-Related Disorders for substance-specific codes)*
Specify if: With Impaired Desire/With Impaired Arousal/With Impaired Orgasm/With Sexual Pain
Specify if: With Onset During Intoxication
302.70 Sexual Dysfunction NOS

Paraphilias

302.4 Exhibitionism
302.81 Fetishism
302.89 Frotteurism
302.2 Pedophilia
Specify if: Sexually Attracted to Males/Sexually Attracted to Females/Sexually Attracted to Both
Specify if: Limited to Incest
Specify type: Exclusive Type/Nonexclusive Type
302.83 Sexual Masochism
302.84 Sexual Sadism
302.3 Transvestic Fetishism
Specify if: With Gender Dysphoria
302.82 Voyeurism
302.9 Paraphilia NOS

Gender Identity Disorders

302.xx Gender Identity Disorder
  .6 in Children
  .85 in Adolescents or Adults
Specify if: Sexually Attracted to Males/Sexually Attracted to Females/Sexually Attracted to Both/Sexually Attracted to Neither
302.6 Gender Identity Disorder NOS
302.9 Sexual Disorder NOS

EATING DISORDERS

307.1 Anorexia Nervosa
Specify type: Restricting Type; Binge-Eating/Purging Type
307.51 Bulimia Nervosa
Specify type: Purging Type/Nonpurging Type
307.50 Eating Disorder NOS

SLEEP DISORDERS

Primary Sleep Disorders

Dyssomnias

307.42 Primary Insomnia
307.44 Primary Hypersomnia
Specify if: Recurrent
347 Narcolepsy
780.59 Breathing-Related Sleep Disorder
307.45 Circadian Rhythm Sleep Disorder
Specify type: Delayed Sleep Phase Type/Jet Lag Type/Shift Work Type/Unspecified Type
307.47 Dyssomnia NOS

Parasomnias

307.47 Nightmare Disorder
307.46 Sleep Terror Disorder
307.46 Sleepwalking Disorder
307.47 Parasomnia NOS

Sleep Disorders Related to Another Mental Disorder

307.42 Insomnia Related to ... *[Indicate the Axis I or Axis II Disorder]*
307.44 Hypersomnia Related to ... *[Indicate the Axis I or Axis II Disorder]*

Other Sleep Disorders

780.xx Sleep Disorder Due to ... *[Indicate the General Medical Condition]*
.52 Insomnia Type
.54 Hypersomnia Type
.59 Parasomnia Type
.59 Mixed Type
___._ Substance-Induced Sleep Disorder (refer to Substance-Related Disorders for substance-specific codes)
Specify type: Insomnia Type/Hypersomnia Type/Parasomnia Type/Mixed Type
Specify if: With Onset During Intoxication/With Onset During Withdrawal

IMPULSE-CONTROL DISORDERS NOT ELSEWHERE CLASSIFIED

312.34 Intermittent Explosive Disorder
312.32 Kleptomania
312.33 Pyromania
312.31 Pathological Gambling
312.39 Trichotillomania
312.30 Impulse-Control Disorder NOS

ADJUSTMENT DISORDERS

309.xx Adjustment Disorder
.0 With Depressed Mood
.24 With Anxiety
.28 With Mixed Anxiety and Depressed Mood
.3 With Disturbance of Conduct
.4 With Mixed Disturbance of Emotions and Conduct
.9 Unspecified
Specify if: Acute/Chronic

PERSONALITY DISORDERS

***Note:** These are coded on Axis II.*

301.0 Paranoid Personality Disorder
301.20 Schizoid Personality Disorder
301.22 Schizotypal Personality Disorder
301.7 Antisocial Personality Disorder
301.83 Borderline Personality Disorder
301.50 Histrionic Personality Disorder
301.81 Narcissistic Personality Disorder
301.82 Avoidant Personality Disorder
301.6 Dependent Personality Disorder
301.4 Obsessive-Compulsive Personality Disorder
301.9 Personality Disorder NOS

OTHER CONDITIONS THAT MAY BE A FOCUS OF CLINICAL ATTENTION

Psychological Factors Affecting Medical Condition

316 *... [Specified Psychological Factor] Affecting ... [Indicate the General Medical Condition] Choose name based on nature of factors:*
Mental Disorder Affecting Medical Condition
Psychological Symptoms Affecting Medical Condition
Personality Traits or Coping Style Affecting Medical Condition
Maladaptive Health Behaviors Affecting Medical Condition
Stress-Related Physiological Response Affecting Medical Condition
Other or Unspecified Psychological Factors Affecting Medical Condition

Medication-Induced Movement Disorders

332.1 Neuroleptic-Induced Parkinsonism
333.92 Neuroleptic Malignant Syndrome
333.7 Neuroleptic-Induced Acute Dystonia

333.99 Neuroleptic-Induced Acute Akathisia
333.82 Neuroleptic-Induced Tardive Dyskinesia
333.1 Medication-Induced Postural Tremor
333.90 Medication-Induced Movement Disorder NOS

Other Medication-Induced Disorder

995.2 Adverse Effects of Medication NOS

Relational Problems

V61.9 Relational Problem Related to a Mental Disorder or General Medical Condition
V61.20 Parent-Child Relational Problem
V61.1 Partner Relational Problem
V61.8 Sibling Relational Problem
V62.81 Relational Problem NOS

Problems Related to Abuse or Neglect

V61.21 Physical Abuse of Child *(code 995.5 if focus of attention is on victim)*
V61.21 Sexual Abuse of Child *(code 995.5 if focus of attention is on victim)*
V61.21 Neglect of Child *(code 995.5 if focus of attention is on victim)*
V61.1 Physical Abuse of Adult *(code 995.81 if focus of attention is on victim)*
V61.1 Sexual Abuse of Adult *(code 995.81 if focus of attention is on victim)*

Additional Conditions That May Be a Focus of Clinical Attention

V15.81 Noncompliance With Treatment
V65.2 Malingering
V71.01 Adult Antisocial Behavior
V71.02 Child or Adolescent Antisocial Behavior
V62.89 Borderline Intellectual Functioning
Note: *This is coded on Axis II.*
780.9 Age-Related Cognitive Decline
V62.82 Bereavement
V62.3 Academic Problem
V62.2 Occupational Problem
313.82 Identity Problem
V62.89 Religious or Spiritual Problem
V62.4 Acculturation Problem
V62.89 Phase of Life Problem

ADDITIONAL CODES

300.9 Unspecified Mental Disorder (nonpsychotic)
V71.09 No Diagnosis or Condition on Axis I
799.9 Diagnosis or Condition Deferred on Axis I
V71.09 No Diagnosis on Axis II
799.9 Diagnosis Deferred on Axis II

MULTIAXIAL SYSTEM

Axis I Clinical Disorders
Other Conditions That May Be a Focus of Clinical Attention
Axis II Personality Disorders
Mental Retardation
Axis III General Medical Conditions
Axis IV Psychosocial and Environmental Problems
Axis V Global Assessment of Functioning

From *Diagnostic and Statistical Manual of Mental Disorders* (4th edition). American Psychiatric Association. (2000). Washington, DC: Author.

APPENDIX B
NANDA-I Nursing Diagnoses 2009–2011

Domain 1
Health Promotion
Ineffective **Health** Maintenance
Ineffective Self **Health** Management
Impaired **Home** Maintenance
Readiness for Enhanced **Immunization** Status
Self **Neglect**
Readiness for Enhanced **Nutrition**
Ineffective Family **Therapeutic** Regimen Management
Readiness for Enhanced **Self Health** Management

Domain 2
Nutrition
Ineffective Infant **Feeding** Pattern
Imbalanced **Nutrition**: Less Than Body Requirements
Imbalanced **Nutrition**: More Than Body Requirements
Risk for Imbalanced **Nutrition**: More Than Body Requirements
Impaired **Swallowing**
Risk for Unstable Blood **Glucose** Level
Neonatal **Jaundice**
Risk for Impaired **Liver** Function
Risk for **Electrolyte** Imbalance
Readiness for Enhanced **Fluid** Balance
Deficient **Fluid** Volume
Excess **Fluid** Volume
Risk for Deficient **Fluid** Volume
Risk for Imbalanced **Fluid** Volume

Domain 3
Elimination and Exchange
Functional Urinary **Incontinence**
Overflow Urinary **Incontinence**
Reflex Urinary **Incontinence**
Stress Urinary **Incontinence**
Urge Urinary **Incontinence**
Risk for Urge Urinary **Incontinence**
Impaired **Urinary** Elimination
Readiness for Enhanced **Urinary** Elimination
Urinary Retention
Bowel Incontinence
Constipation
Perceived **Constipation**
Risk for **Constipation**
Diarrhea
Dysfunctional Gastrointenstinal **Motility**
Risk for Dysfunctional Gastrointestinal **Motility**
Impaired **Gas** Exchange

Domain 4
Activity Rest
Insomnia
Disturbed **Sleep** Pattern
Sleep Deprivation
Readiness for Enhanced **Sleep**
Risk for **Disuse** Syndrome
Deficient **Diversional** Activity
Sedentary **Lifestyle**
Impaired Bed **Mobility**
Impaired Physical **Mobility**
Impaired Wheelchair **Mobility**
Delayed **Surgical** Recovery
Impaired **Transfer** Ability
Impaired **Walking**
Disturbed **Energy** Field
Fatigue
Activity Intolerance
Risk for **Activity** Intolerance
Risk for **Bleeding**
Ineffective **Breathing** Pattern
Decreased **Cardiac** Output
Ineffective Peripheral Tissue **Perfusion**
Risk for Decreased Cardiac Tissue **Perfusion**
Risk for Ineffective Cerebral Tissue **Perfusion**
Risk for Ineffective Gastrointestinal **Perfusion**
Risk for **Ineffective Renal Perfusion**
Risk for **Shock**
Impaired Spontaneous **Ventilation**
Dysfunctional **Ventilatory** Weaning Response
Readiness for Enhanced **Self-Care**
Bathing **Self-Care** Deficit
Dressing **Self-Care** Deficit
Feeding **Self-Care** Deficit
Toileting **Self-Care** Deficit

Domain 5
Perception/Cognition
Unilateral **Neglect**
Impaired **Environmental** Interpretation Syndrome
Wandering
Disturbed **Sensory** Perception (Specify: Visual, Auditory, Kinesthetic, Gustatory, Tactile, Olfactory)
Acute **Confusion**
Chronic **Confusion**
Risk for Acute **Confusion**
Deficient **Knowledge**
Readiness for Enhanced **Knowledge**
Impaired **Memory**
Readiness for Enhanced **Decision-Making**
Ineffective **Activity** Planning
Impaired Verbal **Communication**
Readiness for Enhanced **Communication**

Domain 6
Self-Perception
Risk for Compromised Human **Dignity**
Hopelessness
Disturbed Personal **Identity**
Risk for **Loneliness**
Readiness for Enhanced **Power**
Powerlessness
Risk for **Powerlessness**
Readiness for Enhanced **Self-Concept**
Situational Low **Self-Esteem**
Chronic Low **Self-Esteem**
Risk for Situational Low **Self-Esteem**
Disturbed **Body** Image

Domain 7
Role Relationships
Caregiver Role Strain
Risk for **Caregiver** Role Strain
Impaired **Parenting**
Readiness for Enhanced **Parenting**
Risk for Impaired **Parenting**
Risk for Impaired **Attachment**
Dysfunctional **Family** Processes
Interrupted **Family** Processes
Readiness for Enhanced **Family** Processes
Effective **Breastfeeding**
Ineffective **Breastfeeding**
Interrupted **Breastfeeding**
Parental Role **Conflict**
Readiness for Enhanced **Relationship**
Ineffective **Role** Performance
Impaired **Social** Interaction

Domain 8
Sexuality
Sexual Dysfunction
Ineffective **Sexuality** Pattern
Readiness for Enhanced **Childbearing** Process
Risk for Disturbed **Maternal/Fetal** Dyad

Domain 9
Coping/Stress Tolerance
Post-Trauma Syndrome
Risk for **Post-Trauma** Syndrome
Rape-Trauma Syndrome
Relocation Stress Syndrome
Risk for **Relocation** Stress Syndrome
Anxiety
Death **Anxiety**
Risk-Prone Health **Behavior**
Compromised Family **Coping**
Defensive **Coping**
Disabled Family **Coping**
Ineffective **Coping**
Ineffective Community **Coping**
Readiness for Enhanced **Coping**
Readiness for Enhanced Community **Coping**
Readiness for Enhanced Family **Coping**
Ineffective **Denial**
Fear
Grieving
Complicated **Grieving**
Risk for Complicated **Grieving**
Impaired Individual **Resilience**
Readiness for Enhanced **Resilience**
Risk for Compromised **Resilience**
Chronic **Sorrow**
Stress Overload
Autonomic Dysreflexia
Risk for **Autonomic** Dysreflexia
Disorganized **Infant** Behavior
Risk for Disorganized **Infant** Behavior
Readiness for Enhanced Organized **Infant** Behavior
Decreased **Intracranial** Adaptive Capacity

Domain 10
Life Principles
Readiness for Enhanced **Hope**
Readiness for Enhanced **Spiritual** Well-Being
Decisional **Conflict**
Moral **Distress**
Noncompliance
Impaired **Religiosity**
Readiness for Enhanced **Religiosity**
Risk for Impaired **Religiosity**
Spiritual Distress
Risk for **Spiritual** Distress

Domain 11
Safety/Protection
Risk for **Infection**
Ineffective **Airway** Clearance
Risk for **Aspiration**
Risk for Sudden Infant **Death** Syndrome
Impaired **Dentition**
Risk for **Falls**
Risk for **Injury**
Risk for Perioperative-Positioning **Injury**
Impaired **Oral** Mucous Membrane
Risk for **Peripheral** Neurovascular Dysfunction
Ineffective **Protection**
Impaired **Skin** Integrity
Risk for Impaired **Skin** Integrity
Risk for **Suffocation**
Impaired **Tissue** Integrity
Risk for **Trauma**
Risk for Vascular **Trauma**
Self-Mutilation
Risk for **Suicide**
Risk for Other-Directed **Violence**
Risk for Self-Directed **Violence**
Contamination
Risk for **Contamination**
Risk for **Poisoning**
Latex **Allergy** Response
Risk for Latex **Allergy** Response
Risk for Imbalanced **Body** Temperature
Hyperthermia
Hypothermia
Ineffective **Thermoregulation**

Domain 12
Comfort
Readiness for Enhanced **Comfort**
Impaired **Comfort**
Nausea
Acute **Pain**
Chronic **Pain**
Social Isolation

Domain 13
Growth/Development
Adult **Failure** to Thrive
Delayed **Growth** and Development
Risk for Disproportionate **Growth**
Risk for Delayed **Development**

Source: *NANDA-I Nursing Diagnoses: Definitions & Classifications, 2009–2011,* by North American Nursing Diagnosis Association, 2009. West Sussex, United Kingdom: John Wiley & Sons, Ltd.

APPENDIX C
Nursing Outcomes Classifications (NOC)

Abuse Cessation
Abuse Protection
Abuse Recovery Status
Abuse Recovery: Emotional
Abuse Recovery: Financial
Abuse Recovery: Physical
Abuse Recovery: Sexual
Abusive Behavior Self-Restraint
Acceptance: Health Status
Activity Tolerance
Acute Confusion Control
Adaptation to Physical Disability
Adherence Behavior
Adherence Behavior: Healthy Diet
Aggression Self-Control
Agitation Level
Alcohol Abuse Cessation Behavior
Allergic Response: Localized
Allergic Response: Systematic
Ambulation
Ambulation: Wheelchair
Anxiety Level
Anxiety Self-Control
Appetite
Aspiration Prevention
Asthma Self-Management

Balance
Blood Coagulation
Blood-Glucose Level
Blood Loss Severity
Blood Transfusion Reaction
Body Image
Body Mechanics Performance
Body Positioning: Self-Initiated
Bone Healing
Bowel Continence
Bowel Elimination
Breastfeeding Establishment: Infant
Breastfeeding Establishment: Maternal
Breastfeeding: Maintenance
Breastfeeding: Weaning
Burn Healing
Burn Recovery

Cardiac Disease Self-Management
Cardiac Pump Effectiveness
Cardiopulmonary Status
Caregiver Adaptation to Patient Institutionalization
Caregiver Emotional Health
Caregiver Home Care Readiness
Caregiver Lifestyle Disruption
Caregiver-Patient Relationship
Caregiver Performance: Direct Care
Caregiver Performance: Indirect Care
Caregiver Physical Health
Caregiver Role Support
Caregiver Stressors
Caregiver Well-Being
Caregiving Endurance Potential
Child Adaptation to Hospitalization
Child Development: 1 Month
Child Development: 2 Months
Child Development: 4 Months
Child Development: 6 Months
Child Development: 12 Months
Child Development: 2 Years
Child Development: 3 Years
Child Development: 4 Years
Child Development: Middle Childhood
Child Development: Adolescence
Circulation Status
Client Satisfaction
Client Satisfaction: Access to Care Resources
Client Satisfaction: Caring
Client Satisfaction: Case Management
Client Satisfaction: Communication
Client Satisfaction: Continuity of Care
Client Satisfaction: Cultural Needs Fulfillment
Client Satisfaction: Functional Assistance
Client Satisfaction: Pain Management
Client Satisfaction: Physical Care
Client Satisfaction: Physical Environment
Client Satisfaction: Protection of Rights
Client Satisfaction: Psychological Care
Client Satisfaction: Safety
Client Satisfaction: Symptom Control
Client Satisfaction: Teaching
Client Satisfaction: Technical Aspects of Care
Cognition
Cognitive Orientation
Comfort Status
Comfort Status: Environment
Comfort Status: Physical
Comfort Status: Psychospiritual
Comfort Status: Sociocultural
Comfortable Death

Communication
Communication: Expressive
Communication: Receptive
Community Competence
Community Disaster Readiness
Community Disaster Response
Community Health Status
Community Health Status: Immunity
Community Risk Control: Chronic Disease
Community Risk Control: Communicable Disease
Community Risk Control: Lead Exposure
Community Risk Control: Violence
Community Violence Level
Compliance Behavior
Compliance Behavior: Prescribed Diet
Compliance Behavior: Prescribed Medication
Concentration
Coordinated Movement
Coping

Decision Making
Depression Level
Depression Self-Control
Development: Late Adulthood
Development: Middle Adulthood
Development: Young Adulthood
Diabetes Self-Management
Dignified Life Closure
Discharge Readiness: Independent Living
Discharge Readiness: Supported Living
Discomfort Level
Distorted Thought Self-Control
Drug Abuse Cessation Behavior

Electrolyte and Acid/Base Balance
Elopement Occurrence
Elopement Propensity Risk
Endurance
Energy Conservation

Fall Prevention Behavior
Falls Occurrence
Family Coping
Family Functioning
Family Health Status
Family Integrity
Family Normalization
Family Participation in Professional Care
Family Physical Environment
Family Resiliency
Family Social Climate
Family Support During Treatment
Fatigue Level
Fear Level
Fear Level: Child
Fear Self-Control
Fetal Status: Antepartum
Fetal Status: Intrapartum
Fluid Balance
Fluid Overload Severity

Gastrointestinal Function
Grief Resolution
Growth

Health Beliefs
Health Beliefs: Perceived Ability to Perform
Health Beliefs: Perceived Control
Health Beliefs: Perceived Resources
Health Beliefs: Perceived Threat
Health Orientation
Health-Promoting Behavior
Health-Seeking Behavior
Hearing Compensation Behavior
Heedfulness of Affected Side
Hemodialysis Access
Hope
Hydration
Hyperactivity Level

Identity
Immobility Consequences: Physiological
Immobility Consequences: Psycho-Cognitive
Immune Hypersensitivity Response
Immune Status
Immunization Behavior
Impulse Self-Control
Infection Severity
Infection Severity: Newborn
Information Processing

Joint Movement: Ankle
Joint Movement: Elbow
Joint Movement: Fingers
Joint Movement: Hip
Joint Movement: Knee
Joint Movement: Neck
Joint Movement: Passive
Joint Movement: Shoulder
Joint Movement: Spine
Joint Movement: Wrist
Kidney Function
Knowledge: Arthritis Management
Knowledge: Asthma Management
Knowledge: Body Mechanics
Knowledge: Breastfeeding
Knowledge: Cancer Management
Knowledge: Cancer Threat Reduction
Knowledge: Cardiac Disease Management
Knowledge: Child Physical Safety
Knowledge: Conception Prevention
Knowledge: Congestive Heart Failure Management
Knowledge: Depression Management
Knowledge: Diabetes Management
Knowledge: Diet
Knowledge: Disease Process
Knowledge: Energy Conservation
Knowledge: Fall Prevention
Knowledge: Fertility Promotion
Knowledge: Health Behavior
Knowledge: Health Promotion
Knowledge: Health Resources
Knowledge: Hypertension Management
Knowledge: Illness Care
Knowledge: Infant Care
Knowledge: Infection Control
Knowledge: Labor and Delivery
Knowledge: Medication
Knowledge: Multiple Sclerosis Management
Knowledge: Ostomy Care
Knowledge: Pain Management
Knowledge: Parenting
Knowledge: Personal Safety
Knowledge: Postpartum Maternal Health
Knowledge: Preconception Maternal Health
Knowledge: Pregnancy
Knowledge: Prescribed Activity
Knowledge: Preterm Infant Care
Knowledge: Sexual Functioning
Knowledge: Substance Abuse Control
Knowledge: Treatment Procedure(s)
Knowledge: Treatment Regimen
Knowledge: Weight Management

Leisure Participation
Loneliness Severity

Maternal Status: Antepartum
Maternal Status: Intrapartum
Maternal Status: Postpartum
Mechanical Ventilation Response: Adult
Mechanical Ventilation Weaning Response: Adult
Medication Response
Memory
Mobility
Mood Equilibrium
Motivation
Multiple Sclerosis Self-Management

Nausea & Vomiting Control
Nausea & Vomiting: Disruptive Effects
Nausea & Vomiting Severity
Neglect Cessation
Neglect Recovery
Neurological Status
Neurological Status: Autonomic
Neurological Status: Central Motor Control
Neurological Status: Consciousness
Neurological Status: Cranial Sensory/Motor Function
Neurological Status: Peripheral Sensory/Motor Function
Neurological Status: Spinal Sensory/Motor Function
Newborn Adaptation
Nutritional Status
Nutritional Status: Biochemical Measures
Nutritional Status: Energy
Nutritional Status: Food and Fluid Intake
Nutritional Status: Nutrient Intake

Oral Hygiene
Ostomy Self-Care

Pain: Adverse Psychological Response
Pain Control
Pain: Disruptive Effects
Pain Level
Parent-Infant Attachment
Parenting: Adolescent Physical Safety
Parenting: Early/Middle Childhood Physical Safety
Parenting: Infant/Toddler Physical Safety
Parenting Performance
Parenting: Psychosocial Safety
Participation in Health Care Decisions
Personal Autonomy
Personal Health Status
Personal Safety Behavior
Personal Well-Being
Physical Aging
Physical Fitness
Physical Injury Severity
Physical Maturation: Female
Physical Maturation: Male
Play Participation
Post-Partum Maternal Health Behavior
Post Procedure Recovery Status
Prenatal Health Behavior
Pre-Procedure Readiness
Preterm Infant Organization
Psychomotor Energy
Psychosocial Adjustment: Life Change

Quality of Life

Respiratory Status: Airway Patency
Respiratory Status: Gas Exchange
Respiratory Status: Ventilation
Rest
Risk Control
Risk Control: Alcohol Use
Risk Control: Cancer
Risk Control: Cardiovascular Health
Risk Control: Drug Use
Risk Control: Hearing Impairment
Risk Control: Hyperthermia
Risk Control: Hypothermia
Risk Control: Infectious Process
Risk Control: Sexually Transmitted Diseases (STDs)
Risk Control: Sun Exposure
Risk Control: Tobacco Use
Risk Control: Unintended Pregnancy
Risk Control: Visual Impairment
Risk Detection
Role Performance

Safe Home Environment
Safe Wandering
Seizure Control
Self-Care Status
Self-Care: Activities of Daily Living (ADL)
Self-Care: Bathing
Self-Care: Dressing
Self-Care: Eating
Self-Care: Hygiene
Self-Care: Instrumental Activities of Daily Living (IADL)
Self-Care: Non-parenteral Medication
Self-Care: Oral Hygiene
Self-Care: Parenteral Medication
Self-Care: Toileting
Self-Direction of Care
Self-Esteem
Self-Mutilation Restraint
Sensory Function Status
Sensory Function: Cutaneous
Sensory Function: Hearing
Sensory Function: Proprioception
Sensory Function: Taste and Smell
Sensory Function: Vision
Sexual Functioning
Sexual Identity
Skeletal Function
Sleep
Smoking Cessation Behavior
Social Interaction Skills
Social Involvement
Social Support
Spiritual Health
Stress Level
Student Health Status
Substance Addiction Consequences
Substance Withdrawal Severity
Suffering Severity
Suicide Self-Restraint
Swallowing Status
Swallowing Status: Esophageal Phase
Swallowing Status: Oral Phrase
Swallowing Status: Pharyngeal Phase
Symptom Control
Symptom Severity
Symptom Severity: Perimenopause
Symptom Severity: Premenstrual Syndrome (PMS)
Systemic Toxin Clearance: Dialysis

Thermoregulation
Thermoregulation: Newborn
Tissue Integrity: Skin and Mucous Membranes
Tissue Perfusion: Abdominal Organs
Tissue Perfusion: Cardiac
Tissue Perfusion: Cerebral
Tissue Perfusion: Peripheral
Tissue Perfusion: Pulmonary

Transfer Performance
Treatment Behavior: Illness or Injury

Urinary Continence
Urinary Elmination

Vision Compensation Behavior
Vital Signs

Weight: Body Mass
Weight Gain Behavior

Weight Loss Behavior
Weight Maintenance Behavior
Will to Live
Wound Healing: Primary Intention
Wound Healing: Secondary Intention

From Moorhead, S., Johnson, M., Maas, M., & Swanson, E. *Nursing Outcomes Classifications*, 4th ed., 2008. Reprinted with permission from Elsevier Science.

APPENDIX D
Nursing Interventions Classifications (NIC)

Abuse Protection Support
Abuse Protection Support: Child
Abuse Protection Support: Domestic Partner
Abuse Protection Support: Elder
Abuse Protection Support: Religious
Acid-Base Management
Acid-Base Management: Metabolic Acidosis
Acid-Base Management: Metabolic Alkalosis
Acid-Base Management: Respiratory Acidosis
Acid-Base Management: Respirartory Alkalosis
Acid-Base Monitoring
Active Listening
Activity Therapy
Acupressure
Admission Care
Airway Insertion and Stabilization
Airway Management
Airway Suctioning
Allergy Management
Amnioinfusion
Amputation Care
Analgesic Administration
Analgesic Administration: Intraspinal
Anaphylaxis Management
Anesthesia Administration
Anger Control Assistance
Animal-Assisted Therapy
Anticipatory Guidance
Anxiety Reduction
Area Restruction
Aromatherapy
Art Therapy
Artificial Airway Management
Aspiration Precautions
Assertiveness Training
Asthma Management
Attachment Promotion
Autogenic Training
Autotransfusion

Bathing
Bed Rest Care
Bedside Laboratory Testing
Behavior Management
Behavior Management: Overactivity/ Inattention
Behavior Management: Self-Harm
Behavior Management: Sexual
Behavior Modification
Behavior Modification: Social Skills
Bibliotherapy
Biofeedback
Bioterrorism Preparedness
Birthing
Bladder Irrigation
Bleeding Precautions
Bleeding Reduction
Bleeding Reduction: Antepartum Uterus
Bleeding Reduction: Gastrointestinal
Bleeding Reduction: Nasal
Bleeding Reduction: Postpartum Uterus
Bleeding Reduction: Wound
Blood Products Administration
Body Image Enhancement
Body Mechanics Promotion
Bottle Feeding
Bowel Incontinence Care
Bowel Incontinence Care: Encopresis
Bowel Irrigation
Bowel Management
Bowel Training
Breast Examination
Breastfeeding Assistance

Calming Technique
Capillary Blood Sample
Cardiac Care
Cardiac Care: Acute
Cardiac Care: Rehabilitative
Cardiac Precautions
Caregiver Support
Care Management
Cast Care: Maintenance
Cast Care, Wet
Cerebral Edema Management
Cerebral Perfusion Promotioon
Cesarean Section Care
Chemical Restraint
Chemotherapy Management
Chest Physiotherapy
Childbirth Preparation
Circulatory Care: Arterial Insufficiency
Circulatory Care: Mechanical Assist Device
Circulatory Care: Venous Insufficiency
Circulatory Precautions
Circumcision Care

Code Management
Cognitive Restructuring
Cognitive Stimulation
Communicable Disease Management
Communication Enhancement: Hearing Deficit
Communication Enhancement: Speech Deficit
Communication Enhancement: Visual Deficit
Community Disaster Preparedness
Community Health Development
Complex Relationship Building
Conflict Mediation
Constipation/Impaction Management
Consultation
Contact Lens Care
Controlled Substance Checking
Coping Enhancement
Cost Containment
Cough Enhancement
Counseling
Crisis Intervention
Critical Path Development
Culture Brokerage
Cutaneous Stimulation

Decision-Making Support
Defibrillator Management : External
Defibrillator Management: Internal
Delegation
Delirium Management
Delusion Management
Dementia Management
Dementia Management: Bathing
Deposition/Testimony
Developmental Care
Developmental Enhancement: Adolescent
Developmental Enhancement: Child
Dialysis Access Maintenance
Diarrhea Management
Diet Staging
Discharge Planning
Distraction
Documentation
Dressing
Dying Care
Dysreflexia Management
Dysrhythmia Management

Ear Care
Eating Disorders Management
Electroconvulsive Therapy (ECT) Management
Electrolyte Management
Electrolyte Management: Hypercalcemia
Electrolyte Management: Hyperkalemia
Electrolyte Management: Hypermagnesemia
Electrolyte Management: Hypernatremia
Electrolyte Management: Hyperphosphatemia
Electrolyte Management: Hypocalcemia
Electrolyte Management: Hypokalemia
Electrolyte Management: Hypomagnesemia
Electrolyte Management: Hyponatremia
Electrolyte Management: Hypophosphatemia
Electrolyte Monitoring
Electronic Fetal Monitoring: Antepartum
Electronic Fetal Monitoring: Intrapartum
Elopement Precautions
Embolus Care: Peripheral
Embolus Care: Pulmonary
Embolus Precautions
Emergency Care
Emergency Cart Checking
Emotional Support
Endotracheal Extubation
Energy Management
Enteral Tube Feeding
Environmental Management
Environmental Management: Attachment Process
Environmental Management: Comfort
Environmental Management: Community
Environmental Management: Home Preparation
Environmental Management: Safety
Environmental Management: Violence Prevention
Environmental Management: Worker Safety
Environmental Risk Protection
Examination Assistance
Exercise Promotion
Exercise Promotion: Strength Training
Exercise Promotion: Stretching
Exercise Therapy: Ambulation
Exercise Therapy: Balance
Exercise Therapy: Joint Mobility
Exercise Therapy: Muscle Control
Eye Care
Fall Prevention
Family Integrity Promotion
Family Integrity Promotion: Childbearing Family
Family Involvement Promotion
Family Mobilization
Family Planning: Contraception
Family Planning: Infertility
Family Planning: Unplanned Pregnancy
Family Presence Facilitation
Family Process Maintenance
Family Suppor rt
Family Therapy
Feeding
Fertility Preservation
Fever Treatment
Financial Resource Assistance
Fire-Setting Precautions
First Aid
Fiscal Resource Management
Flatulence Reduction
Fluid/Electrolyte Management
Fluid Management
Fluid Monitoring
Fluid Resuscitation
Foot Care
Forensic Data Collection
Forgiveness Facilitation

Gastrointestinal Intubation
Genetic Counseling
Grief Work Facilitation
Grief Work Facilitation: Perinatal Death
Guided Imagery
Guilt Work Facilitation

Hair Care
Hallucination Management
Health Care Information Exchange
Health Education
Health Literacy Enhancement
Health Policy Monitoring
Health Screening
Health System Guidance
Heat/Cold Application
Heat Exposure Treatment
Hemodialysis Therapy
Hemodynamic Regulation
Hemofiltration Therapy
Hemorrhage Control
High-Risk Pregnancy Care
Home Maintenance Assistance
Hope Installation

Hormone Replacement Therapy
Humor
Hyperglycemia Management
Hypervolemia Management
Hypnosis
Hypoglycemia Management
Hypothermia Treatment
Hypovolemia Management

Immunization/Vaccination Management
Impulse Control Training
Incident Reporting
Incision Site Care
Infant Care
Infection Control
Infection Control: Intraoperative
Infection Protection
Insurance Authorization
Intracranial Pressure (ICP) Monitoring
Intrapartal Care
Intrapartal Care: High-Risk Delivery
Intravenous (IV) Insertion
Intravenous (IV) Therapy
Invasive Hemodynamic Monitoring

Journaling

Kangaroo Care

Labor Induction
Labor Suppression
Laboratory Data Interpretation
Lactation Counseling
Lactation Suppression
Laser Precautions
Latex Precautions
Learning Facilitation
Learning Readiness Enhancement
Leech Therapy
Limit Setting
Lower Extremity Monitoring

Malignant Hyperthermia Precautions
Mechanical Ventilation Management: Invasive
Mechanical Ventilation Management: Non-invasive
Mechanical Ventilatory Weaning
Medication Administration
Medication Administration: Ear
Medication Administration: Enteral
Medication Administration: Eye
Medication Administration: Inhalation
Medication Administration: Interpleural
Medication Administration: Intradermal
Medication Administration: Intramuscular (IM)
Medication Administration: Intraosseous
Medication Administration: Intraspinal
Medication Administration: Intravenous (IV)
Medication Administration: Nasal
Medication Administration: Oral
Medication Administration: Rectal
Medication Administration: Skin
Medication Administration: Subcutaneous
Medication Administration: Vaginal
Medication Administration: Ventricular Reservoir
Medication Management
Medication Prescribing
Medication Reconciliation
Meditation Facilitation
Memory Training
Milieu Therapy
Mood Management
Multidisciplinary Care Conference
Music Therapy
Mutual Goal Setting

Nail Care
Nausea Management
Neurologic Monitoring
Newborn Care
Newborn Monitoring
Nonnutritive Sucking
Normalization Promotion
Nutrition Management
Nutrition Therapy
Nutritional Counseling
Nutritional Monitoring

Oral Health Maintenance
Oral Health Promotion
Oral Health Restoration
Order Transcription
Organ Procurement
Ostomy Care
Oxygen Therapy

Pacemaker Management: Temporary
Pacemaker Management: Permanent
Pain Management
Parent Education: Adolescent
Parent Education: Childrearing Family
Parent Education: Infant
Parenting Promotion
Pass Facilitation
Patient Contracting
Patient Controlled Analgesia (PCA) Assistance
Patients Rights Protection
Peer Review
Pelvic Muscle Exercise
Perineal Care
Peripheral Sensation Management
Peripherally Inserted Central (PIC) Catheter Care
Peritoneal Dialysis Therapy
Pessary Management
Phlebotomy: Arterial Blood Sample
Phlebotomy: Blood Unit Acquisition
Phlebotomy: Cannulated Vessel
Phlebotomy: Venous Blood Sample
Phototherapy: Mood/Sleep Regulation
Phototherapy: Neonate
Physical Restraint
Physician Support
Pneumatic Tourniquet Precautions
Positioning
Positioning: Intraoperative
Positioning: Neurologic
Positioning: Wheelchair
Postanesthesia Care
Postmortem Care
Postpartal Care
Preceptor: Employee
Preceptor: Student
Preconception Counseling
Pregnancy Termination Care
Premenstrual Syndrome (PMS) Management
Prenatal Care
Preoperative Coordination
Prepatory Sensory Information
Presence
Pressure Management
Pressure Ulcer Care
Pressure Ulcer Prevention
Product Evaluation
Program Development
Progressive Muscle Relation
Prompted Voiding
Prosthesis Care
Pruritus Management

Quality Monitoring

Radiation Therapy Management
Rape-Trauma Treatment
Reality Orientation
Recreation Therapy
Rectal Prolapse Management
Referral
Relaxation Therapy
Religious Addiction Prevention
Religious Ritual Enhancement
Relocation Stress Reduction
Reminiscence Therapy
Reproductive Technology Management
Research Data Collection
Resiliency Promotion
Respiratory Monitoring
Respite Care
Resuscitation
Resuscitation: Fetus
Resuscitation: Neonate
Risk Identification
Risk Identification: Childbearing Family
Risk Identification: Genetic
Role Enhancement

Seclusion
Security Enhancement
Sedation Management
Seizure Management
Seizure Precautions
Self-Awareness Enhancement
Self-Care Assistance
Self-Care Assistance: Bathing/Hygiene
Self-Care Assistance: Dressing/Grooming
Self-Care Assistance: Feeding
Self-Care Assistance: Instrumental Activities of Daily Living (IADL)
Self-Care Assistance: Toileting
Self-Care Assistance: Transfer
Self-Efficacy Enhancement
Self-Esteem Enhancement
Self-Hypnosis Facilitation
Self-Modification Assistance
Self-Responsibility Facilitation
Sexual Counseling
Shift Report
Shock Management
Shock Management: Cardiac
Shock Management: Vasogenic
Shock Management: Volume
Shock Prevention
Sibling Support
Simple Guided Imagery
Simple Massage
Simple Relaxation Therapy
Skin Care: Donor Site
Skin Care: Graft Site
Skin Care: Topical Treatments
Skin Surveillance
Sleep Enhancement
Smoking Cessation Assistance
Socialization Enhancement
Social Marketing
Specimen Management
Spiritual Growth Facilitation
Spiritual Support
Splinting
Sports-Injury Prevention: Youth
Staff Development
Staff Supervision
Subarachnoid Hemorrhage Precautions
Substance Use Prevention
Substance Use Treatment
Substance Use Treatment: Alcohol Withdrawal
Substance Use Treatment: Drug Withdrawal
Substance Use Treatment: Overdose
Suicide Prevention
Supply Management
Support Group
Support System Enhancement
Surgical Assistance
Surgical Precautions
Surgical Preparation
Surveillance
Surveillance: Community
Surveillance: Late Pregnancy
Surveillance: Remote Electronic
Surveillance: Safety
Sustenance Support
Suturing
Swallowing Therapy

Teaching: Disease Process
Teaching: Foot Care
Teaching: Group
Teaching: Individual
Teaching: Infant Nutrition: 0–3 months
Teaching: Infant Nutrition: 4–6 months
Teaching: Infant Nutrition: 7–9 months
Teaching: Infant Nutrition: 10–12 months
Teaching: Infant Safety: 0–3 months
Teaching: Infant Safety: 4–6 months
Teaching: Infant Safety: 7–9 months
Teaching: Infant Safety: 10–12 months
Teaching: Infant Stimulation: 0–4 months
Teaching: Infant Stimulation: 5–8 months
Teaching: Infant Stimulation: 9–12 months
Teaching: Preoperative
Teaching: Prescribed Activity/Exercise
Teaching: Prescribed Diet
Teaching: Prescribed Medication
Teaching: Procedure/Treatment
Teaching: Psychomotor Skill
Teaching: Safe Sex
Teaching: Sexuality
Teaching: Toddler Nutrition: 13–18 months
Teaching: Toddler Nutrition: 19–24 months
Teaching: Toddler Nutrition: 25–36 months
Teaching: Toddler Safety: 13–18 months
Teaching: Toddler Safety: 19–24 months
Teaching: Toddler Safety: 25–36 months
Teaching: Toilet Training
Technology Management
Telephone Consultation
Telephone Follow-Up
Temperature Regulation
Temperature Regulation: Intraoperative
Temporary Pacemaker Management
Therapeutic Play
Therapeutic Touch
Therapy Group
Thrombolytic Therapy Management
Total Parenteral Nutrition (TPN) Administration
Touch
Traction/Immobilization Care
Transcutaneous Electrical Nerve Stimulation (TENS)
Transfer: Interfacility
Transfer: Intrafacility
Transport
Trauma Therapy: Child
Triage: Disaster
Triage: Emergency Center
Triage: Telephone
Truth Telling

Tube Care
Tube Care: Chest
Tube Care: Gastrointestinal
Tube Care: Umbilical Line
Tube Care: Urinary
Tube Care: Ventriculostomy/Lumbar Drain

Ultrasonography: Limited Obstetric
Unilateral Neglect Management
Urinary Bladder Training
Urinary Catheterization
Urinary Catheterization: Intermittent
Urinary Elimination Management
Urinary Habit Training
Urinary Incontinence Care
Urinary Incontinence Care: Enuresis
Urinary Retention Care

Validation Therapy
Values Clarification
Vehicle Safety Promotion
Venous Access Device (VAD) Maintenance
Ventilation Assistance
Visitation Facilitation
Vital Signs Monitoring
Vomiting Management

Weight Gain Assistance
Weight Management
Weight Reduction Assistance
Wound Care: Burns
Wound Care: Closed Drainage
Wound Irrigation

APPENDIX E
Critical Pathway for a Client Experiencing Depression

HEALTH CARE TEAM MEMBERS AND THEIR RESPONSIBILITIES

Physician Directs the client's medical care.

Registered Nurse (RN) Provides skilled observation and assessment. Performs nursing procedures as needed. Teaches client and family how to maintain health at home. Plans and coordinates care with the physician. Registered nurses are available 24 hours daily.

Physical Therapists Teach strengthening exercises to increase physical independence.

Occupational Therapists Help the client return to her previous lifestyle with aids to daily living.

Speech Therapists Evaluate communication problems and work with the client and family to improve communication.

Nursing Assistants Provide services under the direction of a Registered Nurse. They assist client and family to achieve independence in daily activities. They also assist with personal hygiene.

Social Workers Assist with family or financial problems.

OVERALL GUIDELINES FOR THE NURSE

Guidelines for the nurse providing education to the depressed client in home health:

- Client will make a written agreement with the nurse to seek help prior to acting on suicidal thoughts. Agreement will be renewed each visit.
- Client verbalizes the importance of eating 60% of meals three times a day.
- Client verbalizes the importance of sleeping at least six hours per night.
- Client is able to demonstrate at least three relaxation techniques.
- Client will name each medication, identify the purpose, describe when it is to be taken, and be able to list two potential side effects caused by each.
- Client will verbalize the importance of compliance with medication.
- Client will verbalize the importance of compliance with follow-up care.
- Client will demonstrate increased energy and motivation by attending one meeting or social function per week.
- Client will increase activity by one activity each week.

Critical Pathway for a Client Experiencing Depression

DRG 426 Anticipated LOS 3 months Admit Date ______________ Discharge Date ______________

DSM-IV Diagnosis ____

Psychiatrist/Physician ______________________ Consultants ______________________

____

Problem: **Suicide Risk**

Nursing Diagnosis: *High risk for self-directed violence* r/t depressed mood, feelings of hopelessness, worthlessness.

Date Initiated ____________ Modified ____________ Resolved ____________

Expected Outcome:
1. Client will not harm herself while in the home environment.
2. Client will comply with taking medications as prescribed.
3. Client will report suicidal thoughts to nurse, counselor, or physician prior to taking action.

Nursing Assessment/ Interventions (practice standards):
1. Establish a therapeutic rapport with client.
2. Establish a contract with client that she will not harm self and if thoughts of self-harm occur, client will inform family, counselor, nurse, or physician prior to acting on such thoughts.
3. Assess safety of environment.

Problem: **Weight Loss, Lack of Energy**

Nursing Diagnosis: *Imbalanced nutrition:* less than body requirements r/t decreased energy levels, poor appetite, lack of motivation to prepare and consume food.

Date Initiated ____________ Modified ____________ Resolved ____________

Expected Outcome:
1. Client will eat at least 60% of three meals daily.
2. Client will maintain current weight.
3. Client will demonstrate increased energy and motivation to prepare and consume meals.

Nursing Assessment/ Interventions (practice standards):
1. Weigh client every visit.
2. Assess ability of client to prepare meals.
3. Assess client's motivation to consume meals.

Problem: ____

Nursing Diagnosis: ____

Date Initiated ____________ Modified ____________ Resolved ____________

Expected Outcome: 1. ____

Nursing Assessment/ Interventions (practice standards):
1.
2.
3.

Path and discharge goals explained to the client/significant other with mutual agreement.

Date ______________ RN Signature ____

Critical Pathway for a Client Experiencing Depression

	Admission VISIT #1	VISIT #2	VISIT #3
Therapeutic Rapport	Prior to visit, call and make an appointment. Arrive on time. Establish trust. Allow time to talk prior to physical assessment. Establish ground rules of the relationship. Encourage client participation in forming plan of treatment. Set mutual goals.	Maintain trusting relationship. Actively listen; clarify; repeat; allow time for client to verbalize feelings. Offer encouragement and support. Promote: positive thinking; increased self esteem; increased sociability.	Maintain trusting relationship. Actively listen; clarify; repeat; allow time for client to verbalize feelings. Offer encouragement and support. Promote: positive thinking; increased self esteem; increased sociability.
Mental Status	**Anxiety Level:** ☐ Moderate ☐ Severe ☐ Panic **Mood:** ☐ WNL ☐ Labile ☐ Angry ☐ Hopeless ☐ Depressed ☐ Euphoric ☐ Guilt ☐ Worthless ☐ Incongruent **Thought Processes:** ☐ Incoherent ☐ Preoccupied ☐ Disorganized **Insight/Judgment:** ☐ WNL ☐ Poor ☐ Dangerous/Reckless **Suicide Potential:** ☐ Yes ☐ No ☐ Plan ☐ Physician Notified **Appearance:** ☐ Clean ☐ Unkempt ☐ Dirty **Behavior:** ☐ Friendly ☐ Evasive ☐ Indifferent **Speech:** ☐ Rate ☐ Cadence ☐ Tone **Orientation:** ☐ Month ☐ Day ☐ Year ☐ Time	**Anxiety Level:** ☐ Moderate ☐ Severe ☐ Panic **Mood:** ☐ WNL ☐ Labile ☐ Angry ☐ Hopeless ☐ Depressed ☐ Euphoric ☐ Guilt ☐ Worthless ☐ Incongruent **Thought Processes:** ☐ Incoherent ☐ Preoccupied ☐ Disorganized **Insight/Judgment:** ☐ WNL ☐ Poor ☐ Dangerous/Reckless **Suicide Potential:** ☐ Yes ☐ No ☐ Plan ☐ Physician Notified **Appearance:** ☐ Clean ☐ Unkempt ☐ Dirty **Behavior:** ☐ Friendly ☐ Evasive ☐ Indifferent **Speech:** ☐ Rate ☐ Cadence ☐ Tone **Orientation:** ☐ Month ☐ Day ☐ Year ☐ Time	**Anxiety Level:** ☐ Moderate ☐ Severe ☐ Panic **Mood:** ☐ WNL ☐ Labile ☐ Angry ☐ Hopeless ☐ Depressed ☐ Euphoric ☐ Guilt ☐ Worthless ☐ Incongruent **Thought Processes:** ☐ Incoherent ☐ Preoccupied ☐ Disorganized **Insight/Judgment:** ☐ WNL ☐ Poor ☐ Dangerous/Reckless **Suicide Potential:** ☐ Yes ☐ No ☐ Plan ☐ Physician Notified **Appearance:** ☐ Clean ☐ Unkempt ☐ Dirty **Behavior:** ☐ Friendly ☐ Evasive ☐ Indifferent **Speech:** ☐ Rate ☐ Cadence ☐ Tone **Orientation:** ☐ Month ☐ Day ☐ Year ☐ Time
Physical Assessment	☐ Past Health History Dietary Needs Met? ☐ Yes ☐ No Wt ________ Fluid Intake ________ N/V ________ LBM ________ **Vital Signs:** BP ___ R ___ P ___ T ___ ☐ Apical Pulse ☐ Lung Sounds ☐ Skin Integrity ☐ Bowel Sounds ☐ Mobility ☐ Edema ☐ Pulses of Extremities ☐ Sleep	Dietary Needs Met? ☐ Yes ☐ No Wt ________ Fluid Intake ________ N/V ________ LBM ________ **Vital Signs:** BP ___ R ___ P ___ T ___ ☐ Apical Pulse ☐ Lung Sounds ☐ Skin Integrity ☐ Bowel Sounds ☐ Mobility ☐ Edema ☐ Pulses of Extremities ☐ Sleep	Dietary Needs Met? ☐ Yes ☐ No Wt ________ Fluid Intake ________ N/V ________ LBM ________ **Vital Signs:** BP ___ R ___ P ___ T ___ ☐ Apical Pulse ☐ Lung Sounds ☐ Skin Integrity ☐ Bowel Sounds ☐ Mobility ☐ Edema ☐ Pulses of Extremities ☐ Sleep
Complete Assessment	☐ Safety ☐ MSW ☐ ADLS		

Critical Pathway continues

	VISIT #1 Admission (continued)	VISIT #2 (continued)	VISIT #3 (continued)
Self-Care		☐ WNL ☐ Needs Assist	☐ WNL ☐ Needs Assist
Diagnostic Studies	☐ Obtain Labs PRN	☐ Obtain Labs PRN	☐ Obtain Labs PRN
Medications	☐ How are you taking your medications? ☐ Have you missed any doses? ☐ Have you had any problems with the medications? ☐ Provide information regarding adverse effects and benefits of medications. ☐ Fill medication box. ☐ Aims	☐ How are you taking your medications? ☐ Have you missed any doses? ☐ Have you had any problems with the medications? ☐ Provide information about side effects and benefits of medications. ☐ Fill medication box. ☐ Aims	☐ How are you taking your medications? ☐ Have you missed any doses? ☐ Have you had any problems with the medications? ☐ Provide information about side effects and benefits of medications. ☐ Fill medication box. ☐ Aims
Discharge Planning	**Assess:** Self-management of medication regimen; caregiver's ability to manage medications; willingness of caregiver; motivation and ability to keep appointments for follow-up. **Teach:** The importance of medication compliance. **Refer:** Support groups; community resources.	**Assess:** Self-management of medication regimen; caregiver's ability to manage medications; willingness of caregiver; motivation and ability to keep appointments for follow-up. **Teach:** The importance of medication compliance. **Refer:** Support groups; community resources.	**Assess:** Self-management of medication regimen; caregiver's ability to manage medications; willingness of caregiver; motivation and ability to keep appointments for follow-up. **Teach:** The importance of medication compliance. **Refer:** Support groups; community resources.
Expected Outcomes	Client will maintain a therapeutic relationship with the HH nurse. Client will be oriented to the benefits of home health care. Client will be able to maintain safety while in a home environment. Client will provide a written contract with nurse to seek help prior to acting on suicidal thoughts. Client will comply with taking medications as ordered by the physician. Client will maintain adequate diet. Client will sleep 6 hours per night. Client will report suicidal thoughts prior to acting on them. Client will keep all follow-up appointments.	Client will be able to maintain safety while in a home environment. Client will comply with taking medications as ordered by the physician. Client will maintain adequate diet. Client will sleep 6 hours per night. Client will report suicidal thoughts prior to acting on them. Client will be able to describe medication regimen.	Client will be able to maintain safety while in a home environment. Client will comply with taking medications as ordered by the physician. Client will maintain adequate diet. Client will sleep 6 hours per night. Client will report suicidal thoughts prior to acting on them. Client will list 3 side effects of medications and how to manage them.
Variances			

Critical Pathway continues

	VISIT #4	VISIT #5	VISIT #6
Therapeutic Rapport	Maintain trusting relationship. Actively listen; be empathetic; redefine; allow time for client to verbalize feelings. Offer encouragement and support. Promote: positive thinking; increased self esteem; increased sociability.	Maintain trusting relationship. Actively listen; be genuine; be nonjudgmental; allow time for client to verbalize feelings. Offer encouragement and support. Promote: positive thinking; increased self esteem; increased sociability.	Maintain trusting relationship. Actively listen; be honest; offer hope; allow time for client to verbalize feelings. Offer encouragement and support. Promote: positive thinking; increased self esteem; increased sociability.
Mental Status	**Anxiety Level:** ☐ Moderate ☐ Severe ☐ Panic **Mood:** ☐ WNL ☐ Labile ☐ Angry ☐ Hopeless ☐ Depressed ☐ Euphoric ☐ Guilt ☐ Worthless ☐ Incongruent **Thought Processes:** ☐ Incoherent ☐ Preoccupied ☐ Disorganized **Insight/Judgment:** ☐ WNL ☐ Poor ☐ Dangerous/Reckless **Suicide Potential:** ☐ Yes ☐ No ☐ Plan ☐ Physician Notified **Appearance:** ☐ Clean ☐ Unkempt ☐ Dirty **Behavior:** ☐ Friendly ☐ Evasive ☐ Indifferent **Speech:** ☐ Rate ☐ Cadence ☐ Tone **Orientation:** ☐ Month ☐ Day ☐ Year ☐ Time	**Anxiety Level:** ☐ Moderate ☐ Severe ☐ Panic **Mood:** ☐ WNL ☐ Labile ☐ Angry ☐ Hopeless ☐ Depressed ☐ Euphoric ☐ Guilt ☐ Worthless ☐ Incongruent **Thought Processes:** ☐ Incoherent ☐ Preoccupied ☐ Disorganized **Insight/Judgment:** ☐ WNL ☐ Poor ☐ Dangerous/Reckless **Suicide Potential:** ☐ Yes ☐ No ☐ Plan ☐ Physician Notified **Appearance:** ☐ Clean ☐ Unkempt ☐ Dirty **Behavior:** ☐ Friendly ☐ Evasive ☐ Indifferent **Speech:** ☐ Rate ☐ Cadence ☐ Tone **Orientation:** ☐ Month ☐ Day ☐ Year ☐ Time	**Anxiety Level:** ☐ Moderate ☐ Severe ☐ Panic **Mood:** ☐ WNL ☐ Labile ☐ Angry ☐ Hopeless ☐ Depressed ☐ Euphoric ☐ Guilt ☐ Worthless ☐ Incongruent **Thought Processes:** ☐ Incoherent ☐ Preoccupied ☐ Disorganized **Insight/Judgment:** ☐ WNL ☐ Poor ☐ Dangerous/Reckless **Suicide Potential:** ☐ Yes ☐ No ☐ Plan ☐ Physician Notified **Appearance:** ☐ Clean ☐ Unkempt ☐ Dirty **Behavior:** ☐ Friendly ☐ Evasive ☐ Indifferent **Speech:** ☐ Rate ☐ Cadence ☐ Tone **Orientation:** ☐ Month ☐ Day ☐ Year ☐ Time
Physical Assessment	Dietary Needs Met? ☐ Yes ☐ No Wt ________ Fluid Intake ________ N/V ________ LBM ________ **Vital Signs:** BP_____ R_____ P_____ T____ ☐ Apical Pulse ☐ Lung Sounds ☐ Skin Integrity ☐ Bowel Sounds ☐ Mobility ☐ Edema ☐ Pulses of Extremities ☐ Sleep	Dietary Needs Met? ☐ Yes ☐ No Wt ________ Fluid Intake ________ N/V ________ LBM ________ **Vital Signs:** BP_____ R_____ P_____ T____ ☐ Apical Pulse ☐ Lung Sounds ☐ Skin Integrity ☐ Bowel Sounds ☐ Mobility ☐ Edema ☐ Pulses of Extremities ☐ Sleep	Dietary Needs Met? ☐ Yes ☐ No Wt ________ Fluid Intake ________ N/V ________ LBM ________ **Vital Signs:** BP_____ R_____ P_____ T____ ☐ Apical Pulse ☐ Lung Sounds ☐ Skin Integrity ☐ Bowel Sounds ☐ Mobility ☐ Edema ☐ Pulses of Extremities ☐ Sleep
Self-Care	☐ WNL ☐ Needs Assist	☐ WNL ☐ Needs Assist	☐ WNL ☐ Needs Assist
Diagnostic Studies	☐ Obtain Labs PRN	☐ Obtain Labs PRN	☐ Obtain Labs PRN

Critical Pathway continues

	VISIT #4 (continued)	VISIT #5 (continued)	VISIT #6 (continued)
Medications	☐ How are you taking your medications? ☐ Have you missed any doses? ☐ Have you had any problems with the medications? ☐ Provide information regarding adverse effects and benefits of medications. ☐ Fill medication box. ☐ Aims	☐ How are you taking your medications? ☐ Have you missed any doses? ☐ Have you had any problems with the medications? ☐ Provide information regarding adverse effects and benefits of medications. ☐ Fill medication box. ☐ Aims	☐ How are you taking your medications? ☐ Have you missed any doses? ☐ Have you had any problems with the medications? ☐ Provide information regarding adverse effects and benefits of medications. ☐ Fill medication box. ☐ Aims
Discharge Planning	**Assess:** Self-management of medication regimen; caregiver's ability to manage medications; willingness of caregiver; motivation and ability to keep appointments for follow-up. **Teach:** Importance of medication compliance. **Refer:** Support groups; community resources.	**Assess:** Self-management of medication regimen; caregiver's ability to manage medications; willingness of caregiver; motivation and ability to keep appointments for follow-up. **Teach:** Importance of medication compliance; relaxation techniques. **Refer:** Support groups; community resources.	**Assess:** Self-management of medication regimen; caregiver's ability to manage medications; willingness of caregiver; motivation and ability to keep appointments for follow-up. **Teach:** Importance of medication compliance; coping strategies. **Refer:** Support groups; community resources; financial support.
Expected Outcomes	Client will maintain a therapeutic relationship. Client will be able to maintain safety while in a home environment. Client will comply with taking medications as ordered by the physician. Client will keep all follow-up appointments. Client will maintain adequate diet. Client will sleep 6 hours per night. Client will report suicidal thoughts prior to acting on them.	Client will maintain a therapeutic relationship. Client will be able to maintain safety while in a home environment. Client will comply with taking medications as ordered by the physician. Client will keep all follow-up appointments. Client will maintain adequate diet. Client will sleep 6 hours per night. Client will report suicidal thoughts prior to acting on them. Client will verbalize three benefits of taking medications.	Client will maintain a therapeutic relationship. Client will be able to maintain safety while in a home environment. Client will comply with taking medications as ordered by the physician. Client will keep all follow-up appointments. Client will maintain adequate diet. Client will sleep 6 hours per night. Client will report suicidal thoughts prior to acting on them. Client will demonstrate one relaxation technique other than medication. Client will attend one support group during the week.
Variances			

Critical Pathway continues

	VISIT #7	VISIT #8	VISIT #9
Therapeutic Rapport	Maintain trusting relationship. Actively listen; clarify; be empathetic; allow time for client to verbalize feelings. Offer encouragement and support. Promote: positive thinking; increased self esteem; increased sociability.	Maintain trusting relationship. Actively listen; be nonjudgmental; offer hope; allow time for client to verbalize feelings. Offer encouragement and support. Promote: positive thinking; increased self esteem; increased sociability.	Maintain trusting relationship. Actively listen; clarify; be accepting; allow time for client to verbalize feelings. Offer encouragement and support. Promote: positive thinking; increased self esteem; increased sociability.
Mental Status	**Anxiety Level:** ☐ Moderate ☐ Severe ☐ Panic **Mood:** ☐ WNL ☐ Labile ☐ Angry ☐ Hopeless ☐ Depressed ☐ Euphoric ☐ Guilt ☐ Worthless ☐ Incongruent **Thought Processes:** ☐ Incoherent ☐ Preoccupied ☐ Disorganized **Insight/Judgment:** ☐ WNL ☐ Poor ☐ Dangerous/Reckless **Suicide Potential:** ☐ Yes ☐ No ☐ Plan ☐ Physician Notified **Appearance:** ☐ Clean ☐ Unkempt ☐ Dirty **Behavior:** ☐ Friendly ☐ Evasive ☐ Indifferent **Speech:** ☐ Rate ☐ Cadence ☐ Tone **Orientation:** ☐ Month ☐ Day ☐ Year ☐ Time	**Anxiety Level:** ☐ Moderate ☐ Severe ☐ Panic **Mood:** ☐ WNL ☐ Labile ☐ Angry ☐ Hopeless ☐ Depressed ☐ Euphoric ☐ Guilt ☐ Worthless ☐ Incongruent **Thought Processes:** ☐ Incoherent ☐ Preoccupied ☐ Disorganized **Insight/Judgment:** ☐ WNL ☐ Poor ☐ Dangerous/Reckless **Suicide Potential:** ☐ Yes ☐ No ☐ Plan ☐ Physician Notified **Appearance:** ☐ Clean ☐ Unkempt ☐ Dirty **Behavior:** ☐ Friendly ☐ Evasive ☐ Indifferent **Speech:** ☐ Rate ☐ Cadence ☐ Tone **Orientation:** ☐ Month ☐ Day ☐ Year ☐ Time	**Anxiety Level:** ☐ Moderate ☐ Severe ☐ Panic **Mood:** ☐ WNL ☐ Labile ☐ Angry ☐ Hopeless ☐ Depressed ☐ Euphoric ☐ Guilt ☐ Worthless ☐ Incongruent **Thought Processes:** ☐ Incoherent ☐ Preoccupied ☐ Disorganized **Insight/Judgment:** ☐ WNL ☐ Poor ☐ Dangerous/Reckless **Suicide Potential:** ☐ Yes ☐ No ☐ Plan ☐ Physician Notified **Appearance:** ☐ Clean ☐ Unkempt ☐ Dirty **Behavior:** ☐ Friendly ☐ Evasive ☐ Indifferent **Speech:** ☐ Rate ☐ Cadence ☐ Tone **Orientation:** ☐ Month ☐ Day ☐ Year ☐ Time
Physical Assessment	Dietary Needs Met? ☐ Yes ☐ No Wt ________ Fluid Intake ________ N/V________ LBM________ **Vital Signs:** BP____ R____ P____ T____ ☐ Apical Pulse ☐ Lung Sounds ☐ Skin Integrity ☐ Bowel Sounds ☐ Mobility ☐ Edema ☐ Pulses of Extremities ☐ Sleep	Dietary Needs Met? ☐ Yes ☐ No Wt ________ Fluid Intake ________ N/V________ LBM________ **Vital Signs:** BP____ R____ P____ T____ ☐ Apical Pulse ☐ Lung Sounds ☐ Skin Integrity ☐ Bowel Sounds ☐ Mobility ☐ Edema ☐ Pulses of Extremities ☐ Sleep	Dietary Needs Met? ☐ Yes ☐ No Wt ________ Fluid Intake ________ N/V________ LBM________ **Vital Signs:** BP____ R____ P____ T____ ☐ Apical Pulse ☐ Lung Sounds ☐ Skin Integrity ☐ Bowel Sounds ☐ Mobility ☐ Edema ☐ Pulses of Extremities ☐ Sleep
Self-Care	☐ WNL ☐ Needs Assist	☐ WNL ☐ Needs Assist	☐ WNL ☐ Needs Assist
Diagnostic Studies	☐ Obtain Labs PRN	☐ Obtain Labs PRN	☐ Obtain Labs PRN *Critical Pathway continues*

	VISIT #7 (continued)	VISIT #8 (continued)	VISIT #9 (continued)
Medications	☐ How are you taking your medications? ☐ Have you missed any doses? ☐ Have you had any problems with the medications? ☐ Ask client to provide information regarding adverse effects and benefits of medications. ☐ Discuss medication names as client fills medication box. ☐ Aims	☐ How are you taking your medications? ☐ Have you missed any doses? ☐ Have you had any problems with the medications? ☐ Request information regarding adverse effects and benefits of medications from client. ☐ Assist as client fills medication box. ☐ Aims	☐ How are you taking your medications? ☐ Have you missed any doses? ☐ Have you had any problems with the medications? ☐ Ask client to verbalize information regarding benefits and adverse effects of medications. ☐ Observe as client fills medication box. ☐ Aims
Discharge Planning	**Assess:** Self-management of medication regimen, caregiver's ability to manage medications; willingness of caregiver; motivation and ability to keep appointments for follow-up. **Teach:** Importance of medication compliance; relaxation techniques. **Refer:** Support groups; community resources.	**Assess:** Self-management of medication regimen; caregiver's ability to manage medications; willingness of caregiver; motivation and ability to keep appointments for follow-up. **Teach:** Importance of medication compliance; relaxation techniques. **Refer:** Support groups; community resources.	**Assess:** Self-management of medication regimen; caregiver's ability to manage medications; willingness of caregiver; motivation and ability to keep appointments for follow-up. **Teach:** Importance of medication compliance; relaxation techniques. **Refer:** Support groups; community resources.
Expected Outcomes	Client will maintain a therapeutic relationship. Client will be able to maintain safety while in a home environment. Client will comply with taking medications as ordered by the physician. Client will keep all follow-up appointments. Client will maintain adequate diet. Client will sleep 6 hours per night. Client will report suicidal thoughts prior to acting on them. Client will demonstrate medication regimen. Client will identify three ways of coping with side effects of medications.	Client will maintain a therapeutic relationship. Client will be able to maintain safety while in a home environment. Client will comply with taking medications as ordered by the physician. Client will keep all follow-up appointments. Client will maintain adequate diet. Client will sleep 6 hours per night. Client will report suicidal thoughts prior to acting on them. Client will exhibit increased energy level by cleaning house. Client will identify three ways of decreasing medication side effects.	Client will maintain a therapeutic relationship. Client will be able to maintain safety while in a home environment. Client will comply with taking medications as ordered by the physician. Client will keep all follow-up appointments. Client will maintain adequate diet. Client will sleep 6 hours per night. Client will report suicidal thoughts prior to acting on them. Client will demonstrate two relaxation techniques other than medication.
Variances			

Critical Pathway continues

	VISIT #10	VISIT #11	VISIT #12
Therapeutic Rapport	Maintain trusting relationship. Actively listen; redefine; repeat for clarification; allow time for client to verbalize feelings. Offer encouragement and support. Promote: positive thinking; increased self-esteem; increased sociability.	Maintain trusting relationship. Actively listen; offer hope; be genuine; allow time for client to verbalize feelings. Offer encouragement and support. Promote: positive thinking; increased self-esteem; increased sociability.	Maintain trusting relationship. Actively listen; be empathetic; nonjudgmental; allow time for client to verbalize feelings. Offer encouragement and support. Promote: positive thinking; increased self-esteem; increased sociability.
Mental Status	**Anxiety Level:** ☐ Moderate ☐ Severe ☐ Panic **Mood:** ☐ WNL ☐ Labile ☐ Angry ☐ Hopeless ☐ Depressed ☐ Euphoric ☐ Guilt ☐ Worthless ☐ Incongruent **Thought Processes:** ☐ Incoherent ☐ Preoccupied ☐ Disorganized **Insight/Judgment:** ☐ WNL ☐ Poor ☐ Dangerous/Reckless **Suicide Potential:** ☐ Yes ☐ No ☐ Plan ☐ Physician Notified **Appearance:** ☐ Clean ☐ Unkempt ☐ Dirty **Behavior:** ☐ Friendly ☐ Evasive ☐ Indifferent **Speech:** ☐ Rate ☐ Cadence ☐ Tone **Orientation:** ☐ Month ☐ Day ☐ Year ☐ Time	**Anxiety Level:** ☐ Moderate ☐ Severe ☐ Panic **Mood:** ☐ WNL ☐ Labile ☐ Angry ☐ Hopeless ☐ Depressed ☐ Euphoric ☐ Guilt ☐ Worthless ☐ Incongruent **Thought Processes:** ☐ Incoherent ☐ Preoccupied ☐ Disorganized **Insight/Judgment:** ☐ WNL ☐ Poor ☐ Dangerous/Reckless **Suicide Potential:** ☐ Yes ☐ No ☐ Plan ☐ Physician Notified **Appearance:** ☐ Clean ☐ Unkempt ☐ Dirty **Behavior:** ☐ Friendly ☐ Evasive ☐ Indifferent **Speech:** ☐ Rate ☐ Cadence ☐ Tone **Orientation:** ☐ Month ☐ Day ☐ Year ☐ Time	**Anxiety Level:** ☐ Moderate ☐ Severe ☐ Panic **Mood:** ☐ WNL ☐ Labile ☐ Angry ☐ Hopeless ☐ Depressed ☐ Euphoric ☐ Guilt ☐ Worthless ☐ Incongruent **Thought Processes:** ☐ Incoherent ☐ Preoccupied ☐ Disorganized **Insight/Judgment:** ☐ WNL ☐ Poor ☐ Dangerous/Reckless **Suicide Potential:** ☐ Yes ☐ No ☐ Plan ☐ Physician Notified **Appearance:** ☐ Clean ☐ Unkempt ☐ Dirty **Behavior:** ☐ Friendly ☐ Evasive ☐ Indifferent **Speech:** ☐ Rate ☐ Cadence ☐ Tone **Orientation:** ☐ Month ☐ Day ☐ Year ☐ Time
Physical Assessment	Dietary Needs Met? ☐ Yes ☐ No Wt ________ Fluid Intake ________ N/V________ LBM________ **Vital Signs:** BP____ R____ P____ T____ ☐ Apical Pulse ☐ Lung Sounds ☐ Skin Integrity ☐ Bowel Sounds ☐ Mobility ☐ Edema ☐ Pulses of Extremities ☐ Sleep	Dietary Needs Met? ☐ Yes ☐ No Wt ________ Fluid Intake ________ N/V________ LBM________ **Vital Signs:** BP____ R____ P____ T____ ☐ Apical Pulse ☐ Lung Sounds ☐ Skin Integrity ☐ Bowel Sounds ☐ Mobility ☐ Edema ☐ Pulses of Extremities ☐ Sleep	Dietary Needs Met? ☐ Yes ☐ No Wt ________ Fluid Intake ________ N/V________ LBM________ **Vital Signs:** BP____ R____ P____ T____ ☐ Apical Pulse ☐ Lung Sounds ☐ Skin Integrity ☐ Bowel Sounds ☐ Mobility ☐ Edema ☐ Pulses of Extremities ☐ Sleep
Self-Care	☐ WNL ☐ Needs Assist	☐ WNL ☐ Needs Assist	☐ WNL ☐ Needs Assist
Diagnostic Studies	☐ Obtain Labs PRN	☐ Obtain Labs PRN	☐ Obtain Labs PRN

Critical Pathway continues

	VISIT #10 (continued)	VISIT #11 (continued)	VISIT #12 (continued)
Medications	☐ How are you taking your medications? ☐ Have you missed any doses? ☐ Have you had any problems with the medications? ☐ Have client list benefits and adverse effects of medications. ☐ Observe as client fills medication box. ☐ Aims	☐ How are you taking your medications? ☐ Have you missed any doses? ☐ Have you had any problems with the medications? ☐ Ask client to name each medication. ☐ Ask client to verbalize two adverse effects of medications. ☐ Observe client as she fills medication box. ☐ Aims	☐ How are you taking your medications? ☐ Have you missed any doses? ☐ Have you had any problems with the medications? ☐ Ask client to name each medication. ☐ Ask client to list two side effects of medications. ☐ Observe client as she fills medication box. ☐ Ask client to verbalize when each medication is due.
Discharge Planning	**Assess:** Self-management of medication regimen; caregiver's ability to manage medications; willingness of caregiver; motivation and ability to keep appointments for follow-up. **Teach:** Importance of medication compliance; relaxation techniques. **Refer:** Support groups; community resources.	**Assess:** Self-management of medication regimen; caregiver's ability to manage medications; willingness of caregiver; motivation and ability to keep appointments for follow-up. **Teach:** Importance of medication compliance. **Refer:** Support groups; community resources.	**Assess:** Self-management of medication regimen; caregiver's ability to manage medications; willingness of caregiver; motivation and ability to keep appointments for follow-up. **Teach:** Importance of medication compliance. **Refer:** Support groups; community resources.
Expected Outcomes	Client will maintain a therapeutic relationship. Client will be able to maintain safety while in a home environment. Client will comply with taking medications as ordered by the physician. Client will keep all follow-up appointments. Client will maintain adequate diet. Client will sleep 6 hours per night. Client will report suicidal thoughts prior to acting on them. Client will demonstrate increased energy by attending two social activities during the week.	Client will maintain a therapeutic relationship. Client will be able to maintain safety while in a home environment. Client will agree not to discontinue or add medications without consulting the physician. Client will verbalize methods of decreasing side effects of medications such as hard candy for dry mouth, drink water, exercise to decrease constipation. Client will keep all follow-up appointments. Client will maintain adequate diet. Client will sleep 6 hours per night. Client will deny suicidal thoughts. Client will demonstrate one relaxation technique other than medication.	Client will maintain a therapeutic relationship. Client will be able to maintain safety while in a home environment. Client will be able to list medications and verbalize purpose for each. Client will keep all follow-up appointments. Client will maintain adequate diet. Client will sleep 6 hours per night. Client will report no suicidal thoughts. Client will demonstrate one relaxation technique other than medication. Client will attend at least three social functions per week. Client will verbalize community resources available for assistance.
Variances			

APPENDIX F
Psychological Tests in Common Use

Psychological tests are assessment tools that provide information to the clinician regarding either the intellectual or cognitive abilities of the client. Psychological tests can also provide an assessment of personality. Formal psychological tests are designed to be administered and scored by a professional psychologist or psychometrician. They are different from brief screening tools or questionnaires of the sort that clinicians frequently use in diagnosis or client follow-up. Examples of screening tools include the CAGE interview, the Michigan Alcohol Screening Test, the Beck Depression Inventory, and the Mini Mental Status Test. These screening tools have been validated in multiple study populations, but they are typically used to suggest diagnoses or to monitor the severity of conditions on repeat visits. In contrast, formal psychological testing is generally used for diagnostic purposes, often in conjunction with psychiatric interview data and direct observations of client behaviors. Because DSM-IV criteria form the basis for most current psychiatric diagnoses, formal testing may be less frequently used than in the past. The following should prove useful when an unfamiliar test is encountered in clinical practice. Formal psychological tests may be of three types: projective tests, objective tests, and intelligence tests (the latter is a variety of objective test designed to assess specific cognitive abilities).

PROJECTIVE TESTS

A projective test uses unstructured stimuli to measure relevant psychological attributes.

Draw-a-Person Test

The client is given a blank piece of paper and asked to first draw any person, then specifically a person of the opposite sex.

Interpretation: There are standardized norms for interpreting the results. This test assesses factors related to self-esteem, body image, and interpersonal relationships. In children, the draw-a-person test can provide important clues to level of psychomotor development.

Rorschach Test

The Rorschach test presents a client with 10 standardized "ink-blot" images. The client is asked to describe what she sees in these black and white forms.

Interpretation: Each image has a set of potential responses, and the test is scored in accord with whatthe client describes seeing. The results are closely tied to psychoanalytic theories of personality development.

Thematic Apperception Test (TAT)

The client is presented with a standardized series of 30 ambiguous pictures and asked to make up a story about each picture.

Interpretation: Scoring is standardized. The person's responses reveal personality dynamics and issues of importance to the client.

Sentence Completion Test (SCT)

The client is presented with 75 to 100 incomplete sentences and asked to complete these sentences with the first idea that comes into his mind, no matter how odd or inappropriate it may seem. An incomplete sentence might be "The nursing student is. . . ." (This sentence is not part of the SCT, but you might want to imagine how you would complete it.)

Interpretation: The test is standardized and can help identify the client's preoccupations, fears, or goals.

OBJECTIVE TESTS

Objective tests present the client with a series of multiple-choice questions regarding values, attitudes, or descriptions of situations for which responses have been normed, so that the individual's responses can be compared to those of others.

Minnesota Multiphasic Personality Inventory (MMPI)

This lengthy test has 567 items designed to measure aspects of personality such as hypomania, paranoia, hypochondriasis, depression, schizophrenia, psychopathic deviation, and degree of masculinity/femininity. The test questions were empirically constructed based on clinical observations. This is one of the most common psychological tests given to adults.

Interpretation: Scores for each scale are compared with norms. Client tendencies for specific behaviors and psychiatric conditions/diagnoses are reported.

California Personality Inventory

This test has 17 separate scales and focuses on factors that seem to reflect personality.

Interpretation: Standardized norms provide indications of personality characteristics and traits, such as responsibility or socialization.

INTELLIGENCE TESTS

Intelligence tests are a type of objective test that provides information about intelligence, normed against a subset of the population. The Wechsler Adult Intelligence Scale (WAIS) and Wechsler Intelligence Scale for Children (WISC) are divided into verbal and nonverbal scales. Although all intelligence tests are culturally biased toward the group from which the norms were calculated, intelligence tests may provide information about a client's strengths or weaknesses. The WAIS has an important role in assessing persons with mental retardation and other developmental disorders presenting in adulthood. It has less value in the assessment of dementia, in which clinical screening (including the Mini Mental Status Examination) is used more often. The WISC is exceedingly important in evaluating developmental problems in children and adolescents.

Wechsler Adult Intelligence Scale (WAIS)

This is a test with subscales covering vocabulary, comprehension, information, similarities, digit span, arithmetic, picture arrangement, picture completion, object assembly, block design, and digit symbol.

Interpretation: Scores yield a measure of intelligence expressed as IQ (intelligence quotient).

Wechsler Intelligence Scale for Children (WISC)

A version of the WAIS that is appropriate for children ages 5 to 15 years.

Interpretation: Scores yield a measure of intelligence expressed as IQ, normed for children.

GLOSSARY

A

Abandonment Negligence in which a client is left in need without alternatives for treatment.

Acquaintance (or Date) Rape Forcible rape or sexual battery that occurs by the victim's acquaintances or dates.

Adaptive Energy Individual's ability to respond to a stressor.

Adaptive Potential Capacity of the person to respond to stressors—to utilize resources to cope.

Adaptive Potential Assessment Model Erickson and colleagues' model describing three states of coping potential: arousal, equilibrium, and impoverishment.

Addiction Inability to abstain from drug use, accompanied by drug tolerance and withdrawal.

Adversity Measure of the strength of a given stimulus for anxiety.

Aggravated Criminal Sexual Assault Criminal sexual assault in which a weapon is used or displayed; the victim's life or someone else's is endangered or threatened; the perpetrator causes bodily harm to the victim; the assault occurs during the commission of another felony; or force is used to threaten or cause physical harm to the victim.

Aggregate Population or defined group.

Agnosia Loss of ability to recognize objects.

Agoraphobia Fear of going out in public places.

Akathisia Subjective sense of restlessness with a perceived need to pace or otherwise move continuously.

Akinesia Reaction involving loss of movement.

Alcoholism Compulsion to drink alcohol.

Alogia Tendency to speak very little and use brief and seemingly empty phrases.

Amnesia Loss of memory.

Anger Control Assistance Nursing intervention aimed at facilitation of the expression of anger in an adaptive and nonviolent manner.

Anhedonia Inability to find enjoyment in daily activities.

Animal-Assisted Therapy Use of animals to provide attention, affection, diversion, and/or relaxation.

Anorexia Nervosa Psychological eating disorder characterized by profound disturbance in body image, failure to maintain minimum weight, and obsession with weight, despite underweight status.

Antipsychotic Drugs Major tranquilizers administered to control symptoms of psychosis.

Antisocial Personality Disorder Behavior pattern characterized by violence, impulsiveness, dishonesty, carelessness, and irresponsibility.

Anxiety State where a person has strong feelings of worry or dread, where the source is nonspecific or unknown.

Aphasia Difficulty or inability to recall words.

Apraxia Loss of motor function.

Arousal Stress state in which an individual possesses coping resources.

Asperger's Syndrome Condition characterized by combination of severe impairments in social interaction and highly repetitive patterns of interests and behaviors.

Asylum Large public hospital of the eighteenth century that provided for treatment of the insane.

Autism Developmental disorder in which children remain emotionally detached, engage in ritualistic behavior, and exhibit delay in acquiring language skills.

Autonomy Individual's right to self-determination and independence.

Avoidant Personality Disorder Behavior pattern characterized by social inhibition, feelings of inadequacy, and shyness.

Avolition Lack of motivation for work or other goal-oriented activities.

B

Battery Any un-consented touching of another person.

Behaviorally Oriented Therapy Process focused on helping an individual gain the tools needed to change behavior and feelings.

Beneficence Belief that all treatments must be for the client's good.

Bipolar Depression Mood disorder characterized by up-and-down swings.

Bipolar Disorder (BPD) Mood disorder characterized by cyclic experiences with both mania and depression.

Blinded Clinical Trial Study in which subjects do not know whether they are receiving an active treatment or a placebo.

Blood-Brain Barrier Capillary barrier between blood and brain.

Borderline Personality Disorder Disorder characterized by unstable interpersonal relationships and self-image, efforts to avoid being abandoned, and impulsive actions.

Breathing-Related Sleep Disorders A group of disorders in which breathing during sleep stops for less than 10 seconds, occurring 20 or more times per hour and causing measurable blood deoxygenation.

Brief Dynamic Therapy Short-term psychotherapy that focuses on resolving core conflicts that derive from personality and living situations.

Brown Report A 1948 report authored by Esther Lucille Brown on the future of nursing. This report advised that psychiatric hospitals be used as agencies for affiliation in teaching of nurses.

Bulimia Nervosa Psychological eating disorder characterized by fasting, binging, purging (by either self-induced vomiting or misuse of laxatives, diuretics, or enemas), and lack of extreme weight loss.

Bullying Hurting or intimidating someone who is smaller or weaker.

Burnout Description for caregivers who find themselves unable to provide the quality of care that is desirable; characterized by depletion of energy, decreased ability to concentrate, and a sense of hopelessness.

C

Capitation Funding mechanism in which all defined services for a specified period of time are provided for an agreed-on single payment.

Case-Control Study Study comparing two groups: the cases (all members have the given disease or condition) and the controls (all members are free of the disease or condition).

Case Group *See* Experimental Group.

Case Management Constellation of services that includes screening, assessment, care planning, arranging for service delivery, monitoring, reassessment, evaluation, and discharge, for the purpose of ensuring continuity of care.

Cataplexy Sudden loss of muscle power at times of sudden emotion.

Catastrophic Reaction Severe overreaction out of proportion to the stimulus.

Catatonia Behavior disorder marked by a decrease in reactivity to the environment, sometimes reaching an extreme degree of complete unawareness.

Catharsis Experience of release that occurs when unconscious thoughts are brought into consciousness.

Child Abuse Any physical or mental injury, sexual abuse, exploitation, negligent treatment, or maltreatment of a child by a parent or caregiver.

Child Molestation Sexual involvement with a child, such as oral-genital contact, genital fondling and viewing, or masturbation in front of a child.

Child Neglect Failing to provide care needed by a child for normal growth and/or development. The definition of neglect is generally established by local laws, but may be based on nationally-focused "model statutes."

Child Soldiers Typically refers to very young children forced or otherwise induced to fight in military conflicts.

Child Pornography Sexually explicit reproduction of a child's image.

Choice Point Time in a person's life when previously successful activities are no longer solving disruptions in one's life patterns.

Chronic Grief Unresolved bereavement.

CINAHL The Cumulative Index of Nursing and Allied Health Literature; a nursing-specific search tool for published literature.

Circadian Rhythm Biorhythm that determines human responses to the environment; refers to attention span in relation to the presence or absence of daylight.

Circular Communication Predictable pattern of communication and response between two people.

Civil Commitment Period of hospitalization requested by a mental health provider following an emergency hospitalization.

Clarification Technique in which an analyst points out a behavior pattern that is not recognized by the client.

Classification System of categorization that allows useful distinctions to be established.

Client-Centered Therapy Process focused on bringing out individual internal resources and understanding.

Closed Group Meeting with a defined number of participants that is not open to new members.
Code of Ethics Positive statements and guidelines of what persons should do.
Codependence Behaviors exhibited by significant others of a substance-abusing individual that serve to enable and protect the abuse at the exclusion of personal fulfillment and self-development.
Cognator Subsystem Higher brain functions that deal with information processing, judgment, emotion, and perception.
Cognition Process by which a person "knows the world" and interacts with it.
Cognitive-Behavior(al) Therapy Treatment approach aimed at helping a client identify stimuli that cause the client's anxiety, develop plans to respond to those stimuli in a nonanxious manner, and problem-solve when unanticipated anxiety-provoking situations arise.
Cognitive Therapy Short-term psychotherapy that focuses on removing symptoms by identifying and correcting perceptual biases in client's thinking and correcting unrecognized assumptions.
Cohort Study *See* Longitudinal Study.
Community Crisis Threat of proportion to affect an entire group of people.
Community Health Nursing Synthesis of nursing and public health practice to promote, maintain, and conserve the health of population aggregates in the community.
Community Mental Health Synthesis of community nursing and public health practice to promote, maintain, and conserve the health of population aggregates in the community, with particular emphasis on mental health.
Community Support System (CSS) Organized network of people committed to helping persons with severe mental illness meet their needs and move toward independence.
Competency to Stand Trial Judgment that an individual is able to understand the nature of legal proceedings and is able to tell his or her own story to an attorney and the court.
Complementary Modalities Those modalities being used as an adjunct to medical care and psychiatric treatment that are thought to have effects on stress, sleep disturbance, anxiety, and/or other emotions.
Compulsion Repetitive behavior or act, the goal of which is to prevent or reduce anxiety or distress.
Computerized Tomography A scan that uses conventional X-rays to form an image that is an actual reconstruction from hundreds of X-rays taken from various angles.
Concept Basic building block of theory; abstraction of reality.
Concept Map A diagrammatic representation of organized knowledge. In nursing care, a diagrammatic representation of the nursing process, illustrating the relationships between and among issues and characteristics that emerge from assessment data.
Conceptual Framework Group of concepts that are linked together to provide a way of organizing or viewing something.
Conduct Disorder Disorder in which children show a pattern of cruelty and disrespect for the rights of others.
Confabulation Intentional efforts to cover up memory losses or gaps.
Confrontation Technique in which an analyst challenges a client's behavior or thought, with the goal of provoking a reaction and overcoming an emotional barrier to change.
Confusion Multidimensional phenomenon incorporating changes in both cognition and behavior.
Conservative-Withdrawal State Psychological response to stress; stage of exhaustion.
Conservator Person appointed to handle the estate of another person who is judged incompetent.
Continuous Cycling Recurrent movement from mania to depression without an intervening normal period.
Control Group Persons receiving no treatment or being free of a given condition or disease under study.
Controlled Clinical Trial Evaluation in which neither the clients nor their caregivers are allowed to know exactly what treatment is being given.
Conversion Disorder Condition in which an individual exhibits physical symptoms that cannot be explained by any medical or neurological conditions.
Cortex The part of the brain consisting of the four lobes: frontal, temporal, parietal, and occipital.
Craving Strong, overpowering urge for drugs felt by an individual who abuses or is dependent on drugs.
Created Environment Mobilization of all system variables.
Criminal Sexual Assault Genital, anal, or oral penetration by a part of the perpetrator's body or by an object using force or without the victim's consent.
Crisis Stressor or life challenge that requires an individual to adjust to the unexpected and to adapt to an unpredicted situation or event.
Cultural Blindness Attempt to treat all persons fairly by ignoring differences and acting as though differences do not exist; misguided attempt to achieve "fairness" by ignoring real cultural differences.
Cultural Crisis Situation of shock resulting from an individual's adaptation to a new culture or return to a previously experienced culture; also known as culture shock.
Cultural Facilitator/Broker Person who can interpret the language, culture, and health care culture of another as a means to bridging the communication barriers between people from different cultures.

Culture Values, beliefs, norms, and lifeways that are learned and shared within a particular group.
Culture Care Facets of culture that deal with individual and group health and well-being, including efforts to improve on the human condition or to deal with illness, handicaps, or death.
Culture Care Accommodation/Negotiation Nursing actions and decisions that involve reshaping the way in which care values are enacted so the actions will better support well-being, dealing with handicaps, recovering from illness, or facing death.
Culture Care Preservation/Maintenance Nursing actions and decisions that help people of a cultural group keep or preserve those care values that are applicable to the current situation to maintain well-being, deal with handicaps, recover from illness, or face death.
Culture Care Repatterning/Restructuring Nursing actions and decisions that involve change in culturally based care practices.
Culture Shock State in which a person is overwhelmed or even immobilized by cultural differences in expectations, communication, and general habits between an individual's culture of origin and a new culture to which the individual is trying to assimilate. (*See* also Cultural Crisis)
Cyclothymic Pattern Cycle of an individual's mood changing back and forth between hypomanic and melancholic states.

D

Defense Mechanisms Unconscious responses used by individuals to protect themselves from internal conflict and external stress.
Deinstitutionalization Movement of clients and mental health services from state mental hospitals into community settings.
Delayed Grief Bereavement that is not accomplished at the time of the loss and remains with the individual.
Delirium Acute change in a person's level of consciousness and cognition that develops during a short period.
Delusion False belief that misrepresents either perceptions or experiences.
Dementia Gradual onset of multiple cognitive changes in memory, abstract thinking, judgment, and perception that often results in a progressive decline in intellectual functioning and decreased capacity to perform daily activities.
Deontology Theory founded on human duties to others and the principles on which these duties are based.
Deoxyribonucleic Acid (DNA) A molecule that carries a genetic code in its sequence of bases.
Dependent Personality Disorder Behavior pattern characterized by clinging and submissiveness.
Depersonalization Persistent or recurrent feelings of being separated from one's normal mental fuctions or feeling as if one is outside one's body.
Depression State wherein an individual experiences a profound sadness.
Derailment Speech that gets off the point or subject.
Descriptive Study Survey to determine the incidence and prevalence of a disease or condition.
Diencephalon The part of the brain consisting of two major structures: the thalamus and the hypothalamus.
Differentiation Process of unfolding, growth, and maturation, leading to a balance between emotional and intellectual components.
Disability Impairment in one or more important areas of functioning.
Dissociative Disorders Disorders characterized by a disruption in the usually integrated functions of consciousness, memory, identity, or perception.
Dissociative Identity Disorder The condition of possessing two or more distinct identities, at least two of which periodically take control of the individual's behavior.
Distress Negative response to stimuli that are perceived as threatening.
Domestic Violence Violence that occurs between intimate partners or parents/caretakers and children or elders.
Double-Blinded Trial Study in which neither subjects nor persons evaluating the outcome know whether subjects are receiving treatment or a placebo.
Drug Dependence Condition occurring when individuals exhibit a set of behaviors associated with inability to control use of a drug.
Drug Use Any taking of a drug.
DSM-IV-TR *Diagnostic and Statistical Manual, Fourth edition-Text Revision;* classification system for mental disorders.
Dyssomnia Condition where there is an abnormality in the amount, quality, or timing of sleep.
Dysthymia Condition of feeling sad or depressed. Persistent state of sadness.
Dystonia Sustained, involuntary muscle spasms.

E

Echolalia An involuntary, parrotlike repetition of words spoken by others.
Ecomap Graphic depiction of family members' interactions with systems outside the family.
Ego Conscious mind governed by the reality principle; controls the impulses of the id.
Elder Abuse Domestic violence involving dependent elderly persons. May include non-physical acts such as financial abuse.

Elder Neglect Failing to provide needed care for a dependent elderly person; typically refers to care provided by responsible family members, though neglect can occur in institutional settings as well.
Electroconvulsive Therapy (ECT) Passage of an electrical stimulus to the brain to produce a seizure.
Emergency Hospitalization Power of states to detain a person in an emergency situation for a limited time until further evaluation and court proceedings can occur.
Emotional Cutoff Children's efforts to distance themselves from their families in order to achieve independence; any family member's efforts to distance self from family and others to reduce anxiety.
Endemic Descriptor for a disease or condition that is constantly or regularly found in the population.
Energy-Based Modalities Techniques for healing grounded in the notion of the human energy field.
Epidemic Descriptor for a disease or condition that spreads or circulates within a population.
Epidemiology Study of the causes and distribution of injuries and diseases in a population.
Equilibrium State of balance following a stress state.
Ethics Branch of philosophy that considers how behavioral principles guiding human interactions can be analyzed and set.
Ethnicity Identification with a socially, culturally, and politically constructed group that holds a common set of characteristics not shared by others with whom its members come in contact.
Ethnocentrism Perception that one's worldview is the only acceptable truth and that the beliefs, values, and behaviors sanctioned by one's culture are superior to all others.
Euthanasia Act of killing or permitting a death for reasons of mercy.
Exaggerated Grief Bereavement that is overwhelming.
Exhibitionism Exposing one's genitals to a stranger.
Experience-Oriented Therapy Process focusing on the client's experiences as an agent for producing change.
Experimental Group Persons receiving treatment or having a given condition or disease under study; also known as Case Group.
External Environment Forces, factors, and influences that occur outside the boundaries of a system.
Extrapersonal Stressor Stimuli from a great distance outside the system boundary.

F

Factitious Disorder Condition marked by physical or psychological symptoms that are intentionally and knowingly produced by an individual in order to gain attention; also known as Munchausen's Syndrome.
Family Social system composed of two or more persons who coexist within the context of some expectations of reciprocal affection, mutual responsibility, and temporal duration.
Family Attachment Diagram Representation of the reciprocal nature and quality of the affectional ties between family members.
Family Projection Process Situation in which adult family members deal with their own anxiety by projecting the anxiety onto a child.
Fear State wherein a person feels a strong sense of dread focused on a specific object or event.
Feedback Response of a receiver of a message to the communicator.
Fetishism Sexual arousal occurring from contact with a nonliving object, often an article of clothing.
Fidelity Individual's obligation to honor commitments and contracts.
Fight-Flight Response Psychological response to stress; state of high anxiety and energy.
Financial Abuse Theft or conversion of money or anything of value belonging to the elderly by their relatives or caregivers.
Fixation Preoccupation with pleasures associated with a previous developmental stage.
Flattened Affect Loss of expressiveness.
Folk System Culturally based acts that respond to apparent or anticipated needs related to living, health, well-being, handicaps, or death.
Forcible Rape Forced intercourse or penetration of a body orifice by a penis or other object by a perpetrator.
Foreclosure One of four identity statuses; refers to the adolescent's lack of thoroughly exploring alternatives before making a commitment to an adult identity.
Frotteurism Recurrent sexual touching of a nonconsenting individual, usually a stranger and usually in a crowded public place.
Fugue Sudden unexpected travel away from home or normal environment, usually associated with confusion about past identity.

G

Gang Rape Sexual acts that proximate in time by multiple perpetrators who are either acquaintances of or strangers to the victim.
Gender Dysphoria Condition existing when an individual has a strong desire to live as the opposite sex.
Gender Identity An individual's subjective feeling associated with being male or female.
Gender Identity Disorder Condition in which an individual feels him- or herself to be a member of the opposite sex and desires gender change.

Gender Role Learned expressions of femaleness and maleness; public recognition of one's gender assignment as male or female and the individual's expression of appropriate social behaviors related to that assignment.
General Adaptation Syndrome Specific, predictable, physiological response to stress involving an alarm reaction, a resistance stage, and an exhaustion stage.
Generalized Anxiety Disorder Psychiatric illness characterized by excessive anxiety or dread.
Genetic Marker Identifiable patterns of DNA structure that can be readily confirmed by laboratory analysis.
Genogram Graphic depiction of a family tree that records information over at least three generations.
Genome Entire complement of heritable information.
Grandiose Delusion Perception of importance, special powers, or religious significance that is not in line with reality.
Gradiosity An inflated appraisal of one's worth, knowledge, power, or importance, often including delusional thinking.
Grief Healthy expression of bereavement.
Group Collection of persons who come together in some way that makes them interdependent.
Group Content Specific problems, topics, or conditions addressed by a group.
Group Dynamics Underlying forces working to produce behavior patterns in groups.
Group Leader/Facilitator Person who invites or selects group members and identifies the purpose and goals of the group.
Group Process Interaction (verbal and nonverbal) between and among group members.
Guided Imagery An unconditional process in which the practitioner leads the subject with specific words, suggestions, symbols, or images to elicit a positive response.

H

Half-Life Time for plasma concentrations of a drug to decrease to half of an initial value.
Hallucination Sensory experiences not perceptible to other nonpsychotic individuals.
Healing Touch Systematic approach to healing using several energy interventions that incorporate a variety of therapeutic maneuvers.
Helicy The movement of human development toward increasing diversity and complexity.
HIPAA The Health Insurance Portability and Accountability Act; federal legislation protecting the privacy of medical records.
Histrionic Personality Disorder Behavior pattern characterized by excesses of emotional expression and a desire to be the center of attention.
Home Health Nursing Delivery of health services in the home under the direction of a health care agency.
Homelessness Condition of being without shelter or a permanent place to live.
Hypnosis Assisting the client to an altered state of consciousness to create an awareness and a directed-focus experience.
Hypoactive Sexual Desire Disorder Significant distress or disturbance in interpersonal relationships when the sexual desire is truly less than would be normal for an individual.
Hypochondriasis Condition marked by preoccupation with fear of having a serious disease, based on misinterpretation of bodily symptoms or functions.
Hypomania Mild form of mania (elevated mood) that lasts for at least 4 days.
Hypothalamus A central brain structure that is primarily involved with the autonomic nervous system and the endocrine system and that plays a role in the nervous mechanisms underlying moods and motivational states.

I

ICD *International Classification of Diseases;* a comprehensive listing of clinical diagnoses, each associated with a unique numerical code.
ICNP The International Classification of Nursing Practice.
Id Unconscious mind; the reservoir of psychic energy or libido.
Identity Achievement One of the four identity statuses in which an adolescent makes a commitment to an adult identity after a period of exploring alternatives.
Identity Diffusion One of the four identity statuses in which an adolescent avoids making a full commitment to an adult identity and does not reach his or her potential; often associated with restricted emotional expression or detachment from others.
Identity Formation An adolescent's process of finding a unique place within the larger society, beyond the boundaries of the family.
Identity Status Style used by an adolescent in resolving issues of adult identity.
Impoverishment Stress state in which an individual's coping resources are depleted.
Incarcerated Condition of being in jail or other correctional institution.
Incest Sexual relations between children and blood relatives or surrogate family members.
Incidence Number of new cases of an illness, condition, or injury that begin within a certain time period.
Incoherence Speech that is not logically connected.
Incompetence State of an individual with a mental disorder that causes inability to make judgments and renders the person unable to handle his or her own affairs.

Insight-Oriented Therapy Process focusing on helping an individual gain understanding of feelings and behaviors.
Insomnia Sleep disorder characterized by difficulty in initiating or maintaining sleep.
Integrality The energy fields of the human being and of the environment are each part of the other's.
Intentionality Consciousness and awareness directed mentally toward an object and involving expectation, belief, action, desire, and the unconscious.
Internal Environment Forces, factors, and influences that occur completely within the boundaries of a system.
Interpersonal Stressor Stimuli from outside the system boundary but proximal to the system.
Interpersonal Therapy Process of gaining insight based on the recognition that psychological distress may occur in conjunction with disturbed human relationships.
Interpretation Technique in which an analyst offers an explanation of a client's unconscious behavior processes.
Interrater Agreement Accord on diagnosis between individuals evaluating the same condition.
Interrater Reliability Accord on diagnosis between different evaluators on the same examination.
Interventive Questions Circular questions used to uncover relationships and connections between individuals, events, ideas, and beliefs.
Intimate Partner Violence (Often referred to as spousal/partner abuse or battering syndrome.) Intentional violent or controlling behavior by a person who is or has been intimate with the victim(s) and may or may not reside in the same household.
Intrapersonal Stressor Stimuli from within the system boundary.
Intrarater Reliability Accord on diagnosis on different examinations by the same evaluator.

J

Justice Principle ensuring fairness, equity, and honesty in decisions.

L

Least Restrictive Alternative Legal principle requiring that clients be treated with the least amount of constraint of liberty consistent with their safety.
Light Therapy (Phototherapy) Provision of artificial indoor lighting, 5 to 10 times brighter than ordinary lighting, to the environment of a person with Seasonal Affective Disorder (SAD).
Longitudinal Study Population-based study conducted over a period of time, typically years; also known as Cohort Study.

M

Magnetic Resonance Imaging An imaging technique that uses no X-rays. The image is produced through use of a magnetic field, radio frequencies, and computerized reconstructions.
Malingering Fabrication of symptoms with the intent of achieving some objective goal.
Malpractice Negligence in the medical field that results in harm.
Managed Care Prepaid health plan in which an identified intermediary is given authority to manage the means and the source from which the client may obtain services.
Mania Mood disorder characterized by an elevated, expansive, or irritable mood.
Manic Episode Distinct period of abnormally and persistently elevated, expansive, or irritable mood, lasting at least 1 week.
Marital Therapy Short-term psychotherapy that attempts to resolve problems that occur within a marriage.
Masked Grief Bereavement that is hidden by either a physical symptom or a maladaptive behavior; the individual is unaware of the connection to the grief or loss.
Massage Stimulation of the skin and underlying tissues for the purposes of increasing circulation and inducing a relaxation response.
Maturational Crisis Stage in an individual's life requiring adjustment or adaptation to new responsibilities or life patterns.
Mental Disorder Behavior or psychological syndrome or pattern associated with distress or disability or increased risk of suffering, death, pain, or loss of freedom.
Mental Health State in which a person has knowledge of self, meets basic needs, assumes responsibility for behavior and self-growth, integrates thoughts and feelings with actions, resolves conflicts, maintains relationships, respects others, communicates directly, and adapts to change in the environment.
Mental Illness State in which an individual shows deficits in functioning, cannot view self clearly or has a distorted image of self, is unable to maintain personal relationships, and cannot adapt to the environment.
Mental Injury Harm to a child's psychological or intellectual functioning; manifested as severe anxiety, depression, withdrawal or outward aggressive behavior, or a combination of these behaviors.
Meta-Analysis Statistical analysis that combines the results of several separate clinical studies.
Mind Modulation Processes by which thoughts, feelings, attitudes, and emotions are converted by the brain into neurohormonal messenger molecules.

M'Naghten Test Legal definition of lack of guilt of a crime by virtue of insanity.
Modeling Assessment with the goal of understanding the client's world from the client's perspective.
Mood Disorder Pattern of mood episodes that results in difficulty functioning in family, work, and social affairs.
Mood Episode Experience of a strong emotion of depression, mania, or a mixture of both for a period of at least 2 weeks.
Moratorium One of the four identity statuses in which an individual delays making a decision about adult identity while exploring various alternatives during adolescence.
Multigenerational Transmission Process Situation in which patterns of dealing with anxiety are passed from one generation to the next.
Munchausen's Syndrome Another term for Factitious Disorder.
Munchausen's Syndrome by Proxy Form of child abuse marked by a caregiver falsely giving reports of a child's illness that result in unnecessary medical investigations or treatments.
Music Therapy Use of specific kinds of music and its ability to affect changes in behavior, emotions, and physiology.
Mutuality Client involvement in the therapeutic relationship.

N

NANDA NANDA International prepared a taxonomy of nursing diagnoses, which are statements of the phenomena of concern to nurses.
Narcissistic Personality Disorder Behavior pattern characterized in part by lack of empathy for others and a grandiose sense of self-importance.
Narcolepsy Sleep disorder characterized by frequent irresistible urges for sleep, hallucinatory dreamlike states, and episodes of cataplexy.
National Mental Health Act Provided federal funds for research and education in all areas of psychiatric care. Act was passed in 1946. Established NIMH.
Negligence Behaving in a way in which a prudent individual would not have behaved or failing to use the diligence and care expected of a reasonable individual in similar circumstances.
Negligent Treatment Failure of a parent or caregiver to provide, for reasons other than poverty, adequate food, clothing, shelter, or medical care, which may lead to serious endangerment of the physical health of the child.
Neologistic Word Invented word, often used by persons suffering from schizophrenia.
Neuroleptic Malignant Syndrome Disorder associated with sudden fever, rigidity, tachycardia, hypertension, and decreased levels of consciousness.
Neurotransmitter A chemical messenger that permits the movement of ions and chemicals across synapses.
NIC *Nursing Interventions Classification;* outlines list of nursing interventions designed to identify activities that nurses perform to assist client status or behavior.
Nightmare Exceedingly vivid dream from which the sleeper wakens in fear, often sweating and with heart racing, and is able to recall the dream.
NIMBY Syndrome Literally, "not in my backyard." Condition of persons or groups who state support for services for the homeless or underprivileged groups but who refuse to allow such services in their own neighborhoods.
NMDS Nursing Minimum Data Set; grouping that identifies the minimum information necessary to meet information demands of nursing practice.
Nonmaleficence Belief that care providers must do no harm.
Nonverbal Communication Messages sent by means other than oral or written.
Normal Sexual Behavior Any sexual act that is consensual, lacks force, is mutually satisfying to both partners, and is conducted in private. [For adults]
Normative Ethics Guidelines and procedures useful in establishing moral decisions and actions.
Norms Learned behaviors that are perceived to be appropriate or inappropriate in a culture.
Nuclear Family Emotional System Process by which a family manages anxiety.
Nurse Agency Nursing activities required to compensate for the client's inability to meet his own self-care needs (Orem's theory).
Nursing Agency Characteristic that allows nurses to act for others in meeting therapeutic self-care demands.
Nursing Care Plan A method of documenting the steps of the nursing process that includes a statement related to each step of the process: assessment, diagnosis, outcomes identification, planning/interventions, and evaluation.
Nursing System The design of care based on the type of self-care deficit.

O

Obsession Recurrent thought, image, or impulse that is experienced as intrusive and inappropriate and that causes marked anxiety or distress.
Obsessive-Compulsive Personality Disorder Behavior pattern characterized by preoccupation with order, cleanliness, control, and perfectionism.
Oculogyric Crisis Reaction in which extraocular muscle spasm forces the eyes into a fixed, usually upward gaze.
Open Group Meeting in which participants are free to come and go, depending on their individual needs.

Oppositional Defiant Disorder Condition characterized by a consistent pattern of rejecting authority.
Orientation The phase of the nurse-patient relationship in which they come to know each other and begin to identify the patient's needs.
Orientation Phase First stage of a relationship, during which the nurse and client get to know one another, establish trust, and outline goals and boundaries.

P

Panic Disorder Psychiatric illness characterized by discrete episodes of intense anxiety (panic attacks) that begin abruptly and peak within 10 minutes.
Paranoid Personality Disorder Behavior pattern characterized by persistent yet unfounded fear of exploitation or harm by others.
Paraphilia Disorder of sexual interest, arousal, and orgasm.
Parasomnia Condition in which the person suffers from profoundly disturbed sleep, most commonly nightmares, sleep terrors, or sleepwalking.
Parasympathetic System Response Nervous system response that works in opposition to the sympathetic nervous system, bringing about a decrease in heart and respiratory rates, dilation of peripheral blood vessels, muscle relaxation, lowered blood pressure, and increased flow of endorphins.
Passive-Aggressive Personality Disorder Behavior pattern characterized by pervasive negativity with passive resistance to social/occupational demands, procrastination, and stubbornness.
Passive Physical Abuse (or Negligence) Conduct that is careless and a breach of duty that results in injury to the person or is a violation of rights; includes the withholding of medication, medical treatment, food, and personal care necessary for the well-being of the elderly person.
Pedophilia Sexual interests directed primarily or exclusively toward children.
Persecutory Delusion Paranoid perception that others are "out to get me."
Personality Habitual patterns and qualities of behavior expressed by physical and mental activities and attitudes; the distinctive individual qualities of a person.
Personality Disorder Pervasive and inflexible pattern of behavior demonstrating unhealthy characteristics that limit the individual's ability to function in society.
Personality Traits Qualities of behavior that make a person unique.
Phobia Persistent fear of a specific object or situation.
Physical Abuse Conduct of violence that results in bodily harm or mental stress; includes a spectrum of violence ranging from assault to murder.
Physical Injury Lacerations, fractured bones, burns, internal injuries, severe bruising, or serious bodily harm.
Physical Restraint Use of an apparatus that significantly inhibits mobility.
Placebo Treatment that has no intended effect on the expected outcome of a trial.
Population Aggregate of persons in the community who share a common characteristic, such as age or diagnosis.
Positron Emission Tomography (PET) A scan that requires the injection of a radioactive contrast that permits visualization of precise areas of the brain where functions like blood flow can be observed.
Post-Traumatic Stress Disorder Anxiety disorder resulting from a frightening event such as a crime, accident, or battle.
Power Influences each family member has on the family processes and functioning.
Presence Activity of being physically present with another person that begins with the nurse's genuine commitment to caring and nurturing the potential of the client.
Prevalence Number of persons in a population who are living with a disease or disorder at any time; includes both new and old cases.
Primary Hypersomnia Severe daytime sleepiness despite normal nighttime sleep patterns that interferes with daily activities; a condition that cannot be explained by any other sleep, medical, or pharmacological cause.
Primary Insomnia Condition in which an individual can fall asleep easily and remain asleep for several hours but does not feel rested on waking.
Primary Prevention Activities directed at reducing the incidence of mental disorder within a population.
Probate Proceedings Judicial hearing to determine the competence of an individual to manage personal affairs.
Process Recording Verbatim account of a communication, with interpretation of techniques used and their effectiveness.
Professional System Acts based on formal preparation for dealing with health, illness, and wellness.
Program for Assertive Community Treatment (PACT) Model providing a full range of medical, psychosocial, and rehabilitation services by a community-based, multidisciplinary team.
Prospective Payment System Reimbursement mechanism based on predetermined payment for a specific period or diagnosis.
Psychiatric Consultation-Liaison Nursing Practice concerned with the study, diagnosis, treatment, and prevention of psychiatric illness in the physically ill and of psychological factors affecting physical conditions.
Psychiatric Mental Health Advanced Practice Registered Nurse A licensed nurse educationally certified at

the masters or doctoral level and nationally certified as a clinical specialist in psychiatric and mental health nursing.
Psychiatric Mental Health Nurse A licensed nurse who has passed a certification exam and is thereby certified within a specialty.
Psychoanalysis Treatment focused on uncovering unconscious memories and processes.
Psychodynamic Therapy Brief process based on psychoanalytic principles, with the goal of improved functioning rather than personality reconstruction.
Psychological Abuse Simple name calling and verbal assaults in a protracted and systematic effort to dehumanize the victim, sometimes with the goal of driving the victim to insanity or suicide; usually exists in combination with one or more other abuses.
Psychological Development Continuum of milestones from infancy through adulthood showing evolution of personal history.
Psychosis State in which an individual has lost the ability to recognize reality.
Psychotherapy Treatment of mental or emotional disorders through psychological rather than physical methods.
Psychotic Mental state involving the loss of rational thought and/or loss of ability to accurately interpret the environment.
Public Health Nursing Field of nursing that addresses the social, economic, and environmental conditions that influence health.
PubMed A public-domain search tool of published medical literature sponsored by the National Library of Medicine (NLM).

Q

Quasi-Experimental Study Analytical study in which a population is studied before and after a given event; usually includes both a case and a control set.

R

Rape Act of sexual intercourse in which the person does not give consent; accomplished against a person's will by means of force or fear of immediate and unlawful bodily injury or threatening to retaliate in the future against the victim or other person.
Rapid Cycling Four or more episodes of mania in a year.
Reactive Depression Adjustment disorder with depressed mood.
Referential Delusion Perception that common events refer specifically to the individual.
Refugee A person who enters a country of which s/he is not a citizen or formal immigrant because of fears of persecution or other harm on returning to a home country. Laws often distinguish between political and economic refugees because the former are often singled out for harm on return.
Regression Reversion to pleasures of a previous developmental stage.
Regulator Subsystem Human processes related to the autonomic nervous system and involving chemical, neural, and endocrine responses.
Relativistic Thinking Process of understanding the contextual nature of the world from multiple perspectives.
Relaxation A psychophysiological state characterized by parasympathetic dominance involving multiple visceral and somatic symptoms, including the absence of physical, mental, and emotional tension.
Reliability Measurement of reproducibility of a testing instrument.
Repression Process in which painful memories, thoughts, or experiences are actively kept out of conscious awareness.
Resonancy The movement of human energy wave patterns from low and slow to high and fast.
Risk Factors Traits that predispose an individual to a disease.
Role-Modeling Developing an individualized plan of care based on the client's world model.

S

Schizoaffective Disorder Condition characterized by elements of schizophrenia and manic-depressive disorder.
Schizoid Personality Disorder Behavior pattern characterized by lack of emotion and close friendships and detachment from persons and events in the immediate environment.
Schizophrenia Mental disorder characterized by disordered thoughts, hallucinations, and delusions.
Schizotypal Personality Disorder Behavior pattern characterized by inability to form close relations and a pattern of cognitive and perceptual distortions and eccentricities.
Search Engines Internet tools that allow the user to find Web sites based on words entered into the engines.
Seclusion State of a client being put in an isolated room or cell.
Secondary Prevention Activities directed at reducing the prevalence of mental disorders by shortening the duration of a sufficient number of established cases.
Self-Awareness Perception of oneself in relation to others and relative to society's expectations.
Self-Care Activities that humans perform for themselves to maintain life, to function, and to develop.
Self-Care Agency Ability to perform self-care in light of gender, age, socioeconomic status, developmental level,

health, family, environment, living patterns, and availability of resources.
Self-Care Deficit State that occurs when an individual's therapeutic self-care demand is greater than the capacity to meet that demand.
Self-Efficacy Ability to organize and manage individual responses to the demands of the environment.
Self-Help Group Persons coming together who are facing a common difficulty.
Separation Anxiety Anxiety and fear experienced by a child when forced to separate from his/her parents.
Serotonergic Syndrome Drug reaction involving agitation, sweating, rigidity, fever, hyperreflexia, tachycardia, and hypotension.
Severe Violence Violence that results in prolonged impairment or death
Sexual Abuse (Child) Employment, use, persuasion, inducement, enticement, or coercion of a child to engage in, or assist another person to engage in sexually implicit conduct; includes rape, molestation, prostitution, or other forms of sexual exploitation of children or incest with children.
Sexual Abuse (Elder) Threat of sexual assault or actual sexual battery, rape, incest, sodomy, oral copulation, penetration of genital or anal opening by a foreign object, coerced nudity, and sexually explicit photographing.
Sexual Battery Activity of a person touching an intimate part (sexual organs, groin, buttocks, breast) of another person, if that touching is against the will of the person touched and is for the purpose of sexual arousal, gratification, or abuse.
Sexual Dysfunction Condition existing when a person experiences a change with any aspect of sexuality that is viewed as unsatisfying, unrewarding, or inadequate.
Sexually Explicit Content In the context of Psychiatric Mental Health Nursing this term often refers to pornography; alternatively, printed material or film that shows sexual content, usually for prurient purposes
Sexual Exploitation Child pornography, sexually explicit reproduction of a child's image, or child prostitution.
Sexual Masochism Disorder characterized by sexual excitement resulting from fantasies or behaviors about being the recipient of physical abuse or humiliation.
Sexual Sadism Disorder characterized by sexual excitement resulting from persistent fantasies or behaviors involving infliction of suffering on others.
Sexually Explicit Conduct Actual or simulated sexual intercourse, bestiality, masturbation, lascivious exhibition of the genitals of a person or animal, or sadistic or masochistic abuse.
Sibling Position Birth order of children.
Situational Crisis Event that poses a threat or challenge to an individual.
Sleep Hygiene Specific activities that assist many persons to achieve restful sleep.
Sleep Latency Time it takes to fall asleep.
Sleep Paralysis Sensation of being unable to move, speak, or breathe during sleep.
Sleep Terrors Parasomnia in which there is *no recall* of the sleep-related event.
Sleepwalking Pattern of sleep behavior usually including getting out of bed, walking around in the bedroom, or on occasion outside of the bedroom, and then returning to bed.
SNOMED Systematized Nomenclature of Medicine; coding system that includes nursing diagnoses, nursing interventions, multiple axes that identify causative factors of illness, and related functional deficits and social factors.
Social Competence Degree to which significant others rate an individual as successful at performing expected social tasks.
Social Phobia Social anxiety, fear of being embarrassed in social settings.
Societal Regression Process of reversion in which anxiety leads to emotionally based decision making.
Somatic Therapies Interventions used in the management of psychiatric symptoms, for example, use of seclusion or physical restraints in control of anger.
Somatization Disorder Somatoform disorder in which there are multiple physical complaints without an apparent physiological cause.
Somatoform Disorder Psychiatric condition manifested in physical rather than psychological symptoms.
Spousal Rape Sexual intercourse against the victim's will by the spouse; accompanied by force, fear of bodily harm, or future retaliation.
Statutory Rape Sexual activity with a person under the age of consent (in most states, under 16 years of age) and considered to have occurred despite the apparent willingness of the underage person.
Stereotyping Assumption that people sharing certain characteristics will think and act similarly.
Stranger Rape Aggravated criminal sexual assault, forcible rape, or sexual battery that is committed against a victim by persons not acquainted with the victim.
Stranger Violence Physical assault or other injury committed against a victim by persons not acquainted with the victim.
Stress Stimulus that an individual perceives as challenging or harmful.
Structural Violence Harm that comes to individuals from political and social structures that lead to exploitation or deprivation; may include direct violence such as war or genocide.
Substance Abuse Maladaptive pattern of use of a drug in situations of real or potential harm.

Suggestion Psychoanalytic technique in which the analyst interprets the client's thoughts, actions, or dreams.
Suicidal Ideation Thoughts of taking one's life.
Suicide Purposefully taking one's own life.
Suicide Potential Person's risk level for completing a suicide.
Suicide Survivor Friend or family member of an individual who dies from suicide.
Superego Conscious mind, governed by conscience and ego ideal.
Supportive-Educative Role Nursing activities that focus on enhancing the client's ability both to carry on effectively without nursing support and to rise above the feelings of depression (Orem's Theory).
Supportive Group Persons coming together to offer support, education, socialization, and/or recreation.
Switch Process Mood changes between mania and depression.
Sympathetic System Response Nervous system responses to stress that include increased heart rate, breathing, and blood pressure; constriction of peripheral blood vessels; muscle tension; gastric hyperacidity; release of adrenaline; and formation of cortisol.
Synapse Structure formed in which axons and dendrites come together.

T

Tangentiality Speech marked by failure to reach a goal or stick to the original point.
Tarasoff Duty to Warn Legal obligation of health care professionals to advise potential victims of violence so that the potential victim may seek protection.
Tardive Dyskinesia Neurological disorder characterized by involuntary movements, usually of the tongue and lips.
Termination The final phase of the nurse-patient relationship in which the relationship is ended after the patient's needs have been met.
Tertiary Prevention Activities directed at reducing the residual defects that are associated with mental disorders.
Thalamus An exceptionally important brain region that serves to relay a wide range of sensory inputs to the cerebral cortex; it is also a critical structure for maintaining consciousness.
Theory A set of interrelated concepts that provide testable relationships and direction or prediction.
Therapeutic Communication Purposeful use of dialogue to bring about the client's insight, control of symptoms, and healing. Communication that builds a trusting relationship.
Therapeutic Imagery The ability to take one's natural thought processes and direct those thoughts in a creative way, potentiating a positive outcome.
Therapeutic Massage Extension of massage techniques, involving deep tissue and advanced massage techniques.
Therapeutic Self-Care Demand Activities needed to meet self-care requisites to fulfill self-care agency.
Therapeutic Touch (TT) Five-step process of touch that involves centering; assessing the client's energy field; smoothing, or "unruffling," the field; modulating or transferring energy; and knowing when to stop.
Therapeutic Window Time for peak effectiveness of a drug.
Therapy Group Persons coming together to receive psychotherapy.
Tolerance Acquired resistance to the effects of a drug.
Trafficking Movement of vulnerable persons across national boundaries, often for sexual purposes, but sometimes to evade immigration legalities.
Trait Anxiety Personality characteristic reflecting susceptibility to anxiety.
Transvestic Fetishism Cross-dressing or fantasies about cross-dressing.
Triangulation Relational pattern among three members.

U

UMLS Unified Medical Language System: thesaurus of all terms included in existing taxonomies.
Unipolar Depression Disorder in which mood swings are always in one direction, toward depression.
Utilitarianism Theory based on the principle that an ethical decision serves to produce the greatest good for the greatest number of persons.

V

Validity Measurement of accuracy of a testing instrument.
Values Learned beliefs about what is held to be good or bad in a culture.
Victim Consciousness Belief that one is at the mercy of circumstances beyond one's control.
Violation of Rights Abuse that occurs when the inalienable rights provided by the U.S. Constitution and federal statutes are violated by a family member or caregiver; includes such rights as not to have one's property taken without due process, the right to adequate appropriate medical treatment, and the right to freedom of assembly, speech, and religion.
Violence The intentional use of physical force or power, threatened or actual, against oneself, another person, or against a group or community, that either results in or has a high likelihood of resulting in injury, death, psychological harm, maldevelopment, or deprivation (WHO definition).
Voyeurism Observing or fantasizing about observing others disrobing, naked, or involved in sexual activity.

W

Withdrawal Condition occurring when cessation of drug use results in a drug-specific set of symptoms that would be relieved by additional doses of the drug.

Word Salad Speech marked by a group of disconnected words.

Working Phase The phase of the nurse-patient relationship in which the nurse and patient work together to meet the patient's needs.

INDEX

Note: Page numbers in italics indicate artwork and movie clips; page numbers followed by "t" indicate tables; page numbers followed by "b" indicate boxed material; page numbers followed by "f" indicate figures.

A

B

C

D

E

H

I

J

K

N

Q

R

T

U

V

W

Y

Z

StudyWARE™ to Accompany Psychiatric Mental Health Nursing, Fourth Edition

Minimum System Requirements

- Operating systems: Microsoft Windows XP w/SP 2, Windows Vista w/ SP 1, Windows 7
- Processor: Minimum required by Operating System
- Memory: Minimum required by Operating System
- Hard Drive Space: 650MB
- Screen resolution: 1024 × 768 pixels
- CD-ROM drive
- Sound card & listening device required for audio features
- Flash Player 10. The Adobe Flash Player is free, and can be downloaded from http://www.adobe.com/products/flashplayer/

Setup Instructions

1. Insert disc into CD-ROM drive. The StudyWARE™ installation program should start automatically. If it does not, go to step 2.
2. From My Computer, double-click the icon for the CD drive.
3. Double-click the *setup.exe* file to start the program.

Technical Support

Telephone: 1-800-648-7450
8:30 A.M.-6:30 P.M. Eastern Time
E-mail: delmar.help@cengage.com

ENGAGE LEARNING HAS PROVIDED YOU WITH HIS PRODUCT FOR YOUR REVIEW AND, TO THE XTENT THAT YOU ADOPT THE ASSOCIATED EXTBOOK FOR USE IN CONNECTION WITH OUR COURSE, YOU AND YOUR STUDENTS WHO URCHASE THE TEXTBOOK MAY USE THE MATE-IALS AS DESCRIBED BELOW.

MPORTANT! READ CAREFULLY: This End User icense Agreement ("Agreement") sets forth the conditions y which Cengage Learning will make electronic access to ie Cengage Learning-owned licensed content and associ-ed media, software, documentation, printed materials, and ectronic documentation contained in this package and/or ade available to you via this product (the "Licensed Con-nt"), available to you (the "End User"). BY CLICKING HE "I ACCEPT" BUTTON AND/OR OPENING THIS ACKAGE, YOU ACKNOWLEDGE THAT YOU HAVE EAD ALL OF THE TERMS AND CONDITIONS, AND HAT YOU AGREE TO BE BOUND BY ITS TERMS, ONDITIONS, AND ALL APPLICABLE LAWS AND EGULATIONS GOVERNING THE USE OF THE LI-ENSED CONTENT.

.0 Scope of License

.1. Licensed Content. The Licensed Content may contain portions of modifiable content ("Modifiable Content") and content which may not be modified or otherwise altered by the End User ("Non-Modifiable Content"). For purposes of this Agreement, Modifiable Content and Non-Modifiable Content may be collectively referred to herein as the "Licensed Content." All Licensed Content shall be considered Non-Modifiable Content, unless such Licensed Content is presented to the End User in a modifiable format and it is clearly indicated that modification of the Licensed Content is permitted.

.2. Subject to the End User's compliance with the terms and conditions of this Agreement, Cengage Learning hereby grants the End User, a nontransferable, nonexclusive, limited right to access and view a single copy of the Licensed Content on a single personal computer system for noncommercial, internal, personal use only, and, to the extent that End User adopts the associated textbook for use in connection with a course, the limited right to provide, distribute, and display the Modifiable Content to course students who purchase the textbook, for use in connection with the course only. The End User shall not (i) reproduce, copy, modify (except in the case of Modifiable Content), distribute, display, transfer, sublicense, prepare derivative work(s) based on, sell, exchange, barter or transfer, rent, lease, loan, resell, or in any other manner exploit the Licensed Content; (ii) remove, obscure, or alter any notice of Cengage Learning's intellectual property rights present on or in the Licensed Content, including, but not limited to, copyright, trademark, and/or patent notices; or (iii) disassemble, decompile, translate, reverse engineer, or otherwise reduce the Licensed Content. Cengage reserves the right to use a hardware lock device, license administration software, and/or a license authorization key to control access or password protection technology to the Licensed Content. The End User may not take any steps to avoid or defeat the purpose of such measures. Use of the Licensed Content without the relevant required lock device or authorization key is prohibited. UNDER NO CIRCUMSTANCES MAY NON-SALEABLE ITEMS PROVIDED TO YOU BY CENGAGE (INCLUDING, WITHOUT LIMITATION, ANNOTATED INSTRUCTOR'S EDITIONS, SOLUTIONS MANUALS, INSTRUCTOR'S RESOURCE MATERIALS AND/OR TEST MATERIALS) BE SOLD, AUCTIONED, LICENSED OR OTHERWISE REDISTRIBUTED BY THE END USER.

2.0 Termination

2.1. Cengage Learning may at any time (without prejudice to its other rights or remedies) immediately terminate this Agreement and/or suspend access to some or all of the Licensed Content, in the event that the End User does not comply with any of the terms and conditions of this Agreement. In the event of such termination by Cengage Learning, the End User shall immediately return any and all copies of the Licensed Content to Cengage Learning.

3.0 Proprietary Rights

3.1. The End User acknowledges that Cengage Learning owns all rights, title and interest, including, but not limited to all copyright rights therein, in and to the Licensed Content, and that the End User shall not take any action inconsistent with such ownership. The Licensed Content is protected by U.S., Canadian and other applicable copyright laws and by international treaties, including the Berne Convention and the Universal Copyright Convention. Nothing contained in this Agreement shall be construed as granting the End User any ownership rights in or to the Licensed Content.

3.2. Cengage Learning reserves the right at any time to withdraw from the Licensed Content any item or part of an item for which it no longer retains the right to publish, or which it has reasonable grounds to believe infringes copyright or is defamatory, unlawful, or otherwise objectionable.

4.0 Protection and Security

4.1. The End User shall use its best efforts and take all reasonable steps to safeguard its copy of the Licensed Content to ensure that no unauthorized reproduction, publication, disclosure, modification, or distribution of the Licensed Content, in whole or in part, is made. To the extent that the End User becomes aware of any such unauthorized use of the Licensed Content, the End

User shall immediately notify Cengage Learning. Notification of such violations may be made by sending an e-mail to infringement@cengage.com.

5.0 Misuse of the Licensed Product

5.1. In the event that the End User uses the Licensed Content in violation of this Agreement, Cengage Learning shall have the option of electing liquidated damages, which shall include all profits generated by the End User's use of the Licensed Content plus interest computed at the maximum rate permitted by law and all legal fees and other expenses incurred by Cengage Learning in enforcing its rights, plus penalties.

6.0 Federal Government Clients

6.1. Except as expressly authorized by Cengage Learning, Federal Government clients obtain only the rights specified in this Agreement and no other rights. The Government acknowledges that (i) all software and related documentation incorporated in the Licensed Content is existing commercial computer software within the meaning of FAR 27.405(b)(2); and (2) all other data delivered in whatever form, is limited rights data within the meaning of FAR 27.401. The restrictions in this section are acceptable as consistent with the Government's need for software and other data under this Agreement.

7.0 Disclaimer of Warranties and Liabilities

7.1. Although Cengage Learning believes the Licensed Content to be reliable, Cengage Learning does not guarantee or warrant (i) any information or materials contained in or produced by the Licensed Content, (ii) the accuracy, completeness or reliability of the Licensed Content, or (iii) that the Licensed Content is free from errors or other material defects. THE LICENSED PRODUCT IS PROVIDED "AS IS," WITHOUT ANY WARRANTY OF ANY KIND AND CENGAGE LEARNING DISCLAIMS ANY AND ALL WARRANTIES, EXPRESSED OR IMPLIED, INCLUDING, WITHOUT LIMITATION, WARRANTIES OF MERCHANTABILITY OR FITNESS FOR A PARTICULAR PURPOSE. IN NO EVENT SHALL CENGAGE LEARNING BE LIABLE FOR: INDIRECT, SPECIAL, PUNITIVE OR CONSEQUENTIAL DAMAGES INCLUDING FOR LOST PROFITS, LOST DATA, OR OTHERWISE. IN NO EVENT SHALL CENGAGE LEARNING'S AGGREGATE LIABILITY HEREUNDER, WHETHER ARISING IN CONTRACT, TORT, STRICT LIABILITY OR OTHERWISE, EXCEED THE AMOUNT OF FEES PAID BY THE END USER HEREUNDER FOR THE LICENSE OF THE LICENSED CONTENT.

8.0 General

8.1. Entire Agreement. This Agreement shall constitute th entire Agreement between the Parties and supercede all prior Agreements and understandings oral or writte relating to the subject matter hereof.

8.2. Enhancements/Modifications of Licensed Conten From time to time, and in Cengage Learning's sole dis cretion, Cengage Learning may advise the End User c updates, upgrades, enhancements and/or improvemen to the Licensed Content, and may permit the End Use to access and use, subject to the terms and conditions c this Agreement, such modifications, upon payment c prices as may be established by Cengage Learning.

8.3. No Export. The End User shall use the Licensed Con tent solely in the United States and shall not transfer c export, directly or indirectly, the Licensed Content ou side the United States.

8.4. Severability. If any provision of this Agreement is in valid, illegal, or unenforceable under any applicable sta ute or rule of law, the provision shall be deeme omitted to the extent that it is invalid, illegal, or uner forceable. In such a case, the remainder of the Agree ment shall be construed in a manner as to give greates effect to the original intention of the parties hereto.

8.5. Waiver. The waiver of any right or failure of either part to exercise in any respect any right provided in thi Agreement in any instance shall not be deemed to be waiver of such right in the future or a waiver of an other right under this Agreement.

8.6. Choice of Law/Venue. This Agreement shall be inte preted, construed, and governed by and in accordanc with the laws of the State of New York, applicable t contracts executed and to be wholly preformed therei without regard to its principles governing conflicts c law. Each party agrees that any proceeding arising out c or relating to this Agreement or the breach or threat ened breach of this Agreement may be commenced an prosecuted in a court in the State and County of Ne York. Each party consents and submits to the nonexclu sive personal jurisdiction of any court in the State an County of New York in respect of any such proceeding

8.7. Acknowledgment. By opening this package and/or b accessing the Licensed Content on this Web site, TH END USER ACKNOWLEDGES THAT IT HA READ THIS AGREEMENT, UNDERSTANDS IT AND AGREES TO BE BOUND BY ITS TERMS AN CONDITIONS. IF YOU DO NOT ACCEPT THES TERMS AND CONDITIONS, YOU MUST NO ACCESS THE LICENSED CONTENT AN RETURN THE LICENSED PRODUCT TO CEN GAGE LEARNING (WITHIN 30 CALENDAR DAY OF THE END USER'S PURCHASE) WITH PROO OF PAYMENT ACCEPTABLE TO CENGAG LEARNING, FOR A CREDIT OR A REFUND. Shoul the End User have any questions/comments regardin this Agreement, please contact Cengage Learning a Delmar.help@cengage.com.